Leukemias: Principles and Practice of Therapy

EDITED BY

Stefan Faderl, MD
Associate Professor
Department of Leukemia
University of Texas
MD Anderson Cancer Center
Houston, TX, USA

Hagop Kantarjian, MD
Chairman & Professor
Department of Leukemia
University of Texas
MD Anderson Cancer Center
Houston, TX, USA

WILEY-BLACKWELL
A John Wiley & Sons, Ltd., Publication

This edition first published 2011, © 2011 by Blackwell Publishing Ltd

Blackwell Publishing was acquired by John Wiley & Sons in February 2007. Blackwell's publishing program has been merged with Wiley's global Scientific, Technical and Medical business to form Wiley-Blackwell.

Registered office: John Wiley & Sons Ltd, The Atrium, Southern Gate, Chichester, West Sussex, PO19 8SQ, UK

Editorial offices: 9600 Garsington Road, Oxford, OX4 2DQ, UK
The Atrium, Southern Gate, Chichester, West Sussex, PO19 8SQ, UK
111 River Street, Hoboken, NJ 07030-5774, USA

For details of our global editorial offices, for customer services and for information about how to apply for permission to reuse the copyright material in this book please see our website at www.wiley.com/wiley-blackwell

This book is published in the following electronic formats: ePDF 9781444327366; Wiley Online Library 9781444327359

ISBN: 978-1-4051-8235-5

A catalogue record for this book is available from the British Library.

Library of Congress Cataloging-in-Publication Data
Leukemias : principles and practice of therapy / edited by Stefan Faderl, Hagop Kantarjian.
p. ; cm.
Includes bibliographical references and index.
ISBN 978-1-4051-8235-5 (alk. paper)
1. Leukemia. I. Faderl, S. H. (Stefan H.) II. Kantarjian, Hagop, 1952–
[DNLM: 1. Leukemia--diagnosis. 2. Leukemia--therapy. WH 250 L65597 2011]
RC643.L433 2011
616.99'419–dc22

2010024070

Set in 9.25/12pt Palatino by Toppan Best-set Premedia Limited
Printed and bound in Singapore by Markono Print Media Pte Ltd.

1 2011

Contents

The color plate section can be found facing p. 86

Contributors

Lionel Ades
Service d'hematologie clinique
Hopital Avicenne (Assistance Publique-Hopitaux de Paris)
and Paris 13 University
Bobigny, France

Gheath Alatrash DO, PhD
Assistant Professor of Medicine
Department of Stem Cell Transplantation and
Cellular Therapy
Division of Cancer Medicine
University of Texas
MD Anderson Cancer Center
Houston, Texas, USA

Maher Albitar
Quest Diagnostics Nichols Institute
San Juan Capistrano
California, USA

Elias Anaissie MD
Professor
Deputy Chair and Head, Division of Supportive Care
Myeloma Institute for Research and Therapy
University of Arkansas for Medical Sciences
Little Rock, Arkansas, USA

John Anastasi MD
Section of Hematopathology
Department of Pathology
University of Chicago
Chicago, Illinois, USA

Ulrike Bacher
Department of Stem Cell Transplantation
University of Hamburg
Hamburg, Germany

David Bowen
Consultant Haematologist and Honorary Professor of
Myeloid Leukaemia Studies
St. James's Institute of Oncology
Leeds Teaching Hospitals
Leeds, UK

Carlos Bueso-Ramos MD, PhD
Professor
Department of Hematopathology
University of Texas
MD Anderson Cancer Center
Houston, Texas, USA

Daniel J DeAngelo MD, PhD
Associate Professor of Medicine
Harvard Medical School;
Clinical Director, Adult Leukemia Program
Department of Medical Oncology
Dana-Farber Cancer Institute
Boston, Massachusetts, USA

Claire Dearden MD, FRCP, FRCPATH
Consultant Haematologist
Royal Marsden NHS Foundation Trust
Surrey, UK

Marcos de Lima, MD
Associate Professor of Medicine
Department of Stem Cell Transplantation and Cellular Therapy
University of Texas
MD Anderson Cancer Center
Houston, Texas, USA

Hartmut Döhner MD
Department of Internal Medicine III
University of Ulm
Ulm, Germany

Barbara Eichhorst, MD
Specialist for Hematology and Oncology
Department I of Internal Medicine
University Clinic of Cologne
Cologne, Germany

Elihu Estey
Clinical Research Department
Fred Hutchinson Cancer Research Center
Division of Hematology
University of Washington School of Medicine
Seattle, Washington, USA

Pierre Fenaux MD, PhD
Service d'hematologie clinique
Hopital Avicenne (Assistance Publique-Hopitaux de Paris)
and Paris 13 University
Bobigny, France

Alessandra Ferrajoli MD
Associate Professor of Medicine
Department of Leukemia
University of Texas
MD Anderson Cancer Center
Houston, Texas, USA

Andrew Fletcher MBChB, MRCPCH
Department of Pediatric Hematology
St. James's University Hospital
Leeds, UK

Olga Frankfurt MD
Assistant Professor of Medicine
Northwestern University Feinberg School of Medicine
Robert H. Lurie Comprehensive Cancer Center
Chicago, Illinois, USA

Guillermo Garcia-Manero MD
Associate Professor of Medicine
Chief, Section of Myelodysplastic Syndromes
Department of Leukemia
University of Texas
MD Anderson Cancer Center
Houston, Texas, USA

Ulrich Germing MD, PhD
Department of Hematology, Oncology and Clinical Immunology
Heinrich-Heine-University
Dusseldorf, Germany

Valentin Goede MD
Resident
Department I of Internal Medicine
University Clinic of Cologne
Cologne, Germany

Nicola Gökbuget MD
Head of Study Center
Goethe University Hospital
Department of Medicine II, Hematology/Oncology
Frankfurt, Germany

Steven D Gore MD
Professor of Oncology
Hematologic Malignancies
Sidney Kimmel Comprehensive Cancer Center
Johns Hopkins
Baltimore, Maryland, USA

John G Gribben MD, DSc, FRCP, FRCPath, FMedSci
Professor
Institute of Cancer
Bart's and the London School of Medicine
London, UK

Sandeep Gurbuxani MBBS, PhD
Section of Hematopathology
Department of Pathology
University of Chicago
Chicago, Illinois, USA

Claudia Haferlach
MLL Munich Leukemia Laboratory
Munich, Germany

Torsten Haferlach
MLL Munich Leukemia Laboratory
Munich, Germany

Simon Hallam MA, MB, BChir, MRCP
Institute of Cancer
Bart's and the London School of Medicine
London, UK

Michael Hallek MD
Director
Department I of Internal Medicine
University Clinic of Cologne
Cologne, Germany

Syed Khizer Hasan PhD
Department of Biopathology
University Tor Vergata
Rome, Italy

Devendra Hiwase MD
Consultant Haematologist
Haematology Division
SA Pathology
Adelaide, Australia

Andreas Hochhaus MD
Professor of Internal Medicine, Hematology and Oncology
Universitatsklinikum Jena, Klinik für Innere Medizin II
Abteilung Hamatolgie und Internistische Onkologie
Jena, Germany

Dieter Hoelzer MD
Professor of Internal Medicine
Onkologikum am Museumsufer
Frankfurt, Germany

Timothy Hughes MD
Professor of Haematology
Haematology Division
SA Pathology, Adelaide, Australia

Judith E Karp MD
Professor of Oncology and Medicine
Director, Leukemia Program
Sidney Kimmel Comprehensive Cancer Center
Johns Hopkins University
Baltimore, Maryland, USA

Partow Kebriaei MD
Associate Professor of Medicine
University of Texas
MD Anderson Cancer Center
Houston, Texas, USA

Wolfgang Kern, MD
MLL Munich Leukemia Laboratory
Munich, Germany

Hartmut Koeppen MD, PhD
Staff Pathologist
Department of Pathology
Genentech, Inc
South San Francisco, California, USA

Sergej Konoplev MD, PhD
Department of Hematopathology
University of Texas
MD Anderson Cancer Center
Houston, Texas, USA

Francesco Lo-Coco MD
Department of Biopathology
University Tor Vergata
Rome, Italy

Junia V Melo MD, PhD, FRCPath
Professor of Haematology
University of Adelaide
Centre for Cancer Biology—SA Pathology
Adelaide, SA, Australia

Ruben Mesa MD
Professor of Medicine
Director, Acute and Chronic Leukemias Program
Mayo Clinic
Scottsdale, Arizona, USA

Bijay Nair MD, MPH
Assistant Professor of Medicine
Myeloma Institute for Research and Therapy
University of Arkansas for Medical Sciences
Little Rock, Arkansas, USA

Marcio Nucci MD
University Hospital
Universidade Federal do Rio de Janeiro
Rio de Janeiro, Brazil;
Myeloma Institute for Research and Therapy
University of Arkansas for Medical Sciences
Little Rock, Arkansas, USA

Nnenna Osuji
Honorary Consultant, Section of Haemato-Oncology
Royal Mardsen NHS Foundation Trust/Institute of Cancer Research
Surrey, UK

Keith W Pratz MD
Assistant Professor of Oncology
Sidney Kimmel Comprehensive Cancer Center
Johns Hopkins University
Baltimore, Maryland, USA

Jerald Radich MD
Clinical Research Division
Fred Hutchinson Cancer Research Center
Seattle, Washington, USA

Farhad Ravandi MD
Associate Professor of Medicine
Department of Leukemia
University of Texas
MD Anderson Cancer Center
Houston, Texas, USA

Paolo Rebulla MD
Director, Center of Transfusion Medicine
Cellular Therapy and Cryobiology
Foundation 'Ca' Granda Ospedale Maggiore Policlinico'
Milano, Italy

Michael Rytting MD
Assistant Professor-Pediatrics and Leukemia
University of Texas
MD Anderson Cancer Center
Houston, Texas, USA

Olga Sala-Torra MD
Clinical Research Division
Fred Hutchinson Cancer Research Center
Seattle, Washington, USA

Eric Schafer MD
Instructor in Pediatrics and Oncology
Sidney Kimmel Comprehensive Cancer Center
Johns Hopkins University
Baltimore, Maryland, USA

Susanna Schnittger
MLL Munich Leukemia Laboratory
Munich, Germany

Donald Small MD, PhD
Kyle Haydock Professor of Oncology
Professor of Oncology, Pediatrics, Cellular and Molecular Medicine
Director, Pediatric Oncology
Sidney Kimmel Comprehensive Cancer Center
Johns Hopkins University
Baltimore, Maryland, USA

William Stevenson MBBS, PhD
Hematologist
Royal North Shore Hospital
Sidney, Australia

Stephan Stilgenbauer MD
Department of Internal Medicine III
University of Ulm
Ulm, Germany

Sylvain Thépot
Service d'hematologie clinique
Hopital Avicenne (Assistance Publique-Hopitaux de Paris) and Paris 13 University
Bobigny, France

Xavier Thomas MD, PhD
Leukemia Unit
Department of Hematology
Edouard Herriot Hospital
Lyon, France

Wei-Gang Tong MD, PhD
Clinical Fellow
Department of Leukemia
University of Texas
MD Anderson Cancer Center
Houston, Texas, USA

Srdan Verstovsek MD, PhD
Associate Professor
University of Texas
MD Anderson Cancer Center
Houston, Texas, USA

Martha Wadleigh, MD
Assistant Professor of Medicine
Harvard Medical School
Department of Medical Oncology
Dana-Farber Cancer Institute
Boston, MA

Erica D. Warlick, MD
Assistant Professor
Division of Hematology, Oncology, and Transplantation
Department of Medicine University of Minnesota
Minneapolis, Minnesota, USA

Meir Wetzler MD, FACP
Professor of Medicine
Chief, Leukemia Section
Department of Medicine
Roswell Park Cancer Institute
Buffalo, New York, USA

Annika Whittle
Specialist Registrar
Department of Hematology
St. James's Institute of Oncology
Leeds, UK

Agnes S M Yong MB BCh, MRCP (UK), PhD, FRCPath
Senior Research Fellow
Hematology Branch
National Institutes of Health
Bethesda, Maryland, USA

Amer Zeidan MD
Academic Hospitalist
Division of Hospital Medicine
General Medicine Unit
Rochester General Hospital
Rochester, New York, USA;
Sidney Kimmel Comprehensive Cancer Center at Johns Hopkins
Baltimore, Maryland, USA

Thorsten Zenz MD
Department of Internal Medicine III
University of Ulm
Ulm, Germany

Preface

Progress in the definition and therapy of hematologic malignancies has been at the forefront of a therapeutic revolution in cancer medicine. The introduction of imatinib mesylate in the management of patients with Philadelphia chromosome-Fl positive chronic myeloid leukemia only 10 years ago has sparked a concerted effort into targeted therapies that extend, by now, far beyond the initial BCR–ABL kinase. Exciting developments in unraveling the biology of leukemic disorders coincide with the availability of an array of drugs never before realized. New prognostic markers, which are being tested in clinical trials, are helping to fine-tune the treatment approaches in many different leukemic disorders. Markers predictive of response to specific therapies are integrated into clinical algorithms, as, for example, the finding of 17p abnormalities in patients with chronic lymphocytic leukemias has demonstrated. As so often is the case, the ever increasing body of knowledge also raises many more new questions. Hence the practicing physician and academician is constantly faced with new challenges and confronted with the frequently daunting task to reconcile the major developments of a specialty that is becoming both more spread out and specialized "within." This book, dedicated exclusively to leukemic disorders, aims to discuss and summarize new pathophysiologic concepts, therapeutic approaches, developments of supportive care, and future investigational strategies. Experts in their respective fields from all over the world have been invited to share their unique insights, vision, and expertise. To compile a book like this is always a trying task as it will struggle with the same challenge as every one of us faces, that is to keep up with all the new information in this incredibly dynamic field, even as it is going through the production process. It is the wish of the editors that this book will be instructive and helpful to its hopefully many readers.

Stefan Faderl

Part 1
Background and Diagnostic

Chapter 1
Stem-cell Biology in Normal and Malignant Hematopoiesis

Amer Zeidan[1] *and Meir Wetzler*[2]
[1] Division of Hospital Medicine, General Medicine Unit, Rochester General Hospital, Rochester, New York, USA
[2] Department of Medicine, Roswell Park Cancer Institute, Buffalo, New York, USA

Introduction

Hematopoiesis is the highly orchestrated process of blood cell production that maintains homeostasis by reproducing billions of white blood cells (WBCs), red blood cells (RBCs), and platelets on a daily basis [1].

Hematopoietic stem cells (HSCs) represent the small population of long-lived, quiescent, undifferentiated, pluripotent cells which are characterized by the capacity of self-renewal, exceptional proliferation potential, resistance to apoptosis, and the ability of multilineage differentiation into all blood cell types mediated by the production of several lineage-committed progenitors [1–5].

The central role of leukemia stem cells (LSCs) in the pathogenesis of some forms of leukemia has become well recognized over the last two decades. LSCs share many basic characteristics with HSCs, including quiescence, self-renewal, extensive proliferative capacity, and the ability to give rise to differentiated progeny in a hierarchical pattern [6–12]. Some scientists even view leukemia as a newly formed, abnormal hematopoietic tissue initiated by a few LSCs that undergo an aberrant and poorly regulated process of organogenesis analogous to that of the normal HSCs [13].

Many researchers believe that the persistence of LSCs, which are resistant to most of the traditional chemotherapeutic agents that kill the bulk of the leukemic cell populations, is a major cause of leukemia relapse after "successful" remission induction. Subsequently, designing effective therapeutic modalities that specifically target the LSCs is likely to reduce the incidence of relapse, and possibly even lead to a cure. As discussed below, the ongoing efforts to develop "magic bullets" targeting the LSCs will continue to face significant challenges because of their similarities to normal HSCs [14]. It is very important to further delineate the differences between normal HSCs and LSCs in order to design novel therapeutic modalities that offer maximal cytotoxicity to LSCs while sparing the normal HSCs [4,14].

In this chapter, we will briefly review the basic principles of the biology of HSCs and LSCs and examine the major scientific advances in this field. We will also discuss some of the ongoing efforts to utilize this growing knowledge for the purpose of developing targeted therapies directed against LSCs that could reduce the frequency of leukemia relapse.

Hematopoietic stem-cell biology in normal hematopoiesis

The HSC is the best-defined somatic stem cell to date [15]. The experimental data support the presence of an HSC compartment that is arranged as a continuum with unidirectional, irreversible progression of cells with decreasing capacities for self-renewal, increasing likelihood for differentiation, and increasing proliferative activity [16]. HSCs generate all the multiple hematopoietic lineages for the entire lifespan through a successive series of intermediate progenitors, known as colony-forming units (CFUs) or colony-forming cells (CFCs) [4,5]. As these intermediate progenitors continue to mature, they become more restricted in terms of the number and type of lineages that they can generate and exhibit a reduced self-renewal capacity [4,5]. Researchers have demonstrated the presence of a common lymphoid progenitor (CLP) and a common myeloid progenitor (CMP), which possibly reflects the earliest branching points between the lymphoid and myeloid lineages [17,18].

Studies on murine hematopoietic stem cells

Studies in mice have contributed considerably to our current understanding of HSC biology. Initially, it was

Leukemias: Principles and Practice of Therapy, 1st edition. Edited by S. Faderl and H. Kantarjian.

demonstrated that bone marrow cells injected into lethally irradiated recipient mice re-established hematopoiesis [19]. Later, it was shown that the first step in this engraftment was the formation of multilineage colonies in the spleen within 10 days of the injection [20]. Each of these spleen multilineage colonies actually arose from a single pluripotent stem cell, the spleen colony-forming unit (CFU-S) [21]. Those spleen colonies containing the CFU-S were capable of giving rise to new colonies in secondary recipients [22]. Subsequent studies demonstrated that the CFU-S actually consists of a heterogeneous population of more advanced progenitor cells that are distinct from the more primitive and more highly renewing HSCs, and that CFU-S are not capable of long-term multilineage hematopoietic reconstitution *in vivo* [23].

Jones *et al.* [24] showed that serial bone marrow transplantations, which eventually failed to reconstitute lethally irradiated mice, dissociated two phases of engraftment. The first unsustained phase was maintained with repeated serial transfer and appeared to be produced by committed progenitors, like granulocyte-macrophage colony-forming units (CFU-GM) and the CFU-S. The second sustained phase was eventually lost with repeated serial transfer, apparently due to decreasing numbers of pluripotent HSCs. Prolonging the time interval between serial transfers reestablished the ability of the serially transplanted marrow to reconstitute hematopoiesis [24], suggesting that the HSCs needed more time to allow long-term engraftment. Thereafter, Morrison *et al.* concluded that marrow reconstitution in mice was deterministic, not stochastic [25].

Studies on human hematopoietic stem cells

Owing to the clear limitations of experimenting on humans, most of our current knowledge about human HSCs was obtained indirectly from *in vitro* studies and xenotransplantation of human cells into immunodeficient animals [1]. Despite the presence of important differences, evidence suggests that the human HSC compartment, although not completely defined, parallels that of the murine counterpart, with a heterogeneous population of primitive cells with varying capacities for differentiation, proliferation, and self-renewal [1,4].

The *in vitro* culture assays [26–29] can evaluate some of the important characteristics of HSCs such as pluripotency and proliferative potential, but cannot accurately measure the bona fide properties of HSCs: the sustained and complete hematopoietic repopulating ability, and the maximal differentiating ability [5,30]. The severe combined immune-deficient (SCID) mice, which lack adaptive immunity, and the non-obese diabetic SCID (NOD/SCID) mice, which lack both innate and adaptive immunity, offered a more accurate reflection of the human HSC function than the *in vitro* culture assays [14,31–33]. The accuracy of these *in vivo* repopulation assays has been further improved by co-injection of distinguishable reference cells [5].

Characteristics of hematopoietic stem cells

In contrast to the morphologically well-defined committed precursors and mature cells, the HSCs are morphologically indistinguishable from the hematopoietic progenitor cells (HPCs). On the other hand, the HSCs can be phenotypically distinguished from the HPCs through multiparameter flow cytometry. The most commonly used surface antigen to enrich for HSCs is cluster designation CD34. Unlike their murine counterparts that are usually negative for the murine homolog of CD34 (mCD34$^-$), primitive human HSCs are usually CD34$^+$ [34]. Terstappen *et al.* [35] demonstrated that 1% of the CD34$^+$ cells did not express the CD38 antigen. The CD34$^+$/CD38$^-$ cells were homogeneous and lacked lineage-commitment specific markers (Lin$^-$), in agreement with what is expected from putative pluripotent HSCs. In contrast, the CD34$^+$/CD38$^+$ cells were heterogeneous and contained myeloblasts and erythroblasts, as well as lymphoblasts, suggesting an upregulation of CD38 antigen upon differentiation of the CD34$^+$/CD38$^-$ cells [35]. Later, the CD34$^+$/CD38$^-$ cell subset was shown to generate long-term, multilineage human hematopoiesis in the human-fetal sheep *in vivo* model. In contrast, the CD34$^+$/CD38$^+$ cells generated only short-term human hematopoiesis, suggesting again that the CD34$^+$/CD38$^+$ cell population contained relatively early multipotent HPCs, but not HSCs [36]. This work proved that the CD34$^+$/CD38$^-$ cell population has a high capacity for long-term multilineage hematopoietic engraftment, indicating the presence of stem cells in this minor adult human marrow cell subset [36].

In addition, HSCs were found to typically express high levels of stem-cell antigen 1 (SCA-1) and permeability glycoprotein (P-gp), a multidrug efflux transporter located in the plasma membrane and encoded by the multidrug resistance 1 gene (*MDR1*) [37,38]. On the other hand, HSCs typically have either absent or low levels of expression of Thy-1.1, CD33, CD71, CD10, CD45RA, and HLA-DR, while the more mature progenitors express one or more of these markers [1,15,35,39]. Finally, Gunji *et al.* [40] showed that the CD34$^+$ cell fraction that exhibited low expression of the c-Kit proto-oncogene protein (c-kit-low) contained CD34$^+$/CD38$^-$ cells that are considered to be the more primitive hematopoietic cells. In comparison, the CD34$^+$/c-Kit-high cell fraction contained many granulocyte-macrophage-committed progenitor cells. Osawa *et al.* [34] showed that injecting a single murine pluripotent HSC (characterized by the phenotype mCD34[lo/$^-$], c-Kit$^+$, SCA1$^+$, lineage markers negative [Lin$^-$]) resulted in long-term reconstitution of the hematopoietic system. These data suggest that all primitive cells are c-Kit$^+$, but HSCs have lower expression of c-Kit than the less primitive progenitors.

The dogma that all HSCs express CD34 has been challenged recently by studies suggesting the existence of an unrecognized population of HSCs that lack the CD34 surface marker and are characterized by their ability to efflux the Hoechst dye [41,42]. These cells were referred to as "side population" (SP) cells [43,44]. These SP cells were found to be highly enriched for long-term culture-initiating cells (LTC-ICs), an indicator of primitive hematopoietic cells [42]. Similarly, Zanjani *et al.* [45] demonstrated that the $CD34^-/Lin^-$ fraction of the normal human bone marrow contained cells which were capable of engraftment and differentiation into $CD34^+$ progenitors and multiple hematopoietic lineages in primary and secondary hosts.

It is evident from the above discussion that we are still facing significant challenges that limit our ability to accurately identify and isolate HSCs. A major goal of future investigations is to determine whether novel markers or marker combinations exist that will allow HSCs to be prospectively identified and isolated from any source [39].

Hematopoietic stem cells and self-renewal

Hematopoiesis encompasses a complex interaction between the HSCs and their microenvironment, which plays a critical role in the maintenance of HSCs. This complex interaction determines whether the HSCs, HPCs, and mature blood cells remain quiescent, proliferate, differentiate, self-renew, or undergo apoptosis [1,46]. While the majority of HSCs are quiescent in the G_0 phase in steady-state bone marrow, many of the stem cells are actually cycling regularly, although slowly, to maintain a constant flow of short-lived HPCs that can generate enough cells to replace those that are constantly lost during normal turnover [15,47].

Self-renewal is the ability of a stem cell to divide, yielding one daughter cell that can differentiate and another that maintains the pluripotent stem-cell function [14,15,48,49]. There are two hypothetical mechanisms by which asymmetric cell division might be achieved: divisional asymmetry and environmental asymmetry [2]. In divisional asymmetry, specific cell-fate determinants redistribute unequally before the onset of or during cell division [2,15]. As a result, only one daughter cell receives those determinants and therefore retains the HSC fate, while the other daughter cell proceeds to differentiation. In environmental asymmetry, a stem cell would first undergo a symmetric division, producing two identical daughter cells [15]. However, only one cell remains in the HSC niche (see below) and conserves its HSC fate, while the other cell enters a different microenvironment and subsequently produces signals initiating differentiation instead of preserving its stem-cell phenotype [2,15].

The longevity of the HSCs is another area of active research. Morrison *et al.* [50] showed that HSCs from old mice were only one-quarter as efficient at homing to and engrafting the bone marrow of irradiated recipients in comparison with HSCs from young mice, suggesting that the self-renewal capacity of HSCs is not infinite. Two of the proposed theories to explain this phenomenon are the progressive telomeric DNA shortening and the accumulation of DNA damage leading to stem-cell exhaustion [51,52].

Despite recent advances in our understanding of the complex molecular mechanisms that underlie the process of HSC self-renewal, there are still many aspects of this process that require further elucidation. Detailed discussion of the proposed molecular regulatory mechanisms controlling self-renewal in normal HSCs is beyond the scope of this review, but it is important to note that a large number of transcription factors, proteins, and signaling pathways have been implicated in the regulation of this process (reviewed in refs 2,5,38).

Hematopoietic stem cells and the microenvironment

The mechanisms of bone and blood formation have traditionally been viewed as distinct unrelated processes, but compelling evidence suggests that they are intertwined [53]. HSCs reside in the bone marrow, close to the endosteal surfaces of the trabecular bone in what is commonly referred to as "the niche" [54]. A stem-cell niche can be defined as a spatial structure in which HSCs are housed for an indefinite period of time and are maintained by allowing progeny production through self-renewal in the absence of differentiation [15,54,55]. There is accumulating evidence indicating that the stromal cells in the niche, especially the endosteal osteoblasts, play a major role in regulating the HSC maintenance, proliferation, and maturation [53,56–58]. Although the osteoblast is one of the main cellular elements of the HSC niche, the exact nature of the factors produced by the osteoblast that participate in the regulatory microenvironment for HSCs are known in only limited detail [15,48,53].

Several cell-surface receptors were implicated in controlling the localization of HSCs to the endosteal niche. One example is the calcium-sensing receptor (CaR) [15,49]. A unique feature of the bone that may contribute to the HSC homing might be the high concentration of calcium ions at the HSC-enriched endosteal surface [48]. It was shown that CaR-deficient HSCs from murine fetal liver failed to engraft in the bone marrow [49]. In addition, these cells were highly defective in localizing anatomically to the endosteal niche following transfer to lethally irradiated wild-type recipients, indicating the importance of CaR in homing of HSCs to the bone marrow niche [49]. Several other cell-surface receptors were described to be involved in the localization of the HSCs to the niche; one additional example, chemokine (C-X-C motif) receptor 4 (CXCR-4), and its ligand, the stromal-cell derived factor 1 (SDF-1), will be discussed later in the chapter.

While the majority of HSCs and HPCs are located in the bone marrow, a significant minority of them that play an important role in the establishment and functioning of the hematopoietic system are found in the peripheral blood under steady-state conditions [60,61]. The realization of the presence of large numbers of HSCs and HPCs in the umbilical cord blood and the ability to mobilize these cells into the circulation with chemotherapy and hematopoietic growth factors led to very significant advances in the fields of stem-cell biology, transplantation, and gene therapies [62–65].

Hematopoietic stem-cell plasticity

A fascinating aspect of the biology of HSCs is their potential plasticity. The term plasticity refers to the ability of organ-specific stem cells to recover their ability to differentiate into cells of other lineages, either *in vitro* or after transplantation *in vivo* [1,66,67]. There have been a number of reports that documented HSCs differentiating into non-hematopoietic cells including myocardium, muscle cells, neurons, and hepatocytes [68–71]. A detailed discussion of this phenomenon is beyond the scope of this review, but the interested reader can refer to some of the many reports published on this subject [1,66–71].

Leukemic stem cells

Two interesting observations suggested the presence of LSCs. First, despite the aggressive course of acute myeloid leukemia (AML), it has long been recognized that most leukemic blasts have limited *in vivo* proliferative capacity and that only a minority of these blasts are capable of forming colonies *in vitro* [72,73]. Second, the leukemic blasts in any individual, despite their morphologic homogeneity, are characterized by significant intercell biologic heterogeneity [74]. While it has long been assumed that stochastic variations related to the genomic instability of the tumor cells are largely responsible for this phenomenon, it has become increasingly evident that intrinsic development processes such as those normally found within stem-cell-based hierarchies also play a significant role [12]. Mounting evidence over the last two decades suggested that the leukemic clone is maintained by a rare population of stem cells—the LSCs, also known as the leukemia-initiating cells (LICs) [75,76]. Some researchers even viewed leukemia as a newly formed abnormal hematopoietic tissue initiated by a few LSCs that undergo an aberrant and poorly regulated process of organogenesis analogous to that of normal HSCs, but the differentiation from the LSC population gives rise to "blast" cells, which represent arrested or aberrant stages of myeloid development [11,13].

The seminal work by John Dick's laboratory in 1994 [75] provided the first proof for the presence of LSCs by isolation of a population of $CD34^+/CD38^-$ cells from patients with AML followed by engraftment of these cells into SCID mice. This resulted in a pattern of dissemination and leukemic cell morphology similar to that seen in the original patients. Work from the same laboratory later demonstrated that fewer $CD34^+/CD38^-$ LSCs were needed to induce AML in NOD/SCID mice than in SCID mice [9]. The authors concluded that the LSCs possess the differentiative and proliferative capacities and the potential for self-renewal seen in HSCs, and that LSCs were able to differentiate *in vivo* into leukemic blasts, indicating that the leukemic clone is organized as a hierarchy [9]. Subsequently, the presence of LSCs has been demonstrated in chronic myeloid leukemia (CML), and also some forms of acute lymphoblastic leukemia (ALL) (see below for more detailed discussion).

LSCs, which constitute a minority of the tumor bulk, are functionally defined on the basis of their ability to transfer leukemia into an immunodeficient recipient animal [14]. LSCs share many of the basic characteristics with normal HSCs including quiescence, self-renewal, extensive proliferative capacity, and the ability to give rise to differentiated progeny in a hierarchical pattern [6–12] (Table 1.1). It was shown that LSCs are not functionally homogeneous but, similar to the normal HSC compartment, comprise distinct hierarchically arranged LSC classes [77]. In a xenotransplantation model, some LSCs emerged only in recipients of serial transplantation, indicating that they divided rarely and underwent self-renewal rather than commitment after cell division within primary recipients. On the other hand, other LSCs gave only short-term leukemic repopulation in secondary recipients. This led to the conclusion that the distinct LSC fates were derived from heterogeneous self-renewal potential, which is analogous to the hierarchy observed in normal HSCs with long and short repopulation potentials [25,77].

Most of the chemotherapeutic agents traditionally used to treat leukemias are cell-cycle active agents, which primarily target dividing cells. These agents are highly unlikely to eradicate the quiescent LSCs [8,78,79]. In addi-

Table 1.1 Common characteristics of hematopoietic stem cells and leukemia stem cells.

Quiescence
Self-renewal
Extensive proliferative capacity
Ability to give rise to a differentiated progeny
Expression of efflux proteins
Survival in a "niche"
Resistance to apoptosis
$CD34^+/CD38^-/CD71^-/HLA\text{-}DR^-$ immunophenotype
Comprising hierarchy-arranged classes
Bmi-1 expression

tion, the LSCs seem to be biologically distinct from their more differentiated progeny, with specific cellular and molecular mechanisms that control their behavior; these mechanisms are quite different from those controlling the more mature leukemic blasts [11]. Therefore, it seems plausible that the agents acting against the more mature blasts will not be as efficient in eradicating the LSCs, possibly significantly contributing to treatment failure and future relapse [11]. In addition, it is highly likely that LSCs, similar to their normal HSC counterparts, possess efflux pumps, such as the P-gp, which confer resistance to traditional chemotherapy by quickly removing the cytotoxic agents from the cells [43,44,80].

Where does the leukemic stem cell come from?

The experimental data from John Dick's laboratory [9,75] led the authors to conclude that, given the homogeneous $CD34^+/CD38^-$ immunophenotype of LSCs and their ability for hierarchical differentiation, proliferation, and self-renewal, leukemic transformation occurred at the level of the normal HSCs rather than the committed progenitor cells. Later, this postulation that LSCs necessarily arise from aberrant HSCs [9,25,81] was challenged. Alternatively, it was suggested that LSCs could arise from more committed progenitors caused by mutations and/or selective expression of genes that enhance their otherwise limited self-renewal capabilities [13,82–86]. In fact, several groups [83–86] reported the ability to induce transformation of committed progenitor cells to LSCs by transducing these cells with the oncogenic fusion genes. Cozzio *et al.* [83] reported similar latencies of developing AML in recipient mice when transducing the leukemogenic chimeric gene *MLL-ENL* (MLL, also known as *ALL1*, mixed-lineage-leukemia, and *ENL*, 11–19–lysine-rich-leukemia) into either HSCs or myeloid progenitors with granulocyte–macrophage differentiation potential (GMPs). Similarly, Krivtsov *et al.* [84] demonstrated that the oncogenic fusion protein MLL-AF9 (*ALL1* fused gene from chromosome 9) can transform GMPs. These findings established the ability of transient repopulating progenitors to initiate myeloid leukemias in response to the *MLL* oncogene, thus supporting the existence of an LSC that overlaps with the multipotent HSC [83]. This led some researchers to propose that the nature of the LSC may vary depending upon the particular stage in normal hematopoiesis during which the insult occurred, resulting in significant pathogenetic and therapeutic differences of the leukemic phenotypes [10,12,74,77].

In addition, Huntly *et al.* [85] showed that while CMPs that were transduced with the oncogene MYST histone acetyltransferase (monocytic leukemia) 3-transcriptional intermediary factor 2 (*MOZ-TIF2*) resulted in an AML *in vivo* that could be serially transplanted, *BCR–ABL* transduction into CMPs conferred none of these properties. These data demonstrated that some, but not all, leukemia oncogenes can transfer properties of LSCs to HPCs destined to undergo apoptotic cell death. Thereafter, Stubbs *et al.* [86] showed that GMPs transduced with *MLL-AF9* and FMS-like tyrosine kinase-internal tandem duplication (*FLT3-ITD*) mutation cooperated to produce a more aggressive AML when compared with AML induced by *MLL-AF9* alone. These observations supported the theory of multistep nature of leukemogenesis where the initial genetic event (first hit) often leads to the expression of chimeric oncogenes (e.g. *MLL-AF9*) encoded by recurrent chromosomal translocations, while subsequent mutations (second hit) may activate specific signaling pathways (e.g. *FLT3-ITD*) [86]. It is important to note that all of the data on the progenitor origin of LSCs come from mouse models.

The terms "LSC" and "cancer stem cell" have caused significant confusion in the literature, partly because they implied that these cells originate from a normal stem cell. Recently, a panel of the American Association for Cancer Research agreed that the term "cancer stem cell" in general does not refer to the cell of origin of the cancer [87,88]. Rather, this term encompasses the notion that the cell type that sustains the growth of many cancers possesses stem-cell properties and lies at the pinnacle of a neoplastic hierarchy, giving rise to a "differentiated" progeny that lacks these same properties [87,88].

Leukemic stem cells in *BCR–ABL*-positive leukemia (CML, AML, and ALL)

In CML the mature leukemic cells and their progenitors are morphologically indistinguishable from their normal counterparts, and the distinction requires proof of the presence or absence of the Philadelphia (Ph) chromosome or the Bcr–Abl transcript in these cells [89]. The Ph chromosome is the cytogenetic hallmark of CML, and it results from the reciprocal translocation between the long arms of chromosomes 9 and 22 that leads to the formation of the chimeric oncogenic tyrosine kinase Bcr–Abl, which is central to the pathogenesis of the disease [90]. The Ph chromosome has been shown to be present in nearly all hematopoietic lineages, indicating that the cell of origin of CML has a multilineage differentiation potential [91]. Researchers were able to transplant $CD34^+$ malignant primitive cells from patients with CML into immunodeficient SCID and NOD/SCID mice, which subsequently were able to proliferate and produce mature Ph^+ progeny with kinetics that recapitulated the phase of the donor's disease, and thus providing an *in vivo* model for CML biology [92–94].

Holyoake *et al.* [95] provided the first direct and definitive evidence of the presence of a reversibly quiescent subpopulation of *BCR–ABL*$^+$/$CD34^+$ leukemic cells that exhibit both *in vivo* and *in vitro* stem-cell properties in patients with CML. In a later study, the same group [95,96] demonstrated that those stem cells were leukemic

(*BCR–ABL*$^+$), expressed the immunophenotype CD34$^+$/CD38$^-$/CD45RA$^-$ /CD71$^-$, and could spontaneously exit G_0 state to enter a continuously cytokine-independent proliferating state to produce a *BCR–ABL*$^+$ progeny.

The development of imatinib mesylate (IM) (Gleevec®, Novartis, Basel, Switzerland), a tyrosine kinase inhibitor (TKI) that targets Bcr–Abl, represented a major advance in the treatment of CML, and is now widely accepted as the standard of care first-line treatment of chronic phase CML (CP-CML) [97]. Despite its impressive results, a significant minority of patients with CP-CML and a majority of the patients with the accelerated phase (AP-CML) and blastic phase (BP-CML) either do not respond (primary resistance) or lose their initial response (secondary resistance) to imatinib [98]. Even among imatinib responders, only a few patients achieve complete molecular remission, that is the complete disappearance of *BCR–ABL* transcripts in highly sensitive reverse transcriptase polymerase chain reaction assays [90,99]. There is accumulating evidence that CML LSCs are not eradicated by IM *in vivo*, with patients in complete cytogenetic response (CCR) still demonstrating Ph$^+$ CD34$^+$ cells, CFUs, and LTC-ICs [100]. This indicates that the disease is not eradicated in the vast majority of patients, which is concerning for the possibility of future relapse. Based on these observations, it has been proposed that the successful targeting of the quiescent CML LSC population might be the "holy grail" for achieving cure for this disease.

The most common mechanism of imatinib resistance in CML is the development of mutations in *ABL* [90,101,102]. An important, recent addition to the arsenal against IM-resistant CML, and Ph$^+$ leukemias in general, was the development of nilotinib (Tasigna®, Novartis, Basel, Switzerland) and dasatinib (Sprycel®, Bristol-Myers Squibb, New York). Nilotinib and dasatinib are second-generation TKIs with greater potency of Bcr–Abl inhibition than imatinib. Both nilotinib and dasatinib were demonstrated to be clinically effective in patients with different phases of imatinib-resistant CML, and both were capable of inhibiting the majority of kinase mutations in imatinib-resistant CML [103–107]. However, none of the TKIs in clinical use for CML target the CML LSC [108–111].

Several possible mechanisms were proposed to explain the resistance of CML LSCs to TKIs in addition to mutations. One such mechanism, which is unique to CML, is the amplification of the Bcr–Abl transcript and Bcr–Abl protein [111,112]. Other mechanisms include increased expression of interleukin (IL) 3 receptor, granulocyte colony-stimulating factor receptor, MDR1, and suppressed expression of organic cation transporter 1 (an influx transporter important for imatinib uptake) [112]. It is not clear whether one of these mechanisms is more important than the others or whether they act in concert.

BMS-214662 is a very promising farnesyl transferase inhibitor (FTI) that has been shown to induce selective apoptosis of CML LSCs *in vitro*, both as a single agent and in combination with imatinib or dasatinib, with little effect on normal HSCs [113,114]. BMS-214662 potently induced apoptosis of both proliferating and quiescent CML stem/progenitor cells with <1% recovery of Ph$^+$ LTC-ICs whether harboring wild-type or mutant *BCR–ABL* [114]. Its mechanism of action involves induction of apoptosis through activation of caspases 3 and 8, inhibition of the mitogen activated protein kinase pathway, the inhibitor of apoptosis protein 1, nuclear factor (NF) κB, and the inducible nitric oxide synthase, in addition to the traditional mechanism of action of FTIs, which involves *RAS* inhibition [113,114]. This agent offers the potential for eradication of CP-CML, and a clinical trial is forthcoming [113,114].

The LIC in Ph$^+$ ALL (for further discussion of LSCs in ALL please see below) seems to be considerably more differentiated than an HSC since the phenotype is almost exclusively of B lineage. Castor *et al.* [115] showed that p210$^{BCR-ABL}$ cells originated from HSCs, whereas p190$^{BCR-ABL}$ cells originated from B-cell progenitors. Their data suggested that p210$^{BCR-ABL}$ and p190$^{BCR-ABL}$ represent largely distinct biologic and clinical entities.

Leukemic stem cells in acute myeloid leukemia

The primitive AML leukemic subpopulation capable of leukemic repopulation into NOD/SCID mice has a distinct immunophenotype that is quite similar across the different AML subtypes except acute promyelocytic leukemia, in which direct assessment of the frequency and immunophenotype of LSCs has not been achieved [9,11,76,116]. While heterogeneity exists between individual patients, most AML LSCs share the CD34$^+$/CD38$^-$/CD71$^-$/HLA-DR$^-$ phenotype with normal HSCs (Table 1.1) [9,76]. Nevertheless, several cell-surface antigens were reported to have differential expression between LSCs and normal HSCs (Table 1.2). AML LSCs, for example, differ from normal HSCs by the lack of Thy-1 (CD90) and c-Kit (CD117) expression, and by the expression of IL-3 receptor α chain (CD123) and the novel antigen C-type lectin-like molecule 1 (CLL-1) [117–121]. Additionally, most AML LSCs express CD33, but some

Table 1.2 Key features that distinguish acute myeloid leukemia leukemic stem cells from normal, non-malignant hematopoietic stem cells.

NF-κB upregulation
PI3K upregualtion
PTEN depletion
Lack of expression of c-Kit (CD117), Thy-1 (CD90)
Expression of IL-3 receptor alpha chain (CD123), C-type lectin-like molecule-1 (CLL-1), and VLA-4
Possible overexpression of CD44 and CD33

normal HSCs may express this antigen as well [81]. Finally, CD44 was reported to be overexpressed in both AML and CML LSCs in comparison with normal HSCs [122,123]. In summary, while AML LSCs share some characteristics with HSCs, they differ from HSCs by others, suggesting that these differences should play a role in targeting the LSCs while sparing the non-malignant HSCs.

Leukemic stem cells in acute lymphoblastic leukemia

The presence of an LSC in ALL is a controversial subject. Similar to AML, ALL is a heterogeneous disease with clinically and genetically different subtypes. Rearrangements of the T-cell receptor (TcR) or the immunoglobulin heavy chain (IgH) genes support the theory that T and B-lineage ALL originate in cells already committed to the T or B-cell lineages [124–126].

The development of ALL from a committed B-cell progenitor was suggested by Castor *et al.* [115], who demonstrated that primary *ETV6-RUNX1* (previously *TEL-AML1*; t[12;21][p13;q22]) fusions and subsequent leukemic transformations were targeted to committed B-cell progenitors. Similarly, Kong *et al.* [127] used a novel *in vivo* xenotransplantation model in which purified CD34$^+$/CD38$^+$/CD19$^+$, CD34$^+$/CD38$^-$/CD19$^+$, and CD34$^+$/CD38$^-$/CD19$^-$ cells from pediatric patients with B-ALL were injected into sublethally irradiated newborn NOD/SCID/IL2rγ(null) mice. The authors found that both CD34$^+$/CD38$^+$/CD19$^+$ and CD34$^+$/CD38$^-$/CD19$^+$ cells initiate B-ALL in primary recipients, whereas the recipients of CD34$^+$/CD38$^-$/CD10$^-$/CD19$^-$ cells showed normal human hematopoietic repopulation. It was noted that the extent of leukemic infiltration into the spleen, liver, and kidney was similar between the recipients transplanted with CD34$^+$/CD38$^+$/CD19$^+$ cells and those transplanted with CD34$^+$/CD38$^-$/CD19$^+$ cells. In addition, transplantation of CD34$^+$/CD38$^+$/CD19$^+$ cells resulted in the development of B-ALL in secondary recipients, demonstrating self-renewal capacity. The authors concluded that the identification of CD34$^+$CD38$^+$CD19$^+$ self-renewing B-ALL cells proposes a hierarchy of LICs distinct from that of AML.

Over the last few years there have been several reports indicating that in some ALL subtypes, the leukemic blasts may arise from a more phenotypically primitive HSC rather than a lymphoid-lineage committed progenitor. For example, cytogenetically aberrant cells have been shown to be present in the CD34$^+$/CD38$^-$/CD33$^-$/CD19$^-$ bone marrow compartment in children with B-cell precursor-ALL (BCP-ALL) indicating that ALL blasts in some patients may evolve from a precursor compartment [128]. Similarly, Cox *et al.* [129,130] have demonstrated the presence of cells capable of long-term proliferation in the CD34$^+$/CD10$^-$/CD19$^-$ subfraction of BCP-ALL samples, and in the CD34$^+$/CD4$^-$ and CD34$^+$/CD7$^-$ subfractions of T-ALL pediatric samples. This suggested that a more primitive phenotype was the target for leukemic transformation in these cases. Finally, le Viseur *et al.* [131] showed that in pediatric ALL, blasts at different stages of immunophenotypic maturation have stem-cell properties. The investigators transplanted human leukemic bone marrow into NOD/SCID mice, and found that blasts representative of all of the different maturational stages (CD34$^+$/CD19$^-$, CD34$^+$/CD19$^+$, and CD34$^-$/CD19$^+$) were able to reconstitute and re-establish the complete leukemic phenotype *in vivo*. This represents the potential malleability or plasticity of LSCs, that is the ability of more differentiated leukemia cells to reacquire the LSC characteristics [132]. It is clear that the ALL story is not as straightforward as the AML story.

Targeting the leukemic stem cell

Many genetic mutations, molecular aberrations, and signaling pathway disruptions have been reported to drive leukemogenesis in AML, but little is known on how these abnormalities affect the LSCs [11]. Given the many similarities between LSCs and HSCs, and the central role that LSCs play in leukemia maintenance, studies have focused on identifying pathways of proliferation, self-renewal, and survival that are differentially active in LSCs rather than HSCs. The clear goal is to introduce drugs that are capable of selective targeting pathways that maintain LSCs while sparing normal HSCs (see Table 1.3 for a summary of the targeted approaches discussed below).

The importance of minimal residual disease (MRD) in causing relapse after achieving complete remission (CR) in leukemia is well established [133]. For example, van Rhenen *et al.* recently showed that phenotypically defined LSCs could be detected in patients with AML who achieved CR, and that the frequency of these LSCs at diagnosis correlates with MRD after chemotherapy and with survival [120,121]. These observations suggest that MRD can be detected at the stem-cell level, which may allow for development of a therapy targeted at these residual cells.

Table 1.3 Agents that target leukemia stem cells and spare the hematopoietic stem cells.

Target	Agent
NF-κB	MG-132
	Bortezomib
	DMAPT
	TDZD-8
PI3K	Rapamycin
	ET-18-OCH
Farnesyl transferase	BMS-214662
Mechanism unknown	Hyperthermia
Niche	AMD3100
	Anti-CD44

Targeting leukemic stem-cell survival pathways

The identification of survival pathways that are preferentially overexpressed in LSCs suggest that differential activation of apoptosis mechanisms in LSCs should be possible, and strategies specifically modulating these pathways are likely to be effective in eradication of LSCs [8,12,79,134–136].

Among the more characterized dysfunctional signal transduction pathways that control cell survival in LSCs are NF-κB and phosphatidyl-inositide-3 kinase (PI3K). While unstimulated normal HSCs do not express NF-κB, AML LSCs exhibit readily detectable NF-κB levels [8]. NF-κB is a transcription factor that often has anti-apoptotic effects which render survival advantage to malignant cells [137,138]. Taking advantage of NF-κB, Guzman *et al.* [8] demonstrated that inhibiting NF-κB with the proteasome inhibitor MG-132 contributed to the rapid induction of death of LSCs, whereas normal HSCs were minimally affected, if at all. The agents targeting NF-κB would be of particular appeal since they are expected to have a quite favorable therapeutic index given the almost undetectable levels of NF-κB in normal HSCs [8,11]. The same group [79] combined MG-132 and the anthracycline idarubicin; this combination induced a rapid and extensive apoptosis of the LSC population while leaving normal HSCs viable. Molecular genetic studies demonstrated that inhibition of NF-κB and activation of p53-regulated genes contributed to LSC apoptosis [79].

Parthenolide (PTL), a recently described agent, was found to preferentially induce robust apoptosis in primary human AML cells, AML progenitor cells, and AML stem-cell populations, while sparing normal HSCs [135]. The molecular mechanism of PTL-mediated apoptosis was shown to be strongly associated with NF-κB inhibition and p53 activation [135]. However, PTL has relatively poor pharmacologic properties that limit its potential clinical use [10,136]. Consequently, the investigators [136] developed an oral analog of PTL, dimethylamino-parthenolide (DMAPT), which was demonstrated to induce rapid death of primary human LSCs from both myeloid and lymphoid leukemias, combined with high cytotoxicity to bulk leukemic cell populations. Another exciting, recently described agent is TDZD-8 (4-benzyl-2-methyl-1,2,4-thiadiazolidine-3,5-dione), a molecule that belongs to a family of compounds with glycogen synthase kinase-3β and NF-κB inhibitory activity [10,139]. TDZD-8 selectively induces the death of primary myeloid LSCs and leukemia progenitor cells without causing significant harm to the normal HSCs [139]. In xenotransplantation assays, TDZD-8 inhibited the engraftment of AML LSCs, but did not significantly inhibit the engraftment of normal HSCs [139]. In addition to killing the myeloid LSCs, this agent exhibited potent cytotoxic activity against the bulk blast populations from both lymphoid and myeloid malignancies [139].

Several groups have studied the targeting the PI3K pathway [140–142]. Xu *et al.* [140] reported that the PI3K pathway was constitutively activated in AML cells. The authors also demonstrated that inhibition of either of two important downstream mediator proteins of PI3K, namely Akt/protein kinase B (PKB) or the mammalian target of rapamycin (mTOR), leads to decreased survival of the malignant cells [140]. The same group [141] demonstrated that the combination of rapamycin, an mTOR inhibitor, and etoposide resulted in significant cytotoxicty against AML blasts and reduced LSC survival. Finally, Wierenga *et al.* [142] showed that LSCs have an increased hyperthermic sensitivity compared with their normal counterparts and that this difference can be further increased in combination with ET-18-OCH, another known PI3K inhibitor.

Phosphatase and tensin homolog deleted on chromosome 10 (*PTEN*) was first described as a tumor suppressor located on chromosome 10q23, and was found to be an important suppressor of the PI3K/Akt/mTOR pathway [143–146]. Yilmaz *et al.* [147] demonstrated that conditionally deleting the *PTEN* gene in mice led to a myeloproliferative disease (MPD) within days that evolved into transplantable leukemias within weeks. *PTEN* gene deletion led to HSC depletion, preventing these cells from stably reconstituting irradiated mice, indicating that, in contrast to LSCs, normal HSCs were unable to maintain themselves without *PTEN* [147]. These effects were mostly mediated by mTOR as they were inhibited by rapamycin, which not only depleted LSCs in mice with established leukemia, but also restored normal HSC function [147].

Based on these observations, Jordan and Guzman [12] proposed a model in which the preferential induction of apoptosis in the LSC population, while sparing the normal HSC population, is achieved by a combination of specific types of cellular stress (e.g. hyperthermia or genotoxic stress caused by idarubicin) and inhibition of survival signals (by NF-κB or PI3K inhibitors).

Targeting leukemic stem cell surface antigens and microenvironment

Another appealing mechanism in the attempts to eradicate the LSCs is the use of monoclonal antibodies directed against some of the surface antigens that are differentially expressed on LSCs. CD44 is a transmembrane glycoprotein that has been implicated in cell homing and migration, and was demonstrated to be expressed on the leukemic blasts from most patients with AML [148]. Recent reports have identified the CD44 receptor as a necessary factor in hematopoietic mobilization/homing of both AML and CML LSCs [125,149]. Anti-CD44 monoclonal antibodies were found to reverse myeloid differentiation blockage in monocytic and non-monocytic AML and to induce apoptosis of AML blasts [148]. Later, Jin *et al.* [122] used the same monoclonal antibody (H90 anti-CD44) in NOD/SCID mice transplanted with human AML. This resulted in marked reduction of leukemic repopulation and in absence of leukemia in serially transplanted mice, indicating that AML LSCs were directly targeted [122]. In addition, these findings indicated that homing is crucial for AML LSCs to maintain their stem-cell functions, suggesting that the leukemogenic process does not completely abrogate niche dependence for AML LSCs [122]. The authors [122] pointed out that AML LSCs were more sensitive to anti-CD44-induced eradication than HSCs, probably as a result of the greater abundance of CD44 on the surface of LSCs as compared with normal HSCs.

SDF-1, produced by stromal cells in the bone marrow niche, and its receptor, CXCR4, expressed on normal HSCs, both play an important role in the survival, homing, and engraftment of human HSCs and their retention in the bone marrow niche [150,151]. Similarly, SDF-1–CXCR4 interactions were found to participate in the migration, repopulation, survival, and development of AML LSCs in the bone marrow, therefore neutralizing the SDF-1–CXCR4 axis can act as a potential treatment for AML [152]. Some experimental data suggested that AML LSCs are more sensitive to anti-CXCR4 treatment than normal human HSCs [152]. AMD3100, a selective antagonist of SDF-1 by binding to its receptor CXCR4, was found to inhibit the transmigration of AML blasts, the outgrowth of leukemic CFUs, and the ability of SDF-1 to induce engraftment of AML cells [152,153]. Future studies will determine the selectivity of AMD3100 to LSCs compared with normal HSCs.

Another important surface antigen, CD33, is expressed on normal immature cells of the myeloid lineage, on many AML blasts, and LSCs, regardless of the AML subtype [81]. Gemtuzumab ozogamicin (Mylotarg®, Wyeth, Maidenhead, UK), an anti-CD33 antibody conjugated with calicheamicin with proven activity against AML blasts, has been postulated to cause some direct killing of $CD33^+$ AML LSCs, possibly explaining its efficacy in some AML cases where the majority of the blasts were $CD33^-$ [81,154]. However, despite relatively good efficacy and certain specificity for LSCs compared with normal HSCs, the drug does not work uniformly in all patients and has significant side-effects [154]. The occurrence of prolonged cytopenias in some patients treated with Gemtucumab suggested that CD33 might be expressed on some normal HSCs [81].

Some of the other surface antigens on LSCs that have been proposed as possible targets for future trials of directed therapy include CLL-1, CD123, and the integrin—very late antigen 4 (VLA-4) [120,121,155–158]. No trials have yet reported on the differential effects of these targeted approaches on non-malignant HSCs.

Targeting DNA repair mechanisms of leukemic stem cells

Radiation therapy and some chemotherapeutic agents target G_0 cells. These modalities are expected to inflict significant damage on normal HSCs as well—in fact, normal HSCs may be more susceptible to these effects than LSCs. DNA-damaged normal stem cells, unlike their malignant counterparts, are likely to inhibit DNA repair pathways, preventing error-prone resynthesis of damaged DNA. This path results in the death of these damaged normal stem cells [159]. LSCs, on the other hand, have dysfunctional DNA repair pathways, possibly resulting in continued ability of these DNA-damaged LSCs to escape apoptosis and continue to proliferate. Approaches exploiting these differences are under way.

Targeting self-renewal pathways in leukemic stem cells

The molecular mechanisms that control self-renewal in normal HSCs and LSCs are poorly understood, and most of our limited knowledge so far stems from the mouse leukemia model [14]. Inhibition of self-renewal in LSCs may merely result in causing the LSCs to become dormant without causing significant cytotoxicity [12]. In addition, inhibition of such pathways is likely to also affect normal HSCs [12,14]. On the other hand, blocking self-renewal may result in increased differentiation pressure, which may in turn deplete the LSC compartment [12].

The Polycomb group gene *Bmi-1* belongs to a group of proteins that regulate cell fate in several tissues through diverse mechanisms that include regulation of self-renewal/proliferation, senescence/immortalization and regulation of cell death [160]. In both humans and mice, *Bmi-1* has been shown to be expressed only in primitive bone marrow cells [161–163]. The expression of *Bmi-1* is required for self-renewal and maintenance of normal HSCs [164]. In addition, *Bmi-1* is expressed in all myeloid leukemias studied to date, including the $CD34^+$-enriched LSC fraction [162,165]. The proliferative potential of LSCs and leukemic progenitor cells lacking *Bmi-1* was shown to be compromised, leading to inability to propagate leukemia in mice [165]. In complementation studies, *Bmi-1* completely rescued these proliferative defects, indicating that it has a direct role in mediating self-renewal and regulating the proliferative activity of LSCs in addition to the normal HSCs [165]. These findings suggest that molecular targeting of *Bmi-1* in leukemic stem/progenitor cells might have potent and specific therapeutic effects [165]. In addition, the data from *Bmi-1* studies reinforced the view that understanding how self-renewal processes are linked to mechanisms of survival in both LSCs and normal HSCs is critical for devising future LSC-targeted therapies [12].

A similar pathway of significance is the wingless-type mouse mammary tumor virus (MMTV) integration site family (Wnt)/β-catenin. Wnt signaling plays an important role in HSC self-renewal and proliferation, and aberrant activation of Wnt signaling and downstream effectors has been demonstrated in several forms of leukemias

[166,167]. These findings suggest that the Wnt signaling pathway is an important target in several leukemogenic pathways and may provide a novel opportunity for targeting LSCs [166]. Detailed discussion of this pathway is beyond the scope of this chapter and the interested reader is referred to references 166–169 for further reading.

Conclusions

The LSCs are the best characterized type of cancer stem cells and serve as a model for our understanding of cancer stem-cell biology in general. The central role of LSCs in the pathogenesis of leukemia has become well established. LSCs share some of the basic characteristics with normal HSCs but also differ from the latter by other characteristics. These differences are the basis for the ongoing efforts to develop "magic bullets" targeted against LSCs that will spare the normal HSCs.

Acknowledgments

Supported partially by a grant from the National Cancer Institute Grant CA16056 (MW) and the Heidi Leukemia Research Fund (Buffalo, NY). We thank Dr. Craig T. Jordan (James P. Wilmot Cancer Center, University of Rochester School of Medicine and Dentistry, Rochester, NY) for his critical review of the chapter.

References

1 Smith C. Hematopoietic stem cells and hematopoiesis. *Cancer Control* 2003;10:9–16.
2 Huang X, Cho S, Spangrude GJ. Hematopoietic stem cells: generation and self-renewal. *Cell Death Differ* 2007;14:1851–9.
3 Guo W, Lasky JL, 3rd, Wu H. Cancer stem cells. *Pediatr Res* 2006;59:59R–64R.
4 Wang JC, Dick JE. Cancer stem cells: lessons from leukemia. *Trends Cell Biol* 2005;15:494–501.
5 Szilvassy SJ. The biology of hematopoietic stem cells. *Arch Med Res* 2003;34:446–60.
6 Terpstra W, Ploemacher RE, Prins A, *et al.* Fluorouracil selectively spares acute myeloid leukemia cells with long-term growth abilities in immunodeficient mice and in culture. *Blood* 1996;88:1944–50.
7 Guan Y, Gerhard B, Hogge DE. Detection, isolation, and stimulation of quiescent primitive leukemic progenitor cells from patients with acute myeloid leukemia (AML). *Blood* 2003;101:3142–9.
8 Guzman ML, Neering SJ, Upchurch D, *et al.* Nuclear factor-κB is constitutively activated in primitive human acute myelogenous leukemia cells. *Blood* 2001;98:2301–7.
9 Bonnet D, Dick JE. Human acute myeloid leukemia is organized as a hierarchy that originates from a primitive hematopoietic cell. *Nat Med* 1997;3:730–7.
10 Jordan CT. The leukemic stem cell. *Best Pract Res Clin Haematol* 2007;20:13–18.
11 Jordan CT. Unique molecular and cellular features of acute myelogenous leukemia stem cells. *Leukemia* 2002;16:559–62.
12 Jordan CT, Guzman ML. Mechanisms controlling pathogenesis and survival of leukemic stem cells. *Oncogene* 2004;23:7178–87.
13 Passegue E, Jamieson CH, Ailles LE, Weissman IL. Normal and leukemic hematopoiesis: are leukemias a stem cell disorder or a reacquisition of stem cell characteristics? *Proc Natl Acad Sci U S A* 2003;100(Suppl.1):11842–9.
14 Krause DS, Van Etten RA. Right on target: eradicating leukemic stem cells. *Trends Mol Med* 2007;13:470–81.
15 Wilson A, Trumpp A. Bone-marrow haematopoietic-stem-cell niches. *Nat Rev Immunol* 2006;6:93–106.
16 Hellman S, Botnick LE, Hannon EC, Vigneulle RM. Proliferative capacity of murine hematopoietic stem cells. *Proc Natl Acad Sci U S A* 1978;75:490–4.
17 Akashi K, Traver D, Miyamoto T, Weissman IL. A clonogenic common myeloid progenitor that gives rise to all myeloid lineages. *Nature* 2000;404:193–7.
18 Manz MG, Miyamoto T, Akashi K, Weissman IL. Prospective isolation of human clonogenic common myeloid progenitors. *Proc Natl Acad Sci U S A* 2002;99:11872–7.
19 Ford CE, Hamerton JL, Barnes DW, Loutit JF. Cytological identification of radiation-chimaeras. *Nature* 1956;177:452–4.
20 Till JE, McCulloch EA. A direct measurement of the radiation sensitivity of normal mouse bone marrow cells. *Radiat Res* 1961;14:213–22.
21 Becker AJ, McCulloch EA, Till JE. Cytological demonstration of the clonal nature of spleen colonies derived from transplanted mouse marrow cells. *Nature* 1963;197:452–4.
22 Siminovitch L, McCulloch EA, Till JE. The distribution of colony-forming cells among spleen colonies. *J Cell Physiol* 1963;62:327–36.
23 Iscove N. Haematopoiesis. Searching for stem cells. *Nature* 1990;347:126–7.
24 Jones RJ, Celano P, Sharkis SJ, Sensenbrenner LL. Two phases of engraftment established by serial bone marrow transplantation in mice. *Blood* 1989;73:397–401.
25 Morrison SJ, Weissman IL. The long-term repopulating subset of hematopoietic stem cells is deterministic and isolatable by phenotype. *Immunity* 1994;1:661–73.
26 Fauser AA, Messner HA. Identification of megakaryocytes, macrophages, and eosinophils in colonies of human bone marrow containing neurtophilic granulocytes and erythroblasts. *Blood* 1979;53:1023–7.
27 Leary AG, Ogawa M, Strauss LC, Civin CI. Single cell origin of multilineage colonies in culture. Evidence that differentiation of multipotent progenitors and restriction of proliferative potential of monopotent progenitors are stochastic processes. *J Clin Invest* 1984;74:2193–7.
28 Nakahata T, Ogawa M. Identification in culture of a class of hemopoietic colony-forming units with extensive capability to self-renew and generate multipotential hemopoietic colonies. *Proc Natl Acad Sci U S A* 1982;79:3843–7.
29 Bhatia M, Bonnet D, Kapp U, Wang JC, Murdoch B, Dick JE. Quantitative analysis reveals expansion of human hematopoietic repopulating cells after short-term ex vivo culture. *J Exp Med* 1997;186:619–24.

30 Harrison DE, Jordan CT, Zhong RK, Astle CM. Primitive hemopoietic stem cells: direct assay of most productive populations by competitive repopulation with simple binomial, correlation and covariance calculations. *Exp Hematol* 1993;21:206–19.

31 Kamel-Reid S, Dick JE. Engraftment of immune-deficient mice with human hematopoietic stem cells. *Science* 1988;242:1706–9.

32 Bhatia M, Wang JC, Kapp U, Bonnet D, Dick JE. Purification of primitive human hematopoietic cells capable of repopulating immune-deficient mice. *Proc Natl Acad Sci U S A* 1997;94: 5320–5.

33 Bhatia M, Bonnet D, Murdoch B, Gan OI, Dick JE. A newly discovered class of human hematopoietic cells with SCID-repopulating activity. *Nat Med* 1998;4:1038–45.

34 Osawa M, Hanada K, Hamada H, Nakauchi H. Long-term lymphohematopoietic reconstitution by a single CD34-low/negative hematopoietic stem cell. *Science* 1996;273:242–5.

35 Terstappen LW, Huang S, Safford M, Lansdorp PM, Loken MR. Sequential generations of hematopoietic colonies derived from single nonlineage-committed CD34+CD38– progenitor cells. *Blood* 1991;77:1218–27.

36 Civin CI, Almeida-Porada G, Lee MJ, Olweus J, Terstappen LW, Zanjani ED. Sustained, retransplantable, multilineage engraftment of highly purified adult human bone marrow stem cells in vivo. *Blood* 1996;88:4102–9.

37 Chaudhary PM, Roninson IB. Expression and activity of P-glycoprotein, a multidrug efflux pump, in human hematopoietic stem cells. *Cell* 1991;66:85–94.

38 Reya T, Morrison SJ, Clarke MF, Weissman IL. Stem cells, cancer, and cancer stem cells. *Nature* 2001;414:105–11.

39 Wognum AW, Eaves AC, Thomas TE. Identification and isolation of hematopoietic stem cells. *Arch Med Res* 2003;34:461–75.

40 Gunji Y, Nakamura M, Osawa H, *et al.* Human primitive hematopoietic progenitor cells are more enriched in KIT-low cells than in KIT-high cells. *Blood* 1993;82:3283–9.

41 Ogawa M, Tajima F, Ito T, Sato T, Laver JH, Deguchi T. CD34 expression by murine hematopoietic stem cells. Developmental changes and kinetic alterations. *Ann N Y Acad Sci* 2001;938: 139–45.

42 Goodell MA, Rosenzweig M, Kim H, *et al.* Dye efflux studies suggest that hematopoietic stem cells expressing low or undetectable levels of CD34 antigen exist in multiple species. *Nat Med* 1997;3:1337–45.

43 Zhou S, Schuetz JD, Bunting KD, *et al.* The ABC transporter Bcrp1/ABCG2 is expressed in a wide variety of stem cells and is a molecular determinant of the side-population phenotype. *Nat Med* 2001;7:1028–34.

44 Scharenberg CW, Harkey MA, Torok-Storb B. The ABCG2 transporter is an efficient Hoechst 33342 efflux pump and is preferentially expressed by immature human hematopoietic progenitors. *Blood* 2002;99:507–12.

45 Zanjani ED, Almeida-Porada G, Livingston AG, Flake AW, Ogawa M. Human bone marrow CD34- cells engraft in vivo and undergo multilineage expression that includes giving rise to CD34+ cells. *Exp Hematol* 1998;26:353–60.

46 Domen J, Weissman IL. Self-renewal, differentiation or death: regulation and manipulation of hematopoietic stem cell fate. *Mol Med Today* 1999;5:201–8.

47 Bradford GB, Williams B, Rossi R, Bertoncello I. Quiescence, cycling, and turnover in the primitive hematopoietic stem cell compartment. *Exp Hematol* 1997;25:445–53.

48 Adams GB, Scadden DT. The hematopoietic stem cell in its place. *Nat Immunol* 2006;7:333–7.

49 Adams GB, Chabner KT, Alley IR, *et al.* Stem cell engraftment at the endosteal niche is specified by the calcium-sensing receptor. *Nature* 2006;439:599–603.

50 Morrison SJ, Wandycz AM, Akashi K, Globerson A, Weissman IL. The aging of hematopoietic stem cells. *Nat Med* 1996;2: 1011–16.

51 Nijnik A, Woodbine L, Marchetti C, *et al.* DNA repair is limiting for haematopoietic stem cells during ageing. *Nature* 2007; 447:686–90.

52 Greenwood MJ, Lansdorp PM. Telomeres, telomerase, and hematopoietic stem cell biology. *Arch Med Res* 2003;34: 489–95.

53 Taichman RS. Blood and bone: two tissues whose fates are intertwined to create the hematopoietic stem-cell niche. *Blood* 2005;105:2631–9.

54 Ohlstein B, Kai T, Decotto E, Spradling A. The stem cell niche: theme and variations. *Curr Opin Cell Biol* 2004;16:693–9.

55 Spradling A, Drummond-Barbosa D, Kai T. Stem cells find their niche. *Nature* 2001;414:98–104.

56 Calvi LM, Adams GB, Weibrecht KW, *et al.* Osteoblastic cells regulate the haematopoietic stem cell niche. *Nature* 2003;425: 841–6.

57 Zhang J, Niu C, Ye L, *et al.* Identification of the haematopoietic stem cell niche and control of the niche size. *Nature* 2003;425: 836–41.

58 Visnjic D, Kalajzic Z, Rowe DW, Katavic V, Lorenzo J, Aguila HL. Hematopoiesis is severely altered in mice with an induced osteoblast deficiency. *Blood* 2004;103:3258–64.

59 Stier S, Ko Y, Forkert R, *et al.* Osteopontin is a hematopoietic stem cell niche component that negatively regulates stem cell pool size. *J Exp Med* 2005;201:1781–91.

60 Fliedner TM. The role of blood stem cells in hematopoietic cell renewal. *Stem Cells* 1998;16(Suppl.1):13–29.

61 Mayani H, Alvarado-Moreno JA, Flores-Guzman P. Biology of human hematopoietic stem and progenitor cells present in circulation. *Arch Med Res* 2003;34:476–88.

62 Wagner JE, Kernan NA, Steinbuch M, Broxmeyer HE, Gluckman E. Allogeneic sibling umbilical-cord-blood transplantation in children with malignant and non-malignant disease. *Lancet* 1995;346:214–19.

63 Little MT, Storb R. History of haematopoietic stem-cell transplantation. *Nat Rev Cancer* 2002;2:231–8.

64 Rosenberg SA. Cellular therapy: an introduction. *Cancer J* 2001;7(Suppl.2):S51–2.

65 Kohn DB, Weinberg KI, Nolta JA, *et al.* Engraftment of gene-modified umbilical cord blood cells in neonates with adenosine deaminase deficiency. *Nat Med* 1995;1:1017–23.

66 Kondo M, Scherer DC, Miyamoto T, *et al.* Cell-fate conversion of lymphoid-committed progenitors by instructive actions of cytokines. *Nature* 2000;407:383–6.

67 Trounson A. Stem cells, plasticity and cancer—uncomfortable bed fellows. *Development* 2004;131:2763–8.

68 Goodell MA, Jackson KA, Majka SM, *et al.* Stem cell plasticity in muscle and bone marrow. *Ann N Y Acad Sci* 2001;938:208–18; discussion 218–20.

69 Lagasse E, Connors H, Al-Dhalimy M, *et al.* Purified hematopoietic stem cells can differentiate into hepatocytes in vivo. *Nat Med* 2000;6:1229–34.

70 Mezey E, Chandross KJ, Harta G, Maki RA, Mckercher SR. Turning blood into brain: cells bearing neuronal antigens generated in vivo from bone marrow. *Science* 2000;290:1779–82.

71 Orlic D, Kajstura J, Chimenti S, Bodine DM, Leri A, Anversa P. Bone marrow cells regenerate infarcted myocardium. *Nature* 2001;410:701–5.

72 Bruce WR, Vander Gaag H. A quantitative assay for the number of murine lymphoma cells capable of proliferation in vivo. *Nature* 1963;199:79–80.

73 Clarkson B, Ohkita T, Ota K, Fried J. Studies of cellular proliferation in human leukemia. I. Estimation of growth rates of leukemic and normal hematopoietic cells in two adults with acute leukemia given single injections of tritiated thymidine. *J Clin Invest* 1967;46:506–29.

74 Griffin JD, Lowenberg B. Clonogenic cells in acute myeloblastic leukemia. *Blood* 1986;68:1185–95.

75 Lapidot T, Sirard C, Vormoor J, *et al.* A cell initiating human acute myeloid leukaemia after transplantation into SCID mice. *Nature* 1994;367:645–8.

76 Blair A, Hogge DE, Sutherland HJ. Most acute myeloid leukemia progenitor cells with long-term proliferative ability in vitro and in vivo have the phenotype CD34(+)/CD71(−)/HLA-DR−. *Blood* 1998;92:4325–35.

77 Hope KJ, Jin L, Dick JE. Acute myeloid leukemia originates from a hierarchy of leukemic stem cell classes that differ in self-renewal capacity. *Nat Immunol* 2004;5:738–43.

78 Costello RT, Mallet F, Gaugler B, *et al.* Human acute myeloid leukemia CD34+/CD38− progenitor cells have decreased sensitivity to chemotherapy and Fas-induced apoptosis, reduced immunogenicity, and impaired dendritic cell transformation capacities. *Cancer Res* 2000;60:4403–11.

79 Guzman ML, Swiderski CF, Howard DS, *et al.* Preferential induction of apoptosis for primary human leukemic stem cells. *Proc Natl Acad Sci U S A* 2002;99:16220–5.

80 Chaudhary PM, Roninson IB. Expression and activity of P-glycoprotein, a multidrug efflux pump, in human hematopoietic stem cells. *Cell* 1991;66:85–94.

81 Taussig DC, Pearce DJ, Simpson C, *et al.* Hematopoietic stem cells express multiple myeloid markers: implications for the origin and targeted therapy of acute myeloid leukemia. *Blood* 2005;106:4086–92.

82 Pardal R, Clarke MF, Morrison SJ. Applying the principles of stem-cell biology to cancer. *Nat Rev Cancer* 2003;3:895–902.

83 Cozzio A, Passegue E, Ayton PM, Karsunky H, Cleary ML, Weissman IL. Similar MLL-associated leukemias arising from self-renewing stem cells and short-lived myeloid progenitors. *Genes Dev* 2003;17, 3029–35.

84 Krivtsov AV, Twomey D, Feng Z, *et al.* Transformation from committed progenitor to leukaemia stem cell initiated by *MLL-AF9*. *Nature* 2006;442:818–22.

85 Huntly BJ, Shigematsu H, Deguchi K, *et al. MOZ-TIF2*, but not *BCR–ABL*, confers properties of leukemic stem cells to committed murine hematopoietic progenitors. *Cancer Cell* 2004;6:587–96.

86 Stubbs MC, Kim YM, Krivtsov AV, *et al. MLL-AF9* and *FLT3* cooperation in acute myelogenous leukemia: development of a model for rapid therapeutic assessment. *Leukemia* 2008;22:66–77.

87 Clarke MF, Dick JE, Dirks PB, *et al.* Cancer stem cells–perspectives on current status and future directions: AACR Workshop on cancer stem cells. *Cancer Res* 2006;66:9339–44.

88 Kennedy JA, Barabe F, Poeppl AG, Wang JC, Dick JE. Comment on 'Tumor growth need not be driven by rare cancer stem cells'. *Science* 2007;318:1722, Author reply 1722.

89 Petzer AL, Gunsilius E. Hematopoietic stem cells in chronic myeloid leukemia. *Arch Med Res* 2003;34:496–506.

90 Hughes T, Branford S. Molecular monitoring of BCR–ABL as a guide to clinical management in chronic myeloid leukaemia. *Blood Rev* 2006;20:29–41.

91 Haferlach T, Winkemann M, Nickenig C, *et al.* Which compartments are involved in Philadelphia chromosome-positive chronic myeloid leukaemia? An answer at the single cell level by combining May–Grunwald–Giemsa staining and fluorescence in situ hybridization techniques. *Br J Haematol* 1997;97:99–106.

92 Sirard C, Lapidot T, Vormoor J, *et al.* Normal and leukemic SCID-repopulating cells (SRC) coexist in the bone marrow and peripheral blood from CML patients in chronic phase, whereas leukemic SRC are detected in blast crisis. *Blood* 1996;87:1539–48.

93 Dazzi F, Capelli D, Hasserjian R, *et al.* The kinetics and extent of engraftment of chronic myelogenous leukemia cells in non-obese diabetic/severe combined immunodeficiency mice reflect the phase of the donor's disease: an in vivo model of chronic myelogenous leukemia biology. *Blood* 1998;92:1390–6.

94 Verstegen MM, Cornelissen JJ, Terpstra W, Wagemaker G, Wagnum AW. Multilineage outgrowth of both malignant and normal hemopoietic progenitor cells from individual chronic myeloid leukemia patients in immunodeficient mice. *Leukemia* 1999;13:618–28.

95 Holyoake T, Jiang X, Eaves C, Eaves A. Isolation of a highly quiescent subpopulation of primitive leukemic cells in chronic myeloid leukemia. *Blood* 1999;94:2056–64.

96 Holyoake TL, Jiang X, Jorgensen HG, *et al.* Primitive quiescent leukemic cells from patients with chronic myeloid leukemia spontaneously initiate factor-independent growth in vitro in association with up-regulation of expression of interleukin-3. *Blood* 2001;97:720–8.

97 Kantarjian HM, Talpaz M, Giles F, O'Brien S, Cortes J. New insights into the pathophysiology of chronic myeloid leukemia and imatinib resistance. *Ann Intern Med* 2006;145:913–23.

98 Baccarani M, Saglio G, Goldman J, *et al.* Evolving concepts in the management of chronic myeloid leukemia: recommendations from an expert panel on behalf of the European LeukemiaNet. *Blood* 2006;108:1809–20.

99 Hughes TP, Kaeda J, Branford S, *et al.* Frequency of major molecular responses to imatinib or interferon alpha plus cytarabine in newly diagnosed chronic myeloid leukemia. *N Engl J Med* 2003;349:1423–32.

100 Bhatia R, Holtz M, Niu N, *et al.* Persistence of malignant hematopoietic progenitors in chronic myelogenous leukemia patients in complete cytogenetic remission following imatinib mesylate treatment. *Blood* 2003;101:4701–7.

101 Nardi V, Azam M, Daley GQ. Mechanisms and implications of imatinib resistance mutations in *BCR–ABL*. *Curr Opin Hematol* 2004;11:35–43.

102 Branford S, Rudzki Z, Walsh S, *et al.* Detection of *BCR–ABL* mutations in patients with CML treated with imatinib is virtually always accompanied by clinical resistance, and mutations in the ATP phosphate-binding loop (P-loop) are associated with a poor prognosis. *Blood* 2003;102:276–83.

103 Cortes J, Rousselot P, Kim DW, *et al.* Dasatinib induces complete hematologic and cytogenetic responses in patients with imatinib-resistant or -intolerant chronic myeloid leukemia in blast crisis. *Blood* 2007;109:3207–13.

104 Hochhaus A, Kantarjian HM, Baccarani M, *et al.* Dasatinib induces notable hematologic and cytogenetic responses in chronic-phase chronic myeloid leukemia after failure of imatinib therapy. *Blood* 2007;109:2303–9.

105 Guilhot F, Apperley J, Kim DW, *et al.* Dasatinib induces significant hematologic and cytogenetic responses in patients with imatinib-resistant or -intolerant chronic myeloid leukemia in accelerated phase. *Blood* 2007;109:4143–50.

106 le Coutre P, Ottmann OG, Giles F, *et al.* Nilotinib (formerly AMN107), a highly selective BCR–ABL tyrosine kinase inhibitor, is active in patients with imatinib-resistant or -intolerant accelerated-phase chronic myelogenous leukemia. *Blood* 2008; 111:1834–9.

107 Kantarjian HM, Giles F, Gattermann N, *et al.* Nilotinib (formerly AMN107), a highly selective BCR–ABL tyrosine kinase inhibitor, is effective in patients with Philadelphia chromosome-positive chronic myelogenous leukemia in chronic phase following imatinib resistance and intolerance. *Blood* 2007;110:3540–6.

108 Graham SM, Jorgensen HG, Allan E, *et al.* Primitive, quiescent, Philadelphia-positive stem cells from patients with chronic myeloid leukemia are insensitive to STI571 in vitro. *Blood* 2002;99:319–25.

109 Jorgensen HG, Allan EK, Graham SM, *et al.* Lonafarnib reduces the resistance of primitive quiescent CML cells to imatinib mesylate in vitro. *Leukemia* 2005;19:1184–91.

110 Jorgensen HG, Allan EK, Jordanides NE, Mountford JC, Holyoake TL. Nilotinib exerts equipotent antiproliferative effects to imatinib and does not induce apoptosis in CD34+ CML cells. *Blood* 2007;109:4016–19.

111 Copland M, Hamilton A, Elrick LJ, *et al.* Dasatinib (BMS-354825) targets an earlier progenitor population than imatinib in primary CML but does not eliminate the quiescent fraction. *Blood* 2006;107:4532–9.

112 Jiang X, Zhao Y, Smith C, *et al.* Chronic myeloid leukemia stem cells possess multiple unique features of resistance to BCR–ABL targeted therapies. *Leukemia* 2007;21:926–35.

113 Jorgensen HG, Holyoake TL. Characterization of cancer stem cells in chronic myeloid leukaemia. *Biochem Soc Trans* 2007; 35:1347–51.

114 Copland M, Pellicano F, Richmond L, *et al.* BMS-214662 potently induces apoptosis of chronic myeloid leukemia stem and progenitor cells and synergizes with tyrosine kinase inhibitors. *Blood* 2008;111:2843–53.

115 Castor A, Nilsson L, Astrand-Grundstrom I, *et al.* Distinct patterns of hematopoietic stem cell involvement in acute lymphoblastic leukemia. *Nat Med* 2005;11:630–7.

116 Grimwade D, Enver T. Acute promyelocytic leukemia: where does it stem from? *Leukemia* 2004;18:375–84.

117 Blair A, Hogge DE, Ailles LE, Lansdorp PM, Sutherland HJ. Lack of expression of Thy-1 (CD90) on acute myeloid leukemia cells with long-term proliferative ability in vitro and in vivo. *Blood* 1997;89:3104–12.

118 Jordan CT, Upchurch D, Szilvassy SJ, *et al.* The interleukin-3 receptor alpha chain is a unique marker for human acute myelogenous leukemia stem cells. *Leukemia* 2000;14:1777–84.

119 Blair A, Sutherland HJ. Primitive acute myeloid leukemia cells with long-term proliferative ability in vitro and in vivo lack surface expression of c-kit (CD117). *Exp Hematol* 2000;28:660–71.

120 van Rhenen A, Moshaver B, Kelder A, *et al.* Aberrant marker expression patterns on the CD34+CD38– stem cell compartment in acute myeloid leukemia allows to distinguish the malignant from the normal stem cell compartment both at diagnosis and in remission. *Leukemia* 2007;21:1700–7.

121 van Rhenen A, van Dongen GA, Kelder A, *et al.* The novel AML stem cell associated antigen CLL-1 aids in discrimination between normal and leukemic stem cells. *Blood* 2007;110: 2659–66.

122 Jin L, Hope KJ, Zhai Q, Smadja-Joffe F, Dick JE. Targeting of CD44 eradicates human acute myeloid leukemic stem cells. *Nat Med* 2006;12:1167–74.

123 Krause DS, Lazarides K, von Andrian UH, van Etten RA. Requirement for CD44 in homing and engraftment of BCR–ABL-expressing leukemic stem cells. *Nat Med* 2006;12:1175–80.

124 Russell NH. Biology of acute leukaemia. *Lancet* 1997;349:118–22.

125 Greaves MF. Stem cell origins of leukaemia and curability. *Br J Cancer* 1993;67:413–23.

126 Campana D, van Dongen JJ, Mehta A, *et al.* Stages of T-cell receptor protein expression in T-cell acute lymphoblastic leukemia. *Blood* 1991;77:1546–54.

127 Kong Y, Yoshida S, Saito Y, *et al.* CD34+CD38+CD19+ as well as CD34+CD38-CD19+ cells are leukemia-initiating cells with self-renewal capacity in human B-precursor ALL. *Leukemia* 2008;6:1207–13.

128 Quijano CA, Moore D, 2nd, Arthur D, Feusner J, Winter SS, Pallavicini MG. Cytogenetically aberrant cells are present in the CD34+CD33–38–19- marrow compartment in children with acute lymphoblastic leukemia. *Leukemia* 1997;11:1508–15.

129 Cox CV, Evely RS, Oakhill A, Pamphilon DH, Goulden NJ, Blair A. Characterization of acute lymphoblastic leukemia progenitor cells. *Blood* 2004;104:2919–25.

130 Cox CV, Martin HM, Kearns PR, Virgo P, Evely RS, Blair A. Characterization of a progenitor cell population in childhood T-cell acute lymphoblastic leukemia. *Blood* 2007;109:674–82.

131 le Viseur C, Hotfilder M, Bomken S, *et al.* In childhood acute lymphoblastic leukemia, blasts at different stages of immunophenotypic maturation have stem cell properties. *Cancer Cell* 2008;14:47–58.

132 Trounson A. Stem cells, plasticity and cancer—uncomfortable bed fellows. *Development* 2004;131:2763–2768.

133 Kern W, Haferlach C, Haferlach T, Schnittger S. Monitoring of minimal residual disease in acute myeloid leukemia. *Cancer* 2008;112:4–16.

134 Guzman ML, Jordan CT. Considerations for targeting malignant stem cells in leukemia. *Cancer Control* 2004;11:97–104.

135 Guzman ML, Rossi RM, Karnischky L, *et al.* The sesquiterpene lactone parthenolide induces apoptosis of human acute myelogenous leukemia stem and progenitor cells. *Blood* 2005;105: 4163–9.

136 Guzman ML, Rossi RM, Neelakantan S, *et al.* An orally bioavailable parthenolide analog selectively eradicates acute myelogenous leukemia stem and progenitor cells. *Blood* 2007;110: 4427–35.

137 Mayo MW, Baldwin AS. The transcription factor NF-kappaB: control of oncogenesis and cancer therapy resistance. *Biochim Biophys Act* 2000;1470:M55–62.

138 Karin M, Cao Y, Green FR, Li ZW. NF-kappaB in cancer: from innocent bystander to major culprit. *Nat Rev Cancer* 2002;2: 301–10.

139 Guzman ML, Li X, Corbett CA, *et al.* Rapid and selective death of leukemia stem and progenitor cells induced by the compound 4-benzyl, 2-methyl, 1,2,4-thiadiazolidine, 3,5 dione (TDZD-8). *Blood* 2007;110:4436–44.

140 Xu Q, Simpson SE, Scialla TJ, Bagg A, Carroll M. Survival of acute myeloid leukemia cells requires PI3 kinase activation. *Blood* 2003;102:972–80.

141 Xu Q, Thompson JE, Carroll M. mTOR regulates cell survival after etoposide treatment in primary AML cells. *Blood* 2005;106:4261–8.

142 Wierenga PK, Setroikromo R, Kamps G, *et al.* Differences in heat sensitivity between normal and acute myeloid leukemic stem cells: feasibility of hyperthermic purging of leukemic cells from autologous stem cell grafts. *Exp Hematol* 2003;31: 421–7.

143 Steck PA, Pershouse MA, Jasser SA, *et al.* Identification of a candidate tumour suppressor gene, *MMAC1*, at chromosome 10q23.3 that is mutated in multiple advanced cancers. *Nat Genet* 1997;15:356–62.

144 Li J, Yen C, Liaw D, *et al.* PTEN, a putative protein tyrosine phosphatase gene mutated in human brain, breast, and prostate cancer. *Science* 1997;275:1943–7.

145 Li DM, Sun H. TEP1, encoded by a candidate tumor suppressor locus, is a novel protein tyrosine phosphatase regulated by transforming growth factor beta. *Cancer Res* 1997;57: 2124–9.

146 Cantley LC, Neel BG. New insights into tumor suppression: PTEN suppresses tumor formation by restraining the phosphoinositide 3-kinase/AKT pathway. *Proc Natl Acad Sci U S A* 1999;96:4240–5.

147 Yilmaz OH, Valdez R, Theisen BK, *et al.* Pten dependence distinguishes haematopoietic stem cells from leukaemia-initiating cells. *Nature* 2006;441:475–82.

148 Charrad RS, Li Y, Delpech B, *et al.* Ligation of the CD44 adhesion molecule reverses blockage of differentiation in human acute myeloid leukemia. *Nat Med* 1999;5:669–76.

149 Avigdor A, Goichberg P, Shivtiel S, *et al.* CD44 and hyaluronic acid cooperate with SDF-1 in the trafficking of human CD34+ stem/progenitor cells to bone marrow. *Blood* 2004;103: 2981–9.

150 Lee Y, Gotoh A, Kwon HJ, *et al.* Enhancement of intracellular signaling associated with hematopoietic progenitor cell survival in response to SDF-1/CXCL12 in synergy with other cytokines. *Blood* 2002;99:4307–17.

151 Peled A, Petit I, Kollet O, *et al.* Dependence of human stem cell engraftment and repopulation of NOD/SCID mice on CXCR4. *Science* 1999;283:845–8.

152 Tavor S, Petit I, Porozov S, *et al.* CXCR4 regulates migration and development of human acute myelogenous leukemia stem cells in transplanted NOD/SCID mice. *Cancer Res* 2004; 64:2817–24.

153 Liesveld JL, Bechelli J, Rosell K, *et al.* Effects of AMD3100 on transmigration and survival of acute myelogenous leukemia cells. *Leuk Res* 2007;31:1553–63.

154 Sperr WR, Florian S, Hauswirth AW, Valent P. CD 33 as a target of therapy in acute myeloid leukemia: current status and future perspectives. *Leuk Lymphoma* 2005;46:1115–20.

155 Bakker AB, van den Oudenrijn S, Bakker AQ, *et al.* C-type lectin-like molecule-1:a novel myeloid cell surface marker associated with acute myeloid leukemia. *Cancer Res* 2004;64: 8443–50.

156 Hogge DE, Feuring-Buske M, Gerhard B, Frankel AE. The efficacy of diphtheria-growth factor fusion proteins is enhanced by co-administration of cytosine arabinoside in an immunodeficient mouse model of human acute myeloid leukemia. *Leuk Res* 2004;28:1221–6.

157 Matsunaga T, Takemoto N, Sato T, *et al.* Interaction between leukemic-cell VLA-4 and stromal fibronectin is a decisive factor for minimal residual disease of acute myelogenous leukemia. *Nat Med* 2003;9:1158–65.

158 Du X, Ho M, Pastan I. New immunotoxins targeting CD123, a stem cell antigen on acute myeloid leukemia cells. *J Immunother* 2007;30:607–13.

159 Cairns J. Somatic stem cells and the kinetics of mutagenesis and carcinogenesis. *Proc Natl Acad Sci U S A* 2002;99:10567–70.

160 Lessard J, Sauvageau G. Polycomb group genes as epigenetic regulators of normal and leukemic hemopoiesis. *Exp Hematol* 2003;31:567–85.

161 Lessard J, Schumacher A, Thorsteinsdottir U, *et al.* Functional antagonism of the Polycomb-Group genes eed and Bmi1 in hemopoietic cell proliferation. *Genes Dev* 1999;13:2691–703.

162 Lessard J, Baban S, Sauvageau G. Stage-specific expression of polycomb group genes in human bone marrow cells. *Blood* 1998;91:1216–24.

163 Park IK, He Y, Lin F, *et al.* Differential gene expression profiling of adult murine hematopoietic stem cells. *Blood* 2002;99: 488–98.

164 Park IK, Qian D, Kiel M, *et al.* Bmi-1 is required for maintenance of adult self-renewing haematopoietic stem cells. *Nature* 2003;423:302–5.

165 Lessard J, Sauvageau G. Bmi-1 determines the proliferative capacity of normal and leukaemic stem cells. *Nature* 2003; 423:255–60.

166 Mikesch JH, Steffen B, Berdel WE, Serve H, Müller-Tidow C. The emerging role of Wnt signaling in the pathogenesis of acute myeloid leukemia. *Leukemia* 2007;21:1638–47.

167 Zhao C, Blum J, Chen A, *et al.* T. Loss of beta-catenin impairs the renewal of normal and CML stem cells in vivo. *Cancer Cell* 2007;12:528–41.

168 Schugar RC, Robbins PD, Deasy BM. Small molecules in stem cell self-renewal and differentiation. *Gene Ther* 2008;15: 126–35.

169 Styczynski J, Drewa T. Leukemic stem cells: from metabolic pathways and signaling to a new concept of drug resistance targeting. *Acta Biochim Pol* 2007;54:717–26.

Chapter 2
Epidemiology and Etiology of Leukemias

Andrew Fletcher[1], Annika Whittle[2], and David Bowen[2]
[1]St James's University Hospital, Leeds, UK
[2]St. James's Institute of Oncology, St James's University Hospital, Leeds, UK

Myelodysplastic syndromes and acute myeloid leukemia

Demographics

The incidence of myelodysplastic syndrome (MDS) is consistent across several population-based studies from diagnostic centers at approximately 4 per 100,000 [1,2; see also http://seer.cancer.gov]. MDS becomes more common with increasing age, such that the incidence rises to >30 per 100,000 for people >70 years old [1–3]. Age distribution is similar across French–American–British (FAB) subtypes, with a median age of 77 years at presentation in a large population-based study [1]. Recent studies suggest a lower age at presentation in patients with MDS in Far East countries [4,5]. Males are more commonly affected than females. Although the incidence of MDS is not increasing [2], an aging population will produce an increased prevalence [6].

MDS in children is considerably less common and has different characteristics to the adult form. Examples of these differences include the spectrum of FAB/World Health Organization (WHO) types (refractory anemia with ringed sideroblast [RARS] and 5q– syndrome are almost never seen in childhood) and the spectrum of chromosome abnormalities (a higher proportion of children have abnormalities of chromosome 7) [7].

For patients with *de novo* MDS, the latency time to disease development is unknown. For cases of MDS developing after exposure to an agent known or presumed to cause MDS, the latency period varies. This may be from 1 to 41 years for different radiation exposures [8] and from 1 to 10 years for alkylator cytotoxic drugs [9,10].

Large-scale population-based demographic study of acute myeloid leukemia (AML) has been a surprisingly neglected area, primarily because of the lack of comprehensive registration programs in most world healthcare systems. The incidence of AML is approximately 3.0–3.6 per 100,000 [1; see also http://seer.cancer.gov], and the median age at diagnosis is 67–71 years, with 6.3% of patients diagnosed when under 20 years of age [1; see also http://seer.cancer.gov]. The incidence in adults increases from 1.3 per 100,000 in adolescence to over 15 per 100,000 in the seventh and eighth decade of life [1]. Most studies indicate a predominance of males with adult AML [11,12], but when corrected for population-based age and sex distribution the male predominance becomes less striking [13]. When age- and sex-corrected, female predominance cannot be identified in any karyotypic subgroup [13].

The distribution of karyotypic subgroups in *de novo* AML drastically varies with age. In children and young adults, the favorable karyotypes represent over 25% of AML cases, but in patients <60 years old, this percentage falls to under 10% [13,14]. In contrast, AML with chromosome 5/7 deletion is more common in older patients than in children or young adults [13].

Geographic variation has not been meaningfully studied, but some evidence suggests that, in the USA, white people have a higher incidence of AML than other racial groups (http://seer.cancer.gov).

Etiology

For the great majority of patients with MDS and AML, no clear causative factor can be identified.

Inherited myelodysplastic syndrome/acute myeloid leukemia

Although rare, families with more than one MDS sufferer are described [15]. There is little evidence that MDS with onset at the typical age in late adulthood has an inherited basis. Thirty percent of children with MDS have other associated abnormalities, and some of these are part of well-recognized syndromes, including Fanconi anemia, dyskeratosis congenita, and Schwachman–Diamond syndrome. *Forme fruste* presentations in adulthood are now recognized with both aplastic anemia and MDS. Telomerase complex gene mutations (*TERC* and *TERT*) are presumed causative in these pedigrees [16,17].

True familial AML is also very rare. Families with inherited mutations in the *RUNX1* and also *CEBP*α genes are described [18]. Inherited *RUNX1* mutation is associated with disordered platelets, both quantitative and qualitative, whereas inherited *CEBP*α mutation produces

Leukemias: Principles and Practice of Therapy, 1st edition. Edited by S. Faderl and H. Kantarjian.

apparently isolated AML with no associated hematopoietic or phenotypic defect. *In utero* initiation of AML is also supported by Guthrie card analysis in children with t(8;21) AML (associated with the *AML1–ETO* fusion gene). Although the fusion gene can be identified at birth, such children may develop AML with a latency of as long as 10 years [19]. Other AML subtypes common in infancy include those associated with *MLL* gene rearrangement and AML associated with Down syndrome, particularly transient myeloproliferative disease and acute megakaryoblastic leukemia [20]. No direct evidence for an *in utero* initiation of these tumors has yet been established.

Low penetrance genetic predisposition

Frequently appearing characteristics of MDS and AML include large-scale genomic abnormalities (aneuploidy, predominantly deletional), chromosomal translocations, and a spectrum of more localized genomic damage, namely point mutations, tandem duplications, and small deletions, among many others. The mechanisms underlying aneuploidy, and indeed chromosomal translocation, remain poorly understood.

Murine models indicate an inherited component for predisposition to both benzene- [21] and radiation-induced [22] genomic instability. This creates a paradigm for lower penetrance genetic predisposition, which in turn may produce a weak propensity to leukemogenesis. Theoretically, this predisposition could evolve from functional genetic polymorphisms in key defense genes within detoxification, antioxidant, DNA repair, and genome stabilization pathways, or indeed from the recently proposed quantitative trait loci that govern the number of target (hematopoietic stem) cells (Figure 2.1) [22].

The larger cohorts reported thus far are from patients with AML entered into clinical trials [23] or a relatively young, non-selected AML population [24,25]. Relatively large cohorts of patients with MDS are beginning to be studied [26]. Some studies have correlated polymorphic variant frequency with biologic (cytogenetic) subgroups, and include associations between inv(16) and *NQO1* C609T variant [25], and between cytochrome P450 1A1*2B variant and *NRAS* gene mutation [27]. These subgroup analyses require verification within larger cohorts.

Case–control studies

Attempts to study the environmental/occupational etiology of MDS have focused mainly on case–control studies, although there is little consistency between these studies. Exposure to radiation, halogenated organics, and metals is implicated in one large study [28], while another large study implicated a family history of hematopoietic cancer, smoking, exposure to agricultural chemicals, and exposure to solvents [29]. Several small to medium-sized case–control studies of occupational and environmental exposures are reported for AML [30–33]. Although no consistent exposures are identified across all studies, two studies highlight pesticide exposure as a risk factor [30,31]—one implicates solvent exposure [32], and another emphasizes tobacco smoke exposure [33].

Others

Limited data weakly support an excess of leukemias in painters [34], seamen on tankers [35], and synthetic rubber workers [36], with an excess of myeloid leukemia or AML in meat industry workers [37] and embalmers/funeral directors [38].

Cytotoxic chemotherapeutic agents

Prior exposure to cytotoxic chemotherapy is the most consistent and well-known risk factor for the development of

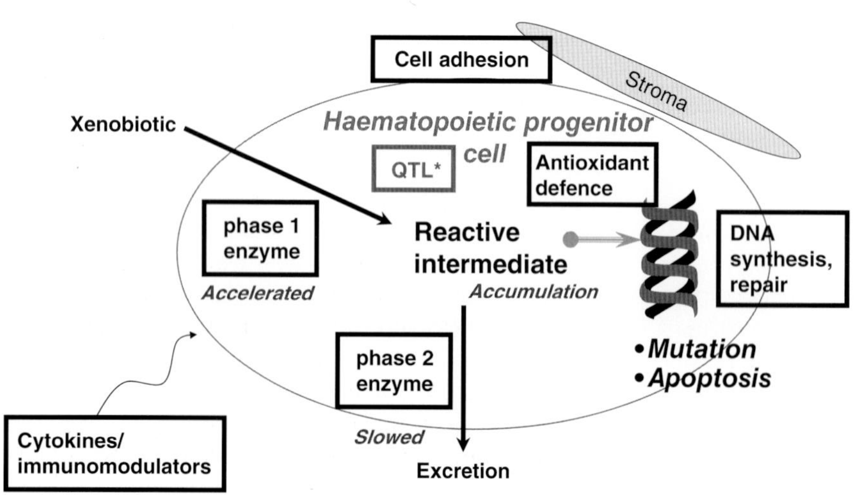

Figure 2.1 Map of physiologic pathways that include predisposition genes with allelic variants that may have been implicated in the initiation of AML and/or MDS. QTL; quantitative trait loci.

AML and MDS. These cases account for approximately 13% of adult patients with AML [10] but less than 10% of all cases of adult MDS. The similarities between the more common karyotypic abnormalities in therapy-related MDS/AML (t-MDS/AML) and poor risk *de novo* MDS/AML have prompted the hypothesis that exposure to environmental genotoxic agents may be implicated in these *de novo* subtypes. Separate genetic pathways to t-MDS/AML can now be defined [39] and these are also observed in *de novo* AML [13,40]. Subtypes of t-MDS/AML have also been distinguished by gene expression profiles [41]. t-MDS/AML following exposure to alkylating agents is characterized by abnormalities of chromosomes 5 and 7, and perhaps most closely mirrors the poorer-prognosis *de novo* AML in the elderly. The latency of onset from the start of previous therapy to the development of t-MDS/AML following exposure to alkylating agent chemotherapy was 63 months (range 7–173 months) in a recent large series [10]. In contrast, t-AML with a short latency and no preceding MDS phase is a rare complication of exposure to topisomerase II inhibitors, and is often associated with *MLL* gene rearrangement and balanced translocations [10]. The increased risk following autologous stem-cell transplantation may be more a function of prior exposure to relevant cytotoxic therapy than of the pathology of transplantation, and the cumulative incidence of t-MDS/AML may be no higher than for conventional chemotherapy alone [42–44].

Several small studies now indicate that genetic predisposition to t-MDS/AML may result from polymorphic variants in genes encoding xenobiotic detoxification pathways, specifically cytochrome P450, glutathione-S transferases T1, M1, and P1, and NADP(H) quinine oxidoreductase-1, but the data are inconsistent [45]. There is stronger evidence for the role of polymorphic variants in genes encoding DNA synthesis and repair pathway proteins as predisposition factors to t-AML. These genes and pathways include methyl tetrahydrofolate reductase [46], nucleotide excision repair [47], homologous recombination [48], and mismatch repair [49,50]. Moreover, allelic variants in genes controlling genomic stability, namely *MDM2* and *TP53*, have recently been shown to predispose to t-AML when combined, but not in isolation [51].

Ionizing radiation

Cases of MDS are reported in cohorts of people exposed to radiation, either for treatment of diseases such as ankylosing spondylitis [52] or following exposure to the atomic bomb in Hiroshima and Nagasaki [53]. Mauritzson *et al.* identified a longer latency period for the development of t-MDS/AML following radiotherapy exposure (median 207 months) compared with alkylating agent chemotherapy plus or minus radiotherapy (median 63 months) [10]. The incidence of t-MDS/AML does not appear to be increased following local radiotherapy for lymphoma, but is probably increased following total body irradiation exposure at autologous stem-cell transplant [54]. There is clear evidence from atomic bomb survivors that relatively high-dose exposure to ionizing radiation can cause AML, with an increased risk that peaked 10 years after exposure and persisted for approximately 15 years after exposure [55].

Prior to 1940, occupational exposure to high doses of radiation also increased the risk of AML, but such a risk no longer appears to be identifiable [56,57]. Radiotherapy for non-malignant conditions can increase the risk of subsequent AML [58–62], but this treatment is no longer offered. Local radiotherapy for cancer is probably not a significant risk factor for AML development when used as the sole treatment, but this remains uncertain [63,64]. While direct genotoxic effects of ionizing radiation are well described [65], a significant contribution may arise from bystander damage to cells adjacent to the hematopoietic stem cell [66]. The most authoritative recent report indicates a lifetime-attributable risk for the development of leukemia following exposure to low-dose ionizing radiation (0.1 Gy) of 1 per 1000 exposed cases [67].

Benzene

Early observations on the link between high-concentration benzene exposure and leukemia/bone marrow failure in Turkish shoe workers identified a preleukemic pancytopenia phase in 13 of 51 patients [68]. In a later follow-up from this cohort ($n = 44$), approximately half of these pancytopenic patients had probable aplastic anemia and the remainder had normo- or hypercellular marrows [69]. A recent prospective cohort study has suggested a high incidence of morphologic dysplasia with subsequent development of MDS or AML in individuals exposed to benzene [70]. The same cohort of benzene-exposed shoe workers (74,828 individuals) showed a significantly elevated relative risk for the development of MDS of ∞ (95% confidence interval, 1.7 ∞) compared with a non-exposed cohort (35,805 individuals) [71].

These data for occupational exposure to high concentrations of benzene indicate a cause and effect for the development of AML. This is supported by data from a seminal study of benzene exposure to employees in Pliofilm manufacture [72]. These exposures are now historic, with strict exposure limits now imposed upon modern western industry. The data for the relationship between exposure to low doses of benzene and the development of AML are contentious, and usually rely on models of linear extrapolation from high-dose exposure studies [73,74]. Environmental exposure to benzene predominantes in tobacco smoke (see below) and unleaded gas. No consistent increased risk of developing AML has been identified for car users, gas station employees, vehicle mechanics [75], or exposure to diesel exhaust [76].

Inflammatory/infectious disorders

Many paradigms exist linking cancer to inflammatory or infectious disease. Although no definite associations can be identified for AML, there are weak associations reported with inflammatory bowel disease [77,78]. There appears to be no clear link between infectious disease and AML.

Lifestyle factors

Although not extensively studied, there is no evidence to implicate diet in the etiology of MDS or AML [79,80]. Exposure to tobacco smoke is a consistent but weak risk factor for the development of AML. The largest reported studies are from a relatively younger cohort of patients, aged 16–69 years [81], and from a Scandinavian cohort with a median age of 62 years [82]. The risk appears strongest in current smokers, and probably declines to baseline in ex-smokers up to 10 years after quitting. The only carcinogen present in tobacco smoke that is implicated in the etiology of AML is benzene. However, the estimated exposure levels to benzene for smokers are considerably lower than those observed in individuals with occupational benzene poisoning. Nevertheless, the leukemogenic effects of low-level benzene exposure remain unclear, and some authors believe that benzene exposure is responsible for up to 60% of smoking-related AML mortality [83].

Acute lymphoblastic leukemia

Demographics

There are three distinct age groups for acute lymphoblastic leukemia (ALL): adulthood (>19 years old), childhood (1–19 years old), and infancy (less than 1 year old), with the highest incidence of ALL in children between the ages of 1 and 10 years. The National Cancer Institute's (NCI) Surveillance Epidemiology and End Results (SEER) cancer statistics analysis estimated that in 2008 there would be almost 5500 new cases of ALL diagnosed in adults in the USA. Sixty percent of these would be male. The age adjusted incidence of ALL is 1.6 per 100,000 per year. The incidence rises steadily from the third decade from 0.7 to 1.8 per 100,000 at an age of >85 years [84].

The commonest childhood cancer is ALL, with 2400 new patients diagnosed in the USA each year. The incidence rate of ALL peaks at 80 cases per 100,000 between 2 and 3 years of age, drops rapidly to 20 per 100,000 at 10 years of age, then slowly decreases through adolescence. There is a slight gender difference in childhood, with boys having a 20% higher incidence than girls. Adolescence (15–29 years of age) is a true transition from pediatric to adult ALL incidence and subtypes [85]. Within this age group the incidence of all malignancies is 2.7 times greater than in childhood, but much less common than in adulthood. The incidence of ALL drops from 1.2 per 100,000 in 15–19 year olds to less than 0.5 per 100,000 in 25–29 year olds. The difference in incidence between genders is more marked between the ages of 15 and 19 years than in adults or children. ALL in infants has an incidence of 4.4 per 100,000, with approximately 200 new cases per year in the USA [84].

The incidence of ALL in all age groups has been gradually rising over the past 25 years [2]. The reasons for this are poorly understood but it is suggested that increasing population mixing, as discussed below, may be contributing to this [85].

Etiology

The search for the etiology of ALL has focused on childhood disease because this is where its incidence is highest. Investigations have shown that prenatal genetic translocations are the first step in leukemogenesis followed by postnatal events leading to further genetic mutations and then overt disease [86].

Genetic disorders that have been shown to increase the risk of ALL include Down syndrome, Bloom syndrome, Fanconi anemia, and ataxia telangiectasia [87–90]. Down syndrome is probably the most investigated, and there are now proven links with the biology of Down syndrome and leukemia. However, the common genetic abnormalities seen in ALL are less frequent in Down syndrome and it is postulated that other factors may play a role in leukemogenesis in these children [88].

Cytogenetic abnormalities are seen in more than 75% of patients with ALL [91]. Different translocations and genetic changes are seen at the various stages of life, each with varying impact on leukemogenesis.

The high incidence of ALL in childhood points directly to there being an initiating event *in utero* on the background of a genetic predisposition [92]. The prenatal origin of ALL is supported by the concordance rates in identical twins, analysis of neonatal Guthrie card blood spots, and analysis of umbilical cord blood samples of children developing leukemia. Concordance rates in twins developing ALL vary with the age at diagnosis. Concordance rates for infant ALL, childhood ALL, and adult ALL are >50%, 10%, and <1%, respectively. Siblings of those with ALL have a risk that is twice that of the general population. Guthrie card analysis of children developing ALL has shown that the genetic lesions can be detected within days of birth, supporting the suggestion that these changes occur *in utero*. Genetic alterations are detectable in Guthrie card tests for all children with mixed lineage leukemia (MLL) rearrangements, and in 75% of those with the *TEL–AML1* fusion gene [93–99]. Hyperdiploid is the other common genetic change seen in childhood ALL. Evidence that this is also a prenatal event in the majority of cases comes from analysis of cord blood samples collected at birth. Although these genetic events occur *in utero*, a latency period of up to 14 years must follow before overt leukemia is detected [95]. However, the fact that not all pairs of twins show concordant development of ALL supports the notion that additional later events must bring about genetic alterations leading to leukemogenesis [96–100].

Significant evidence for postnatal events, which trigger the development of ALL, include the high incidence of *TEL–AML1* fusion genes detectable in neonatal blood spots that far exceed the rate of ALL. One percent of newborns have this fusion gene detectable 100 times more frequently than ALL with this translocation [101]. This is further supported by the discovery that the majority of adults have transient circulation of cells with the *BCR–ABL* translocation but never develop chronic myeloid leukemia or ALL. These cells are either not present in large enough numbers or more likely require further transforming events to generate clinically significant disease [102].

The search for factors other than genetic predisposition has focused on the demographic epidemiology of ALL. The most likely cooperating candidates are infections, and investigation into these as a causative factor has given rise to two closely related hypotheses that cannot be mutually exclusive.

Kinlen's hypothesis that population mixing bringing common infective agents, most likely viruses, into a new community increases the incidence of ALL. This hypothesis came about through investigation of the increased incidence of ALL and non-Hodgkin lymphoma in the localities near two nuclear power stations in the UK. The evidence was against direct exposure to radioactive material, and Kinlen proposed that the influx of specialist workers to previously isolated communities had brought about exposure to new pathogens [107]. This has been demonstrated in a number of studies within the United Kingdom and elsewhere, all of which demonstrate time–space clustering in populations that undergo frequent alterations and mixing [104–110]. It has been suggested that population mixing can be implicated in up to 50% of cases of childhood ALL [104]. The mechanism translating the population mixing hypothesis into cases of ALL is postulated to be an abnormal immune response giving rise to an abnormal lymphoid leukemia clone.

The second hypothesis by Greaves suggests that a delayed exposure to common infective agents brings about a mutation within the normal immune response, which could act as a "second hit" to cause ALL in those who are already genetically predisposed [111]. Greaves suggests that increased cleanliness, or protection against pathogens, reduces the stimulation of the normal immune system responses that allow its effectiveness and efficiency to develop [86]. Support for this hypothesis is seen in work demonstrating that increasing attendance at preschool day care has an inverse relationship to developing ALL, as it does for those in areas of higher socioeconomic status [112–114]. This association may be significant in up to 75% of ALL cases diagnosed between the ages of 2 and 5 years [111,115].

The hypotheses of Greaves and Kinlen complement rather than contradict each other. Population mixing leads to an increase in exposure to infections in a previously protected group, and this leads to a delayed immune stimulation, bringing about leukemogenesis.

Infection exposure as a risk for ALL can be seen when the number of infections within the first year of life are counted. Those who have had more infections have a higher risk of developing ALL [116]. However, investigations into specific viral genomes (e.g. herpes viruses, polyoma viruses [JC and BK], parvovirus B19, and TT viruses) within leukemia cells in blood or marrow have not found a direct causative agent [117]. Direct viral transformation is therefore unlikely to cause ALL, suggesting an indirect immunologic mechanism.

Ionizing radiation is commonly known for having leukemogenic effects in some diseases. However, these direct effects leading to ALL have been challenged. Since the 1940s, descriptions of an increased risk of leukemia in radiologists have been published. Exposure to ionizing radiation in any form, including X-rays, radiotherapy, and the aftermath of the atomic bombs of Hiroshima and Nagasaki, have all been shown to increase the risk of leukemia [118]. Ionizing radiation effects random DNA damage, mutations, and genetic instability within affected cells. There is also increasing evidence that intracellular communication and inflammation contribute to the development of malignant cells [119]. Following radiation exposure, the risk of developing hematologic malignancy is greatest for AML and MDS, followed by ALL and chronic myeloid leukemia [120]. Because the genetic changes in ALL are not random, ionizing radiation is now less likely to be considered as a direct effect, but rather as a factor for developing secondary genetic changes in those with primary predisposing mutations in the same way as the indirect effect of infection, as described above [121].

The risk of exposure to non-ionizing radiation has been a controversial topic of discussion. Initial studies reported a twofold increased risk of ALL in those exposed to electromagnetic fields greater than 0.4 μT [122]. This has been challenged by statistically more robust work detailing that there was no link with electromagnetic fields measured in the houses of those diagnosed with ALL compared with those of matched controls [123].

Other environmental exposures considered to increase the risk of ALL include smoking, alcohol intake, and exposure to benzene, gas, and pesticides. All of these have been reported to increase the risk of infant ALL after exposure when in the womb [124]. Some of these associations, especially smoking, are subject to considerable controversy, but the common link is the presence of topoisomerase inhibitors [125]. The topoisomerase enzymes play a central role in DNA repair. The most carefully studied drugs that inhibit this repair system are cancer therapies, including epipodophyllotoxins (etoposide) and anthracyclines (doxorubicin), and some quinolone antibiotics (ciprofloxacin).The anticancer drugs are intensively investigated and known to be involved in causing secondary cancers, seen after therapy for germ cell tumors, ALL, and lymphoma [126]. It has therefore not been difficult to extrapolate a link between ALL in infants and maternal topoisomerase-inhibitor exposure, and further work in this area continues [94,125].

Other factors being investigated as potentially causative for ALL include birth weight and parental age. A meta-analysis has concluded that an increased birth weight (above 4000 g) was associated with a greater risk of ALL. This shows a dose–response-like effect [127]. Swedish and Italian investigators have demonstrated an increased risk of ALL with increasing maternal age, but no direct biologic reason can be determined [128].

Polycythemia rubra vera

The incidence of polycythemia vera (PV) in southern England was 1.08 per 100,000 in 1999–2000 [1]. However, the reported rates worldwide vary from 0.2 per 100,000 per year in Japan [129] to 28 per 100,000 per year in Goteborg, Sweden [130], and SEER reports an incidence for all chronic myeloproliferative disorders of 2 per 100,000 for the period of 2000–2005 (http://seer.cancer.gov). The 15-year survival was 65% for patients with PV in Italy, with a significantly higher mortality risk of 1.6 as compared with the general population [131]. An American study described the prevalence as 22 per 100,000 in the state of Connecticut, with values of less than 10 in the under 40 age group and 400 in over 75 year olds [132]. PV presents at a median age of 60–70 years, and the incidence is the same in men and women [1].

Several families with clonal polycythemia rubra vera (PRV) have been described in the literature, as identified by erythropoietin-independent erythroid colony and X chromosome linkage studies [133,134]. Strong evidence now supports a familial predisposition to all myeloproliferative disorders (MPDs), with an increased risk in first-degree relatives [135]. One recent paper presents a statistical model, which may allow only one event (insult) to produce PRV with a very long latency [136]. Occupational toxins, ionizing radiation, and viruses have all occasionally been suggested as causes [137,138].

Essential thrombocythemia

The incidence of essential thrombocythemia (ET) is 1.65 per 100,000 in southern England [1]. In the state of Connecticut, the prevalence was described as 24 per 100,000, with a steep rise in prevalence with age from 42 in the under 40 year olds to 339 in the over 75 year olds [132]. The median age at diagnosis is 73 years (range 21–99 years), and there are no significant gender differences [1]. There are two peaks of incidence, one in young women and one in later adult life.

Families with a history of clonal myeloproliferative disorders often display ET, with some pedigrees including cases of both PV and ET [134]. There are no meaningful studies of environmental etiology.

Idiopathic myelofibrosis

The incidence of chronic idiopathic myelofibrosis (IMF) was 0.37 per 100,000 in south-east England in 2000 [1], and the WHO quotes rates of 0.5–1.5 per 100,000 [139]. The peak incidence is in the 7th decade, with no difference between genders [139].

Idiopathic myelofibrosis is a clonal myeloproliferative disorder, which can be primary (idiopathic) or secondary to PV or ET. The etiology of IMF remains poorly researched, but some familial cases have been reported [134]. As regards environmental epidemiology, ionizing radiation and occupational exposure to toxins in gas refinery and chemical-plant workers have been linked to IMF [137–139].

Chronic myeloid leukemia

Chronic myeloid leukemia (CML) has a worldwide incidence of 1–1.5 per 100,000 [139–141]. CML constitutes 15–20% of all leukemias. SEER reports age-adjusted rates of around 0.7 for patients <65 years old, and seven for patients >65 years old (http://seer.cancer.gov). The median age at diagnosis is 40–60 years, and although it is rare below the age of 20, all age groups can be affected. The incidence of CML increases exponentially with age. There is no geographic variation, but it is slightly more common in white and black people than in Hispanic or Asian people in the USA (http://seer.cancer.gov). CML has a slight male predominance [142].

The latent phase between the transforming event and diagnosis is not known, but in atomic bomb survivors incidence of CML increased around 7 years after exposure, and the median latent period was 11 years (range 20–25 years) [143]. In patients irradiated for ankylosing spondylitis, the latent phase was shorter at 3.6 years (range 1–6 years) [143].

Therapeutic and diagnostic radiation exposure has been well described as a causative factor for CML, as has a higher incidence of CML in atomic bomb survivors [144]. A recent review concluded that there was some evidence for increased risk in farmers and agricultural workers exposed to pesticides [141], but most papers state that, bar radiation, no predisposing factors have been identified. There is no obvious familial association or predisposing human leukocyte antigen (HLA) type. No link with infectious agents has been established.

Chronic lymphocytic leukemia

The incidence of B chronic lymphocytic leukemia (CLL) is 3–5 per 100,000 per year [145–147]. Although some report a stable [147] or decreasing incidence [145], others point at delayed reporting due to early diagnoses being made by immunophenotyping only [148,149]. Supporting this latter hypothesis, a recently published study detected monoclonal CLL-phenotype B cells in 5.1% (78/1520) of adults with a normal blood count and 13.9% (309/2228) of adults with lymphocytosis [150]. CLL is the commonest type of leukemia in the western world, accounting for 30–40% of leukemias in those over 65 years of age [148], and it represents two-thirds of B-cell lymphocytoses. It is 20–30 times more common in Europe, Australasia, and North America than in India, China, and Japan [151]. Age-adjusted incidence rates for CLL/small lymphocytic lymphoma are 25–28% and 69–80% lower among African-Americans and Asian/Pacific islanders, respectively, in comparison with white people [146,147,149,152]. Interestingly, the low incidence rates persist among emigrants to the USA from Asian countries and their descendants, excluding an environmental or lifestyle influence [153,154].

It is twice as common in men than in women in all populations [145,146]. The median age at presentation is 60–65 years, and it is rare below the age of 30–40 years [155]. Most current figures include pre-WHO diagnoses (e.g. other chronic lymphoproliferative disorders), and are therefore, to an extent, inaccurate [148]. In approximately 50% of patients, the disease is a chance finding on a full blood count done for another reason.

The etiology of CLL is still unclear, although age, race, and family history of CLL or other lymphoproliferative malignancies are risk factors for CLL [145,148,151]. A familial component can be detected in 5–10% of patients [156]. There is an increase in both lymphoid malignancies, including CLL, and subclinical monoclonal B-cell expansion in first- and second-degree relatives of patients with CLL [157,158]; the relative risk of developing the disease has been quoted as twofold to sevenfold in relatives of patients with CLL [159]. Some families with CLL also show the phenomenon of anticipation, in which the disease presents earlier and in a more severe form in successive generations [156]. Despite these data supporting a genetic basis, and the identification of a number of candidate genes, specific susceptibility genes have not been replicated in follow-up studies [160].

Beside genetic and familial factors predisposing to CLL, very little is known in terms of causal factors determining the onset of the disease [146]. Cigarette smoking, diet, and viral infections have not been convincingly linked to CLL [161]. While radiation is linked to other types of leukemia, no convincing association has been found for CLL [162]. Some studies have linked exposure to chemical agents, especially pesticides and solvents, to CLL, but the evidence to date remains inconclusive [163]. Although autoimmune disorders such as hemolytic anemia are strongly linked with CLL, these occur as a consequence of the immune deregulation and are not causal factors [164,165]. CLL is not more frequent in patients affected by immunodeficiencies [155]. The incidence of second malignancies is increased both in treated and untreated CLL.

Several biologic, molecular, and functional factors support the possibility that an antigenic stimulation (either by self-antigens or foreign elements) might play a relevant role in the natural history of the disease [155,161,165]. In one study, rheumatic valve disease (associated with antibiotic use) had a lower CLL risk, while patients with pneumonia and sinusitis had a borderline increased risk of CLL [164,166].

Most studies point at two main difficulties when investigating the etiology of CLL. Firstly, classification has changed multiple times, and often includes other leukemias or B-cell lymphomas. Secondly, the rarity of CLL requires very large patient numbers in order to reach statistical significance.

References

1 Phekoo KJ, Richards MA, Moller H, Schey SA. The incidence and outcome of myeloid malignancies in 2,112 adult patients in South East-England. *Haematologica* 2006;91:1400–4.
2 Germing U, Strupp C, Kundgen A, *et al.* No increase in age-specific incidence of myelodysplastic syndromes. *Haematologica* 2004;89:905–10.
3 Williamson PJ, Kruger AR, Reynolds PJ, Hamblin TJ, Oscier DG. Establishing the incidence of myelodysplastic syndrome. *Br J Haematol* 1994;87:743–5.
4 Chen B, Zhao WL, Jin J, *et al.* Clinical and cytogenetic features of 508 Chinese patients with myelodysplastic syndrome and comparison with those in Western countries. *Leukemia* 2005;19: 767–75.
5 Irons RD, Wang X, Gross SA, *et al.* Prevalence of MDS subtypes in Shanghai, China: a comparison of the World Health Organization and French American British classifications. *Leuk Res* 2006;30:769–75.
6 Aul C, Germing U, Gattermann N, Minning H. Increasing incidence of myelodysplastic syndromes: real or fictitious? *Leuk Res* 1998;22:93–100.
7 Niemeyer CM, Hasle H. Myelodysplastic syndrome and juvenile myelomonocytic leukemia in children. In: Bennett JM, editor. *The Myelodysplastic Syndromes*. New York: Marcel Dekker Inc, 2002. p.299.
8 Moloney WC. Radiogenic leukemia revisited. *Blood* 1987;70: 905–8.
9 Pedersen-Bjergaard J, Andersen MK, Christiansen DH, Nerlov C. Genetic pathways in therapy-related myelodysplasia and acute myeloid leukemia. *Blood* 2002;99:1909–12.

10 Mauritzson N, Albin M, Rylander L, *et al.* Pooled analysis of clinical and cytogenetic features in treatment-related and de novo adult acute myeloid leukemia and myelodysplastic syndromes based on a consecutive series of 761 patients analyzed 1976–1993 and on 5098 unselected cases reported in the literature 1974–2001. *Leukemia* 2002;16:2366–78.
11 Cartwright RA, Gurney KA, Moorman AV. Sex ratios and the risks of haematological malignancies. *Br J Haematol* 2002;118: 1071–7.
12 Preiss BS, Kerndrup GB, Schmidt KG, *et al.* Cytogenetic findings in adult de novo acute myeloid leukaemia. A population-based study of 303/337 patients. *Br J Haematol* 2003;123:219–34.
13 Sanderson RN, Johnson PR, Moorman AV, *et al.* Population-based demographic study of karyotypes in 1709 patients with adult acute myeloid leukemia. *Leukemia* 2006;20:444–50.
14 Pui CH, Schrappe M, Ribeiro RC, Niemeyer CM. Childhood and adolescent lymphoid and myeloid leukemia. *Hematology Am Soc Hematol Educ Program* 2004;118–45.
15 Lucas GS, West RR, Jacobs A. Familial myelodysplasia. *BMJ* 1989;299:551.
16 Marrone A, Sokhal P, Walne A, *et al.* Functional characterization of novel telomerase *RNA* (*TERC*) mutations in patients with diverse clinical and pathological presentations. *Haematologica* 2007;92:1013–20.
17 Xin ZT, Beauchamp AD, Calado RT, *et al.* Functional characterization of natural telomerase mutations found in patients with hematologic disorders. *Blood* 2007;109:524–32.
18 Owen C, Barnett M, Fitzgibbon J. Familial myelodysplasia and acute myeloid leukaemia-a review. *Br J Haematol* 2008;140: 123–32.
19 Wiemels JL, Xiao Z, Buffler PA, *et al.* In utero origin of t(8;21) AML1-ETO translocations in childhood acute myeloid leukemia. *Blood* 2002;99:3801–5.
20 Zwaan MC, Reinhardt D, Hitzler J, Vyas P. Acute leukemias in children with Down syndrome. *Pediatr Clin North Am* 2008;55:53–70, x.
21 Gowans ID, Lorimore SA, McIlrath JM, Wright EG. Genotype-dependent induction of transmissible chromosomal instability by gamma-radiation and the benzene metabolite hydroquinone. *Cancer Res* 2005;65:3527–30.
22 Boulton E, Cole C, Knight A, Cleary H, Snowden R, Plumb M. Low-penetrance genetic susceptibility and resistance loci implicated in the relative risk for radiation-induced acute myeloid leukemia in mice. *Blood* 2003;101:2349–54.
23 Seedhouse C, Faulkner R, Ashraf N, Das-Gupta E, Russell N. Polymorphisms in genes involved in homologous recombination repair interact to increase the risk of developing acute myeloid leukemia. *Clin Cancer Res* 2004;10:2675–80.
24 Sibley K, Rollinson S, Allan JM, *et al.* Functional FAS promoter polymorphisms are associated with increased risk of acute myeloid leukemia. *Cancer Res* 2003;63:4327–30.
25 Smith MT, Wang Y, Kane E, *et al.* Low NAD(P)H: quinone oxidoreductase 1 activity is associated with increased risk of acute leukemia in adults. *Blood* 2001;97:1422–6.
26 Jankowska AM, Gondek LP, Szpurka H, Nearman ZP, Tiu RV, Maciejewski JP. Base excision repair dysfunction in a subgroup of patients with myelodysplastic syndrome. *Leukemia* 2008;22:551–8.
27 Bowen DT, Frew ME, Rollinson S, *et al.* CYP1A1*2B (Val) allele is overrepresented in a subgroup of acute myeloid leukemia patients with poor-risk karyotype associated with *NRAS* mutation, but not associated with *FLT3* internal tandem duplication. *Blood* 2003;101:2770–4.
28 West RR, Stafford DA, Farrow A, Jacobs A. Occupational and environmental exposures and myelodysplasia: a case–control study. *Leuk Res* 1995;19:127–39.
29 Strom SS, Gu Y, Gruschkus SK, Pierce SA, Estey EH. Risk factors of myelodysplastic syndromes: a case–control study. *Leukemia* 2005;19:1912–18.
30 Richardson S, Zittoun R, Bastuji Garin S, *et al.* Occupational risk factors for acute leukaemia: a case–control study. *Int J Epidemiol* 1992;21:1063–73.
31 Ciccone G, Mirabelli D, Levis A, *et al.* Myeloid leukemias and myelodysplastic syndromes: chemical exposure, histologic subtype and cytogenetics in a case–control study. *Cancer Genet Cytogenet* 1993;68:135–9.
32 Lazarov D, Waldron HA, Pejin D. Acute myeloid leukaemia and exposure to organic solvents—a case–control study. *Eur J Epidemiol* 2000;16:295–301.
33 Speer SA, Semenza JC, Kurosaki T, Anton-Culver H. Risk factors for acute myeloid leukemia and multiple myeloma: a combination of GIS and case–control studies. *J Environ Health* 2002;64:9–16.
34 Chen R, Seaton A. A meta-analysis of painting exposure and cancer mortality. *Cancer Detect Prev* 1998;22:533–9.
35 Nilsson RI, Nordlinder R, Horte LG, Jarvholm B. Leukaemia, lymphoma, and multiple myeloma in seamen on tankers. *Occup Environ Med* 1998;55:517–21.
36 Sathiakumar N, Delzell E, Hovinga M, *et al.* Mortality from cancer and other causes of death among synthetic rubber workers. *Occup Environ Med* 1998;55:230–5.
37 Metayer C, Johnson ES, Rice JC. Nested case–control study of tumors of the hemopoietic and lymphatic systems among workers in the meat industry. *Am J Epidemiol* 1998;147: 727–38.
38 Hayes RB, Blair A, Stewart PA, Herrick RF, Mahar H. Mortality of U.S. embalmers and funeral directors. *Am J Ind Med* 1990; 18:641–52.
39 Pedersen-Bjergaard J, Andersen MK, Andersen MT, Christiansen DH. Genetics of therapy-related myelodysplasia and acute myeloid leukemia. *Leukemia* 2008;22:240–8.
40 Schoch C, Kern W, Kohlmann A, Hiddemann W, Schnittger S, Haferlach T. Acute myeloid leukemia with a complex aberrant karyotype is a distinct biological entity characterized by genomic imbalances and a specific gene expression profile. *Genes Chromosomes Cancer* 2005;43:227–38.
41 Qian Z, Fernald AA, Godley LA, Larson RA, Le Beau MM. Expression profiling of CD34+ hematopoietic stem/progenitor cells reveals distinct subtypes of therapy-related acute myeloid leukemia. *Proc Natl Acad Sci U S A* 2002;99:14925–30.
42 Metayer C, Curtis RE, Vose J, *et al.* Myelodysplastic syndrome and acute myeloid leukemia after autotransplantation for lymphoma: a multicenter case–control study. *Blood* 2003;101: 2015–23.
43 Pedersenbjergaard J, Pedersen M, Myhre J, Geisler C. High risk of therapy-related leukemia after beam chemotherapy and autologous stem cell transplantation for previously treated lymphomas is mainly related to primary chemotherapy and not to the beam-transplantation procedure. *Leukemia* 1997;11:1654–60.

44 Barlogie B, Tricot G, Haessler J, *et al.* Cytogenetically defined myelodysplasia after melphalan-based autotransplantation for multiple myeloma linked to poor hematopoietic stem-cell mobilization: the Arkansas experience in more than 3,000 patients treated since 1989. *Blood* 2008;111:94–100.

45 Seedhouse C, Russell N. Advances in the understanding of susceptibility to treatment-related acute myeloid leukaemia. *Br J Haematol* 2007;137:513–29.

46 Guillem VM, Collado M, Terol MJ, *et al.* Role of MTHFR (677, 1298) haplotype in the risk of developing secondary leukemia after treatment of breast cancer and hematological malignancies. *Leukemia* 2007;21:1413–22.

47 Allan JM, Smith AG, Wheatley K, *et al.* Genetic variation in XPD predicts treatment outcome and risk of acute myeloid leukemia following chemotherapy. *Blood* 2004;104:3872–7.

48 Jawad M, Seedhouse CH, Russell N, Plumb M. Polymorphisms in human homeobox HLX1 and DNA repair RAD51 genes increase the risk of therapy-related acute myeloid leukemia. *Blood* 2006;108:3916–8.

49 Rund D, Krichevsky S, Bar-Cohen S, *et al.* Therapy-related leukemia: clinical characteristics and analysis of new molecular risk factors in 96 adult patients. *Leukemia* 2005;19:1919–28.

50 Worrillow LJ, Smith AG, Scott K, *et al.* Polymorphic MLH1 and risk of cancer after methylating chemotherapy for Hodgkin lymphoma. *J Med Genet* 2008;45:142–6.

51 Ellis NA, Huo D, Yildiz O, *et al.* MDM2 SNP309 and TP53 Arg72Pro interact to alter therapy-related acute myeloid leukemia susceptibility. *Blood* 2008;112:741–9.

52 Brown WM, Doll R. Mortality from cancer and other causes after radiotherapy for ankylosing spondylitis. *Br Med J* 1965;5474:1327–32.

53 Matsuo T, Tomonaga M, Bennett JM, *et al.* Reclassification of leukemia among A-bomb survivors in Nagasaki using French-American-British (FAB) classification for acute leukemia. *Jpn J Clin Oncol* 1988;18:91–6.

54 Armitage JO, Carbone PP, Connors JM, Levine A, Bennett JM, Kroll S. Treatment-Related Myelodysplasia and Acute leukemia in Non-Hodgkin's Lymphoma Patients. *J Clin Oncol* 2003;21:897–906.

55 Shimizu Y, Schull WJ, Kato H. Cancer risk among atomic bomb survivors. The RERF Life Span Study. Radiation Effects Research Foundation. *JAMA* 1990;264:601–4.

56 Doody MM, Mandel JS, Lubin JH, Boice JD, Jr. Mortality among United States radiologic technologists, 1926–90. *Cancer Causes Control* 1998;9:67–75.

57 Cardis E, Gilbert ES, Carpenter L, *et al.* Effects of low doses and low dose rates of external ionizing radiation: cancer mortality among nuclear industry workers in three countries. *Radiat Res* 1995;142:117–32.

58 Weiss HA, Darby SC, Fearn T, Doll R. Leukemia mortality after X-ray treatment for ankylosing spondylitis. *Radiat Res* 1995;142:1–11.

59 Inskip PD, Monson RR, Wagoner JK, *et al.* Leukemia following radiotherapy for uterine bleeding. *Radiat Res* 1990;122:107–19.

60 Urowitz MB, Rider WD. Myeloproliferative disorders in patients with rheumatoid arthritis treated with total body irradiation. *Am J Med* 1985;78:60–4.

61 Inskip PD, Kleinerman RA, Stovall M, *et al.* Leukemia, lymphoma, and multiple myeloma after pelvic radiotherapy for benign disease. *Radiat Res* 1993;135:108–24.

62 Griem ML, Kleinerman RA, Boice JD, Jr., Stovall M, Shefner D, Lubin JH. Cancer following radiotherapy for peptic ulcer. *J Natl Cancer Inst* 1994;86:842–9.

63 Travis LB, Curtis RE, Storm H, *et al.* Risk of second malignant neoplasms among long-term survivors of testicular cancer. *J Natl Cancer Inst* 1997;89:1429–39.

64 Curtis RE, Boice JD, Jr., Stovall M, *et al.* Risk of leukemia after chemotherapy and radiation treatment for breast cancer. *N Engl J Med* 1992;326:1745–51.

65 Reynolds TY, Rockwell S, Glazer PM. Genetic instability induced by the tumor microenvironment. *Cancer Res* 1996; 56:5754–7.

66 Lorimore SA, Coates PJ, Scobie GE, Milne G, Wright EG. Inflammatory-type responses after exposure to ionizing radiation in vivo: a mechanism for radiation-induced bystander effects? *Oncogene* 2001;20:7085–95.

67 BEIR. Health risks from exposure to low levels of ionizing radiation BEIR VII phase 2. 2006.

68 Aksoy M, Dincol K, Erdem S, Dincol G. Acute leukemia due to chronic exposure to benzene. *Am J Med* 1972;52:160–6.

69 Aksoy M, Erdem S. Followup study on the mortality and the development of leukemia in 44 pancytopenic patients with chronic exposure to benzene. *Blood* 1978;52:285–92.

70 Travis LB, Li CY, Zhang ZN, *et al.* Hematopoietic malignancies and related disorders among benzene-exposed workers in China. *Leuk Lymphoma* 1994;14:91–102.

71 Yin SN, Hayes RB, Linet MS, *et al.* An expanded cohort study of cancer among benzene-exposed workers in china. *Environ Health Perspect* 1996;104:1339–41.

72 Paustenbach DJ, Bass RD, Price P. Benzene toxicity and risk assessment, 1972–1992: implications for future regulation. *Environ Health Perspect* 1993;101(Suppl.6):177–200.

73 Smith MT. Mechanistic studies of benzene toxicity—implications for risk assessment. *Adv Exp Med Biol* 1996;387: 259–66.

74 Zeise L, McDonald TA. California perspective on the assessment of benzene toxicological risks. *J Toxicol Environ Health A* 2000;61:479–83 2000;61:479–83.

75 Hotz P, Lauwerys RR. Hematopoietic and lymphatic malignancies in vehicle mechanics. *Crit Rev Toxicol* 1997;27:443–94.

76 Boffetta P. Risk of acute myeloid leukemia after exposure to diesel exhaust: a review of the epidemiologic evidence. *J Occup Environ Med* 2004;46:1076–83.

77 Caspi O, Polliack A, Klar R, Ben Yehuda D. The association of inflammatory bowel disease and leukemia-coincidence or not? *Leuk Lymphoma* 1995;17:255–62.

78 Askling J, Brandt L, Lapidus A, *et al.* Risk of haematopoietic cancer in patients with inflammatory bowel disease. *Gut* 2005;54:617–22.

79 Ross JA, Kasum CM, Davies SM, Jacobs DR, Folsom AR, Potter JD. Diet and risk of leukemia in the Iowa Women's Health Study. *Cancer Epidemiol Biomarkers Prev* 2002;11:777–81.

80 Hursting SD, Margolin BH, Switzer BR. Diet and human leukemia—an analysis of international data. *Preventive Medicine* 1993;22:409–22.

81 Kane EV, Roman E, Cartwright R, Parker J, Morgan G. Tobacco and the risk of acute leukaemia in adults. *Br J Cancer* 1999;81: 1228–33.

82 Bjork J, Albin M, Mauritzson N, Stromberg U, Johansson B, Hagmar L. Smoking and acute myeloid leukemia: associations

with morphology and karyotypic patterns and evaluation of dose-response relations. *Leuk Res* 2001;25:865–72.

83 Korte JE, Hertz-Picciotto I, Schulz MR, Ball LM, Duell EJ. The contribution of benzene to smoking-induced leukemia. *Environ Health Perspect* 2000;108:333–9.

84 Bleyer A, O'Leary M, Barr R, Ries L, (eds). *Cancer Epidemiology in Older Adolescents and Young Adults 15 to 29 Years of Age, Including SEER Incidence and Survival: 1975–2000*. Bethesda, MD: National Cancer Institute: No. 06–5767, 2006.

85 Ries L, Smith M, Gurney J, *et al.*, (eds). *Cancer Incidence and Survival among Children and Adolescents: United States SEER Program 1975–1995*. Bethesda, MD: National Cancer Institute: No. 99–4649, 1999.

86 Greaves M. Infection, immune responses and the aetiology of childhood leukaemia. *Nat Rev Cancer* 2006;6:193.

87 Miller RW. Relation between cancer and congenital defects: an epidemiologic evaluation. *J Natl Cancer Inst* 1968;40: 1079–85.

88 Ravindranath Y. Down syndrome and leukemia: new insights into the epidemiology, pathogenesis, and treatment. *Pediatr Blood Cancer* 2005;44:1–7.

89 Swift M. Fanconi's anaemia in the genetics of neoplasia. *Nature* 1971;230:370–3.

90 Toledano SR, Lange BJ. Ataxia-telangiectasia and acute lymphoblastic leukemia. *Cancer* 1980;45:1675–8.

91 Pui CH, Crist WM, Look AT. Biology and clinical significance of cytogenetic abnormalities in childhood acute lymphoblastic leukemia. *Blood* 1990;76:1449–63.

92 Greaves MF, Maia AT, Wiemels JL, Ford AM. Leukemia in twins: lessons in natural history. *Blood* 2003;102:2321–33.

93 Gill Super HJ, Rothberg PG, Kobayashi H, *et al.* Clonal, nonconstitutional rearrangements of the *MLL* gene in infant twins with acute lymphoblastic leukemia: in utero chromosome rearrangement of 11q23. *Blood* 1994;83:641–4.

94 Ford AM, Bennett CA, Price CM, *et al.* Fetal origins of the *TEL–AML1* fusion gene in identical twins with leukemia. *Proc Natl Acad Sci U S A* 1998;95:4584–8.

95 Wiemels JL, Ford AM, Van Wering ER, Postma A, Greaves M. Protracted and variable latency of acute lymphoblastic leukemia after *TEL-AML1* gene fusion in utero. *Blood* 1999;94: 1057–62.

96 Maia AT, Ford AM, Jalali GR, *et al.* Molecular tracking of leukemogenesis in a triplet pregnancy. *Blood* 2001;98: 478–82.

97 Yagi T, Hibi S, Tabata Y, *et al.* Detection of clonotypic IGH and TCR rearrangements in the neonatal blood spots of infants and children with B-cell precursor acute lymphoblastic leukemia. *Blood* 2000;96:264–8.

98 Fasching K, Panzer S, Haas OA, *et al.* Presence of clone-specific antigen receptor gene rearrangements at birth indicates an in utero origin of diverse types of early childhood acute lymphoblastic leukemia. *Blood* 2000;95:2722–4.

99 Hjalgrim LL, Madsen HO, Melbye M, *et al.* Presence of clone-specific markers at birth in children with acute lymphoblastic leukaemia. *Br J Cancer* 2002;87:994–9.

100 Wiemels JL, Leonard BC, Wang Y, *et al.* Site-specific translocation and evidence of postnatal origin of the t(1;19) E2A–PBX1 fusion in childhood acute lymphoblastic leukemia. *Proc Natl Acad Sci* 2002;99:15101–6.

101 Mori H, Colman SM, Xiao Z, *et al.* Chromosome translocations and covert leukemic clones are generated during normal fetal development. *Proc Natl Acad Sci* 2002;99:8242–7.

102 Biernaux C, Loos M, Sels A, Stryckmans P. Detection of major *BCR-ABL* gene expression at a very low level in blood cells of some healthy individuals. *Blood* 1995;86:3118–22.

103 Kinlen L. Evidence for an infective cause of childhood leukaemia: comparison of a Scottish new town with nuclear reprocessing sites in Britain. *Lancet* 1988;2:1323–7.

104 McNally RJQ, Eden TOB. An infectious aetiology for childhood acute leukaemia: a review of the evidence. *Br J Haematol* 2004;127:243–63.

105 Steinmaus C, Lu M, Todd RL, Smith AH. Probability estimates for the unique childhood leukemia cluster in Fallon, Nevada, and risks near other U.S. Military aviation facilities. *Environ Health Perspect* 2004;112:766–71.

106 Alexander FE. Space-time clustering of childhood acute lymphoblastic leukaemia: indirect evidence for a transmissible agent. *Br J Cancer* 1992;65:589–92.

107 Kinlen LJ. Epidemiological evidence for an infective basis in childhood leukaemia. *Br J Cancer* 1995;71:1–5.

108 Dickinson HO, Parker L. Quantifying the effect of population mixing on childhood leukaemia risk: the Seascale cluster. *Br J Cancer* 1999;81:144–51.

109 Alexander FE, Chan LC, Lam TH, *et al.* Clustering of childhood leukaemia in Hong Kong: association with the childhood peak and common acute lymphoblastic leukaemia and with population mixing. *Br J Cancer* 1997;75:457–63.

110 Kinlen L, Doll R. Population mixing and childhood leukaemia: Fallon and other US clusters. *Br J Cancer* 2004;91:1–3.

111 Greaves MF. Speculations on the cause of childhood acute lymphoblastic leukemia. *Leukemia* 1988;2:120–5.

112 Perrillat F, Clavel J, Auclerc MF, *et al.* Day-care, early common infections and childhood acute leukaemia: a multicentre French case–control study. *Br J Cancer* 2002;86:1064–9.

113 Kamper-Jorgensen M, Woodward A, Wohlfahrt J, *et al.* Childcare in the first 2 years of life reduces the risk of childhood acute lymphoblastic leukemia. *Leukemia* 2007;22:189.

114 Gilham C, Peto J, Simpson J, *et al.* Day care in infancy and risk of childhood acute lymphoblastic leukaemia: findings from UK case–control study. *BMJ* 2005;330:1294.

115 Greaves MF. Aetiology of acute leukaemia. *Lancet* 1997;349: 344–9.

116 Roman E, Simpson J, Ansell P, *et al.* Childhood acute lymphoblastic leukemia and infections in the first year of life: a report from the united kingdom childhood cancer study. *Am J Epidemiol* 2007;165:496–504.

117 MacKenzie J, Greaves MF, Eden TO, *et al.* The putative role of transforming viruses in childhood acute lymphoblastic leukemia. *Haematologica* 2006;91:240–3.

118 Doll R. Hazards of ionising radiation: 100 years of observations on man. *Br J Cancer* 1995;72:1339–49.

119 Wright EG. Ionizing radiation and leukaemia: more questions than answers. *Hematol Oncol* 2005;23:119–26.

120 Rund D, Ben-Yehuda D. Therapy-related leukemia and myelodysplasia: evolving concepts of pathogenesis and treatment. *Hematology* 2004;9:179–87.

121 Nakmura N. A hypothesis: radiation-related leukemia is mainly attributable to the small number of people who carry

pre-existing clonally expanded preleukemic cells. *Radiat Res* 2005;163:258–65.

122 Ahlbom A, Day N, Feychting M, *et al.* A pooled analysis of magnetic fields and childhood leukaemia. *Br J Cancer* 2000;83:692–8.

123 Skinner J, Mee TJ, Blackwell RP, *et al.* Exposure to power frequency electric fields and the risk of childhood cancer in the UK. *Br J Cancer* 2002;87:1257–66.

124 Shu XO, Ross JA, Pendergrass TW, *et al.* Parental alcohol consumption, cigarette smoking, and risk of infant leukemia: a Childrens Cancer Group study. *J Natl Cancer Inst* 1996;88: 24–31.

125 Ross JA, Potter JD, Reaman GH, Pendergrass TW, Robison LL. Maternal exposure to potential inhibitors of DNA topoisomerase II and infant leukemia (United States): a report from the Children's Cancer Group. *Cancer Causes Control* 1996;7: 581–90.

126 Howard R, Gilbert E, Lynch CF, *et al.* Risk of leukemia among survivors of testicular cancer: a population-based study of 42,722 patients. *Ann Epidemiol* 2008;18:416–21.

127 Hjalgrim LL, Westergaard T, Rostgaard K, *et al.* Birth weight as a risk factor for childhood leukemia: a meta-analysis of 18 epidemiologic studies. *Am J Epidemiol* 2003;158:724–35.

128 Maule MM, Merletti F, Pastore G, Magnani C, Richiardi L. Effects of maternal age and cohort of birth on incidence time trends of childhood acute lymphoblastic leukemia. *Cancer Epidemiol Biomarkers Prev* 2007;16:347–51.

129 Kurita S. [Epidemiological studies of polycythemia vera in Japan (Author's transl.)]. *Nippon Ketsueki Gakkai Zasshi* 1974;37: 793–5.

130 Kutti J, Ridell B. Epidemiology of the myeloproliferative disorders: essential thrombocythaemia, polycythaemia vera and idiopathic myelofibrosis. *Pathol Biol (Paris)* 2001;49: 164–6.

131 Passamonti F, Rumi E, Pungolino E, *et al.* Life expectancy and prognostic factors for survival in patients with polycythemia vera and essential thrombocythemia. *Am J Med* 2004;117: 755–61.

132 Ma X, Vanasse G, Cartmel B, Wang Y, Selinger HA. Prevalence of polycythemia vera and essential thrombocythemia. *Am J Hematol* 2008;83:359–62.

133 Kralovics R, Stockton DW, Prchal JT. Clonal hematopoiesis in familial polycythemia vera suggests the involvement of multiple mutational events in the early pathogenesis of the disease. *Blood* 2003;102:3793–6.

134 Rumi E, Passamonti F, Pietra D, *et al.* *JAK2* (*V617F*) as an acquired somatic mutation and a secondary genetic event associated with disease progression in familial myeloproliferative disorders. *Cancer* 2006;107:2206–11.

135 Landgren O, Goldin LR, Kristinsson SY, Helgadottir EA, Samuelsson J, Bjorkholm M. Increased risks of polycythemia vera, essential thrombocythemia, and myelofibrosis among 24 577 first-degree relatives of 11 039 patients with myeloproliferative neoplasms in Sweden. *Blood* 2008;112: 2199–204.

136 Vickers MA. JAK2 617V>F positive polycythemia rubra vera maintained by approximately 18 stochastic stem-cell divisions per year, explaining age of onset by a single rate-limiting mutation. *Blood* 2007;110:1675–80.

137 Marsh GM, Enterline PE, McCraw D. Mortality patterns among petroleum refinery and chemical plant workers. *Am J Ind Med* 1991;19:29–42.

138 Kaplan SD. Update of a mortality study of workers in petroleum refineries. *J Occup Med* 1986 Jul;28:514–16.

139 Jaffe ES, Harris NL, Stein H, Vardiman J, (eds). *Tumours of Haematopoietic and Lymphoid Tissues*. IARC Press: Lyon, 2001.

140 Faderl S, Talpaz M, Estrov Z, Kantarjian HM. Chronic myelogenous leukemia: biology and therapy. *Ann Intern Med* 1999;131:207–19.

141 Van Maele-Fabry G, Duhayon S, Lison D. A systematic review of myeloid leukemias and occupational pesticide exposure. *Cancer Causes Control* 2007;18:457–78.

142 Berger U, Maywald O, Pfirrmann M, *et al.* Gender aspects in chronic myeloid leukemia: long-term results from randomized studies. *Leukemia* 2005;19:984–9.

143 Moloney WC. Radiogenic leukemia revisited. *Blood* 1987;70: 905–8.

144 Corso A, Lazzarino M, Morra E, *et al.* Chronic myelogenous leukemia and exposure to ionizing radiation–a retrospective study of 443 patients. *Ann Hematol* 1995;70:79–82.

145 Morton LM, Wang SS, Devesa SS, Hartge P, Weisenburger DD, Linet MS. Lymphoma incidence patterns by WHO subtype in the United States, 1992–2001. *Blood* 2006;107:265–76.

146 Dores GM, Anderson WF, Curtis RE, *et al.* Chronic lymphocytic leukaemia and small lymphocytic lymphoma: overview of the descriptive epidemiology. *Br J Haematol* 2007;139:809–19.

147 Surveillance, epidemiology and end result (SEER). 2008.

148 Zent CS, Kyasa MJ, Evans R, Schichman SA. Chronic lymphocytic leukemia incidence is substantially higher than estimated from tumor registry data. *Cancer* 2001;92:1325–30.

149 Linet MS, Schubauer-Berigan MK, Weisenburger DD, *et al.* Chronic lymphocytic leukaemia: an overview of aetiology in light of recent developments in classification and pathogenesis. *Br J Haematol* 2007;139:672–86.

150 Rawstron AC, Bennett FL, O'Connor SJ, *et al.* Monoclonal B-cell lymphocytosis and chronic lymphocytic leukemia. *N Engl J Med* 2008;359:575–83.

151 Herrinton LJ. Epidemiology of the revised European-American lymphoma classification subtypes. *Epidemiol Rev* 1998;20: 187–203.

152 Linet MS, Van Natta ML, Brookmeyer R, *et al.* Familial cancer history and chronic lymphocytic leukemia. A case–control study. *Am J Epidemiol* 1989;130:655–64.

153 Gale RP, Cozen W, Goodman MT, Wang FF, Bernstein L. Decreased chronic lymphocytic leukemia incidence in Asians in Los Angeles County. *Leuk Res* 2000;24:665–9.

154 Herrinton LJ, Goldoft M, Schwartz SM, Weiss NS. The incidence of non-Hodgkin's lymphoma and its histologic subtypes in Asian migrants to the United States and their descendants. *Cancer Causes Control* 1996;7:224–30.

155 Rozman C, Montserrat E. Chronic lymphocytic leukemia. *N Engl J Med* 1995;333:1052–7.

156 Yuille MR, Houlston RS, Catovsky D. Anticipation in familial chronic lymphocytic leukaemia. *Leukemia* 1998;12:1696–8.

157 Rawstron AC, Yuille MR, Fuller J, *et al.* Inherited predisposition to CLL is detectable as subclinical monoclonal B-lymphocyte expansion. *Blood* 2002;100:2289–90.

158 Houlston RS, Catovsky D, Yuille MR. Genetic susceptibility to chronic lymphocytic leukemia. *Leukemia* 2002;16:1008–14.

159 Capalbo S, Trerotoli P, Ciancio A, *et al.* Increased risk of lymphoproliferative disorders in relatives of patients with B-cell chronic lymphocytic leukemia: relevance of the degree of familial linkage. *Eur J Hematol* 2000;85:114–17.

160 Slager SL, Kay NE, Fredericksen ZS, *et al.* Susceptibility genes and B-chronic lymphocytic leukaemia. *Br J Haematol* 2007; 139:762–71.

161 Linet MS, Schubauer-Berigan MK, Weisenburger DD, *et al.* Chronic lymphocytic leukaemia: an overview of aetiology in light of recent developments in classification and pathogenesis. *Br J Haematol* 2007;139:672–86.

162 Schubauer-Berigan MK, Daniels RD, Fleming DA, *et al.* Chronic lymphocytic leukaemia and radiation: findings among workers at five US nuclear facilities and a review of the recent literature. *Br J Haematol* 2007;139:799–808.

163 Blair A, Purdue MP, Weisenburger DD, Baris D. Chemical exposures and risk of chronic lymphocytic leukaemia. *Br J Haematol* 2007;139:753–61.

164 Landgren O, Engels EA, Caporaso NE, *et al.* Patterns of autoimmunity and subsequent chronic lymphocytic leukemia in Nordic countries. *Blood* 2006;108:292–6.

165 Rosenblatt KA, Koepsell TD, Daling JR, *et al.* Antigenic stimulation and the occurrence of chronic lymphocytic leukemia. *Am J Epidemiol* 1991;134:22–8.

166 Landgren O, Gridley G, Check D, Caporaso NE, Morris BL. Acquired immune-related and inflammatory conditions and subsequent chronic lymphocytic leukaemia. *Br J Haematol* 2007;139:791–8.

Chapter 3
Traditional Diagnostic Approaches

Hartmut Koeppen[1], *Carlos E. Bueso-Ramos*[2], *and Sergej N. Konoplev*[2]
[1]Genentech, Inc., South San Francisco, California, USA
[2]The University of Texas M. D. Anderson Cancer Center, Houston, Texas, USA

Myeloproliferative neoplasms

Chronic myeloproliferative neoplasms (MPNs) are a heterogeneous group of disorders that share the clonal proliferation of one or more myeloid lineages as a common characteristic. The classification of these disorders is currently in flux, reflecting the recent progress made in the understanding of the pathobiology and identification of genetic changes relevant to them.

For a long time, MPNs have been recognized as distinct disease entities. William Dameshek frequently receives credit for establishing the unifying concept of myeloproliferative disorders, and for recognizing that individual disease entities such as chronic myeloid leukemia (CML), polycythemia vera (PV), essential thrombocythemia (ET) or "megakaryocytic leukemia", and primary myelofibrosis (PMF) or "idiopathic myeloid metaplasia of the spleen" may represent variations of the theme of a proliferation "en masse" of bone marrow precursors in response to an unidentified stimulus [1]. While Dameshek may have been the first to formulate this hypothesis in the absence of sound experimental data, other investigators have recognized that the proliferation of more than just one particular cell type was frequently seen in myeloproliferative disorders [2].

The World Health Organization (WHO) classification [3] recognizes MPN as one of five categories of myeloid neoplasms, which also include myelodysplastic syndromes (MDS), myelodysplastic syndrome/myeloproliferative neoplasms (MDS/MPN), myeloid/lymphoid neoplasms with eosinophilia and abnormalities of platelet-derived growth factor receptor α (PDGFR-α), PDGFR-β, and fibroblast growth factor receptor 1 (FGFR-1), and acute myeloid leukemia (AML). In this particular classification scheme, MPNs cover CML, PV, ET, and PMF, as well as chronic neutrophilic leukemia (CNL), chronic eosinophilic leukemia (CEL), mastocytosis, and an "unclassifiable" category of MPNs. While at first sight this appears to be a heterogeneous group of conditions, certain common features have been recognized that distinguish them from other myeloid disorders, such as MDS, MDS/MPN, and acute leukemia. MPNs represent a clonal proliferation of one or more lineages characterized by effective and progressive maturation, which results in an increased number of mature granulocytes, erythrocytes, and/or platelets in the peripheral blood. This symptomatology is in contrast to the ineffective, dysplastic hematopoietic maturation seen in MDS and the proliferation of immature cells without the maturation characteristic of acute leukemias.

While the distinction from other myeloid disorders might be evident on the basis of clinical and morphologic criteria, there is considerable overlap between individual MPNs in their clinicopathologic features. Elevated counts of granulocytes, erythrocytes, and platelets, as well as hepatosplenomegaly, are frequently seen in all of the MPNs. However, the increased availability of cytogenetic—including fluorescence *in situ* hybridization (FISH)—and molecular testing has streamlined the diagnostic approach to MPNs (Figure 3.1). This section of the chapter will cover in some detail the diagnostic approach to CML, and briefly highlight the characteristic morphologic features of *BCR–ABL1*$^-$ gene MPNs.

Chronic myeloid leukemia

Initially described in 1845, CML has evolved into a disease where molecular techniques are essential for establishing diagnosis, defining responses to therapy, and evaluating the basis for resistance to therapy. Nowell and Hungerford [4] identified the Philadelphia chromosome as the karyotypic abnormality in CML, while Rowley [5] determined its nature as a reciprocal translocation between chromosomes 9 and 22, involving the *BCR* gene on chromosome 22 and the *ABL1* gene on chromosome 9 (reviewed in ref. 6).

The close association between the presence of a *BCR–ABL* rearrangement and the development of CML has led to a shift in the definition of CML, such that a diagnosis of CML is now rendered exclusively when the characteristic morphologic, cytogenetic, and/or molecular features

Leukemias: Principles and Practice of Therapy, 1st edition. Edited by S. Faderl and H. Kantarjian.

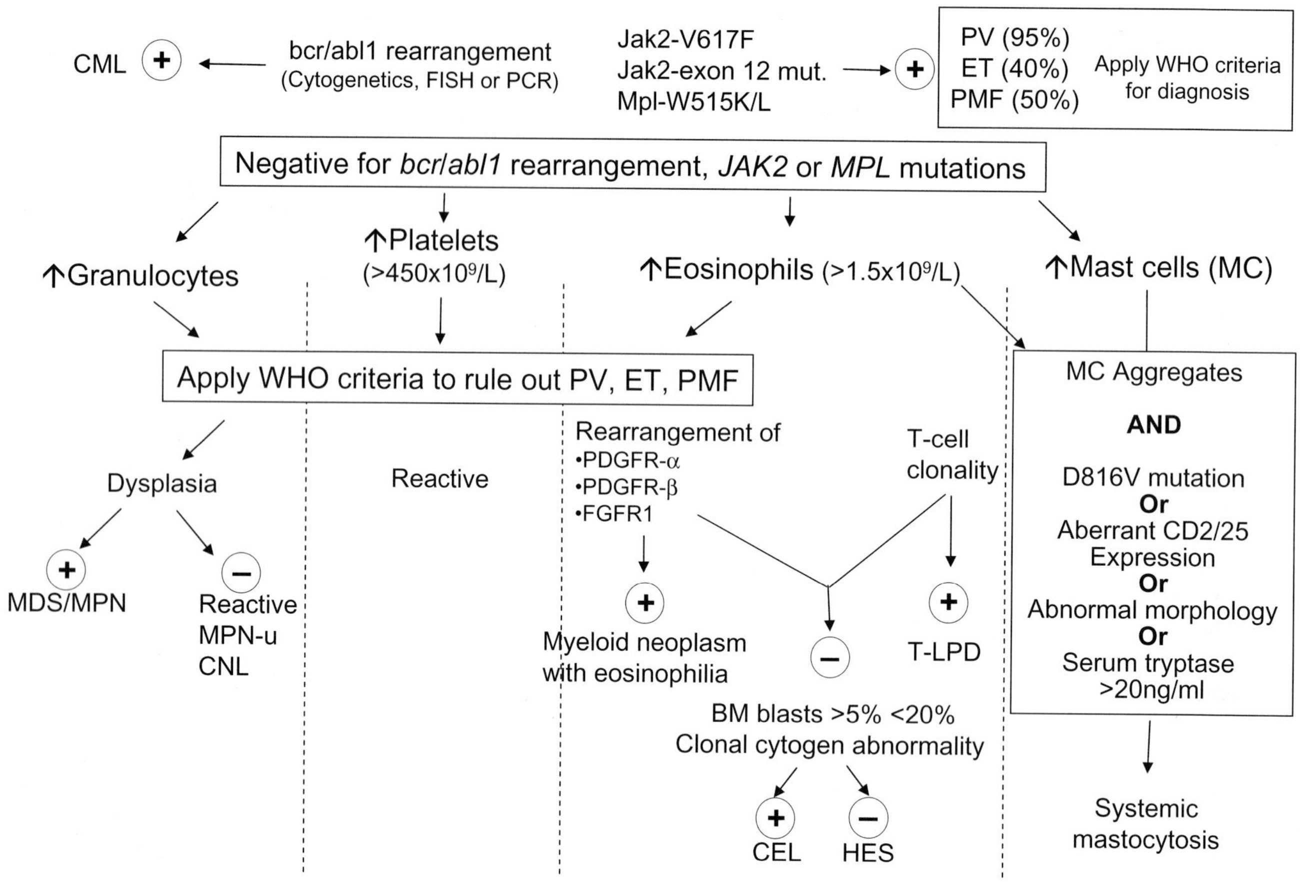

Figure 3.1 Suspected myeloproliferative neoplasm (MPN). Abnormal peripheralblood film or bone marrow biopsy.

are present. The WHO currently defines CML as a myeloproliferative disease that originates in an abnormal pluripotent bone marrow stem cell and is consistently associated with the *BCR–ABL1* fusion gene [7]. By applying this definition, CML can be distinguished from all benign or neoplastic disorders that may mimic CML morphologically.

The most common myeloproliferative disease is CML, which constitutes 15–20% of all leukemia cases [7–9]. CML can occur at any age, but is rare under the age of 20, and has a slight predominance in males. Similar to other myeloproliferative disorders, CML is usually triphasic with a chronic, accelerated, and blast phase [10]. The precise definition of these phases is still a subject of debate, but regardless of the definition or treatment used, patients whose CML is in chronic phase do better than patients with CML in blast or accelerated phase [7,11,12].

The main laboratory finding in patients with chronic-phase CML is peripheral blood leukocytosis with absolute neutrophilia, basophilia, and frequently eosinophilia [13]. The granulocytes in the peripheral blood represent all maturation stages, including occasional blasts; dysplastic features are typically not conspicuous (Figure 3.1). Platelet counts range from thrombocytopenia to thrombocytosis. Anemia is frequently encountered. The peripheral blood findings change with disease progression as the proportion of immature elements increase. Quantifying the proportion of blasts, basophils, or platelets in the peripheral blood is important because some of the staging criteria are based on peripheral blood parameters [14]. The reduced activity of leukocyte alkaline phosphatase (LAP) can be used to distinguish CML from reactive leukocytoses that are typically associated with higher LAP scores, which indicate a functional deficit of CML granulocytes [15].

The bone marrow in chronic-phase CML is typically hypercellular with marked myeloid predominance [16]. In paratrabecular areas, increased numbers of immature cells create thick cuffs of immature progenitors. Most cells in the intertrabecular spaces consist of myeloid cells. The number of megakaryocytes may be increased, and are typically small and hypolobated. Histiocytes with abundant foamy cytoplasm (pseudo-Gaucher cells) are sometimes encountered as a consequence of increased cell turnover [17,18]. Bone marrow basophilia and eosinophilia are frequently present. The number of blasts is within normal limits, and increases only as the disease progresses. Bone marrow smears typically confirm the lack of dysplastic features in granulocytic and erythroid progenitors. The extent of bone marrow fibrosis is highly variable but tends to be minimal in early stages.

Various diagnostic criteria for accelerated-phase CML have been proposed, including persistent and therapy-refractory leukocytosis, thrombocytosis, thrombocytopenia or splenomegaly, and increased basophils (≥20%) or blasts (10–19%) [7]. Given the change in therapy of CML over the last few years, the clinical significance of at least some of these criteria is still controversial. A diagnosis of blast phase is generally accepted when blasts represent 20% or more of the peripheral blood or bone marrow-nucleated elements, or in the case of an extramedullary blast proliferation. Also, intertrabecular sheets of blasts and extramedullary proliferations of blasts are essentially diagnostic of the blast phase [7]. The morphology of blasts varies according to lineage; in most cases, blasts show evidence of myeloid differentiation (approximately 70%) followed by lymphoid differentiation (20%). Bilineal or biphenotypic myeloblasts, megakaryoblasts, or erythroblasts are identified in approximately 10% of cases [19–21]. Flow cytometry—while of limited value for the diagnosis of chronic-phase CML—is critical for determining the immunophenotype of the blasts in the accelerated and blast phases; lineage assignment can usually be accomplished by determining the expression of myeloid (CD13, CD33, myeloperoxidase), monocytic (CD14, CD64), lymphoid (TdT, CD10, cCD3, CD7, CD19, CD20), megakaryocytic (CD41, CD42, CD61), or erythroid (CD71, hemoglobin A) differentiation markers.

Karyotypic analysis and molecular analysis to demonstrate the pathognomonic t(9;22)(q34;q11) and a *BCR–ABL* fusion transcript, respectively, are mandatory for a diagnosis of CML; the translocation can be identified by cytogenetic analysis or FISH in 90–95% of patients. The remaining patients may have variant or cryptic translocations; their presence can be inferred by using polymerase chain reaction (PCR)-based techniques to demonstrate fusion genes or transcripts [22]. Conventional cytogenetic analysis is valuable for identifying additional abnormalities of potential clinical significance, including trisomy 8, i(17q), an additional Philadelphia chromosome, and trisomy 19. Less commonly identified anomalies that have also been described include the loss of chromosomes 7, 17, and Y, trisomy of chromosomes 17 and 21, as well as translocations involving chromosomes 3 and 21 [23–25].

BCR–ABL1-negative myeloproliferative neoplasms

There is considerable overlap in the morphologic features between the various entities in this category of MPN, and proper diagnostic classification frequently depends on clinical and molecular characterization (Figure 3.1). The text below summarizes morphologic features for individual MPNs that may aid in the differential diagnosis, and also refers to molecular alterations unique to individual entities.

Chronic neutrophilic leukemia

This rare MPN is characterized by peripheral leukocytosis ($>25 \times 10^9$/L) with a predominance of mature neutrophils, but without an increase in circulating myeloblasts, eosinophils, or basophils and without dysplastic features in any of the lineages [26,27]. The bone marrow is hypercellular with an increased myeloid:erythroid (M:E) ratio. Granulocytic maturation is morphologically unremarkable, and blasts are not increased. Some cases may show increased numbers of erythroid precursors and megakaryocytes; unlike PV, ET, and PMF, the megakaryocyte morphology is unremarkable in CNL and reticulin fibrosis is typically absent [28]. The vast majority of cases of CNL are karyotypically normal, lacking *BRC-ABL1* rearrangements in particular. An association between CNL and concurrent multiple myeloma has been described by some investigators [29–31].

Primary myelofibrosis, polycythemia vera, and essential thrombocythemia

PMF, PV, and ET are clonal MPNs with proliferation of one or more hematopoietic lineages and, particularly for PMF and PV, a stepwise evolution and progression of the disease (reviewed in ref. 32). Overlap is seen not only in clinical and morphologic features but also in genetic abnormalities: a mutation at codon 617 of the *JAK2* gene is seen in >90% of cases of PV, 50% of cases of PMF, and 40% of cases of ET [33–35]. Other changes, such as *JAK2* exon 12 mutations (PV) or mutations in the *MPL* gene (primarily codon 515; PMF and ET), are much less frequent [36–38]. These mutational changes represent one of the major diagnostic criteria for PV, PMF, and ET as outlined by the WHO [39–41]. The other major diagnostic criterion for a diagnosis of PV is evidence of an increased red blood cell volume in the presence of a decreased serum level of erythropoietin (minor criteria). Major diagnostic criteria for PMF and ET include the failure to meet WHO-defined diagnostic criteria for other myeloid neoplasms, such as *BCR–ABL1*$^+$ CML or MDS, as well as megakaryocytic (ET) or megakaryocytic and granulocytic proliferation (PMF). The reader is referred to the current WHO classification of hematopoietic malignancies for a more detailed review of the diagnostic criteria for MPNs [42]. The bone marrow cellularity is highly variable: early stages of PV and PMF are characterized by a hypercellular marrow caused by panmyelosis (PV) or prominent granulocytic and megakaryocytic hyperplasia (PMF). Cellularity in later stages is more variable owing to reticulin or collagen fibrosis [43–45]. Megakaryocytic hyperplasia leading to a sustained thrombocytosis in the peripheral blood (>450 × 10^9/L) is the morphologic hallmark of ET [46,47]. In ET, the megakaryocytes are large, mature-appearing forms with often hyperlobulated nuclei; the bone marrow in PV and PMF typically shows clusters of atypical megakaryocytes that vary in size and nuclear morphology (hyperlobulated and frequently hyperchromatic nuclei) with frequent "naked" megakaryocyte nuclei. The degree of megakaryocytic atypia and clustering of megakaryocytes is typically more pronounced in PMF than in PV [48,49]. Dysplastic changes in erythroid or granulocytic precursors are typically inconspicuous in PV, PMF, or ET and, if present, are more consistent with a diagnosis of MDS than MPN. Increased numbers of myeloblasts—a finding not present in the chronic phase of PV, PMF, or ET—may indicate a transformation to acute leukemia. This is a more commonly observed event for patients with PV and PMF than for patients with ET [50–52].

Mastocytosis

Clonal proliferations of mast cells can manifest as several distinct entities; bone marrow involvement is typically seen in the systemic form of mastocytosis (SM) or mast cell leukemia (MCL). The diagnosis of bone marrow involvement by SM requires the presence of multifocal mast-cell aggregates of ≥15 cells (major criterion) and/or atypical (spindle-shaped) morphology, a codon 816 mutation in the *KIT* gene, immunophenotypic aberrancies (coexpression of CD2 and CD25), or an elevated serum tryptase level (all minor criteria) [53]. Mast-cell aggregates are frequently associated with reticulin fibrosis [54,55]. The association of SM with another hematolymphoid neoplasm of non-mast cell lineage disease (SM-AHNMD) is a well-recognized phenomenon; this second malignancy—most frequently CML—can occur in any temporal relationship with a diagnosis of SM [56–58].

MCL is a rare, clinically aggressive disorder characterized by the presence of >20% mast cells in bone marrow aspirate smears and with variable numbers of circulating mast cells [59,60]. The neoplastic cells in MCL and in the even rarer entity of mast cell sarcoma show signs of cellular atypia, and immunohistochemistry (IHC) for tryptase and CD117 is often required for a definitive diagnosis [61].

Myeloid and lymphoid neoplasms with eosinophilia and abnormalities of *PDGFRA*, *PDGFRB*, or *FGFR-1*

Each of these three disorders is characterized by a specific genetic abnormality involving the genes for PDGFRA, PDGFRB, or FGFR-1; the manifestation of the disease is to a certain degree dictated by the underlying genetic change. Forms with rearrangements of the *PDGFRA* and *PDGFRB* genes typically present as MPNs; chronic eosinophilic leukemia is most commonly seen in PDGFRA-associated disorders whereas the MPN associated with PDGFRB rearrangements most closely resembles a chronic myelomonocytic leukemia (CMML) with eosinophilia [62–65]. Increased numbers of mast cells can be seen in either form. The FGFR-1-associated form shows the highest incidence of lymphoid malignancies, most commonly T-lymphoblastic leukemia/lymphoma (T-LBL); the vast majority of patients with this form demonstrate eosinophilia and neutrophilia. Monocytosis is less commonly observed [66]. Classical cytogenetic analysis will reveal in most cases the PDGFRB- and FGFR-1-associated rearrangements, but numerous fusion partners have been observed [64,66]. The genetic alteration with involvement of the *PDGFRA* gene is in most cases a cryptic interstitial deletion on the long arm of chromosome 4 leading to elimination of the *CHIC2* gene; real time-PCR- or FISH-based assays are needed to reveal the PDGFRA rearrangement [67,68].

Acute leukemias

Acute leukemias are defined as clonal proliferations of hematopoietic precursors with limited potential to mature and differentiate into functional granulocytes, monocytes, lymphocytes, red blood cells, or platelets [69], leading to an increased population of immature cells or "blasts." Based on the lineage of these blasts, acute leukemias are generally categorized into precursor B- or T-cell acute lymphoblastic leukemia (B-/T-ALL) and AML, all of which represent a heterogeneous group of disorders [70,71]. Infrequently, blasts have a phenotype representative of two or more lineages and are then classified as acute leukemias of ambiguous lineage.

Treatment decisions for patients with acute leukemia are based on the accurate classification of the disease. In addition to morphologic evaluation, ancillary studies are almost always needed to properly classify an acute leukemia; the additional studies routinely include immunophenotyping by flow cytometry, cytochemistry, cytogenetics, and frequently molecular studies. All of these studies place demands on the type of specimen needed and/or handling of the specimen; the reader is referred to additional texts for a discussion of the technical aspects of laboratory work-up of acute leukemias [72]. This section will focus on the morphologic aspects in the diagnosis of acute leukemias, and diagnostic algorithms utilized for the accurate classification of these disorders.

The current WHO classifications of AML and precursor lymphoid neoplasms are shown in Tables 3.1 and 3.2, respectively. Morphologic as well as clinical, immunophenotypic, cytogenetic, and molecular parameters contribute to, and are required for, appropriate classification [42,70,71,73]. A workflow diagram for the diagnostic work-up of acute leukemias is presented in Figure 3.2.

Table 3.1 World Health Organization classification of acute myeloid leukemias.

AML with recurrent genetic abnormalities
AML with t(8;21)(q22;q22); *RUNX1-RUNX1T1*
AML with inv(16)(p13.1q22) or t(16;16)(p13.1;q22); CBFB-MYH11
APL with t(15;17)(q22;q12); *PML-RARA*
AML with t(9;11)(p22;q23); MLLT3-MLL
AML with t(6;9)(p23;q34); *DEK-NUP214*
AML with inv(3)(q21q26.2) or t(3;3)(q21;q26.2);RPN1-EVI1
AML (megakaryoblastic) with t(1;22)(p13;q13);*RBM15-MKL1*
AML with mutated *NPM1*
AML with mutated CEBPA
AML with myelodysplasia-related changes
Therapy-related myeloid neoplasms
AML, NOS
AML with minimal differentiation
AML without maturation
AML with maturation
Acute myelomonocytic leukemia
Acute monoblastic and monocytic leukemia
Acute erythroid leukemia
Acute megakaryoblastic leukemia
Acute basophilic leukemia
Acute panmyelosis with myelofibrosis
Myeloid sarcoma
Myeloid proliferations related to Down syndrome
Transient abnormal myelopoiesis
Myeloid leukemia associated with Down syndrome
Blastic plasmacytoid dendritic cell neoplasm

AML, acute myeloid leukemia; NOS, not otherwise specified.

Table 3.2 World Health Organization classifications of precursor lymphoid neoplasms.

B lymphoblastic leukemia/lymphoma, NOS
B lymphoblastic leukemia/lymphoma with recurrent genetic abnormalities
B lymphoblastic leukemia/lymphoma with t(9;22)(q34;q11.2); *BCR–ABL1*
B lymphoblastic leukemia/lymphoma with t(v;11q23); MLL rearranged
B lymphoblastic leukemia/lymphoma with t(12;21)(p13;q22); *TEL-AML1 (ETV6-RUNX1)*
B lymphoblastic leukemia/lymphoma with hyperdiploidy
B lymphoblastic leukemia/lymphoma with hypodiploidy (hypodiploid ALL)
B lymphoblastic leukemia/lymphoma with t(5;14)(q31;q32); *IL3-IGH*
B lymphoblastic leukemia/lymphoma with t(1;19) (q23;p13.3); E2A-PBX1 (TCF3-PBX1)
T lymphoblastic leukemia/lymphoma

NOS, not otherwise specified.

Acute myeloid leukemia

The current WHO classification for AML includes four major categories: AML with recurrent genetic abnormalities, AML with myelodysplasia-related changes, therapy-related myeloid neoplasms, and AML not otherwise specified (NOS) [42]. A preliminary diagnosis of AML-NOS is typically given with emphasis on morphologic features and degree of maturation and differentiation, as outlined by the previous French–American–British (FAB) classification [73]. As the results of molecular and cytogenetic studies become available in the later stages of the diagnostic work-up, a more definitive classification using the WHO criteria might be possible.

Using the WHO criteria, the diagnosis of AML requires a peripheral blood or bone marrow blast count of more than 20%; if one of the established recurring genetic abnormalities can be demonstrated, a diagnosis of AML should be made regardless of the blast count. If the bone marrow contains >50% erythroid progenitors, the percentage of blasts is calculated based on the number of non-erythroid cells. This is critical to establish a diagnosis of acute erythroid leukemia.

In AML, blasts are classified as myeloblasts, monoblasts, erythroblasts, or megakaryoblasts. Three types (I–III) of myeloid blasts have previously been reported in the literature. This distinction—no longer observed by the WHO classification—was based on the absence (type I) or presence (≤20 for type II, >20 for type III) of azurophilic cytoplasmic granules. Promyelocytes and promonocytes are considered "blast equivalents" in cases with the recurring cytogenetic abnormality t(15;17) and AML with monocytic differentiation, respectively, and need to be included in the overall blast count in such cases.

Bone marrow biopsy and aspirate smears

The bone marrow biopsy sections of patients with AML typically show a hypercellular marrow with replacement of normal hematopoiesis by blasts to a variable degree. Approximately 5% of adult AML cases present with a hypocellular (<30% cellularity) bone marrow. Focal marrow involvement by leukemia can be seen. Myeloblasts may be distributed uniformly throughout the bone marrow interstitium or may be present in large aggregates or sheets. In most cases, blasts present as a relatively uniform, monotonous population of small or medium-sized cells with round or oval, sometimes indented or lobed, nuclei, variably prominent nucleoli, and variable amounts of cytoplasm. The cytologic appearance of myeloblasts on bone marrow aspirate smears is variable as far as cellular size, amount of cytoplasm, and nuclear shapes are concerned. More often than not, blasts have finely distributed nuclear chromatin and feature one or several distinct nucleoli. One characteristic feature of myeloblasts in AML is the presence of Auer rods, which represent aggregated azurophilic, granular material and occur

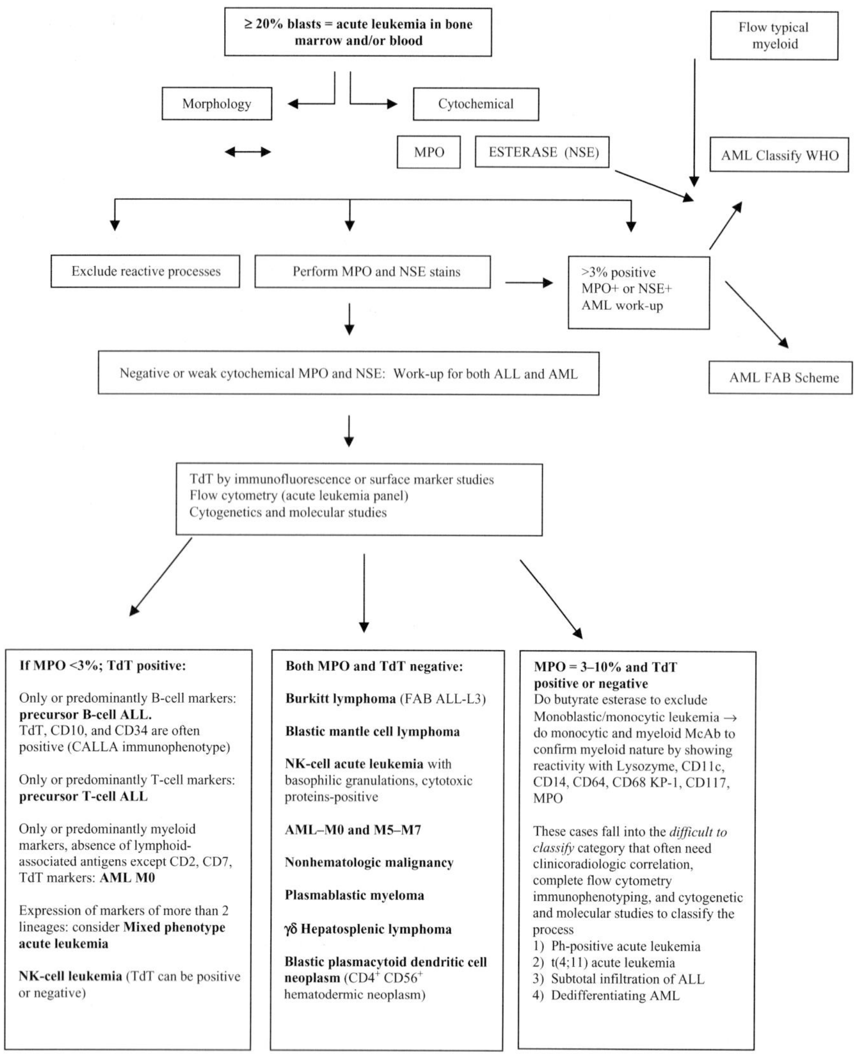

Figure 3.2 MDACC system for defining acute leukemias.

more frequently in AML with the recurring cytogenetic abnormalities t(15;17)(q22;q12) or t(8;21)(q22;q22). Monoblasts are, on average, larger than myeloblasts and have round, oval, or sometimes folded nuclei, finely dispersed nuclear chromatin, and rather prominent nucleoli; cytoplasm is typically basophilic and present in moderate or abundant amounts. Delicate azurophilic cytoplasmic granules and/or cytoplasmic vacuoles are frequently seen. Promonocytes show mildly basophilic or amphophilic, sometimes vacuolated, cytoplasm, and lobation or nuclear folds are more prominent than those seen in monoblasts. Erythroblasts have deeply basophilic, agranular cytoplasm; cytoplasmic projections or vacuoles are variably present. The nuclei are round with variably condensed chromatin and distinct nucleoli. The morphologic features of megakaryoblasts are highly variable, ranging from small, undifferentiated blasts to cells with abundant cytoplasm showing pseudopods or blebs. The biopsy section in megakaryoblastic leukemia may demonstrate marked reticulin fibrosis causing a "dry tap" on the aspirate smear; IHC on the biopsy sections is frequently needed in these cases to establish a diagnosis.

In addition to evaluating blasts and blast equivalents, mature and maturing hematopoietic elements need to be examined for signs of dysplasia or morphologic features uniquely associated with specific cytogenetic abnormalities. Granulocytic dysplasia manifests itself as hypogranular cells, or cells with hyposegmented nuclei (pseudo-Pelger–Huët), or pseudo-Chédiak–Higashi-type giant granules. Dysplastic megakaryocytes are small forms with hypolobated nuclei (micromegakaryocytes) or forms with widely separated nuclei. Morphologic criteria for dyserythropoiesis are nuclear-cytoplasmic dyssynchrony, irregular nuclear contours, multinuclearity, cytoplasmic vacuolization, or aberrant positive staining with periodic acid-Schiff (PAS). In acute promyelocytic leukemia (APL) with t(15;17)(q22;q12) the atypical promyelocytes are characteristically densely granulated and may contain numerous Auer rods (hypergranular variant). The microgranular variant shows cells with bilobed or folded nuclei and sparse cytoplasmic granules [74]. AML with inv(16)(p13q22) or t(16;16)(p13;q22) features eosinophils with prominent, purple-colored granules that are seen primarily in eosinophilic promyelocytes or myelocytes. The absolute number of eosinophils may be either increased or within normal limits [75]. Characteristic morphologic features of AML with t(8;21)(q22;q22) are seen in the neutrophils and neutrophilic precursors and include salmon-colored cytoplasm, pseudo-Pelger–Huët nuclei, and pseudo-Chédiak–Higashi granules [76].

Cytochemistry

An important aspect of the classification of acute leukemia is the cytochemical reactivity shown by the blasts. A positive cytochemical reaction for myeloperoxidase in more than 3% of the blasts proves myeloid lineage of the leukemia; cytochemical reactions for α-naphthyl butyrate or α-naphthyl acetate esterase are tools to establish monocytic differentiation. If the blasts are negative for myeloperoxidase but show reactivity for butyrate or non-specific esterase, acute monocytic leukemia is diagnosed. Minimally differentiated leukemia shows a lack of reactivity for myeloperoxidase but expresses myeloid antigens, as demonstrated by flow cytometry.

Flow cytometry

Immunophenotyping by flow cytometry (FCM) is now an integral part of the laboratory work-up of acute leukemias, and results are frequently available prior to IHC or even cytochemical results. In most cases of acute leukemia (>90%), FCM will unequivocally determine the lineage (myeloid vs. lymphoid) and also the differentiation of the blasts (monocytic, erythroid, megakaryoblastic). However, the enumeration of immature cells by FCM does not replace a blast count based on morphology because a hemodilute specimen submitted for FCM is not representative of the cellular composition of the marrow. The European Group for the Immunological Characterisation of Leukaemias (EGIL) originally proposed a scoring system for lineage assignment for leukemias with an ambiguous phenotype [77,78]; recently, this has been revised by the WHO classification. In the revised scoring system, expression of CD3 (cytoplasmic or surface) indicates T-lymphoid lineage, CD19 in conjunction with CD79a, CD22 (cytoplasmic), or CD10 indicates B-lymphoid lineage, and expression of myeloperoxidase or monocytic markers (NSE, CD14, CD64, CD11c, or lysozyme) indicates myeloid lineage.

Immunohistochemistry

In the laboratory work-up of acute leukemias, IHC can be an invaluable tool if a representative bone marrow aspirate sample is not available for morphologic evaluation (blast count) or for phenotyping by cytochemistry or FCM. The proportion of blasts among nucleated marrow elements can be ascertained by stains for CD34 and CD117 with the caveat that blasts can lack expression of CD34 in a significant proportion of cases of AML [79]. Antibodies suitable for paraffin section IHC are available for most lineage-specific markers including myeloperoxidase (myeloid), lysozyme (monocytic), glycophorin A (erythroid), and CD61 (megakaryocytic). Availability of antibodies against megakaryocytic markers for IHC has essentially eliminated the need for electronmicroscopy, which, in the past, was used to demonstrate platelet peroxidase to confirm a diagnosis of megakaryoblastic leukemia.

The utility of cytogenetic and molecular analysis of acute leukemias lies in the identification of prognostic and predictive markers; furthermore, several subtypes of AML are now recognized as distinct entities by the most recent WHO classification on the basis of unique karyotypic or mutational events [42,71]. Therefore, the laboratory work-up of new cases of acute leukemias is incomplete without karyotypic and molecular evaluation. However, the reader is referred to other chapters in this book for a more extensive discussion of this highly relevant topic.

Acute lymphoblastic leukemia

According to the recently revised WHO Classification of Tumours of Haematopoietic and Lymphoid Tissues [80], ALL is an aggressive neoplasm that is defined by the presence of >20% lymphoblasts in bone marrow or peripheral blood. This classification of ALL identifies three categories: B lymphoblastic leukemia/lymphoma NOS, B lymphoblastic leukemia/lymphoma with recurrent genetic abnormalities, and T lymphoblastic leukemia/lymphoma.

Bone marrow biopsy and aspirate smears

The bone marrow in ALL is typically hypercellular with extensive replacement of normal hematopoiesis by a monotonous population of leukemic cells. A hypocellular bone marrow with lymphoblasts being the most prevalent cellular elements is an unusual presentation [81]. Cases of ALL-L3 frequently show a "starry-sky" pattern due to the presence of numerous macrophages with ingested karyorrhectic material.

Occasionally, ALL is associated with prominent eosinophilia. In these cases, myeloid disorders may enter the differential diagnosis [82], and cytogenetic analysis may reveal t(5;14)(q31;q32) translocation that juxtaposes the interleukin 3 (IL-3) gene with the immunoglobulin heavy-chain (IGH) gene cluster or the t(5;9)(q31;p24) [83].

In the FAB system, three morphologic types (L1, L2, and L3) were recognized based on the cytologic features of the lymphoblasts in Wright–Giemsa-stained bone marrow smears [84]. Type L1 lymphoblasts are homogeneous and small in size with a high nuclear–cytoplasmic ratio and inconspicuous nucleoli. The lymphoblasts of the L2 type are morphologically more variable with a lower nuclear–cytoplasmic ratio owing to more abundant cytoplasm, and have distinct nucleoli. The morphologic features associated with the L1 or L2 phenotype do not predict immunophenotype, karyotype, or clinical outcome. Therefore, the distinction between the L1 and the L2 phenotype is no longer observed in the current WHO classification [80,85]. The L3 type (Burkitt leukemia/lymphoma) remains a separate entity defined by its unique combination of morphologic, genetic, and immunophenotypic features. The cells typically show limited morphologic variability, are of medium size with deeply basophilic, vacuolated cytoplasm, and feature nuclei with several distinct nucleoli. However, it is important to remember that L1/L2 blasts may show basophilic, vacuolated cytoplasm [86,87] and that L3 blasts with t(8;14) may have very few vacuoles, although they generally retain the deep basophilia of the cytoplasm and the multiple nucleoli.

Cytochemistry

While there is not a single cytochemical reaction that defines ALL, the combination of lack of reactivity for myeloperoxidase (MPO) and non-specific esterase and the presence of terminal deoxynucleotidyl transferase (TdT) is typical. However, rare cases of ALL may show weak immunoreactivity for MPO or MPO-ribonucleic acid (RNA) [88,89], and expression of TdT is a well-recognized phenomenon for a minority of AML cases [90–92]. Nevertheless, >95% of L1 and L2 ALLs are positive for TdT [93]. In contrast, L3 ALL is generally but not universally TdT^- [94]. Detection of TdT is useful in distinguishing reactive lymphocytosis from ALL of L1 type, a not uncommon diagnostic dilemma: L1-ALL cells may morphologically mimic a reactive lymphocytosis but are usually TdT^+, whereas reactive lymphocytes are TdT^-. This feature is particularly useful for limited specimens such as cerebrospinal fluid [95].

Flow cytometry

Most cases of ALL are of B-cell lineage, which is typically established by demonstrating expression of CD19 and cytoplasmic expression of CD22 and CD79a. The immunophenotypic profile correlates with the maturational stage of the neoplastic cells: early precursor B-ALL (pro-B-ALL) is positive for the B-lineage markers above and nuclear TdT, while ALL of intermediate maturational stage acquires expression of CD10. Expression of cytoplasmic immunoglobulin M (IgM) is seen only in the most mature forms of pre-B-ALL and expression of surface immunoglobulin is seen only in rare cases. Expression of CD34 is variable, as is expression of CD20. By contrast, mature B cells express surface immunoglobulin and CD20, and lack TdT reactivity. Rare exceptions to these rules do exist [94].

Approximately 15% of ALLs are of T-cell lineage. T-cell ALL has been subclassified according to normal thymocyte development. The early subtype is negative for surface CD3 (but positive for cytoplasmic CD3) and is either double positive or double negative for CD4 and CD8. The subtype corresponding to later stages of T-cell development is positive for surface (and cytoplasmic) CD3, negative for CD1a, and positive for either CD4 or CD8 but not both.

It is not uncommon to see expression of myeloid-associated markers in ALL. It has been reported more frequently in patients with translocations t(9;22) and t(4;11) [96]. CD13 and CD33 are among the most frequently expressed myeloid-associated antigens; expression of CD117 is rarely seen. Although earlier studies had shown a worse outcome, with coexpression of myeloid markers [97], recent studies have not shown any prognostic significance [98–100]. While expression of CD117 might be associated with lower complete response rates, it has been suggested that these patients may benefit from AML therapy [101,102].

Immunohistochemistry

Antigen retrieval techniques allow routinely fixed, paraffin-embedded bone marrow biopsy sections to be used for immunophenotypic characterization by IHC [103,104]. When fresh bone marrow aspirate and peripheral blood samples are not available, this method is useful in classifying acute leukemias. The following markers are typically included in the IHC panel: (i) Myeloid-associated markers—myeloperoxidase, CD117, CD68, lysozyme. (ii) T-cell associated markers: CD3, CD5, CD4, CD8. (iii) B-cell associated markers—CD20, CD22, CD79a, Pax-5, kappa and lambda light chains. Antibodies against TdT, CD10, and CD34 are also useful in this setting. Although myeloperoxidase mRNA is expressed in a subset of ALL [89], the presence of a significant protein level of myeloperoxidase strongly argues against a diagnosis of ALL.

Cytogenetic and molecular markers

Recurrent cytogenetic and molecular abnormalities occur in about 80% of children and 60–70% of adults with ALL. The frequency and prognostic significance of common recurrent cytogenetic and molecular abnormalities in pediatric and adult ALL have recently been reviewed [105] and will be discussed in other chapters of this book.

Chronic lymphocytic leukemia and related lymphoproliferative disorders

Chronic lymphoproliferative disorders are typically considered as clonal proliferations of morphologically mature-appearing lymphoid cells. Diagnostic accuracy and a meaningful classification of these entities require the integration of morphologic, immunologic, cytogenetic, molecular, and clinical data. The focus of this section is on chronic lymphocytic leukemia (CLL), but reference will be made to other lymphoid neoplasms with potential disease manifestations in bone marrow or peripheral blood if pertinent for differential diagnostic consideration.

For older adults, CLL is the most common type of leukemia with 90% of all cases occuring in patients >50 years old. CLL is a clonal proliferation of B lymphocytes (B-CLL). The key laboratory feature of, and diagnostic criteria for, CLL are persistent (>3 months) peripheral blood lymphocytosis ($>5 \times 10^9$/L) with evidence of clonality and expression of a distinct immunophenotype [106–108]. Morphologically, the neoplastic cells of CLL are frequently indistinguishable from normal mature lymphocytes on a routinely stained blood smear. In some cases of CLL, the leukemic lymphocytes show prominent clumping of nuclear chromatin with dark-staining chromatin aggregates separated by light-staining areas of parachromatin, giving rise to a "soccer ball" appearance. Morphologic heterogeneity does occur, and some cases of CLL show lymphoid cells with increased variability in nuclear shape and size and/or in the amount of cytoplasm [109]. It is important to determine the proportion of prolymphocytes (larger cells with a less condensed chromatin pattern and a single, prominent nucleolus); typical CLL shows <5% prolymphocytes, but cases with increased numbers of prolymphocytes may behave more aggressively (see definition of prolymphocytic leukemia below). The peripheral blood film in CLL may show isolated or combined cytopenias due to extensive marrow or splenic involvement or due to autoimmune mechanisms.

The extent and pattern of bone marrow infiltration are highly variable in CLL. Three patterns of involvement or combinations thereof can be identified: nodular, interstitial, and diffuse [110,111]. The nodular pattern is characterized by distinct, randomly distributed aggregates of small lymphocytes. In the interstitial pattern, the lymphocytes infiltrate the marrow to a variable degree without forming distinct nodules or displacement of adipocytes. In both of these patterns, residual hematopoiesis is present in affected areas. In the diffuse pattern, normal hematopoietic cells are replaced by sheets formed by the atypical lymphoid infiltrate. The morphologic distinction between the various patterns of marrow involvement by CLL is prognostically relevant: patients with a nodular or an interstitial pattern have a better clinical outcome than patients with a diffuse pattern [112].

Immunophenotypic analysis by flow cytometry is critical for the diagnosis of B-CLL. The typical finding is a distinct population of B lymphocytes with faint expression of cell-surface light-chain-restricted immunoglobulin (sIg) of IgM or IgD isotype and coexpression of CD5, CD19, CD20, CD23, CD79a, CD43, CD52, and CD11c. The levels of expression of CD20 and CD11c are variable, but are low in most cases of typical CLL. The cells are typically negative for CD10 and FMC7. CD20 and CD52 are potential targets for antibody therapeutics and the level of expression may relate to therapy response. Expression of CD38 and ζ-chain-associated protein kinase 70 (ZAP-70) are now routinely measured in new cases of CLL for prognostic relevance; expression of CD38 is typically measured by flow cytometry, and expression of ZAP-70 is measured by flow or IHC. Expression of either or both markers has been associated with a more aggressive clinical course [108]. Other poor prognostic indicators (discussed in other chapters) include cytogenetic abnormalities such as deletions of 11q, 17p, and 6q, as well as a lack of somatic hypermutation of the expressed immunoglobulin variable chain gene.

Transformation of B-CLL into an aggressive diffuse large B-cell lymphoma (Richter's transformation) accounts for up to 5% of all deaths in CLL [109,113]; transformation to acute leukemia is very unusual. A significant number of cases will show a slowly progressive increase in proportion of prolymphocytes; however, transformation to B-prolymphocytic leukemia is rare.

As the diagnosis of CLL rests on the integration of clinical morphologic, immunophenotypic, and molecular data, this type of information and the same techniques are used to distinguish CLL from other LPD.

1 ALL: the clinical presentation of patients with ALL is in most cases very different from that of patients with CLL; therefore, ALL rarely enters the differential diagnosis for CLL. Morphologically, the chromatin pattern of ALL blasts is not as condensed as that seen in CLL lymphoid cells, but rather reticular with variably prominent nucleoli. Bone marrow involvement by ALL tends to be extensive with frequently >90% blasts; immunophenotypically, most cases of ALL express CD19, cytoplasmic CD22 and cytoplasmic CD79a, CD10 and TdT with variable expression of CD20 and CD34. The vast majority of cases are negative for sIg [80].

2 Prolymphocytic leukemia (PLL): the diagnosis of PLL requires that prolymphocytes constitute >55% of the peripheral blood leukocytes. Prolymphocytes are often identified as cells larger than small lymphocytes with a single, prominent nucleolus [114–116]. Immunophenotypically, B-PLL shows stronger expression of sIg and other B-cell antigens than CLL; expression of CD5 and CD23 is seen in significantly fewer cases of B-PLL than B-CLL.

3 Mantle cell lymphoma (MCL): bone marrow and peripheral blood involvement are frequently seen in MCL and can mimic B-PLL. Morphologically, MCL cells tend to display more irregular nuclear membranes than typically seen in CLL. Immunophenotypically, MCL shows strong expression of B-cell markers CD19, CD20, FMC-7, and sIgM/D; most cases are positive for CD5, whereas expression of CD23 is variable and in most cases weak or negative. MCL is defined by the t(11;14) leading to overexpression of cyclin D1, which can be demonstrated immunohistochemically.

4 Follicular lymphoma (FL): leukemic presentation of FL is uncommon, and bone marrow involvement by FL typically manifests itself in the form of paratrabecular lymphoid aggregates. The centrocytes of FL have markedly irregular nuclear contours. The immunophenotype is distinct from CLL by bright expression of CD19, CD20, CD22, CD79a, expression of CD10, and lack of expression of CD5 and CD43. Most cases of FL show strong expression of Bcl-6 and Bcl-2, the latter owing to the t(14;18).

5 Hairy cell leukemia (HCL): the characteristic appearance of lymphoid cells with fine hair-like, irregular cytoplasmic projections typical for HCL can be appreciated on well-prepared peripheral blood and bone marrow aspirate smears. Peripheral blood involvement is typically sparse despite significant marrow involvement, usually in the form of a loose interstitial infiltrate associated with reticulin fibrosis. In addition to the characteristic morphologic features, HCL has a distinct immunophenotype with strong expression of CD19, CD20, CD22, CD25, CD11c, CD103, and CD123; most cases are negative for CD5 and CD10 [117,118]. Cytochemically, the cells are strongly positive for acid phosphatase in the presence of tartrate.

6 Splenic B-cell marginal zone lymphoma (SMZL): involvement of bone marrow and peripheral blood is common in this entity, which is characterized by the presence of lymphoid cells with polar cytoplasmic projections. The pattern of bone marrow involvement—unlike HCL—is nodular. Immunophenotypically, the cells express sIgM/D, CD19, CD20, and CD79a, and are negative for CD5, CD10, CD23, and CD43. Most cases are negative for CD103 and cyclin D1 [119].

7 Several T- and natural killer (NK)-lineage lymphoproliferative disorders can give rise to peripheral blood and/or bone marrow lymphocytosis. The expression of antigens indicating T- or NK-lineage is most easily determined by flow cytometry of peripheral blood or bone marrow aspirate specimens, or by IHC on solid-tissue specimens.

T-cell prolymphocytic leukemia (T-PLL) is a rare disorder characterized by lymphadenopathy, hepatosplenomegaly, and prominent lymphocytosis; the circulating lymphocytes are of small or medium size with mildly to markedly irregular nuclear outlines and a variably prominent nucleolus. Immunophenotypically, the cells are positive for the pan-T-cell markers CD2, CD3, and CD7 and most cases are also positive for CD4; coexpression of CD4 and CD8 is observed in some cases, and expression of CD8 without expression of CD4 is seen infrequently [120]. Molecular studies in these cases show typically clonal rearrangements of the T-cell receptor β and γ genes.

Sézary syndrome is the leukemic phase of the most common cutaneous T-cell lymphoma, mycosis fungoides, and is characterized by abnormal circulating lymphocytes, called Sézary cells [121]. The morphologic hallmark of Sézary cells is the hyperchromatic nuclear chromatin pattern with numerous nuclear folds and grooves, giving rise to a "cerebriform" appearance best appreciated at the ultrastructural level. The bone marrow is infrequently involved. Immunophenotyping of Sézary cells typically shows expression of markers indicating a mature T-lineage phenotype such as CD2, CD3, and CD4.

Adult T-cell leukemia/lymphoma (ATLL), common in Japan and the Caribbean, is caused by human T-cell leukemia/lymphoma virus 1 (HTLV-1) and is characterized by generalized lymphadenopathy, hypercalcemia, bone and skin lesions, and atypical lymphocytosis in blood and bone marrow [122]. A convoluted nuclear envelope causes a "cloverleaf" appearance in abnormal lymphocytes. As in T-PLL and Sézary syndrome, ATLL cells show reactivity with the T-lineage antigens CD2, CD3, and CD5; most cases express CD4 and CD25 but typically lack CD7. Mutation in the tumor suppressor gene p53 is seen in 30–50% of patients with ATLL [123].

Chronic T-cell large granular lymphocytic leukemia (LGL) has the morphologic distinction of persistent circulating lymphocytes that have abundant pale-blue cytoplasm with azurophilic granules. Three distinct clinical syndromes are now recognized in patients with increased numbers of circulating LGL cells [124,125]. When LGL carries a phenotype of T-LGL leukemia (a clonal proliferation of $CD3^+$ LGL), then chronic neutropenia and autoimmune disorders, most commonly rheumatoid arthritis, are characteristic [126,127]. Natural killer LGL leukemia is characterized by a clonal, $CD3^-$ LGL proliferation with an aggressive clinical course and multiorgan involvement. The majority of patients with increased numbers of $CD3^-$ cells do not have features of NK-LGL leukemia but rather demonstrate a more indolent clinical course. Quantitative changes in the LGL population are common and their presence in peripheral blood may represent a transient reactive phenomenon. It is therefore important to perform immunophenotyping and molecular studies, and to correlate these data with the clinical course.

Reactive lymphocytoses are self-limiting occurrences and are most commonly associated with viral infections; counts rarely exceed 5×10^9 cells/L [109]. The reactive lymphocytes are large cells with abundant, variably basophilic cytoplasm of T-cell lineage and polyclonal in origin.

References

1 Dameshek W. Some speculations on the myeloproliferative syndromes. *Blood* 1951;6:372–5.

2 Tefferi A. The history of myeloproliferative disorders: before and after Dameshek. *Leukemia* 2008;22:3–13.
3 Swerdlow S, Campo E, Harris N, *et al. WHO Classification of Tumours of Haematopoietic and Lymphoid tissues.* IARC Press: Lyon, 2008.
4 Nowell PC, Hungerford DA. Chromosome studies on normal and leukemic human leukocytes. *J Natl Cancer Inst* 1960;25: 85–109.
5 Rowley JD. Letter: A new consistent chromosomal abnormality in chronic myelogenous leukaemia identified by quinacrine fluorescence and Giemsa staining. *Nature* 1973;243: 290–3.
6 Kurzrock R, Gutterman JU, Talpaz M. The molecular genetics of Philadelphia chromosome-positive leukemias. *N Engl J Med* 1988;319:990–8.
7 Vardiman JW, Melo JV, Baccarani M, Thiele J. Chronic myelogenous leukaemia, *BCR-ABL1* positive. In: Swerdlow SH, Campo E, Harris NL, *et al* (eds). IARC Press: Lyon, 2008. pp.32–7.
8 Gunz FW. The epidemiology and genetics of the chronic leukaemias. *Clin Haematol* 1977;6:3–20.
9 Young JL, Jr., Percy CL, Asire AJ, *et al.* Cancer incidence and mortality in the United States, 1973–77. *Natl Cancer Inst Monogr* 1981;57:1–187.
10 Faderl S, Talpaz M, Estrov Z, Kantarjian HM. Chronic myelogenous leukemia: biology and therapy. *Ann Intern Med* 1999;131:207–19.
11 Baccarani M, Saglio G, Goldman J, *et al.* Evolving concepts in the management of chronic myeloid leukemia: recommendations from an expert panel on behalf of the European LeukemiaNet. *Blood* 2006;108:1809–20.
12 Jabbour E, Cortes J, Kantarjian H. Novel tyrosine kinase inhibitors in chronic myelogenous leukemia. *Curr Opin Oncol* 2006;18:578–83.
13 Spiers AS, Bain BJ, Turner JE. The peripheral blood in chronic granulocytic leukaemia. Study of 50 untreated Philadelphia-positive cases. *Scand J Haematol* 1977;18:25–38.
14 Savage DG, Szydlo RM, Goldman JM. Clinical features at diagnosis in 430 patients with chronic myeloid leukaemia seen at a referral centre over a 16-year period. *Br J Haematol* 1997;96:111–16.
15 Rosner F, Schreiber ZR, Parise F. Leukocyte alkaline phosphatase. Fluctuations with disease status in chronic granulocytic leukemia. *Arch Intern Med* 1972;130:892–4.
16 Lorand-Metze I, Vassallo J, Souza CA. Histological and cytological heterogeneity of bone marrow in Philadelphia-positive chronic myelogenous leukaemia at diagnosis. *Br J Haematol* 1987;67:45–9.
17 Anastasi J, Musvee T, Roulston D, Domer PH, Larson RA, Vardiman JW. Pseudo-Gaucher histiocytes identified up to 1 year after transplantation for CML are BCR/ABL-positive. *Leukemia* 1998;12:233–7.
18 Hayhoe FG, Flemans RJ, Cowling DC. Acquired lipidosis of marrow macrophages: birefringent blue crystals and Gaucher-like cells, sea-blue histiocytes, and grey-green crystals. *J Clin Pathol* 1979;32:420–8.
19 Khalidi HS, Brynes RK, Medeiros LJ, *et al.* The immunophenotype of blast transformation of chronic myelogenous leukemia: a high frequency of mixed lineage phenotype in "lymphoid" blasts and A comparison of morphologic, immunophenotypic, and molecular findings. *Mod Pathol* 1998;11: 1211–21.
20 Nair C, Chopra H, Shinde S, *et al.* Immunophenotype and ultrastructural studies in blast crisis of chronic myeloid leukemia. *Leuk Lymphoma* 1995;19:309–13.
21 Saikia T, Advani S, Dasgupta A, *et al.* Characterisation of blast cells during blastic phase of chronic myeloid leukaemia by immunophenotyping–experience in 60 patients. *Leuk Res* 1988; 12:499–506.
22 Hughes T, Deininger M, Hochhaus A, *et al.* Monitoring CML patients responding to treatment with tyrosine kinase inhibitors: review and recommendations for harmonizing current methodology for detecting Bcr-Abl transcripts and kinase domain mutations and for expressing results. *Blood* 2006;108: 28–37.
23 Faderl S, Talpaz M, Estrov Z, O'Brien S, Kurzrock R, Kantarjian HM. The biology of chronic myeloid leukemia. *N Engl J Med* 1999;341:164–72.
24 Mitelman F. The cytogenetic scenario of chronic myeloid leukemia. *Leuk Lymphoma* 1993;11(Suppl.1):11–15.
25 Mitelman F, Nilsson PG, Levan G, Brandt L. Non-random chromosome changes in acute myeloid leukemia. Chromosome banding examination of 30 cases at diagnosis. *Int J Cancer* 1976;18:31–8.
26 Bohm J, Schaefer HE. Chronic neutrophilic leukaemia: 14 new cases of an uncommon myeloproliferative disease. *J Clin Pathol* 2002;55:862–4.
27 Elliott MA, Hanson CA, Dewald GW, Smoley SA, Lasho TL, Tefferi A. WHO-defined chronic neutrophilic leukemia: a long-term analysis of 12 cases and a critical review of the literature. *Leukemia* 2005;19:313–17.
28 You W, Weisbrot IM. Chronic neutrophilic leukemia. Report of two cases and review of the literature. *Am J Clin Pathol* 1979;72:233–42.
29 Cehreli C, Undar B, Akkoc N, Onvural B, Altungoz O. Coexistence of chronic neutrophilic leukemia with light chain myeloma. *Acta Haematol* 1994;91:32–4.
30 Dincol G, Nalcaci M, Dogan O, *et al.* Coexistence of chronic neutrophilic leukemia with multiple myeloma. *Leuk Lymphoma* 2002;43:649–51.
31 Standen GR, Steers FJ, Jones L. Clonality of chronic neutrophilic leukaemia associated with myeloma: analysis using the X-linked probe M27 beta. *J Clin Pathol* 1993;46:297–8.
32 Tefferi A, Vardiman JW. Classification and diagnosis of myeloproliferative neoplasms: the 2008 World Health Organization criteria and point-of-care diagnostic algorithms. *Leukemia* 2008;22:14–22.
33 Baxter EJ, Scott LM, Campbell PJ, *et al.* Acquired mutation of the tyrosine kinase JAK2 in human myeloproliferative disorders. *Lancet* 2005;365:1054–61.
34 Kralovics R, Passamonti F, Buser AS, *et al.* A gain-of-function mutation of *JAK2* in myeloproliferative disorders. *N Engl J Med* 2005;352:1779–90.
35 Levine RL, Wadleigh M, Cools J, *et al.* Activating mutation in the tyrosine kinase JAK2 in polycythemia vera, essential thrombocythemia, and myeloid metaplasia with myelofibrosis. *Cancer Cell* 2005;7:387–97.
36 Pardanani AD, Levine RL, Lasho T, *et al. MPL515* mutations in myeloproliferative and other myeloid disorders: a study of 1182 patients. *Blood* 2006;108:3472–3476.

37 Pardanani A, Lasho TL, Finke C, Hanson CA, Tefferi A. Prevalence and clinicopathologic correlates of *JAK2* exon 12 mutations in *JAK2V617F*-negative polycythemia vera. *Leukemia* 2007, 21:1960–3.

38 Scott LM, Tong W, Levine RL, Scott MA, Beer PA, Stratton MR, *et al.* *JAK2* exon 12 mutations in polycythemia vera and idiopathic erythrocytosis. *N Engl J Med* 2007;356:459–68.

39 Thiele J, Kvasnika HM, Orazi A, Tefferi A, Birgegard G. Polycythemia vera. In: Swerdlow SH, Campo E, Harris NL, *et al* (eds). IARC Press: Lyon, 2008. pp.40–3.

40 Thiele J, Kvasnika HM, Tefferi A, Barosi G, Orazi A, Vardiman JW. Primary myelofibrosis. In: Swerdlow SH, Campo E, Harris NL, *et al* (eds). IARC Press: Lyon, 2008. pp.44–7.

41 Thiele J, Kvasnika HM, Orazi A, Tefferi A, Gisslinger H. Essential thrombocythaemia. In: Swerdlow SH, Campo E, Harris NL, *et al* (eds). IARC Press: Lyon, 2008. pp.48–50.

42 Vardiman JW, Brunning RD, Arber DA, *et al.* Introduction and overview of the classification of the myeloid neoplasms. In: Swerdlow SH, Campo E, Harris NL, *et al* (eds). IARC Press: Lyon, 2008. pp.18–30.

43 Ellis JT, Peterson P, Geller SA, Rappaport H. Studies of the bone marrow in polycythemia vera and the evolution of myelofibrosis and second hematologic malignancies. *Semin Hematol* 1986;23:144–55.

44 Georgii A, Buesche G, Kreft A. The histopathology of chronic myeloproliferative diseases. *Baillieres Clin Haematol* 1998;11: 721–49.

45 Thiele J, Kvasnicka HM. Diagnostic impact of bone marrow histopathology in polycythemia vera (PV). *Histol Histopathol* 2005;20:317–28.

46 Finazzi G, Harrison C. Essential thrombocythemial. *Semin Hematol* 2005;42:230–8.

47 Gisslinger H. Update on diagnosis and management of essential thrombocythemia. *Semin Thromb Hemost* 2006;32:430–6.

48 Thiele J, Kvasnicka HM, Zankovich R, Diehl V. Relevance of bone marrow features in the differential diagnosis between essential thrombocythemia and early stage idiopathic myelofibrosis. *Haematologica* 2000;85:1126–34.

49 Thiele J, Kvasnicka HM. Clinicopathological criteria for differential diagnosis of thrombocythemias in various myeloproliferative disorders. *Semin Thromb Hemost* 2006;32:219–30.

50 Dupriez B, Morel P, Demory JL, *et al.* Prognostic factors in agnogenic myeloid metaplasia: a report on 195 cases with a new scoring system. *Blood* 1996;88:1013–18.

51 Harrison CN, Green AR. Essential thrombocythemia. *Hematol Oncol Clin North Am* 2003;17:1175–90.

52 Passamonti F, Rumi E, Pungolino E, *et al.* Life expectancy and prognostic factors for survival in patients with polycythemia vera and essential thrombocythemia. *Am J Med* 2004;117: 755–61.

53 Horny HP, Metcalfe DD, Bennett JM, *et al.* Mastocytosis. In: Swerdlow SH, Campo E, Harris NL, *et al* (eds). IARC Press: Lyon, 2008. pp.54–63.

54 Horny HP, Parwaresch MR, Lennert K. Bone marrow findings in systemic mastocytosis. *Hum Pathol* 1985;16:808–14.

55 Krokowski M, Sotlar K, Krauth MT, Fodinger M, Valent P, Horny HP. Delineation of patterns of bone marrow mast cell infiltration in systemic mastocytosis: value of CD25, correlation with subvariants of the disease, and separation from mast cell hyperplasia. *Am J Clin Pathol* 2005;124:560–8.

56 Stellmacher F, Sotlar K, Balleisen L, Valent P, Horny HP. Bone marrow mastocytosis associated with IgM kappa plasma cell myeloma. *Leuk Lymphoma* 2004;45:801–5.

57 Horny HP, Sotlar K, Sperr WR, Valent P. Systemic mastocytosis with associated clonal haematological non-mast cell lineage diseases: a histopathological challenge. *J Clin Pathol* 2004;57: 604–8.

58 Ault P, Lynn A, Tam CS, Medeiros LJ, Keating MJ. Systemic mastocytosis in association with chronic lymphocytic leukemia: a rare diagnosis. *Leuk Res* 2007;31:1755–8.

59 Brunning RD, McKenna RW, Rosai J, Parkin JL, Risdall R. Systemic mastocytosis. Extracutaneous manifestations. *Am J Surg Pathol* 1983;7:425–38.

60 Valent P, Horny HP, Escribano L, *et al.* Diagnostic criteria and classification of mastocytosis: a consensus proposal. *Leuk Res* 2001;25:603–25.

61 Horny HP, Parwaresch MR, Kaiserling E, *et al.* Mast cell sarcoma of the larynx. *J Clin Pathol* 1986;39:596–602.

62 Burgstaller S, Kreil S, Waghorn K, *et al.* The severity of *FIP1L1-PDGFRA*-positive chronic eosinophilic leukaemia is associated with polymorphic variation at the IL5RA locus. *Leukemia* 2007;21:2428–32.

63 Metzgeroth G, Walz C, Score J, *et al.* Recurrent finding of the *FIP1L1-PDGFRA* fusion gene in eosinophilia-associated acute myeloid leukemia and lymphoblastic T-cell lymphoma. *Leukemia* 2007;21:1183–8.

64 Bain BJ, Fletcher SH. Chronic eosinophilic leukemias and the myeloproliferative variant of the hypereosinophilic syndrome. *Immunol Allergy Clin North Am* 2007;27:377–88.

65 Steer EJ, Cross NC. Myeloproliferative disorders with translocations of chromosome 5q31–35: role of the platelet-derived growth factor receptor Beta. *Acta Haematol* 2002;107: 113–22.

66 Macdonald D, Reiter A, Cross NC. The 8p11 myeloproliferative syndrome: a distinct clinical entity caused by constitutive activation of FGFR1. *Acta Haematol* 2002;107:101–7.

67 Tashiro H, Shirasaki R, Noguchi M, Gotoh M, Kawasugi K, Shirafuji N. Molecular analysis of chronic eosinophilic leukemia with t(4;10) showing good response to imatinib mesylate. *Int J Hematol* 2006;83:433–8.

68 Cools J, DeAngelo DJ, Gotlib J, *et al.* A tyrosine kinase created by fusion of the PDGFRA and FIP1L1 genes as a therapeutic target of imatinib in idiopathic hypereosinophilic syndrome. *N Engl J Med* 2003;348:1201–14.

69 Fialkow PJ, Singer JW, Adamson JW, *et al.* Acute nonlymphocytic leukemia: heterogeneity of stem cell origin. *Blood* 1981;57:1068–73.

70 Vardiman JW, Harris NL, Brunning RD. The World Health Organization (WHO) classification of the myeloid neoplasms. *Blood* 2002;100:2292–302.

71 Arber D, Brunning RD, LeBeau MM, *et al.* Acute Myeloid Leukaemia. In: Jaffe ES, Harris NL, Stein H, Vardiman JW (eds). *World Health Organization Classification of Tumours: Pathology and Genetics of Tumors of Haematopoietic and Lymphoid Tissues*. IARC Press: Lyon, 2008. pp.75–107.

72 Foucar K. *Bone Marrow Pathology*. ASCP Press: Chicago, 2001.

73 Bennett JM, Catovsky D, Daniel MT, *et al.* Proposed revised criteria for the classification of acute myeloid leukemia. A report of the French-American-British Cooperative Group. *Ann Intern Med* 1985;103:620–5.

74 Golomb HM, Rowley JD, Vardiman JW, Testa JR, Butler A. "Microgranular" acute promyelocytic leukemia: a distinct clinical, ultrastructural, and cytogenetic entity. *Blood* 1980;55: 253–9.
75 Le Beau MM, Larson RA, Bitter MA, Vardiman JW, Golomb HM, Rowley JD. Association of an inversion of chromosome 16 with abnormal marrow eosinophils in acute myelomonocytic leukemia. A unique cytogenetic-clinicopathological association. *N Engl J Med* 1983;309:630–6.
76 Nucifora G, Dickstein JI, Torbenson V, Roulston D, Rowley JD, Vardiman JW. Correlation between cell morphology and expression of the AML1/ETO chimeric transcript in patients with acute myeloid leukemia without the t(8;21). *Leukemia* 1994;8:1533–8.
77 Bene MC, Castoldi G, Knapp W, *et al*. Proposals for the immunological classification of acute leukemias. European Group for the Immunological Characterization of Leukemias (EGIL). *Leukemia* 1995;9:1783–6.
78 The value of c-kit in the diagnosis of biophenotypic acute leukemia. EGIL (European Group for the Immunological Classification of Leukaemias). *Leukemia* 1998;12:2038.
79 Kanda Y, Hamaki T, Yamamoto R, *et al*. The clinical significance of CD34 expression in response to therapy of patients with acute myeloid leukemia: an overview of 2483 patients from 22 studies. *Cancer* 2000;88:2529–33.
80 Borowitz MJ, Chan JKC. B lymphoblastic leukaemia/lymphoma, not otherwise specified. In: Swerdlow SH, Campo E, Harris NL, *et al* (eds). IARC Press: Lyon, 2008. pp.168–78.
81 Wegelius R. Preleukaemic states in children. *Scand J Haematol Suppl* 1986;45:133–9.
82 Spitzer G, Garson OM. Lymphoblastic leukemia with marked eosinophilia: a report of two cases. *Blood* 1973;42:377–84.
83 Nunez CA, Zipf TF, Roberts WM, Medeiros LJ, Hayes K, Bueso-Ramos CE. Molecular monitoring of cerebrospinal fluid can predict clinical relapse in acute lymphoblastic leukemia with eosinophilia. *Arch Pathol Lab Med* 2003;127:601–5.
84 Bennett JM, Catovsky D, Daniel MT, *et al*. Proposals for the classification of the acute leukaemias. French-American-British (FAB) co-operative group. *Br J Haematol* 1976;33: 451–8.
85 Harris NL, Jaffe ES, Stein H, *et al*. A revised European-American classification of lymphoid neoplasms: a proposal from the International Lymphoma Study Group. *Blood* 1994; 84:1361–92.
86 Lilleyman JS, Hann IM, Stevens RF, Richards SM, Eden OB. Blast cell vacuoles in childhood lymphoblastic leukaemia. *Br J Haematol* 1988;70:183–6.
87 Potter VP, Sorell M, Baglivo JA, Sather H, Miller DR. Prognostic significance of vacuoles in L1 lymphoblasts in childhood acute lymphoblastic leukaemia: a report from Children's Cancer Study Group. *Br J Haematol* 1984;56:215–22.
88 Ferrari S, Mariano MT, Tagliafico E, *et al*. Myeloperoxidase gene expression in blast cells with a lymphoid phenotype in cases of acute lymphoblastic leukemia. *Blood* 1988;72: 873–6.
89 Serrano J, Roman J, Sanchez J, Torres A. Myeloperoxidase gene expression in acute lymphoblastic leukaemia. *Br J Haematol* 1997;97:841–3.
90 Huh YO, Smith TL, Collins P, *et al*. Terminal deoxynucleotidyl transferase expression in acute myelogenous leukemia and myelodysplasia as determined by flow cytometry. *Leuk Lymphoma* 2000;37:319–31.
91 Khalidi HS, Medeiros LJ, Chang KL, Brynes RK, Slovak ML, Arber DA. The immunophenotype of adult acute myeloid leukemia: high frequency of lymphoid antigen expression and comparison of immunophenotype, French-American-British classification, and karyotypic abnormalities. *Am J Clin Pathol* 1998;109:211–20.
92 Stass SA, Pui CH, Melvin S, *et al*. Sudan black B positive acute lymphoblastic leukaemia. *Br J Haematol* 1984;57:413–21.
93 Janossy G, Hoffbrand AV, Greaves MF, *et al*. Terminal transferase enzyme assay and immunological membrane markers in the diagnosis of leukaemia: a multiparameter analysis of 300 cases. *Br J Haematol* 1980;44:221–34.
94 Vasef MA, Brynes RK, Murata-Collins JL, Arber DA, Medeiros LJ. Surface immunoglobulin light chain-positive acute lymphoblastic *Leukemia* of FAB L1 or L2 type: a report of 6 cases in adults. *Am J Clin Pathol* 1998;110:143–9.
95 Desai K, Fallon MA, Willard-Smith D, Wilbur DC. Improving the diagnostic accuracy of cytologic cerebrospinal fluid examinations in acute lymphoblastic leukemia using high-power microscopy and terminal deoxynucleotidyl transferase determinations. *Diagn Cytopathol* 1997;16:413–19.
96 Greaves MF, Chan LC, Furley AJ, Watt SM, Molgaard HV. Lineage promiscuity in hemopoietic differentiation and leukemia. *Blood* 1986;67:1–11.
97 Wiersma SR, Ortega J, Sobel E, Weinberg KI. Clinical importance of myeloid-antigen expression in acute lymphoblastic leukemia of childhood. *N Engl J Med* 1991;324:800–8.
98 Thalhammer-Scherrer R, Mitterbauer G, Simonitsch I, *et al*. The immunophenotype of 325 adult acute leukemias: relationship to morphologic and molecular classification and proposal for a minimal screening program highly predictive for lineage discrimination. *Am J Clin Pathol* 2002;117:380–89.
99 Uckun FM, Sather HN, Gaynon PS, *et al*. Clinical features and treatment outcome of children with myeloid antigen positive acute lymphoblastic leukemia: a report from the Children's Cancer Group. *Blood* 1997;90:28–35.
100 Putti MC, Rondelli R, Cocito MG, *et al*. Expression of myeloid markers lacks prognostic impact in children treated for acute lymphoblastic leukemia: Italian experience in AIEOP-ALL 88–91 studies. *Blood* 1998;92:795–801.
101 Preti HA, Huh YO, O'Brien SM, *et al*. Myeloid markers in adult acute lymphocytic leukemia. Correlations with patient and disease characteristics and with prognosis. *Cancer* 1995;76: 1564–70.
102 Tsao AS, Kantarjian H, Thomas D, *et al*. C-kit receptor expression in acute leukemias-association with patient and disease characteristics and with outcome. *Leuk Res* 2004;28:373–8.
103 Chuang SS, Li CY. Useful panel of antibodies for the classification of acute leukemia by immunohistochemical methods in bone marrow trephine biopsy specimens. *Am J Clin Pathol* 1997;107:410–18.
104 Pileri SA, Ascani S, Milani M, *et al*. Acute leukaemia immunophenotyping in bone-marrow routine sections. *Br J Haematol* 1999;105:394–401.
105 Pui CH, Relling MV, Downing JR. Acute lymphoblastic leukemia. *N Engl J Med* 2004;350:1535–48.
106 Chronic lymphocytic Leukemia: recommendations for diagnosis, staging, and response criteria. International Workshop

on Chronic Lymphocytic Leukemia. *Ann Intern Med* 1989;110:236–38.

107 Cheson BD, Bennett JM, Grever M, *et al.* National Cancer Institute-sponsored Working Group guidelines for chronic lymphocytic leukemia: revised guidelines for diagnosis and treatment. *Blood* 1996;87:4990–7.

108 Mueller-Hermelink HK, Montserrat E, Catovsky D, Campo E, Harris NL, Stein H. Chronic lymphocytic leukaemia/small lymphocytic lymphoma. In: Swerdlow SH, Campo E, Harris NL, *et al.* IARC Press: Lyon, 2008. pp.180–4.

109 Bennett JM, Catovsky D, Daniel MT, *et al.* Proposals for the classification of chronic (mature) B and T lymphoid leukaemias. French-American-British (FAB) Cooperative Group. *J Clin Pathol* 1989;42:567–84.

110 Montserrat E, Sanchez-Bisono J, Vinolas N, Rozman C. Lymphocyte doubling time in chronic lymphocytic leukaemia: analysis of its prognostic significance. *Br J Haematol* 1986;62: 567–75.

111 Rozman C, Montserrat E, Rodriguez-Fernandez JM, *et al.* Bone marrow histologic pattern–the best single prognostic parameter in chronic lymphocytic leukemia: a multivariate survival analysis of 329 cases. *Blood* 1984;64:642–8.

112 Geisler C, Ralfkiaer E, Hansen MM, Hou-Jensen K, Larsen SO. The bone marrow histological pattern has independent prognostic value in early stage chronic lymphocytic leukaemia. *Br J Haematol* 1986;62:47–54.

113 Tsimberidou AM, Keating MJ. Richter syndrome: biology, incidence, and therapeutic strategies. *Cancer* 2005;103:216–28.

114 Galton DA, Goldman JM, Wiltshaw E, Catovsky D, Henry K, Goldenberg GJ. Prolymphocytic leukaemia. *Br J Haematol* 1974;27:7–23.

115 Katayama I, Aiba M, Pechet L, Sullivan JL, Roberts P, Humphreys RE. B-lineage prolymphocytic leukemia as a distinct clinicopathologic entity. *Am J Pathol* 1980;99:399–412.

116 Schlette E, Bueso-Ramos C, Giles F, Glassman A, Hayes K, Medeiros LJ. Mature B-cell leukemias with more than 55% prolymphocytes. A heterogeneous group that includes an unusual variant of mantle cell lymphoma. *Am J Clin Pathol* 2001;115:571–81.

117 Jaffe ES, Harris NL, Stein H, Vardiman JW (eds). *World Health Organization Classification of Tumours: Pathology and Genetics of Tumours of Haematopoietic and Lymphoid Tissues.* IARC Press: Lyon, 2001.

118 Jennings CD, Foon KA. Recent advances in flow cytometry: application to the diagnosis of hematologic malignancy. *Blood* 1997;90:2863–92.

119 Matutes E, Morilla R, Owusu-Ankomah K, Houlihan A, Catovsky D. The immunophenotype of splenic lymphoma with villous lymphocytes and its relevance to the differential diagnosis with other B-cell disorders. *Blood* 1994;83: 1558–62.

120 Matutes E, Brito-Babapulle V, Swansbury J, *et al.* Clinical and laboratory features of 78 cases of T-prolymphocytic leukemia. *Blood* 1991;78:3269–74.

121 Flandrin G, Brouet JC. The Sezary cell: cytologic, cytochemical, and immunologic studies. *Mayo Clin Proc* 1974;49: 575–83.

122 Shimoyama M. Diagnostic criteria and classification of clinical subtypes of adult T-cell leukaemia-lymphoma. A report from the Lymphoma Study Group (1984–87). *Br J Haematol* 1991; 79:428–37.

123 Sakashita A, Hattori T, Miller CW, Suzushima H, Asou N, Takatsuki K, *et al.* Mutations of the *p53* gene in adult T-cell leukemia. *Blood* 1992;79:477–80.

124 Loughran TP, Jr. Clonal diseases of large granular lymphocytes. *Blood* 1993;82:1–14.

125 Scott CS, Richards SJ, Sivakumaran M. Disorders of large granular lymphocytes and natural killer-associated cells. *Blood* 1994;83:301–3.

126 Shastri KA, Logue GL. Autoimmune neutropenia. *Blood* 1993; 81:1984–95.

127 Tefferi A, Li CY, Witzig TE, Dhodapkar MV, Okuno SH, Phyliky RL. Chronic natural killer cell lymphocytosis: a descriptive clinical study. *Blood* 1994;84:2721–5.

Chapter 4
Diagnosis of Leukemias: New Diagnostic Modalities and Implications for Classification

Maher Albitar
Quest Diagnostics Nichols Institute, San Juan Capistrano, California, USA

Introduction

The diagnosis and classification of leukemias is becoming increasingly dependent on the underlying molecular abnormalities. The development of new therapeutic agents that target specific molecular abnormalities necessitates methods for diagnosis and classification of these specific aberrations—for all types of cancers, not only leukemia. Progress in various molecular techniques is also providing discovery tools for better defining new diagnostic entities that previously were classified under other diseases. Karyotyping and fluorescence *in situ* hybridization (FISH) studies, along with flow cytometry and morphologic examination, remain at the cornerstone of any leukemia diagnosis and classification scheme. However, for more precise and detailed subclassification, numerous important diagnostic and prognostic molecular abnormalities need to be evaluated using relatively sophisticated molecular testing. Various high-throughput nucleic acid-, protein array-, and mass spectrometry-based platforms are being used in research settings and have been extremely helpful in drug discovery and for finding novel molecular abnormalities. However, the use of such high-throughput approaches and the evaluation of large numbers of variables leads to inherent problems in terms of quality assurance and reproducibility. These techniques are not ready for use in day-to-day clinical laboratory testing, and thus are not being used in the diagnosis or classification of leukemias.

This chapter will focus on technologic advances and new tests that are being used in clinical laboratories for the diagnosis and classification of leukemias. It will briefly discuss some of the common technologies used in the diagnosis of leukemias, with a focus on the new technologies that are making or have made their way to the clinical laboratory. Additionally, individual leukemias will be discussed and I will review recent discoveries that may prove to be of benefit for classification.

Technology

Sample-type and plasma-based testing for molecular abnormalities in leukemic cells

Traditionally, cells from bone marrow or peripheral blood have been used for the detection of molecular abnormalities in leukemic cells. Because leukemic cells frequently do not circulate and cannot be detected in the peripheral blood, bone marrow samples are often required. Bone marrow aspirates are subject to numerous drawbacks: they are often diluted by peripheral blood; leukemic cells are sometimes "patchy" and are missed; and samples are often not representative.

It is now becoming evident that DNA, RNA, and proteins from leukemic cells can easily be detected as cell-free circulating molecules in the plasma or serum [1–12]. This is particularly relevant in leukemias and hematologic diseases because leukemic cells are immersed in blood. In addition, tumor cells have a high turnover and therefore pour their DNA, RNA, and protein into the circulation—not as free molecules, but rather as apoptotic bodies or cellular debris. Purified free nucleic acids are degraded immediately by various enzymes when added to plasma. In contrast, the endogenous DNA, RNA, and proteins are most likely protected by forming protein–protein, protein–DNA, or protein–RNA complexes. Therefore, plasma is an ideal sample type for testing because it is less diluted by products from normal cells and less affected by sampling bias. For example, in early stage chronic myeloproliferative neoplasms (MPNs), *JAK2* mutations may be present in only a small subpopulation of cells or megakaryocytes and will thus not be detectable when cells are used; the mutation is detected more easily when plasma is used [2].

Another advantage to using plasma is ease of quantification: we can quantify molecular abnormalities and

Leukemias: Principles and Practice of Therapy, 1st edition. Edited by S. Faderl and H. Kantarjian.

express levels in a specific quantity of plasma, facilitating a comparison of results between patients. More importantly, this approach allows us to introduce the concept of "tumor load," quantify the volume of the tumor, and monitor the response to therapy. For example, our previous studies quantifying *BCR–ABL1* fusion RNA [4] or protein [12] molecules in 10 µL of plasma demonstrated significant interindividual variation among newly diagnosed patients, reflecting differences in tumor loads. While we do not yet know how to use this information to stratify patients or adjust dosing, new studies correlating these findings with clinical behavior promise to yield improved care and better understanding of the individuality of patients (ie, personalized medicine).

The use of plasma allows detection of adverse abnormalities in subclones even when there is heterogeneity in the leukemic cells [5]. Evolving clones are usually more aggressive and have higher rates of growth and turnover; therefore, they pour their contents into circulation at a higher rate than the rest of the leukemic cells [3]. Such clones can thus be detected more easily in the plasma. This is particularly seen in patients with chronic myeloid leukemia (CML) being treated with imatinib mesylate. Emerging resistant clones are detected in plasma earlier than in bone marrow samples [5].

Clearly, more studies are needed to confirm and expand on the use of plasma as a replacement for bone marrow and peripheral blood cells in detecting molecular abnormalities and monitoring hematologic diseases. More importantly, further studies are needed to determine how to incorporate the new information that is being generated from plasma-based testing of tumor load or minimal residual disease (MRD) into clinical practice.

Nucleic acid-based techniques

Detection of mutations

Multiple methods are used to detect mutations in leukemic samples. Sequencing remains the gold standard and the most accurate approach. However, the sensitivity of direct sequencing is low (5–20%) when conventional methods are used. New sequencers, or so called "next-generation" sequencers, hold the promise of high throughput with higher sensitivity, but these instruments remain in the research phase and are not yet adaptable to the clinical laboratory in a cost-effective fashion. Nevertheless, numerous additional methods are currently used for the detection of mutations, most of which are based on primer-specific hybridization and polymerase chain reaction (PCR) amplification of target sequences in RNA or DNA. Methods based on high performance liquid chromatography (HPLC) are also used for screening, but mutations detected by HPLC generally should be confirmed using conventional methods. Mutations that generate a new restriction enzyme site can be efficiently detected with restriction fragment length analysis. When the mutations are in the form of deletion or duplication of a segment of DNA, rather than a point mutation, simple amplification and resolution of the amplification product can be an adequate approach. Additional promising new approaches that have made their way to the clinical laboratory are described in greater detail below.

Pyrosequencing

Pyrosequencing is a sequencing approach based on measuring the release of pyrophosphate (PPi) by nucleotide incorporation during DNA synthesis. Briefly, a PCR-amplified, single-stranded DNA template is hybridized with a specific primer in the presence of DNA polymerase, luciferase, adenosine triphosphate (ATP) sulfurylase, apyrase, luciferin, and adenosine 5′ phosphosulfate. Deoxynucleotides (dNTPs) are then added one at a time. If the added dNTP is complementary to the template strand, DNA polymerase catalyzes its incorporation into the DNA strand with the release of PPi. Light emission is achieved by converting the released PPi to ATP by way of ATP sulfurylase, thus providing energy to oxidize luciferin. The amount of light generated is proportional to the number of incorporated nucleotides. The next dNTP is added after the unincorporporated dNTPs are degraded by apyrase, and the process repeats. The most important advantage of pyrosequencing is its potential for quantification. It is also reported to be slightly more sensitive than conventional sequencing (5% sensitivity) and may also be helpful in sequencing DNA with difficult secondary structures [13].

Single-nucleotide polymorphism analysis

Single-nucleotide polymorphism (SNP) is based on DNA polymerase-mediated single-base extension. First, PCR amplification of genomic DNA containing the regions of interest is performed in a single tube. A multiplex single-base extension (minisequencing) reaction is then performed using primers immediately upstream of the mutation site. Resolving these extended products on capillary electrophoresis allows for the detection of the specific mutation based on the type of the labeled incorporated nucleotide. For multiplexing, amplification products for each region of interest should have different sizes to allow detection of multiple mutations in different sites or genes. This approach is sensitive and reproducible.

mRNA expression and quantification

Measurement of gene expression levels is now used extensively in clinical laboratories, most often to detect abnormal expression secondary to chromosomal translocations. The quantification methodology used most frequently is real-time PCR, which is based on determining the rate of release of a dye during the amplification of the target sequence. The most common approaches used with real-time PCR are SYBR Green 1 (or other dyes) and Taqman® probes. Numerous questions regarding the standardization and robustness of these real-time PCR methods remain unanswered and need to be addressed if results from one laboratory are to be compared with results from others. However, this approach remains the most widely used in molecular testing for monitoring patients, especially those with chromosomal translocations.

Methylation profiling

DNA methylation plays an important role in the regulation of expression and imprinting of genes. DNA methylation typically occurs in the CpG islands, which are usually in the CG-rich region upstream of the promoter region of genes. Numerous approaches can be used to study DNA methylation, and no single method is appropriate for every application; method selection requires understanding of the type of information needed and the potential for bias and artifacts associated with each approach. Bisulfite modification of DNA is the foundation for the majority of assays geared toward clinical testing. The differences in bisulfite-based methylation assays arise from the manner in which bisulfite-modified DNA is analyzed. Bisulfite modification converts non-methylated cytosines to uracils, which are then converted to thymines during DNA amplification by PCR, whereas methylated cytosines are protected from bisulfite modification. DNA sequencing and the use of methylation-sensitive primers are the two most commonly used techniques to analyze bisulfite-treated DNA. The extension of an oligonucleotide to the 5′ end of a CpG site using dideoxycytidine (ddCTP) or dideoxythymidine (ddTTP), followed by real-time PCR, allows for a quantitative assessment of methylation patterns and can be applied to multiple sites simultaneously. Digesting the DNA with methylation-sensitive restriction enzymes and analyzing the digestion products by PCR or Southern blots remains a viable and reliable approach, but is less used because of its relative complexity. The current new-generation sequencers allow for high-throughput genome-wide methylation analysis. Measuring levels of methylation in a particular tissue or plasma is increasingly used for the diagnosis and prediction of prognosis in various tumor types, including leukemias [14–17].

Protein-based techniques

Immunologic techniques

Antibody-based assays are extensively used to detect and measure protein expression in intact cells, in cell lysates, and in circulation. Flow cytometry and analysis of surface or intracellular markers are widely used to evaluate and classify leukemias and to detect MRD. Recent technologic advances have also made it possible to monitor changes in expression and modification (eg, phosphorylation and acetylation) of intracellular proteins during therapy, particularly proteins that are targeted by the therapeutic agent(s). Enzyme-linked immunosorbent assays (ELISA) remain a cornerstone of immunologic testing and have been used to establish the clinical utility of various new biomarkers in leukemia. Immunologic techniques such as ELISA also lend themselves to multiplex analysis of various targets in a single assay using a single aliquot, which can provide important information.

However, one of the major advances in immunologic techniques relating to leukemias is the recently reported ability to detect chromosomal translocations resulting in the expression of fusion proteins using simple sandwich ELISA-like methods. This approach employs a "capture" antibody targeting the product of one of the two fused genes, and a "detection" antibody targeting the product of the second fused gene. Sandwich immunoassays such as this have been used to detect Bcr–Abl in cells and in plasma of patients with CML [12]. The advantages of using such an approach is better precision relative to real-time PCR assays and the potential for standardization for interlaboratory comparisons.

Mass spectrometry for protein analysis

Mass spectrometry (MS) has emerged in recent years as a powerful tool for the analysis of proteins. Recent improvements in the measurement of large proteins are moving MS closer to the clinical laboratory. MS is expected to provide a highly specific tool for detecting and measuring proteins that were difficult to measure in the past.

Molecules can be separated by MS based on their charges and size as they travel in electric and magnetic fields. The molecule of interest is first transferred into gas phase and ionized, and the ratio of the mass to the charge (m/z) is measured. The protein or peptide is first evaporated and bombarded with a laser (adding protons or removing electrons). This is facilitated using matrix-assisted laser desorption/ionization (MALDI) or electrospray ionization (ESI). The current MS instruments are based mainly around time of flight (TOF), quadrupole, and ion resonance. The TOF instruments are usually adapted for MALDI and work simply by energizing ions with a laser, allowing them to accelerate in the electric field until they reach a detector where the time of their flight, which is proportional to their m/z, is measured. The linear quadrupole is compatible with pulsed ion source. It is based on applying voltage to four rod filters. This results in focusing forces that act in traverse direction, which allows specific m/z to be stable and excludes other m/z. By changing the voltage and electric fields successively, various m/z can be separated. Linear quadrupole is usually used for scanning. Quadrupole ion and three-dimensional quadrupole ion trap work around the same principle, except they trap the ions upon collision with helium gas then release them into an electron multiplier.

Currently, MS is used for numerous tests in clinical laboratories but has yet to be utilized in the context of leukemia. With further research, MS is expected to become an important technology for the diagnosis and classification of leukemias in the near future.

Acute myeloid leukemia

The following diagnostic subgroups of acute myeloid leukemia (AML) are particularly important because of their clinical course and therapeutic implications.

Core binding factor abnormalities

Core binding factors (CBFs) are protein heterodimers that bind to DNA and act as transcription factors; three genes (*CBFA1, CBFA2, CBFA3)* encode α subunits, which bind DNA, and one gene, *CBFB*, encodes the non-DNA-binding β subunit. The t(8;21)(q22;q22) translocation fuses *CBFA2* (also called *AML1* and *RUNX1*) to *ETO*, and inv(16)(p13q22)/t(16;16)(p13;q22) similarly disrupts *CBFB* by fusing the N-terminal portion of the CBF beta subunit to the carboxy terminal of the MYH11 (also called SMMHC) protein. These abnormalities are associated with good outcomes [18–20], but other translocations involving *CBFA2* and additional genes have been reported in AML. For example, t(3;21)(q26;q22) results in fusion of *CBFA2* to *EAP, MDS1*, or *EVI1* [21,22] and is associated with poor outcome. In addition, mutations in the *CBFA2* gene have been reported in rare cases of AML, and germline *CBFA2* mutations have been reported in rare autosomal dominant familial platelet disorders with predisposition to AML [23].

Translocation of the *CBFA2* gene to the *TEL* gene in t(12;21)(p13;q22) leads to acute lymphoblastic leukemia (ALL), rather than AML, and represents the most common abnormality in pediatric ALL.

Abnormalities involving CBFα/β are thought to require additional complementary molecular abnormalities to cause a leukemic phenotype. Mutations in exons 8 of *c-Kit* have been reported at a relatively high frequency (approximately 22%) in leukemias with *AML1* translocation, and varied (from 9% to 29%) in leukemias with CBFβ translocations [24]. Patients with CBFβ abnormalities have a relatively high rate of mutations in the *RAS* oncogene, similar to that reported in acute monocytic leukemias. *FLT3* mutations also have been reported in cases with CBFβ abnormality [24]. The presence of these mutations in this group of patients is also associated with adverse outcome. All translocations can be detected using real-time PCR as well as FISH approaches. Mutations are best detected using direct sequencing, but other approaches are also acceptable.

Retinoic acid receptor alpha abnormalities

The retinoic acid receptor alpha (RARα) class of leukemia is characterized by the presence of translocations that involve juxtaposition of *RARA* with downstream genes by means of translocation. The most common fusion partner gene (90–95%) is *PML* [25–27], located on chromosome 15, which is fused to *RARA* as a result of t(15;17)(q21;q22). The resulting deregulation of the *RARA* gene is believed to cause maturation arrest of myeloid cells at the promyelocyte state, leading to manifestations of morphologic and immunophenotypic characteristics of acute promyelocytic leukemia (APL). In 5–10% of APL cases, the partner gene is not PML. APL cases with t(11;17)(q23;q21), t(5;17)(q35;q21), and t(11;17)(q13;q21) have been reported [27,28] in which the *RARA* is fused to the *PLZF* (promyelocytic leukemia zinc finger) [29], *NPM* (nucleophosmin) [30], and *NuMA* (nuclear mitotic apparatus) [31] genes, respectively. Translocations of *RARA* to the *STAT5b* gene on 17q21 [32] and the *PRKAR1A* gene on 17q22-24 [33] have also been reported. *PRKAR1A* encodes the regulatory subunit type I-α (RIα) of cyclic adenosine monophosphate (cAMP)-dependent protein kinase (PKA).

Distinguishing these cases is important because combination therapy for APL with all-trans-retinoic acid (ATRA) and arsenic trioxide (ATO) is successful except in the presence of *PLZF–RARA* or *STAT5b* fusion genes [32,34]. Mutations in the FMS-like tyrosine kinase 3 (*FLT3*) have been reported to be more frequent in APL and to be associated with a higher white blood cell count [24,35].

11q23 (*MLL*) abnormalities

The *MLL* gene has been reported to translocate into almost all chromosomes, and a number of *MLL* abnormalities can be seen in ALL as well as AML. Some of the translocations cannot be detected by routine karyotyping, so FISH or molecular studies are required. In addition, about 10% of patients with AML with a normal karyotype may have partial internal tandem duplications in the *MLL* gene [36,37], which can be detected only by molecular testing. *MLL* abnormalities are associated with more aggressive disease, frequently with monocytic differentiation [37–39]. This abnormality is also more frequent in therapy-related leukemia.

Normal cytogenetics and intermediate cytogenetic abnormalities

Patients with AML and intermediate cytogenetic abnormalities are a very heterogeneous group. Some will respond well to therapy and have a relatively long survival, while others will have a more aggressive disease with very short survival. This group of patients has thus been the focus of intense research in the hope of identifying specific molecular abnormalities that correlate with specific clinical courses. AML with intermediate cytogenetics usually encompasses all patients who do not have anomalies associated with a favorable outcome (RARα or CBF) or with a poor outcome (–5, –7, inv(3q) or complex abnormalities); most have normal karyotypes. Patients with trisomy 8 are included in this group [40], although some studies suggest that trisomy 8 should be included as an unfavorable cytogenetic abnormality [19].

The most common molecular abnormalities that are potentially associated with the outcome in patients with intermediate cytogenetics are *FLT3* internal tandem duplication (ITD) (~30%), *NPM1* mutations (~25%), and *CEBPA* (CCAAT/enhancer binding protein α) mutations (22%) [41,42]. *NPM1* [41,43–45] and *CEBPA* [46,47] mutations have been reported to be associated with better survival. Wilms tumor 1 (*WT1*) gene mutations have been reported in about 10–13% of patients with AML with normal cytogenetics, and are associated with significantly shorter survival [48,49]. However, one study found the negative prognostic value to hold true only in the presence of *FLT3* mutation [50].

Increased levels of the *BAALC* gene (brain and acute leukemia, cytoplasmic) [51] and *ERG* (ETS-related gene) [52] mRNA in peripheral blood samples are also reported to be associated with more aggressive disease in patients with normal cytogenetics. However, these findings are based on a PCR expression technique and should not be applied in a clinical laboratory setting without full clinical validation, because results could be influenced by the number of blasts, selection of primers, and internal controls among other variables.

Recently, large-scale profiling of RNA, DNA, microRNA, and protein has been used to further subclassify patients with AML [42,53–59]. However, such approaches have questionable practicality, reliability, and reproducibility, and cannot yet be used in the day-to-day management of patients.

Unfavorable cytogenetic abnormalities

Unfavorable cytogenetic abnormalities in AML include –5/del(5q), –7/del(7q), inv(3q), complex karyotype (≥3 karyotypic abnormalities), or 11q23. For practical and clinical purposes, this group of patients can be grouped together given their similar clinical course. The survival rate in these patients is approximately 10%. Most of the recent data suggest that trisomy 8 is associated with an unfavorable outcome only when accompanied with other unfavorable cytogenetic abnormalities [40,60]. These abnormalities are more frequent in older age groups and in therapy-related leukemias.

Acute lymphoblastic leukemia

Acute lymphoblastic leukemia is diagnosed by the presence of clonal precursor lymphoid cells (lymphoblasts) that are negative for myeloperoxidase and positive for TdT (terminal deoxynucleotidyl transferase). Despite some biologic overlap between pediatric and adult ALL, the clinical behavior and outcome differ significantly between the two. Even in the pediatric group, children aged 1–9 years have a significantly better outcome than children aged >10 years, and older children in turn have a better outcome than adults. Numerous studies have indicated the ability of DNA/RNA or protein profiling to classify ALL on the basis of various biologic characteristics [61–71]. However, these approaches are considered as not yet ready for implementation in clinical laboratories.

The following subcategories of ALL should be distinguished based on their specific therapeutic approach and clinical outcome.

Philadelphia-positive acute lymphoblastic leukemia

Translocation (9;22), or Philadelphia chromosome, is the most frequent primary abnormality in ALL, and expression of the resulting Bcr–Abl fusion protein is associated with more aggressive disease. Therapy with kinase inhibitors (imatinib, nilotinib, or dasatinib) in patients with Bcr–Abl translocation may lead to the development of Abl kinase mutations associated with drug resistance. Testing for Abl kinase mutations is thus a key consideration when treating patients with kinase inhibitors. However, most laboratories design their Abl kinase domain mutation analysis around the expression of the P210 protein, which is expressed in CML, and some of these procedures may not adequately amplify the P190 fusion transcript, which is expressed in ALL [72]. Therefore, the assay should be designed specifically to encompass the P190 transcript.

IKZF1 abnormalities

A recent report suggested that the *IKZF1* gene, which codes for the lymphoid transcription factor Ikaros, is abnormal (deleted or mutated) in 28.6% of pediatric patients with ALL, and that patients with this abnormality have higher rates of failure and relapse [73]. While these data need further confirmation, this abnormality should be considered in patients with ALL.

Burkitt-type acute lymphoblastic leukemia

ALL with B-cell immunophenotype is usually associated with t(8;14)(q24.1;q32) or t(8;22)(q24.1;q11.2). Patients with Burkitt-type lymphoma typically have a very aggressive disease course and short survival. CD20 expression is more common in these patients, and the addition of rituximab to chemotherapy has been shown to improve outcome [74].

IL3-IgH translocation [t(5;14)(q31;q32)]

Patients with this abnormality should be distinguished because they may present with eosinophilia and a slight increase in blasts [75–77]. Therefore, the diagnosis can be confusing or missed. High levels of IL3 are detected in these patients and are considered the cause of the eosinophilia.

Cytogenetics

Several cytogenetic abnormalities are associated with a relatively favorable outcome in ALL. These include hyperdiploidy (>50 chromosomes/leukemic cell) [78], t(12;21)–TEL-AML1 fusion [78], t(1;19)–E2A-PBX1 fusion [78], and trisomy 4, 10, and 17 [79–81]. Other cytogenetic findings are associated with unfavorable outcome. These include t(4;11)–MLL-AF4 fusion [78] and hypodiploidy (<44 chromosomes per leukemic cell) [78].

HOX gene family

There are four clusters of highly conserved homeobox (*HOX*) genes, each encoding 61 amino acids: the *HOXA* cluster on chromosome 7, *HOXB* on chromosome 17, *HOXC* on chromosome 12, and *HOXD* on chromosome 2. These *HOX* genes constitute a highly conserved family of DNA-binding genes that play a significant role in hematopoiesis. In addition, deregulation of *HOX* genes and the more divergent homeobox genes scattered throughout the genome are involved in leukemogenesis in myeloid and lymphoid cells [82–84]. For example, the homeobox gene *PBX1* is translocated to the *E2A* gene in precursor B-cell ALL with t(1;19) [85], and the *HOX11* gene is involved in the translocation t(10;14) in precursor T-cell ALL [86,87]. ALL with t(1;19) rarely expresses CD34 and is, in general, considered to be more aggressive [88–90].

NOTCH gene and precursor acute lymphoblastic leukemia

The NOTCH signaling pathway is important for cell–cell interaction and is involved in the control of cell differentiation and survival. NOTCH receptors are transmembrane glycoproteins that heterodimerize to be stable on the surface. When activated by the ligand, the intracytoplasmic domain is cleaved and translocated into the nucleus where it activates the transcription of target genes. *NOTCH1*, a member of the *NOTCH* gene family, contains activating mutations in 50–70% of precursor T-cell ALL [91,92]. Most of the mutations in ALL involve the heterodimerization domain. Available data suggest that *NOTCH1* gain-of-function mutations correlate with a good outcome in children and adult T-ALL [93–96]. The *NOTCH* gene pathway is also affected by abnormalities in the Ikaros gene *IKZF1*; the Ikaros protein is a direct repressor of NOTCH target genes [97]. However, additional data are necessary before implementing testing of these genes in the diagnosis and classification of ALL.

Pharmacogenomics in acute lymphoblastic leukemia

Genomic variability and single-nucleotide polymorphisms play an increasing role in evaluating drug susceptibility and pharmacogenomics. For example, polymporphisms in the gene encoding thiopurine methyltransferase (TPMT), which catalyzes S-methylation of thiopurines, have been associated with decreased enzyme activity and increased hematopoietic toxicity in patients receiving thiopurines. About 10% of the total population inherits one wild-type *TPMT* allele and one nonfunctional variant allele, resulting in intermediate enzyme activity; 1 in 300 people inherit two nonfunctional variant alleles, with no enzyme activity [98,99]. When treated with conventional doses of thiopurines, up to half of patients with the heterozygous deficiency and all homozygous-deficient patients develop hematopoietic toxicity effects, which can be fatal in the homozygous group. The enzyme deficiency also confers a high risk of developing therapy-related AML and radiation-induced brain tumors (in the context of intensive thiopurine treatment) [100]. Conversely, patients with high levels of enzyme activity might be at greater risk of relapse owing to decreased exposure of leukemic cells to active drug metabolites. Studies of thiopurine methyltransferase activity can be helpful in patients with poor tolerance [99,101,102] to antimetabolite-based therapy and should be used to guide drug dosing.

Chronic myeloid leukemia

Chronic myeloid leukemia is characterized by the proliferation of maturing myeloid cells and the presence of the t(9;22)(q34;q11) chromosomal translocation, resulting in a shortened chromosome 22 (Philadelphia chromosome). This translocation fuses the *BCR* gene with the *ABL1* gene, leading to the expression of a fusion mRNA and protein. Although rare, translocations fusing *ABL1* to a gene other than *BCR* have been described, and t(9;12)(q34;p13) resulting in an *ETV6-ABL1* gene rearrangement/fusion has been reported in patients with a disease similar to CML [103]. In addition, cases with *BCR–JAK2* fusion with t(9;22)(p24;q11) [104–106] have been reported. Unusual t(8;9)(p22;p24) translocation with a molecular abnormality involving the *PCM1* and *JAK2* genes were reported in patients presenting with chronic MPN. However, this disease did not respond to standard kinase inhibitor therapy, which suggests a different clinical entity [107,108].

The development of imatinib and next-generation kinase inhibitors has changed the course of the CML disease. Five-year survival is now greater than 80%. However, some patients demonstrate primary or secondary resistance and some progress to accelerated or blast phase. The major diagnostic issues to be considered in this disease are summarized below.

Monitoring disease and determining molecular response

In addition to cytogenetic and FISH data, it is important to use reverse transcriptase/PCR (RT/PCR)-based testing to monitor patients with CML being treated with imatinib or the new kinase inhibitors. Unfortunately, despite some attempts, there is no standardization for Bcr–Abl1 mRNA testing and results are difficult to compare between one laboratory and another. More importantly, the coefficient of variation (CV) of such assays is too high (30–40%) for clinical decisions to be based on a single measurement; trends and patterns of changes should be evaluated before making a clinical decision when RT/PCR results are used. However, taking log change from one laboratory and comparing it with log changes from other laboratories has proven to be useful. Protein-based assays that are currently under development for assessing disease response promise to change the practice when specificity is improved [12].

Treatment resistance and Bcr–Abl1 kinase mutation

Determination of imatinib resistance should be based on lack or loss of hematologic, cytogenetic, or molecular responses rather than on the detection of mutation alone. Some *ABL1* kinase domain mutations can be detected transiently during therapy and do not always imply resistance [109]. However, some mutations, such as Y253H, E255K/V, and T315I, when detected using direct sequencing, are usually indicative of resistance [110–112]. *ABL1* mutations are detected in 30–40% of resistant patients [113–116]. However, early detection of resistance is important. Switching to one of the newly available kinase inhibitors at an early sign of resistance, or even increasing dosage of imatinib, may prevent overt resistance [113,117–120]. Recent findings indicate that an alternatively spliced Bcr–Abl1 mRNA, causing insertion of 35 nucleotides between exons 8 and 9, leads to the expression of a truncated but very resistant Bcr–Abl1 protein [121]. Low-level expression of this alternatively spliced Bcr–Abl1 could allow some cells to evade kinase inhibitor therapy, providing more opportunity to develop additional mutations and overtly resistant disease. One method for detecting Abl1 kinase mutations at early stages without compromising specificity is to test plasma rather than cells from bone marrow or peripheral blood.

Chronic lymphocytic leukemia

The diagnosis of chronic lymphocytic leukemia (CLL) requires the presence of ≥5000 clonal B lymphocytes/μL in the peripheral blood [78]. CLL should be distinguished from prolymphocytic leukemia, a morphologic distinction based on the presence of prolymphocytes comprising at least 55% of the blood lymphocytes [78]. More importantly, CLL should be distinguished from a new entity called "monoclonal B-lymphocytosis" (MBL). MBL is defined by the presence of clonal B cells, but <5000 B lymphocytes/μL of blood in the absence of lymphadenopathy or organomegaly [122]. MBL is considered analogous to monoclonal gammopathy of undetermined significance (MGUS) and is believed to progress to frank CLL at a rate of 1–2% per year [123].

Subclassification based on *IgVH* mutation status

Although CLL is a chronic disease, most patients die from other causes. However, in some patients, CLL may progress relatively rapidly and prove lethal within 4–5 years. Patients with CLL expressing unmutated (<3% mutation rate) *IgVH* show aggressive disease and should be distinguished from those expressing a mutated *IgVH* gene [124–126]. All patients with CLL should be tested for *IgVH* mutation for subclassification [127].

Subclassification based on cytogenetic abnormalities

Cytogenetic abnormalities are helpful for evaluating prognosis in patients with CLL, and FISH testing for 13q14, 11q22, 6q21, and 17p13 deletion and trisomy 12 is considered standard of care. However, given the prognostic importance of *IgVH* mutation status, only 17p13 and 11q22 are independent prognostic factors, and these two abnormalities should be evaluated to stratify patients. Conventional cytogenetic studies rarely add additional information to that obtained with FISH [128].

Deletion of 13q14 leads to abnormalities in micro-RNAs (miRNAs) [129], which repress the translation and degrade the transcription of a variety of genes. Both miR-15a and miR-16-1 are deleted with 13q14. Data show that these two genes act as tumor suppressors by downregulating the translation of AU-rich elements found in oncogenes such as *MCL1*, *BCL2*, *ETS1*, and *JUN*, which are involved in apoptosis and cell cycle regulation [130]. While evaluating the expression of these miRNAs is logical, testing for the 13q14 deletion using the FISH approach remains the gold standard at this time.

Minimal residual disease

Multiple reports have indicated that evaluating minimal residual disease (MRD) in patients with CLL is clinically useful for predicting relapse and progression [131–136]. Flow cytometry remains a reliable means for detecting MRD in CLL, with a sensitivity between 0.01% and 0.1%. However, using a PCR-based assay (allele specific or ligation specific) for the detection of immunoglobulin (CDR3) rearrangement is also a very reliable approach, with 0.01–0.001% sensitivity for the detection of MRD [135,137]. However, the need for such sensitivity in managing CLL is questionable, and flow cytometry is a simple, relatively inexpensive approach.

Chronic myeloproliferative diseases (other than CML)

Because of the specific molecular abnormality in CML (ie, Philadelphia chromosome), the term chronic myeloproliferative disease or neoplasia (MPD or MPN) frequently refers to chronic myeloproliferative diseases excluding CML. MPNs include polycythemia vera (PV), primary myelofibrosis (PMF), essential thrombocythemia (ET), hypereosinophilic syndrome (HES) and chronic eosinophilic leukemia, mastocytosis, and chronic neutrophilic leukemia (CNL). The various MPNs exhibit significant similarity at the clinical, morphologic, and molecular levels. CNL remains a distinct entity with an aggressive course, but without a specific defined molecular abnormality. However, diagnosis is relatively straightforward based on morphology and clinical presentation. PV, ET, and PMF show significant overlap, and most affected patients develop marrow fibrosis.

Subclassification according to *JAK2* mutation status

JAK2 mutations in exons 12, 13, 14, and 15 are the most common mutations in this group of diseases. All reported mutations are in the pseudokinase domain and are expected to relieve the autoinhibitory function of this domain on *JAK2* kinase activity. When screening for *JAK2* mutations, the use of plasma rather than cells for RNA extraction may allow more timely detection of disease. Early signs of disease, in which platelets are the main neoplastic cell type, can be missed if cells rather than plasma are used for testing [2,138].

Among *JAK2* mutations, V617F represents the most common abnormality and is present in 80–90% of patients with PV, 35–45% of those with ET, and 35–45% of those with PMF. *JAK2* mutations other than V617F are rare, only accounting for about 1–2% of *JAK2* mutations. Most other *JAK2*-reported mutations are in exon 12 [139], but rare mutations in exons 13, 14, and 15 have also been described [140].

MPL mutations

It has been estimated that 5% of patients with PV, ET, or PMF without *JAK2* mutation may have mutation in the thrombopoietin receptor MPL (myeloproliferative leukemia virus oncogene) [141,142]. The W515L/K mutation has been reported in sporadic cases [142], and the S505N [143] as well as P106L [144] have been reported in familial forms of MPD. These mutations typically occur in the absence of *JAK2* V617F mutation [145,146] and should be tested for after *JAK2* mutations have been ruled out in patients whose clinical presentation suggests MPD. However, in some cases, recent studies have demonstrated concurrence of *MPL* and *JAK2* V617F mutations [147,148]. Our data suggest that *MPL* mutations are twice as common as *JAK2* exon 12 and 13 mutations in patients with *JAK2* V617F$^-$ non-CML MPNs.

FGFR1 abnormalities

Translocations affecting the *FGFR1* gene are associated with 8p11 myeloproliferative syndrome, a specific disease that usually presents with eosinophilia and myeloproliferative features but may also progress to AML or ALL. Multiple *FGFR1* fusion partners have been reported, and the most common translocations are t(8;13)(p11;q12), t(8;9)(p11;q33), t(6;8)(q27;p11), t(8;22)(p11;q11), t(8;17)(p11;q23), t(8;19)(p11;q13), and t(7;8)(q34;p11) [78]. Frequently, these abnormalities are detected by routine karyotype analysis.

FIP1L1–PDGFRA fusion

Patients with eosinophilia and increased mast cells have a specific class of MPN that is frequently associated with the *FIP1L1–PDGFRA* (FIP1-like-1 platelet-derived growth-factor receptor α) fusion, formed by a cryptic deletion at 4q12. These patients should be distinguished because they respond to imatinib therapy [149]. However, some of the patients with this abnormality may also present with AML and ALL [150]. This abnormality cannot be seen by routine karyotyping, but can be detected by FISH as well as RT/PCR-based molecular testing.

PDGFRB rearrangement

The *PDGFRB* (platelet-derived growth factor receptor β) gene is located on 5q31~33 and can be translocated and fused with one of multiple genes. The most common translocation is t(5;12)(q32;p12), resulting in fusion with the *ETV6* gene [151–153]. Some patients with MPN and eosinophilia may present with this abnormality, but *PDGFRB* rearrangement can also be seen in acute leukemia, myelodysplasia, and CMML. Given the possibility of multiple fusion partners when the *PDGFRB* is involved, break-apart FISH testing is recommended when *PDGFRB* rearrangement is suspected and conventional karyotyping is negative.

References

1 Yeh CH, Tseng R, Albitar M. Plasma-based detection of clonality in lymphoid malignancies. *Eur J Haematol* 2009. [Epub ahead of print.]

2 Ma W, Kantarjian H, Zhang X, *et al*. Higher detection rate of *JAK2* mutation using plasma. *Blood* 2008;111:3906–7.

3 Giles FJ, Albitar M. Plasma-based testing as a new paradigm for clinical testing in hematologic diseases. *Expert Rev Mol Diagn* 2007;7:615–23.

4 Ma W, Tseng R, Gorre M, *et al*. Plasma RNA as an alternative to cells for monitoring molecular response in patients with chronic myeloid leukemia. *Haematologica* 2007;92:170–5.

5 Ma W, Kantarjian H, Jilani I, *et al.* Heterogeneity in detecting Abl kinase mutations and better sensitivity using circulating plasma RNA. *Leukemia* 2006;20:1989–91.

6 Ma W, Jilani I, Gorre M, *et al.* Plasma as a source of mRNA for determining *IgV(H)* mutation status in patients with chronic lymphocytic leukaemia. *Br J Haematol* 2006;133:690–2.

7 Ma W, Kantarjian H, O'Brien S, *et al.* Enzymatic activity of circulating proteasomes correlates with clinical behavior in patients with chronic lymphocytic leukemia. *Cancer* 2008; 112:1306–12.

8 Jilani I, Wei C, Bekele BN, *et al.* Soluble syndecan-1 (sCD138) as a prognostic factor independent of mutation status in patients with chronic lymphocytic leukemia. *Int J Lab Hematol* 2009;31:97–105.

9 Albitar M, Johnson M, Do KA, *et al.* Levels of soluble HLA-I and beta2M in patients with acute myeloid leukemia and advanced myelodysplastic syndrome: association with clinical behavior and outcome of induction therapy. *Leukemia* 2007;21:480–8.

10 Rogers A, Joe Y, Manshouri T, *et al.* Relative increase in leukemia-specific DNA in peripheral blood plasma from patients with acute myeloid leukemia and myelodysplasia. *Blood* 2004;103:2799–801.

11 Ahmed M, Giles F, Joe Y, *et al.* Use of plasma DNA in detection of loss of heterozygosity in patients with multiple myeloma. *Eur J Haematol* 2003;71:174–8.

12 Jilani I, Kantarjian H, Faraji H, *et al.* An immunological method for the detection of BCR-ABL fusion protein and monitoring its activation. *Leuk Res* 2008;32:936–43.

13 Ronaghi M, Nygren M, Lundeberg J, Nyrén P. Analyses of secondary structures in DNA by pyrosequencing. *Anal Biochem* 1999;267:65–71.

14 Garcia-Manero G, Yang H, Kuang SQ, O'Brien S, Thomas D, Kantarjian H. Epigenetics of acute lymphocytic leukemia. *Semin Hematol* 2009;46:24–32.

15 Yang H, Kadia T, Xiao L, *et al.* Residual DNA methylation at remission is prognostic in adult Philadelphia chromosome-negative acute lymphocytic leukemia. *Blood* 2009;113:1892–8.

16 Grövdal M, Khan R, Aggerholm A, *et al.* Negative effect of DNA hypermethylation on the outcome of intensive chemotherapy in older patients with high-risk myelodysplastic syndromes and acute myeloid leukemia following myelodysplastic syndrome. *Clin Cancer Res* 2007;13:7107–12.

17 Strathdee G, Holyoake TL, Sim A, *et al.* Inactivation of *HOXA* genes by hypermethylation in myeloid and lymphoid malignancy is frequent and associated with poor prognosis. *Clin Cancer Res* 2007;13:5048–55.

18 Marcucci G, Mrózek K, Ruppert AS, *et al.* Prognostic factors and outcome of core binding factor acute myeloid leukemia patients with t(8;21) differ from those of patients with inv(16): a Cancer and Leukemia Group B study. *J Clin Oncol* 2005; 23:5705–17.

19 Byrd JC, Mrózek K, Dodge RK, *et al.* Cancer and Leukemia Group B (CALGB 8461). Pretreatment cytogenetic abnormalities are predictive of induction success, cumulative incidence of relapse, and overall survival in adult patients with de novo acute myeloid leukemia: results from Cancer and leukemia Group B (CALGB 8461). *Blood* 2002;100:4325–4336.

20 Grimwade D, Walker H, Harrison G, *et al.* Medical Research Council Adult Leukemia Working Party. The predictive value of hierarchical cytogenetic classification in older adults with acute myeloid leukemia (AML): analysis of 1065 patients entered into the United Kingdom Medical Research Council AML11 trial. *Blood* 2001;98:1312–20.

21 Nucifora G, Begy CR, Kobayashi H, *et al.* Consistent intergenic splicing and production of multiple transcripts between AML1 at 21q22 and unrelated genes at 3q26 in (3;21)(q26;q22) translocations. *Proc Natl Acad Sci U S A* 1994;91:4004–8.

22 Zent C, Kim N, Hiebert S, *et al.* Rearrangement of the *AML1/CBFA2* gene in myeloid leukemia with the 3;21 translocation: expression of co-existing multiple chimeric genes with similar functions as transcriptional repressors, but with opposite tumorigenic properties. *Curr Top Microbiol Immunol* 1996;211: 243–52.

23 Michaud J, Wu F, Osato M, *et al.* *In vitro* analyses of known and novel *RUNX1/AML1* mutations in dominant familial platelet disorder with predisposition to acute myelogenous leukemia: implications for mechanisms of pathogenesis. *Blood* 2002;99:1364–72.

24 Boissel N, Leroy H, Brethon B, *et al.* Acute Leukemia French Association (ALFA); Leucémies Aiguës Myéloblastiques de l'Enfant (LAME) Cooperative Groups. Incidence and prognostic impact of *c-Kit*, *FLT3*, and *RAS* gene mutations in core binding factor acute myeloid leukemia (CBF-AML). *Leukemia* 2006;20:965–70.

25 Rowley JD, Golomb HM, Dougherty C. 15/17 translocation, a consistent chromosomal change in acute promyelocytic leukaemia. *Lancet* 1977;1:549–50.

26 Larson RA, Kondo K, Vardiman JW, Butler AE, Golomb HM, Rowley JD. Evidence for a 15;17 translocation in every patient with acute promyelocytic leukemia. *Am J Med* 1984;76: 827–41.

27 Grimwade D, Biondi A, Mozziconacci M-J, *et al.* Characterization of acute promyelocytic leukemia cases lacking the classic t(15;17): results of the European Working Party. *Blood* 2000; 96:1297–308.

28 Redner RL. Variations on a theme: the alternate translocations in APL. *Leukemia* 2002;16:1927–32.

29 Chen SJ, Zelent A, Tong JH, *et al.* Rearrangements of the retinoic acid receptor alpha and promyelocytic zinc finger genes resulting from t(11;17)(q23;q21) in a patient with acute promyelocytic leukaemia. *J Clin Invest* 1993;91:2260–7.

30 Redner RL, Rush EA, Faas S, Rudert WA, Corey SJ. The t(5;17) variant of acute promyelocytic leukemia expresses a nucleophosmin-retinoic acid receptor fusion. *Blood* 1996;87: 882–6.

31 Wells RA, Catzavelos C, Kamel-Reid S. Fusion of retinoic acid receptor α to NuMA, the nuclear mitotic apparatus protein, by a variant translocation in acute promyelocytic leukaemia. *Nat Genet* 1997;17:109–13.

32 Arnould C, Philippe C, Bourdon V, Grégoire MJ, Berger R, Jonveaux P. The signal transducer and activator of transcription *STAT5b* gene is a new partner of retinoic acid receptor α in acute promyelocytic-like leukemia. *Hum Mol Genet* 1999; 8:1741–9.

33 Catalano A, Dawson MA, Somana K, *et al.* The *PRKAR1A* gene is fused to *RARA* in a new variant acute promyelocytic leukemia. *Blood* 2007;110:4073–6.

34 Guidez F, Ivins S, Zhu J, Soderstrom M, Waxman S, Zelent A. Reduced retinoic acid-sensitivities of nuclear receptor

corepressor binding to PML- and PLZF-RAR alpha underlie molecular pathogenesis and treatment of acute promyelocytic leukemia. *Blood* 1998;91:2634–42.

35 Gale RE, Hills R, Pizzey AR, *et al.* NCRI Adult Leukaemia Working Party. Relationship between *FLT3* mutation status, biologic characteristics, and response to targeted therapy in acute promyelocytic leukemia. *Blood* 2005;106:2768–76.

36 Caligiuri MA, Strout MP, Lawrence D, *et al.* Rearrangement of ALL1 (*MLL*) in acute myeloid leukemia with normal cytogenetics. *Cancer Res* 1998;58:55–9.

37 Döhner K, Tobis K, Ulrich R, *et al.* Prognostic significance of partial tandem duplications of the *MLL* gene in adult patients 16 to 60 years old with acute myeloid leukemia and normal cytogenetics: a study of the Acute Myeloid Leukemia Study Group Ulm. *J Clin Oncol* 2002;20:3254–61.

38 Shiah HS, Kuo YY, Tang JL, *et al.* Clinical and biological implications of partial tandem duplication of the *MLL* gene in acute myeloid leukemia without chromosomal abnormalities at 11q23. *Leukemia* 2002;16:196–202.

39 Muñoz L, Nomdedéu JF, Villamor N, *et al.* Spanish CETLAM Group. Acute myeloid leukemia with *MLL* rearrangements: clinicobiological features, prognostic impact and value of flow cytometry in the detection of residual leukemic cells. *Leukemia* 2003;17:76–82.

40 Wolman SR, Gundacker H, Appelbaum FR, Slovak ML. Impact of trisomy 8 (+8) on clinical presentation, treatment response, and survival in acute myeloid leukemia: a Southwest Oncology Group study. *Blood* 2002;100:29–35.

41 Schlenk RF, Döhner K, Krauter J, *et al.* German-Austrian Acute Myeloid Leukemia Study Group. Mutations and treatment outcome in cytogenetically normal acute myeloid leukemia. *N Engl J Med* 2008;358:1909–18.

42 Mrózek K, Marcucci G, Paschka P, Whitman SP, Bloomfield CD. Clinical relevance of mutations and gene-expression changes in adult acute myeloid leukemia with normal cytogenetics: are we ready for a prognostically prioritized molecular classification? *Blood* 2007;109:431–48.

43 Döhner K, Schlenk RF, Habdank M, *et al.* Mutant nucleophosmin (*NPM1*) predicts favorable prognosis in younger adults with acute myeloid leukemia and normal cytogenetics: interaction with other gene mutations. *Blood* 2005;106:3740–6.

44 Schnittger S, Schoch C, Kern W, *et al.* Nucleophosmin gene mutations are predictors of favorable prognosis in acute myelogenous leukemia with a normal karyotype. *Blood* 2005;106: 3733–9.

45 Verhaak RG, Goudswaard CS, van Putten W, *et al.* Mutations in nucleophosmin (*NPM1*) in acute myeloid leukemia (AML): association with other gene abnormalities and previously established gene expression signatures and their favorable prognostic significance. *Blood* 2005;106:3747–54.

46 Marcucci G, Maharry K, Radmacher MD, *et al.* Prognostic significance of, and gene and microRNA expression signatures associated with, *CEBPA* mutations in cytogenetically normal acute myeloid leukemia with high-risk molecular features: a Cancer and Leukemia Group B Study. *J Clin Oncol* 2008;26:5078–87, erratum in *J Clin Oncol* 2008;26:6021.

47 Wouters BJ, Löwenberg B, Erpelinck-Verschueren CA, van Putten WL, Valk PJ, Delwel R. Double *CEBPA* mutations, but not single *CEBPA* mutations, define a subgroup of acute myeloid leukemia with a distinctive gene expression profile that is uniquely associated with a favorable outcome. *Blood* 2009;113:3088–91.

48 Paschka P, Marcucci G, Ruppert AS, *et al.* Wilms' tumor 1 gene mutations independently predict poor outcome in adults with cytogenetically normal acute myeloid leukemia: a cancer and leukemia group B study. *J Clin Oncol* 2008;26:4595–602.

49 Virappane P, Gale R, Hills R, *et al.* Mutation of the Wilms' tumor 1 gene is a poor prognostic factor associated with chemotherapy resistance in normal karyotype acute myeloid leukemia: the United Kingdom Medical Research Council Adult Leukaemia Working Party. *J Clin Oncol* 2008;26:5429–35.

50 Gaidzik VI, Schlenk RF, Moschny S, *et al.* Prognostic impact of *WT1* mutations in cytogenetically normal acute myeloid leukemia (AML): a study of the German-Austrian AML Study Group (AMLSG). *Blood* 2009. [Epub ahead of print.]

51 Baldus CD, Tanner SM, Ruppert AS, *et al.* BAALC expression predicts clinical outcome of de novo acute myeloid leukemia patients with normal cytogenetics: a Cancer and leukemia Group B Study. *Blood* 2003;102:1613–18.

52 Marcucci G, Baldus CD, Ruppert AS, *et al.* Overexpression of the ETS-related gene, *ERG*, predicts a worse outcome in acute myeloid leukemia with normal karyotype: a Cancer and Leukemia Group B study. *J Clin Oncol* 2005;23:9234–42.

53 Suela J, Alvarez S, Cifuentes F, *et al.* DNA profiling analysis of 100 consecutive de novo acute myeloid leukemia cases reveals patterns of genomic instability that affect all cytogenetic risk groups. *Leukemia* 2007;21:1224–31.

54 Bullinger L, Döhner K, Bair E, *et al.* Use of gene-expression profiling to identify prognostic subclasses in adult acute myeloid leukemia. *N Engl J Med* 2004;350:1605–16.

55 Valk PJ, Verhaak RG, Beijen MA, *et al.* Prognostically useful gene-expression profiles in acute myeloid leukemia. *N Engl J Med* 2004;350:1617–28.

56 Radmacher MD, Marcucci G, Ruppert AS, *et al.* Cancer and Leukemia Group B. Independent confirmation of a prognostic gene-expression signature in adult acute myeloid leukemia with a normal karyotype: a Cancer and Leukemia Group B study. *Blood* 2006;108:1677–83.

57 Baldus CD, Bullinger L. Gene expression with prognostic implications in cytogenetically normal acute myeloid leukemia. *Semin Oncol* 2008;35:356–64.

58 Balkhi MY, Trivedi AK, Geletu M, *et al.* Proteomics of acute myeloid leukaemia: Cytogenetic risk groups differ specifically in their proteome, interactome and post-translational protein modifications. *Oncogene* 2006;25:7041–58.

59 Ross ME, Mahfouz R, Onciu M, *et al.* Gene expression profiling of pediatric acute myelogenous leukemia. *Blood* 2004; 104:3679–87.

60 Jaff N, Chelghoum Y, Elhamri M, Tigaud I, Michallet M, Thomas X. Trisomy 8 as sole anomaly or with other clonal aberrations in acute myeloid leukemia: impact on clinical presentation and outcome. *Leuk Res* 2007;31:67–73.

61 Yeoh EJ, Ross ME, Shurtleff SA, *et al.* Classification, subtype discovery, and prediction of outcome in pediatric acute lymphoblastic leukemia by gene expression profiling. *Cancer Cell* 2002;1:133–43.

62 Kohlmann A, Schoch C, Schnittger S, *et al.* Pediatric acute lymphoblastic leukemia (ALL) gene expression signatures classify an independent cohort of adult ALL patients. *Leukemia* 2004;18:63–71.

63 Bhojwani D, Kang H, Menezes RX, *et al*; Children's Oncology Group Study; Dutch Childhood Oncology Group; German Cooperative Study Group for Childhood Acute Lymphoblastic Leukemia. Gene expression signatures predictive of early response and outcome in high-risk childhood acute lymphoblastic leukemia: A Children's Oncology Group Study [corrected]. *J Clin Oncol* 2008;26:4376–84, erratum in *J Clin Oncol* 2008;26:5142.

64 Den Boer ML, van Slegtenhorst M, De Menezes RX, *et al.* A subtype of childhood acute lymphoblastic leukaemia with poor treatment outcome: a genome-wide classification study. *Lancet Oncol* 2009;10:125–34.

65 Willenbrock H, Juncker AS, Schmiegelow K, Knudsen S, Ryder LP. Prediction of immunophenotype, treatment response, and relapse in childhood acute lymphoblastic leukemia using DNA microarrays. *Leukemia* 2004;18:1270–7.

66 Hegedus CM, Gunn L, Skibola CF, *et al.* Proteomic analysis of childhood leukemia. *Leukemia* 2005;19:1713–18.

67 Cario G, Stanulla M, Fine BM, *et al.* Distinct gene expression profiles determine molecular treatment response in childhood acute lymphoblastic leukemia. *Blood* 2005;105:821–6.

68 Flotho C, Coustan-Smith E, Pei D, *et al.* A set of genes that regulate cell proliferation predicts treatment outcome in childhood acute lymphoblastic leukemia. *Blood* 2007;110:1271–7.

69 Andersson A, Ritz C, Lindgren D, *et al.* Microarray-based classification of a consecutive series of 121 childhood acute leukemias: prediction of leukemic and genetic subtype as well as of minimal residual disease status. *Leukemia* 2007;21: 1198–203.

70 Albitar M, Potts SJ, Giles FJ, *et al.* Proteomic-based prediction of clinical behavior in adult acute lymphoblastic leukemia. *Cancer* 2006;106:1587–94.

71 Shi L, Zhang J, Wu P, *et al.* Discovery and identification of potential biomarkers of pediatric acute lymphoblastic leukemia. *Proteome Sci* 2009;7:7.

72 Jones CD, Yeung C, Zehnder JL. Comprehensive validation of a real-time quantitative bcr-abl assay for clinical laboratory use. *Am J Clin Pathol* 2003;120:42–8.

73 Mullighan CG, Su X, Zhang J, *et al.* Children's Oncology Group. Deletion of IKZF1 and prognosis in acute lymphoblastic leukemia. *N Engl J Med* 2009;360:470–80.

74 Thomas DA, Faderl S, O'Brien S, *et al.* Chemoimmunotherapy with hyper-CVAD plus rituximab for the treatment of adult Burkitt and Burkitt-type lymphoma or acute lymphoblastic leukemia. *Cancer* 2006;106:1569–80.

75 Hogan TF, Koss W, Murgo AJ, Amato RS, Fontana JA, VanScoy FL. Acute lymphoblastic leukemia with chromosomal 5;14 translocation and hypereosinophilia: case report and literature review. *J Clin Oncol* 1987;5:382–90.

76 Tono-oka T, Sato Y, Matsumoto T, *et al.* Hypereosinophilic syndrome in acute lymphoblastic leukemia with a chromosome translocation [t(5q;14q)]. *Med Pediatr Oncol* 1984;12: 33–7.

77 Grimaldi JC, Meeker TC. The t(5;14) chromosomal translocation in a case of acute lymphocytic leukemia joins the interleukin-3 gene to the immunoglobulin heavy chain gene. *Blood* 1989;73:2081–5.

78 Swerdlow SH, Campo E, Harris NL, *et al* (eds). *WHO Classification of Tumours of Haematopoietic and Lymphoid Tissues.* IARC Press: Lyon;2008:109–38.

79 Harris MB, Shuster JJ, Carroll A, *et al.* Trisomy of leukemic cell chromosomes 4 and 10 identifies children with B-progenitor cell acute lymphoblastic leukemia with a very low risk of treatment failure: a Pediatric Oncology Group study. *Blood* 1992;79:3316–24.

80 Sharathkumar A, DeCamillo D, Bhambhani K, *et al.* Children with hyperdiploid but not triple trisomy (+4,+10,+17) acute lymphoblastic leukemia have an increased incidence of extramedullary relapse on current therapies: a single institution experience. *Am J Hematol* 2008;83:34–40.

81 Sutcliffe MJ, Shuster JJ, Sather HN, *et al.* High concordance from independent studies by the Children's Cancer Group (CCG) and Pediatric Oncology Group (POG) associating favorable prognosis with combined trisomies 4, 10, and 17 in children with NCI Standard-Risk B-precursor Acute Lymphoblastic leukemia: a Children's Oncology Group (COG) initiative. *Leukemia* 2005;19:734–40.

82 Argiropoulos B, Humphries RK. *HOX* genes in hematopoiesis and leukemogenesis. *Oncogene* 2007;26:6766–76.

83 Chiba S. Homeobox genes in normal hematopoiesis and leukemogenesis. *Int J Hematol* 1998;68:343–53.

84 Owens BM, Hawley RG. *HOX* and non-*HOX* homeobox genes in leukemic hematopoiesis. *Stem Cells* 2002;20:364–79.

85 Hunger SP, Galili N, Carroll AJ, Crist WM, Link MP, Cleary ML. The t(1;19)(q23;p13) results in consistent fusion of E2A and PBX1 coding sequences in acute lymphoblastic leukemias. *Blood* 1991;77:687–93.

86 Hatano M, Roberts CW, Minden M, Crist WM, Korsmeyer SJ. Deregulation of a homeobox gene, *HOX11*, by the t(10;14) in T cell leukemia. *Science* 1991;253:79–82.

87 Kennedy MA, Gonzalez-Sarmiento R, Kees UR, *et al. HOX11*, a homeobox-containing T-cell oncogene on human chromosome 10q24. *Proc Natl Acad Sci U S A* 1991;88:8900–4.

88 Borowitz MJ, Hunger SP, Carroll AJ, *et al.* Predictability of the t(1;19)(q23;p13) from surface antigen phenotype: implications for screening cases of childhood acute lymphoblastic leukemia for molecular analysis: a Pediatric Oncology Group study. *Blood* 1993;82:1086–91.

89 Foa R, Vitale A, Mancini M, *et al.* E2A-PBX1 fusion in adult acute lymphoblastic leukaemia: biological and clinical features. *Br J Haematol* 2003;120:484–7.

90 Privitera E, Kamps MP, Hayashi Y, *et al.* Different molecular consequences of the 1;19 chromosomal translocation in childhood B-cell precursor acute lymphoblastic leukemia. *Blood* 1992;79:1781–8.

91 Weng AP, Ferrando AA, Lee W, *et al.* Activating mutations of *NOTCH1* in human T cell acute lymphoblastic leukemia. *Science* 2004;306:269–71.

92 Mansour MR, Linch DC, Foroni L, Goldstone AH, Gale RE. High incidence of *NOTCH-1* mutations in adult patients with T-cell acute lymphoblastic leukemia. *Leukemia* 2006;20:537–9.

93 Joshi I, Minter LM, Telfer J, *et al.* Notch signaling mediates G1/S cell-cycle progression in T cells via cyclin D3 and its dependent kinases. *Blood* 2009;113:1689–98.

94 Breit S, Stanulla M, Flohr T, *et al.* Activating *NOTCH1* mutations predict favorable early treatment response and long-term outcome in childhood precursor T-cell lymphoblastic leukemia. *Blood* 2006;108:1151–7.

95 van Grotel M, Meijerink JP, van Wering ER, *et al.* Prognostic significance of molecular-cytogenetic abnormalities in

pediatric T-ALL is not explained by immunophenotypic differences. *Leukemia* 2008;22:124–31.
96 Park MJ, Taki T, Oda M, *et al.* *FBXW7* and *NOTCH1* mutations in childhood T cell acute lymphoblastic leukaemia and T cell non-Hodgkin lymphoma. *Br J Haematol* 2009. [Epub ahead of print]
97 Kathrein KL, Chari S, Winandy S. Ikaros directly represses the notch target gene *HES1* in a leukemia T cell line: implications for CD4 regulation. *J Biol Chem* 2008;283:10476–84.
98 Weinshilboum RM, Sladek SL. Mercaptopurine pharmacogenetics: monogenic inheritance of erythrocyte thiopurine methyltransferase activity. *Am J Hum Genet* 1980;32:651–62.
99 McLeod HL, Siva C. The thiopurine S-methyltransferase gene locus–implications for clinical pharmacogenomics. *Pharmacogenomics* 2002;3:89–98.
100 Relling MV, Rubnitz JE, Rivera GK, *et al.* High incidence of secondary brain tumours after radiotherapy and antimetabolites. *Lancet* 1999;354:34–9.
101 McLeod HL, Coulthard S, Thomas AE, *et al.* Analysis of thiopurine methyltransferase variant alleles in childhood acute lymphoblastic leukaemia. *Br J Haematol* 1999;105:696–700.
102 Evans WE, Hon YY, Bomgaars L, *et al.* Preponderance of thiopurine S-methyltransferase deficiency and heterozygosity among patients intolerant to mercaptopurine or azathioprine. *J Clin Oncol.* 2001;19:2293–301.
103 Andreasson P, Johansson B, Carlsson M, *et al.* BCR/ABL-negative chronic myeloid *Leukemia* with ETV6/ABL fusion. *Genes Chromosomes Cancer* 1997;20:299–304.
104 Griesinger F, Hennig H, Hillmer F, *et al.* A *BCR-JAK2* fusion gene as the result of a t(9;22)(p24;q11.2) translocation in a patient with a clinically typical chronic myeloid leukemia. *Genes Chromosomes Cancer* 2005;44:329–33.
105 Cirmena G, Aliano S, Fugazza G, *et al.* A *BCR-JAK2* fusion gene as the result of a t(9;22)(p24;q11) in a patient with acute myeloid leukemia. *Cancer Genet Cytogenet* 2008;183:105–8.
106 Lane SW, Fairbairn DJ, McCarthy C, Nandini A, Perry-Keene J, Kennedy GA. Leukaemia cutis in atypical chronic myeloid leukaemia with a t(9;22) (p24;q11.2) leading to *BCR-JAK2* fusion. *Br J Haematol* 2008;142:503.
107 Reiter A, Walz C, Watmore A, *et al.* The t(8;9)(p22;p24) is a recurrent abnormality in chronic and acute leukemia that fuses *PCM1* to *JAK2*. *Cancer Res* 2005;65:2662–7.
108 Bousquet M, Quelen C, De Mas V, *et al.* The t(8;9)(p22;p24) translocation in atypical chronic myeloid leukaemia yields a new *PCM1-JAK2* fusion gene. *Oncogene* 2005;24:7248–52.
109 Apperley JF. Part I: mechanisms of resistance to imatinib in chronic myeloid leukaemia. *Lancet Oncol* 2007;8:1018–29.
110 Corbin AS, Buchdunger E, Pascal F, Druker BJ. Analysis of the structural basis of specificity of inhibition of the Abl kinase by STI571. *J Biol Chem* 2002;277:32214–19.
111 Hochhaus A, Kreil S, Corbin AS, *et al.* Molecular and chromosomal mechanisms of resistance to imatinib (STI571) therapy. *Leukemia* 2002;16:2190–6.
112 Branford S, Rudzki Z, Walsh S, *et al.* Detection of *BCR-ABL* mutations in patients with CML treated with imatinib is virtually always accompanied by clinical resistance, and mutations in the ATP phosphate-binding loop (P-loop) are associated with a poor prognosis. *Blood* 2003;102:276–83.
113 Talpaz M, Shah NP, Kantarjian H, *et al.* Dasatinib in imatinib-resistant Philadelphia chromosome-positive leukemias. *N Engl J Med* 2006;354:2531–41.
114 Jabbour E, Kantarjian H, Jones D, *et al.* Frequency and clinical significance of *BCR-ABL* mutations in patients with chronic myeloid leukemia treated with imatinib mesylate. *Leukemia* 2006;20:1767–73.
115 Soverini S, Colarossi S, Gnani A, *et al.* GIMEMA Working Party on Chronic Myeloid Leukemia. Contribution of ABL kinase domain mutations to imatinib resistance in different subsets of Philadelphia-positive patients: by the GIMEMA Working Party on Chronic Myeloid Leukemia. *Clin Cancer Res* 2006;12:7374–9.
116 Shah NP, Nicoll JM, Nagar B, *et al.* Multiple Bcr-Abl kinase domain mutations confer polyclonal resistance to the tyrosine kinase inhibitor imatinib (STI571) in chronic phase and blast crisis chronic myeloid leukemia. *Cancer Cell* 2002;2:117–25.
117 Gruber FX, Lamark T, Anonli A, *et al.* Selecting and deselecting imatinib-resistant clones: observations made by longitudinal, quantitative monitoring of mutated *BCR-ABL*. *Leukemia* 2005;19:2159–65.
118 O'Hare T, Walters DK, Stoffregen EP, *et al.* Combined Abl inhibitor therapy for minimizing drug resistance in chronic myeloid leukemia: Src/Abl inhibitors are compatible with imatinib. *Clin Cancer Res.* 2005;11:6987–93.
119 Weisberg E, Manley PW, Cowan-Jacob SW, Hochhaus A, Griffin JD. Second generation inhibitors of BCR-ABL for the treatment of imatinib-resistant chronic myeloid leukaemia. *Nat Rev Cancer* 2007;7:345–56.
120 Martinelli G, Iacobucci I, Soverini S, *et al.* Monitoring minimal residual disease and controlling drug resistance in chronic myeloid leukaemia patients in treatment with imatinib as a guide to clinical management. *Hematol Oncol* 2006;24:196–204.
121 Lee TS, Ma W, Zhang X, *et al.* BCR-ABL alternative splicing as a common mechanism for imatinib resistance: evidence from molecular dynamics simulations. *Mol Cancer Ther* 2008;7:3834–41.
122 Marti GE, Rawstron AC, Ghia P, *et al.* The International Familial CLL Consortium. Diagnostic criteria for monoclonal B-cell lymphocytosis. *Br J Haematol* 2005;130:325–32.
123 Rawstron AC, Bennett FL, O'Connor SJ, *et al.* Monoclonal B-cell lymphocytosis and chronic lymphocytic leukemia. *N Engl J Med* 2008;359:575–83.
124 Damle RN, Wasil T, Fais F, *et al.* *Ig V* gene mutation status and CD38 expression as novel prognostic indicators in chronic lymphocytic leukemia. *Blood* 1999;94:1840–7.
125 Hamblin TJ, Davis Z, Gardiner A, Oscier DG, Stevenson FK. Unmutated *Ig V(H)* genes are associated with a more aggressive form of chronic lymphocytic leukemia. *Blood* 1999;94:1848–54.
126 Kharfan-Dabaja MA, Chavez JC, Khorfan KA, Pinilla-Ibarz J. Clinical and therapeutic implications of the mutational status of IgVH in patients with chronic lymphocytic leukemia. *Cancer* 2008;113:897–906.
127 Lin KI, Tam CS, Keating MJ, *et al.* Relevance of the immunoglobulin VH somatic mutation status in patients with chronic lymphocytic leukemia treated with fludarabine, cyclophosphamide, and rituximab (FCR) or related chemoimmunotherapy regimens. *Blood* 2008. [Epub ahead of print.]

128 Dohner H, Stilgenbauer S, Benner A, *et al.* Genomic aberrations and survival in chronic lymphocytic leukemia. *N Engl J Med* 2000;343:1910–16.

129 Calin GA, Dumitru CD, Shimizu M, *et al.* Frequent deletions and down-regulation of micro- RNA genes miR15 and miR16 at 13q14 in chronic lymphocytic leukemia. *Proc Natl Acad Sci U S A* 2002;99:15524–9.

130 Calin GA, Cimmino A, Fabbri M, *et al.* MiR-15a and miR-16-1 cluster functions in human leukemia. *Proc Natl Acad Sci U S A* 2008;105:5166–71.

131 Cabezudo E, Matutes E, Ramrattan M, Morilla R, Catovsky D. Analysis of residual disease in chronic lymphocytic leukemia by flow cytometry. *Leukemia* 1997;11:1909–14.

132 Provan D, Bartlett-Pandite L, Zwicky C, *et al.* Eradication of polymerase chain reaction detectable chronic lymphocytic leukemia cells is associated with improved outcome after bone marrow transplantation. *Blood* 1996;88:2228–35.

133 Rawstron AC, Kennedy B, Evans PA, *et al.* Quantitation of minimal disease levels in chronic lymphocytic leukemia using a sensitive flow cytometric assay improves the prediction of outcome and can be used to optimize therapy. *Blood* 2001; 98:29–35.

134 Moreton P, Kennedy B, Lucas G, *et al.* Eradication of minimal residual disease in B-cell chronic lymphocytic leukemia after alemtuzumab therapy is associated with prolonged survival. *J Clin Oncol* 2005;23:2971–9.

135 Moreno C, Villamor N, Colomer D, *et al.* Clinical significance of minimal residual disease, as assessed by different techniques, after stem cell transplantation for chronic lymphocytic leukemia. *Blood* 2006;107:4563–9.

136 Rawstron AC, Villamor N, Ritgen M, *et al.* International standardized approach for flow cytometric residual disease monitoring in chronic lymphocytic leukaemia. *Leukemia* 2007; 21:956–64.

137 Bottcher S, Ritgen M, Pott C, *et al.* Comparative analysis of minimal residual disease detection using four-color flow cytometry, consensus IgH-PCR, and quantitative IgH PCR in CLL after allogeneic and autologous stem cell transplantation. *Leukemia* 2004;18:1637–45.

138 Ma W, Kantarjian H, Verstovsek S, *et al.* Hemizygous/homozygous and heterozygous *JAK2 m*utation detected in plasma of patients with myeloproliferative diseases: correlation with clinical behaviour. *Br J Haematol* 2006;134:341–3.

139 Pardanani A, Lasho TL, Finke C, *et al.* Prevalence and clinicopathologic correlates of *JAK2* exon 12 mutations in *JAK2V617F*-negative polycythemia vera. *Leukemia* 2007;21:1960–3.

140 Ma W, Kantarjian H, Zhang X, *et al.* Mutation profile of JAK2 transcripts in patients with chronic myeloproliferative neoplasias. *J Mol Diagn* 2009;11:49–53.

141 Pancrazzi A, Guglielmelli P, Ponziani V, *et al.* A sensitive detection method for *MPLW515L* or *MPLW515K* mutation in chronic myeloproliferative disorders with locked nucleic acid-modified probes and real-time polymerase chain reaction. *J Mol Diagn* 2008;10:435–41.

142 Pikman Y, Lee BH, Mercher T, *et al. MPLW515L* is a novel somatic activating mutation in myelofibrosis with myeloid metaplasia. *PLoS Med* 2006;3:1140–51.

143 Ding J, Komatsu H, Wakita A, *et al.* Familial essential thrombocythemia associated with a dominant-positive activating mutation of the c-*MPL* gene, which encodes for the receptor for thrombopoietin. *Blood* 2004;103: 4198–200.

144 El-Harith el-HA, Roesl C, Ballmaier M, *et al.* Familial thrombocytosis caused by the novel germ-line mutation *p.Pro106Leu* in the *MPL* gene. *Br J Haematol* 2009;144:185–94.

145 Beer PA, Campbell PJ, Scott LM, *et al. MPL* mutations in myeloproliferative disorders: analysis of the PT-1 cohort. *Blood* 2008;112:141–9.

146 Schnittger S, Bacher U, Haferlach C, *et al.* Characterization of 35 new cases with four different *MPLW515* mutations and essential thrombocytosis or primary myelofibrosis. *Haematologica* 2009;94:141–4.

147 Vannucchi AM, Antonioli E, Guglielmelli P, *et al.* Characteristics and clinical correlates of *MPL 515W>L/K* mutation in essential thrombocythemia. *Blood* 2008;112:844–7.

148 Lasho TL, Pardanani A, McClure RF, *et al.* Concurrent *MPL515* and *JAK2V617F m*utations in myelofibrosis: chronology of clonal emergence and changes in mutant allele burden over time. *Br J Haematol* 2006;135:683–7.

149 Cools J, DeAngelo DJ, Gotlib J, *et al.* A tyrosine kinase created by fusion of the *PDGFRA* and *FIP1L1* genes as a therapeutic target of imatinib in idiopathic hypereosinophilic syndrome. *N Engl J Med* 2003;348:1201–14.

150 Metzgeroth G, Walz C, Score J, *et al.* Recurrent finding of the *FIP1L1-PDGFRA* fusion gene in eosinophilia-associated acute myeloid leukemia and lymphoblastic T-cell lymphoma. *Leukemia* 2007; 21:1183–8.

151 Golub TR, Barker GF, Lovett M, *et al.* Fusion of PDGF receptor beta to a novel ETS-like gene, *TEL*, in chronic myelomonocytic leukemia with t(5;12) chromosomal translocation. *Cell* 1994;77:307–16.

152 Steer EJ, Cross NC. Myeloproliferative disorders with translocations of chromosome 5q31–35: role of the platelet-derived growth factor receptor Beta. *Acta Haematol* 2002;107: 113–22.

153 Bain BJ, Fletcher SH. Chronic eosinophilic leukemias and the myeloproliferative variant of the hypereosinophilic syndrome. *Immunol Allergy Clin North Am* 2007;27:377–88.

Chapter 5
Non-cytogenetic Markers and Their Impact on Prognosis

Eric Schafer and Donald Small
Sidney Kimmel Comprehensive Cancer Center at Johns Hopkins, Baltimore, Maryland, USA

Introduction

It is known that all cancers are aberrant cellular expansions that grow by a process of clonal evolution driven by mutation [1]. As cancers of the hematopoietic system, acute leukemias are no exception to this rule. Over the last several decades, roughly two-thirds of leukemias have been characterized by non-random, somatically acquired chromosomal translocations or inversions [2]. This phenomenon is seen in both lymphoid and myeloid malignancies, and is present in tumors of both pediatric and adult origin (pediatric acute myeloid leukemia [AML], ~75%; adult AML, ~55%; pediatric acute lymphoblastic leukemia [ALL], ~65%; adult ALL, ~75%) (Figure 5.1) [3–12]. However, a single chromosomal genetic abnormality is almost never sufficient to cause leukemogenesis and appears to be "one hit" in a multistep pathway, which includes mutations at the subchromosomal level [13]. The discovery of a number of these recurrent somatic mutations have revolutionized the field of leukemia biology by providing new insights into leukemogenesis, risk, and treatment stratification, and are forming the basis for development of molecularly targeted therapies.

Molecular diagnostics and molecular monitoring of disease

In 1971, Hart *et al.* were the first to correlate the karyotypic cytogenetic characteristics of acute leukemias with clinical features and prognosis when they noted that hypoploidy portends a poor response to treatment and survival while hyperploidy is a positive prognositic indicator in both ALL and AML [14]. In 1976, the French–American–British (FAB) cooperative group attempted to combine the expanding knowledge of clinical cytogenetics and the new science of immunophenotyping with classical morphology to better codify the latest knowledge in hematologic malignancies [15]. While this FAB classification of acute leukemias was originally designed to be both diagnostic and prognostic [16], it was eventually shown to have major flaws in both goals [17–20]. To more closely meet original classification objectives, in 1997 the World Health Organization (WHO) created new criteria by which to distinguish the neoplastic diseases of the hematopoietic and lymphoid tissues [21]. The WHO classification reflected a major paradigm shift from previous schemes in that, for the first time, genetic information was formally incorporated and combined with morphology, immunophenotype, and clinical information in order that entities could both be recognized by pathologists and have clinical relevance [22,23]. Using the WHO classification system as a touchstone, cooperative leukemia study groups were able to develop systems of risk stratification that were greatly influenced by genetic markers [24–27]. As such, patients with "favorable" or "low-risk" disease could be treated in a way that minimized toxicities, while patients with "unfavorable" or "high-risk" disease could be identified early and considered for intensified treatments (Table 5.1). While this system greatly improved care, it failed to fully describe the 15–30% of ALL cases [29] and the 40–50% of AML [30] cases considered as "normal karyotype" (NK) leukemias because they lack macroscopic chromosomal abnormalities. In addition, both oncogenesis and the treatment response of leukemias are dependent on more than a single alteration, and therefore, even within diseases with abnormal karyotypes, much is learned by identifying additional molecular alterations [31,32].

Since the 1997 WHO classification, a large body of literature has begun to emerge that identifies subchromosomal mutations in both ALL and AML as markedly influential in determining disease type, risk stratification, therapy delivery, and future drug development [33–36]. This information has begun to be incorporated into decision making for clinical practice. For example, the Children's Oncology Group began to use submicrosomal aberrations in upfront risk stratification when patients with NK-AML with internal tandem duplication (ITD)

Leukemias: Principles and Practice of Therapy, 1st edition. Edited by S. Faderl and H. Kantarjian.

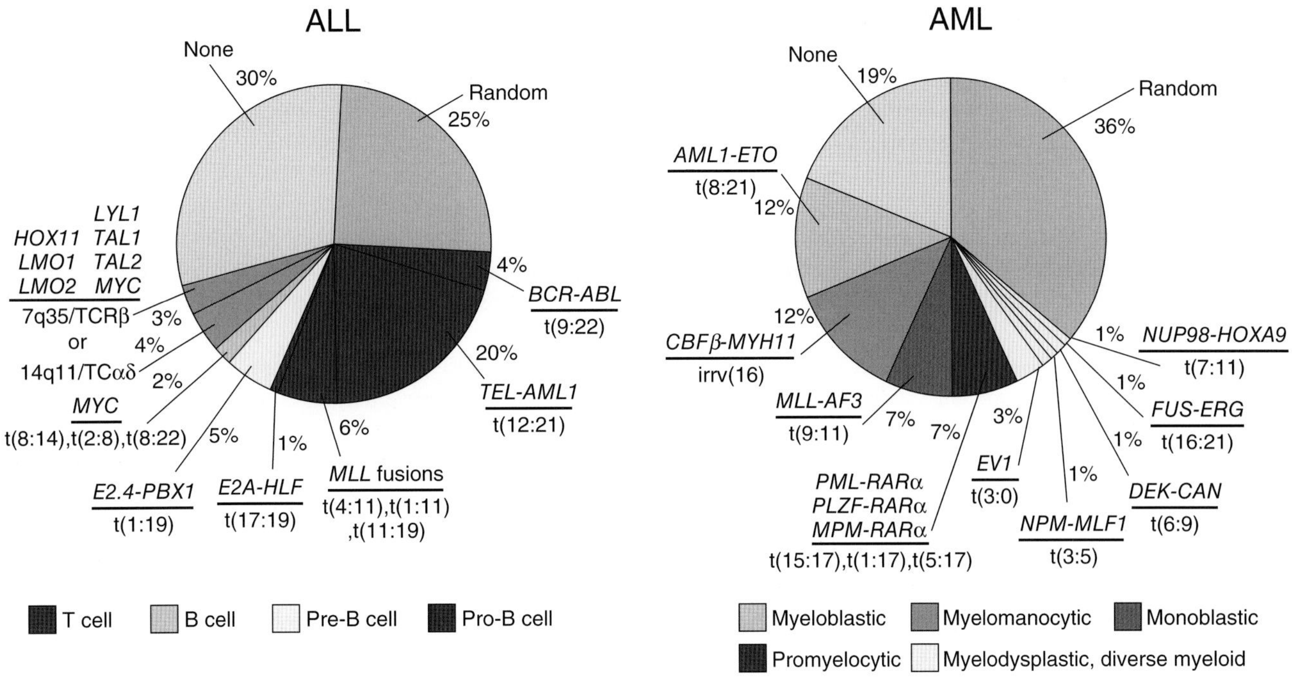

Figure 5.1 Distribution of cytogenetic alterations in acute leukemias. (Adapted from Look 1997 [2].)

Table 5.1 Hierarchical cytogenetics-based AML risk stratification system of major cooperative oncology research groups.

Risk level	MRC	SWOG/ECOG	CALGB	COG
Favorable/ low risk	t(8;21) inv(16)/t(16;16) t(15;17)	t(8;21) without del(9q) or complex karyotype inv(16)/t(16;16)/del(16q) t(15;17)	t(8;21) inv(16)/t(16;16) del(9q)	t(8;21)[a] inv(16)/t(16;16)[a]
Intermediate	NK-AML del(7q) +8 del(9q) abn(11q23) +21 +22	NK-AML +8 +6 –Y del(12p)	NK-AML del(7q) +21 –Y abn(12p) del(5q) t(9;11) +11 del(11q) +13 del(20)q	Mostly NK-AML The COG considers patients with features defined as neither low risk disease nor high risk disease to be intermediate risk; in addition, this group includes patients for whom cytogenetics are unable to be performed
Unfavorable/ high risk	abn(3q) –5/del(5q) –7 >/=5 aberrations	abn(3q) –5/del(5q) –7/del(7q) t(6;9) >/=3 aberrations abn(9q) abn(11q) abn(17p) abn(20q) abn(21q)	inv(3)/t(3;3) –7 t(6;9) >/=3 aberrations t(6;11) +8 t(11;19)	–5/del(5q) –7 *FLT3*/ITD-AR > 0.4

Adapted from Frohling S, Scholl C, Gilliland DG and Levine RL (2005) [28], with additional information adapted from COG AAML0531.

CALGB, Cancer and Leukemia Group B; COG, Children's Oncology Group; *FLT3*/ITD-AR, FMS-like tyrosine kinase 3 internal tandem duplication-allelic ratio; MRC, Medical Research Council; NK-AML, normal karyotype AML; SWOG/ECOG, Southwest Oncology Group/Eastern Cooperative Oncology Group.

[a]The COG considers these patients low risk regardless of the coexpression of the adverse characteristics monosomy 7 or –5/del(5q); however, patients having coexpression of *FLT3* high ITD-allelic ratio (>0.4) are moved to the high risk category.

mutations in the FMS-like tyrosine kinase 3 (*FLT3*) were classified as "high risk" in a recent phase III protocol for *de novo* AML (Table 5.1). The WHO revised the classification of neoplastic diseases of the hematopoietic and lymphoid tissues in 2008. In that classification it included *JAK2, MPL,* and *KIT* mutations in organizing myeloproliferative neoplasms (MPN), *NRAS, KRAS, NF1,* and *PTPN11* in organizing myelodysplastic syndrome (MDS)/MPN, *NPM1, CEBPα, FLT3, RUNX1, WT1,* and *MLL* in organizing AML, and *GATA1* in organizing myeloid proliferation in Down syndrome [23].

The treatment of patients with leukemia is becoming increasingly reliant on both early identification of the disease and on longitudinal assessment of disease burden, and the assays used to make these determinations have very closely paralleled developments in diagnostic technology [37]. Using morphology alone, it was estimated that a tumor burden of as many as 10^{10} cells (approximately 1%) could go unnoticed [38]. In 1990, it was demonstrated that double marker immunofluoresence flow cytometry performed on both ALL and AML samples known to be in full morphologic remission could not only detect disease burden as low as 0.01%, but was also prognositically significant in predicting relapse [39]. There have since been myriad studies that have demonstrated strong correlations of minimal residual disease (MRD) with disease outcome [40–42]. The two major tools used in following potential MRD are the identification of leukemia-associated aberrant immunophenotypes (LAIPs) by multiparameter flow cytometry (MFC) and quantitative polymerase chain reaction (qPCR) [43]. MRD monitoring was originally performed exclusively by MFC. Because normal bone marrow features reproducible patterns of antigen expression during differentiation that are often not recapitulated in leukemic blasts, normal and aberrant populations of cells can be differentiated [44]. By focusing on blasts with the use of CD45$^+$ gating, most MFC-based MRD studies cite sensitivity of approximately 0.05–0.01% [45]. In that range, detectable MRD was found as significantly related to relapse risk in AML and ALL [46]. Despite its potential use for treatment selection in leukemias, MFC-based MRD has several limitations. First, LAIPs are not identified in all leukemic populations [47]; second, LAIPs have been seen to change between diagnosis and relapse [48]; and third, the current ceiling of sensitivity seems to be about 0.01% [49]. For these reasons, qPCR assays of molecular markers are now being extensively studied in an attempt to overcome the limitations of MFC. Because qPCR measures levels of a single altered molecular target (relative to a housekeeping gene) instead of characterizing general cell surface markers, the sensitivity of such assays generally exceeds that of MFC by a log or more [50,51] and can reach levels of less than 1:10,000,000 [42]. Of note, while the ability to detect MRD to the level of 0.01% in acute leukemia has provided valuable prognostic information [39,52], it is not yet clear whether being able to detect MRD at levels below 0.01% provides any additional prognostic sensitivity [50]. An additional advantage of qPCR over MFC is that the genotypes of leukemia cells are generally stable between diagnosis and relapse [42]. Despite this, an obvious disadvantage to molecular MRD assays is their lack of universal inclusivity. However, as more leukemia-specific translocations and mutations are discovered, the number of possible PCR-based MRD targets increases, as does the percentage of hematologic malignancies eligible for molecular MRD monitoring.

Some of the best targets used to date are fusion-gene transcripts. In 1992, Miller *et al.* described the initial use of reverse transcription (RT)-PCR for the fusion transcript *PML–RARα* in the detection and monitoring of MRD in patients with acute promyelocytic leukemia (APL) [53]. Since then, multiple fusion genes have been described as useful in MRD monitoring including *E2A–PBX1, MLL–AF4, AML1–ETO, BCR–ABL, TEL–AML1,* and *CBFβ–MYH11* [54]. Because of the great diversity of breakpoints within fusion partner pairs between individual patients, the technical aspects of PCR can be challenging [55]. In addition, only about 25% of cases of leukemia have fusion genes amenable to molecular MRD detection [51].

Subchromosomal genetic alterations in leukemia may also serve as MRD-PCR amplicons and have become very attractive, not only because the targets are patient-specific and related to oncogenesis, but also because of the relative simplicity of the technical assays [55]. Several well-characterized gene mutations in AML, such as the *FLT3*/ITD, the mixed lineage leukemia (*MLL*) partial tandem duplication (PTD), *CEBPα* and nucleophosmin (*NPM1*), have been studied in PCR-based assays and found to be extremely reliable and sensitive MRD targets [42,55,56]. However, like leukemias characterized by fusion genes, to date only 25% of patients have known recurrent gene mutations [57]. There are also exceptions to the stability of these alterations in the leukemic clone. In ALL, one example is seen in the analysis of Ig/TCR gene rearrangements [58], and in AML this can be seen in the analysis of *FLT3* mutations [59]. Data from the study of *TEL-AML1* rearranged childhood leukemia have shown that late relapses likely result from changes occurring in a preexisting preleukemic clone and not from recurrence of the original tumor [60]. Therefore, these relapses have different Ig and TCR gene rearrangements, and consequently would not be picked up on a molecular MRD PCR assay [61]. *FLT3* mutations in AML sometimes occur as late mutations in a subclone of the disease and not always in the leukemic stem cell. Kottaridis *et al.* [62] showed that, in a sample of 44 patients with AML, of 20 with *FLT3*/

ITD mutations at diagnosis, five lost those mutations at relapse, and of 24 patients with *FLT3*-wild-type (WT) at diagnosis, five were found to have an *FLT3*/ITD mutation at relapse [62]. In addition, Schnittger *et al.* [63] discovered that while *FLT3* kinase domain mutations are more stable between diagnosis and relapse than are *FLT3*/ITD mutations, there were still several patient samples that were mutants at diagnosis which became wild type at relapse [63]. Thus, to improve the accuracy of PCR-based MRD studies, the development of alternative targets are necessary.

In an effort to take advantage of the simplicity of single-gene mRNA/cDNA PCR but overcome the fact that only a small fraction of leukemias carry gene mutations, many researchers have looked to overexpressed genes as a new method of MRD detection. The genes of interest in these studies have focused on those coding for tumor-associated antigens (TAA) and are selected based on the observations that they are either entirely silenced or expressed in extremely low levels in normal hematopoietic cells, while they are easily detectible in tumor cells [64]. By biostatistical analysis, certain expression levels or fold changes throughout the monitoring of the disease have been correlated with various outcome measurements. For example, *WT1* is overexpressed in 80–90% of AML and 70–80% of ALL, and, with the exception of pediatric ALL [65], its use in MRD testing has been well established [66–68]. Additionally, *MDS-EVI1/EVI1* [69] and *PRAME* have been explored as detectors of MRD in AML [70]. The major drawback to using overexpressed genes in MRD testing is its lack of sensitivity, which is reported as between 1:100 and just over 1:10,000 [42]. However, using gene expression profiles and microarray technology, Steinbach *et al.* identified a panel of seven overexpressed genes (*WT1, PRAME, CCL23, GAGED2, MSLN, SPAG6,* and *ST18*) in pediatric AML that could be analyzed together, partially overcoming this limitation [71].

In recent years, many groups have begun to look at high-throughput microarray-based assays to try to improve on leukemia diagnosis, risk stratification, and surveillance. In 1999, Golub *et al.* introduced the concept by showing that AML could be differentiated from ALL based on their individual genome-wide "genetic fingerprints" [72]. Since then, microarray signatures have been developed that stratify leukemias into previously known risk categories. Taking the technology one step further, Wilson *et al.* reported an unsupervised gene expression analysis of adults with AML that was able to distinguish six groups not predicted by traditional studies [73]. Additionally, Bullinger *et al.* showed that an *FLT3* gene-expression signature outperformed *FLT3*/ITD mutation status in predicting clinical outcome [74]. Even greater gene profiling sensitivity has been introduced with high-density single nucleotide polymorphism (SNP) arrays [75,76]. In addition, the recent discovery of the influence that micro-RNAs (miRNAs)—which are small, non-coding segments of RNA that hybridize to complementary mRNA targets and consequently inhibit translation—have on malignant transformation has led to the publication of miRNA signatures of leukemia [77]. Over the past 30 years, the tools available in leukemia pathology have evolved from simple cellular morphology and cytogenetics to differentiating cancers based on mutational analysis, gene expression, SNPs, and miRNAs. The ability to accurately diagnose and follow the disease response of acute leukemias will not only allow clinicians to predict outcome, identify relapse risk, and better tailor individual therapy, but will also allow researchers to gain a better understanding of leukemogenesis and more quickly and accurately assess the efficacy of new molecular-targeted therapies.

Major subchromosomal mutations in leukemia

Acute myeloid leukemia

It is becoming increasingly apparent that the genetic events underlying leukemogenesis in AML seem to fall into two broadly defined complementation groups [28]. The first group (class I mutations) comprises mutations that activate signal transduction pathways, resulting primarily in enhanced proliferation and/or survival of hematopoietic progenitors. The second group (class II mutations) comprises mutations that usually involve transcription factors and primarily result in impaired hematopoietic differentiation [37]. Interestingly, in mouse models, lesions from a single class are not enough to cause frank leukemia [78–81]. In addition, in human leukemia cells, lesions from different classes occur together more often than lesions from the same class, lending evidence to a "two hit" model of AML [82,83]. The recent sequencing of the entire cancer genome from a patient with AML adds additional complexity to this model, as two mutations which frequently occur together in AML (*NPM1* and *FLT3*) were observed along with eight novel mutated genes that were not seen in 180 additional samples tested [84]. It is unclear if these eight other mutations are "drivers", which actively participate in transformation, or "passengers", which are simply random mutations that do not contribute to oncogenesis. Alternatively, it could be reasoned that there is a huge pool of potentially mutable genes that contribute minimally by themselves, but that together contribute as much of a signal as more powerful oncogenes. Similar findings were observed from sequencing results of the pancreatic [85], glioblastoma multiformae [86], breast, and colon cancer genomes [87].

Class I mutations

FLT3

FMS-like tyrosine kinase 3 (*FLT3*) is a membrane-bound receptor tyrosine kinase (RTK) subclass III family member (along with *FMS, KIT*, and *PDGFR*α and β), which is coded for on chromosome 13q12 [88]. *FLT3* is normally expressed by myeloid and lymphoid progenitor cells, and its expression is usually lost as hematopoietic cells differentiate [89]. *FLT3* plays an important role in the proliferation, differentiation, and survival of multipotent stem/progenitor cells and is overexpressed at the mRNA and protein level in a large percentage of AML and ALL blasts [90], precursor B-cell infant leukemia blasts [91], and a small percentage of T-cell ALL blasts and CML cells in blast crisis [90,92,93]. *FLT3* mutations result in the constitutive activation of the *FLT3* RTK, and thus the phosphorylation of its downstream targets (which include GAB1, GAB2, SHP-2, AKT, FOXO3a, CBL, STAT5a, ERK1/2, GRB2, SHC, VAV, LYN, GAP, p90RSK, BAD, C/EBPα and SHIP) as well as *FLT3* itself by means of autophosphorylation. *FLT3* mutations are found in approximately one-third of patients with AML and appear as two major types [94]. The first type (seen in 23% of adult and 15% of pediatric patients with AML) is an in-frame exon 14 and/or 15 internal tandem duplication (ITD) mutation of 3–399 bp, which maps to the intracellular juxtamembrane region [95]. The second type (seen in 8–12% of adult and pediatric patients with AML) is defined by missense point mutations that most frequently involve aspartic acid 835 or isoleucine 836 of the activation loop of the tyrosine kinase domain (TKD) [96]. Most affected patients with AML have only one type of *FLT3* mutation, but patients carrying multiple TKD mutations or both TKD and ITD mutations have been observed [97,98].

While *FLT3* mutations have been frequently observed in association with t(15;17) and less frequently with t(8;21) and inv(16) positive AML [99], they are most often found in NK-AML and as such were originally risk stratified as "intermediate prognosis." However, there have been many studies showing that *FLT3*/ITD mutations in children and adults carry an independently poor prognosis because of reduced disease-free survival (DFS) and overall survival (OS) (Table 5.2) [127]. Despite the overall poor prognosis that *FLT3* mutations predict, the molecular characteristics of each individual mutant leukemia are quite different. For example, while it is known that a particularly poor prognostic subgroup are patients who have completely lost the wild-type allele of *FLT3* [128], patients with a low allelic ratio (AR) ($FLT3_{mutant}$:$FLT3_{WT}$ < 0.4:1) appear to have a survival rate comparable to patients without *FLT3* mutations [101,129].

FLT3 mutational status often changes between diagnosis and relapse, with about 9% of patients losing their *FLT3*/ITD mutation, 6% acquiring a new *FLT3*/ITD mutation, and 6% showing a change in the length of their original mutation [59]. It has also been shown that the AR often increases between diagnosis and relapse [130]. In addition, more than 50% of *FLT3*/TKD mutations are lost at relapse [131]. This provides some evidence for the argument that, in many patients, *FLT3* mutations are not the first, but most likely are later events in leukemogenesis, despite both its high prevalence and poor prognostic implications in AML.

c-KIT

KIT is highly expressed in approximately 80% of primary AML blasts but, unlike in the case of *FLT3, KIT* mutations are found almost exclusively in association with core binding factor (CBF) AML [132]. The *KIT* proto-oncogene is located on chromosome 4q12 and encodes a type III RTK family transmembrane glycoprotein whose ligand is stem-cell factor (SCF) [133]. Gain of function mutations may affect either the extracellular portion of the *c-KIT* receptor (coded for on exon 8), the juxtamembrane domain (which results from an ITD of exon 11), or the activation loop of the TKD (most commonly involving D816V of exon 17, which is the homologous amino acid so frequently mutated in *FLT3*/TKD AML) [134]. Extracellular *KIT* mutations have been shown to result in spontaneous receptor dimerization and subsequent activation of downstream targets such as MAP-kinase and PI3K [135]. D816V mutations induce constitutive activation of STAT3 and its downstream targets such as Bcl_{XL}, MYC, and the PI3K/AKT pathway [138]. The ultimate outcome of these effects in *KIT*-mutated AML is to increase the risk of relapse and decrease the overall survival of the normally good prognosis CBF AMLs (Table 5.2) [137].

RAS, *PTPN11, and NF1*

RAS oncogenes encode a family of guanine nucleotide-binding proteins that regulate signal transduction when activated by a variety of membrane receptors such as the RTKs FLT3 and *c-KIT*. As such, *RAS* plays an important role in the differentiation and survival of hematopoietic progenitors [138]. This family of proteins includes KRAS, NRAS, and HRAS. Ras proteins normally exist in an equilibrium between the active (GTP-bound) and inactive (GDP-bound) states [139]. However, mutations in *RAS*, which are usually single base changes in codons 12, 13, or 61, abrogate intrinsic Ras GTPase activity and lead to constitutive Ras activation and subsequent activation of its downstream effectors, such as RAF and MAP kinase/ERK [140]. *RAS* mutations are found in approximately 20% of patients with AML. However, less a single study that showed a significant survival disadvantage in NRAS mutant AML [141], the presence of *RAS* mutations, in most leukemia studies, does not seem to have any prognostic significance (Table 5.2) [105]. This is in contrast to myelodysplastic syndrome, where mutant *RAS* is a

Table 5.2 Incidence and prognostic significance of major somatic mutations in acute leukemias.

Molecular alteration	Age group	Incidence (%)	Prognostic significance	Source
AML				
FLT3/ITD	Adult	23	No difference in CR; significantly decreased survival CR: 65% vs. 76% ($P = 0.27$) OS: 19% vs. 45% ($P = 0.001$)	[100]
	Pediatric	12	Significantly decreased survival 4 year PFS: 31% vs. 55%	[101]
$FLT3_{mutant}$:$FLT3_{WT}$	Adult	50	Significantly decreased survival $FLT3/ITD_{mutant}$:$FLT3_{wt}$>0.78:1 OR for OS: 1.8 ($P = 0.002$) OR for DFS: 3.2 ($P < 0.001$)	[102]
	Pediatric	9	Significantly decreased PFS FLT3/ITD mutant:FLT3-wt >0.4:1 4 year PFS: 16% vs. 55% ($P < 0.001$)	[101]
FLT3/ALM (TKD)	Adult	14	No significant difference in either CR or OS CR: 82% vs. 65% ($P = 0.27$) OS: 39% vs. 45% ($P = 0.63$)	[100]
	Pediatric	6.7	No significant impact on survival	[101]
KIT mutations (in CBF)	Adult	46	Significantly increased risk of relapse and decreased OS RR: 76–90% vs. 35% ($P = 0.002$) 24 month OS: 25% vs. 76.5% ($P = 0.006$)	[103]
	Pediatric	17	Significantly negative impact in t(8;21) in KIT^+ vs. *KIT*– 4 year OS: 50% vs. 97.4% ($P = 0.001$) DFS: 37.5% vs. 97.4% ($P < 0.001$) RR: 47% vs. 2.7% ($P < 0.001$)	[104]
NRAS mutations	Adult	10.3	No significant difference in CR or OS CR: 60% vs. 57% ($P = 0.34$) OS: 1460 days vs. 604 days ($P = 0.96$) OS: 424 days vs. 335 days ($P = 0.146$)	[105]
	Pediatric	18	No significant impact on survival (possibly less likely to relapse) 5 year EFS: 59% vs. 41% 5 year OS: 67% vs. 54% RR: (22% vs. 45%, $P = 0.08$)	[106]
CEBPα mutations	Adult	11%	No significant difference in CR; significantly increased survival CR: 87% vs. 78% ($P = 0.74$) OS: 53% vs. 25% ($P = 0.04$)	[107]
	Young adults[a]	15	Significantly increased overall survival at 109 months OS: 61% vs. 38% ($P = 0.05$)	[108]
	Pediatric	6	No prognostic information	[109]
MLL/PTD	Adult	5	Significantly decreased survival 8 year OS: 0% vs.42%	[110]
	Pediatric	13.3	Significantly decreased survival 3 year OS: 56.3% vs. 83.2% DFS: 41.7% vs. 69.6% RR: 54.3% vs. 27.6%	[111]
NPM1 mutations	Adult	47	Overall: no impact on survival CR: 86% vs. 88% 6 year EFS: 43% vs. 37% ($P = 0.83$) 6 year OS: 32% vs. 26% ($P = 0.64$)	[112]
		27.5	In *FLT3*/ITD^- patients: significantly improved survival EFS: 19 months vs. 14 months OS: 16 months vs.11 months	[113]
	Pediatric	8	Overall: no significant impact on survival 5 year EFS: 50% vs. 33% 5 year OS: 55% vs. 49%	[114]
		4.7	In *FLT3*/ITD^- patients: significantly improved survival 5 year EFS: 69% vs. 35% (ITD^b–/NPMc–) vs. 21% (ITD^{+b}/NPMc–) vs. 25% (ITD^{+b}/$NPMc^+$) 5 year OS: 77% vs. 51% (ITD^b–/NPMc–) vs. 34% (ITD^{+b}/NPMc–) vs. 25% (ITD^{+b}/$NPMc^+$)	[114]

Table 5.2 *Continued*

Molecular alteration	Age group	Incidence (%)	Prognostic significance	Source
High *ERG* expression[c]	Adult	25	Significantly increased survival 2 year EFS: 71% vs. 34%	[115]
High *MN1* expression[d]	Adult	50	Significantly decreased CR and OS CR: 71% vs. 87% ($P = 0.02$) 3 year OS: 38% vs. 58% ($P = 0.03$)	[116]
High *BAALC* expression[d]	Adult	50	Significantly decreased OS 3 year OS: 36% vs. 54% ($P = 0.001$)	[117]
High *Bcl2* expression[d]	Adult	50	Significantly negative impact on survival CR: 45% vs. 79% ($P = 0.0001$) 4 year DSF: 0% vs. 26% ($P = 0.019$) 4 year OS: 0% vs. 18% ($P = 0.0001$)	[118]
High *Bax:Bcl2* ratio[d]	Pediatric	50	No significant impact on survival	[119]
WT1	Young adult[a]	12	No significant impact on survival	[120]
	Pediatric	12	Significantly negative impact on survival 5 year EFS: 22% vs. 46% ($P < 0.001$) 5 year OS: 35% vs. 66% ($P = 0.002$)	[121]
High *EVI1* expression[e]	Adult	6	Significantly negative impact on survival 5 year EFS: 3% vs. 29% ($P < 0.001$) 5 year OS: 13% vs. 39% ($P < 0.001$)	[122]
High BCRP expression[f]	Adult	33% (NK-AML)	Significantly negative impact on survival DFS: 8 months vs. 27 months (p = 0.027)	[123]
ALL				
B cell				
IKZF1 mutations	Pediatric	7 (28.6% in HR ALL)	Significantly negative impact on survival (in cohort of HR ALL) 10 year incidence of relapse: 46% vs. 22% ($P = 0.002$)	[124]
T cell				
NOTCH1 mutations	Adult	46	Significantly decreased survival 2 year RFS: 0% vs. ~50% ($P = 0.0015$ for RFS and $P = 0.0041$ for OS)	[125]
	Pediatric	34	No significant impact on survival	[125]
High *ERG* expression[d]	Adult	50	Significantly negative impact on survival 5 year RFS: 34% vs. 72% ($P = 0.003$) 5 year OS: 26% vs. 58% ($P = 0.02$)	[126]
High *BAALC* expression[d]	Adult	50	Significantly decreased impact on survival 4 year RFS: 21% vs. 65% ($P = 0.001$) 4 year OS: 18% vs. 58% ($P = 0.001$)	[126]

CBF, core binding factor; DFS, disease-free survival; EFS, event-free survival; *FLT3*/AML(TKD), FMS-like tyrosine kinase 3/activation loop domain (tyrosine kinase domain); *FLT3*/ITD, FMS-like tyrosine kinase 3/internal tandem duplication; *MLL*/PTD, mixed lineage leukemia gene/partial tandem duplication; NPMc, aberrant cytoplasmic localization of the NMP protein; *NPM1,* nucleophosmin gene; OS, overall survival; PFS, progression-free survival; RFS, relapse-free survival; RR, relapse rate; OR, odds ratio; WT, wild type.

[a]Young adults: 16–60 years.

[b]Refers to *FLT3*/ITD status.

[c]To distinguish "high-expression values" from "low-expression values", expression levels were dichotomized into quartiles with "high expressors" constituting the highest quartile and "low expressors" constituting the lowest quartile.

[d]To distinguish "high expression values" from "low expression values", expression levels were dichotomized into two groups at the median value.

[e]"High expressors" were defined as having a "gene expression value">50 (gene expression level calculated by $2^{(-\delta\delta Ct)}$ with δCt1: [normal bone marrow Ct_{EVI1}–CtP_{BGD}] and δCt2: [AML Ct_{EVI1}–Ct_{PBGD}]).

[f]"High expressors" were defined as patients whose blasts had a mean fluorescence intensity ratio (BCRP antibody: background fluorescence) >/=5 : 1.

negative prognostic indicator [142]. Despite the equivocal outcome that *RAS* mutant AML has to RAS_{WT} AML, *RAS* is recognized as a rational target for molecular therapy [36,105].

Mutations in SHP-2 and NF1 have also been reported to be leukemogenic, and like *RAS* mutations also affect the RAF and MAP kinase/ERK pathway. *PTPN11* encodes a protein tyrosine phosphatase (SHP-2) whose autoinhibitory properties are weakened with mutations and therefore its downstream signaling targets, which are thought to influence cell growth and development, are overactivated [143]. Recently, gain of function mutations in SHP-2 were shown to drastically increase the spreading and migration of various cell types including hematopoietic cells [144] and be associated with both hyperactivation of the ERK, AKT, and STAT5 pathways [145] and cytokine hypersensitivity [146].

The *NF1* gene on chromosome 17q11.2 encodes for the protein neurofibromin, which is a GTPase activating protein that inhibits Ras signaling by hydrolysis of active Ras-GTP into inactive Ras-GDP [147]. Both intragenic mutations of and microdeletions in the *NF1* gene inactivate neurofibromin and lead to the clinical syndrome of neurofibromatosis (NF1) [148,149]. While patients with NF1 have long been known to have a predisposition for both solid and liquid tumors [150], the *NF1* gene is now thought to be an independent tumor-suppressor gene and type 1 leukemogenic somatic mutation with reports of *NF1* mutations in juvenile myelomonocytic leukemia (JMML) [151], AML [152], and pediatric T-cell ALL [153] in patients with no clinical stigmata of neurofibromatosis.

Class II mutations

C/EBP*α*

C/EBPα, located on chromosome 19q13.1, codes for a transcription factor belonging to the CCAAT/enhancer-binding protein family and plays a critical role during the differentiation of various cell types, including hematopoietic cells [154]. *C/EBPα* is thought to affect blood cell development by upregulation of both granulocyte lineage-specific genes including CBF complex genes and PU.1 [155], and by downregulation of the proto-oncogene *c-MYC*, thus enabling differentiation to take place [156]. In addition, the *C/EBPα* protein inhibits cell proliferation by activating the transcription of the tumor suppressor p21/waf1 [157], by stabilizing p21 and by inhibiting CDK2 and CDK4, thus promoting myeloblast cell cycle withdrawal and terminal differentiation [158]. *C/EBPα* alterations occur by genomic mutation (leading to dominant negative-mutant proteins), transcriptional suppression by leukemic fusion proteins, translational inhibition by activated RNA-binding proteins, and functional inhibition by phosphorylation or increased proteasomal-dependent degradation [159]. Mutations in the *C/EBPα* gene in AML have been universally noted to be a positive prognostic indicator for survival in both pediatric and adult patients (Table 5.2) [107,109]. This conclusion has been made not only in the 9% of patients with AML harboring somatic *C/EBPα* mutations but also in a family carrying a germ line 212delC *C/EBPα* mutation [160].

MLL/*PTD*

The *MLL* (also called *ALL1*) gene is located at band 11q23 and encodes a 4230 kDa protein with histone methyltransferase activity that regulates *HOX* gene expression during the development of hematopoietic stem cells [161]. Most abnormalities of the *MLL* gene involve a translocation of the N-terminus of the MLL protein, which contains an AT-hook region functioning as a DNA-binding domain and two transcriptional repressor domains that are of DNA methyltransferase and histone deacetylase homology, with the C-terminus of one of over 60 known fusion partner genes [162]. *MLL* translocations have been identified in multiple hematopoietic malignancies including infant, childhood, and adult ALL, *de novo* AML, and therapy-related AML [163]. In addition to these chromosomal translocations, the *MLL* gene can also undergo partial tandem duplication (*MLL*/PTD), spanning exons 2 to 6 [164]. *MLL*/PTD has been identified in 8% of adults and 13% of children with *de novo* AML [111,165]. The negative prognostic significance of *MLL*/PTD in patients with AML has been well established. Explanations include both its strong association with other negative prognostic normal karyotype cytogenetic markers such as mutations in *FLT3* [110,165,166] and its upregulation of target genes, such as *HOXa9*, in a dominant, gain-of-function fashion [167]. In addition, Whitman *et al.* [128] showed that, as a result of epigenetic silencing, the other allele potentially coding for the MLL_{WT} transcript is not expressed in AML blasts harboring *MLL*/PTD [128]. Because of proper epigenetic signaling being central to both wild-type MLL and mutant MLL pathways, histone deacetylase and/or DNA methyltransferase inhibitors may have a therapeutic efficacy in patients with AML with this subgroup of poor prognosis mutation [168].

Nucleophosmin mutations (*NPM1* mutations)

Nucleophosmin (also called protein B23) is a multifunctional phosphoprotein that is localized primarily in the nucleolus but shuttles rapidly between the nucleus and cytoplasm in its role as a molecular chaperone [169]. The NPM1 protein has been shown to contribute to many basic cellular processes, including biosynthesis of ribosomes [170], preventing nucleolar protein aggregation [171] and initiating centrosome duplication through cyclin E/cyclin-dependent kinase 2 phosphorylation [172]. In addition, it has been found to be a stress-induced regulator of p53 function [173] and is a nucleolar binding partner of *ARF* (a tumor-suppressor gene widely regarded as an upstream activator of p53 dependent apoptosis)

[174]. The nucleophosmin gene (*NPM1*) is located at chromosome band 5q35 and mutations in its sequence have been implicated in the pathogenesis of a number of hematopoietic malignancies in addition to AML. For example, a large fraction of anaplastic large cell lymphomas are known to arise from the t(2;5)(p23;q35) translocation, resulting in expression of the oncogenic NPM1–ALK fusion protein [175]. The exact role of *NPM1* mutations described to date in oncogenesis remains controversial, as it has been credited with both oncogenic and tumor-suppressive properties [176]. However, it is clear that each of the 40 different *NPM1* mutations causes both the loss of trytophan residues 288 and 290 (which are critical for its nuclear localization) and the acquision of a C-terminal nuclear export signal motif, leading to the aberrant expression of nucleophosmin in the cytoplasm and likely explaining its altered cellular function [177].

In AML, *NPM1* mutations are known to be a positive prognostic indicator (Table 5.2) [178]. However, it was also shown that not only is the presence of an *NPM1* mutation highly associated with *FLT3*/ITD mutations (at a rate of 40%), but that the existence of *NPM1* mutations does not affect the poor prognosis of patients with *FLT3*/ITD mutations [179]. Subsequent studies with multivariate analyses confirmed that the favorable affect *NPM1* mutations have in AML only applies in the absence of *FLT3*/ITD mutations [113,180].

WT1

The *WT1* gene, which is located on chromosome 11p13, encodes a zinc finger transcription regulator. Around 12% of both children and adults with AML are found to have mutations in the gene, which usually cluster in exons 7 and 9 [120]. These mutations are thought to promote stem-cell proliferation and induce a differentiation block of hematopoietic cells through PU.1, which is a hematopoietic-specific ETS-family transcription factor required for normal blood cell development [134]. In AML, the *WT1* gene has been found to be a useful marker of MRD [181]. Prognostic studies showed that while mutations in *WT1* had no impact on survival in adults [120], they had a significantly negative impact on survival in children (Table 5.2) [121].

Overexpressed genes

ERG

The v-ets erythroblastosis virus E26 oncogene homolog (*ERG*) gene is a member of the ETS family of transcription factors, which are downstream effectors of mitogenic signaling transduction pathways and are involved in key steps in the regulation of cell proliferation, apoptosis, and differentiation [182]. Located on band 21q22, *ERG* was initially isolated as part of the fusion product in Ewing sarcoma tumors harboring t(21;22)(q22;q12). High levels of *ERG* are frequently expressed in leukemia. When patients with leukemia were divided into "low *ERG* expressor" and "high *ERG* expressor" groups, increased expression was found to independently predict worse DFS and OS in both T-cell ALL (when the higher expressing half of patients were compared with the lower expressing half) [117] and AML (when the highest expressing quartile was compared with the lowest expressing quartile) (Table 5.2) [115]. It is also overexpressed in several solid tumors including prostate [183], ovarian, and breast cancer [184].

MN1

The meningioma (disrupted in balanced translocation) 1 (*MN1*) gene, which is located at 22q11, is associated with poor response to induction chemotherapy when overexpressed in AML [185]. A follow-up study confirmed that when 142 patients with NK-AML were divided into two groups based on *MN1* expression, the half with higher *MN1* expression had a worse relapse rate and a poorer overall survival (Table 5.2) [116]. This occurs even when associated with the normally good prognosis inv(16) AML [186]. It is not yet clear how MN1 influences leukemogenesis. However, it is thought that MN1, which functions as a transcriptional co-activator, is recruited to and regulates the transcriptional activity of RAR/RXR and VDR/RXR through p300/CBP, and therefore affects differentiation of myeloid progenitors by means of up and downregulation of target genes [187]. Because of its clear association with poor prognosis, the MN1 protein has been proposed as a therapeutic target [188].

BAALC

Overexpression of the brain and acute leukemia cytoplasmic (*BAALC*) gene is another marker of poor prognosis (when patients were divided into two groups based on the mean *BAALC* expression level within the study group) in normal karyotype AML [117,189,190] and in T-cell ALL (Table 5.2) [126]. The gene is located on chromosome 8 at q22.3 but has no homology to known proteins [191]. It encodes at least eight alternatively spliced transcripts and, as it is expressed in normal $CD34^+$ bone marrow cells, is thought to represent a marker of early hematopoietic progenitor cells [189]. While the exact role of *BAALC* in leukemogenesis is unclear, a study by Langer *et al.* [192] showed that leukemic cells with high BAALC levels are characterized by an miRNA gene-expression signature consistent with less-differentiated and chemotherapy-resistant AML blasts, possibly correlating with the lower complete remission rate and worse survival for those with high *BAALC* expression [192].

BCL-2

BCL-2 is a gene located at chromosome 18q21.3 [193]. The gene was isolated by three groups studying the most common cytogenetic abnormality in follicular lymphoma, the translocation t(14;18)(q32;21) [194–196]. It was found to be a novel type of oncogene in that it functions as a repressor of programmed cell death instead of specifically conferring a proliferative advantage [197]. *BCL-2* and its family proteins can be divided into suppressers (eg, Bcl-2, Bcl_{XL}, and Mcl-1) and inducers (eg, Bax, Bad, Bak, and Bid) of apoptosis [198,199]. The central pathway involved in programmed cell death in most tissues involves mitochondria and several Bcl-2 family proteins, both antiapoptotic and proapoptotic have C-terminal transmembrane domains which insert in the outer membrane of mitochondria [200]. The proapoptotic family members Bax and Bak induce mitochondrial outer-membrane permeabilization, initiating a cascade that leads to programmed cell death. In contrast, antiapoptotic proteins such as Bcl-2 serve as guardians against apoptosis by opposing Bax and Bak either by direct blockade through heterodimerization or through its phosphorylation and activation of cytoplasmic signal transducers and activators of transcription [198,201,202]. High levels of Bcl-2 expression, relative to its proapoptotic family member Bax, have been associated with poor prognosis AML in adults (Table 5.2) [118].

BCRP

The breast cancer resistance protein (BCRP) is overexpressed in 33% of adult AML [123]. BCRP is encoded by the *ABCG2* gene on chromosome 4q22. It belongs to the ATP-binding cassette superfamily of membrane transporters and has been shown to confer resistance to many chemotherapeutic compounds including mitaxantrone, doxorubicin, daunorubicin, and topoisomerase II inhibitors through its action as an efflux pump [203].

Others (JAK2, EVI1)

Less common class I cytogenetic mutations seen in AML include mutations in Janus kinase 2 (*JAK2*). JAK2 is a cytoplasmic protein-tyrosine kinase that catalyzes the transfer of the gamma-phosphate group of ATP to the hydroxyl groups of specific tyrosine residues in signal transduction molecules and mediates signaling downstream of cytokine receptors after ligand-induced autophosphorylation of both the receptor and enzyme [204]. The mutation enhances the kinase activity of JAK2 and leads to hyperactivation of the downstream signaling components STAT5, PI3K/AKT, and ERK [205]. *JAK2V617F* is common in myeloproliferative disorders (MPD) as it is isolated in 90–95% of patients with polycythemia vera and 50–60% of patients with essential thrombocythemia and myelofibrosis [206]. *JAK2V617F* is also seen in 70% of AML arising from MPD but is seen in only 1.6% of *de novo* AML [207].

Less common class II overexpressed gene changes include the ectopic virus integration site 1 (*EVI1*) gene. Inappropriate expression of *EVI1* has been implicated as a marker of high-risk AML. *EVI1*, which codes for a zinc finger protein, is known to play an important role in normal development and is also known to be a proto-oncogene [208]. Most patients with AML with high *EVI1* expression have a reciprocal translocation at 3q26 (either t[3;3][q21;q26] or inv3[q21;q26]), but 6% of patients with NK-AML have been found to be high wild-type *EVI1* expressors (based on a relative gene expression by real-time PCR). In adult patients this high expression portended a significantly worse outcome (Table 5.2) [122,209].

Acute lymphoblastic leukemias

Even more so than in AML, ALLs are largely defined by gross chromosomal translocations such as t(12;21) or *TEL-AML1*, t(9;22) or *BCR–ABL*, 11q23 or *MLL* rearrangements, and t(1;19) or *E2A-PBX1* [210] (Figure 5.1). However, recent studies have uncovered several key subchromosomal mutations that also play important roles in lymphoid leukemogenesis.

Precursor B-cell acute lymphoblastic leukemia

PAX5

PAX5 is a transcription factor located at chromosome 9q13 that regulates the expression of B-cell specific genes, including *BLNK*, *CD19*, *LEF-1*, *BLK*, and *MB-1*, and thus plays a central role in B-cell differentiation [211]. In addition, PAX5 is important for maintaining the identity and function of mature B cells in late lymphopoiesis [212]. In a recent genome-wide SNP analysis, subchromosomal deletions, amplifications, point mutations, and structural rearrangements were found in 40% of 242 pediatric ALL cases [75]. In that study, the *PAX5* gene was the most frequent target of somatic mutation, being altered in 31.7% of cases [75]. These mutations were noted in and relatively evenly distributed among most genetic subtypes of ALL, with the exception of a low representation in *MLL* rearranged and high hyperdiploid subtypes [75]. A similar study of 45 adolescent and adult ALL samples found similar results, with 33% of samples showing a mutation in *PAX5* [213]. Another finding from both the pediatric and adult SNP array studies was that the microdeletions noted did not correlate with any other leukemic markers such as chromosomal translocations, age, sex, morphologic, or clinical features. Thus, microdeletions of key genes appear to be a feature of ALL that is shared among different clinical, morphologic, and cytogenetic subgroups [75,213]. In addition, while *PAX5* mutations did not seem to be an independent indicator of prognosis [75], a subsequent study identified a new poor prognosis pediatric precursor B-cell ALL subgroup that has 5-year DFS similar to that of $BCR–ABL^+$ disease, of which 36% had mutations in *PAX5* [214].

Ikaros (IKZF1)

Ikaros (LyF-1) is a transcription factor and the founding member of a family of highly homologous zinc finger nuclear proteins (which includes Aiolos, Eos, Helios, and Pegasus) required for normal lymphoid development [215]. The Ikaros gene (*IKZF1*), located on chromosome 7p12.2, encodes a protein consisting of two functionally distinct domains of Krupple-like zinc fingers. Ikaros has a central role in the regulation of hematopoiesis and appears to act as both a repressor and activator of transcription [216]. However, certain deletional mutations of Ikaros disrupt the proper binding activities of the zinc fingers and cause it to become a dominant negative repressor of transcription [217]. Mouse models with these deletions develop lymphoproliferative disorders and eventually die of leukemias and lymphomas [216]. Recently, Ikaros was shown to be one of the most common microdeletions in both pediatric and adult ALL (7% and 18%, respectively) [75,213]. In addition, alterations in *IKZF1* were shown to be an independent prognostic factor associated with an increased risk of relapse and adverse events in a cohort of children with high-risk ALL (Table 5.2) [124].

T-cell acute lymphoblastic leukemia

NOTCH1

The *NOTCH* genes encode single-pass transmembrane receptors that are involved in apoptosis, proliferation, and cell fate determination [218]. *NOTCH1*, which is located at chromosome 9q34, is mutated in more than 50% of patients with T-cell ALL [219]. The mature NOTCH1 receptor consists of an extracellular and a transmembrane subunit, which are non-covalently bound by a heterodimerization domain [220]. Binding of the δ-serrate-lag 2 (DSL) family of ligands to the extracellular subunit results in activation of the NOTCH1 receptor, which initiates a cascade of proteolytic cleavages of the transmembrane subunit [220]. The final cleavage is catalyzed by the gamma secretase complex and generates intracellular NOTCH1 [220]. Intracellular NOTCH1 subsequently translocates to the nucleus where it associates with other proteins to form a transcription activator complex [220]. Studies of downstream signaling initiated by NOTCH1 in T-cell ALL have demonstrated important connections between NOTCH1 and the MYC, NFKβ, and the PI3K/AKT signaling pathways [125]. One study showed that, in adults, the presence of this mutation significantly decreased survival while no impact was noted in pediatric patients with ALL with similar mutations (Table 5.2) [125].

CDKN2A

Alterations of the 9p21 locus, which inactivate the tumor suppressor gene cyclin-dependent kinase inhibitor 2A (*CDKN2A*), have been reported in both B-cell (20% in adult and 21% in pediatric) and T-cell (60% in adult and 50% in pediatric) ALL [221,222]. The *CDKN2A* gene encodes $p16^{INK4A}$ and $p14^{ARF}$, which specifically inhibits cyclin–CDK-4/6 complexes that block cell division during the G_1/S phase of the cell cycle [223]. Interestingly, there are several reported mechanisms by which *CDKN2A* is inactivated, including loss of heterozygosity, mutation, and silencing by gene promoter hypermethylation [222].

Others (JAK2, NF1, *and* ERG)

Two groups recently reported that a *JAK2R683* mutation, which is distinct from the V617F mutation seen in MPD and AML, is present in 18–28% of ALL associated with Down syndrome, as well as a smaller fraction of patients with high-risk ALL [224,225]. In addition, mutations in the developmental genes *EBF1*, *LEF1*, and *IKZF3* (Aiolos) have also been reported [26]. As mentioned in the section on *RAS* mutations, there was a recent report of three pediatric patients with T-cell ALL noted to have cryptic *NF1* mutations when 103 such patients were screened using a high-resolution 44K oligoarray-CGH platform [153]. High *ERG* expression (discussed in the AML section) has been shown to be a negative prognostic indicator in T-cell ALL as well as in AML (Table 5.2) [226].

Therapeutic targeting of molecular abnormalities

The desired endpoint of the study of leukemia molecular alterations is to improve patient outcome. Toward that goal, new drug development serves to either improve long-term survival, decrease the toxicity of current therapeutic regimens, or both. Classic chemotherapies are general tissue poisons [227], and while the mastering of their use has greatly improved cure rates in some tumor types, in others a limit in the effectiveness of chemotherapy intensification appears to have been reached as a result of offsetting increases in toxicity [228]. Using modern chemotherapeutic regimens, roughly 20% of children and 60% of adults with ALL will not achieve long-term remission [229], and in AML 50% of children [230], 70% of adults, and 90% of patients over 60 years old will not survive their disease [231]. Rationally designed targeted therapies aim to disrupt the underlying molecular genetic lesions responsible for the establishment or maintenance of the malignant clone while limiting toxicity to normal tissues, and therefore should cooperate with traditional chemotherapy to improve outcome [232].

To date, there are two success stories in targeted therapy of leukemias. In 1985, all-trans-retinoic acid (ATRA) was introduced into clinical practice after discovering that it could induce differentiation in APL cells [233]. Since then, it has improved the long-term survival rate of patients with promyelocytic leukemia (PML) from 35–40% to 75–80% [234]. It was years after the discovery of its effect on APL cells that the translocation defining most cases of PML, t(15;17), was shown to involve the retinoic acid receptor, thus explaining ATRA's mechanism of action

[232]. Imatinib mesylate (originally CGP57148B and then STI571) was reported as a small molecule inhibitor of ATP binding to the Bcr–Abl oncoprotein derived from the Philadelphia chromosome t(9;22) found in CML and ALL [235]. In the phase I study of this drug for patients with chronic-phase CML, imatinib was shown to induce a complete hematologic response in 53 of 54 patients and a complete cytogenetic response in 29 of 54 patients [236]. While the dramatic results of ATRA in APL and imatinib in chronic-phase CML have yet to be duplicated in other leukemias, many therapies have been discovered that hold the promise of at least improving the outcome for patients with these diseases (Table 5.3).

Table 5.3 Examples of targeted therapies being developed for specific mutations.

FLT3
Tyrosine kinase inhibitors
Lestaurtinib (CEP701)
Semaxinib (SU5416)
Sunitinib (SU11248)
Tandutinib (MLN518)
Midostaurin (PKC412)
Sorafenib (BAY43–9006)
c-KIT
Tyrosine kinase inhibitors
Semaxinib (SU5416)
Sunitinib (SU11248)
Imatinib (STI571)
Tandutinib (MLN518)
Sorafenib (BAY43–9006)
(PKC412)
(PTK787)
High Bcl-2 to Bax ratio
Apoptosis inhibitors/Bcl-2 antisense oligonucleotides
Oblimersen sodium (G3139)
Small molecule direct Bcl-2 protein inhibitors
Ascenta/gossypol (AT101)
Gemin X/obatoclax (GX15–070)
ABT737
ABT263
Aurora kinase inhibitors
VX680
RAS
Farnesyl transferase inhibitors
Tipifarnib/Zarnestra (R115777)
(BMS214662)
NOTCH1
Gamma secretase inhibitors
LY450139 (tested in phase I studies in patients with Alzheimer disease)
L885458

Immunotherapy has shown promise in the arena of targeted leukemia treatment. It is now well known that leukemias have unique immunophenotypic signatures (LAIPs). This phenomenon has been exploited by designing targeted therapeutics against surface antigens specific to hematologic malignancies. There are currently three classes of surface-targeted biologic therapies. The first is unlabeled monoclonal antibodies (MAbs). Examples are rituximab (MAb targeted against CD20) and alemtuzumab (MAb targeted against CD52), which are agents used almost exclusively in lymphomas. They exert their effect by causing apoptosis induction through enhancing antibody dependent cellular-mediated cytotoxicity (ADCC) and through complement-dependent cytotoxicity [237]. IMC-EB10 is another example of a "naked" antibody that is targeted to *FLT3* and is entering clinical trials. IMC-EB10 proves effective against both AML and ALL because of the high-level expression of *FLT3* in those diseases [238,239].

The second class is radiolabeled MAbs that target radiation therapy to malignant cells. The best studied agents in this class are both targets of CD20. The first is ^{90}Y-ibritumomab tiuxetan (Zevalin) and the second is ^{131}I-tositumomab (Bexxar) [240]. While currently Food and Drug Administration (FDA) approved only for non-Hodgkin lymphoma, these drugs have also been explored as part of preparative regimens for bone marrow transplants for both AML and ALL [241].

Finally, MAbs may be conjugated to toxins. Directed cell killing is achieved when the targeted cell internalizes the drug through receptor-mediated endocytosis and the drug's highly cytotoxic agent is released intracellularly [232]. One example of immunotoxic therapy is gemtuzumab ozogamicin, which is a humanized anti-CD33 MAb conjugated to the highly potent antitumor antibiotic calicheamicin. Phase I studies in AML showed a complete remission (CR) rate of 13%, with an additional 13% achieving a CR with inadequate platelet recovery. It had a tolerable safety profile other than the involvement of veno-occlusive disease in transplanted patients [242]. Encouraging studies have continued and it is currently being incorporated into phase III studies in pediatric and adult AML during upfront therapy in combination with standard chemotherapy [243,244]. Other immunotoxins in development for treatment of leukemias have conjugated MAbs with *Pseudomonas* exotoxin. BL22, which is an anti-CD22 Mab-PE conjugate, has shown some efficacy against chemotherapy-resistant hairy cell leukemia [245].

Constitutive activation of protein kinases through somatic mutation have been documented in a wide variety of human cancers, including leukemias, and interrupting this process with small molecule tyrosine kinase inhibitors (TKIs) has already been shown to be an effective targeted therapy in chronic-phase CML. The major focus in AML has been on *FLT3* because of the frequency of the *FLT3*/ITD mutation and the poor prognosis that it portends (Table 5.3). There are currently eight known chemical classes to which FLT3 inhibitors belong, but for the most part they work by competing with ATP for binding to the ATP-binding pocket of the kinase domain of the FLT3 receptor [94]. Most FLT3 inhibitors in clinical trials have shown favorable tolerance and safety profiles [246]. Two FLT3 inhibitors that are the furthest advanced in clinical trials in *FLT3* mutant AML are the idolocarbazole compounds PKC412 (midostaurin) and CEP701 (lestaurtinib). PKC412 has been shown to selectively induce G_1 cell cycle arrest and apoptosis in cell lines expressing mutant *FLT3* by directly inhibiting its kinase activity [247]. A phase II clinical trial in a small cohort of patients showed a 50% decrease in peripheral blast counts in most patients with mutated *FLT3* [248]. It is now in a phase III randomized trial in newly diagnosed patients with AML [249]. CEP701 has shown potent activity against autophosphorylation of WT and constitutively activated FLT3 receptors [250]. In preclinical trials, CEP701 was shown to be highly effective against both pediatric and adult AML cells *in vitro* [251,252]. In a phase II trial of CEP701 in patients with refractory or relapsed AML expressing *FLT3*-activating mutations, measurable clinical response with significant reduction in peripheral blasts was seen in many patients if the blasts were sensitive to the induction of apoptosis by the drug *in vitro* and adequate *FLT3* inhibition was achieved *in vivo* [246]. CEP701 is also now in phase III trials in both relapsed and newly diagnosed patients with AML with *FLT3* mutations [249].

Several TKIs have reported activity against constitutively active *c-KIT*, which occurs in a small fraction of AML. For example, imatinib has been shown to inhibit *c-KIT* autophosphorylation [253], although it showed only marginal effects on *c-KIT* positive primary AML patient blasts [254]. A possible explanation for this is that imatinib does not inhibit the kinase activity of the *D816V KIT* isoform [255]. However, TKIs such as PKC412 [256] and SU5416 [257] are active against the D816V mutant. In a phase II trial of SU5416 in Europe, five of eight patients who received a full 4-week course showed a partial response [258]. Additional clinical studies with this and other TKIs are under way for treatment of *c-KIT* positive AML [258].

Farnesyl transferase inhibitors (FTIs) are specific competitive inhibitors of the intracellular enzyme farnesyl protein transferase (FTase). This enzyme catalyzes the transfer of a farnesyl moiety to the cysteine terminal residue of substrate proteins, including Ras, resulting in their localization to the cell membrane. This has led to the investigation of FTIs as "*RAS* targeted" therapy for AML (Table 5.3) [259,260]. While FTIs have shown some activity against AML cells [261,262], the responses have not correlated biologically either with the mutational status of *RAS* or its ability to inhibit the downstream targets of Ras, p-ERK, and p-AKT, suggesting that there may be other important targets of FTIs other than Ras [263]. A phase II study of the FTI tipifarnib/zarnestra (R115777) in previously untreated adult patients with poor-risk AML showed a 23% overall response rate, with minimal adverse effects [264].

Several strategies are under investigation for targeting genetic mutations in AML that render cells resistant to apoptosis (Table 5.3). Downregulation of Bcl-2 by antisense oligonucleotides *in vitro* has been shown to sensitize AML cell lines to standard chemotherapeutic agents [265]. Several phase I trials have shown safety and efficacy of combining oblimersen sodium (G3139), an intravenously administered Bcl-2 antisense oligonucleotide, with standard chemotherapy [116,266]. The studies have shown that the toxicities were little different than with chemotherapy alone and have correlated clinical response to decreased Bcl-2 mRNA and protein levels, suggesting a targeted response. Phase III studies are currently being planned [267]. In addition, several small molecule drugs that directly interact with and inhibit Bcl-2 proteins are in various phases of development [268]. Finally, a recent study has shown that the aurora kinase inhibitor VX-680 induces apoptosis in AML cell lines with a concomitant increase in the Bax:Bcl-2 ratio (decreased Bcl-2 activity), suggesting a potential third possible Bcl-2 targeted therapy [269].

With regards to T-cell ALL, excitement has been generated for exploring the possible benefit of gamma secretase inhibitors to target *NOTCH1* mutations (Table 5.3). By inhibiting the final proteolytic cleavage of the *NOTCH1* receptor, the upregulated action of mutated *NOTCH1* is tempered [270]. Gamma secretase inhibitors were originally developed in an effort to target the production of amyloidogenic peptides in Alzheimer disease, which is also reliant on gamma secretase activity [271]. Several phase I studies of the oral gamma secretase inhibitor LY450139 have been conducted in patients with Alzheimer disease that have shown good tolerability and have been encouraging for translation to treatment in patients with T-cell leukemia [272,273]. Thus far, gamma secretase inhibitors have been shown to be effective in human *NOTCH1* mutant cell lines [274] and in *NOTCH1* mutant mouse model cell lines [275]—prompting interest in the future study of this targeted therapy.

Other examples of targeted therapy under investigation include proteosome inhibitors that interrupt the NF-κB transcriptional activator known to be constitutively activated in many primary AML specimens [276,277], mTOR inhibitors that target the overactivation of the mammalian target of rapamycin (mTOR) seen in 70% of AML samples and which have shown antitumor effects in several model systems [278], and epigenetic therapies such as histone deacetylase inhibitors (HDACIs) and DNA methyltransferase inhibitors (DNMTIs), which have shown activity in AML by unsilencing repressed tumor-suppressor genes [279]. The list of targeted therapies under investigation continues to increase as the understanding of the genetic mechanisms underlying leukemogenesis improves. This expanding armamentarium of treatment options holds the promise of prolonged survival, improved quality of life, and, potentially, outright cure for patients battling leukemia.

References

1 Vogelstein B, Kinzler KW. The multistep nature of cancer. *Trends Genet* 1993;9:138–41.

2 Look AT. Oncogenic transcription factors in the human acute leukemias. *Science* 1997;278:1059–64.

3 Leverger G, Bernheim A, Daniel MT, Flandrin G, Schaison G, Berger R. Cytogenetic study of 130 childhood acute nonlymphocytic leukemias. *Med Pediatr Oncol* 1988;16:227–32.

4 Raimondi SC, Kalwinsky DK, Hayashi Y, Behm FG, Mirro J, Jr., Williams DL. Cytogenetics of childhood acute nonlymphocytic leukemia. *Cancer Genet Cytogenet* 1989;40:13–27.

5 Heim S, Mitelman F. Cytogenetic analysis in the diagnosis of acute leukemia. *Cancer* 1992;70(Suppl.6):1701–9.

6 Chessels JM, Swansbury GJ, Reeves B, Bailey CC, Richards SM. Cytogenetics and prognosis in childhood lymphoblastic leukemia: results of MRC UKALL X. Medical Research Council Working Party in Childhood Leukemia. *Br J Haematol* 1997;99: 93–100.

7 Chessells JM, Hall E, Prentice HG, *et al.* The impact of age on outcome in lymphoblastic *Leukemia*; MRC UKALL X and XA compared: a report from the MRC Pediatric and Adult Working Parties. *Leukemia* 1998;12:463–73.

8 Grimwade D, Walker H, Oliver F, *et al.* The importance of diagnostic cytogenetics on outcome in AML: analysis of 1,612 patients entered into the MRC AML 10 trial. The Medical Research Council Adult and Children's Leukemia Working Parties. *Blood* 1998;92:2322–33.

9 Heerema NA, Nachman JB, Sather HN, *et al.* Hypodiploidy with less than 45 chromosomes confers adverse risk in childhood acute lymphoblastic leukemia: a report from the children's cancer group. *Blood* 1999;94:4036–45.

10 Slovak ML, Kopecky KJ, Cassileth PA, *et al.* Karyotypic analysis predicts outcome of preremission and postremission therapy in adult acute myeloid leukemia: a Southwest Oncology Group/Eastern Cooperative Oncology Group Study. *Blood* 2000;96:4075–83.

11 Thomas X, Danaila C, Le QH, *et al.* Long-term follow-up of patients with newly diagnosed adult acute lymphoblastic leukemia: a single institution experience of 378 consecutive patients over a 21-year period. *Leukemia* 2001;15:1811–22.

12 Byrd JC, Mrozek K, Dodge RK, *et al.* Pretreatment cytogenetic abnormalities are predictive of induction success, cumulative incidence of relapse, and overall survival in adult patients with de novo acute myeloid leukemia: results from Cancer and Leukemia Group B (CALGB 8461). *Blood* 2002;100:4325–36.

13 Gilliland DG, Jordan CT, Felix CA. The molecular basis of leukemia. *Hematology Am Soc Hematol Educ Program* 2004; 80–97.

14 Hart JS, Trujillo JM, Freireich EJ, George SL, Frei E, 3rd. Cytogenetic studies and their clinical correlates in adults with acute leukemia. *Ann Intern Med* 1971;75:353–60.

15 Bennett JM, Catovsky D, Daniel MT, *et al.* Proposals for the classification of the acute leukaemias. French-American-British (FAB) co-operative group. *Br J Haematol* 1976;33:451–8.

16 Miller DR, Leikin S, Albo V, Sather H, Hammond D. Prognostic importance of morphology (FAB classification) in childhood acute lymphoblastic leukemia (ALL). *Br J Haematol* 1981;48: 199–206.

17 Burns CP, Armitage JO, Frey AL, Dick FR, Jordan JE, Woolson RF. Analysis of the presenting features of adult acute leukemia: the French-American-British classification. *Cancer* 1981;47: 2460–9.

18 Ffrench M, Manel AM, Magaud JP, *et al.* Adult acute lymphoblastic leukemia: is cell proliferation related to other clinical and biological features? *Br J Haematol* 1987;65:419–23.

19 Lilleyman JS, Hann IM, Stevens RF, *et al.* Cytomorphology of childhood lymphoblastic leukemia: a prospective study of 2000 patients. United Kingdom Medical Research Council's Working Party on Childhood Leukemia. *Br J Haematol* 1992;81:52–7.

20 Shanta V, Maitreyan V, Sagar TG, Gajalakshmi CK, Rajalekshmy KR. Prognostic variables and survival in pediatric acute lymphoblastic leukemias: cancer institute experience. *Pediatr Hematol Oncol* 1996;13:205–16.

21 Bennett JM. World Health Organization classification of the acute leukemias and myelodysplastic syndrome. *Int J Hematol* 2000;72:131–3.

22 Harris NL, Jaffe ES, Diebold J, *et al.* The World Health Organization classification of neoplastic diseases of the hematopoietic and lymphoid tissues. Report of the Clinical Advisory Committee meeting, Airlie House, Virginia, November, 1997. *Ann Oncol* 1999;10:1419–32.

23 Vardiman JW, Thiele J, Arber DA, *et al.* The 2008 revision of the WHO classification of myeloid neoplasms and acute leukemia: rationale and important changes. *Blood* 2009;114:937–51.

24 Milligan DW, Grimwade D, Cullis JO, *et al.* Guidelines on the management of acute myeloid leukemia in adults. *Br J Haematol* 2006;135:450–74.

25 Apostolidou E, Swords R, Alvarado Y, Giles FG. Treatment of acute lymphoblastic leukemia: a new era. *Drugs* 2007;67:2153–71.

26 Pui CH, Robison LL, Look AT. Acute lymphoblastic leukemia. *Lancet* 2008;371:1030–43.

27 Rubnitz JE, Gibson B, Smith FO. Acute myeloid leukemia. *Pediatr Clin North Am* 2008;55:21–51.

28 Frohling S, Scholl C, Gilliland DG, Levine RL. Genetics of myeloid malignancies: pathogenetic and clinical implications. *J Clin Oncol* 2005;23:6285–95.

29 Ferrando AA, Look AT. Clinical implications of recurring chromosomal and associated molecular abnormalities in acute lymphoblastic leukemia. *Semin Hematol* 2000;37:381–95.

30 Gaidzik V, Dohner K. Prognostic implications of gene mutations in acute myeloid leukemia with normal cytogenetics. *Semin Oncol* 2008;35:346–55.

31 Pui CH, Relling MV, Downing JR. Acute lymphoblastic leukemia. *N Engl J Med* 2004;350:1535–48.

32 Marcucci G, Mrozek K, Bloomfield CD. Molecular heterogeneity and prognostic biomarkers in adults with acute myeloid leukemia and normal cytogenetics. *Curr Opin Hematol* 2005;12: 68–75.

33 Armstrong SA, Look AT. Molecular genetics of acute lymphoblastic leukemia. *J Clin Oncol* 2005;23:6306–15.

34 Kuiper RP, Schoenmakers EF, van Reijmersdal SV. High-resolution genomic profiling of childhood ALL reveals novel recurrent genetic lesions affecting pathways involved in lymphocyte differentiation and cell cycle progression. *Leukemia* 2007;21:1258–66.

35 Mrozek K, Dohner H, Bloomfield CD. Influence of new molecular prognostic markers in patients with karyotypically normal acute myeloid leukemia: recent advances. *Curr Opin Hematol* 2007;14:106–14.

36 Schlenk RF, Dohner K, Krauter J. Mutations and treatment outcome in cytogenetically normal acute myeloid leukemia. *N Engl J Med* 2008;358:1909–18.

37 Estey E, Dohner H. Acute myeloid leukemia. *Lancet* 2006; 368:1894–907.

38 Visser JW, Martens AC, Hagenbeek A. Detection of minimal residual disease in acute leukemia by flow cytometry. *Ann N Y Acad Sci* 1986;468:268–75.

39 Campana D, Coustan-Smith E, Janossy G. The immunologic detection of minimal residual disease in acute leukemia. *Blood* 1990;76:163–71.

40 Coustan-Smith E, Behm FG, Sanchez J, *et al.* Immunological detection of minimal residual disease in children with acute lymphoblastic leukemia. *Lancet* 1998;351:550–4.

41 Borowitz MJ, Devidas M, Hunger SP. Clinical significance of minimal residual disease in childhood acute lymphoblastic leukemia and its relationship to other prognostic factors: a Children's Oncology Group study. *Blood* 2008;111:5477–85.

42 Kern W, Haferlach C, Haferlach T, Schnittger S. Monitoring of minimal residual disease in acute myeloid leukemia. *Cancer* 2008;112:4–16.

43 Cheson BD, Bennett JM, Kopecky KJ, *et al.* Revised recommendations of the International Working Group for Diagnosis, Standardization of Response Criteria, Treatment Outcomes, and Reporting Standards for Therapeutic Trials in Acute Myeloid Leukemia. *J Clin Oncol* 2003;21:4642–9.

44 Macedo A, Orfao A, Gonzalez M. Immunological detection of blast cell subpopulations in acute myeloblastic leukemia at diagnosis: implications for minimal residual disease studies. *Leukemia* 1995;9:993–8.

45 Kern W, Voskova D, Schnittger S, Schoch C, Hiddemann W, Haferlach T. Four-fold staining including CD45 gating improves the sensitivity of multiparameter flow cytometric assessment of minimal residual disease in patients with acute myeloid leukemia. *Hematol J* 2004;5:410–8.

46 Haferlach T, Kern W, Schnittger S, Schoch C. Modern diagnostics in acute leukemias. *Crit Rev Oncol Hematol* 2005;56: 223–34.

47 Griesinger F, Piro-Noack M, Kaib N, *et al.* Leukemia-associated immunophenotypes (LAIP) are observed in 90% of adult and childhood acute lymphoblastic leukemia: detection in remission marrow predicts outcome. *Br J Haematol* 1999;105:241–55.

48 Voskova D, Schoch C, Schnittger S, Hiddemann W, Haferlach T, Kern W. Stability of leukemia-associated aberrant immunophenotypes in patients with acute myeloid leukemia between diagnosis and relapse: comparison with cytomorphologic, cytogenetic, and molecular genetic findings. *Cytometry B Clin Cytom* 2004;62:25–38.

49 Malec M, van der Velden VH, Bjorkland E, *et al.* Analysis of minimal residual disease in childhood acute lymphoblastic leukemia: comparison between RQ-PCR analysis of Ig/TcR gene rearrangements and multicolor flow cytometric immunophenotyping. *Leukemia* 2004;18:1630–6.

50 Neale GA, Coustan-Smith E, Stow P, *et al.* Comparative analysis of flow cytometry and polymerase chain reaction for the detection of minimal residual disease in childhood acute lymphoblastic leukemia. *Leukemia* 2004;18:934–8.

51 van der Velden VH, Boeckx N, van Wering ER, van Dongen JJ. Detection of minimal residual disease in acute leukemia. *J Biol Regul Homeost Agents* 2004;18:146–54.

52 San Miguel JF, Vidriales MB, Lopez-Berges C, *et al.* Early immunophenotypical evaluation of minimal residual disease in acute myeloid leukemia identifies different patient risk groups and may contribute to postinduction treatment stratification. *Blood* 2001;98:1746–51.

53 Miller WH Jr., Kakizuka A, Frankel SR, *et al.* Reverse transcription polymerase chain reaction for the rearranged retinoic acid receptor alpha clarifies diagnosis and detects minimal residual disease in acute promyelocytic leukemia. *Proc Natl Acad Sci U S A* 1992;89:2694–8.

54 van Dongen JJ, Macintyre EA, Gabert JA, *et al.* Standardized RT-PCR analysis of fusion gene transcripts from chromosome aberrations in acute leukemia for detection of minimal residual disease. Report of the BIOMED-1 Concerted Action: investigation of minimal residual disease in acute leukemia. *Leukemia* 1999;13:1901–28.

55 van der Velden VH, Hochhaus A, Cazzaniga G, Szczepanski T, Gabert J, van Dongen JJ. Detection of minimal residual disease in hematologic malignancies by real-time quantitative PCR: principles, approaches, and laboratory aspects. *Leukemia* 2003;17:1013–34.

56 Cazzaniga G, Gaipa G, Rossi V, Biondi A. Monitoring of minimal residual disease in leukemia, advantages and pitfalls. *Ann Med* 2006;38:512–21.

57 Kern W, Schoch C, Haferlach T, Schnittger S. Monitoring of minimal residual disease in acute myeloid leukemia. *Crit Rev Oncol Hematol* 2005;56:283–309.

58 Germano G, del Giudice L, Palatron S, *et al.* Clonality profile in relapsed precursor-B-ALL children by GeneScan and sequencing analyses. Consequences on minimal residual disease monitoring. *Leukemia* 2003;17:1573–82.

59 Shih LY, Huang CF, Wu JH, *et al.* Internal tandem duplication of FLT3 in relapsed acute myeloid leukemia: a comparative analysis of bone marrow samples from 108 adult patients at diagnosis and relapse. *Blood* 2002;100:2387–92.

60 Ford AM, Fasching K, Panzer-Grümayer ER, Koenig M, Haas OA, Greaves MF. Origins of "late" relapse in childhood acute lymphoblastic leukemia with TEL–AML1 fusion genes. *Blood* 2001;98:558–64.

61 Peham M, Konrad M, Harbott J, König M, Haas OA, Panzer-Grümayer ER. Clonal variation of the immunogenotype in relapsed ETV6/RUNX1-positive acute lymphoblastic leukemia indicates subclone formation during early stages of leukemia development. *Genes Chromosomes Cancer* 2004;39: 156–60.

62 Kottaridis PD, Gale RE, Langabeer SE, Frew ME, Bowen DT, Linch DC. Studies of FLT3 mutations in paired presentation and relapse samples from patients with acute myeloid leukemia: implications for the role of FLT3 mutations in leukemogenesis, minimal residual disease detection, and possible therapy with FLT3 inhibitors. *Blood* 2002;100:2393–8.

63 Schnittger S, Schoch C, Kern W, Hiddemann W, Haferlach T. FLT3 length mutations as marker for follow-up studies in acute myeloid leukemia. *Acta Haematol* 2004;112:68–78.

64 Greiner J, Schmitt M, Li L, *et al.* Expression of tumor-associated antigens in acute myeloid leukemia: Implications for specific immunotherapeutic approaches. *Blood* 2006;108:4109–17.

65 Boublikova L, Kalinova M, Ryan J, *et al.* Wilms' tumor gene 1 (WT1) expression in childhood acute lymphoblastic leukemia: a wide range of WT1 expression levels, its impact on prognosis and minimal residual disease monitoring. *Leukemia* 2006;20: 254–63.

66 Weisser M, Kern W, Rauhut S, *et al.* Prognostic impact of RT-PCR-based quantification of WT1 gene expression during MRD monitoring of acute myeloid leukemia. *Leukemia* 2005;19: 1416–23.

67 Cilloni D, Gottardi E, Saglio G. WT1 overexpression in acute myeloid leukemia and myelodysplastic syndromes. *Methods Mol Med* 2006;125:199–211.

68 Lapillonne H, Renneville A, Auvrignon A, *et al.* High WT1 expression after induction therapy predicts high risk of relapse and death in pediatric acute myeloid leukemia. *J Clin Oncol* 2006;24:1507–15.

69 Weisser M, Kern W, Schoch C, *et al.* Reverse transcriptase-polymerase chain reaction based quantification of the combined MDS-EVI1/EVI1 gene in acute myeloid leukemia. *Leuk Lymphoma* 2006;47:2645–7.

70 Matsushita M, Yamazaki R, Kawakami Y. Quantitative analysis of PRAME for detection of minimal residual disease in leukemia. *Methods Mol Med* 2004;97:267–75.

71 Steinbach D, Schramm A, Eggert A, *et al.* Identification of a set of seven genes for the monitoring of minimal residual disease in pediatric acute myeloid leukemia. *Clin Cancer Res* 2006;12:2434–41.

72 Golub TR, Slonim DK, Tamayo P, *et al.* Molecular classification of cancer: class discovery and class prediction by gene expression monitoring. *Science* 1999;286:531–7.

73 Wilson CS, Davidson GS, Martin SB, *et al.* Gene expression profiling of adult acute myeloid leukemia identifies novel biologic clusters for risk classification and outcome prediction. *Blood* 2006;108:685–96.

74 Bullinger L, Dohner K, Kranz R, *et al.* An FLT3 gene-expression signature predicts clinical outcome in normal karyotype AML. *Blood* 2008;111:4490–5.

75 Mullighan CG, Goorha S, Radtke I, *et al.* Genome-wide analysis of genetic alterations in acute lymphoblastic leukemia. *Nature* 2007;446:758–64.

76 Gondek LP, Tiu R, O'Keefe CL, Sekeres MA, Theil KS, Maciejewski JP. Chromosomal lesions and uniparental disomy detected by SNP arrays in MDS, MDS/MPD, and MDS-derived AML. *Blood* 2008;111:1534–42.

77 Calin GA, Croce CM. Micro RNA signatures in human cancers. *Nat Rev Cancer* 2006;6:857–66.

78 Kelly LM, Gilliland DG. Genetics of myeloid leukemias. *Annu Rev Genomics Hum Genet* 2002;3:179–98.

79 Downing JR. The core-binding factor leukemias: lessons learned from murine models. *Curr Opin Genet Dev* 2003;13:48–54.

80 Chan IT, Gilliland DG. Oncogenic K-ras in mouse models of myeloproliferative disease and acute myeloid leukemia. *Cell Cycle* 2004;3:536–7.

81 Li L, Piloto O, Nguyen HB, *et al.* Knock-in of an internal tandem duplication mutation into murine FLT3 confers myeloproliferative disease in a mouse model. *Blood* 2008;111: 3849–58.

82 Cammenga J, Horn S, Bergholz U, *et al.* Extracellular KIT receptor mutants, commonly found in core binding factor AML, are constitutively active and respond to imatinib mesylate. *Blood* 2005;106:3958–61.

83 Schnittger S, Kohl TM, Haferlach T, *et al.* KIT-D816 mutations in AML1-ETO-positive AML are associated with impaired event-free and overall survival. *Blood* 2006;107:1791–9.

84 Ley TJ, Mardis ER, Ding L, *et al.* DNA sequencing of a cytogenetically normal acute myeloid leukemia genome. *Nature* 2008;456:66–72.

85 Jones S, Zhang X, Parsons DW, *et al.* Core signaling pathways in human pancreatic cancers revealed by global genomic analyses. *Science* 2008;321:1801–6.

86 Parsons DW, Jones S, Zhang X, *et al.* An integrated genomic analysis of human glioblastoma multiforme. *Science* 2008;321: 1807–12.

87 Leary RJ, Lin JC, Gummins J, *et al.* Integrated analysis of homozygous deletions, focal amplifications, and sequence alterations in breast and colorectal cancers. *Proc Natl Acad Sci U S A* 2008;105:16224–9.

88 Carow CE, Kim E, Hawkins AL, *et al.* Localization of the human stem cell tyrosine kinase-1 gene (FLT3) to 13q12–>q13. *Cytogenet Cell Genet* 1995;70:255–7.

89 Lyman SD, Jacobsen SE. c-kit ligand and Flt3 ligand: stem/progenitor cell factors with overlapping yet distinct activities. *Blood* 1998;91:1101–34.

90 Carow CE, Levenstein M, Kaufmann SH, *et al.* Expression of the hematopoietic growth factor receptor FLT3 (STK-1/Flk2) in human leukemias. *Blood* 1996;87:1089–96.

91 Stam RW, den Boer ML, Schneider P, *et al.* Targeting FLT3 in primary MLL-gene-rearranged infant acute lymphoblastic leukemia. *Blood* 2005;106:2484–90.

92 Birg F, Courcoul M, Rosnet O, *et al.* Expression of the FMS/KIT-like gene FLT3 in human acute leukemias of the myeloid and lymphoid lineages. *Blood* 1992;80:2584–93.

93 George P, Bali P, Annavarapu S, *et al.* Combination of the histone deacety-lase inhibitor LBH589 and the hsp90 inhibitor 17-AAG is highly active against human CML-BC cells and AML cells with activating mutation of FLT3. *Blood* 2005;105:1768–76.

94 Small D. FLT3 mutations: biology and treatment. *Hematology Am Soc Hematol Educ Program* 2006;178–84.

95 Reilly JT. FLT3 and its role in the pathogenesis of acute myeloid leukemia. *Leuk Lymphoma* 2003;44:1–7.

96 Yamamoto Y, Kiyoi H, Nakano Y, *et al.* Activating mutation of D835 within the activation loop of FLT3 in human hematologic malignancies. *Blood* 2001;97:2434–9.

97 Bagrintseva K, Geisenhof S, Kern R, *et al.* FLT3-ITD-TKD dual mutants associated with AML confer resistance to FLT3 PTK inhibitors and cytotoxic agents by overexpression of Bcl-x(L). *Blood* 2005;105:3679–85.

98 Mead AJ, Linch DC, Hills RK, Wheatley K, Burnett AK, Gale RE. FLT3 tyrosine kinase domain mutations are biologically distinct from and have a significantly more favorable prognosis than FLT3 internal tandem duplications in patients with acute myeloid leukemia. *Blood* 2007;110:1262–70.

99 Kainz B, Heintel D, Marculescu R, *et al.* Variable prognostic value of FLT3 internal tandem duplications in patients with de novo AML and a normal karyotype, t(15;17), t(8;21) or inv(16). *Hematol J* 2002;3:283–9.

100 Frohling S, Schlenk RF, Breitruck J, *et al.* Prognostic significance of activating FLT3 mutations in younger adults (16 to 60 years) with acute myeloid leukemia and normal cytogenetics: a study of the AML Study Group Ulm. *Blood* 2002;100:4372–80.
101 Meshinchi S, Alonzo TA, Stirewalt DL, *et al.* Clinical implications of FLT3 mutations in pediatric AML. *Blood* 2006;108:3654–61.
102 Thiede C, Steudel C, Mohr B, *et al.* Analysis of FLT3-activating mutations in 979 patients with acute myelogenous leukemia: association with FAB subtypes and identification of subgroups with poor prognosis. *Blood* 2002;99:4326–35.
103 Cairoli R, Beghini A, Grillo G, *et al.* Prognostic impact of c-KIT mutations in core binding factor leukemias: an Italian retrospective study. *Blood* 2006107(9):3463–8.
104 Shimada A, Taki T, Tabuchi K, *et al.* KIT mutations, and not FLT3 internal tandem duplication, are strongly associated with a poor prognosis in pediatric acute myeloid leukemia with t(8;21): a study of the Japanese Childhood AML Cooperative Study Group. *Blood* 2006;107:1806–9.
105 Bacher U, Haferlach T, Schoch C, Kern W, Schnittger S. Implications of NRAS mutations in AML: a study of 2502 patients. *Blood* 2006;107:3847–53.
106 Goemans BF, Zwaan CM, Miller M, *et al.* Mutations in KIT and RAS are frequent events in pediatric core-binding factor acute myeloid leukemia. *Leukemia* 2005;19:1536–42.
107 Preudhomme C, Sagot C, Boissel N, *et al.* Favorable prognostic significance of CEBPA mutations in patients with de novo acute myeloid leukemia: a study from the Acute Leukemia French Association (ALFA). *Blood* 2002;100:2717–23.
108 Frohling S, Schlenk RF, Stolze I, *et al.* CEBPA mutations in younger adults with acute myeloid leukemia and normal cytogenetics: prognostic relevance and analysis of cooperating mutations. *J Clin Oncol* 2004;22:624–33.
109 Liang DC, Shih LY, Huang CF, *et al.* CEBP alpha mutations in childhood acute myeloid leukemia. *Leukemia* 2005;19:410–4.
110 Dohner K, Tobis K, Ulrich R, *et al.* Prognostic significance of partial tandem duplications of the MLL gene in adult patients 16 to 60 years old with acute myeloid leukemia and normal cytogenetics: a study of the Acute Myeloid Leukemia Study Group Ulm. *J Clin Oncol* 2002;20:3254–61.
111 Shimada A, Taki T, Tabuchi K, *et al.* Tandem duplications of MLL and FLT3 are correlated with poor prognoses in pediatric acute myeloid leukemia: a study of the Japanese childhood AML Cooperative Study Group. *Pediatr Blood Cancer* 2008;50:264–9.
112 Boissel N, Renneville A, Biggio V, *et al.* Prevalence, clinical profile, and prognosis of NPM mutations in AML with normal karyotype. *Blood* 2005;106:3618–20.
113 Thiede C, Koch S, Creutzig E, *et al.* Prevalence and prognostic impact of NPM1 mutations in 1485 adult patients with acute myeloid leukemia (AML). *Blood* 2006;107:4011–20.
114 Brown P, McIntyre E, Rau R, *et al.* The incidence and clinical significance of nucleophosmin mutations in childhood AML. *Blood* 2007;110:979–85.
115 Marcucci G, Baldus CD, Ruppert AS, *et al.* Overexpression of the ETS-related gene, ERG, predicts a worse outcome in acute myeloid leukemia with normal karyotype: a Cancer and Leukemia Group B study. *J Clin Oncol* 2005;23:9234–42.
116 Heuser M, Beutel G, Krauter J, *et al.* High meningioma 1 (MN1) expression as a predictor for poor outcome in acute myeloid leukemia with normal cytogenetics. *Blood* 2006;108:3898–905.
117 Baldus CD, Thiede C, Soucek S, Bloomfield CD, Thiel E, Ehninger G. BAALC expression and FLT3 internal tandem duplication mutations in acute myeloid leukemia patients with normal cytogenetics: prognostic implications. *J Clin Oncol* 2006;24:790–7.
118 Del Poeta G, Venditti A, Del Principe MI, *et al.* Amount of spontaneous apoptosis detected by Bax/Bcl-2 ratio predicts outcome in acute myeloid leukemia (AML). *Blood* 2003;101:2125–31.
119 Tamm I, Richter S, Oltersdorf D, *et al.* High expression levels of x-linked inhibitor of apoptosis protein and survivin correlate with poor overall survival in childhood de novo acute myeloid leukemia. *Clin Cancer Res* 2004;10:3737–44.
120 Gaidzik VI, Schlenk RF, Moschny S, *et al.* Prognostic impact of WT1 mutations in cytogenetically normal acute myeloid leukemia: a study of the German-Austrian AML Study Group. *Blood* 2009;113:4505–11.
121 Hollink IH, van den Heuvel-Eibrink MM, Zimmermann M, *et al.* Clinical relevance of Wilms' tumor 1 gene mutations in childhood acute myeloid leukemia. *Blood* 2009;113:5951–60.
122 Lugthart S, van Drunen E, van Norden Y, *et al.* High EVI1 levels predict adverse outcome in acute myeloid leukemia: prevalence of EVI1 overexpression and chromosome 3q26 abnormalities underestimated. *Blood* 2008;111:4329–37.
123 Damiani D, Tiribelli M, Calistri E, *et al.* The prognostic value of P-glycoprotein (ABCB) and breast cancer resistance protein (ABCG2) in adults with de novo acute myeloid leukemia with normal karyotype. *Haematologica* 2006;91:825–8.
124 Mullighan CG, Su X, Zhang J, *et al.* Deletion of IKZF1 and prognosis in acute lymphoblastic leukemia. *N Engl J Med* 2009;360:470–80.
125 Zhu YM, Zhao WL, Fu JF, *et al.* NOTCH1 mutations in T-cell acute lymphoblastic leukemia: prognostic significance and implication in multifactorial leukemogenesis. *Clin Cancer Res* 2006;12:3043–9.
126 Baldus CD, Martus P, Burmeister T, *et al.* Low ERG and BAALC expression identifies a new subgroup of adult acute T-lymphoblastic leukemia with a highly favorable outcome. *J Clin Oncol* 2007;25:3739–45.
127 Cloos J, Goemans BF, Hess CJ, *et al.* Stability and prognostic influence of FLT3 mutations in paired initial and relapsed AML samples. *Leukemia* 2006;20:1217–20.
128 Whitman SP, Archer KJ, Feng L, *et al.* Absence of the wild-type allele predicts poor prognosis in adult de novo acute myeloid leukemia with normal cytogenetics and the internal tandem duplication of FLT3: a cancer and leukemia group B study. *Cancer Res* 2001;61:7233–9.
129 Liang DC, Shih LY, Hung IJ, *et al.* Clinical relevance of internal tandem duplication of the FLT3 gene in childhood acute myeloid leukemia. *Cancer* 2002;94:3292–8.
130 Tiesmeier J, Muller-Tidow C, Westermann A, *et al.* Evolution of FLT3-ITD and D835 activating point mutations in relapsing acute myeloid leukemia and response to salvage therapy. *Leuk Res* 2004;28:1069–74.
131 Shih LY, Huang CF, Wu JH, *et al.* Heterogeneous patterns of FLT3 Asp(835) mutations in relapsed de novo acute myeloid leukemia: a comparative analysis of 120 paired diagnostic and relapse bone marrow samples. *Clin Cancer Res* 2004;10:1326–32.

132 Schwartz S, Heinecke A, Zimmerman M, *et al.* Expression of the C-kit receptor (CD117) is a feature of almost all subtypes of de novo acute myeloblastic leukemia (AML), including cytogenetically good-risk AML, and lacks prognostic significance. *Leuk Lymphoma* 1999;34:85–94.

133 Williams DE, Eisenman J, Baird A, *et al.* Identification of a ligand for the c-kit proto-oncogene. *Cell* 1990;63:167–74.

134 Renneville A, Roumier C, Biggio V, *et al.* Cooperating gene mutations in acute myeloid leukemia: a review of the literature. *Leukemia* 2008;22:915–31.

135 Kohl TM, Schnittger S, Ellwart JW, Hiddemann W, Spiekermann K. KIT exon 8 mutations associated with core-binding factor (CBF)-acute myeloid leukemia (AML) cause hyperactivation of the receptor in response to stem cell factor. *Blood* 2005;105:3319–21.

136 Ning ZQ, Li J, McGuinness M, Arceci RJ. STAT3 activation is required for Asp(816) mutant c-Kit induced tumorigenicity. *Oncogene* 2001;20:4528–36.

137 Beghini A, Ripamonti CB, Cairoli R, *et al.* KIT activating mutations: incidence in adult and pediatric acute myeloid leukemia, and identification of an internal tandem duplication. *Haematologica* 2004;89:920–5.

138 Downward J. Targeting RAS signaling pathways in cancer therapy. *Nat Rev Cancer* 2003;3:11–22.

139 Ayllon V, Rebollo A. Ras-induced cellular events (review). *Mol Membr Biol* 2000;17:65–73.

140 Reuter CW, Morgan MA, Bergmann L. Targeting the Ras signaling pathway: a rational, mechanism-based treatment for hematologic malignancies? *Blood* 2000;96:1655–69.

141 Kiyoi H, Naoe T, Nakano Y, *et al.* Prognostic implication of FLT3 and N-RAS gene mutations in acute myeloid leukemia. *Blood* 1999;93:3074–80.

142 Padua RA, Guinn BA, Al-Sabah AI, *et al.* RAS, FMS and p53 mutations and poor clinical outcome in myelodysplasias: a 10-year follow-up. *Leukemia* 1998;12:887–92.

143 Tartaglia M, Niemeyer CM, Fragale A, *et al.* Somatic mutations in PTPN11 in juvenile myelomonocytic leukemia, myelodysplastic syndromes and acute myeloid leukemia. *Nat Genet* 2003;34:148–50.

144 Wang S, Yu WM, Zhang W, McCrae KR, Neel BG, Qu CK. Noonan syndrome/leukemia-associated gain-of-function mutations in SHP-2 phosphatase (PTPN11) enhance cell migration and angiogenesis. *J Biol Chem* 2009;284:913–20.

145 Mohi MG, Williams IR, Dearolf CR, *et al.* Prognostic, therapeutic, and mechanistic implications of a mouse model of leukemia evoked by Shp2 (PTPN11) mutations. *Cancer Cell* 2005;7:179–91.

146 Chan RJ, Leedy MB, Munugalavadla V, *et al.* Human somatic PTPN11 mutations induce hematopoietic-cell hypersensitivity to granulocyte-macrophage colony-stimulating factor. *Blood* 2005;105:3737–42.

147 Phillips RA, Hunter JL, Eccleston JF, Webb MR. The mechanism of Ras GTPase activation by neurofibromin. *Biochemistry* 2003;42:3956–65.

148 Jenne DE, Tinschert S, Reimann H, *et al.* Molecular characterization and gene content of breakpoint boundaries in patients with neurofibromatosis type 1 with 17q11.2 microdeletions. *Am J Hum Genet* 2001;69:516–27.

149 Theos A, Korf BR. Pathophysiology of neurofibromatosis type 1. *Ann Intern Med* 2006;144:842–9.

150 Korf BR. Malignancy in neurofibromatosis type 1. *Oncologist* 2000;5:477–85.

151 Side LE, Emanuel PD, Taylor B, *et al.* Mutations of the NF1 gene in children with juvenile myelomonocytic leukemia without clinical evidence of neurofibromatosis, type 1. *Blood* 1998;92:267–72.

152 Akagi T, Ogawa S, Dugas M, *et al.* Frequent genomic abnormalities in acute myeloid leukemia/myelodysplastic syndrome with normal karyotype. *Haematologica* 2009;94:213–23.

153 Balgobind BV, Van Vlierberghe P, van den Ouweland AM, *et al.* Leukemia-associated NF1 inactivation in patients with pediatric T-ALL and AML lacking evidence for neurofibromatosis. *Blood* 2008;111:4322–8.

154 Mueller BU, Pabst T. C/EBP alpha and the pathophysiology of acute myeloid leukemia. *Curr Opin Hematol* 2006;13:7–14.

155 Friedman AD. Transcriptional regulation of granulocyte and monocyte development. *Oncogene* 2002;21:3377–90.

156 Johansen LM, Iwama A, Lodie TA, *et al.* c-Myc is a critical target for c/EBPalpha in granulopoiesis. *Mol Cell Biol* 2001;21: 3789–806.

157 Timchenko NA, Wilde M, Nakanishi M, Smith JR, Darlington GJ. CCAAT/enhancer-binding protein alpha (C/EBP alpha) inhibits cell proliferation through the p21 (WAF-1/CIP-1/SDI-1) protein. *Genes Dev* 1996;10:804–15.

158 Wang H, Iakova P, Wilde M, *et al.* C/EBPalpha arrests cell proliferation through direct inhibition of Cdk2 and Cdk4. *Mol Cell* 2001;8:817–28.

159 Pabst T, Mueller BU. Transcriptional dysregulation during myeloid transformation in AML. *Oncogene* 2007;26:6829–37.

160 Smith ML, Cavenagh JD, Lister TA, Fitzgibbon J. Mutation of CEBPA in familial acute myeloid leukemia. *N Engl J Med* 2004;351:2403–7.

161 Hess JL. MLL: a histone methyltransferase disrupted in leukemia. *Trends Mol Med* 2004;10:500–7.

162 Daser A, Rabbitts TH. The versatile mixed lineage *Leukemia* gene MLL and its many associations in leukemogenesis. *Semin Cancer Biol* 2005;15:175–88.

163 De Braekeleer M, Morel F, Le Bris MJ, Herry A, Douet-Guilbert N. The MLL gene and translocations involving chromosomal band 11q23 in acute leukemia. *Anticancer Res* 2005;25:1931–44.

164 Shiah HS, Kuo YY, Tang JL, *et al.* Clinical and biological implications of partial tandem duplication of the MLL gene in acute myeloid leukemia without chromosomal abnormalities at 11q23. *Leukemia* 2002;16:196–202.

165 Caligiuri MA, Strout MP, Lawrence D, *et al.* Rearrangement of ALL1 (MLL) in acute myeloid leukemia with normal cytogenetics. *Cancer Res* 1998;58:55–9.

166 Libura M, Asnafi V, Tu A, *et al.* FLT3 and MLL intragenic abnormalities in AML reflect a common category of genotoxic stress. *Blood* 2003;102:2198–204.

167 Dorrance AM, Liu S, Chong A, *et al.* The Mll partial tandem duplication: differential, tissue-specific activity in the presence or absence of the wild-type allele. *Blood* 2008;112:2508–11.

168 Whitman SP, Liu S, Vukosavljevic T, *et al.* The MLL partial tandem duplication: evidence for recessive gain-of-function in acute myeloid leukemia identifies a novel patient subgroup for molecular-targeted therapy. *Blood* 2005;106:345–52.

169 Cordell JL, Pulford KA, Bigerna B, *et al.* Detection of normal and chimeric nucleophosmin in human cells. *Blood* 1999;93: 632–42.

170 Huang N, Negi S, Szebeni A, Olson MO. Protein NPM3 interacts with the multifunctional nucleolar protein B23/nucleophosmin and inhibits ribosome biogenesis. *J Biol Chem* 2005; 280:5496–502.

171 Szebeni A, Olson MO. Nucleolar protein B23 has molecular chaperone activities. *Protein Sci* 1999;8:905–12.

172 Okuda M, Horn HF, Tarapore P, *et al.* Nucleophosmin/B23 is a target of CDK2/cyclin E in centrosome duplication. *Cell* 2000;103:127–40.

173 Colombo E, Marine JC, Danovi D, Falini B, Pelicci PG. Nucleophosmin regulates the stability and transcriptional activity of p53. *Nat Cell Biol* 2002;4:529–33.

174 Brady SN, Yu Y, Maggi LB, Jr., Weber JD. ARF impedes NPM/B23 shuttling in an Mdm2-sensitive tumor suppressor pathway. *Mol Cell Biol* 2004;24:9327–38.

175 Morris SW, Kirstein MN, Valentine MB, *et al.* Fusion of a kinase gene, ALK, to a nucleolar protein gene, NPM, in non-Hodgkin's lymphoma. *Science* 1994;263:1281–4.

176 Grisendi S, Mecucci C, Falini B, Pandolfi PP. Nucleophosmin and cancer. *Nat Rev Cancer* 2006;6:493–505.

177 Falini B, Bolli N, Shan J, *et al.* Both carboxy-terminus NES motif and mutated tryptophan(s) are crucial for aberrant nuclear export of nucleophosmin leukemic mutants in NPMc+ AML. *Blood* 2006;107:4514–23.

178 Dohner K, Schlenk RF, Habdank M, *et al.* Mutant nucleophosmin (NPM1) predicts favorable prognosis in younger adults with acute myeloid leukemia and normal cytogenetics: interaction with other gene mutations. *Blood* 2005;106:3740–6.

179 Falini B, Nicoletti I, Martelli MF, Mecucci C. Acute myeloid leukemia carrying cytoplasmic/mutated nucleophosmin (NPMc+ AML): biologic and clinical features. *Blood* 2007;109: 874–85.

180 Schnittger S, Schoch C, Kern W, *et al.* Nucleophosmin gene mutations are predictors of favorable prognosis in acute myelogenous leukemia with a normal karyotype. *Blood* 2005;106: 3733–9.

181 Willasch AM, Gruhn B, Coliva T, *et al.* Standardization of WT1 mRNA quantitation for minimal residual disease monitoring in childhood AML and implications of WT1 gene mutations: a European multicenter study. *Leukemia* 2009;23:1472–9.

182 Seth A, Watson DK. ETS transcription factors and their emerging roles in human cancer. *Eur J Cancer* 2005;41:2462–78.

183 Rouzier C, Haudebourg J, Carpentier X, *et al.* Detection of the TMPRSS2–ETS fusion gene in prostate carcinomas: retrospective analysis of 55 formalin-fixed and paraffin-imbedded samples with clinical data. *Cancer Genet Cytogenet* 2008;183:21–7.

184 Davidson B, Goldberg I, Tell L, *et al.* The clinical role of the PEA3 transcription factor in ovarian and breast carcinoma in effusions. *Clin Exp Metastasis* 2004;21:191–9.

185 Heuser M, Wingen LU, Steinemann D, *et al.* Gene-expression profiles and their association with drug resistance in adult acute myeloid leukemia. *Haematologica* 2005;90:1484–92.

186 Ross ME, Mahfouz R, Onciu M, *et al.* Gene expression profiling of pediatric acute myelogenous leukemia. *Blood* 2004;104: 3679–87.

187 van Wely KH, Molijn AC, Buijs A, *et al.* The MN1 oncoprotein synergizes with coactivators RAC3 and p300 in RAR-RXR-mediated transcription. *Oncogene* 2003;22:699–709.

188 Grosveld GC. MN1, a novel player in human AML. *Blood Cells Mol Dis* 2007;39:336–9.

189 Baldus CD, Tanner SM, Kusewitt DF, *et al.* BAALC, a novel marker of human hematopoietic progenitor cells. *Exp Hematol* 2003;31:1051–6.

190 Bienz M, Ludwig M, Lei-bundgut EO, *et al.* Risk assessment in patients with acute myeloid leukemia and a normal karyotype. *Clin Cancer Res* 2005;11:1416–24.

191 Tanner SM, Austin JL, Leone G, *et al.* BAALC, the human member of a novel mammalian neuroectoderm gene lineage, is implicated in hematopoiesis and acute leukemia. *Proc Natl Acad Sci U S A* 2001;98:13901–6.

192 Langer C, Radmacher MD, Ruppert AS, *et al.* High BAALC expression associates with other molecular prognostic markers, poor outcome, and a distinct gene-expression signature in cytogenetically normal patients younger than 60 years with acute myeloid leukemia: a Cancer and Leukemia Group B (CALGB) study. *Blood* 2008;111:5371–9.

193 Schimmer AD. Apoptosis in leukemia: from molecular pathways to targeted therapies. *Best Pract Res Clin Haematol* 2008; 21:5–11.

194 Tsujimoto Y, Finger LR, Yunis J, Nowell PC, Croce CM. Cloning of the chromosome breakpoint of neoplastic B cells with the t(14;18) chromosome translocation. *Science* 1984;226: 1097–9.

195 Bakhshi A, Jensen JP, Goldman P, *et al.* Cloning the chromosomal breakpoint of t(14;18) human lymphomas: clustering around JH on chromosome 14 and near a transcriptional unit on 18. *Cell* 1985;41:899–906.

196 Cleary ML, Sklar J. Nucleotide sequence of a t(14;18) chromosomal breakpoint in follicular lymphoma and demonstration of a breakpoint-cluster region near a transcriptionally active locus on chromosome 18. *Proc Natl Acad Sci U S A* 1985;82: 7439–43.

197 Galteland E, Sivertsen EA, Svendsrud DH, *et al.* Translocation t(14;18) and gain of chromosome 18/BCL2: effects on BCL2 expression and apoptosis in B-cell non-Hodgkin's lymphomas. *Leukemia* 2005;19:2313–23.

198 Deng X, Kornblau SM, Ruvolo PP, May WS, Jr. Regulation of Bcl2 phosphorylation and potential significance for leukemic cell chemoresistance. *J Natl Cancer Inst Monogr* 2001;28:30–7.

199 Cory S, Huang DC, Adams JM. The Bcl-2 family: roles in cell survival and oncogenesis. *Oncogene* 2003;22:8590–607.

200 Green DR, Kroemer G. The pathophysiology of mitochondrial cell death. *Science* 2004;305:626–9.

201 Mahajan NP, Linder K, Berry G, Gordon GW, Heim R, Herman B. Bcl-2 and Bax interactions in mitochondria probed with green fluorescent protein and fluorescence resonance energy transfer. *Nat Biotechnol* 1998;16:547–52.

202 Reed JC. Bcl-2-family proteins and hematologic malignancies: history and future prospects. *Blood* 2008;111:3322–30.

203 Plasschaert SL, Van Der Kolk DM, De Bont ES, Vellenga E, Kamps WA, de Vries EG. Breast Cancer Resistance protein (BCRP) in acute leukemia. *Leuk Lymphoma* 2004;45:649–54.

204 Tefferi A, Gilliland DG. The JAK2V617F tyrosine kinase mutation in myeloproliferative disorders: status report and immediate implications for disease classification and diagnosis. *Mayo Clin Proc* 2005;80:947–58.

205 Winston LA, Hunter T. JAK2, Ras, and Raf are required for activation of extracellular signal-regulated kinase/mitogen-activated protein kinase by growth hormone. *J Biol Chem* 1995;270:30837–40.

206 Koppikar P, Levine RL. JAK2 and MPL mutations in myeloproliferative neoplasms. *Acta Haematol* 2008;119:218–25.
207 Levine RL, Loriaux M, Huntly BJ, *et al.* The JAK2V617F activating mutation occurs in chronic myelomonocytic leukemia and acute myeloid leukemia, but not in acute lymphoblastic leukemia or chronic lymphocytic leukemia. *Blood* 2005;106:3377–9.
208 Wieser R. The oncogene and developmental regulator EVI1: expression, biochemical properties, and biological functions. *Gene* 2007;396:346–57.
209 Barjesteh van Waalwijk van Doorn-Khosrovani S, Erpelinck C, van Putten WL, *et al.* High EVI1 expression predicts poor survival in acute myeloid leukemia: a study of 319 de novo AML patients. *Blood* 2003;101:837–45.
210 Greaves MF, Wiemels J. Origins of chromosome translocations in childhood leukemia. *Nat Rev Cancer* 2003;3:639–49.
211 Schebesta M, Heavey B, Busslinger M, *et al.* Transcriptional control of B-cell development. *Curr Opin Immunol* 2002;14: 216–23.
212 Horcher M, Souabni A, Busslinger M. Pax5/BSAP maintains the identity of B cells in late B lymphopoiesis. *Immunity* 2001; 14:779–90.
213 Paulsson K, Cazier JB, Macdougall F, *et al.* Microdeletions are a general feature of adult and adolescent acute lymphoblastic leukemia: Unexpected similarities with pediatric disease. *Proc Natl Acad Sci U S A* 2008;105:6708–13.
214 Den Boer ML, van Slegtenhorst M, De Menezes RX, *et al.* A subtype of childhood acute lymphoblastic leukemia with poor treatment outcome: a genome-wide classification study. *Lancet Oncol* 2009;10:125–34.
215 Ng SY, Yoshida T, Georgopoulos K. Ikaros and chromatin regulation in early hematopoiesis. *Curr Opin Immunol* 2007;19: 116–22.
216 Winandy S, Wu P, Georgopoulos K. A dominant mutation in the Ikaros gene leads to rapid development of leukemia and lymphoma. *Cell* 1995;83:289–99.
217 Mullighan C, Downing J. Ikaros and acute leukemia. *Leuk Lymphoma* 2008;49:847–9.
218 Nefedova Y, Cheng P, Alsina M, Dalton WS, Gabrilovich DI. Involvement of Notch-1 signaling in bone marrow stroma-mediated de novo drug resistance of myeloma and other malignant lymphoid cell lines. *Blood* 2004;103:3503–10.
219 Jundt F, Schwarzer R, Dorken B. Notch signaling in *Leukemias* and lymphomas. *Curr Mol Med* 2008;8:51–9.
220 Aster JC, Pear WS, Blacklow SC. Notch signaling in leukemia. *Annu Rev Pathol* 2008;3:587–613.
221 Ruas M, Peters G. The p16INK4a/CDKN2A tumor suppressor and its relatives. *Biochim Biophys Acta* 1998;1378:F115–77.
222 Sulong S, Moorman AV, Irving JA, *et al.* A comprehensive analysis of the CDKN2A gene in childhood acute lymphoblastic leukemia reveals genomic deletion, copy number neutral loss of heterozygosity, and association with specific cytogenetic subgroups. *Blood* 2009;113:100–7.
223 Drexler HG. Review of alterations of the cyclin-dependent kinase inhibitor INK4 family genes p15, p16, p18 and p19 in human leukemia-lymphoma cells. *Leukemia* 1998;12:845–59.
224 Bercovich D, Ganmore I, Scott LM, *et al.* Mutations of JAK2 in acute lymphoblastic leukaemias associated with Down's syndrome. *Lancet* 2008;372:1484–92.
225 Kearney L, Gonzalez De Castro D, Yeung J, *et al.* Specific JAK2 mutation (JAK2R683) and multiple gene deletions in Down syndrome acute lymphoblastic leukemia. *Blood* 2009;113: 646–8.
226 Baldus CD, Burmeister T, Martus P, *et al.* High expression of the ETS transcription factor ERG predicts adverse outcome in acute T-lymphoblastic leukemia in adults. *J Clin Oncol* 2006;24: 4714–20.
227 Watt J. The use of cytotoxic drugs in the surgery of malignant disease. *J Bone Joint Surg Br* 1968;50:511–23.
228 Brown P, Smith FO. Molecularly targeted therapies for pediatric acute myeloid leukemia: progress to date. *Paediatr Drugs* 2008;10:85–92.
229 Sallan SE. Myths and lessons from the adult/pediatric interface in acute lymphoblastic leukemia. *Hematology Am Soc Hematol Educ Program* 2006;128–32.
230 Woods WG. Curing childhood acute myeloid leukemia (AML) at the half-way point: promises to keep and miles to go before we sleep. *Pediatr Blood Cancer* 2006;46:565–9.
231 Rowe JM. Innovative approaches in the treatment and support of patients with acute myelogenous leukemia. *Oncologist* 2007; 12(Suppl.2):1.
232 Downing JR. Targeted therapy in leukemia. *Mod Pathol* 2008; 21(Suppl.2):S2–7.
233 Breitman T, Selonick SE, Collins SJ. Induction of differentiation of the human promyelocytic leukemia cell line (HL-60) by retinoic acid. *Proc Natl Acad Sci U S A* 1980;77:2936–40.
234 Wang ZY, Chen Z. Acute promyelocytic leukemia: from highly fatal to highly curable. *Blood* 2008;111:2505–15.
235 Druker BJ, Tamura S, Buchdunger E, *et al.* Effects of a selective inhibitor of the Abl tyrosine kinase on the growth of Bcr-Abl positive cells. *Nat Med* 1996;2:561–6.
236 Druker BJ, Talpaz M, Resta DJ, *et al.* Efficacy and safety of a specific inhibitor of the BCR-ABL tyrosine kinase in chronic myeloid leukemia. *N Engl J Med* 2001;344:1031–7.
237 Fanale MA, Younes A. Monoclonal antibodies in the treatment of non-Hodgkin's lymphoma. *Drugs* 2007;67:333–50.
238 Piloto O, Levis M, Huso D, *et al.* Inhibitory antiFLT3 antibodies are capable of mediating antibody-dependent cell-mediated cytotoxicity and reducing engraftment of acute myelogenous leukemia blasts in nonobese diabetic/severe combined immunodeficient mice. *Cancer Res* 2005;65:1514–22.
239 Piloto O, Nguyen B, Huso D, *et al.* IMC-EB10, an antiFLT3 monoclonal antibody, prolongs survival and reduces nonobese diabetic/severe combined immunodeficient engraftment of some acute lymphoblastic leukemia cell lines and primary leukemic samples. *Cancer Res* 2006;66:4843–51.
240 Park SI, Press OW. Radioimmunotherapy for treatment of B-cell lymphomas and other hematologic malignancies. *Curr Opin Hematol* 2007;14:632–8.
241 Bethge WA, Wilbur DS, Sandmaier BM, *et al.* Radioimmunotherapy as non-myeloablative conditioning for allogeneic marrow transplantation. *Leuk Lymphoma* 2006;47:1205–14.
242 Stasi R, Evangelista ML, Buccisano F, Venditti A, Amadori S. Gemtuzumab ozogamicin in the treatment of acute myeloid leukemia. *Cancer Treat Rev* 2008;34:49–60.
243 Gleissner B, Schlenk R, Bornhauser M, Berdel WE. Gemtuzumab ozogamicin (mylotarg) for the treatment of acute myeloid leukemia–ongoing trials. *Onkologie* 2007;30:657–62.
244 Aplenc R, Alonzo TA, Gerbing RB, *et al.* Safety and efficacy of gemtuzumab ozogamicin in combination with chemotherapy for pediatric acute myeloid leukemia: a report from

the Children's Oncology Group. *J Clin Oncol* 2008;26:2390–3295.

245 Kreitman RJ, Wilson WH, Bergeron K, *et al.* Efficacy of the antiCD22 recombinant immunotoxin BL22 in chemotherapy-resistant hairy-cell leukemia. *N Engl J Med* 2001;345:241–7.

246 Smith BD, Levis M, Beran M, *et al.* Single-agent CEP-701, a novel FLT3 inhibitor, shows biologic and clinical activity in patients with relapsed or refractory acute myeloid leukemia. *Blood* 2004;103:3669–76.

247 Weisberg E, Boulton C, Kelly LM, *et al.* Inhibition of mutant FLT3 receptors in leukemia cells by the small molecule tyrosine kinase inhibitor PKC412. *Cancer Cell* 2002;1:433–43.

248 Stone RM, DeAngelo DJ, Klimek V, *et al.* Patients with acute myeloid leukemia and an activating mutation in FLT3 respond to a small-molecule FLT3 tyrosine kinase inhibitor, PKC412. *Blood* 2005;105:54–60.

249 Knapper S. FLT3 inhibition in acute myeloid leukemia. *Br J Haematol* 2007;138:687–99.

250 Levis M, Allebach J, Tse KF, *et al.* A FLT3-targeted tyrosine kinase inhibitor is cytotoxic to leukemia cells *in vitro* and *in vivo*. *Blood* 2002;99:3885–91.

251 Brown P, Meshinchi S, Levis M, *et al.* Pediatric AML primary samples with FLT3/ITD mutations are preferentially killed by FLT3 inhibition. *Blood* 2004;104:1841–9.

252 Levis M, Pham R, Smith BD, Small D. *In vitro* studies of a FLT3 inhibitor combined with chemotherapy: sequence of administration is important to achieve synergistic cytotoxic effects. *Blood* 2004;104:1145–50.

253 Heinrich MC, Griffith DJ, Druker BJ, Wait CL, Ott KA, Zigler AJ. Inhibition of c-kit receptor tyrosine kinase activity by STI 571, a selective tyrosine kinase inhibitor. *Blood* 2000;96:925–32.

254 Scappini B, Onida F, Kantarjian HM, *et al.* Effects of signal transduction inhibitor 571 in acute myelogenous leukemia cells. *Clin Cancer Res* 2001;7:3884–93.

255 Frost MJ, Ferrao PT, Hughes TP, Ashman LK. Juxtamembrane mutant V560GKit is more sensitive to Imatinib (STI571) compared with wild-type c-kit whereas the kinase domain mutant D816VKit is resistant. *Mol Cancer Ther* 2002;1:1115–24.

256 Roberts KG, Odell AF, Byrnes EM, *et al.* Resistance to c-KIT kinase inhibitors conferred by V654A mutation. *Mol Cancer Ther* 2007;6:1159–66.

257 Smolich BD, Yuen HA, West KA, Giles FJ, Albitar M, Cherrington JM. The antiangiogenic protein kinase inhibitors SU5416 and SU6668 inhibit the SCF receptor (c-kit) in a human myeloid leukemia cell line and in acute myeloid leukemia blasts. *Blood* 2001;97:1413–21.

258 Heinrich MC, Blanke CD, Druker BJ, Corless CL. Inhibition of KIT tyrosine kinase activity: a novel molecular approach to the treatment of KIT-positive malignancies. *J Clin Oncol* 2002; 20:1692–703.

259 Lancet JE, Karp JE. Farnesyl transferase inhibitors in myeloid malignancies. *Blood Rev* 2003);17:123–9.

260 Braun T, Fenaux P. Farnesyltransferase inhibitors and their potential role in therapy for myelodysplastic syndromes and acute myeloid leukemia. *Br J Haematol* 2008;141:576–86.

261 Morgan MA, Dolp O, Reuter CW. Cell-cycle-dependent activation of mitogen-activated protein kinase kinase (MEK-1/2) in myeloid leukemia cell lines and induction of growth inhibition and apoptosis by inhibitors of RAS signaling. *Blood* 2001; 97:1823–34.

262 Korycka A, Smolewski P, Robak T. The influence of farnesyl protein transferase inhibitor R115777 (Zarnestra) alone and in combination with purine nucleoside analogs on acute myeloid leukemia progenitors *in vitro*. *Eur J Haematol* 2004;73:418–26.

263 Martinelli G, Iacobucci I, Paolini S, Ottaviani E. Farnesyl-transferase inhibition in hematologic malignancies: the clinical experience with tipifarnib. *Clin Adv Hematol Oncol* 2008;6: 303–10.

264 Lancet JE, Gojo I, Gotlib J, *et al.* A phase 2 study of the farnesyltransferase inhibitor tipifarnib in poor-risk and elderly patients with previously untreated acute myelogenous leukemia. *Blood* 2007;109:1387–94.

265 Konopleva M, Tari AM, Estrov Z, *et al.* Liposomal Bcl-2 antisense oligonucleotides enhance proliferation, sensitize acute myeloid leukemia to cytosine-arabinoside, and induce apoptosis independent of other antiapoptotic proteins. *Blood* 2000; 95:3929–38.

266 Marcucci G, Byrd JC, Dai G, *et al.* Phase 1 and pharmacodynamic studies of G3139, a Bcl-2 antisense oligonucleotide, in combination with chemotherapy in refractory or relapsed acute leukemia. *Blood* 2003;101:425–32.

267 Tallman MS, Gilliland DG, Rowe JM. Drug therapy for acute myeloid leukemia. *Blood* 2005;106:1154–63.

268 Kang MH, Reynolds CP. Bcl-2 inhibitors: targeting mitochondrial apoptotic pathways in cancer therapy. *Clin Cancer Res* 2009;15:1126–32.

269 Huang XF, Luo SK, Xu J, *et al.* Aurora kinase inhibitory VX-680 increases Bax/Bcl-2 ratio and induces apoptosis in Aurora-A-high acute myeloid leukemia. *Blood* 2008;111:2854–65.

270 Weng AP, Ferrando AA, Lee W, *et al.* Activating mutations of NOTCH1 in human T cell acute lymphoblastic leukemia. *Science* 2004;306:269–71.

271 Kukar TL, Ladd TB, Bann MA, *et al.* Substrate-targeting gamma-secretase modulators. *Nature* 2008;453:925–9.

272 Siemers ER, Quinn JF, Kaye J, *et al.* Effects of a gamma-secretase inhibitor in a randomized study of patients with Alzheimer disease. *Neurology* 2006;66:602–4.

273 Siemers ER, Dean RA, Friedrich S, *et al.* Safety, tolerability, and effects on plasma and cerebrospinal fluid amyloid-beta after inhibition of gamma-secretase. *Clin Neuropharmacol* 2007; 30:317–25.

274 De Keersmaecker K, Lahortiga I, Mentens N, *et al.* *In vitro* validation of gamma-secretase inhibitors alone or in combination with other anticancer drugs for the treatment of T-cell acute lymphoblastic leukemia. *Haematologica* 2008;93:533–42.

275 O'Neil J, Calvo J, McKenna K, *et al.* Activating Notch1 mutations in mouse models of T-ALL. *Blood* 2006;107:781–5.

276 Guzman ML, Neering SJ, Upchurch D, *et al.* Nuclear factor-kappaB is constitutively activated in primitive human acute myelogenous leukemia cells. *Blood* 2001;98:2301–7.

277 Guzman ML, Swiderski CF, Howard DS, *et al.* Preferential induction of apoptosis for primary human leukemic stem cells. *Proc Natl Acad Sci U S A* 2002;99:16220–5.

278 Recher C, Beyne-Rauzy O, Demur C, *et al.* Antileukemic activity of rapamycin in acute myeloid leukemia. *Blood* 2005;105: 2527–34.

279 Melnick A. Predicting the effect of transcription therapy in hematologic malignancies. *Leukemia* 2005;19:1109–17.

Part 2
Myelodysplastic Syndromes

Chapter 6
Myelodysplastic Syndromes: Pathophysiology

Steve D. Gore[1] *and Erica Warlick*[2]
[1]Sidney Kimmel Comprehensive Cancer Center, Johns Hopkins, Baltimore, Maryland, USA
[2]University of Minnesota Medical School, Minneapolis, Minnesota, USA

Introduction

Myelodysplastic syndrome (MDS) pathogenesis begins with an inciting genetic (chromosomal, epigenetic, molecular) event within a hematopoietic stem cell in an inflammatory bone marrow microenvironment resulting in an initial proapoptotic/proliferative state and creating a hypercellular marrow with peripheral cytopenias. Further genetic changes lead to progressive disease in which the apoptotic/proliferative balance is tipped and the proliferative advantage dominates. This chapter explores MDS pathogenesis theories in terms of the MDS cell of origin, genetic alterations within the cell of origin, alterations in bone marrow microenvironment and apoptosis, alterations in immune surveillance, and functional cellular abnormalities.

Cell of origin

Although MDS has long been considered a clonal bone marrow disorder, data pointing toward the actual cell of origin has only recently emerged. Central to the ongoing debate regarding the MDS cell of origin is whether the originating cell is a primitive hematopoietic stem cell (HSC) or a myeloid lineage-restricted stem-cell progenitor (MSC). The known characteristic MDS chromosomal abnormalities present a powerful tool for identifying the cell of origin. Early work suggested the cell of origin to be an MSC [1–4] highlighting the presence of chromosomal markers (del)5q, monosomy 7, and trisomy 8 solely in myeloid progeny with absence in lymphoid progenitors. As FACS (fluorescence-activated cell sorting) became more available and the field of stem-cell biology became more developed, elegant studies aimed at pinpointing the cell of origin have suggested that different cytogenetic-defined cases of MDS may originate in different cells.

These studies use disease-specific clonal cytogenetic abnormalities to track the presence of the abnormal genotype in various cellular subsets, relying on the assumption that the cytogenetic abnormality being tracked represents an early, if not the earliest, genetic abnormality inducing the MDS. However, this assumption may not be true in many cases of MDS. Using the $5q^-$ aberration to track the origin of the MDS stem cell, Nilsson *et al.* were the first to show that the chromosomal abnormality was present in the majority of myeloid cells as well as in a significant percentage of B-lineage cells, suggesting a more primitive cell of origin ($CD34^+$, $CD38^-$) [5]. Further evaluations in patients with trisomy 8 showed that while only a varying percentage (0–71%) of the primitive $CD34^+$, $CD38^-$, and Thy-1^+ cells harbored the $^+8$ genotype, the functional capacity of these primitive stem cells as measured by long-term culture-initiating cells (LTC-ICs) and repopulation studies demonstrated an intrinsic deficiency. These data suggest that trisomy 8 is likely to be a later event in MDS pathogenesis and that an event occurs prior to that at the HSC level ($CD34^+$, $CD38^-$, Thy-1^+) [6].

The Nilsson group recently supplied more support for the $CD34^+$, $CD38^-$, and Thy-1^+ cell-of-origin theory using gene profile expression studies. These showed that in the $5q^-$ syndrome the gene profile signature of the $CD34^+$, $CD38^-$, and Thy-1^+ $5q^-$ cells more closely resembled normal hematopoietic stem cells than more differentiated progenitor cells from normal or $5q^-$ bone marrows. While no consensus has been reached, there are accumulating data to suggest that a multipotent hematopoietic stem cell ($CD34^+$, $CD38^-$, Thy-1^+) is the cell of origin in at least the $5q^-$ syndrome [7]. Further investigation into other cytogenetic subsets will be crucial to determine if this is true across other subsets of MDS.

Genetic alterations within the cell of origin

Exogenous toxic exposure

Epidemiologic study of MDS has offered instructive links between various environmental exposures and the

Leukemias: Principles and Practice of Therapy, 1st edition. Edited by S. Faderl and H. Kantarjian. © 2011 Blackwell Publishing Ltd.

development of disease, specifically the accumulation of DNA damage. Numerous environmental exposures have been associated with MDS development, including tobacco [8], alcohol [9], infections [10], or autoimmune disorders [11]. However, the classic causative example linking an environmental toxin exposure to MDS development is highlighted from observational studies involving benzene [12]. Bone marrow failure states noted after exposure to benzene in Turkish shoe workers [13] led to a prospective cohort study involving 74,828 benzene-exposed individuals in China. This revealed a relative risk of MDS approaching infinity [14], noting both genotoxic and non-genotoxic mechanisms of damage: (i) genotoxic mechanisms, characterized by a generation of oxygen-free radicals causing DNA damage and apoptosis [15,16], supported by the presence of chromosomal abnormalities, oncogene mutations, and somatic mutations in benzene-exposed patients with MDS [17–19]; and (ii) non-genotoxic mechanisms, characterized by altered bone marrow microenvironment and immune function, supported by findings of reduced immunoglobulin and complement levels [19].

Radiation and prior chemotherapy are additional known exposures directly linked to MDS development [19–21]. Chemotherapy-associated MDS has been associated with treatment using topoisomerase II inhibitors, anthracyclines, and alkylating agents. While topoisomerase II inhibitors and anthracyclines produce an earlier onset MDS within 1–3 years, typically with balanced genetic alterations often involving 11q23 (mixed lineage leukemia [MLL] gene) [22], these clonal disorders typically progress to and are more akin to acute leukemias. Conversely, alkylating agents yield a later onset, more traditional MDS within 5–10 years, with unbalanced chromosomal alterations often involving chromosomes 5 and 7 [23,24]. Radiation-induced MDS is associated with specific effects and chromosomal abnormalities similar to those seen with alkylating agent exposure [25]. Alkylator and radiation-induced MDS recapitulate the biology and clinical behavior of *de novo* MDS to a much greater extent than MLL-rearranged myeloid neoplasms, which happen to present with less than 20% blasts and are thus categorized as "MDS."

Cytogenetic alterations

A common end result of exposure to environmental toxins is DNA damage and the loss or alteration of gene expression; however, chromosomal abnormalities are often detected in patients with MDS in the absence of such exposures. Clonal chromosomal abnormalities are noted in 30–70% of patients with *de novo* MDS and in the majority (>80%) of treatment-related MDS (t-MDS), and remain the most powerful individual prognostic tool [26–29]. International Prognostic Scoring System (IPSS) cytogenetic risk stratifications include low risk (normal, isolated 5q or 20q), intermediate risk (trisomy 8, others), and high risk (abnormalities of 7 and complex) [26,27,30]. Recent retrospective observational reports now suggest a more refined description of cytogenetic risk profiles and are challenging some previously held beliefs [31]. Further prospective investigation will be needed to validate these findings in order to change practice. Interestingly, while specific cytogenetic abnormalities within MDS do not typically correlate with WHO or French–American–British (FAB) classifications, it is clear that there are characteristic syndromes, $5q^-$ and $17p^-$ syndromes [28,32], with unique clinical and prognostic outcomes. It is also clear that the frequency of cytogenetic abnormalities increases with the severity of disease.

The majority of the chromosomal abnormalities in *de novo* MDS involve unbalanced losses [26,29], suggesting the possible loss or inactivation of critical tumor-suppressor proteins. Until recently, investigating the commonly deleted segments (CDS) in 5q [33–38], 20q deletions [29,39–42], and monosomy 7 [43–45] revealed no specific gene losses of cell-cycle regulators or tumor-suppressor genes. However, recent reports have suggested that haploinsufficiency (mechanism whereby uniallelic inactivation leads to disease) of a specific gene, *RPS14*, encoding for a ribosomal protein may underlie the phenotypically described $5q^-$ syndrome [46]. Additionally, abnormalities in the 17p region include the other cytogenetic alteration linked to a known specific functional alteration—loss of tumor suppressor p53—and are noted in >70% of patients with this cytogenetic abnormality [39].

While few specific correlations between chromosomal loss and functional alteration are documented, numerous specific gene mutations are described. Recently reviewed by Pedersen-Bjergaard *et al.* [22], these alterations fall into two major classes. Class I alterations typically involve receptor tyrosine kinases or other genes that are downstream of the Ras-BRAF-MEK-ERK pathway and lead to continued cell cycling and proliferation. Class II alterations typically involve transcription factors, such as AML1 (RUNX1), EVI1, MLL, and lead to abnormal differentiation and increased self-renewal. The data would suggest that, in many cases, class II alterations are the primary event and class I alterations are a later event in MDS pathogenesis [47]. Runt-related transcription factor 1 (RUNX-1), also known as AML1, represents one example. Alterations in RUNX1, required for hematopoietic differentiation, while reported with a higher frequency in t-MDS (range 22–50%), have an incidence approximating 12% in primary MDS according to newer reports [48]. *RUNX1* mutations are also more prevalent in higher-grade MDS and are often associated with other alterations such as *NRAS* mutations, SOCS1 hypermethylation, and monosomy 7/7q, all of which have been linked with leukemic transformation and inferior overall survival [48].

Epigenetic alterations

In addition to structural chromosomal alterations documented in MDS, epigenetic modification through DNA methylation and post-translational histone modifications can lead to altered gene expression by way of gene silencing despite absence of mutation or deletion. The hypermethylation of cytosines in CpG dinucleotides in the promoter regions of numerous genes has been noted in MDS, with $p15^{INK4B}$ being one of the most studied [49,50]. $p15^{INK4B}$ can act as a tumor suppressor and inhibit cell-cycle progression from G1 to S phase by inhibiting CDK4/6. Hypermethylation prevents the suppressive function of $p15^{INK4B}$, allowing uncontrolled cell-cycle progression and proliferation [51]. $p15^{INK4B}$ hypermethylation has been noted in >50% of primary MDS, specifically high-risk MDS, and even higher rates have been found in t-MDS [50,52,53]. Given *p15*'s crucial role in normal granulocytic differentiation, numerous reports showing its hypermethylation in MDS, and work showing increased incidence of *p15* hypermethylation with advancing disease, highlight the likely importance of $p15^{INK4B}$ hypermethylation in the pathogenesis of MDS.

Hypermethylation of numerous other genes have been described in MDS pathogenesis: calcitonin gene, *SOCS1* (suppressor of cytokine signaling 1), *CDH1* (E-cadherin), and *HIC1* (hypermethylated in cancer 1). Calcitonin gene hypermethylation has been found in up to 65% of MDS cases, typically in those with normal cytogenetics [54], and is reported to be a possible marker of transformation from MDS to acute myeloid leukemia (AML) [55–57]. While hypermethylation of *SOCS1* has also been noted in up to 50% of patients with MDS, with a higher percentage in those with advanced disease, the presence of associated *NRAS* mutations is cited as the main factor promoting progression to AML [58]. Additionally, hypermethylated $p15^{INK4B}$, *CDH1*, and *HIC1* are associated with higher risk MDS, progression to AML, and poorer overall survival compared with unmethylated status with $p15^{INK4B}$ hypermethylation appearing to be the primary event [52]. More recently, tumor suppressors *RASSF1A* [59], associated with transcriptional regulation, and *RIL* [60], mapped to chromosome 5q31.1, have also shown hypermethylation in MDS, and may give further insight into pathogenesis. Conformational alterations of the DNA histone complex also play an important role in the abnormal gene silencing seen in many cancers, with acetylation status altering a number of cellular processes including transcription factors, nuclear-import proteins, signal-transduction proteins, DNA-repair enzymes, and heat-shock proteins [61–65]. These changes lead to altered expression of proapoptotic and cell-cycle proteins [65], potentially resulting in growth arrest, altered differentiation, and altered apoptosis [66,67].

Altered bone marrow microenvironment/apoptotic pathways

Bone marrow microenvironment alterations in the form of altered cytokine milieu, apoptosis rates, and changes in vascular microdensity have also been cited as central to MDS pathogenesis and produce a common pathway of increased apoptosis of $CD34^{+}$ progenitors in early stage MDS and decreased apoptosis in later-stage disease. As MDS progresses toward AML, these pathways become less defined and additional proliferative genetic events play a more important role [68–70].

TNF-α

Elevated tumor necrosis factor (TNF)-α levels are well described in MDS, leading to numerous cellular implications. A hallmark of MDS pathogenesis, apoptotic alterations are explained in part by altered cytokine levels. Specifically, increased apoptosis is mostly associated with early stage MDS (RA/RARS) and decreased apoptosis is more characteristic of advanced disease (RAEB2/AML) [68,70], with TNF-α playing a crucial role [68,71,72]. TNF-α alters apoptosis by engaging either TNF receptor (R) 1 or 2 (TNFRI or TNFRII). TNFRI engagement mediates apoptosis by direct binding with TNFR 1-associated protein with a death domain (TRADD), subsequent indirect binding with Fas-associated protein with a death domain (FADD), and terminal activation of the caspase cascade. Interaction with TNFRII leads to direct interaction with TNFR-associated factor 2 (TRAF-2) and subsequent activation of NF-κB and JNK, ultimately promoting antiapoptotic effects [71,73,74]. Given the differential effects of TNFRI and TNFRII stimulation, the ratio of these receptors impacts the rates of apoptosis: low-risk disease—increased TNFRI and increased apoptosis, and high-risk disease—increased TNFRII and decreased apoptosis leading to the potential for proliferative advantage and disease progression [71].

TNF-α overproduction in MDS may also lead to hematopoietic suppression through abnormal activation of the p38 MAPK pathway, which plays a role in apoptosis, transcription factor activation, transcriptional regulation, and subsequent activation of a downstream effector kinase of p38 named MSK1 (mitogen and stress activated kinase 1). MSK1 or p38 MAPK inhibitor studies revealed release of the hematopoietic suppression induced by these pathways and highlight that both play partial roles in the impaired hematopoiesis of MDS [75,76].

TNF-α levels may have a dual impact on MDS by means of contrary stimulatory and inhibitory effects:

stimulation of primitive progenitor cells, yielding the classic hypercellularity of MDS, in the setting of an apoptotic influence on more mature cells correlating with the peripheral cytopenias [77]. The etiology of these cytokine alterations, and defining the cells from which they originate (macrophages, fibroblasts, or other), remain unanswered questions [78–81].

NF-κB

NF-κB represents another cellular pathway altered in MDS. Functionally, NF-κB has numerous cellular effects, including regulation of inflammation, proliferation, angiogenesis, metastasis, and antiapoptosis via effects on cytokines, chemokines, apoptotic machinery, and adhesion molecules [82]. While NF-κB is required for normal immune function and inflammation, constitutive activation can lead to uncontrolled inflammation and potential tumorigenesis [82] with constitutive activation of NF-κB noted in MDS. NF-κB (p65) is upregulated in high-risk MDS, with the presence of p65 correlating with the percentage of blasts confined to the cells harboring MDS-related cytogenetic abnormality, and is associated with apoptosis suppression and disease progression [83]. Levels of NF-κB activation correlate with IPSS risk category with undetectable or attenuated levels in patients with low/INT-1 disease compared with constitutive activation in patients with INT-2/high-risk disease [83].

Fas/Bcl-2

Altered Fas and Bcl-2 pathways also contribute to apoptotic levels in MDS. Abnormal signals related to the Fas receptor have been described showing a TNF-like increased Fas expression in low-risk disease and decreased Fas expression in high-risk disease [84], with reports correlating increased expression with increased apoptosis [85]. While increased apoptosis is an important component in MDS pathogenesis (primarily in early stage disease), the mechanism is not explained by one pathway alone [68,69]. Conversely, the decreased apoptosis rates implicated in high-risk disease and progression to AML are linked with alterations in antiapoptotic machinery such as Bcl-2, Bcl-x, NF-κB , and Bax [68,69,83,85].

Bone marrow microenvironment: angiogenesis

The role of angiogenesis in hematologic malignancies is slowly being defined with the altered cytokine milieu in MDS, including a variety of angiogenic factors such as vascular endothelial growth factor (VEGF), basic fibroblast growth factor (bFGF), angiogenin, hepatic growth factor (HGF), epidermal growth factor (EGF), and transforming growth factor β (TGF-β). Coupled with the direct evidence of the increased microvascular density (MVD) documented in MDS marrow biopsies, these findings highlight the development of early blood vessels in MDS [86–89] with both plasma VEGF levels and increased MVD, correlating with advanced MDS FAB class [90–92]. These findings may simply represent an epiphenomenon in response to cytokine alterations, or may represent a true process important for pathogenesis.

Altered immune surveillance

B- and T-cell alterations

The role of immune dysregulation in the pathogenesis of MDS is evident from the clinical responses to immune-modulating drugs (cyclosporine [CSA], antithymocyte globulin [ATG]) as well as the potential curative effects with allogeneic bone marrow transplantation. Much of the previous attention on immune dysregulation has been focused on B- and T-cell abnormalities noted in MDS citing increased correlations with autoimmune disorders [93,94] and notable findings of V-β and J region skewing in oligoclonal T-cell populations, suggestive of chronic antigenic stimulation [95–97] as potential contributors to disease.

Natural killer-cell alterations

More recently, alterations in natural killer (NK)-cell mediated killing have been described in patients with MDS. NK cells house a number of both activating and inhibitory receptors that mediate their cytotoxicity. Natural cytotoxicity receptors (NCRs) NKp46 and NKp30, as well as activating receptor NKG2D, are constitutively active receptors, which, in balance with a number of both activating and inhibitory KIRs (killer-cell inhibitory receptors), mediate NK cell-mediated cytotoxicty.

Two groups have investigated the role of NK-cell function in MDS, with alternative suggestions explaining the etiology of diminished NK-cell cytolytic activity. Kiladjian *et al.* showed that, despite normal numbers of NK cells and activating receptors NKp46, NKp30, and NKG2D, both cytolytic function and response to IL-2 stimulation are diminished [98], raising the possibility of soluble or humoral factors affecting cytotoxicity. Alternatively, Epling-Burnette's group [99], while again finding normal numbers of NK cells, noted that MDS NK cells fell into two categories of cytotoxicity: low function and normal function. The low-function NK group was most notably present in the patients with high-risk MDS: (i) INT2 or high risk by IPSS, (ii) those with abnormal cytogenetics, and (iii) those in the RAEB-1, RAEB-2, and AML by WHO categories. Additionally, they noted decreased activating receptors NKp30 and NKG2D in patients with MDS with only NKG2D alterations correlating with decreased cytotoxicity. Epling-Burnette's group evaluated for soluble MICA and MICB (the ligands for NKG2D) as the cause of decreased NK cell cytotoxicity and found no evidence.

Additionally, in contrast to Kiladjian's reports, Epling-Burnette found that IL-2 treatment was able to increase the presence of the activating receptors and increase NK cell-mediated cytotoxicity. In summary, the data for NK-cell alterations in MDS reveal discrepant results citing either soluble/humoral factors [98] versus decreased activating receptors (NKp30, NKp46, NKG2D), with NKG2D the primary effector [99] leading to decreased NK-cell cytotoxicity. Further work is required to substantiate and characterize the NK-cell changes inherent to MDS.

Altered cellular functions/aberrant differentiation

Abnormal differentiation and altered growth characteristics represent the dominant morphologic features of MDS. Exhaustive analysis of cellular signaling pathways to define the key abnormalities in differentiation has led to the finding that this process is linked to studies of the cell cycle. Specifically, the cell's ability to initiate normal cellular division, the speed of the cell cycle, and regulation of cell-cycle checkpoints, are all required for normal differentiation, proliferation, and self-renewal. As described in the sections above, numerous cytogenetic, epigenetic, and molecular abnormalities have been noted in the cell-cycle machinery within MDS and contribute to the structural (dysplastic cells) and functional (impaired granulocytic function leading to increased infections) abnormalities that define MDS.

References

1 Gerritsen WR, Donohue J, Bauman J, *et al.* Clonal analysis of myelodysplastic syndrome: monosomy 7 is expressed in the myeloid lineage, but not in the lymphoid lineage as detected by fluorescent in situ hybridization. *Blood* 1992;80:217–24.

2 Kibbelaar RE, van Kamp H, Dreef EJ, *et al.* Combined immunophenotyping and DNA in situ hybridization to study lineage involvement in patients with myelodysplastic syndromes. *Blood* 1992;79:1823–8.

3 Kroef MJ, Fibbe WE, Mout R, *et al.* Myeloid but not lymphoid cells carry the 5q deletion: polymerase chain reaction analysis of loss of heterozygosity using mini-repeat sequences on highly purified cell fractions. *Blood* 1993;81:1849–54.

4 Saitoh K, Miura I, Takahashi N, Miura AB. Fluorescence in situ hybridization of progenitor cells obtained by fluorescence-activated cell sorting for the detection of cells affected by chromosome abnormality trisomy 8 in patients with myelodysplastic syndromes. *Blood* 1998;92:2886–92.

5 Nilsson L, Astrand-Grundstrom I, Arvidsson I, *et al.* Isolation and characterization of hematopoietic progenitor/stem cells in 5q-deleted myelodysplastic syndromes: evidence for involvement at the hematopoietic stem cell level. *Blood* 2000;96:2012–21.

6 Nilsson L, Astrand-Grundstrom I, Anderson K, *et al.* Involvement and functional impairment of the CD34(+)CD38(−) Thy-1(+) hematopoietic stem cell pool in myelodysplastic syndromes with trisomy 8. *Blood* 2002;100:259–67.

7 Nilsson L, Eden P, Olsson E, *et al.* The molecular signature of MDS stem cells supports a stem-cell origin of 5q myelodysplastic syndromes. *Blood* 2007;110:3005–14.

8 Pasqualetti P, Festuccia V, Acitelli P, Collacciani A, Giusti A, Casale R. Tobacco smoking and risk of haematological malignancies in adults: a case–control study. *Br J Haematol* 1997; 97:659–62.

9 Ido M, Nagata C, Kawakami N, *et al.* A case–control study of myelodysplastic syndromes among Japanese men and women. *Leuk Res* 1996;20:727–31.

10 Mundle S, Allampallam K, Aftab Rashid K, *et al.* Presence of activation-related m-RNA for EBV and CMV in the bone marrow of patients with myelodysplastic syndromes. *Cancer Lett* 2001;164:197–205.

11 Dalamaga M, Petridou E, Cook FE, Trichopoulos D. Risk factors for myelodysplastic syndromes: a case–control study in Greece. *Cancer Causes Control* 2002;13:603–8.

12 Kuang S, Liang W. Clinical analysis of 43 cases of chronic benzene poisoning. *Chem Biol Interact* 2005; 129–35:153–4.

13 Aksoy M, Dincol K, Erdem S, Dincol G. Acute leukemia due to chronic exposure to benzene. *Am J Med* 1972;52:160–6.

14 Yin SN, Hayes RB, Linet MS, *et al.* A cohort study of cancer among benzene-exposed workers in China: overall results. *Am J Ind Med* 1996;29:227–35.

15 Hiraku Y, Kawanishi S. Oxidative DNA damage and apoptosis induced by benzene metabolites. *Cancer Res* 1996;56:5172–8.

16 Yardley-Jones A, Anderson D, Parke DV. The toxicity of benzene and its metabolism and molecular pathology in human risk assessment. *Br J Ind Med* 1991;48:437–44.

17 Smith MT. The mechanism of benzene-induced leukemia: a hypothesis and speculations on the causes of leukemia. *Environ Health Perspect* 1996;104(Suppl. 6):1219–25.

18 Rothman N, Haas R, Hayes RB, *et al.* Benzene induces gene-duplicating but not gene-inactivating mutations at the glycophorin A locus in exposed humans. *Proc Natl Acad Sci U S A* 1995;92:4069–73.

19 Aul C, Bowen DT, Yoshida Y. Pathogenesis, etiology and epidemiology of myelodysplastic syndromes. *Haematologica* 1998; 83:71–86.

20 Catenacci DV, Schiller GJ. Myelodysplasic syndromes: a comprehensive review. *Blood Rev* 2005;19:301–19.

21 Mufti GJ. Pathobiology, classification, and diagnosis of myelodysplastic syndrome. *Best Pract Res Clin Haematol* 2004;17:543–57.

22 Pedersen-Bjergaard J, Philip P, Larsen SO, *et al.* Therapy-related myelodysplasia and acute myeloid leukemia. Cytogenetic characteristics of 115 consecutive cases and risk in seven cohorts of patients treated intensively for malignant diseases in the Copenhagen series. *Leukemia* 1993;7:1975–86.

23 Rund D, Ben-Yehuda D. Therapy-related leukemia and myelodysplasia: evolving concepts of pathogenesis and treatment. *Hematology* 2004;9:179–87.

24 Pedersen-Bjergaard J, Andersen MK, Christiansen DH, Nerlov C. Genetic pathways in therapy-related myelodysplasia and acute myeloid leukemia. *Blood* 2002;99:1909–12.

25 Moloney WC. Radiogenic leukemia revisited. *Blood* 1987;70: 905–8.

26 Hirai H. Molecular mechanisms of myelodysplastic syndrome. *Jpn J Clin Oncol* 2003;33:153–60.

27 Look AT. Molecular Pathogenesis of MDS. *Hematology Am Soc Hematol Educ Program* 2005:156–60.

28 Nimer SD. Clinical management of myelodysplastic syndromes with interstitial deletion of chromosome 5q. *J Clin Oncol* 2006 Jun;24:2576–82.

29 Olney HJ, Le Beau MM. The cytogenetics of myelodysplastic syndromes. *Best Pract Res Clin Haematol* 2001;14:479–95.

30 Greenberg P, Cox C, LeBeau MM, *et al.* International scoring system for evaluating prognosis in myelodysplastic syndromes. *Blood* 1997;89:2079–88.

31 Haase D, Germing U, Schanz J, *et al.* New insights into the prognostic impact of the karyotype in MDS and correlation with subtypes: evidence from a core dataset of 2124 patients. *Blood* 2007;110:4385–95.

32 Jary L, Mossafa H, Fourcade C, Genet P, Pulik M, Flandrin G. The 17p-syndrome:a distinct myelodysplastic syndrome entity? *Leuk Lymphoma* 1997;25:163–8.

33 Fairman J, Chumakov I, Chinault AC, Nowell PC, Nagarajan L. Physical mapping of the minimal region of loss in 5q- chromosome. *Proc Natl Acad Sci U S A* 1995;92: 7406–10.

34 Zhao N, Stoffel A, Wang PW, *et al.* Molecular delineation of the smallest commonly deleted region of chromosome 5 in malignant myeloid diseases to 1–1.5 Mb and preparation of a PAC-based physical map. *Proc Natl Acad Sci U S A* 1997;94: 6948–53.

35 Jaju RJ, Boultwood J, Oliver FJ, *et al.* Molecular cytogenetic delineation of the critical deleted region in the 5q- syndrome. *Genes Chromosomes Cancer* 1998;22:251–6.

36 Horrigan SK, Arbieva ZH, Xie HY, *et al.* Delineation of a minimal interval and identification of 9 candidates for a tumor suppressor gene in malignant myeloid disorders on 5q31. *Blood* 2000;95:2372–7.

37 Le Beau MM, Espinosa R, 3rd, Neuman WL, *et al.* Cytogenetic and molecular delineation of the smallest commonly deleted region of chromosome 5 in malignant myeloid diseases. *Proc Natl Acad Sci U S A* 1993;90:5484–8.

38 Boultwood J, Fidler C, Strickson AJ, *et al.* Transcription mapping of the 5q- syndrome critical region: cloning of two novel genes and sequencing, expression, and mapping of a further six novel cDNAs. *Genomics* 2000 15;66:26–34.

39 Vallespi T, Imbert M, Mecucci C, Preudhomme C, Fenaux P. Diagnosis, classification, and cytogenetics of myelodysplastic syndromes. *Haematologica* 1998;83:258–75.

40 Wattel E, Lai JL, Hebbar M, *et al.* De novo myelodysplastic syndrome (MDS) with deletion of the long arm of chromosome 20:a subtype of MDS with distinct hematological and prognostic features? *Leuk Res* 1993;17:921–6.

41 Davis MP, Dewald GW, Pierre RV, Hoagland HC. Hematologic manifestations associated with deletions of the long arm of chromosome 20. *Cancer Genet Cytogenet* 1984;12:63–71.

42 Asimakopoulos FA, Green AR. Deletions of chromosome 20q and the pathogenesis of myeloproliferative disorders. *Br J Haematol* 1996;95:219–26.

43 Liang H, Fairman J, Claxton DF, Nowell PC, Green ED, Nagarajan L. Molecular anatomy of chromosome 7q deletions in myeloid neoplasms: evidence for multiple critical loci. *Proc Natl Acad Sci U S A* 1998;95:3781–5.

44 Pasquali F, Bernasconi P, Casalone R, *et al.* Pathogenetic significance of "pure" monosomy 7 in myeloproliferative disorders. Analysis of 14 cases. *Hum Genet* 1982;62:40–51.

45 Le Beau MM, Espinosa R, 3rd, Davis EM, Eisenbart JD, Larson RA, Green ED. Cytogenetic and molecular delineation of a region of chromosome 7 commonly deleted in malignant myeloid diseases. *Blood* 1996;88:1930–5.

46 Ebert BL, Pretz J, Bosco J, *et al.* Identification of RPS14 as a 5q- syndrome gene by RNA interference screen. *Nature* 2008;451:335–9.

47 Pedersen-Bjergaard J, Andersen MK, Andersen MT, Christiansen DH. Genetics of therapy-related myelodysplasia and acute myeloid leukemia. *Leukemia* 2008;22:240–8.

48 Chen CY, Lin LI, Tang JL, *et al.* *RUNX1* gene mutation in primary myelodysplastic syndrome–the mutation can be detected early at diagnosis or acquired during disease progression and is associated with poor outcome. *Br J Haematol* 2007;139:405–14.

49 Herman JG, Civin CI, Issa JP, Collector MI, Sharkis SJ, Baylin SB. Distinct patterns of inactivation of *p15INK4B* and *p16INK4A* characterize the major types of hematological malignancies. *Cancer Res* 1997;57:837–41.

50 Quesnel B, Guillerm G, Vereecque R, *et al.* Methylation of the *p15(INK4b)* gene in myelodysplastic syndromes is frequent and acquired during disease progression. *Blood* 1998;91: 2985–90.

51 Leone G, Teofili L, Voso MT, Lubbert M. DNA methylation and demethylating drugs in myelodysplastic syndromes and secondary leukemias. *Haematologica* 2002;87:1324–41.

52 Aggerholm A, Holm MS, Guldberg P, Olesen LH, Hokland P. Promoter hypermethylation of p15INK4B, HIC1, CDH1, and ER is frequent in myelodysplastic syndrome and predicts poor prognosis in early-stage patients. *Eur J Haematol* 2006;76: 23–32.

53 Christiansen DH, Andersen MK, Pedersen-Bjergaard J. Methylation of p15INK4B is common, is associated with deletion of genes on chromosome arm 7q and predicts a poor prognosis in therapy-related myelodysplasia and acute myeloid leukemia. *Leukemia* 2003;17:1813–19.

54 Dhodapkar M, Grill J, Lust JA. Abnormal regional hypermethylation of the calcitonin gene in myelodysplastic syndromes. *Leuk Res* 1995;19:719–26.

55 Wu S, Xie G, Bai R, Wang Y, Zhu P. Semi-quantitative study of calcitonin gene methylation in myelodysplastic syndrome. *Chin Med J (Engl)* 1998;111:690–3.

56 Bai R, Wu S, Zhu P, Xue H, Xu Y, Qin X. Quantitative study of calcitonin gene methylation in myelodysplastic syndromes. *Zhonghua Xue Ye Xue Za Zhi* 1997;18:17–20.

57 Li G, Zou D, Bai R. Clinical significance of human calcitonin and gene-related peptide in the serum of myelodysplastic syndromes patients. *Zhonghua Xue Ye Xue Za Zhi* 1999;20:79–81.

58 Wu SJ, Yao M, Chou WC, *et al.* Clinical implications of SOCS1 methylation in myelodysplastic syndrome. *Br J Haematol* 2006;135:317–23.

59 Johan MF, Bowen DT, Frew ME, Goodeve AC, Reilly JT. Aberrant methylation of the negative regulators RASSFIA, SHP-1 and SOCS-1 in myelodysplastic syndromes and acute myeloid leukemia. *Br J Haematol* 2005;129:60–5.

60 Boumber YA, Kondo Y, Chen X, *et al.* RIL, a LIM gene on 5q31, is silenced by methylation in cancer and sensitizes cancer cells to apoptosis. *Cancer Res* 2007;67:1997–2005.

61 Haggarty SJ, Koeller KM, Wong JC, Grozinger CM, Schreiber SL. Domain-selective small-molecule inhibitor of histone deacetylase 6 (HDAC6)-mediated tubulin deacetylation. *Proc Natl Acad Sci U S A* 2003;100:4389–94.

62 Wolf D, Rodova M, Miska EA, Calvet JP, Kouzarides T. Acetylation of beta-catenin by CREB-binding protein (CBP). *J Biol Chem* 2002;277:25562–7.

63 Bannister AJ, Miska EA, Gorlich D, Kouzarides T. Acetylation of importin-alpha nuclear import factors by CBP/p300. *Curr Biol* 2000;10:467–70.

64 Cohen HY, Lavu S, Bitterman KJ, *et al.* Acetylation of the C terminus of Ku70 by CBP and PCAF controls Bax-mediated apoptosis. *Mol Cell* 2004;13:627–38.

65 Morgan MA, Reuter CW. Molecularly targeted therapies in myelodysplastic syndromes and acute myeloid *leukemias*. *Ann Hematol* 2006;85:139–63.

66 Marks P, Rifkind RA, Richon VM, Breslow R, Miller T, Kelly WK. Histone deacetylases and cancer: causes and therapies. *Nat Rev Cancer* 2001;1:194–202.

67 Johnstone RW, Licht JD. Histone deacetylase inhibitors in cancer therapy: is transcription the primary target? *Cancer Cell* 2003;4:13–18.

68 Parker JE, Mufti GJ. Ineffective haemopoiesis and apoptosis in myelodysplastic syndromes. *Br J Haematol* 1998;101:220–30.

69 Parker JE, Mufti GJ, Rasool F, Mijovic A, Devereux S, Pagliuca A. The role of apoptosis, proliferation, and the Bcl-2-related proteins in the myelodysplastic syndromes and acute myeloid leukemia secondary to MDS. *Blood* 2000;96:3932–8.

70 Rajapaksa R, Ginzton N, Rott LS, Greenberg PL. Altered oncoprotein expression and apoptosis in myelodysplastic syndrome marrow cells. *Blood* 1996;88:4275–87.

71 Sawanobori M, Yamaguchi S, Hasegawa M, *et al.* Expression of TNF receptors and related signaling molecules in the bone marrow from patients with myelodysplastic syndromes. *Leuk Res* 2003;27:583–91.

72 Kitagawa M, Saito I, Kuwata T, *et al.* Overexpression of tumor necrosis factor (TNF)-alpha and interferon (IFN)-gamma by bone marrow cells from patients with myelodysplastic syndromes. *Leukemia* 1997;11:2049–54.

73 Hsu H, Huang J, Shu HB, Baichwal V, Goeddel DV. TNF-dependent recruitment of the protein kinase RIP to the TNF receptor-1 signaling complex. *Immunity* 1996;4:387–96.

74 Hsu H, Xiong J, Goeddel DV. The TNF receptor 1-associated protein TRADD signals cell death and NF-kappa B activation. *Cell* 1995;81:495–504.

75 Katsoulidis E, Li Y, Yoon P, *et al.* Role of the p38 mitogen-activated protein kinase pathway in cytokine-mediated hematopoietic suppression in myelodysplastic syndromes. *Cancer Res* 2005;65:9029–37.

76 Navas TA, Mohindru M, Estes M, *et al.* Inhibition of overactivated p38 MAPK can restore hematopoiesis in myelodysplastic syndrome progenitors. *Blood* 2006;108:4170–7.

77 Raza A, Mundle S, Shetty V, *et al.* Novel insights into the biology of myelodysplastic syndromes: excessive apoptosis and the role of cytokines. *Int J Hematol* 1996;63:265–78.

78 Flores-Figueroa E, Gutierrez-Espindola G, Montesinos JJ, Arana-Trejo RM, Mayani H. *In vitro* characterization of hematopoietic microenvironment cells from patients with myelodysplastic syndrome. *Leuk Res* 2002;26:677–86.

79 Wetzler M, Kurzrock R, Estrov Z, Estey E, Talpaz M. Cytokine expression in adherent layers from patients with myelodysplastic syndrome and acute myelogenous leukemia. *Leuk Res* 1995;19:23–34.

80 Deeg HJ, Beckham C, Loken MR, *et al.* Negative regulators of hemopoiesis and stroma function in patients with myelodysplastic syndrome. *Leuk Lymphoma* 2000;37: 405–14.

81 Koike M, Ishiyama T, Tomoyasu S, Tsuruoka N. Spontaneous cytokine overproduction by peripheral blood mononuclear cells from patients with myelodysplastic syndromes and aplastic anemia. *Leuk Res* 1995;19:639–44.

82 Aggarwal BB. Nuclear factor-kappaB: the enemy within. *Cancer Cell* 2004;6:203–8.

83 Braun T, Carvalho G, Coquelle A, *et al.* NF-kappaB constitutes a potential therapeutic target in high-risk myelodysplastic syndrome. *Blood* 2006;107:1156–65.

84 Bouscary D, De Vos J, Guesnu M, *et al.* Fas/Apo-1 (CD95) expression and apoptosis in patients with myelodysplastic syndromes. *Leukemia* 1997;11:839–45.

85 Claessens YE, Bouscary D, Dupont JM, *et al.* *In vitro* proliferation and differentiation of erythroid progenitors from patients with myelodysplastic syndromes: evidence for Fas-dependent apoptosis. *Blood* 2002;99:1594–601.

86 Estey EH. Modulation of angiogenesis in patients with myelodysplastic syndrome. *Best Pract Res Clin Haematol* 2004;17: 623–39.

87 Aguayo A, Kantarjian H, Manshouri T, *et al.* Angiogenesis in acute and chronic leukemias and myelodysplastic syndromes. *Blood* 2000;96:2240–5.

88 Brunner B, Gunsilius E, Schumacher P, Zwierzina H, Gastl G, Stauder R. Blood levels of angiogenin and vascular endothelial growth factor are elevated in myelodysplastic syndromes and in acute myeloid leukemia. *J Hematother Stem Cell Res* 2002;11:119–25.

89 Zorat F, Shetty V, Dutt D, *et al.* The clinical and biological effects of thalidomide in patients with myelodysplastic syndromes. *Br J Haematol* 2001;115:881–94.

90 Wimazal F, Krauth MT, Vales A, *et al.* Immunohistochemical detection of vascular endothelial growth factor (VEGF) in the bone marrow in patients with myelodysplastic syndromes: correlation between VEGF expression and the FAB category. *Leuk Lymphoma* 2006;47:451–60.

91 Pruneri G, Bertolini F, Soligo D, *et al.* Angiogenesis in myelodysplastic syndromes. *Br J Cancer* 1999;81:1398–401.

92 Korkolopoulou P, Apostolidou E, Pavlopoulos PM, *et al.* Prognostic evaluation of the microvascular network in myelodysplastic syndromes. *Leukemia* 2001;15:1369–76.

93 Marisavljevic D, Kraguljac N, Rolovic Z. Immunologic abnormalities in myelodysplastic syndromes: clinical features and characteristics of the lymphoid population. *Med Oncol* 2006;23:385–92.

94 Billstrom R, Johansson H, Johansson B, Mitelman F. Immune-mediated complications in patients with myelodysplastic syndromes–clinical and cytogenetic features. *Eur J Haematol* 1995;55:42–8.

95 Epperson DE, Nakamura R, Saunthararajah Y, Melenhorst J, Barrett AJ. Oligoclonal T cell expansion in myelodysplastic syn-

drome: evidence for an autoimmune process. *Leuk Res* 2001;25:1075–83.

96 Molldrem JJ, Jiang YZ, Stetler-Stevenson M, Mavroudis D, Hensel N, Barrett AJ. Haematological response of patients with myelodysplastic syndrome to antithymocyte globulin is associated with a loss of lymphocyte-mediated inhibition of CFU-GM and alterations in T-cell receptor Vbeta profiles. *Br J Haematol* 1998;102:1314–22.

97 Melenhorst JJ, Eniafe R, Follmann D, Nakamura R, Kirby M, Barrett AJ. Molecular and flow cytometric characterization of the CD4 and CD8 T-cell repertoire in patients with myelodysplastic syndrome. *Br J Haematol* 2002;119:97–105.

98 Kiladjian JJ, Bourgeois E, Lobe I, *et al.* Cytolytic function and survival of natural killer cells are severely altered in myelodysplastic syndromes. *Leukemia* 2006;20:463–70.

99 Epling-Burnette PK, Bai F, Painter JS, *et al.* Reduced natural killer (NK) function associated with high-risk myelodysplastic syndrome (MDS) and reduced expression of activating NK receptors. *Blood* 2007;109:4816–24.

(a)

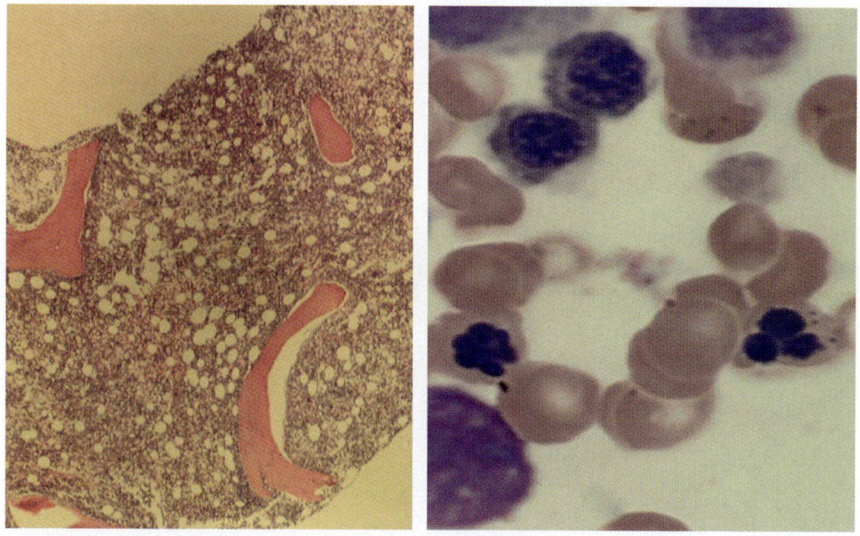

(b)

Plate 8.1 Morphologic features of MDS. (a) The bone marrow biopsy is hypercellular, reflecting ineffective hematopoiesis. (b) Erythroid cells in the bone-marrow aspirate are dysplastic with marked nuclear abnormalities present.

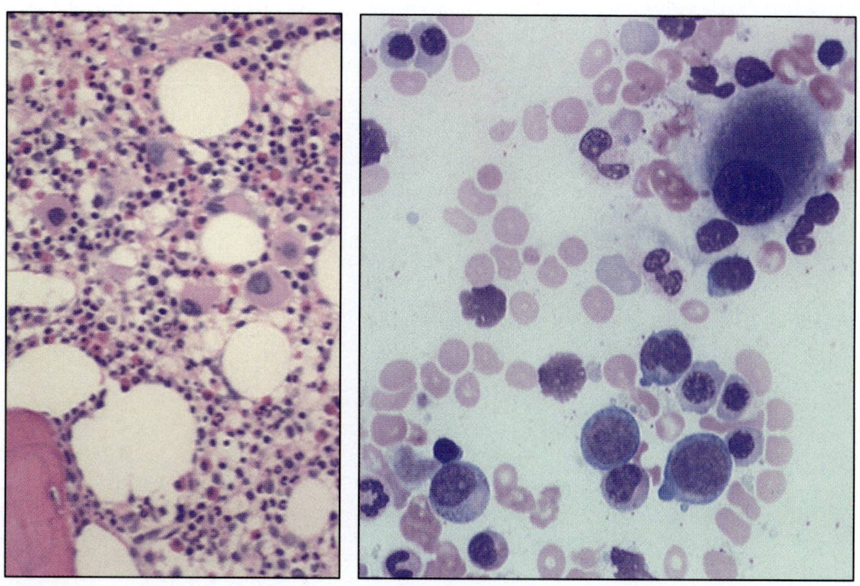

Plate 8.2 Morphologic appearance of a bone marrow specimen of a patient with $5q^-$ syndrome.

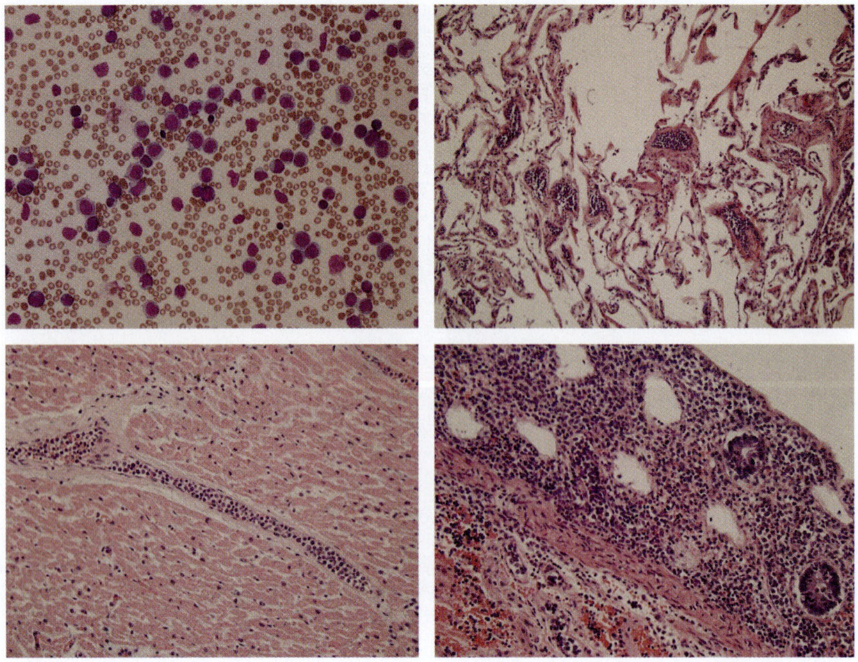

(a) (b) (c) (d)

Plate 31.1 Diffuse infiltration of the parenchyma and vasculature of various organs of a patient presenting with M5 acute myeloid leukemia, presenting with hyperleukocytosis (white blood cell count 116,000/μL) and leukostasis. (a) Peripheral smear demonstrating a high number of myeloid blasts. (b) Lung parenchyma. (c) Left ventricle. (d) Intestine.

Chapter 7
Myelodysplastic Syndromes: The Role of Cytogenetic and Molecular Abnormalities for Classification and Risk Assignment

Ulrich Germing
Heinrich-Heine-University, Düsseldorf, Germany

Introduction

Myelodysplastic syndromes (MDS) belong to the most frequent hematologic disorders, especially in elderly people [1]. Owing to the heterogeneity of the clinical presentation and course of the disease, it is necessary to separate the different types of MDS. The classification and prognostication of MDS is still mainly based on traditional hematologic and morphologic features [2–4], and chromosomal analyses are increasingly used in the diagnostic work-up in patients with MDS. Clonal karyotypic abnormalities are found in about 50% of patients [5–7]. Even more frequent are chromosomal aberrations in treatment-related MDS [8]. However, chromosomal findings are not only useful with regard to diagnosis, but also play a major role in classification, prognostication, and, with growing evidence, in clinical decision making. In contrast to chromosomal examinations, molecular findings have not yet been introduced into clinical procedures. However, there are some molecular findings that also might be helpful with regard to diagnosis and classification. This chapter gives an overview on the different aspects of karyotyping in MDS, illustrating that this technique should be performed in virtually every patient with MDS and highlighting the potential role of molecular examinations in a subset of patients. Beginning with the role of chromosomal and molecular findings with regard to diagnosis, conclusions on classification are discussed later on, followed by a description on how molecular and chromosomal findings can be used in prognostication. Finally, the possible role of molecular and chromosomal findings in clinical decision making and clinical practice is presented.

Leukemias: Principles and Practice of Therapy, 1st edition. Edited by S. Faderl and H. Kantarjian.

Diagnosis and classification

Chromosomal aberrations probably are late events in the pathogenesis of MDS, reflecting the progressive genomic instability of the dysplastic premalignant clone. Although it has not been possible to identify genetic lesions specific to MDS, anomalies are non-random changes, as the majority of the changes are characterized by loss or gain of chromosomal material. This fact has led to the hypothesis that loss of tumor-suppressor genes or specific regulatory genes of hematopoietic cell proliferation and differentiation may cause malignant transformation of stem cells in MDS [9].

Although the diagnosis of MDS still is primarily based on morphologic features in blood and bone marrow, including dysplastic signs and the presence of blasts, cytogenetic findings may influence the diagnostic work-up in patients with MDS. Table 7.1 shows the current World Health Organization (WHO) classification [10]. The WHO classification has been validated by means of different independent patient samples [11,12]. Strictly speaking, an examination of the chromosomes should be performed in every single patient to allow for the correct use of the WHO classification. Although the vast majority of patients can be diagnosed without cytogenetics, karyotyping is strongly recommended in order to avoid missing patients with MDS and del(5q).

The diagnostic procedure in patients with refractory anemia (RA) is often complicated by the fact that the dysplastic features are not only restricted to erythropoiesis, but may also only be subtle. This is the reason why, in some cases, the diagnosis of RA cannot be made without showing clonality by means of cytogenetics or molecular findings. Very recently, the category of these patients showing RA not secondary to other conditions has been defined more exactly and named idiopathic cytopenia of unknown significance (ICUS) [Mufti, personal communication; 13]. This term should only be used if there are no

Table 7.1 Definition of types of myelodysplastic syndromes and mixed myelodysplastic/myeloproliferative neoplasms according to the World Health Organization proposals.

Type	Blood	Marrow
Refractory cytopenia (RC) Refractory granulocytopenia Refractory thrombocytopenia Refractory anemia	≤1% blasts	<5% blasts Dyserythropoiesis only <15% ringed sideroblasts
Refractory anemia with ringed sideroblasts (RARS)	≤1% blasts	<5% blasts Dyserythropoiesis only ≥15% ringed sideroblasts
Refractory cytopenia with multilineage dysplasia (RCMD) with or without ringed sideroblasts	≤1% blasts <1000/μL monocytes	<5% blasts Dysplasia in >10% of other cell lines >/<15 ringed sideroblasts No single del(5q) No Auer rods
Myelodysplastic syndromes (MDS) unclassifiable MDS-U	Rare blasts	<5% blasts No Auer rods Dysplasia in one myeloid cell line
Refractory anemia with excess of blasts I (RAEB I)	Cytopenia <5% blasts No Auer rods <1000/μL monocytes	Unilineage or multilineage dysplasia 5–9% blasts No Auer rods
Refractory anemia with excess of blasts II (RAEB II)	Cytopenia <19% blasts Auer rods + or – <1000/μL monocytes	Unilineage or multilineage dysplasia 10–19% blasts Auer rods + or –
Chronic myelomonocytic leukemia I (CMML I)	<5% blasts ≥1000/μL monocytes	<10% blasts Dysplasia in 1–2 cell lines No t(9;22) No *BCR–ABL*
Chronic myelomonocytic leukemia II (CMML II)	<20% blasts ≥1000/μL monocytes	<20% blasts Dysplasia in 1–2 cell lines No t(9;22) No *BCR–ABL*
Refractory anemia with ringed sideroblasts and thrombocytosis (RARS-T)	<1% blasts	<5% blasts Dysplasia of 1–3 cell lines ≥15% ringed sideroblasts platelets >450.000/μl

chromosomal aberrations and no molecular findings indicating that clonality has been seen. Clonality shown by the human androgen receptor (HUMARA) also can be used to confirm the diagnosis of a real MDS RA and therefore can serve as a molecular classification tool [14].

In some cases it is not easy to distinguish between unilineage and multilineage dysplasia by means of morphology. There is evidence for the fact that *RAS* mutations are not present on unilineage dysplastic patients but can be seen in some multilineage dysplastic patients [15].

Recently, a category of mixed myeloproliferative/myelodysplastic neoplasms has been defined by the WHO (Table 7.1) [16]. Cytogenetic and molecular examinations are absolutely essential for the correct use of this category, as the subtypes often harbor specific molecular features that help to identify the patients. There are some prerequisites to classify a patient into this group. In order to distinguish chronic myelomonocytic leukemia (CMML) from chronic myeloid leukemia (CML), all patients should be screened for *BCR–ABL*, as the presence of this abnormality automatically leads to the diagnosis of CML. Going beyond this exclusion parameter, there are two other molecular abnormalities which should be looked for in order to characterize the biology of the disease as precisely as possible. The group of patients with CMML sometimes harbors mutations of platelet-derived growth factor receptor (PDGFR) α or β. These findings are typical for a small subset of patients and may have consequences for treatment with regard to the use of imatinib. Another entity within the mixed myeloproliferative/myelodysplastic neoplasms is the group of RA with ringed sideroblasts with thrombocytosis (RARS-T) (Table 7.1), which is characterized by morphologic features resembling essential thrombocythemia with hyperplasia of megakaryopoiesis, the presence of ringed sideroblasts, and platelet counts of >600.000/μL. Recently, several groups could show that the vast majority of these patients harbor mutations of *Jak2* (V617F) [17–19]. Recent studies showed that RARS-T is not related to overexpression of c-Mpl [18,19]. Taken together with screening for *BCR–ABL*, PDGFR-α or -β and *JAK2* mutations are mandatory for classification reasons.

Risk assessment

Risk assessment in patients with MDS is mainly based on features characterizing the biology of the disease, although the biology of the patient, particularly their age, also substantially influences the prognosis. The reason for this is the lack of high-quality data on comorbidity in MDS. In the last decades, numerous factors influencing the expected survival and the risk of acute myeloid leukemia (AML) progression have been identified, such as cell counts in blood, medullary blast counts, lactate dehydrogenase (LDH) values, degree of dysplasia, and cytogenetic findings (Figure 7.1). Regarding the last two, some typical chromosomal aberrations are clearly associated with a distinct prognostic pattern.

On the one hand, there is an extreme variability in cytogenetic findings in MDS, and there are no pathognomonic cytogenetic findings. On the other hand, every chromosome can show aberrations either alone or in combination with other chromosomal abnormalities. However, there are some chromosomes that are more frequently involved than others regarding MDS. The most common cytogenetic abnormalities in MDS are del(5q), monosomy 7/del(7q), and trisomy 8, which account for more than 60% of cases with abnormal metaphases [20]. Other recurrent anomalies are translocations involving 1q, rearrangements of 3q, del(11q23), del(12p), deletions of 17p, isochromosome 17q, del(20q), trisomy 21, monosomy 21, and loss of Y chromosomes. The MDS del(5q) anomaly is associated with characteristic hematologic and morphologic findings and was first described by van den Berghe *et al.* [21]. It preferentially occurs in female patients and is associated with macrocytic anemia, normal or elevated platelet counts, erythroid hypoplasia, and a presence of hypolobulated megakaryocytes in the bone marrow. These characteristics have prompted the WHO group to define it as a separate entity. It has since become clear that patients belonging to this category also have typical prognostic features and high response rates to lenalidomide [22–24]. In addition, Giagounidis *et al.* [25] demonstrated that as soon as a del(5q) anomaly occurs within a complex karyotype, or medullary blasts increase, the prognosis worsens.

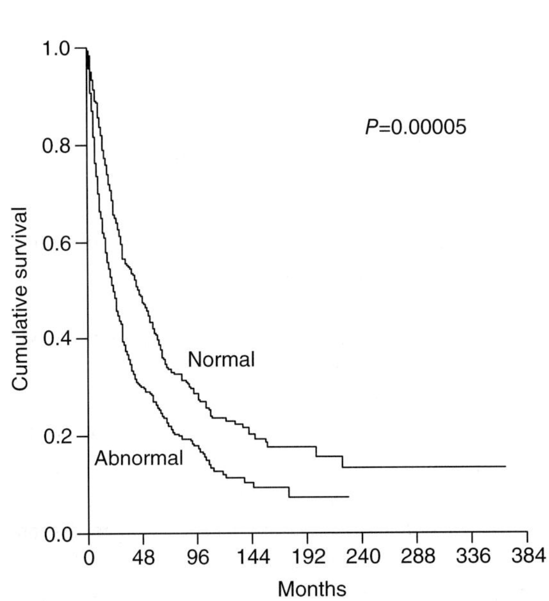

Figure 7.1 Impact of cytogenetic abnormalities on survival (n = 825).

Complex aberrations, involving three or more chromosomes and often involving chromosomes 5 and 7, are three times as frequent in therapy-related MDS as in primary MDS [26,27]. Other unfavorable findings, such as monosomy 7, also occur more frequently in secondary MDS than in primary MDS [28]. The presence of rearrangements typical of AML, such as t(8;21), inv(16), or t(15;17), nowadays defines a patient as having AML [4] even if the medullary and/or peripheral blast count is not significantly increased. As the frequency of chromosomal abnormalities generally increases with progression of MDS (Table 7.2), it has long been questioned whether the karyotype constitutes an independent prognostic factor for survival and leukemic transformation. Various studies could show that chromosomal analysis adds independent prognostic value to the medullary blast count and other conventional hematologic parameters.

It was Morel *et al.* [29] who first performed a large prognostic factor analysis of 408 cases of *de novo* MDS, finding that patients with an abnormal karyotype have a shorter survival than patients with a normal karyotype and that among patients with abnormal cytogenetics, prognosis is poorer for those with complex aberrations. Other studies have confirmed these findings, although no agreement has been reached on the exact definition of a high-risk karyotype. Table 7.3 presents some large studies with differing definitions of cytogenetic risk groups, but showing agreement on the high-risk character of chromosome 7 anomalies as well as complex karyotypes. In a series of patients in the Düsseldorf MDS Registry who were karyotyped at the time of diagnosis (n = 825), those

Table 7.2 World Health Organization (WHO) types and number of cytogenetic aberrations, data from the Düsseldorf MDS Registry.

WHO classification	Abnormal karyotype (%)	Complex karyotype (%)
Refractory anemia (RA)	35	7
Refractory anemia with ringed sideroblasts (RARS)	22	0
Refractory cytopenia with multilineage dysplasia (RCMD)	53	13
Refractory cytopenia with multilineage dysplasia with ringed sideroblasts (RCMD-RS)		
Refractory anemia with excess of blasts I (RAEB I)	53	22
Refractory anemia with excess of blasts II (RAEB II)	52	23
Myedysplastic syndromes (MDS) with del(5q)	100	0
Chronic myelomonocytic leukemia I (CMML I)	38	6
Chronic myelomonocytic leukemia II (CMML II)	33	6
Refractory anemia with ringed sideroblasts and thrombocytosis (RARS-T)	50	0

Table 7.3 Cytogenetic prognostic findings in large series of patients.

Reference	*n*	Abnormal karyotype	Low risk	Intermediate risk	High risk
Morel [29]	408	151	NN, $5q^-$, −Y, −7/$7q^-$, $20q^-$	+8	Complex
Greenberg [31]	816	327	NN, $5q^-$, $20q^-$, −Y	All others	Complex, abnormal #7
Solé[5]	968	500	NN, $5q^-$, $20q^-$, −Y, $11q^-$, $12p^-$	Rea 3q, +8, +9, t11q, $17p^-$	Complex, −7/$7q^-$, i17q
Haase [7]	2072	1080	NN, +1/+1q, t(1q), $5q^-$, t(7q), $9q^-$, $12p^-$, abnormal #15, t(17q), $20q^-$, −21, +21, −X, −Y,	Rea 3q, −7, $7q^-$, +8, $11q^-$, t(11q23), +19, complex (=3)	Complex (>3), t(5q)

with an abnormal karyotype had a median survival of 25 months compared with 44 in patients with a normal karyotype (Figure 7.1). This difference is also present with regard to the risk of AML evolution. Similar data have also been reported by Verhoef *et al.* [30].

A milestone in the assessment of prognosis with regard to cytogenetic findings was the development of the International Prognostic Scoring System (IPSS) [31]. By evaluating 816 patients with primary MDS, the International MDS Risk Consensus Group was able to establish the importance of cytogenetic subgroups regarding survival and risk of evolution to AML. This study defined three subgroups with differing prognoses: (i) a favorable group including patients with a normal karyotype, loss of the Y chromosome, del(5q), or del(20q); (ii) an unfavourable group including patients with complex chromosomal defects (over three anomalies), and any abnormalities of chromosome 7; and (iii) an intermediate-risk group including all other abnormalities. Reliable information on the prognosis of rare cytogenetic risk groups was not available for the large number of different single or double cytogenetic aberrations. These types of aberrations were allocated into the intermediate-risk group. Patients with at least 10 metaphases were included into the study. Sixty percent of the patients had a normal karyotype. Seventy percent of patients, including those with a normal karyotype, were assigned into the low-risk group, 16% into the high-risk group, and 14% into the intermediate-risk group. The median survival times of patients in the low-risk, high-risk, and intermediate-risk cytogenetic subgroups were 3.8, 0.8, and 2.4 years, respectively. AML transformation affected 25% of the patients, with a median time to transformation of 5.6 years for the low-risk group, 0.9 years for the high-risk group, and 1.6 years for the intermediate-risk group. Figures 7.2 and 7.3 demonstrate the prognostic impact of the IPSS cytogenetic categories with regard to survival as well as the risk of AML evolution when the score was assessed in the Düsseldorf data set.

In a new study of 640 patients with *de novo* MDS, Solé *et al.* confirmed the prognostic usefulness of the IPSS cytogenetic subgroups [5]. The authors were able to identify additional subgroups with either a good prognosis (12p deletions) or a very poor prognosis (single 1q abnor-

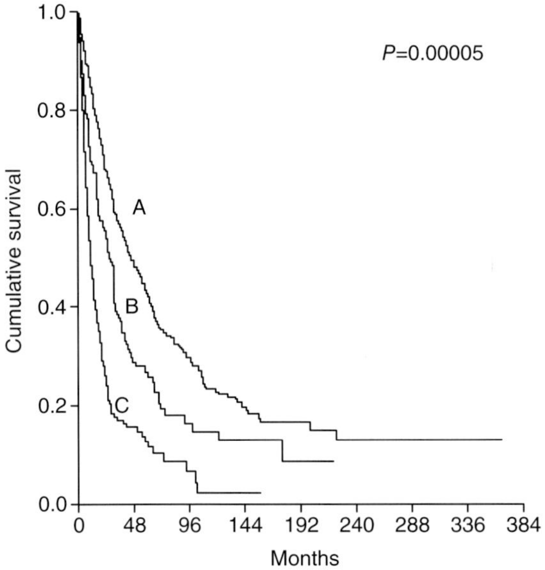

Figure 7.2 Impact of cytogenetic abnormalities according to the IPSS on survival (n = 825).

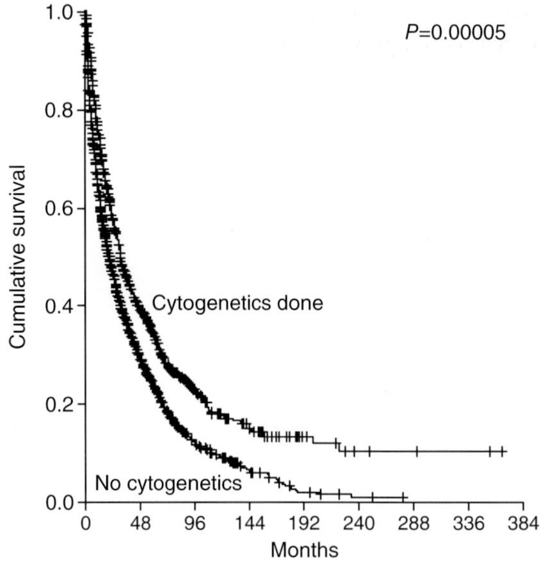

Figure 7.4 Impact of availability of cytogenetic findings on survival.

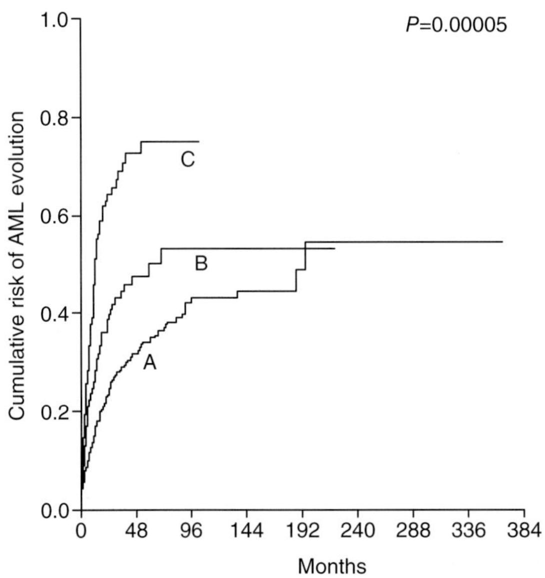

Figure 7.3 Impact of cytogenetic abnormalities according to the IPSS on risk of AML (n = 825).

malities). In addition, the authors described that patients with trisomy 8, one of the most frequent defects in MDS, have a short median survival time of about 1 year and a high risk of leukemic transformation, with a cumulative risk of AML evolution of 34% 1 year after diagnosis. Therefore, the authors proposed to transfer patients with trisomy 8 into the high-risk subgroup.

Clonal evolution with the acquisition of additional karyotypic anomalies during the course of MDS or the development of an abnormal karyotype in patients who originally had a normal karyotype has been shown to be associated with a poor prognosis [32–34]. It is still unknown if the number of residual normal metaphases in a patient with a cytogenetic aberration have any prognostic impact.

To summarize, cytogenetic findings play an increasing role in evaluating the prognosis for MDS and therefore chromosomal analyses should be performed in all patients with MDS. A major problem is that karyotyping is not performed in many patients, either for economic considerations or because of the reluctance of patients and physicians to perform a second bone marrow puncture if the diagnosis of MDS has been made by the first puncture. This fact is reflected in the Düsseldorf MDS Registry, which stores data for around 3300 patients diagnosed between 1975 and 2008. Although the number of karyotyped patients is growing extensively, only 1100 patients had been karyotyped at the time of diagnosis. With regard to the prognostic meaning of cytogenetic findings, we could show that patients who have been karyotyped at the time of diagnosis have a better median survival as compared with those who have not been karyotyped (Figure 7.4). The reason for this finding is that the median age of those who have been karyotyped is 10 years lower that those who have not (64 years vs. 74 years). This implies that physicians feel that cytogenetic examination is not worthwhile in older patients. Developing the essence of these findings, one can speculate that all the data driven from studies of patients who have been karyotyped do not reflect reality and neglect older patients with a poorer prognosis.

The independent prognostic significance of chromosomal analysis in MDS has now been confirmed by multivariate analyses [7,35]. Table 7.4 shows the multivariate analysis of survival performed on 697 patients in the Düsseldorf MDS Registry.

Table 7.4 Multivariate analysis of prognostic parameters including cytogenetic risk factors, data from the Düsseldorf MDS Registry ($n = 697$).

Variable	χ^2	*P*-value
Medullary blast count >5%	52.6	0.00005
Complex karyotype	37.5	0.00005
Lactate dehydrogenase elevated	24.1	0.00005
Hemoglobin <10g/dL	23.0	0.00005
Platelets <100.000/μL	12.6	0.00005

Driven by cytogenetic findings, the IPSS (Table 7.5) has been introduced into clinical practice. This scoring system not only enables improved clinical decision making, but also serves as an excellent tool for planning and conducing clinical trials by making patient groups more distinct. It has been recently validated by the German–Austrian MDS group [35], and Figures 7.5 and 7.6 clearly demonstrate that the IPSS is able to subdivide the patients into groups with different survival times as well as risk of AML evolution. More recently, the WHO-adapted Prognostic Scoring System (WPSS) (Table 7.6) has been developed by an Italian–German cooperation [36], which substitutes medullary blasts for WHO classification and cell counts for transfusion need. The categorization of the cytogenetic findings remained the same as in the IPSS.

Table 7.5 Definition of the International Prognostic Scoring System (IPSS).

Score	0	0.5	1	1.5	2.0
Medullary blasts (%)	0–4	5–10	—	11–20	21–29
Number of cytopenias[a]	0–1	2–3	—	—	—
Cytogenetic risk group[b]	Low	Intermediate	High	—	—
Risk groups	Score				
Low risk	0				
Intermediate risk I	0.5–1				
Intermediate risk II	1.5–2				
High risk	≥2.5				

High risk: complex karyotype (≥three anomalies), chromosome 7 anomalies.
Intermediate risk: all other aberrations.
[a]Platelets <100,000/μL, hemoglobin <10 g/dL, absolute neutrophile count <1800/μL.
[b]Low-risk: normal karyotype, 5q⁻, 20q⁻, –Y.

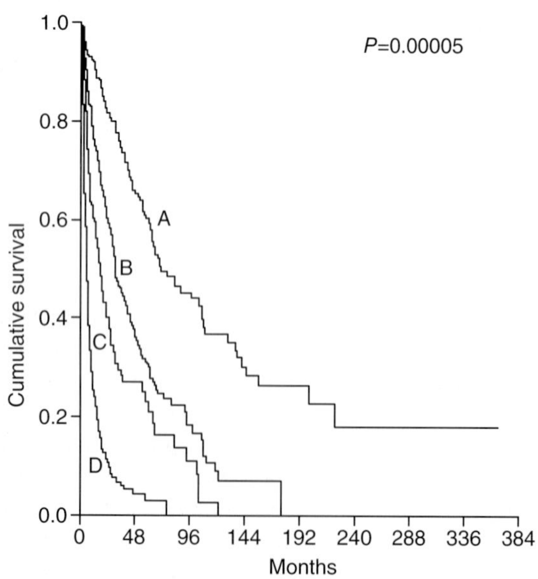

Figure 7.5 Survival of patients with MDS according to the IPSS ($n = 825$).

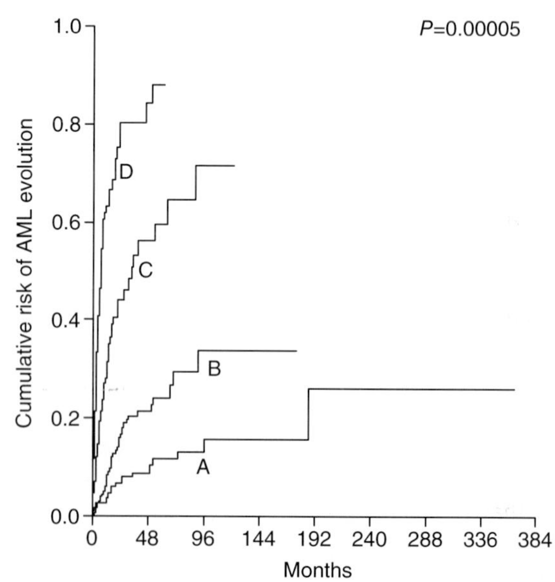

Figure 7.6 Risk of patients with AML and MDS according to the IPSS ($n = 825$).

Table 7.6 Definition of World Health Organization (WHO) adapted Prognostic Scoring System.

Score	0	1	2	3
WHO type	RA/RARS/5q$^-$	RCMD/RSCMD	RAEB I	RAEBII
Karoytype risk[a]	Low	Intermediate	High	—
Transfusion[b]	No	Yes	—	—
Risk groups	Score			
Very low risk	0			
Low risk	1			
Intermediate risk	2			
High risk	3–4			
Very high risk	5–6			

[a]Low: normal, -Y, del(5q), del(20q); high: complex, chromosome 7 anomalies; intermediate: all other abnormalities.
[b]Transfusion requirement: at least one transfusion every 8 weeks over a period of 3 months.

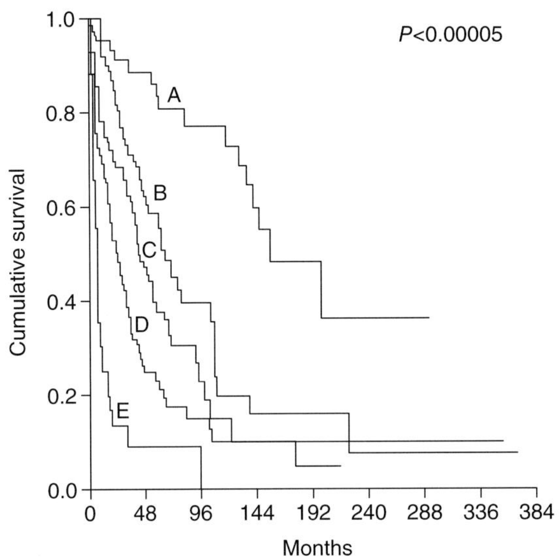

Figure 7.7 Survival of patients with MDS according to the WPSS (n = 713).

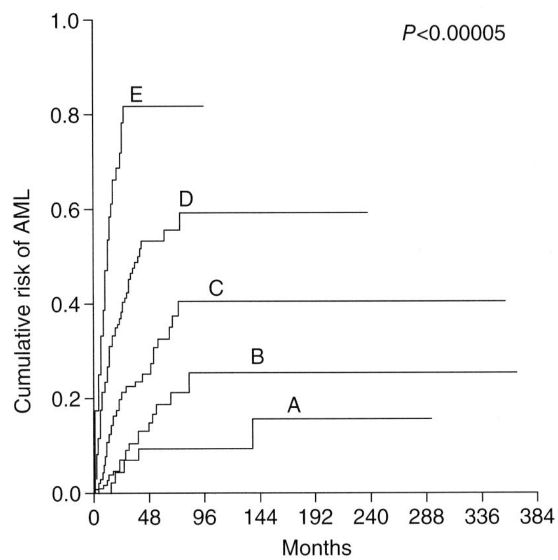

Figure 7.8 Risk of patients with AML and MDS according to the WPSS (n = 713).

This score ends up with five different risk groups that differ in terms of survival and risk of AML evolution. Figures 7.7 and 7.8 present the risk groups when applying the WPSS to the patients of the Düsseldorf MDS registry. In addition, it has been shown that the WPSS can be applied at any given time during the course of the disease. It has been validated in independent data sets of untreated and treated patients [37,38]. However, the IPSS as well as the WPSS have shortcomings, and will be refined in the near future as more is learnt about the prognostic meaning of rare cytogenetic aberrations by pooling large databases. In a multicentric attempt, the German–Austrian MDS Group examines rare cytogenetic findings by combining data from eight centers, resulting in a data set of more than 2000 patients who have been karyotyped at the time of diagnosis [39]. The group proposed a refined categorization of karyotypes with regard to prognosis (Table 7.7). Patients with 12p$^-$, 9q$^-$, t(15q), 15q$^-$, +21, –X, t(1q), t(7q), t(17q), and –21 have a good prognosis comparable to the low-risk group as proposed by the IPSS, and therefore should be added into the low-risk cytogenetic group. Patients with 11q$^-$ and trisomy 8 should form an intermediate-I risk group; patients with t(11q23), any 3q$^-$ abnormality, +19, 7q$^-$, complex anomalies with three chromosomes involved, and –7 should form an intermediate-II risk group; and patients with t(5q) and complex karyotypes involving four or more chromosomes should be defined as a high-risk group. Although this study is the largest so far, these proposals have to be validated in independent data sets. In addition, data from the same group suggest that the weight of cytogenetic findings may be underestimated in the IPSS and WPSS [40], especially in comparison to medullary blast counts. New international approaches are on the way to solve these problems. It remains to be seen if reliable information can be obtained with regard to rare cytogenetic anomalies from other large registries.

Table 7.7 New cytogenetic prognostic subgroups of the German–Austrian MDS study group in 1202 patients treated with supportive care only.

Cytogenetic risk	Cytogenetic findings	n = (%)	Median survival (months)
Good	12p-	7 (0.6)	n.r.
	9q-	6 (0.5)	n.r.
	t(15q)	6 (0.5)	n.r.
	15q⁻	5 (0.4)	n.r.
	+21	13 (1.1)	100.8
	5q⁻	132 (11)	77.2
	20q-	24 (2)	71.0
	-X	6 (0.5)	56.4
	Normal karyotype	622 (51.7)	53.4
	-Y	33 (2.8)	39.4
	t(1q)	7 (0.6)	34.7
	t(7q)	7 (0.6)	34.7
	t(17q)	6 (0.5)	32.1
	−21	6 (0.5)	32.0
Intermediate-1	11q-	11 (0.9)	26.1
	+8	64 (5.3)	23.0
Intermediate-2	t(11q23)	6 (0.5)	20.0
	Any 3q-abnormality	16 (1.3)	19.9
	+19	5 (0.4)	19.8
	7q-	11 (0.9)	19.0
	Complex (=3 anomalies)	32 (2.7)	17.0
	−7	42 (3.5)	14.0
Poor	Complex (>3 anomalies)	134 (11.1)	8.7
	t(5q)	7 (0.6)	4.4

n.r.:median survival not reached.

Molecular genetic findings

A number of proto-oncogene mutations have been described in patients with MDS, although the percentage of mutations in the patient's cohort is low and no molecular findings are pathognomonic. Molecular findings have not been introduced in prognostication of patients with MDS until now because there are no factors that have been shown to be useful in addition to other prognostic factors, such as cytogenetic findings, cell counts, and medullary blast count.

RAS

There is evidence that mutations in the *RAS* gene family may play a role in the pathogenesis of MDS and potentially have prognostic impact. *RAS* genes code for GTP-binding proteins, which play a major role in the signal transduction from membrane receptors to the nucleus. Impaired GTPase activity of defective Ras proteins may lead to increased intracellular GTP levels, which confer a growth advantage upon affected cells. The incidence of *RAS* mutations in patients with MDS is low and differs significantly between studies [41,42]. The highest percentage of *RAS* mutations can be found in CMML [42]. Reviewing published data from 624 patients with MDS, Parker and Mufti have found an overall incidence of 16%, whereas 39% of samples from patients with CMML scored positive. A study by Paquette *et al.* [43] has examined whether *NRAS* mutation has impact on prognosis. Patients with *NRAS* mutations have a shorter median survival time and a high risk of AML evolution. Interestingly, there was no correlation between cytogenetic findings and medullary blast count. Some studies confirmed these findings, whereas others did not [44–47].

FMS

The *FMS* proto-oncogene encodes the receptor for colony-stimulating factor 1 (MCSF-1). *FMS* mutations are rare in MDS, but may play a role in the prognostication. Padua *et al.* [48] found that patients with *FMS* mutations had a higher risk of AML evolution and a shorter survival time. Unfortunately, these data have not been assessed together with other prognostic parameters.

c-MPL

The overexpression of the *c-MPL* gene has been reported in about 40% of RA with excess blasts (RAEB), RA with excess blasts in transformation (RAEB-T), or patients with CMML [49], whereas in non-blastic MDS, overexpression could not be found. As expected, *c-MPL* overexpression was associated with a higher risk of AML evolution and shorter survival, but again it is not known if this is related to the higher medullary blast count or to *c-MPL* directly.

P53

The p53 tumor-suppressor gene (*TP53*), which is located on the short arm of chromosome 17 (band 17p13), plays a key role in the regulation of the cell cycle. Mutations of p53 have been reported in 0–25% of patients with MDS, dependent on the detection method and composition of the patient sample [50,51]. Their presence is strongly correlated with complex chromosome changes including $-5/5q^-$, $-7/7q^-$, and $17p^-$ [52]. It has been speculated that *TP53* mutations reflect previous exposure to carcinogens because there is a relatively high frequency of *TP53* mutations in patients with therapy-related MDS [53,54]. As expected, *TP53* mutations have been shown by some authors to predict short survival and an increased risk of AML transformation, but these data have not been correlated with other parameters.

Other molecular findings

In the last couple of years, very interesting data regarding molecular findings using new technologies have been published, some of which are possibly related to prognosis. Allelic imbalances detected by SNP in patients with MDS potentially are associated with an adverse prognosis [55,56]. Data on gene expression profiling as well as proteomic data on MDS also possibly have impact on the assessment on the prognosis of patients [57,58]. The deciphering of gene with pathophysiologic relevance in MDS may lead to predictive tools in the future [59]. Finally, flow cytometry [60] can serve as an additional tool to detect dysplasia as well as clonal evolution and thereby provide valuable information on the prognosis of the patients.

In summary, some molecular genetic findings, including those mentioned above possibly are associated with prognosis. Up to now, none of these parameters have been introduced in clinical work-up of patients with MDS. For prognostic purposes, they may play a role in the future, but still they can not substitute conventional hematologic and cytogenetic parameters.

Consequences for treatment decisions in the light of old and new compounds

Cytogenetic and molecular findings can be used not only with regard to classification and prognostication, but also with regard to the selection of appropriate treatment for patients with MDS. Although our knowledge about predictive parameters is still very limited, there is growing evidence that specific cytogenetic findings are associated with response to different treatment options. These findings are described in more detail below.

Patients with a normal karyotype are more likely to respond to immunosuppressive treatment with ATG [61], and therefore should be considered to be candidates for such a therapy unless they present with other adverse parameters such as an increased medullary blast count or very old age. The reasons for this correlation are unclear. Patients presenting with a normal karyotype are more likely to achieve complete remission after induction chemotherapy, and have a lower relapse rate and longer disease-free survival compared with patients who show adverse cytogenetic findings [62]. This also translates into a better outcome for these patients after allografting.

The presence of monosomy 7 is strongly related to a better response to hypomethylating agents [63–65]. Again, there is no explanation for this yet, but monosomy 7 should prompt physicians to consider the use of either Vidaza® or Dacogen®.

Even more impressive is the strong correlation of the presence of del(5q) in low and intermediate-I-risk patients and the response to lenalidomide [66–69]. A substantial proportion of patients with normal karyotypes also show hematologic improvement, but do not reach such high remission rates compared with MDS with del(5q). More than 60% of this particular patient group achieve hematologic remission as well as sustained cytogenetic remission within about 4–5 weeks. Although the exact mechanism of action is still unknown, one of the main reasons for the good response could be the stimulation of the *SPARC* gene in these patients.

If patients present with a translocation (5;10) or (5;12) they should be considered to be candidates for treatment with imatinib. These translocations lead to PDGFR-α or -β activation, and have been shown to be predictive of response to imatinib [70]. However, t(5;12) and t(5;10) are infrequent and seen in CMML only.

There are examples that do not show a correlation between a special kind of molecular finding and a response that has been expected to be obvious from the molecular point of view. The farnesyl transferase inhibitors, in particular tipifarnib, showed promising results in intermediate-II-risk and high-risk patients [71,72]. As it acts by inhibiting downstream pathways via Ras, it has been assumed that the compound would lead to the best results in patients with *RAS* mutations, but it has since become clear that this is not the case.

The growing knowledge on molecular findings and the development of new targeted compounds hopefully will lead to the prediction of response and selection of the best drug for each patient.

Cytogenetic and molecular examination during the course of the disease in patients who underwent a special treatment should be regarded as essential in some other patients as well. Remission control after induction therapy must not be restricted to cytology but should include cytogenetics and/or fluorescence *in situ* hybridization (FISH) in patients who initially present with an abnormal karyotype. Patients who do not achieve cytogenetic remission after induction should be considered as high risk and therefore undergo intensified post-induction treatment, including allografting [73,74].

In patients with del(5q), the use of lenalidomide could be monitored by conventional cytogenetics as well as by FISH [75,76] in order to make it possible to interrupt, and possibly restart, treatment, with particular attention given to del(5q).

In the near future, molecular characteristics are going to be assessed and used for decision making in clinical practice with regard to diagnosis, prognostication, selection of treatment, monitoring of response, and minimal residual disease. Hopefully, modern techniques like single-nucelotide polymorphism arrays, gene expression profiling, and proteomics will help substantially.

References

1 Germing U, Strupp C, Kundgen A, *et al.* No increase in age-specific incidence of myelodysplastic syndromes. *Haematologica* 2004;89:905–10.

2 Bennett JM, Catovsky D, Daniel MT, *et al.* Proposals for the classification of the myelodysplastic syndromes. *Br J Haematol* 1982;51:189–99.

3 Bennett JM. World Health Organization classification of the acute leukemias and myelodysplastic syndrome. *Int J Hematol* 2000;72:131–3.

4 Harris NL, Jaffe ES, Diebold J, *et al.* World Health Organization classification of neoplastic diseases of the hematopoietic and lymphoid tissues: report of the Clinical Advisory Committee meeting-Airlie House, Virginia, November 1997. *J Clin Oncol.* 1999;17:3835–49.

5 Solé F, Luno E, Sanzo C, *et al.* Identification of novel cytogenetic markers with prognostic significance in a series of 968 patients with primary myelodysplastic syndromes. *Haematologica* 2005; 90:1168–78.

6 Haase D, Feuring-Buske M, Schäfer C, *et al.* Cytogenetic analysis of CD34+ subpopulations in AML and MDS characterized by the expression of CD38 and CD117. *Leukemia* 1997;11: 674–9.

7 Haase D, Germing U, Schanz J, *et al.* New insights into the prognostic impact of the karyotype in MDS and correlation with subtypes: evidence from a core dataset of 2124 patients. *Blood* 2007;110:4385–95.

8 Pedersen-Bjergaard J, Philip P, Larsen SO, Jensen G, Byrsting K. Chromosome aberrations and prognostic factors in therapy-related myelodysplasia and acute non-lymphocytic leukemia. *Blood* 1990;76:1083–91.

9 Mittelman MM, Lessin LS. Oncogenes and growth factor genes in myelodysplasia. *Hematol Pathol* 1991;5:37–41.

10 Swerdlow SH, Campo E, Harris NL, *et al. WHO Classification of Tumors: Tumors of Hematopoietic and Lymphoid Tissues.* IARC Press: Lyon, 2008.

11 Germing U, Gattermann N, Strupp C, *et al.* Validation of the WHO proposals for a new classification of primary myelodysplastic syndromes: a retrospective analysis of 1600 patients. *Leuk Res* 2000;24:983–92.

12 Germing U, Strupp C, Kuendgen A, *et al.* Prospective validation of the WHO proposals for the classification of myelodysplastic syndromes. *Haematologica* 2006;91:1596–604.

13 Valent P, Horny HP, Bennett JM, *et al.* Definitions and standards in the diagnosis and treatment of the myelodysplastic syndromes: Consensus statements and report from a working conference. *Leuk Res* 2007;31:727–36.

14 Schroeder T, Ruf L, Bernhardt A, *et al.* Distinguishing myelodysplastic syndromes (MDS) from idiopathic cytopenia of undetermined significance (ICUS): HUMARA unravels clonality in a subgroup of patients. *Ann Oncol* 2010, epub ahead of print.

15 Rong A, Gattermann N, Germing U, Aul C, Aivado M. *RAS* mutations are rare in acquired idiopathic sideroblastic anemia (AISA) and apparently absent in pure sideroblastic anemia (PSA). *Onkologie* 2000;23(Suppl. 7):A181.

16 Orazi A, Germing U. The myelodysplastic/myeloproliferative neoplasms: myeloproliferative diseases with dysplastic features. *Leukemia* 2008;22:1308–19.

17 Gattermann N, Billiet J, Kronenwett R, *et al.* High frequency of the *JAK2 V617F* mutation in patients with thrombocytosis (platelet count >600 × 109/L) and ringed sideroblasts more than 15% considered as MDS/MPD, unclassifiable. *Blood* 2007; 109:1334–5.

18 Zipperer E, Wulfert M, Germing U, Haas R, Gattermann N. *MPL 515* and *JAK2* mutation analysis in MDS presenting with a platelet count of more than 500 × 10(9)/l. *Ann Hematol* 2007;87:413–15.

19 Schmitt-Graeff AH, Teo SS, Olschewski M, *et al. JAK2V617F* mutation status identifies subtypes of refractory anemia with ringed sideroblasts associated with marked thrombocytosis. *Haematologica* 2008;93:34–40.

20 Solé F, Espinet B, Sanz GF, *et al.* Grupo Cooperative Espanol de Citogenetica Hematologica. Incidence, characterization and prognostic significance of chromosomal abnormalities in 640 patients with primary myelodysplastic syndromes. *Br J Haematol* 2000;108:346–56.

21 Van den Berghe H, Cassiman J-J, David G, Fryns J-P, Michaux JL, Sokal G. Distinct hematological disorder with the deletion of long arm of no. 5 chromosome. *Nature* 1974;251:437–8.

22 Van den Berghe H, Vermaelen K, Mecucci C, Barbieri D, Tricot G. The 5q- anomaly. *Cancer Genet Cytogenet* 1985;17: 189–255.

23 Mathew P, Tefferi A, Dewald GW, *et al.* The 5q- syndrome: a single-institution study of 43 consecutive patients. *Blood* 1993; 81:1040–5.

24 Boultwood J, Lewis S, Wainscoat JS. The 5q-syndrome. *Blood* 1994;84:3252–60.

25 Giagounidis AA, Germing U, Haase S, *et al.* Clinical, morphological, cytogenetic, and prognostic features of patients with myelodysplastic syndromes and del(5q) including band q31. *Leukemia* 2004;18:113–99.

26 Estey EH. Prognosis and therapy of secondary myelodysplastic syndromes. *Haematologica* 1998;83:543–9.

27 Le Beau MM, Albain KS, Larson RA, *et al*. Clinical and cytogenetic correlations in 63 patients with therapy-related myelodysplastic syndromes and acute nonlymphocytic leukemia: further evidence for characteristic abnormalities of chromosomes no. 5 and 7. *J Clin Oncol* 1986;4:325–45.

28 Heim S. Cytogenetic findings in primary and secondary MDS. *Leuk Res* 1992;16:43–6.

29 Morel P, Hebbar M, Lai JL, *et al*. Cytogenetic analysis has strong independent prognostic value in de novo myelodysplastic syndromes and can be incorporated in a new scoring system: a report on 408 cases. *Leukemia* 1993;7:1315–23.

30 Verhoef G, De Wolf-Peeters C, Kerim S, *et al*. Update on the prognostic implication of morphology, histology, and karyotype in primary myelodysplastic syndromes. *Hematol Pathol* 1991;5:163–75.

31 Greenberg P, Cox C, LeBeau MM, *et al*. International scoring system for evaluating prognosis in myelodysplastic syndromes. *Blood* 1997;89:2079–88.

32 Bernasconi P, Klersy C, Boni M, *et al*. World Health Organization classification in combination with cytogenetic markers improves the prognostic stratification of patients with de novo primary myelodysplastic syndromes. *Br J Haematol* 2007;137: 193–205.

33 Tricot G, Boogaerts MA, De Wolf-Peeters C, Van den Berghe, Verwilghen RL. The myelodysplastic syndromes: different evolution patterns based on sequential morphological and cytogenetic investigations. *Br J Haematol* 1985;59:659–70.

34 Benitez J, Carbonell F, Sanchez Fayos F, Heimpel H. Karyotypic evolution in patients with myelodysplastic syndromes. *Cancer Genet Cytogenet* 1985;16:157–67.

35 Germing U, Hildebrandt B, Pfeilstöcker M, *et al*. Refinement of the international prognostic scoring system (IPSS) by including LDH as an additional prognostic variable to improve risk assessment in patients with primary myelodysplastic syndromes (MDS). *Leukemia* 2005;19:2223–31.

36 Malcovati L, Germing U, Kuendgen A, *et al*. Time-dependent prognostic scoring system for predicting survival and leukemic evolution in myelodysplastic syndromes. *J Clin Oncol* 2007;25: 3503–10.

37 Alessandrino EP, Della Porta MG, Bacigalupo A, *et al*. Gruppo Italiano Trapianto di Midollo Osseo (GITMO). WHO classification and WPSS predict posttransplantation outcome in patients with myelodysplastic syndrome: a study from the Gruppo Italiano Trapianto di Midollo Osseo (GITMO). *Blood* 2008; 112:895–902.

38 Park MJ, Kim HJ, Kim SH, *et al*. Is International Prognostic Scoring System (IPSS) still standard in predicting prognosis in patients with myelodysplastic syndrome? External validation of the WHO Classification-Based Prognostic Scoring System (WPSS) and comparison to IPSS. *Eur J Haematol* 2008;81:364–73.

39 Schanz J, Estey EH, Steidl C, *et al*. Multivariate Analysis Suggests That the Prognostic Impact of Poor Cytogenetics Is Potentially Underestimated in the IPSS. *Blood* (ASH Annual Meeting Abstracts) 2007;110:248.

40 Steidl C, Schanz J, Pfeilstöcker M, *et al*. Growing evidence for an underestimation of poor-risk cytogenetics in the international prognostic scoring system in myelodysplastic syndromes. *Clinical Leukemia* 2008;6:353–6.

41 van Kamp H, de Pijper C, Verlaan-de Vries M, *et al*. Longitudinal analysis of point mutations of *N-ras* proto-oncogene in patients with myelodysplastia using archived blood smears. *Blood* 1992; 79:1266–70.

42 Parker J, Mufti GJ. Ras and myelodysplasia: lessons from the past decade. *Semin Hematol* 1996;33:206–24.

43 Paquette RL, Landaw EM, Pierre RV, *et al*. *N-ras* mutations are associated with poor prognosis and increased risk of leukemia in myelodysplastic syndrome. *Blood* 1993;82:590–9.

44 Constantinidou M, Chalevelakis G, Economopoulos T, *et al*. Codon 12 *RAS* mutations in patients with myelodysplastic syndrome: incidence and prognostic value. *Ann Hematol* 1997;74: 11–14.

45 Padua RA, Guinn BA, Al-Sabah AI, *et al*. *RAS*, *FMS* and *p53* mutations and poor clinical outcome in myelodysplasias: a 10-year follow up. *Leukemia* 1998;12:887–92.

46 Neubauer A, Greenberg P, Negrin R, Ginzton N, Liu E. Mutations in the *RAS* proto-oncogenes in patients with myelodysplastic syndromes. *Leukemia* 1994;8:638–41.

47 Lyons J, Janssen JW, Bartram C, Layton M, Mufti GJ. Mutation of *Ki-ras* and *N-ras* oncogenes in myelodysplastic syndromes. *Blood* 1988;71:1707–12.

48 Ridge SA, Worwood M, Oscier D, Jacobs A, Padua RA. *FMS* mutations in myelodysplastic, leukemic and normal subjects. *Proc Natl Acad Sci U S A* 1990;87:1377–80.

49 Bouscary D, Preudhomme C, Ribrag V, *et al*. Prognostic value of c-mpl expression in myelodysplastic syndromes. *Leukemia* 1995;9:783–8.

50 Tsushita K, Hotta T, Ichikawa A, Saito H. Mutation of *p53* gene does not play a critical role in myelodysplastic syndrome and its transformation to acute leukemia. *Br J Hematol* 1992;81:456–7.

51 Sugimoto K, Hirano N, Toyoshima H, *et al*. Mutations of the *p53* gene in myelodysplastic syndromes (MDS) and MDS-derived *Leukemia*. *Blood* 1993;81:3022–6.

52 Kaneko H, Misawa S, Horiike S, Nakai H, Kashima K. *TP53* mutations emerge at early phase of myelodysplastic syndrome and are associated with complex chromosomal abnormalities. *Blood* 1995;85:2189–93.

53 Jonveaux P, Fenaux P, Quiquandon I, *et al*. Mutations in the *p53* gene in myelodysplastic syndromes. *Oncogene* 1991;6:2243–7.

54 Orazi A, Cattoretti G, Heerema NA, Sozzi G, John K, Neiman RS. Frequent *p53* overexpression in therapy related myelodysplastic syndromes and acute myeloid leukemia: an immunohistochemical study of bone marrow biopsies. *Mod Pathol* 1993,6:521–5.

55 Mohamedali A, Gäken J, Twine NA, *et al*. Prevalence and prognostic significance of allelic imbalance by single-nucleotide polymorphism analysis in low-risk myelodysplastic syndromes. *Blood* 2007;110:3365–73.

56 Gondek LP, Tiu R, O'Keefe, Sekeres MA, Theil KS, Maciejewski JP. Chromosomal lesions and uniparental disomy detected by SNP arrays in MDS, MDS/MPD and MDS-derived AML. *Blood* 2008;111:1534–42.

57 Hofmann WK, de Vos S, Komor M, Hoelzer D, Wachsman W, Koeffler HP. Characterization of gene expression of CD34+ cells from normal and myelodysplastic bone marrow. 2002;100: 3553–60.

58 Aivado M, Spentzos D, Germing U, *et al*. Serum proteome profiling detects myelodysplastic syndromes and identifies CXC chemokine ligands 4 and 7 as markers for advanced disease. *Proc Natl Acad Sci U S A* 2007;104:1307–12.

59 Ebert BL, Pretz J, Bosco J, *et al.* Identification of RPS14 as the 5q-syndrome gene by RNA interference screen. *Nature* 2008; 451:335–340.

60 van de Loosdrecht AA, Westers TM, Westra AH, Dräger AM, van der Velden VH, Ossenkoppele GJ. Identification of distinct prognostic subgroups in low- and intermediate-1-risk myelodysplastic syndromes by flow cytometry. *Blood* 2008;111: 1067–77.

61 Lim ZY, Killick S, Germing U, *et al.* Low IPSS score and bone marrow hypocellularity in MDS patients predict hematological responses to antithymocyte globulin. *Leukemia* 2007;21: 1436–41.

62 Knipp S, Hildebrandt B, Kündgen A, *et al.* Intensive chemotherapy is not recommended for patients aged >60 years who have myelodysplastic syndromes or acute myeloid leukemia with high-risk karyotypes. *Cancer* 2007;25:3503–10.

63 Lübbert M, Wijermanns P, Kunzmann R, *et al.* Cytogenetic responses in high-risk myelodysplastic syndrome following low-dose treatment with the DNA methylation inhibitor 5-aza-2′-deoxycytidine. *Br J Haematol* 2001;114:349–57.

64 Rüter B, Wijermanns P, Claus R, Kunzmann R, Lübbert M. Preferentially cytogenetic response to continuous intravenous low-dose decitabine (DAC) administration in myelodysplastic syndrome with monosomy 7. *Blood* 2007;110: 1080–2.

65 Raj K, John A, Ho A, *et al.* CDKN2B methylation status and isolated chromosome 7 abnormalities predict responses to treatment with 5-azacytidine. *Leukemia* 2007;21:1937–44.

66 List A, Kurtin S, Roe DJ, *et al.* Efficacy of Lenalidomide in Myelodysplastic Syndromes. *New Engl J Med* 2005;352: 549–57.

67 List A, Dewald G, Bennett J, *et al;* Myelodysplastic Syndrome-003 study investigators. Lenalidomide in the myelodysplastic syndrome with chromosome 5q deletion. *New Engl J Med* 2006; 355:1456–65.

68 Giagounidis AAN, Germing U, Strupp C, Hildebrandt B, Heinsch M, Aul C. Prognosis of patients with del(5q) and complex karyotype and the possible role of lenalidomide in this patient subgroup. *Ann Hematol* 2005;84:569–71.

69 Giagounidis AAN, Germing U, Aul C. Biological and prognostic significance of chromosome 5q deletions in myeloid malignancies. *Clin Cancer Res* 2006;12:5–10.

70 Drechsler M, Hildebrandt B, Kündgen A, Germing U, Royer-Pokora B. Fusion of H4/D10S170 to PDGFR? in a patient with chronic myelomonocytic leukemia and long-term responsiveness to imatinib. *Ann Hematol* 2007;86:353–4.

71 Kurzrock R, Kantarjian HM, Blascovich MA, *et al.* Phase I study of alternate-week administration of tipifarnib in patients with myelodysplastic syndrome. *Clin Cancer Res* 2008;14:509–14.

72 Fenaux P, Raza A, Mufti GJ, *et al.* A multicenter phase 2 study of the farnesyltransferase inhibitor tipifarnib in intermediate-to high-risk myelodysplastic syndrome. *Blood* 2007;109: 4158–63.

73 Marcucci G, Mrozek K, Ruppert AS, *et al.* Abnormal cytogenetics at date of morphologic complete remission predicts short overall and disease-free survival, and higher relapse rate in adult acute myeloid leukemia: results from cancer and leukemia group B study 8461. *J Clin Oncol* 2004;22:2410–18.

74 Balleisen S, Hildebrandt B, Royer-Pokora B, *et al.* Persisting Karyotype Abnormalities after Induction Chemotherapy in AML and High Risk MDS Predict Poor Outcome. *Onkologie* 2004;27(Suppl. 3):560.

75 Strupp C, Hildebrandt B, Germing U, Haas R, Gattermann N. Cytogenetic response to thalidomide treatment in three patients with myelodysplastic syndrome. *Leukemia* 2003;17:1200–2.

76 Braulke F, Schanz J, Steidl C, Truemper LH, Haase D. FISH-analyses of circulating $CD34^+$ cells in MDS-patients—A suitable method to measure and predict response to 5-azacytidine. *Blood* (ASH Annual Meeting Abstracts) 2007;110:2466.

Chapter 8
Myelodysplastic Syndromes

William Stevenson[1] *and Guillermo Garcia-Manero*[2]
[1] Royal North Shore Hospital, Sydney, Australia
[2] Department of Leukemia, University of Texas M. D. Anderson Cancer Center, Houston, Texas, USA

Epidemiology and etiology

The incidence of myelodysplastic syndromes (MDS) increases with age. Most patients diagnosed with this condition are more than 60 years old, with a median age at diagnosis in the USA of 75 years [1]. The incidence is higher in males than in females, with an annual incidence rate in men of 4.5 per 100,000 compared with 2.7 per 100,000 in women [1]. A recent analysis of several US Cancer Registries reported an incidence of 3–3.5 individuals/10^5 affected by MDS in the US population, with a relative annual increase, probably related to increased awareness of the disease and reporting efforts [2].

The risk of developing MDS may be dependent upon an individual's racial background. In the USA, MDS incidence is highest in the white population with a low incidence in American Indians, Asians and Pacific Islanders [1]. Geographic differences are evident when patients with MDS in different parts of the world are studied, with patients from Asia tending to present at a younger age. Japanese patients with a diagnosis of refractory anemia (RA) present at a median age of 57 years compared with 71 years for patients from Germany [3]. The Japanese cohort had more severe cytopenia at presentation but an overall better prognosis with a decreased risk of transformation to acute myeloid leukemia (AML). The underlying cause of this discrepancy is not known, but it may reflect subtle differences in the distribution of genetic pathology in MDS between different racial groups. In Asia, patients with MDS appear to have a similar frequency of karyotype abnormality as patients in European and American cohorts, although they may have fewer cases with abnormalities of chromosome 5 and 7 [3–7]. This combination of younger age at diagnosis and lack of chromosome 7 abnormalities are recognized as favorable prognostic features that may explain the longer survival observed in the study groups from Asia.

The majority of patients who present with MDS have no identifiable etiologic cause of the disease. A small number of patients do appear to have a risk factor that may be either genetic or environmental in origin. Genetic syndromes such as Down syndrome, Bloom syndrome, and Fanconi anemia are associated with an increased risk of MDS, which often presents earlier in life than would be expected in the general population [8,9]. Such specific genetic risk factors are rare, but an individual's genetic background, including race, may predispose them to the disease. Genetic polymorphisms influence the activity of enzymes responsible for metabolizing toxic chemicals and chemotherapy drugs in the body and this may influence an individual's predisposition to MDS. Polymorphisms have been described in the cytochrome p450 3A, glutathione-S-transferase, and NAD(P)H quinine oxidoreductase enzyme systems that increase the risk of developing myeloid malignancy [10–12].

Environmental agents may contribute to the development of MDS by causing toxic damage to hematopoietic stem cells. A causal relationship between occupational exposures to benzene and radiation and the development of myeloid malignancy has been demonstrated [13]. Exposure to organic solvents and pesticides has also been implicated in the development of MDS [14–16], and an occupational history of exposure to these chemicals may be associated with an increased incidence of the cytogenetic abnormalities associated with a poor prognosis [17]. There is no known correlation between MDS and socioeconomic status [15].

The most significant risk factor for the development of MDS is previous exposure to chemotherapy or radiotherapy used to treat antecedent hematologic malignancy or solid-organ cancer. This treatment-related MDS (t-MDS) constitutes a minority of MDS diagnoses but may be increasing in prevalence with improved survival rates after successful cancer therapies. t-MDS most commonly presents 5–6 years after the initial cancer treatment and generally has a poor prognosis [18]. Patients treated for lymphoma are at risk of this long-term complication of cancer treatment, with up to 2% of survivors from Hodgkin disease developing treatment-related myeloid malignancy [19,20]. Lymphoma patients who receive

Leukemias: Principles and Practice of Therapy, 1st edition. Edited by S. Faderl and H. Kantarjian.

high-dose chemotherapy associated with autologous hematopoietic stem-cell transplantation appear to be at a particularly high risk of t-MDS or AML, with incidence rates in some centers of up to 10% [21,22].

Clinical and laboratory features

Anemia is the most common clinical manifestation of myelodysplasia, with progressive fatigue being a typical presenting complaint. Fewer patients present for investigation of bleeding or bruising secondary to thrombocytopenia or an infection related to neutropenia. Some patients are diagnosed after cytopenia was discovered in a blood count performed for a non-hematologic indication and are asymptomatic at initial assessment. Physical examination is often normal, with the liver and spleen typically not enlarged. Some patients present with signs of chronic anemia or bruising, which provide a clue to the underlying diagnosis. During follow-up of a patient, a change in the severity of cytopenia or rapid worsening of symptoms may indicate disease transformation. Patients suspected of transformation require prompt investigation as 20% of patients develop acute leukemia throughout their disease course [23].

Initial assessments of patients suspected to have MDS should include a complete blood count (CBC), reticulocyte count, and complete serum chemistry including B_{12}, folate, iron studies, and erythropoietin level. A bone marrow aspirate and biopsy with samples taken for an iron stain and cytogenetic studies is required. MDS is primarily diagnosed by the assessment of morphologic changes in hematopoietic cells present in the peripheral blood and bone marrow smear. Cytogenetic studies may confirm the presence of clonal hematopoiesis and provide additional important prognostic information.

Morphology of the blood and bone marrow

Morphologic classification of MDS is based on a 500 cell differential count on the bone marrow aspirate and a leukocyte differential performed on the blood smear [24]. This analysis determines the percentage of blasts present in the blood and bone marrow and provides an assessment of the number of myeloid lineages involved in the dysplastic process, and the iron stain determines the presence and number of ring sideroblasts [24].

Blood-cell abnormalities on the peripheral blood smear are variable [24,25]. Red cells may be macrocytic and frequently display anisopoikilocytosis. Polychromasia or basophilic stippling may be present. Dysplastic granulocytes may show abnormal folding of the nucleus, and cytoplasmic granules are often reduced or absent. Platelets are of variable size and may also be hypogranular. The presence of circulating blast cells or an excess of monocytes are important for the classification of high-risk MDS and monocytic leukemias, respectively.

Definitive diagnosis requires a bone marrow aspirate and biopsy. The bone marrow is usually normocellular or hypercellular, reflecting that hematopoiesis is ineffective. Abnormal maturation of hematopoietic cells results in a variable proportion of myeloblasts that are significantly increased in the more aggressive forms of the disorder. Morphologic abnormalities found in the nucleus of erythroblasts include nuclear budding, internuclear bridging, karyorrhexis, multinuclearity, and megaloblastoid changes (Plate 8.1). Cytoplasmic features include the presence of ring sideroblasts and abnormal vacuolization. Abnormal or absent granulation is a common feature of a dysplastic granulocyte series. Aberrant nuclear folding of the neutrophil precursor can produce a dysplastic bilobed nucleus, the pseudo-Pelger–Huët anomaly. Megakaryocytes may have an extremely variable morphology, and a small dysplastic form called the micromegakaryocyte is a typical finding in myelodysplasia. A normal megakaryocyte has a polyploid nucleus that can be altered with dysplasia to produce hypolobulation or nuclei that are dispersed throughout the cell. The bone marrow biopsy provides the best assessment of the overall cellularity of the bone marrow and allows examination of the architecture of the marrow and surrounding bone. The presence of fibrosis can be assessed on the biopsy, with specific stains for reticulin and collagen. In normal bone marrow, the immature blast cells are frequently located near the endosteal surface. In MDS, these cells may be distant to this site and form aberrant clusters referred to as abnormal localization of immature precursors (ALIPs). Immunohistochemical staining of biopsies can aid diagnosis, with CD34 staining to identify blast and progenitor cells and CD42 or CD62 for quantitation and assessment of megakaryocytes [26].

Non-clonal diseases may cause dysplastic morphologic changes in blood cells; these secondary causes of dysplasia can potentially complicate the diagnosis of the disease and should be excluded in the initial assessment of a patient. Blood-cell dysplasia is seen with exposure to heavy metals or antituberculous therapies, B_{12} and folate deficiency, HIV infection, excessive alcohol consumption [24], and occasionally with aging [27]. Dysplastic features on blood cells are very commonly observed after chemotherapy or with the therapeutic use of granulocyte colony-stimulating factor (G-CSF). These alternate diagnoses should be assessed in the patients' history and may require exclusion with further laboratory testing. Diagnostic difficulties may occur in patients with marked hypocellularity of the bone marrow and in patients with prominent fibrosis as there are often very few cells in the aspirate sample to allow morphologic assessment of dysplasia.

Patients with prominent hypocellularity of the marrow may be difficult to distinguish from aplastic anemia, in which morphologic dysplasia of the erythroid lineage may also be observed. In cases of marked fibrosis, bone marrow aspiration is often unsuccessful. Some patients with mild dysplastic changes in the bone marrow and a diploid karyotype may be difficult to definitively diagnose at their initial presentation and may require a period of observation to confirm the underlying diagnosis. These patients require review with repeat investigations performed at 3–6 months.

Cytogenetic and molecular analysis

Cytogenetic analysis of hematopoietic cells derived from the bone marrow aspirate provides important additional information in the assessment of a patient with MDS. A karyotype abnormality provides definitive evidence for the presence of a clonal blood disorder, which may be particularly important if the morphologic changes are subtle. The karyotype also provides the clinician with prognostic information, and may guide therapy in situations where a drug appears to have specific activity in a cytogenetic subgroup of the disease. Typically, cytogenetic analysis will assess 20 bone marrow metaphases and can be repeated every 6–12 months to examine for clonal evolution [26].

A cytogenetic abnormality is found in 40–50% of primary MDS. These syndromes are genetically diverse and many hundreds of different cytogenetic abnormalities have been described [28]. The most common karyotype abnormalities involve the gain or loss of genetic material, and the incidence of the most common of these abnormalities is outlined in Figure 8.1. These common cytogenetic abnormalities are not specific for MDS as many are also observed in AML and other myeloid malignancy. Unlike AML and chronic myeloid leukemia (CML), genetic translocations are rare in MDS.

The presence or absence of a cytogenetic abnormality has a marked influence on the overall prognosis of a patient [28]. There is a stark difference in median survival between a patient with a normal diploid karyotype (53 months) and a patient with a complex karyotype of three or more cytogenetic abnormalities (9 months). The genetic context of an individual cytogenetic abnormality is also important. Del(5q) and del(20q) are commonly observed karyotypic abnormalities in MDS and when present in isolation suggest a favorable prognosis. However, when these abnormalities are present in association with other cytogenetic abnormalities, particularly as a component of a complex karyotype, the prognosis for the patient is poor. In contrast, abnormalities of chromosome 7 are associated with a poor prognosis regardless of the presence or absence of other genetic abnormalities. Complex cytogenetic abnormalities are more frequently observed in patients with increased numbers of blasts in the bone marrow, and there is an overall correlation between prognosis and the extent of complexity. Median survival is 35 months for one karyotypic abnormality, 38 months for two abnormalities, and 17 months for three abnormalities. Patients with an increasing complexity of more than six abnormalities have a progressively worse prognosis, with a median survival of 5 months [28]. Complex karyotypes contain a vast array of different cytogenetic abnormalities, but the majority of cases include changes involving chromosomes 5 and 7.

Treatment-related MDS has a particularly high incidence of cytogenetic abnormalities, with karyotypic changes observed in 70–90% of cases [18,28,29]. There is a high incidence of abnormalities associated with an unfavorable prognosis contributing to the overall poor outlook for this group of patients. Abnormalities of chromosome 5 and 7 are frequently observed after exposure to alkylating agents [29,30], and a variety of translocations involving 11q23 are seen after treatment with topoisomerase II inhibitors [29].

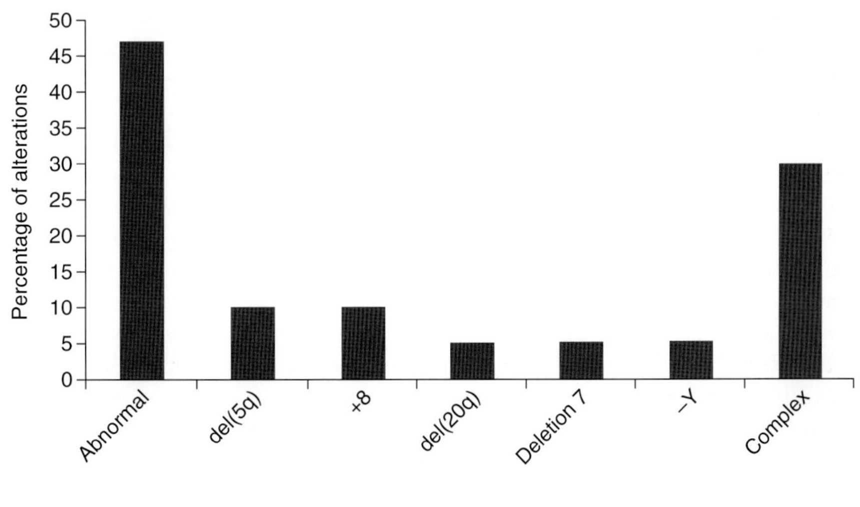

Figure 8.1 Frequency of chromosomal alterations in MDS.

Chromosomal deletion is the most frequent cytogenetic abnormality observed in MDS, suggesting that loss of tumor-suppressor function may be important in the development and progression of the disease.

Despite the identification of frequent deletions sites in MDS, specific gene defects that are causative of dysplastic cell maturation in the bone marrow have not been conclusively identified. Mutations in *RAS* genes and the transcription factor RUNX1 are frequently identified in MDS, occurring in up to 10% of patients [31–33]. These gene defects occur almost exclusively in patients with MDS who have increased marrow blast counts, and *RUNX1* mutations are more frequent in t-MDS and AML. Mutations in other genes associated with AML occur very infrequently in MDS, with only small numbers of patients described with mutations in *FLT3, KIT, MLL,* and *NPM1* [33,34]. Recently, mutations in *TET2* have been reported to occur in approximately 20% of patients with MDS. The prognostic significance of this event is not currently understood [35]. The low frequency of genetic alterations so far reported and the high frequency of chromosomal deletions have prompted interest in the identification of epigenetic repressive alterations such as aberrant DNA methylation in MDS. Although large scale methylation studies are yet to be reported, it is likely that these alterations are also common in MDS. Because of the relative lack of numbers in the identification of frequent dominant genetic lesions in MDS, several groups have used large-scale single-nucleotide polymorphism (SNP) arrays in MDS [36]. This has allowed the identification of areas of microdeletions and uniparenteral disomy in MDS. It is likely that these genomic regions harbor important genes in this disease, as has been recently shown for C-CBL [37].

An association between a genetic abnormality and disease phenotype is reported in a few specific MDS. A minority of patients with an interstitial deletion of chromosome 5q display an indolent anemia with relative preservation of the platelet count associated with hypolobated megakaryocytes in the bone marrow. This array of findings is called the $5q^-$ syndrome [38] and is recognized as a separate diagnostic entity in the current World Health Organization (WHO) classification. The genetic defect within the deleted region that is responsible for the disease is not known; however, recent research has focused on one candidate gene, *SPARC*, which may potentially contribute to the malignant phenotype [39]. *CTNNA1* is another gene on chromosome 5q that has been identified to be important in patients with MDS and AML with deletion of the long arm of this chromosome but without specific features of $5q^-$ syndrome [40]. More recently, Ebbert *et al.* have reported the identification of *RPS14* as haploinsufficient in $5q^-$ MDS. *RPS14* is involved in ribosomal biogenesis and its deficiency has a role in anemia in this syndrome [41]. It is likely that a complex network of genes cooperate in the pathogenesis of this syndrome.

A small number of patients have been described with a deletion of 17p associated with abnormalities in the *p53* gene. This specific disorder has a poor prognosis and may be suspected when morphologic characteristics of prominent dysgranulopoiesis including neutrophils exhibiting the Pelger–Huët anomaly and abnormal vacuolization are present [42,43]. Acquired hemoglobin H disease produces red cell changes on the blood smear reminiscent of α-thalassemia. This red-cell phenotype is secondary to decreased expression of α-globin within the bone marrow MDS clone and is, in most cases, associated with a mutation in the *ATRX* gene [44,45]. Unfortunately, these rare syndromes represent a small minority of patients with MDS, and specific gene defects are not identified in most patients.

Ancillary studies

Flow cytometry is not required for the routine diagnosis of MDS but it may sometimes provide valuable supplementary information. Flow cytometry can confirm the presence of specific myeloid lineages within the marrow, and may also identify aberrant expression of cell-surface markers that are indicative of a clonal-cell population. This may have diagnostic significance in confirming abnormal hematopoiesis, particularly in the setting of a normal diploid karyotype and inconclusive morphologic changes [26]. Quantitation of the number of $CD34^+$ cells in the bone marrow may also assist in the differentiation of hypoplastic MDS from aplastic anemia. In MDS, the number of CD34 cells is usually normal or increased compared with aplastic anemia, where it is frequently reduced [46].

The use of fluorescence *in situ* hybridization (FISH) techniques using probes specific for particular chromosomes (ie, covering chromosomes 5, 7, 20, and 8) have not been fully standardized in MDS—their use should not be considered as a standard of care in MDS and cannot yet replace conventional cytogenetics.

Diagnosis

The classification systems used to group different myelodysplastic syndromes has evolved over time with increased understanding of the biology and genetics of the disease. The first widely accepted classification system was that proposed by the French–American–British (FAB) study group [47]. The FAB categorized MDS primarily on the percentage of blasts in the peripheral blood and bone marrow, with disease entities defined by increased numbers of blasts associated with a more aggressive clinical course. In this system, patients with a bone marrow blast percentage greater than 30% were considered to have AML. This classification system used only morphologic criteria to define disease groups and provided a framework that allowed the study of the natural history of MDS and its response to therapy.

The WHO classification of MDS was developed with the stated intent to utilize all features of disease biology including morphology, genetic abnormalities, immunophenotype, and clinical behavior [24,48]. This classification was updated in 2008 [49]. In the original WHO classification, the importance of morphologic assessment of blast percentage within the bone marrow and peripheral blood was retained, although the threshold level for the diagnosis of acute leukemia was altered such that patients with a bone marrow blast percentage greater than 20% are considered to have AML. This was primarily because patients with 20–29% blasts in the marrow were found to have a similar response to therapy and survival rate as patients with >30% blasts [50]. Within the WHO MDS categories with an increased blast percentage, the magnitude of the blast elevation was quantified between refractory anemia with excess blasts 1 and 2 (RAEB-1 and -2), reflecting the worse prognosis of patients with an elevated blast count [23]. In patients with a normal proportion of blast cells within the bone marrow, the relatively indolent RA and RA with ring sideroblasts (RARS) introduced in the FAB system were further delineated by assessment for the presence of multilineage dysplasia. Patients with dysplastic maturation limited to the erythroid lineage have a more favorable prognosis than patients with cytopenia and dysplasia present in multiple myeloid lineages. The WHO also introduced the $5q^-$ syndrome as a separate diagnostic entity primarily on the basis of a genetic abnormality rather than morphologic features alone. Deletions involving chromosome 5q are relatively common in MDS, and the WHO classification tightly defined the syndrome as an isolated del(5q) associated with anemia, a preserved or increased platelet count, and hypolobated megakaryocytes on the bone marrow biopsy (Plate 8.2). The WHO classification has been widely accepted and validated by a number of independent groups [51–53]. The most recent WHO classification [49] includes the following changes: (i) specific guidelines for the requirement of specimen collection, blast and blast lineage assessment, as well as for the analysis of genetic alterations; (ii) an effort to report new changes in the diagnosis and classification of MDS/myeloproliferative neoplasm (MPN); (iii) major changes specific for MDS included the inclusion of patients with cytopenias but not clear morphologic evidence of MDS in the bone marrow as presumptive MDS; (iv) the inclusion of refractory cytopenia with unilineage dysplasia; and (v) disappearance of the category of refractory cytopenia with multilineage dysplasia and ring sideroblasts (RCMD-RS) [49].

Prognosis

A spectrum of diseases are formed by MDS from chronic disorders with indolent low blood counts to high-risk disease with rapidly progressive cytopenia and transformation to acute leukemia. The development of clinical systems that allow accurate prognostication of individual patients into low and high-risk categories has proven essential to guide rational management decisions and allow the introduction of investigational drug protocols.

The International Prognostic Scoring System (IPSS) [23] is the most widely used system for the assessment of prognosis and treatment planning. It provides an assessment of the prognosis of patients with primary MDS at the time of initial diagnosis. It was designed by the retrospective analysis of a large pool of 816 patients with MDS and followed the natural history of the disease to determine important factors related to patient outcome. Overall survival and the risk of transformation to acute leukemia were found to be related to the number of blood cytopenias, the percentage of myeloblasts in the bone marrow, and the presence of specific cytogenetic abnormalities. The risk associated with cytogenetic abnormalities was determined to be good if a normal diploid karyotype, isolated del(5q), isolated del(20q), or isolated −Y were present. High-risk abnormalities were defined as abnormalities involving chromosome 7 or complex karyotypes with the presence of three or more karyotypic abnormalities. All other cytogenetic abnormalities were considered to be of intermediate risk. The IPSS weights these different variables to produce a score that stratifies patients into four separate risk groups: low, intermediate-I, intermediate-II and high-risk (Table 8.1). Patient survival and the risk of transformation to acute leukemia are then predicted from cohorts of different ages as illustrated in Table 8.1(b). IPSS low and intermediate-I patients are generally considered as low-risk MDS, and intermediate-II and high patients are grouped into high-risk MDS.

Low-risk MDS are typically treated more conservatively than higher risk MDS. Prognostication in this low-risk group may be particularly important as it is unclear at this time whether some low-risk patients may benefit from early therapeutic intervention. To determine which low-risk patients should be considered for treatment protocols investigating early intervention, patients with low-risk MDS at the M. D. Anderson Cancer Center were analyzed to further stratify prognosis in low and intermediate-1 IPSS groupings [54]. Factors associated with a worse prognosis in this low-risk group include thrombocytopenia (platelets $<50 \times 10^9/L$), anemia (hemoglobin concentration <10g/dL), age (>60 years), blast count >4%, and a karyotype that was not diploid or del(5q). This model stratified low-risk patients into three subgroups with a median survival of 80 months, 27

Table 8.1 The International Prognostic Scoring System (IPSS)[22].

(a) IPSS score is the sum of the three listed prognostic factors

Score	0	0.5	1	1.5	2
BM blasts (%)	<5	5–10	—	11–20	21–30
Karyotype[a]	Good	Intermediate	Poor		
Cytopenias	0/1	2/3			

[a]Good: normal, -Y, del(5q), del(20q); Intemediate: other abnormalities; Poor: complex (≥3 abnormalities) or chromosome 7 anomalies. Cytopenias defined as hemoglobinconcentration <10 g/dL, neutrophils <1.5 × 10^9/L, and platelets <100 × 10^9/L.

(b) Prognosis determined by IPSS score

Risk group	IPSS score	Median survival (years)			
Age (years)		≤60	>60	≤70	>70
Low	0	11.8	4.8	9	3.9
Intermediate-1	0.5–1.0	5.2	2.7	4.4	2.4
Intermediate-2	1.5–2.0	1.8	1.1	1.3	1.2
High	≥2.5	0.3	0.5	0.4	0.4

Table 8.2 A low-risk MDS specific model.

(a)

Adverse Factor	Coefficient	*P*-value	Assigned score
Unfavorable cytogenetics	0.203	<0.0001	1
Age ≥60 years	0.348	<0.0001	2
Hgb <10 (g/dL)	0.216	<0.0001	1
Plt <50 × 10^9/L	0.498	<0.0001	2
50–200 × 10^9/L	0.277	0.0001	1
BM blasts ≥4%	0.195	0.0001	1

(b)

Score	Number of patients	Median survival (months)	4-year survival (%)
0	11	NR	78
1	58	83	82
2	113	51	51
3	185	36	40
4	223	22	27
5	166	14	9
6	86	16	7
7	13	9	NA

The score is calculated in patients with MDS and an IPSS score of low or intermediate 1. (a) Significant characteristics by multivariate analysis. Each one has an assigned score. The calculated total score can then be used in (b) to predict median and 4-year survivals.

months, and 14 months, respectively. Increased ferritin and β2 microglobulin were also associated with worse survival in these patients but these factors were not included in the prognostic model. As patient survival was significantly different between these low-risk categories, investigation of early intervention protocols in these low-risk patients with relatively poor survival may be warranted (Table 8.2).

The IPSS determines risk at the time of initial diagnosis but it does not provide information regarding changes in risk as patients progress through the course of their disease. A dynamic prognostication system has been developed to address this deficiency and provides a score that is predictive of survival and leukemic transformation over time. The WHO classification-based prognostic scoring system (WPSS) weights three variables: WHO diagnostic classification, karyotype abnormalities categorized according to the IPSS criteria, and transfusion requirement [55]. This stratifies patients into five disease groups that demonstrate different survival and risk of evolution to acute leukemia over time. Very low-risk patients in this classification were found to have an overall mortality rate that was not different to the general population. This model incorporates changes in the disease-risk profile over time, allowing further refinement in the prediction of survival and leukemic transformation as the disease progresses.

The presence of fibrosis on the bone marrow biopsy occurs in a minority of patients with MDS but this pathologic feature is not incorporated into routine diagnostic classifications or prognostic systems. Fibrosis is more frequently observed in patients with multilineage dysplasia or with karyotype abnormalities, and when present it is associated with a more rapid progression to severe bone marrow failure and shortened survival [56]. In younger patients, it may warrant early consideration of transplant therapies.

Therapy

The number of effective drug treatments available to treat MDS has increased in recent years providing the clinician with a range of management alternatives. Some of these treatments improve hematopoietic function and alleviate symptoms related to blood cytopenia, whereas other therapies alter the natural history of the disease and improve survival. Both approaches may be appropriate in different clinical contexts and many patients receive different combinations of treatments throughout their disease course.

The goals of therapy in MDS vary in different patient populations, and a management plan should consider the patient's age, comorbidities, and disease risk. Patients with low-risk MDS most commonly experience problems related to chronic anemia, and the disease may remain stable for prolonged periods. If these patients are elderly, they may best be managed with relatively non-toxic therapies that aim to maintain quality of life. Treatment options include transfusions of blood products, growth factor therapies (erythropoietin with or without colony-stimulating factors) and non-growth factor therapies with immunomodulators (lenolidamide), and epigenetic drug treatment (azacytidine and decitabine). High-risk MDS has a poor prognosis and forms a continuum with AML. Aggressive therapies may be warranted in these high-risk patients to eradicate the malignant clone and improve survival. Intensive therapies may include high-dose chemotherapy and consideration of allogeneic bone marrow transplantation in younger patients. Intensive treatment protocols are not suitable for all patients because they expose the patient to significant risks of treatment-related morbidity and mortality. An algorithm for treatment approaches at the M. D. Anderson Cancer Center is shown in Figure 8.2.

Accurately assessing response to treatment can be complex as treatment goals in low-risk and high-risk disease may be different. Clinical response criteria in low-risk disease usually measure improvements in peripheral blood cell counts and quality-of-life factors. Response in high-risk disease is typically more stringent, with measures of resolution of bone marrow changes by morphologic and cytogenetic criteria. Standardized criteria are available to assess response to treatment in MDS and are particularly useful to allow comparisons between drug trials [57,58].

Supportive care

Chronic blood cytopenia is a principal characteristic of MDS so therapies aimed at alleviating problems related to anemia, neutropenia, and thrombocytopenia are an essential component of management. Tissue oxygenation is readily improved by red-cell transfusion or more slowly improved with hematopoietic growth-factor support. Bacterial infections require aggressive treatment with antibiotics. Platelet transfusions are administered for episodes of bleeding or for prophylaxis in patients with severe thrombocytopenia. Additional hemostatic support with the use of antifibrinolytic agents may be considered for problematic mucosal bleeding or for surgical procedures.

Symptomatic anemia is often the major clinical problem in patients with low-risk MDS. In this group, red-cell transfusion is effective symptomatic therapy, but a prolonged transfusion program may cause problems with transfusion-related hemosiderosis, alloantibody formation, and volume overload in patients with impaired cardiac function. Repeated blood transfusions cause iron deposition in the heart, liver, and endocrine organs with subsequent impairment of left ventricular function, development of portal fibrosis in the liver, and impaired glucose tolerance [59]. Patients with MDS are often elderly and this pathologic iron deposition is often superimposed on organs with pre-existing dysfunction. The impact of these changes is frequently seen in the heart. Both chronic anemia and iron deposition adversely impact on cardiac function, and cardiac failure is found to be a common cause of death in the MDS patient population [53].

Deposition of iron in body tissues is treated with iron chelation. The efficacy of iron-chelation therapy is best demonstrated in thalassemia major, where regular deferoxamine therapy reduces iron deposition in organs and improves survival [60,61]. In MDS it is hypothesized to have similar advantages [62]. The parenteral administration of deferoxamine is inconvenient for patients, and the development of effective oral iron-chelating drugs, like deferasirox, has allowed iron chelation to be performed

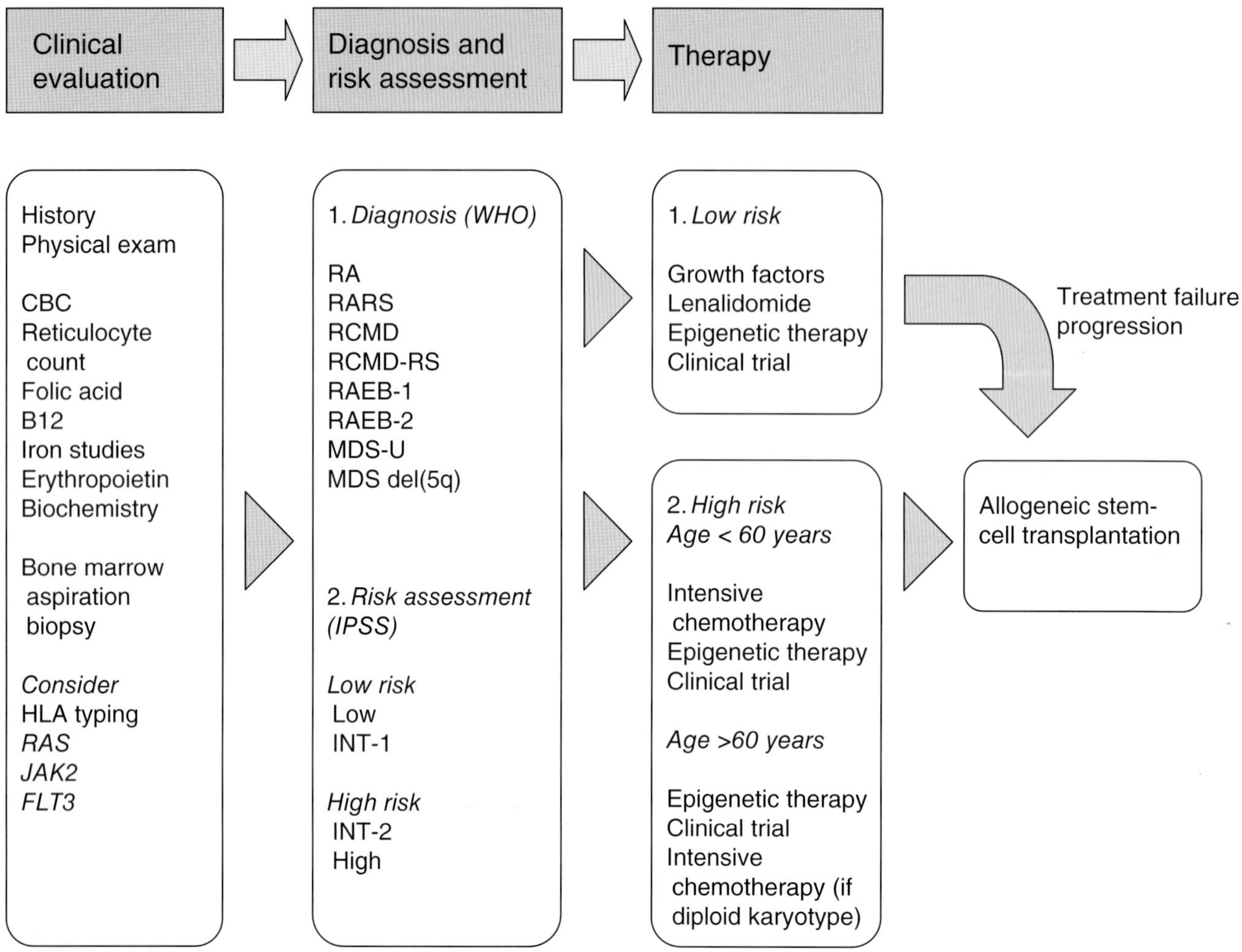

Figure 8.2 Management approach for the MDS.

more easily [63–65]. Iron chelation should commence with parenteral deferoxamine or oral deferasirox after 20–40 units of red cells have been administered, particularly if there is an expectation of prolonged survival and continued transfusion therapy [28]. Serum ferritin may be used as a guide to chelation therapy with a ferritin concentration greater than 1000 μg/L typically attained after transfusion of 20 red-cell units [53]. Iron-chelation therapy should also be considered in younger patients who may be candidates for allogeneic transplantation. An elevated pretransplant ferritin has been associated with a lower overall survival after allogeneic transplantation and an increase in the hepatic transplant complication of veno-occlusive disease [66].

Hematopoietic growth factors

Hematopoietic growth factors are the primary regulators of blood progenitor-cell proliferation and are used therapeutically to promote effective hematopoiesis from myelodysplastic bone marrow. Erythopoietin (EPO) therapy has been explored as an alternative to red-cell transfusion in patients with low-risk MDS. Recombinant erythropoietin (rEPO) in various forms including epoetin α, epoetin β, and the long-acting darbepoetin has been studied in different cohorts of patients. Overall, erythroid responses in unselected patients with MDS are modest in the range of 10–20% [67]. Within these cohorts, the best responses were identified in patients with low-risk MDS, a low-serum EPO level (<200 IU/L) and no red-cell transfusion requirement [67,68]. In this favorable subgroup of patients with MDS, an erythroid response to rEPO therapy is observed in 40–60% of patients [67–69]. The median duration of response is approximately 2 years, and therapy is associated with improved quality of life [69]. Recent data suggest that patients who respond to growth-factor therapy have better survival than historic control cohorts who received supportive care alone [68].

When combined with G-CSF, EPO is also an effective treatment for anemia, with response rates of approximately 40–50% in selected cohorts [70–72]. The combination of these two hematopoietic cytokines appears to offer synergistic benefit in promoting effective erythropoiesis and allows improvements in hemoglobin concentration in some patients who fail to respond to EPO monotherapy [70,73]. There is some evidence that the benefit of this combination therapy is most marked in the diagnostic categories of RARS and RCMD; however, this has not been confirmed in all studies [68]. Disease transformation is a theoretic risk in patients receiving chronic hematopoietic growth-factor therapy, but long-term observation of these patients suggests that these cytokines do not promote leukemic transformation [68,72].

Hematopoietic growth-factor therapy should be considered to treat anemia in patients with low-risk MDS associated with a low-serum EPO. EPO can be initiated as monotherapy with the addition of G-CSF if there is no objective response in 2–3 months.

Thrombopoietin has been used to promote platelet production and minimize the bleeding complications related to severe thrombocytopenia. Initial trials with recombinant thrombopoietin were disappointing [74], and new second-generation thrombomimetic agents are now being tested in the clinic to improve hemostatic function in patients with MDS. Initial trial data for one agent, AMG 531, is encouraging, with sustained improvements in platelet counts in about 40% of patients treated for severe thrombocytopenia related to MDS [75].

Lenalidomide

Lenalidomide is a chemical analog of thalidomide with diverse biologic actions that encompass immune modulation and antiangiogenic effects. Selective activity of lenalidomide against MDS associated with an interstitial deletion on the long arm of chromosome 5 was first suggested in a single-center study examining the effects of this drug on anemia in patients with low-risk MDS [76]. Erythroid responses were noted in 56% of the cohort, with the most significant response found in the subgroup with a del(5q) abnormality. This observation was then confirmed in a larger multicenter phase II study of lenalidomide [77]. This second trial demonstrated an overall erythroid response in 76% of patients with the del(5q) abnormality. Responses were prolonged and occurred rapidly with a median time to a hematologic response of 4–5 weeks. A cytogenetic response was documented in 73% of patients, with almost half of this group developing a cytogenetic remission. Cytogenetic responses were observed in patients with the del(5q) abnormality alone and in patients with the del(5q) abnormality associated with additional cytogenetic defects. This clearly demonstrates that the activity of lenalidomide was not limited to patients with the $5q^-$ syndrome as classified by the WHO, but was observed in patients with low-risk MDS with a variety of WHO classifications associated with a del(5q) abnormality on cytogenetic studies.

Lenalidomide therapy is usually commenced at 10 mg daily to treat myelodysplasia. A favorable response is typically characterized by normalization of blood cytopenias and resolution of morphologic abnormalities on bone marrow biopsy [77]. The most important early side-effect of therapy with lenalidomide is myelosuppression that may necessitate dose reduction in patients with persistent thrombocytopenia and neutropenia. Thrombocytopenia at diagnosis (platelet count $<100 \times 10^9$/L) has been associated with a worse response to lenalidomide treatment in published drug trials. This may reflect repeated or prolonged treatment interruption of the drug therapy secondary to myelosuppression.

Lenalidomide and thalidomide also demonstrate activity in low-risk MDS without the del(5q) abnormality. Lenalidomide has been studied in a group of 214 patients with low-risk MDS (IPSS low and int-1) and a predominantly normal karyotype [78]. In this cohort, 26% of patients achieved transfusion independence, with a further 17% developing a reduction in transfusion requirement. The median duration of transfusion independence while on therapy was 41 weeks, and cytogenetic responses were documented in 19% of patients with karyotypic abnormalities. A minority of patients with low-risk MDS also demonstrated an erythroid response with thalidomide [79]; however, the side-effect profile of this drug is unfavorable compared to lenalidomide, with treated patients commonly experiencing problematic fatigue, constipation, and limb paresthesia.

Epigenetic therapies

5-azacytidine and 5-aza-2′-deoxycytidine (decitabine) are chemical-related drugs with a spectrum of activity that includes both low-risk and high-risk MDS. The mechanism of action of these drugs is uncertain although both agents appear to reverse abnormal DNA methylation that surrounds the promoter of some tumor-suppressor genes in cancer cells. Aberrant promoter methylation is associated with transcriptional repression, or silencing, and may contribute to the loss of tumor-suppressor gene function in MDS. Decitabine and 5-azacytidine are both cytidine analogs that incorporate into DNA and form covalent bonds with DNA methyltransferase enzymes. Depletion of methyltransferase activity within the cell then causes newly synthesized DNA to be hypomethylated compared to the parent strand. After a few rounds of cell division, DNA becomes globally hypomethylated with alteration in gene expression within the leukemic cell. Both agents display cytotoxicity at high doses while hypomethylating activity remains prominent at lower doses. These biochemical changes are an attractive target for drug therapy as normal tissues have little gene-promoter methylation, so hypomethylating therapy may have some degree of specificity for the malignant clone.

Azacytidine was the first drug that demonstrated broad spectrum activity in MDS. Comparison of azacytidine therapy (75 mg/m^2 subcutaneously for 7 days every 28 days) to best supportive care in a randomized control trial demonstrated an overall response rate of 48% for the hypomethylating drug compared to 5% in the supportive care arm [80,81]. In this trial, therapy with azacytidine was associated with a prolongation in the time to leukemic transformation and a better quality of life, with an improvement in symptoms of fatigue and physical function. The median time-to-response was three cycles after commencing azacytidine therapy, and response rates were independent of MDS classification. Complete responses were observed in relatively few patients (10%), with most patients in the trial experiencing hematologic improvement. A report of a multicenter phase III study of azacytidine in patients with high-risk MDS has demonstrated an increase in overall survival of approximately 9 months for patients receiving azacytidine compared with other standard therapies [82]. This is a particularly significant finding as it is the first drug trial that has demonstrated a survival advantage in MDS.

Decitabine has similar clinical activity to azacytidine and has been studied in various dose regimes in predominantly high-risk MDS and AML. Comparison of decitabine (45 mg/m^2 in three divided doses administered for 3 consecutive days every 6 weeks) to best supportive care in a randomized control trial demonstrated an overall response rate of 17%, with complete remissions observed in 9% of patients with predominantly high-risk MDS [83]. Subgroup analysis revealed that patients who received decitabine had a longer median time to transformation to AML or death if they were treatment naïve or had high-risk MDS. Myelosuppression was the major drug toxicity. Data from this trial may underestimate the efficacy of the drug as a significant proportion of patients on the therapy arm received a small number of treatment cycles that may have been insufficient to demonstrate a response. This notion is supported by previous phase II trial data that suggest decitabine has an overall response rate similar to azacytidine [84]. Subsequent clinical trial development with decitabine has focused on improving response rates by lowering the daily dose and lengthening administration schedules. One such schedule of intravenous administration of decitabine for 5 days every 4 weeks demonstrated a complete response rate of 39% in a high-risk MDS cohort [85,86]. Subgroup analysis of trial data suggests that decitabine may have significant activity in MDS associated with abnormalities in chromosome 7. This observation is important and will need to be confirmed in other studies as this cytogenetic abnormality is usually associated with a very poor outcome [87]. It is recognized that improvements in hematopoietic function are often delayed after the initiation of azacytidine or decitabine therapy and drug treatment should continue for four to six cycles before cessation because of poor response. Early problems of myelosuppression may resolve over this time period and should not necessarily initiate dose reduction. Recently, a preliminary report of a randomized study of decitabine did not show any improvement in survival.

Chemical modification of histone proteins by acetylation contribute to the regulation of gene expression and probably interact with abnormal DNA methylation to cause transcriptional suppression of tumor-suppressor genes. Histone deacetylase inhibitors alter chromatin structure to promote gene transcription, and their combination with hypomethylating agents demonstrates significant *in vitro* synergies in cancer cells [88]. Clinical drug trials in MDS and AML are starting to examine this potentially exciting combination of drugs. Trials initiated at the M. D. Anderson Cancer Center have examined decitabine with valproic acid [89] and 5-azacytidine with the combination of valproic acid and all-trans-retinoic acid [90]. Other investigators have examined 5-azacytidine with sodium phenylbutyrate [91]. All of these early trials demonstrate activity of combined hypomethylating drugs and HDAC inhibition with favorable response rates of up to 50% in elderly patients with low induction-related mortality. Significant decreases in global DNA methylation and increases in histone acetylation were observed in these studies but these changes did not correlate with clinical response to drug therapy.

Cytotoxic chemotherapy

The relatively poor prognosis associated with high-risk MDS has initiated intensive treatment strategies incorporating high-dose chemotherapy in the same protocols used to treat AML. In patients diagnosed with high-risk MDS, AML-type treatment protocols produce a complete response rate of about 40–60%, although remissions are usually brief [50,92–95]. Unfortunately, these patients with MDS also experience a shorter period of survival after intensive chemotherapy compared with patients treated for AML. This poor response to high-dose chemotherapy is due to, at least in part, the relatively greater proportion of patients diagnosed with RAEB having poor prognosis cytogenetics involving complex changes of chromosome 5 and 7 [50]. Selection of patients for this treatment approach is important as elderly patients with significant comorbidities poorly tolerate high-dose chemotherapy.

Patients with high-risk MDS have been administered a variety of intensive chemotherapy regimens in the clinical trial setting at the M. D. Anderson Cancer Center [95,96]. Clinical trial protocols have examined using intermediate to high-dose cytosine arabinoside (Ara-C) in various combinations with idarubucin (I), cyclophosphamide (C), fludarabine (F), and topotecan (T), as regimens: IA, FA, FAI, TA, and CAT. The overall complete response rate for these antileukemic chemotherapy protocols was 55–58%, with activity demonstrated against all high-risk MDS diagnostic categories. A short antecedent history of hematologic disorder, a normal karyotype, performance status, age, and treatment in a laminar air-flow environment were all predictive of attaining a complete response. This intensive approach is beneficial in some patients as those who developed a complete response within 6 weeks of commencing chemotherapy obtained a survival advantage. However, these regimens were toxic with significant treatment-related mortality in the first 6 weeks, ranging from 5% with TA to 21% with FAI. Consolidation chemotherapy was used in most cases where a remission was achieved with a regimen containing the drugs used in induction, but at a reduced intensity of 50–66% of the initial dose. Survival of patients treated with IA and TA therapies were comparable and superior to those patients treated with FA, FAI, and CAT regimens, but prognosis with this intensive treatment approach remains poor with a 5 year overall survival rate of 8% [18]. Nevertheless, this approach does benefit some patients with younger individuals (<65 years) with a normal karyotype achieving an encouraging 5-year survival rate of 27% with intensive treatment. For older patients, the TA combination can be considered as it has a relatively low treatment-related mortality and it does not contain anthracycline drugs that are relatively contraindicated in the presence of heart disease.

Low-dose cytarabine (5–20 mg/m^2 per day) as a single agent has been used in myeloid malignancy, particularly in those patients unable to tolerate more intensive regimens. In MDS, low-dose cytarabine has an overall response rate of about 30%, with a complete response observed in up to 20% of patients [97–99]. Duration of response is relatively short with a median duration of complete response of about 10 months. Despite the relatively low dose, myelosuppression is still observed in this group of patients with MDS presumably because of poor bone marrow reserve.

Investigation of new agents as monotherapy or incorporated into protocols with other cytotoxic agents promises improved outcomes for patients with MDS in the future. Clofarabine is a nucleoside analog with significant activity in AML and MDS and is currently being explored in drug trials [100]. Other agents that target specific oncogenic pathways are also being investigated. Tipifarnib, a farnesyl transferase inhibitor that modulates Ras signaling, has demonstrated overall responses of 32% in high-risk MDS [101].

Immunosuppressive therapy

Immune dysfunction contributes to blood cytopenia in some patients with MDS, producing a clinical overlap with aplastic anemia [102]. Immunosuppressive therapy with antithymocyte globulin (ATG), with or without the addition of cyclosporine, has been explored in small numbers of patients with MDS to determine if modulation of the immune system can improve hematopoietic function as demonstrated in therapy for aplastic anemia. Disease response rates of 30–50% have been observed in selected cohorts of patients with low-risk MDS who have been administered a course of ATG, with a minority of patients experiencing a prolonged remission [103–105]. A range of features have been described that predict a good response to immunosuppressive therapy, including younger age, HLA-DR status, shorter duration of red-cell transfusion, low-risk IPSS, and bone marrow hypocellularity [105–107]. Selection of appropriate patients for immunosuppression is important, as ATG therapy is poorly tolerated in an older population with low-risk MDS [105,108].

Hematopoietic stem-cell transplantation

Allogeneic hematopoietic stem-cell transplantation (HSCT) is a potentially curative treatment modality for MDS but the therapy carries significant risk associated with treatment toxicity, prolonged cytopenia, infection, and graft versus host disease. In the small proportion of patients with MDS who are young with a suitable donor, the transplant procedure offers the best chance of cure with a long-term disease-free survival of 30–50% [109–113]. Given the risks associated with this procedure, patient suitability and timing of the transplant are important issues to consider.

Allogeneic transplantation with myeloablative conditioning has been examined exclusively in younger patients with a median age in the mid thirties in most studies. Patients with low-risk disease (RA/RARS) have experienced the best survival rate; however, this is also the subgroup of patients who are predicted to experience prolonged survival without aggressive therapies. This procedure is associated with significant mortality risk, with a treatment related mortality of up to 30–50% in some studies [111,112]. Relapse of the disease after transplantation occurs in approximately 20% of cases, and the relapsed disease has a relatively poor response to donor lymphocyte infusion [111,112,114]. Increased risk of allogeneic transplantation in MDS has been associated with older age, poor-risk cytogenetics, particularly abnormalities of chromosome 7 or a complex karyotype, the presence of excess blasts in the bone marrow, and longer duration of disease [111,115,116]. Patients with treatment-related MDS are also recognized to have a poor transplant outcome, but analysis of this subgroup suggests that this poor survival is related to the frequency of high-risk cytogenetic changes in this group and does not specifically reflect the underlying treatment-related etiology of the disease [116,117].

The development of non-myeloablative allogeneic transplantation with reduced-intensity conditioning has allowed allogeneic transplantation to be considered in older patients with MDS and in patients whose comorbities or organ dysfunction would exclude them from myeloablative treatment [118,119]. This procedure has reduced the transplant-related mortality associated with allogeneic transplantation, which has been the major problem limiting the availability of this potentially curative therapy to older patients with MDS. This therapy aims to minimize organ toxicity related to initial chemo- or radiotherapy but allow stable engraftment of donor cells that provide curative potential by the graft versus leukemia effect. Comparison of reduced-intensity conditioning transplantation with standard myeloablative conditioning has found reduced transplant-related mortality but increased relapse rate, resulting in comparable rates of overall survival between the two transplantation strategies [115,120,121]. Considering that the patients who have received non-myeloablative conditioning have been older with more significant comorbidities, this result is encouraging and has allowed the possibility of cure by means of allogeneic transplantation to be extended to a greater proportion of the MDS population.

Statistical modeling based on historic allogeneic transplantation outcomes for matched sibling transplantation suggests that the maximal overall survival is achieved by different transplant strategies in different MDS risk groups [122]. Patients with low-risk disease (IPSS low and intermediate-1 groups) maximize overall survival by delaying transplantation after diagnosis until a time when there is evidence of disease progression but before the development of overt acute leukemia. This delayed transplant approach provided greatest survival benefit to younger patients aged <40 years. Specific features of disease progression have not been defined, but evidence of new cytogenetic abnormalities, progressive cytopenia, and increasing blast percentage in the bone marrow are suggested as potential triggers for transplantation. Patients with high-risk disease (IPSS intermediate-2 and high) should ideally receive the transplant as soon as possible after diagnosis. The presence of bone marrow fibrosis delays engraftment in allogeneic transplantation and its presence is an additional risk factor in transplant outcome in high-risk MDS. In this group, fibrosis considerably increases transplantation risk and therefore early consideration of transplantation is suggested in a younger patient with significant MDS associated fibrosis [123].

Autologous stem-cell transplantation has been studied in younger patients with MDS who lack a stem-cell donor. This procedure has a relatively low treatment-related mortality of <10% but is associated with a high relapse rate of >50%, with consequent survival at 3 years of 30–40% [124,125]. This procedure can be difficult to perform in some patients because of an inability to collect autologous cells and is not routinely recommended therapy for MDS outside of a clinical-trial setting.

References

1 Ma X, Does M, Raza A, Mayne ST. Myelodysplastic syndromes: incidence and survival in the United States. *Cancer* 2007;109:1536–42.

2 Rollison DE, Howlader N, Smith MT, *et al.* Epidemiology of myelodysplastic syndromes and chronic myeloproliferative disorders in the United States, 2001–2004, using data from the NAACCR and SEER programs. *Blood*, 2008;112:45–52.

3 Matsuda A, Germing U, Jinnai I, *et al.* Difference in clinical features between Japanese and German patients with refractory anemia in myelodysplastic syndromes. *Blood* 2005;106: 2633–40.

4 Morel P, Hebbar M, Lai JL, *et al.*, Cytogenetic analysis has strong independent prognostic value in de novo myelodysplastic syndromes and can be incorporated in a new scoring system: a report on 408 cases. *Leukemia* 1993;7:1315–23.

5 Chen B, Zhao WL, Jin J, *et al.* Clinical and cytogenetic features of 508 Chinese patients with myelodysplastic syndrome and comparison with those in Western countries. *Leukemia* 2005;19: 767–75.

6 Toyama K, Ohyashiki K, Yoshida Y, *et al.* Clinical implications of chromosomal abnormalities in 401 patients with myelodysplastic syndromes: a multicentric study in Japan. *Leukemia* 1993;7:499–508.

7 Sole F, Luno E, Sanzo C, *et al.* Identification of novel cytogenetic markers with prognostic significance in a series of 968 patients with primary myelodysplastic syndromes. *Haematologica* 2005;90:1168–78.

8 Poppe B, Van Limbergen H, Van Roy N, *et al.* Chromosomal aberrations in Bloom syndrome patients with myeloid malignancies. *Cancer Genet Cytogenet* 2001;128:39–42.

9 Luna-Fineman S, Shannon KM, Atwater SK, *et al.* Myelodysplastic and myeloproliferative disorders of childhood: a study of 167 patients. *Blood* 1999;93:459–66.

10 Allan JM, Wild CP, Rollinson S, *et al.* Polymorphism in glutathione S-transferase P1 is associated with susceptibility to chemotherapy-induced leukemia. *Proc Natl Acad Sci U S A* 2001;98:11592–7.

11 Felix CA, Walker AH, Lange BJ, *et al.* Association of CYP3A4 genotype with treatment-related leukemia. *Proc Natl Acad Sci U S A* 1998;95:13176–81.

12 Larson RA, Wang Y, Banerjee M, *et al.* Prevalence of the inactivating 609C→T polymorphism in the NAD(P)H: quinone oxidoreductase (*NQO1*) gene in patients with primary and therapy-related myeloid leukemia. *Blood* 1999;94:803–7.

13 Descatha A, Jenabian A, Conso F, Ameille J. Occupational exposures and haematological malignancies: overview on human recent data. *Cancer Causes Control* 2005;16:939–53.

14 West RR, Stafford DA, Farrow A, Jacobs A. Occupational and environmental exposures and myelodysplasia: a case–control study. *Leuk Res* 1995;19:127–39.

15 Rigolin GM, Cuneo A, Roberti MG, *et al.* Exposure to myelotoxic agents and myelodysplasia: case–control study and cor-

relation with clinicobiological findings. *Br J Haematol* 1998;103: 189–97.

16 Nagata C, Shimizu H, Hirashima K, *et al.* Hair dye use and occupational exposure to organic solvents as risk factors for myelodysplastic syndrome. *Leuk Res* 1999;23:57–62.

17 Golomb HM, Alimena G, Rowley JD, Vardiman JW, Testa JR, Sovik C. Correlation of occupation and karyotype in adults with acute nonlymphocytic leukemia. *Blood* 1982;60:404–11.

18 Kantarjian HM, Keating MJ, Walters RS, *et al.* Therapy-related leukemia and myelodysplastic syndrome: clinical, cytogenetic, and prognostic features. *J Clin Oncol* 1986;4:1748–57.

19 Josting A, Weidenmann S, Franklin J, *et al.* Secondary myeloid leukemia and myelodysplastic syndromes in patients treated for Hodgkin's disease: a report from the German Hodgkin's Lymphoma Study Group. *J Clin Oncol* 2003;21:3440–6.

20 Devereux S, Selassie TG, Vaughan Hudson G, Vaughan Hudson B, Linch DC. Leukemia complicating treatment for Hodgkin's disease: the experience of the British National Lymphoma Investigation. *BMJ* 1990;301:1077–80.

21 Traweek ST, Slovak ML, Nademanee AP, Brynes RK, Niland JC, Forman SJ. Clonal karyotypic hematopoietic cell abnormalities occurring after autologous bone marrow transplantation for Hodgkin's disease and non-Hodgkin's lymphoma. *Blood* 1994;84:957–63.

22 Stone RM, Neuberg D, Soiffer R, *et al.* Myelodysplastic syndrome as a late complication following autologous bone marrow transplantation for non-Hodgkin's lymphoma. *J Clin Oncol* 1994;12:2535–42.

23 Greenberg P, Cox C, LeBeau MM, *et al.* International scoring system for evaluating prognosis in myelodysplastic syndromes. *Blood* 1997;89:2079–88.

24 Jaffe ES, Harris NL, Stein R, Vardiman J. *Pathology and Genetics of Tumors of Hematopoietic and Lymphoid Tissues.* Lyon: IARC Press, 2001.

25 Gralnick HR, Gatton DA, Catovsky D, Sultan C, Bennett JM. Classification of acute leukemia. *Ann Intern Med* 1977;87: 740–53.

26 Valent P, Horny HP, Bennett JM, *et al.* Definitions and standards in the diagnosis and treatment of the myelodysplastic syndromes: Consensus statements and report from a working conference. *Leuk Res* 2007;31:727–36.

27 Bain BJ. The bone marrow aspirate of healthy subjects. *Br J Haematol* 1996;94:206–9.

28 Haase D, Guming U, Schanz J, *et al.* New insights into the prognostic impact of the karyotype in MDS and correlation with subtypes: evidence from a core dataset of 2124 patients. *Blood* 2007;110:4385–95.

29 Pedersen-Bjergaard J, Pedersen M, Roulston D, Philip P. Different genetic pathways in leukemogenesis for patients presenting with therapy-related myelodysplasia and therapy-related acute myeloid leukemia. *Blood* 1995;86:3542–52.

30 Rowley JD, Golomb HM, Vardiman JW. Nonrandom chromosome abnormalities in acute leukemia and dysmyelopoietic syndromes in patients with previously treated malignant disease. *Blood* 1981;58:759–67.

31 Harada H, Harada Y, Niimi H, Kyo T, Kimura A, Inaba T. High incidence of somatic mutations in the *AML1/RUNX1* gene in myelodysplastic syndrome and low blast percentage myeloid leukemia with myelodysplasia. *Blood* 2004;103: 2316–24.

32 Harada H, Harada Y, Tanaka H, Kimura A, Inaba T. Implications of somatic mutations in the *AML1* gene in radiation-associated and therapy-related myelodysplastic syndrome/acute myeloid leukemia. *Blood* 2003;101:673–80.

33 Bacher U, Haferlach T, Kern W, Haferlach C, Schnittger S. A comparative study of molecular mutations in 381 patients with myelodysplastic syndrome and in 4130 patients with acute myeloid leukemia. *Haematologica* 2007;92:744–52.

34 Caudill JS, Sternberg AJ, Li CY, Tefferi A, Lasho TL, Steensma DP. C-terminal nucleophosmin mutations are uncommon in chronic myeloid disorders. *Br J Haematol* 2006;133:638–41.

35 Langemeijer SM, Kuiper RP, Berends M, *et al.* Acquired mutations in *TET2* are common in myelodysplastic syndromes. *Nat Genet* 2009;41:838–42.

36 Maciejewski JP, Mufti GJ. Whole genome scanning as a cytogenetic tool in hematologic malignancies. *Blood* 2008;112: 965–74.

37 Dunbar AJ, Gondek LP, O'Keefe CL, *et al.* 250K single nucleotide polymorphism array karyotyping identifies acquired uniparental disomy and homozygous mutations, including novel missense substitutions of c-Cbl, in myeloid malignancies. *Cancer Res* 2008;68:10349–57.

38 Sokal G, Michaux JL, Van Den Berghe H, *et al.* A new hematologic syndrome with a distinct karyotype: the 5 q–chromosome. *Blood* 1975;46:519–33.

39 Pellagatti A, Jadersten M, Forsblom AM, *et al.* Lenalidomide inhibits the malignant clone and up-regulates the *SPARC* gene mapping to the commonly deleted region in 5q- syndrome patients. *Proc Natl Acad Sci U S A* 2007;104:11406–11.

40 Liu TX, Becker MW, Jelinek J, *et al.* Chromosome 5q deletion and epigenetic suppression of the gene encoding alpha-catenin (*CTNNA1*) in myeloid cell transformation. *Nat Med* 2007;13:78–83.

41 Ebert BL, Pretz J, Bosco J, *et al.* Identification of *RPS14* as a 5q- syndrome gene by RNA interference screen. *Nature* 2008;451:335–9.

42 Lai JL, Preudhomme C, Zandecki M, *et al.* Myelodysplastic syndromes and acute myeloid leukemia with 17p deletion. An entity characterized by specific dysgranulopoiesis and a high incidence of *P53* mutations. *Leukemia* 1995;9: 370–81.

43 Soenen V, Preudhomme C, Roumier C, Daudignon A, Lai JL, Fenaux P. 17p Deletion in acute myeloid leukemia and myelodysplastic syndrome. Analysis of breakpoints and deleted segments by fluorescence in situ. *Blood* 1998;91:1008–15.

44 Gibbons RJ, Pellagatti A, Garrick D, *et al.* Identification of acquired somatic mutations in the gene encoding chromatin-remodeling factor ATRX in the alpha-thalassemia myelodysplasia syndrome (ATMDS). *Nat Genet* 2003;34:446–9.

45 Steensma DP, Gibbons RJ, Higgs DR. Acquired alpha-thalassemia in association with myelodysplastic syndrome and other hematologic malignancies. *Blood* 2005;105: 443–52.

46 Matsui WH, Brodsky RA, Smith BD, Borowitz MJ, Jones RJ. Quantitative analysis of bone marrow CD34 cells in aplastic anemia and hypoplastic myelodysplastic syndromes. *Leukemia* 2006;20:458–62.

47 Bennett JM, Catovsky D, Daniel MT, *et al.* Proposals for the classification of the myelodysplastic syndromes. *Br J Haematol* 1982;51:189–99.

48 Vardiman JW, Harris NL, Brunning RD. The World Health Organization (WHO) classification of the myeloid neoplasms. *Blood* 2002;100:2292–302.

49 Vardiman JW, Thiele J, Arber DA, *et al.* The 2008 revision of the World Health Organization (WHO) classification of myeloid neoplasms and acute leukemia: rationale and important changes. *Blood* 2009;114:937–51.

50 Estey E, Thall P, Beran M, Kantarjian H, Pierce S, Keating M. Effect of diagnosis (refractory anemia with excess blasts, refractory anemia with excess blasts in transformation, or acute myeloid leukemia [AML]) on outcome of AML-type chemotherapy. *Blood* 1997;90:2969–77.

51 Germing U, Gattermann N, Strupp C, Aivado M, Aul C. Validation of the WHO proposals for a new classification of primary myelodysplastic syndromes: a retrospective analysis of 1600 patients. *Leuk Res* 2000;24:983–92.

52 Howe RB, Porwitt-MacDonald A, Wanat R, Tehranchi R, Hellstrom-Lindberg E. The WHO classification of MDS does make a difference. *Blood* 2004;103:3265–70.

53 Malcovati L, Porta MG, Pascutto C, *et al.* Prognostic factors and life expectancy in myelodysplastic syndromes classified according to WHO criteria: a basis for clinical decision making. *J Clin Oncol* 2005;23:7594–603.

54 Garcia-Manero G, Shan J, Federl S, *et al.* A prognostic score for patients with lower risk myelodysplastic syndrome. *Leukemia* 2008;22:538–43.

55 Malcovati L, Germing U, Kuendgen A, *et al.* Time-dependent prognostic scoring system for predicting survival and leukemic evolution in myelodysplastic syndromes. *J Clin Oncol* 2007;25:3503–10.

56 Buesche G, Teoman H, Wilczak W, *et al.* Marrow fibrosis predicts early fatal marrow failure in patients with myelodysplastic syndromes. *Leukemia* 2008;22:313–22.

57 Cheson BD, Bennett JM, Kantarjian H, *et al.* Report of an international working group to standardize response criteria for myelodysplastic syndromes. *Blood* 2000;96:3671–4.

58 Cheson BD, Greenberg PL, Bennett JM, *et al.* Clinical application and proposal for modification of the International Working Group (IWG) response criteria in myelodysplasia. *Blood* 2006;108:419–25.

59 Schafer AI, Cheron RG, Dluhy R, *et al.* Clinical consequences of acquired transfusional iron overload in adults. *N Engl J Med* 1981;304:319–24.

60 Olivieri NF, Nathan DG, MacMillan JH, *et al.* Survival in medically treated patients with homozygous beta-thalassemia. *N Engl J Med* 1994;331:574–8.

61 Brittenham GM, Griffith PM, Neinhuis AW, *et al.* Efficacy of deferoxamine in preventing complications of iron overload in patients with thalassemia major. *N Engl J Med* 1994;331: 567–73.

62 Jensen PD, Heickendorff L, Pedersen B, *et al.* The effect of iron chelation on haemopoiesis in MDS patients with transfusional iron overload. *Br J Haematol* 1996;94:288–99.

63 Nisbet-Brown E, Olivieri NF, Giardina PJ, *et al.* Effectiveness and safety of ICL670 in iron-loaded patients with thalassaemia: a randomized, double-blind, placebo-controlled, dose-escalation trial. *Lancet* 2003;361:1597–602.

64 Cappellini MD, Cohen A, Piga A, *et al.* A phase 3 study of deferasirox (ICL670), a once-daily oral iron chelator, in patients with beta-thalassemia. *Blood* 2006;107:3455–62.

65 Neufeld EJ. Oral chelators deferasirox and deferiprone for transfusional iron overload in thalassemia major: new data, new questions. *Blood* 2006;107:3436–41.

66 Armand P, Kim HT, Cutler CS, *et al.* Prognostic impact of elevated pretransplantation serum ferritin in patients undergoing myeloablative stem cell transplantation. *Blood* 2007;109: 4586–8.

67 Hellstrom-Lindberg E. Efficacy of erythropoietin in the myelodysplastic syndromes: a meta-analysis of 205 patients from 17 studies. *Br J Haematol* 1995;89:67–71.

68 Park S, Grabar S, Kelaidi C, *et al.* Predictive factors of response and survival in myelodysplastic syndrome treated with erythropoietin and G-CSF: the GFM experience. *Blood* 2008;111: 574–82.

69 Hellstrom-Lindberg E, Gulbrandsen N, Lindberg G, *et al.* A validated decision model for treating the anemia of myelodysplastic syndromes with erythropoietin + granulocyte colony-stimulating factor: significant effects on quality of life. *Br J Haematol* 2003;120:1037–46.

70 Negrin RS, Stein R, Doherty K, *et al.* Maintenance treatment of the anemia of myelodysplastic syndromes with recombinant human granulocyte colony-stimulating factor and erythropoietin: evidence for in vivo synergy. *Blood* 1996;87: 4076–81.

71 Casadevall N, Durieux P, Dubois S, *et al.* Health, economic, and quality-of-life effects of erythropoietin and granulocyte colony-stimulating factor for the treatment of myelodysplastic syndromes: a randomized, controlled trial. *Blood* 2004;104: 321–7.

72 Jadersten M, Montgomery SM, Dybedal I, Porwit-MacDonald A, Hellstrom-Lindberg E. Long-term outcome of treatment of anemia in MDS with erythropoietin and G-CSF. *Blood* 2005;106: 803–11.

73 Hellstrom-Lindberg E, Ahlgren T, Beguin Y, *et al.* Treatment of anemia in myelodysplastic syndromes with granulocyte colony-stimulating factor plus erythropoietin: results from a randomized phase II study and long-term follow-up of 71 patients. *Blood* 1998;92:68–75.

74 Kuter DJ, Begley CG. Recombinant human thrombopoietin: basic biology and evaluation of clinical studies. *Blood* 2002; 100:3457–69.

75 Kantarjian H, Fenaux P, Sekeres MA, *et al.* Phase 1/2 study of AMG 531 in thrombocytopenic patients with low-risk myelodysplastic syndrome (MDS): Update including extended treatment. *Am Soc Hematol* 2007;110:250.

76 List A, Kurtin S, Roe DJ, *et al.* Efficacy of lenalidomide in myelodysplastic syndromes. *N Engl J Med* 2005;352:549–57.

77 List A, Dewald G, Bennett J, *et al.* Lenalidomide in the myelodysplastic syndrome with chromosome 5q deletion. *N Engl J Med* 2006;355:1456–65.

78 Raza A, Reeves JA, Feldman EJ, *et al.* Phase II study of lenalidomide in transfusion-dependent, low- and intermediate-1-risk myelodysplastic syndromes with karyotypes other than deletion 5q. *Blood* 2008;111:86–93.

79 Raza A, Meyer P, Dutt D, *et al.* Thalidomide produces transfusion independence in long-standing refractory anemias of patients with myelodysplastic syndromes. *Blood* 2001;98: 958–65.

80 Silverman LR, Demakos EP, Peterson BL, *et al.* Randomized controlled trial of azacitidine in patients with the myelodys-

plastic syndrome: a study of the cancer and leukemia group B. *J Clin Oncol* 2002;20:2429–40.

81 Silverman LR, McKenzie DR, Peterson BL, *et al.* Further analysis of trials with azacitidine in patients with myelodysplastic syndrome: studies 8421, 8921, and 9221 by the Cancer and Leukemia Group B. *J Clin Oncol* 2006;24:3895–903.

82 Fenaux P, Mufti GJ, Hellstrom-Lindberg E, *et al.* Efficacy of azacitidine compared with that of conventional care regimens in the treatment of higher-risk myelodysplastic syndromes: a randomized, open-label, phase III study. *Lancet Oncol* 2009; 10:223–32.

83 Kantarjian H, Issa JP, Rosenfeld CS, *et al.* Decitabine improves patient outcomes in myelodysplastic syndromes: results of a phase III randomized study. *Cancer* 2006;106:1794–803.

84 Wijermans P, Lubbert M, Verhoef G, *et al.* Low-dose 5-aza-2′-deoxycytidine, a DNA hypomethylating agent, for the treatment of high-risk myelodysplastic syndrome: a multicenter phase II study in elderly patients. *J Clin Oncol* 2000;18: 956–62.

85 Issa JP, Garcia-Manero G, Giles FJ, *et al.* Phase 1 study of low-dose prolonged exposure schedules of the hypomethylating agent 5-aza-2′-deoxycytidine (decitabine) in hematopoietic malignancies. *Blood* 2004;103:1635–40.

86 Kantarjian H, Oki Y, Garcia-Manero G, *et al.* Results of a randomized study of 3 schedules of low-dose decitabine in higher-risk myelodysplastic syndrome and chronic myelomonocytic leukemia. *Blood* 2007;109:52–7.

87 Ruter B, Wijermans P, Claus R, Kunzmann R, Lubbert M. Preferential cytogenetic response to continuous intravenous low-dose decitabine (DAC) administration in myelodysplastic syndrome with monosomy 7. *Blood* 2007;110:1080–2; author reply 1083.

88 Cameron EE, Bachman KE, Myohanen S, Herman JG, Baylin SB. Synergy of demethylation and histone deacetylase inhibition in the re-expression of genes silenced in cancer. *Nat Genet* 1999;21:103–7.

89 Garcia-Manero G, Kantarjian HM, Sanchez-Gonzalez B, *et al.* Phase 1/2 study of the combination of 5-aza-2′-deoxycytidine with valproic acid in patients with leukemia. *Blood* 2006;108: 3271–9.

90 Soriano AO, Yang H, Faderl S, *et al.* Safety and clinical activity of the combination of 5-azacytidine, valproic acid, and all-trans retinoic acid in acute myeloid leukemia and myelodysplastic syndrome. *Blood* 2007;110:2302–8.

91 Maslak P, Chanel S, Camacho LH, *et al.* Pilot study of combination transcriptional modulation therapy with sodium phenylbutyrate and 5-azacytidine in patients with acute myeloid leukemia or myelodysplastic syndrome. *Leukemia* 2006;20: 212–17.

92 Wattel E, De Botton S, Luc Lai J, *et al.* Long-term follow-up of de novo myelodysplastic syndromes treated with intensive chemotherapy: incidence of long-term survivors and outcome of partial responders. *Br J Haematol* 1997;98:983–91.

93 Parker JE, Pagliuca A, Mijovic A, *et al.* Fludarabine, cytarabine, G-CSF and idarubicin (FLAG-IDA) for the treatment of poor-risk myelodysplastic syndromes and acute myeloid leukemia. *Br J Haematol* 1997;99:939–44.

94 Bernasconi C, Alessandrino EP, Bernasconi P, *et al.* Randomized clinical study comparing aggressive chemotherapy with or without G-CSF support for high-risk myelodysplastic syndromes or secondary acute myeloid leukemia evolving from MDS. *Br J Haematol* 1998;102:678–83.

95 Kantarjian H, Beran M, Cortes J, *et al.* Long-term follow-up results of the combination of topotecan and cytarabine and other intensive chemotherapy regimens in myelodysplastic syndrome. *Cancer* 2006;106:1099–109.

96 Beran M, Shen Y, Kantarjian H, *et al.* High-dose chemotherapy in high-risk myelodysplastic syndrome: covariate-adjusted comparison of five regimens. *Cancer* 2001;92:1999–2015.

97 Cheson BD, Jasperse DM, Simon R, Friedman MA, *et al.* A critical appraisal of low-dose cytosine arabinoside in patients with acute non-lymphocytic leukemia and myelodysplastic syndromes. *J Clin Oncol* 1986;4:1857–64.

98 Hellstrom-Lindberg E, Robert KH, Gahrton G, *et al.* A predictive model for the clinical response to low dose ara-C: a study of 102 patients with myelodysplastic syndromes or acute leukemia. *Br J Haematol* 1992;81:503–11.

99 Zwierzina H, Suciu S, Loeffler-Ragg J, *et al.* Low-dose cytosine arabinoside (LD-AraC) vs LD-AraC plus granulocyte/macrophage colony stimulating factor vs LD-AraC plus Interleukin-3 for myelodysplastic syndrome patients with a high risk of developing acute leukemia: final results of a randomized phase III study (06903) of the EORTC Leukemia Cooperative Group. *Leukemia* 2005;19:1929–33.

100 Kantarjian H, Gandhi V, Cortes J, *et al.* Phase 2 clinical and pharmacologic study of clofarabine in patients with refractory or relapsed acute leukemia. *Blood* 2003;102: 2379–86.

101 Fenaux P, Raza A, Mufti GJ, *et al.* A multicenter phase 2 study of the farnesyltransferase inhibitor tipifarnib in intermediate-to high-risk myelodysplastic syndrome. *Blood* 2007;109: 4158–63.

102 Sloand EM, Mainwaring L, Fuhrer M, *et al.* Preferential suppression of trisomy 8 compared with normal hematopoietic cell growth by autologous lymphocytes in patients with trisomy 8 myelodysplastic syndrome. *Blood* 2005;106:841–51.

103 Molldrem JJ, Caples M, Mavroudis D, Plante M, Young NS, Barrett AJ. Antithymocyte globulin for patients with myelodysplastic syndrome. *Br J Haematol* 1997;99:699–705.

104 Killick SB, Mufti G, Cavenagh JD, *et al.* A pilot study of antithymocyte globulin (ATG) in the treatment of patients with 'low-risk' myelodysplasia. *Br J Haematol* 2003;120:679–84.

105 Lim ZY, Killick S, Germing U, *et al.* Low IPSS score and bone marrow hypocellularity in MDS patients predict hematological responses to antithymocyte globulin. *Leukemia* 2007;21: 1436–41.

106 Saunthararajah Y, Nakamura R, Nam JM, *et al.* HLA-DR15 (DR2) is overrepresented in myelodysplastic syndrome and aplastic anemia and predicts a response to immunosuppression in myelodysplastic syndrome. *Blood* 2002;100:1570–4.

107 Saunthararajah Y, Nakamura R, Wesley R, Wang QJ, Barrett AJ. A simple method to predict response to immunosuppressive therapy in patients with myelodysplastic syndrome. *Blood* 2003;102:3025–7.

108 Steensma DP, Dispenzieri A, Moore SB, Schroeder G, Tefferi A. Antithymocyte globulin has limited efficacy and substantial toxicity in unselected anemic patients with myelodysplastic syndrome. *Blood* 2003;101:2156–8.

109 Arnold R, de Witte T, van Bienzen A, *et al.* Unrelated bone marrow transplantation in patients with myelodysplastic syndromes and secondary acute myeloid leukemia: an EBMT

survey. European Blood and Marrow Transplantation Group. *Bone Marrow Transplant* 1998;21:1213–16.

110 Runde V, de Witte T, Arnold R, *et al.* Bone marrow transplantation from HLA-identical siblings as first-line treatment in patients with myelodysplastic syndromes: early transplantation is associated with improved outcome. Chronic Leukemia Working Party of the European Group for Blood and Marrow Transplantation. *Bone Marrow Transplant* 1998;21:255–61.

111 Sierra J, Perez WS, Rozman C, *et al.* Bone marrow transplantation from HLA-identical siblings as treatment for myelodysplasia. *Blood* 2002;100:1997–2004.

112 Castro-Malaspina H, Harris RE, Gajewski J, *et al.* Unrelated donor marrow transplantation for myelodysplastic syndromes: outcome analysis in 510 transplants facilitated by the National Marrow Donor Program. *Blood* 2002;99:1943–51.

113 Deeg HJ, Storer B, Slattery JT, *et al.* Conditioning with targeted busulfan and cyclophosphamide for hemopoietic stem cell transplantation from related and unrelated donors in patients with myelodysplastic syndrome. *Blood* 2002;100:1201–7.

114 Campregher PV, Gooley T, Scott BL, *et al.* Results of donor lymphocyte infusions for relapsed myelodysplastic syndrome after hematopoietic cell transplantation. *Bone Marrow Transplant* 2007;40:965–71.

115 Martino R, Iacobelli S, Brand R, *et al.* Retrospective comparison of reduced-intensity conditioning and conventional high-dose conditioning for allogeneic hematopoietic stem cell transplantation using HLA-identical sibling donors in myelodysplastic syndromes. *Blood* 2006;108:836–46.

116 Armand P, Kim HT, De Angelo DJ, *et al.* Impact of cytogenetics on outcome of de novo and therapy-related AML and MDS after allogeneic transplantation. *Biol Blood Marrow Transplant* 2007;13:655–64.

117 Chang C, Storer BE, Scott BL, *et al.* Hematopoietic cell transplantation in patients with myelodysplastic syndrome or acute myeloid leukemia arising from myelodysplastic syndrome: similar outcomes in patients with de novo disease and disease following prior therapy or antecedent hematologic disorders. *Blood* 2007;110:1379–87.

118 Giralt S, Estey E, Albitar M, *et al.* Engraftment of allogeneic hematopoietic progenitor cells with purine analog-containing chemotherapy: harnessing graft-versus-leukemia without myeloablative therapy. *Blood* 1997;89:4531–6.

119 Giralt S, Thall PF, Khouri I, *et al.* Melphalan and purine analog-containing preparative regimens: reduced-intensity conditioning for patients with hematologic malignancies undergoing allogeneic progenitor cell transplantation. *Blood* 2001;97:631–7.

120 Scott BL, Sandmaier BM, Storer B, *et al.* Myeloablative vs non-myeloablative allogeneic transplantation for patients with myelodysplastic syndrome or acute myelogenous leukemia with multilineage dysplasia: a retrospective analysis. *Leukemia* 2006;20:128–35.

121 Sorror ML, Sandmaier BM, Storer BE, *et al.* Comorbidity and disease status based risk stratification of outcomes among patients with acute myeloid leukemia or myelodysplasia receiving allogeneic hematopoietic cell transplantation. *J Clin Oncol* 2007;25:4246–54.

122 Cutler CS, Lee SJ, Greenberg P, *et al.* A decision analysis of allogeneic bone marrow transplantation for the myelodysplastic syndromes: delayed transplantation for low-risk myelodysplasia is associated with improved outcome. *Blood* 2004; 104:579–85.

123 Scott BL, Storer BE, Greene JE, Hackman RC, Appelbaum FR, Deeg HJ. Marrow fibrosis as a risk factor for posttransplantation outcome in patients with advanced myelodysplastic syndrome or acute myeloid leukemia with multilineage dysplasia. *Biol Blood Marrow Transplant* 2007;13:345–54.

124 Al-Ali HK, Brand R, van Biezen A, *et al.* A retrospective comparison of autologous and unrelated donor hematopoietic cell transplantation in myelodysplastic syndrome and secondary acute myeloid leukemia: a report on behalf of the Chronic Leukemia Working Party of the European Group for Blood and Marrow Transplantation (EBMT). *Leukemia* 2007;21: 1945–51.

125 De Witte T, Van Biezen A, Hermans J, *et al.* Autologous bone marrow transplantation for patients with myelodysplastic syndrome (MDS) or acute myeloid leukemia following MDS. Chronic and Acute Leukemia Working Parties of the European Group for Blood and Marrow Transplantation. *Blood* 1997;90: 3853–7.

Part 3
Acute Myeloid Leukemia

Chapter 9
Presentation and Diagnosis: Novel Molecular Markers and their Role in the Prognosis and Therapy of Acute Myeloid Leukemia

Wolfgang Kern[1], *Torsten Haferlach*[1], *Susanne Schnittger*[1], *Claudia Haferlach*[1], *and Ulrike Bacher*[2]
[1]MLL Munich Leukemia Laboratory, Munich, Germany
[2]Department of Stem Cell Transplantation, University of Hamburg, Hamburg, Germany

Introduction

Acute myeloid leukemia (AML) represents a very heterogeneous disorder, comprising various morphologic, immunologic, and genetic subtypes. As these subtypes are associated to very diverse clinical profiles and treatment results, the definition of prognostic parameters as being suitable for individual risk stratification plays an increasing role. In 55% of patients with AML, chromosome-banding analyses in combination with diverse fluorescence *in situ* hybridization (FISH) techniques reveal clonal cytogenetic abnormalities. These chromosomal aberrations span a wide spectrum that ranges from numeric to structural aberrations, and represent strong prognostic parameters. Examples are the prognostically favorable reciprocal rearrangements t(8;21)/*AML1–ETO*, inv(16)/*CBFB–MYH11*, and t(15;17)/*PML–RARA* where long-term survival of >70%, depending on the subentity, is achieved, whereas in cases with complex aberrations or chromosome 7 abnormalities, the outcome is inferior irrespective of the intensity of treatment [1]. Thus, chromosomal markers play a central role for risk stratification and are highly relevant for therapeutic decisions, for example for the selection of patients who might benefit from an early allogeneic stem-cell transplantation.

Further efforts were also made to subclassify the 45% patients with AML who have a normal karyotype and in whom cytogenetic analyses reveal no abnormalities. Descriptions of a variety of recurrent molecular mutations allows the determination of prognosis-defining parameters in >85% of all patients with a normal karyotype [2]. These molecular markers are very diverse because they include mutations of receptor tyrosine kinases such as the *FLT3*-LM/ITD [3], mutations of proto-oncogenes, for example *RAS* [4], or mutations of transcription factors, for example the *CEBPA* or *AML1/RUNX*. The recent description of *Nucleophosmin (NPM1)* mutations in AML cases with normal karyotypes as the currently known most frequent molecular marker is a further breakthrough [5–8]. These mutations are very heterogeneous: they can be characterized by the insertion of hundreds of base pairs, as in the case of *FLT3*-LM/ITD, by point mutations, as in the case of *RAS*, or by a variety of deletions or insertions, as in the case of *AML1/RUNX* mutations.

For most of these markers, the prognostic impact is clearly defined. For example, it is known that both *FLT3*-LM [3,9,10] and *MLL*-PTD (partial tandem duplications of the *MLL* gene) [11,12] have an adverse influence on the chance of survival. In contrast, the *NPM1* mutations are prognostically favorable when they are seen in isolation in a normal karyotype. For other mutations, such as the *NRAS* mutations [13,14], the prognostic impact is still in discussion or can be defined only in coincidence with other molecular markers.

Schlenk *et al.* [15] performed a retrospective correlation of the molecular markers with the outcome in patients with AML who had a normal karyotype. Patients with *FLT3*-ITD or *MLL*-PTD benefitted from an allogeneic stem-cell transplant in first remission, while those with an isolated *NPM1* or *CEBPA* mutation had a better outcome with conservative treatment. Thus, molecular analyses can by now be used as basis for therapeutic decisions in AML with a normal karyotype.

Also, minimal residual disease (MRD) analyses for the evaluation of the response to therapy during the course of AML has gained in importance. For some markers,

Leukemias: Principles and Practice of Therapy, 1st edition. Edited by S. Faderl and H. Kantarjian.

such as the *PML-RARA* in acute promyelocytic leukemia (APL) with the t(15;17), the prognostic value of the MRD load after therapy has been proven in large studies [16,17]. For other mutations, the relevance for postremission strategies is still being defined, for example in case of the *NPM1* mutations [18,19], where quantitative polymerase chain reaction (PCR) seemed to represent a valid follow-up parameter in some studies.

Thus, molecular markers are currently highly relevant for therapeutic decisions in AML at diagnosis and also during follow-up of the disease. This chapter provides an overview on the panel of recurrent molecular markers in AML, on their prognostic impact, and on their value for therapeutic decisions.

Involvement of transcription

Experiments in the animal model and coincidence studies in large cohorts were the basis for models of cooperation in leukemogenesis. Gilliland *et al.*'s "two hit model" is one such model of cooperation based on these studies and experiments [20]. According to this model, mutations mediating a block in differentiation ("class I mutations") cooperate in leukemogenesis with mutations mediating proliferation ("class II mutations"). The first category either directly or indirectly affects the function of transcription factors [21].

Core binding factor leukemia

With respect to the class I mutations, the core binding factor (CBF) leukemias have to be mentioned first. They are represented by inversion inv(16)/t(16;16) with the *CBFB–MYH11* fusion transcript and by the reciprocal translocation t(8;21) with the *AML1–ETO* fusion transcript. AML with inv(16) is characterized by abnormal eosinophils in the bone marrow and has a separate category in the French–American–British (FAB) classification system, the "M4eo". The t(8;21) shows multiple long Auer rods and is mostly correlated with the FAB subtype M2. Both CBF leukemias are found in 6–10% of all AML cases.

The CBF complex is essential for normal hematopoiesis and consists of the CBFα and CBFβproteins. These proteins are encoded by the *AML1* and *CBFB* genes. Rearrangements of *AML1* and *CBFB* with other genes because of the above chromosomal rearrangements lead to chimeric proteins, which disrupt the CBF complex. Consequently, activation of transcription (the process of copying DNA to RNA) is repressed [22]. With standard chemotherapy, a survival rate of >60% can be achieved.

Acute promyelocytic leukemia

"Faggot cells" with multiple Auer rods and dark granulation characterize APL. These atypic promyelocytes result from a differentiation stop in granulopoiesis. According to the FAB classification, APL can be divided into two distinct morphologic subtypes: M3 and M3v. Whereas the M3 subtype represents the "classical APL", the M3v shows binuclear cells. The M3v subtype can sometimes act as an obstacle in the differentiation of APL from other AML subtypes. The clinical picture of APL is characterized by life-threatening coagulopathy.

On the molecular level, the translocation t(15;17) finds correspondence in the *PML–RARA* fusion. This gene fusion disrupts the normal interaction of *RARA* and retinoic acid. This prevents the normal conversion of *RARA* into an activator of transcription [23]. Highly dosed all-trans-retinoic acid (ATRA) is able to overcome the differentiation stop caused by the *PML–RARA* fusion [23], and when in combination with anthracycline-based chemotherapy >80% of patients achieve stable remissions. ATRA is also able to prevent the occurrence of thromboembolic or bleeding complications. Diagnosis of the *PML–RARA* gene fusion should therefore be performed as quickly as possible, either by PCR or by interphase FISH. With both techniques, results can be available after just a few hours.

Another effective compound is arsenic trioxide, which induces degradation of the fusion protein encoded by the *PML–RARA* oncogene and differentiation of leukemic cells [24].

Owing to the favorable prognosis with conservative treatment [25], allogeneic stem-cell transplantation (SCT) was eliminated from first-line strategies in APL and the CBF leukemias in first remission. However, prognosis is worse when the respective mutations occur in coincidence with other molecular markers—the t(15;17)/*PML–RARA* is frequently detected in combination with *FLT3*-ITD mutations [26] and t(8;21)/*AML1–ETO* and inv(16)/*CBFB–MYH11* with *KIT*-D816 mutations [27]. Therefore, combinations of genetic markers are also relevant for the definition of prognosis and for therapeutic decisions.

Quantitative assessment of fusion-gene expression by quantitative PCR represents an ideal parameter in APL and in the CBF leukemias for MRD monitoring. The ratios of gene expression following consolidation compared to initial manifestation correlate significantly with prognosis [17,28]. This allows earlier detection of relapse, with the chance of therapeutic intervention before the clinical manifestation.

Mutations of genes encoding transcription factors

Mutations of genes that encode transcription factors can interfere with transcription. Here, the *CEPBA* and the *RUNX1* gene mutations (*AML1*), both with a strong association to normal karyotype AML, have to be mentioned. The *CEPBA* gene encodes a transcription factor (CAAT/enhancer-binding protein) and regulates the differentiation of granulopoiesis. There are two subtypes of *CEPBA* mutations that interfere with the normal function of the CEBPA protein [29]. As isolated mutations in AML with a normal karyotype, *CEBPA* indicates a favorable prognosis [30,31]. Schlenk *et al.* found that patients with an isolated *CEBPA* mutation gained no benefit from allotransplantation in first remission owing to the favorable outcome with standard chemotherapy [15].

The *RUNX/AML1* gene can be affected by a variety of point mutations, insertions, or deletions (*RUNX* mutations). Their prognostic impact still needs to be clarified.

Alterations of the *MLL* gene

The rearrangements of the *MLL* (mixed lineage leukemia) gene on chromosome 11q23 represent a further mutational subtype that shows interference with transcription. A variety of partner genes can be involved in these rearrangements [32]. They block the normal functions of the *MLL* gene, which regulates transcription [33]. *MLL* rearrangements are frequent in patients with therapy-associated AML (t-AML) after previous application of topoisomerase-II-inhibitors such as etoposide or other cytotoxic compounds. They are closely associated to the monocytic FAB subtype M5a.

Intragenic mutations of the *MLL* gene (partial tandem duplications; *MLL*-PTD) are seen in 5–10% of cases of normal karyotype AML as another mutation subtype [11]. Both the interchromosomal and the intragenic *MLL* abnormalities confer an unfavorable prognostic impact [12,34,35].

Dysregulation of *HOX* genes

HOX (homeobox) genes are classified into several groups localized on four chromosomes. They encode a complex network of proteins that are essential for the regulation of transcription and hematopoiesis. Dysregulation of homeobox-containing genes has a role in different hematologic malignancies. In AML, multiple *HOX* genes are overexpressed in cases with poor prognosis, whereas the expression of these genes is characteristically low in cases with prognostically favorable cytogenetics, for example in APL [36,37].

Activation of proliferation

Involvement of tyrosine kinases

The second category of mutations is represented by activating mutations that frequently involve receptor tyrosine kinases. Stimulation of these kinases leads to increased activation of signaling pathways, which is followed by increased cell proliferation.

Most frequent in this category are mutations within the *FLT3* gene, which encodes the class III receptor FLT3 kinase. *FLT3* mutations are found in ~35% of all patients with AML, thus they belong to the most frequently occurring known genetic alterations in AML. The mutations lead to autophosphorylation of the FLT3 receptor, tyrosine kinase. This results in increased cell proliferation in the inhibition of apoptosis and in the activation of signaling pathways [38].

The *FLT3*-ITD/-LM (internal tandem duplications/ length mutations) are represented by insertions of variable length of up to 200 base pairs. They are localized in the region that encodes the juxtamembranous region of the FLT3 receptor [39]. Mutational screening can be performed by the gene-scan technique, which allows higher sensitivity than conventional PCR. The determination of the specific *FLT3*-ITD requires the performance of sequencing.

Mutations of *FLT3*-ITD have a clear unfavorable prognostic impact, with a long-term survival of <10% of all affected patients [40]. Owing to the high relapse risk, allogeneic SCT should be integrated in therapeutic considerations from the beginning. In part of every case, *FLT3*-ITD mutations are found in combination with other mutations, for example with *NPM1* [6–8] or *MLL*-PTD [41], where they confer an inferior prognostic impact.

At this time, a variety of FLT3 tyrosine kinase inhibitors are being investigated in basic research and clinical studies, with the aim to develop targeted treatment concepts for this large, prognostically adverse subgroup [42,43].

Less frequent are mutations of the *FLT3* tyrosine kinase domain (*FLT3*-TKD). They are localized in the region encoding the activation loop of the receptor kinase. Whether they influence prognosis is still a controversial topic [44].

Involvement of another receptor, class III kinase, is represented by mutations of the *KIT* tyrosine kinase domain. In adult patients with AML, these mutations are mostly localized in the activation loop [45]. Although they are rare in total AML, they are found in 10–25% of all cases of CBF leukemias [27,46]. This coincidence confers a deterioration of prognosis in the otherwise prognostically favorable CBF leukemias. The tyrosine kinase inhibitor imatinib, which is primarily known for its inhibition of the *BCR–ABL* fusion in chronic myeloid leukemia (CML), also has inhibitory effects on the Kit tyrosine kinase and therefore might represent an option for such commutated cases [45]. Additionally, a subset of pediatric patients might benefit from imatinib therapy, as juxtamembrane mutations in *KIT* were reported in 7% of children with AML [47] (in contrast to adults where the mutations are localized in the kinase domain).

The V617F mutation of the *JAK2* gene, which activates the *JAK2* non-receptor tyrosine kinase, and the JAK-STAT pathway are known for their close association to various chronic myeloproliferative disorders (CMPD) [48,49].

However, this mutation is also observed in a low incidence of <8% of AML cases. Mutated cases are mostly found in secondary AML after a preceeding CMPD [50,51] and seem to be associated with the t(8;21)/*AML1–ETO*. This coincidence can be interpreted as a further example of a cooperation of class I and II mutations in accordance with the two-hit model [50,52].

Mutations of oncogenes

Mutations of *RAS* oncogenes are found in many malignancies, in solid tumors as well as in hematologic disorders. *RAS* genes have a central role in the regulation of cell cycle and differentiation. Through the RAS proteins, they lead to constitutive activation of the RAS signaling pathway [53]. There are different subtypes of *RAS* mutations—*NRAS*, *KRAS*, and *HRAS*. In AML, the *NRAS* subtypes are most frequent. Screening for *RAS* (point) mutations can be performed by melting-based PCR assays, and the identification of the exact mutational subtype is possible by sequencing [13].

NRAS mutations are detected in 11–25% of cases of AML, whereas *KRAS* and *HRAS* mutations are less frequently observed. There appear to be specific interactions with distinct genetic subgroups, for example the inv(16)/*CBFB–MYH11*, as suggested by coincidence studies. However, the *NRAS* mutations seem to be prognostically relevant in some genetic subgroups only [13].

Interference with cell cycle and apoptosis

The recent description of *NPM1* mutations led to the definition of a third category of mutations that are involved in cell-cycle regulation and apoptosis.

Mutations of the *NPM1* gene are found in 35% of all AML cases. They are closely linked to normal karyotype AML, where 55% of all cases have mutations. In most cases, they consist of four base-pair insertions [5]. They induce a structural alteration of the NPM1 protein. Normally, the respective protein functions as a shuttle between the nucleus and cytoplasm, which is essential for its participation in a tumor-suppressor pathway. In the case of the respective mutation, the protein is dislocalized to the cytoplasm, which blocks its function in the tumor-suppressor pathway. When it occurs as the sole mutation, *NPM1* is prognostically favorable [5–8,15]. The frequency is age-dependent; children are less frequently affected, and so far the mutation has not been observed in children younger than 3 years old.

NPM1 mutations can occur either solely or in combination with other molecular markers such as *FLT3*-ITD [6–8] or *MLL*-PTD. Such coincidence is associated with a significant deterioration of prognosis [41]. The mechanisms of interaction between the *NPM1* mutations and the partner mutations still remain to be clarified.

Studies on the validation of *NPM1* mutations for follow-up diagnostics are still ongoing, but it seems that these mutations are ideal markers for MRD diagnostics. They provide high stability from the first manifestation to relapse, and they show a rather homogeneous structure that makes them ideal candidates for quantitative PCR [18,54].

Recently, it was demonstrated that the outcome of patients with AML and isolated *NPM1* mutations may be improved by the addition of ATRA to chemotherapy [55]. All other subgroups—those with *NPM1* wild type and those with *FLT3* mutations or *MLL*-PTD—did not benefit from additional ATRA when compared with standard-treated patients. The relevant mechanism of this interaction still has to be defined.

Deletions of the *TP53* tumor-suppressor gene on 17p are rare in *de novo* AML, but they are detected in higher frequencies in secondary or therapy-associated AML and in elderly patients [56]. Also, the p53 deletions are strongly linked to abnormalities of the chromosomes 5q, 7q, and complex aberrations [56,57]. They confer a high risk of relapse and are associated with resistance against chemotherapy. Diagnosis can be performed by chromosome-banding analysis, but in some cases the deletions are detectable only by PCR or interphase FISH.

Other molecular markers

For some recurrent molecular mutations that have been investigated in recent years, the definite role in AML still has to be clarified. One example is the mutation of the *WT1* tumor gene. The *WT1* gene has a coding function for a DNA binding protein. It might act as a tumor-suppressor gene or as an oncogene, which suggests functional duality. *WT1* mutations are detectable in 10% of patients with AML, often in patients with a normal karyotype. There seems to be an association between these mutations and a low response to therapy [58]. Also, expression of the *WT1* gene is increased in AML as in various other leukemias [59]. It is still being investigated whether *WT1* gene expression by quantitative PCR might be suitable for follow-up diagnostic strategies in AML.

The *BAALC* gene is primarily expressed in neuroectoderm-derived tissues and in hematopoietic precursors. It encodes a protein with unclear function. Overexpression was found in diverse hematologic malignancies. In AML, high expression of the *BAALC* gene was suggested to be associated with a poor prognosis in normal karyotype AML [60].

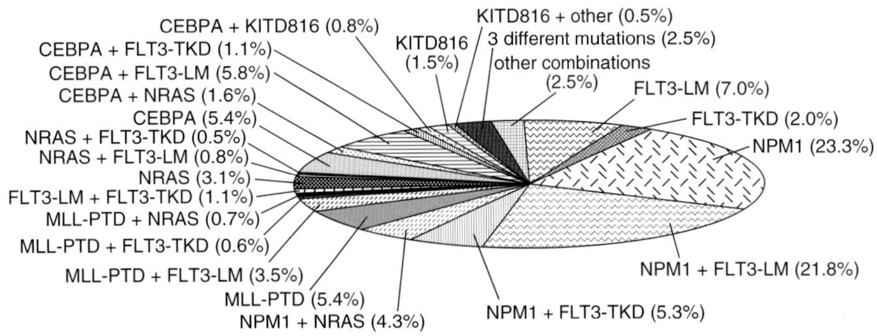

Figure 9.1. Frequency of molecular subtypes in normal karyotype AML according to an analysis of 1441 patients (own data).

Molecular risk stratification in acute myeloid leukemia with normal karyotype

In patients with a normal karyotype, molecular methods allow detailed subclassification in >85% of all cases. A limited panel of markers is sufficient to reach the majority of cases [2,61] (Figure 9.1). Most frequent are the *NPM1* mutations with a frequency of ~55% in normal karyotype cases. This is followed by the *FLT3*-ITD in ~40% of cases. The *MLL*-PTD, *NRAS*, *CEBPA*, and *FLT3*-TKD mutations show frequencies between 6% and 10% in normal-karyotype AML [9,11–13,30,31,34,44,62,63]. These markers can be found either as isolated mutations or in combinations. *FLT3*-ITD mutations are frequently observed in conjunction with *NPM1* [6–8,64] or *MLL*-PTD [41,65] mutations.

The study by Schlenk *et al.* on normal-karyotype AML, where patients with isolated *NPM1* mutations received no benefit from early allogeneic SCT in contrast to those with *NPM1* mutated cases with additional *FLT3*-ITD, who had a clear survival advantage when allogeneic SCT was performed, emphasizes the value of molecular subclassification in normal-karyotype AML. Also, patients with the prognostically unfavorable *MLL*-PTD had a significant benefit from SCT [15].

Planning of molecular diagnostics in acute myeloid leukemia

Given the need for time, labor, and material for the diverse molecular techniques, an appropriate planning of analysis is necessary. This is particularly emphasized when the increasing variety of known molecular mutations in AML are considered. Also, the detection and complete characterization of these mutations require a combination of diverse molecular techniques. These techniques cover a wide spectrum and include conventional PCR, melting point-based PCR assays, or sequencing approaches. Thus, the importance of guiding the molecular techniques in dependence on the results of less specific methods such as morphology and chromosome-banding analyses increases in AML.

First, in those cases where cytomorphology raises suspiscions of the FAB subtypes M4eo (which is associated with inv(16)/*CBFB–MYH11*), M3/M3v (for APL with the t(15;17)/*PML–RARA*), or of the t(8;21)/*AML–ETO*, molecular screening by PCR might be initiated for the underlying gene fusions. This is not only relevant for the confirmation of the respective subtypes, but also provides the basis for further MRD strategies. When the monocytic subtype M5a is detected, molecular screening might be performed for *MLL* rearrangements, as these are often associated with this cytomorphologic subtype.

When chromosome banding analyses show a normal karyotype, screening for the most relevant markers, such as *NPM1*, *FLT3*-ITD, *CEBPA* mutations, or the *MLL*-PTD, might be initiated. These examples demonstrate how molecular analyses can be integrated in the panel of diagnostic methods in AML.

Origin and sequence of molecular mutations in acute myeloid leukemia

It was demonstrated that different fusion transcript types that are specific for diverse AML subtypes can already originate *in utero*. The *AML1–ETO*, *PML-RARA*, and *MLL* rearrangements were retrospectively detected in the blood from Guthrie cards that had been preserved from children who had developed the respective acute leukemia subtypes at a young age [66].

The long intervals between birth and the manifestation of leukemia—>10 years in some of the respective patients—indicates that the above fusion transcripts are not able to cause leukemia on their own but need cooperation with additional secondary genetic alterations.

Also, the *AML1–ETO* gene fusion is detected in a 100-fold higher frequency in newborns when compared with the lifelong risk of the respective AML subtypes. In contrast to these early leukemogenic events, other mutations, such as *FLT3*-LM and *NRAS*, are probably late events in leukemogenesis. Both show considerable instability from diagnosis to relapse [62].

It can thus be hypothesized that the mutation sequence in AML probably starts with reciprocal gene fusions such as *AML1–ETO* or *PML–RARA* and might be followed by activating mutations such as the *FLT3*-LM or the *NRAS* mutations.

Gene expression profiling

Gene expression profiling analyses on the basis of microarrays allow the simultaneous characterization of thousands of genes. This technique has achieved increasing importance in leukemia research in recent years.

An increasing number of AML subclasses can be predicted based on their gene signatures: examples are the t(8;21)/*AML1–ETO*, t(15;17)/*PML–RARA*, inv(16)/*CBFB–MYH*11, and *MLL*/11q23 rearrangements, which can all be separated by specific gene-expression profiles underlining a disease-defining function [67–70]. Other markers, such as *CEBPA* [70] or *NPM*1 [71] mutations, also show specific gene-expression patterns. These are just a few examples of predictable molecular subclasses in AML. The predictability of chemosensitivity on the basis of gene expression analyses opens new horizons for therapeutic strategies in AML [72].

Conclusions

The picture of molecular markers in AML has become more complex in recent years. By now, detailed knowledge of various mutational subtypes and their cooperation processes allows an improved biologic subclassification and improved prognostic predictions. Additionally, molecular techniques allow exact follow-up procedures in many subtypes, as quantitative PCR is able to determine the residual leukemic cell load exactly. Thus, improvement in molecular subclassification—especially in patients with a normal karyotype—in combination with advanced MRD diagnostic techniques now permit a better adaptation of the intensity of treatment to the individual patient's risk profile. Understanding of the pathogenesis of AML has also significantly increased owing to improved insights in the interaction of different mutation types. Hopefully, the next step will be the translation of these new insights in the molecular basis of AML into new treatment concepts in accordance to the individual mutation status in the near future.

References

1 Schoch C, Haferlach T, Haase D, *et al.* Patients with de novo acute myeloid leukemia and complex karyotype aberrations show a poor prognosis despite intensive treatment: a study of 90 patients. *Br J Haematol* 2001;112:118–26.

2 Marcucci G, Mrozek K, Bloomfield CD. Molecular heterogeneity and prognostic biomarkers in adults with acute myeloid leukemia and normal cytogenetics. *Curr Opin Hematol* 2005;12:68–75.

3 Schnittger S, Schoch C, Dugas M, *et al.* Analysis of *FLT3* length mutations in 1003 patients with acute myeloid leukemia: correlation to cytogenetics, FAB subtype, and prognosis in the AMLCG study and usefulness as a marker for the detection of minimal residual disease. *Blood* 2002;100:59–66.

4 Kiyoi H, Naoe T, Nakano Y, *et al.* Prognostic implication of *FLT3* and *N-RAS* gene mutations in acute myeloid leukemia. *Blood* 1999;93:3074–80.

5 Falini B, Mecucci C, Tiacci E, *et al.* Cytoplasmic nucleophosmin in acute myelogenous leukemia with a normal karyotype. *N Engl J Med* 2005;352:254–66.

6 Schnittger S, Schoch C, Kern W, *et al.* Nucleophosmin gene mutations are predictors of favorable prognosis in acute myelogenous leukemia with a normal karyotype. *Blood* 2005;106:3733–9.

7 Dohner K, Schlenk RF, Habdank M, *et al.* Mutant nucleophosmin (NPM1) predicts favorable prognosis in younger adults with acute myeloid leukemia and normal cytogenetics: interaction with other gene mutations. *Blood* 2005;106:3740–6.

8 Verhaak RG, Goudswaard CS, van PW, *et al.* Mutations in nucleophosmin (*NPM1*) in acute myeloid leukemia (AML): association with other gene abnormalities and previously established gene expression signatures and their favorable prognostic significance. *Blood* 2005;106:3747–54.

9 Thiede C, Steudel C, Mohr B, *et al.* Analysis of *FLT3*-activating mutations in 979 patients with acute myelogenous leukemia: association with FAB subtypes and identification of subgroups with poor prognosis. *Blood* 2002;99:4326–35.

10 Yanada M, Matsuo K, Suzuki T, Kiyoi H, Naoe T. Prognostic significance of *FLT3* internal tandem duplication and tyrosine kinase domain mutations for acute myeloid leukemia: a meta-analysis. *Leukemia* 2005;19:1345–9.

11 Schichman SA, Caligiuri MA, Strout MP, *et al.* ALL-1 tandem duplication in acute myeloid leukemia with a normal karyotype involves homologous recombination between Alu elements. *Cancer Res* 1994;54:4277–80.

12 Schnittger S, Kinkelin U, Schoch C, *et al.* Screening for *MLL* tandem duplication in 387 unselected patients with AML identify a prognostically unfavorable subset of AML. *Leukemia* 2000;14:796–804.

13 Bacher U, Haferlach T, Schoch C, Kern W, Schnittger S. Implications of *NRAS* mutations in AML: a study of 2502 patients. *Blood* 2006 15;107:3847–53.

14 Bowen DT, Frew ME, Hills R, *et al. RAS* mutation in acute myeloid leukemia is associated with distinct cytogenetic subgroups but does not influence outcome in patients younger than 60 years. *Blood* 2005;106:2113–19.

15 Schlenk RF, Dohner K, Krauter J, *et al.* Mutations and treatment outcome in cytogenetically normal acute myeloid leukemia. *N Engl J Med* 2008;358:1909–18.

16 Grimwade D. The significance of minimal residual disease in patients with t(15;17). *Best Pract Res Clin Haematol* 2002;15: 137–58.

17 Schnittger S, Weisser M, Schoch C, Hiddemann W, Haferlach T, Kern W. New score predicting for prognosis in PML-RARA+, AML1-ETO+, or CBFBMYH11+ acute myeloid leukemia based on quantification of fusion transcripts. *Blood* 2003; 102:2746–55.

18 Chou WC, Tang JL, Wu SJ, *et al.* Clinical implications of minimal residual disease monitoring by quantitative polymerase chain reaction in acute myeloid leukemia patients bearing nucleophosmin (*NPM1*) mutations. *Leukemia* 2007;21:998–1004.

19 Scholl S, Loncarevic IF, Krause C, Kunert C, Clement JH, Hoffken K. Minimal residual disease based on patient specific *Flt3-ITD* and *-ITT* mutations in acute myeloid leukemia. *Leuk Res* 2005;29:849–53.

20 Gilliland DG. Hematologic malignancies. *Curr Opin Hematol* 2001;8:189–91.

21 Gilliland DG, Jordan CT, Felix CA. The molecular basis of leukemia. *Hematology Am Soc Hematol Educ Program* 2004;1: 80–97.

22 Miyoshi H, Shimizu K, Kozu T, Maseki N, Kaneko Y, Ohki M. t(8;21) breakpoints on chromosome 21 in acute myeloid leukemia are clustered within a limited region of a single gene, *AML1*. *Proc Natl Acad Sci U S A* 1991;88:10431–4.

23 Lin RJ, Evans RM. Acquisition of oncogenic potential by RAR chimeras in acute promyelocytic leukemia through formation of homodimers. *Mol Cell* 2000;5:821–30.

24 Lallemand-Breitenbach V, Jeanne M, Benhenda S, *et al.* Arsenic degrades PML or PML-RARalpha through a SUMO-triggered RNF4/ubiquitin-mediated pathway. *Nat Cell Biol* 2008;10:547–55.

25 Grimwade D, Walker H, Oliver F, *et al.* The importance of diagnostic cytogenetics on outcome in AML: analysis of 1,612 patients entered into the MRC AML 10 trial. The Medical Research Council Adult and Children's Leukemia Working Parties. *Blood* 1998;92:2322–33.

26 Kuchenbauer F, Schoch C, Kern W, Hiddemann W, Haferlach T, Schnittger S. Impact of *FLT3* mutations and promyelocytic leukemia-breakpoint on clinical characteristics and prognosis in acute promyelocytic leukemia. *Br J Haematol* 2005;130: 196–202.

27 Schnittger S, Kohl TM, Haferlach T, *et al. KIT-D816* mutations in *AML1-ETO*-positive AML are associated with impaired event-free and overall survival. *Blood* 2006;107:1791–9.

28 Grimwade D, Howe K, Langabeer S, Burnett A, Goldstone A, Solomon E. Minimal residual disease detection in acute promyelocytic leukemia by reverse-transcriptase PCR: evaluation of PML-RAR alpha and RAR alpha-PML assessment in patients who ultimately relapse. *Leukemia* 1996;10:61–6.

29 Pabst T, Mueller BU, Zhang P, *et al.* Dominant-negative mutations of *CEBPA*, encoding CCAAT/enhancer binding protein-alpha (C/EBPalpha), in acute myeloid leukemia. *Nat Genet* 2001;27:263–70.

30 Preudhomme C, Sagot C, Boissel N, *et al.* Favorable prognostic significance of *CEBPA* mutations in patients with de novo acute myeloid leukemia: a study from the Acute Leukemia French Association (ALFA). *Blood* 2002;100:2717–23.

31 Frohling S, Schlenk RF, Stolze I, *et al. CEBPA* mutations in younger adults with acute myeloid leukemia and normal cytogenetics: prognostic relevance and analysis of cooperating mutations. *J Clin Oncol* 2004;22:624–33.

32 Shih LY, Liang DC, Fu JF, *et al.* Characterization of fusion partner genes in 114 patients with de novo acute myeloid leukemia and *MLL* rearrangement. *Leukemia* 2006;20: 218–23.

33 Armstrong SA, Staunton JE, Silverman LB, *et al. MLL* translocations specify a distinct gene expression profile that distinguishes a unique leukemia. *Nat Genet* 2002;30:41–7.

34 Dohner K, Tobis K, Ulrich R, *et al.* Prognostic significance of partial tandem duplications of the *MLL* gene in adult patients 16 to 60 years old with acute myeloid leukemia and normal cytogenetics: a study of the Acute Myeloid Leukemia Study Group Ulm. *J Clin Oncol* 2002;20:3254–61.

35 Schoch C, Schnittger S, Klaus M, Kern W, Hiddemann W, Haferlach T. AML with 11q23/*MLL* abnormalities as defined by the WHO classification: incidence, partner chromosomes, FAB subtype, age distribution, and prognostic impact in an unselected series of 1897 cytogenetically analyzed AML cases. *Blood* 2003;102:2395–402.

36 Drabkin HA, Parsy C, Ferguson K, *et al.* Quantitative *HOX* expression in chromosomally defined subsets of acute myelogenous leukemia 1. *Leukemia* 2002;16:186–95.

37 Thompson A, Quinn MF, Grimwade D, *et al.* Global down-regulation of *HOX* gene expression in *PML-RARalpha* + acute promyelocytic leukemia identified by small-array real-time PCR 1. *Blood* 2003;101:1558–65.

38 Gilliland DG, Griffin JD. Role of *FLT3* in leukemia. *Curr Opin Hematol* 2002;9:274–81.

39 Kiyoi H, Towatari M, Yokota S, *et al.* Internal tandem duplication of the *FLT3* gene is a novel modality of elongation mutation which causes constitutive activation of the product. *Leukemia* 1998;12:1333–7.

40 Whitman SP, Ruppert AS, Radmacher MD, *et al. FLT3 D835/I836* mutations are associated with poor disease-free survival and a distinct gene-expression sig*Nature* among younger adults with de novo cytogenetically normal acute myeloid leukemia lacking *FLT3* internal tandem duplications. *Blood* 2008;111: 1552–9.

41 Olesen LH, Nyvold CG, Aggerholm A, Norgaard JM, Guldberg P, Hokland P. Delineation and molecular characterization of acute myeloid leukemia patients with coduplication of *FLT3* and *MLL*. *Eur J Haematol* 2005;75:185–92.

42 Tallman MS. New agents for the treatment of acute myeloid leukemia. *Best Pract Res Clin Haematol* 2006;19:311–20.

43 Illmer T, Ehninger G. FLT3 kinase inhibitors in the management of acute myeloid leukemia. *Clin Lymphoma Myeloma* 2007;8(Suppl.1):S24-S34.

44 Bacher U, Haferlach C, Kern W, Haferlach T, Schnittger S. Prognostic relevance of *FLT3-TKD* mutations in AML: the combination matters—an analysis of 3082 patients. *Blood* 2008; 111:2527–37.

45 Cairoli R, Grillo G, Beghini A, *et al. C-Kit* point mutations in core binding factor leukemias: correlation with white blood cell count and the white blood cell index. *Leukemia* 2003; 17:471–2.

46 Paschka P, Marcucci G, Ruppert AS, *et al.* Adverse prognostic significance of *KIT* mutations in adult acute myeloid leukemia with inv(16) and t(8;21): a Cancer and Leukemia Group B Study. *J Clin Oncol* 2006;24:3904–11.

47 Corbacioglu S, Kilic M, Westhoff MA, Reinhardt D, Fulda S, Debatin KM. Newly identified c-KIT receptor tyrosine kinase ITD in childhood AML induces ligand-independent growth and is responsive to a synergistic effect of imatinib and rapamycin. *Blood* 2006;108:3504–13.
48 Baxter EJ, Scott LM, Campbell PJ, *et al.* Acquired mutation of the tyrosine kinase JAK2 in human myeloproliferative disorders. *Lancet* 2005;365:1054–61.
49 Tefferi A, Lasho TL, Gilliland G. *JAK2* mutations in myeloproliferative disorders. *N Engl J Med* 2005;353:1416–17.
50 Schnittger S, Bacher U, Kern W, Haferlach T, Haferlach C. *JAK2V617F* as progression marker in CMPD and as cooperative mutation in AML with trisomy 8 and t(8;21): a comparative study on 1103 CMPD and 269 AML cases. *Leukemia* 2007; 21:1843–5.
51 Steensma DP, McClure RF, Karp JE, *et al.* *JAK2 V617F* is a rare finding in de novo acute myeloid leukemia, but STAT3 activation is common and remains unexplained. *Leukemia* 2006; 20:971–8.
52 Dohner K, Du J, Corbacioglu A, Scholl C, Schlenk RF, Dohner H. *JAK2V617F* mutations as cooperative genetic lesions in t(8;21)-positive acute myeloid leukemia. *Haematologica* 2006; 91:1569–70.
53 Stirewalt DL, Kopecky KJ, Meshinchi S, *et al.* *FLT3*, *RAS*, and *TP53* mutations in elderly patients with acute myeloid leukemia. *Blood* 2001;97:3589–95.
54 Gorello P, Cazzaniga G, Alberti F, *et al.* Quantitative assessment of minimal residual disease in acute myeloid leukemia carrying nucleophosmin (*NPM1*) gene mutations. *Leukemia* 2006;20: 1103–8.
55 Schlenk RF, Frohling S, Hartmann F, *et al.* Phase III study of all-trans retinoic acid in previously untreated patients 61 years or older with acute myeloid leukemia. *Leukemia* 2004;18: 1798–803.
56 Christiansen DH, Andersen MK, Pedersen-Bjergaard J. Mutations of *AML1* are common in therapy-related myelodysplasia following therapy with alkylating agents and are significantly associated with deletion or loss of chromosome arm 7q and with subsequent leukemic transformation. *Blood* 2004;104:1474–81.
57 Schoch C, Kern W, Kohlmann A, Hiddemann W, Schnittger S, Haferlach T. Acute myeloid leukemia with a complex aberrant karyotype is a distinct biological entity characterized by genomic imbalances and a specific gene expression profile. *Genes Chromosomes Cancer* 2005;43:227–38.
58 Summers K, Stevens J, Kakkas I, *et al.* Wilms' tumor 1 mutations are associated with FLT3-ITD and failure of standard induction chemotherapy in patients with normal karyotype AML. *Leukemia* 2007;21:550–1.
59 Weisser M, Kern W, Rauhut S, *et al.* Prognostic impact of RT-PCR-based quantification of *WT1* gene expression during MRD monitoring of acute myeloid leukemia. *Leukemia* 2005;19: 1416–23.
60 Baldus CD, Tanner SM, Ruppert AS, *et al.* BAALC expression predicts clinical outcome of de novo acute myeloid leukemia patients with normal cytogenetics: a Cancer and Leukemia Group B Study. *Blood* 2003;102:1613–18.
61 Haferlach T, Bacher U, Haferlach C, Kern W, Schnittger S. Insight into the molecular pathogenesis of myeloid malignancies. *Curr Opin Hematol* 2007;14:90–7.
62 Schnittger S, Schoch C, Kern W, Hiddemann W, Haferlach T. *FLT3* length mutations as marker for follow-up studies in acute myeloid leukemia. *Acta Haematol* 2004;112:68–78.
63 Steudel C, Wermke M, Schaich M, *et al.* Comparative analysis of *MLL* partial tandem duplication and *FLT3* internal tandem duplication mutations in 956 adult patients with acute myeloid leukemia. *Genes Chromosomes Cancer* 2003;37: 237–51.
64 Falini B, Nicoletti I, Martelli MF, Mecucci C. Acute myeloid leukemia carrying cytoplasmic/mutated nucleophosmin (NPMc + AML): biologic and clinical features. *Blood* 2007;109: 874–85.
65 Libura M, Asnafi V, Tu A, *et al.* *FLT3* and *MLL* intragenic abnormalities in AML reflect a common category of genotoxic stress. *Blood* 2003 15;102:2198–204.
66 McHale CM, Wiemels JL, Zhang L, *et al.* Prenatal origin of childhood acute myeloid leukemias harboring chromosomal rearrangements t(15;17) and inv(16) 1. *Blood* 2003;101: 4640–1.
67 Haferlach T, Kohlmann A, Schnittger S, *et al.* Global approach to the diagnosis of leukemia using gene expression profiling. *Blood* 2005;106:1189–98.
68 Ross ME, Zhou X, Song G, *et al.* Classification of pediatric acute lymphoblastic leukemia by gene expression profiling 1. *Blood* 2003;102:2951–9.
69 Kohlmann A, Schoch C, Schnittger S, *et al.* Molecular characterization of acute leukemias by use of microarray technology. *Genes Chromosomes Cancer* 2003;37:396–405.
70 Valk PJ, Verhaak RG, Beijen MA, *et al.* Prognostically useful gene-expression profiles in acute myeloid leukemia. *N Engl J Med* 2004;350:1617–28.
71 Wilson CS, Davidson GS, Martin SB, *et al.* Gene expression profiling of adult acute myeloid leukemia identifies novel biologic clusters for risk classification and outcome prediction 1. *Blood* 2006;108:685–96.
72 Heuser M, Wingen LU, Steinemann D, *et al.* Gene-expression profiles and their association with drug resistance in adult acute myeloid leukemia. *Haematologica* 2005;90:1484–92.

Chapter 10
Induction Therapy of Acute Myeloid Leukemia

Martha Wadleigh and Daniel J. DeAngelo
Dana-Farber Cancer Institute, Boston, Massachusetts, USA

Acute myeloid leukemia (AML) is a clonal hematopoietic stem-cell disorder for which the treatment—in fact, cure—hinges upon the successful eradication of the leukemic clone. To this end, induction chemotherapy is given to reduce the level of the leukemic burden below the level of detection and to restore normal hematopoiesis. Postremission consolidation, alone or followed by an autologous or allogeneic stem-cell transplant, is then used to further reduce the leukemic burden. For the past three decades, the backbone of remission induction therapy in younger patients (<60 years of age), as well as for a subset of older patients deemed fit enough to undergo such treatment, has consisted of 7 days of continuous-infusion cytarabine combined with 3 days of anthracycline, otherwise known as the "7 plus 3" regimen. Remission rates with induction therapy vary, and depend upon many factors including patient age, cytogenetics, antecedent hematologic disorder, prior chemotherapy, and type of leukemia. Over the past several decades, induction therapy has been intensified with the aim of improving remission rates, extending disease-free survival, and ultimately overall survival. Strategies to improve upon standard therapy have included using different anthracyclines, intensifying the dose of anthracycline, intensifying the dose of cytarabine, using a time-sequence approach, and priming with growth factors, as well as adding other agents to the standard backbone of "7 plus 3." For elderly patients (>60 years of age), induction strategies have concentrated on less toxic induction strategies employing monoclonal antibodies, nucleoside analogs, hypomethylating agents, and other novel compounds.

Pre-treatment evaluation

Once a diagnosis of AML is established, induction chemotherapy is typically given with the goal of inducing a rapid remission—remission being defined as the absence of immature blast cells within the peripheral blood, <5% on a bone marrow aspirate, and the absence of any signs of extramedullary disease. The restoration of normal hematopoiesis is essential to the definition of remission, and the International Working Group has revised the response criteria for the treatment of patients with AML and now define hematopoietic recovery as an absolute neutrophil count of 1000/μL and a platelet count of 100,000/μL regardless of duration [1] (Table 10.1).

Although age is a continuous variable, most studies define "young adults" as <60 years of age. The initial treatment of young adults with *de novo* AML aims at reducing the total body leukemia-cell burden from 10^{12} to 10^{13} cells to a level that is morphologically undetectable, which typically corresponds to appropriately 10^{9} blast cells. Although this is a substantial reduction in the overall tumor burden, patients in complete remission still have a significant tumor burden. Therefore, postremission strategies are equally important in the treatment of patients with AML. Nevertheless, a cure cannot be achieved with the attainment of a complete-remission status.

Induction chemotherapy is a complicated and rigorous process that is required in order to obtain clinical remission [2]. Prior to the initiation of induction chemotherapy, it is important to establish the presence of comorbid conditions, which could potentially complicate the management of the patient. It is clear that all elements of the patient's history and physical status are important. However, particular attention needs to be paid to history of a hematologic disorder, for example a myelodysplastic or myeloproliferative disorder, prior therapy for malignancies including chemotherapy or radiation therapy, as well as a family history of disease. Patients with secondary or treatment-related AML have a significantly worse prognosis, which is predominantly influenced by the higher incidence of unfavorable cytogenetic abnormalities. A history of cardiac disease, such as congestive heart failure, would mandate careful monitoring and potential alteration of induction chemotherapy, as anthracycline-based regimens are standard. Patients typically receive large amounts of intravenous fluids that accompany

Leukemias: Principles and Practice of Therapy, 1st edition. Edited by S. Faderl and H. Kantarjian.

Table 10.1 Response criteria in acute myeloid leukemia.

Response criterion	Time of assessment	Neutrophils (μL)	Platelets (μL)	Bone marrow blasts (%)	Other
Early treatment assessment	7–10 days after therapy	NA	NA	<5	
Morphologic leukemia-free state	Varies by protocol	NA	NA	<5	No EMD
Morphologic CR	Varies by protocol	>1000	>100,000	<5	No transfusions, no EMD
Cytogenetic CR	Varies by protocol	>1000	>100,000	<5	Cytogenics—normal, no EMD
Molecular CR	Varies by protocol	>1000	>100,000	<5	Molecular studies—negative, no EMD
Partial remission	Varies by protocol	>1000	>100,000	>50 decrease or to 5–25%	Blasts <5% if Auer-rod positive

AML, acute myeloid leukemia; CR, complete remission; EMD, extramedullary disease; NA, not applicable.

initial chemotherapy as well as antibiotics and blood and platelet transfusions, and therefore patients with cardiac abnormalities at the time of diagnosis need rigorous and careful monitoring.

Alloimmunization is typically seen in patients with prior transfusions or multiple previous pregnancies, and can significantly complicate induction therapy. In addition, careful appraisal of drug allergies and prior viral infections such as herpes simplex is also important.

Prior to initiation of any induction therapy, it is important to obtain a complete blood count with differential chemistries, including liver and renal function, electrolytes, and glucose, as well as coagulation parameters with a prothrombin time (PT) and activated partial thromboplastin time (aPTT), fibrinogen, lactate dehydrogenase (LDH), calcium phosphorus, uric acid, albumin, and total protein. Serum lysozyme can be useful in patients with monocytic leukemias, as they tend to have significant potassium and magnesium wasting. In addition, one should consider performing serologic testing for antibodies for prior herpes simplex virus (HSV) and cytomegalovirus (CMV) infection. Human leukocyte antigen (HLA) typing should be obtained in all patients who are candidates for hematopoietic stem-cell transplant. In addition, HLA typing will facilitate obtaining HLA-restricted platelets in patients who develop alloimmunization.

Prior to the initiation of chemotherapy, it is common to insert a central venous access device typically with two or three independent ports, which can facilitate the management of transfusions, chemotherapy, antibiotics, intravenous fluids, and other support. For patients with poor dental hygiene, a dental evaluation may be important prior to initiation of chemotherapy. It is important to obtain a standard chest radiograph as a baseline parameter as well as an electrocardiogram (ECG). An echocardiogram (Echo) or technetium labeled radionucleotide study (multigated acquisition [MUGA] scan) is important to establish baseline cardiac function, especially in patients with a history of cardiac disease or prior anthracycline exposure.

All fertile men and women of childbearing potential should receive counseling about the potential effect of the treatment on fertility as well as options for fertility preserving measures. Most patients receiving standard induction chemotherapy and postremission therapy will maintain their fertility. However, those patients who proceed toward stem-cell transplantation will often become permanently sterile. Therefore, there is an urgent need for fertility preserving measures in appropriate candidates. Options for women are unfortunately limited, but men can participate in sperm banking prior to initiation of chemotherapy.

For those patients with neurologic signs and symptoms of leptomeningeal disease, imaging studies such as an MRI with gadolinium may help evaluate for meningeal disease or for the presence of a myeloid sarcoma (chloroma). In addition, one may need to rule out a central nervous system (CNS) hemorrhage, especially in patients with significant coagulopathies. Patients for whom imaging is unhelpful but who have a high index of suspicion for meningeal disease, a lumbar puncture with cerebrospinal fluid (CSF) examination for leukemic involvement is important. CSF should be sent for flow cytometric analysis and/or fluorescence *in situ* hybridization (FISH) analysis, especially for patients with cytogenetic abnormalities. A lumbar puncture, however, is not routinely performed in asymptomatic patients given the risk of bleeding as well as the theoretic possibility of the introduction of malignant cells from the peripheral blood into the CNS. The CNS is a sanctuary site with an active blood–brain barrier, and many of the common chemotherapeutics do not cross this barrier. However, if a lumbar puncture is performed, one should strongly consider the administration of intrathecal chemotherapy with either cytarabine or methotrexate.

There is much debate about the speed at which initiation of induction chemotherapy needs to take place [3]. It is imperative that a treatment plan be initiated at the time of admission. However, it is often more important to stabilize the patient's condition and correct or control comorbidities such as infection, bleeding, hyperuricemia, or renal failure. In addition, laboratory abnormalities such as anemia or thrombocytopenia should also be corrected prior to the initiation of chemotherapy. Oral hydroxyurea can be used for cytoreduction in patients with an elevated peripheral blast count and for patients with symptomatic leukostasis such as pulmonary dysfunction or encephalopathy [4]. Cytoreduction using a pheresis process can rapidly, although transiently, reduce the elevated peripheral blast count. Typically, leukostasis does not occur until the absolute peripheral blast count reaches >50,000.

Choice of anthracycline

The standard choice of anthracycline in the treatment of AML is daunorubicin. Early studies of daunorubicin given as a single agent in patients with AML demonstrated a superior complete remission (CR) rate when given at a dosage of 60 mg/m^2 per day for 5 days compared with intermittent weekly or twice weekly schedules [5]. It was then combined with cytarabine continuous infusion, which generated remission rates of >50% in patients <60 years of age [6]. Initially, daunorubicin was the only anthracycline used for induction chemotherapy; however, in the 1980s other anthracyclines and anthracenediones were introduced. Several randomized trials have been conducted to determine if the choice of anthracycline is important in induction therapy (see Table 10.2).

The bulk of studies have compared daunorubicin with idarubicin, but other agents, including adriamycin [7], aclarubicin [8], mitoxantrone [9], and amascrine [10] have also been studied. An early study by the Cancer and Leukemia Group B (CALGB) demonstrated that daunorubicin administered at a dosage of 45 mg/m^2 daily for 3 days in combination with cytarabine at 100 mg/m^2 daily for 7 days was as effective and less toxic than the same daily dose of adriamycin at 30 mg/m^2 for 3 days, with a CR rate of 72% versus 58% [7]. This is in contrast to other studies in which daunorubicin was not superior to the comparator arm. In a Danish study comparing daunorubicin at 45 mg/m^2 per day for 3 days to aclarubicin at 75 mg/m^2 per day each in combination with cytarabine, the CR rate was significantly higher in the aclarubicin arm (66% vs. 50%, $P = 0.043$). Hematologic toxicity was equivalent in the two arms, and no survival benefit was demonstrated after 4 years [8]. Similarly, mitoxantrone administered at 12mg/m^2 per day for 3 days combined with cytarabine induced remission in 63% (62 of 98 patients) compared with 53% (54 of 102) of patients treated with daunorubicin at 45 mg/m^2 per day combined with cytarabine [9]. Furthermore, 89% of those in the mitoxantrone arm entered remission after only one course of treatment compared with 68% of those in the daunorubicin arm. In another randomized trial from Memorial Sloan Kettering, amascrine given at 190 mg/m^2 per day on days 1–3 with cytarabine and 6-TG was compared with daunorubicin administered at a dosage of 50 mg/m^2 per day on days 1–3 with the same doses and schedules of cytarabine and 6-TG [10]. In this study, the non-daunorubicin arm had a higher CR rate (70% vs. 54%, $P = 0.13$) and more patients entered CR after only one induction course.

Six randomized trials have been conducted comparing idarubicin with daunorubicin when given in conjunction with cytarabine for induction therapy [11–16]. The dose of daunorubicin varied between 45 and 50 mg/m^2 as compared to idarubicin, which varied between 12 and 13 mg/m^2, with the exception of the study by Rieffers *et al.* that compared idarubicin given at a dose of 8 mg/m^2 over 5 days to 3 days of daunorubicin. In each study, the CR rate was better in the idarubicin-treated arm in the non-elderly populations. A meta-analysis of these studies confirmed that the CR rate with idarubicin was significantly better than that of daunorubicin (62% vs. 53%, $P = 0.002$) [17]. In this meta-analysis, early induction failures were similar in the two groups, but after day 40 the later induction failures were less in the idarubicin-treated arm. There was no benefit in disease-free survival, but 5-year overall survival was better in the idarubicin-treated arm compared with the daunorubicin arm (13% vs. 9%, $P = 0.03$). These results indicate that idarubicin may be somewhat more effective given at a dose of 12 mg/m^2 than daunorubicin at 45 mg/m^2 during induction therapy, without increased toxicity as measured by early induction deaths. This meta-analysis also highlighted a higher induction death rate for idarubicin compared with daunorubicin for those patients >40 years old. In a study by Rowe *et al.*, for patients >55 years of age with newly diagnosed AML, the benefit of idarubicin over daunorubicin on the CR rate was only seen in those patients <70 years of age [16].

Dose of anthracycline

It is unclear from these data if these other agents are biologically superior to daunorubicin or if daunorubicin dosed at 45 mg/m^2 is suboptimal. Studies from the large cooperative groups have demonstrated higher CR rates when higher doses of daunorubicin are used. In a trial from the Eastern Cooperative Oncology Group (ECOG) [18], daunorubicin given at a dose of 60 mg/m^2 during induction led to a CR rate of 70%, which was comparable to a successor trial from the same group using idarubicin at 12 mg/m^2 in a similar patient population [19]. Other

Table 10.2 Clinical trials comparing anthracyclines.

Study	Regimen (dose)	Complete remission (%)	*P*-value	Comments
Yates [7]	D (45)	72		Daunorubicin 45 was better than daunorubicin 30 and adriamycin 30, but only in patients <60 years of age
	A (100)			
	D (30)	59		
	A (100)			
	AD (30)	58		
	A (100)			
Hansen [8]	D (45)	50	0.043	Similar hematologic toxicity profiles in the two arms.
	A (100)			No survival benefit after 4 years of follow-up
	ACL (75)	66		
	A (100)			
Arlin [9]	D (45)	53		More patients in CR after one cycle of mitoxantrone compared to daunorubicin (89% vs. 68%)
	A (100)			
	M (12)	63		
	A (100)			
Berman [10]	D (50)	70	0.13	More patients in CR after one course of therapy with amsacrine
	A(25, 160)			
	6-TG (100)			Slightly improved survival with amasacrine
				Comparable non-heme toxicity
	AMS (190)	54		
	A(25, 160)			
	6-TG (100)			
MSKCC/Berman [11]	D (50)	58	<0.005	Induction death rates similar
	A (200)			
	I (12)	80		
	A (200)			
GIMEMA/Mandelli [12]	D	39		No benefit to idarubicin over daunorubicin
	A	40		
	I			
	A			
SECSG/Vogler [13]	D (45)	58	0.03	No significant difference in median survival, median remission duration or induction death rate
	A (100)	71		
	I (12)			
	A (100)			
Einstein/Wiernik [15]	D (45)	59	0.035	Significant difference in CR rate for those <60 years of age
	A (100)	70		
	I (13)			
	A (100)			
BGMT/Rieffers [14]	D (50 x 3)	61	0.3	Overall survival and DFS similar
	A (100)	68		CR rate was significantly better in the IDA group ages 55–65
	I (8 x 5)			
	A (100)			
SWOG/Rowe [16]	D (45)	46	0.04	Difference seen in those <70 years of age
	A (100)			
	I (12)	55		
	A (100)			
	M (12)	51		
	A 9100)			

A, ara-C (cytarabine); AD, adriamycin; ACL, aclarubicin; AMS, amsacrine; CR, complete response; D, daunorubicin; DFS, disease-free survival; I, idarubicin; M, mitoxantrone; 6-TG, 6-thioguanine.

studies by ECOG, the Southwestern Oncology Group (SWOG), and CALGB have demonstrated higher CR rates when the daunorubicin dose is increased to >45 mg/m^2 in patients <60 years of age (Table 10.2).

Based on these intriguing results, the ECOG conducted a prospective randomized trial in patients <60 years of age with newly diagnosed AML, comparing the standard daunorubicin dosage of 45 mg/m^2 per day for 3 days with cytarabine at 100 mg/m^2 continuous infusion for 7 days versus high-dose daunorubicin at 90 mg/m^2 for 3 days also with cytarabine at the same dose and schedule [20]. The CR rate for the high-dose daunorubicin arm was 70.6% compared with 57.3% for the standard-dose daunorubicin arm ($P = 0.001$). There was no difference in induction death rate. Median overall survival was superior in the high-dose arm compared with the standard-dose daunorubicin arm (23.7 vs. 15.7 months, respectively; $P = 0.003$). The benefit of the high-dose daunorubicin was limited to patients <50 years old, and cytogenetics is also important, as patients with unfavorable cytogenetic profiles had a poor outcome regardless of treatment assignment. The high-dose strategy did not significantly improve overall survival for patients with either the *FLT3*-ITD or the *MLL*-PTD mutation.

The difficulty in the widespread extrapolation of this study is that, although the Food and Drug Administration (FDA)-approved dose of daunorubicin in the USA is 45 mg/m^2, the dose that is widely used in the USA is 60 mg/m^2. Whether standard-dose cytarabine with 90 mg/m^2 of daunorubicin is superior to cytarabine plus the 60 mg/m^2 dose of daunorubicin remains to be studied. However, this is the first prospective randomized trial to demonstrate that intensifying induction therapy by increasing the anthracycline dose results not only in improved remission rates but also in improved overall survival. Therefore, for patients <60 years of age, the appropriate dose of daunorubicin is >45 mg/m^2, and there is little evidence supporting the continued use of daunorubicin at 45 mg/m^2 as the standard induction dose for AML in this age population.

A similar randomized study was conducted by the Dutch–Belgian Cooperative Trial Group (Hovon) along with the Swiss Group for Clinical Cancer Research (SAKK) comparing high-dose daunorubicin at 90 mg/m^2 with cytarabine at 200 mg/m^2 versus conventionally dosed daunorubicin at 45 mg/m^2 plus cytarabine at 200 mg/m^2 in patients aged 60–83 years [21]. The CR was 64% in the group that received the escalated dose of daunorubicin versus 54% in the conventional-dose group, and there was no significant difference between the two groups with respect to hematologic toxicity or 30-day mortality. In addition, the overall survival did not differ between the two groups. However, in subset analysis, patients aged 60–65 years fared better in the higher dose anthracycline treatment group with a higher CR (73% vs. 51%), event-free survival (29% vs. 14%), and overall survival (38% vs. 23%). This result contradicts the analysis from the ECOG trial, suggesting that patients >50 years old did not benefit from high-dose daunorubicin.

Dose of cytarabine

Cytarabine is the other agent partnered with anthracyclines in induction chemotherapy, and similar to anthracyclines, attempts have been made to intensify induction therapy and improve remission rates and survival rate by modulating the dose of cytarabine during induction (Table 10.3). Early studies demonstrated that a continuous infusion was superior to bolus or subcutaneous administration [6]. Doses of 100 mg/m^2 continuous infusion have been compared with 200 mg/m^2 and have demonstrated no significant difference in terms of CR rate or toxicity [26]. A study from the University of California, Los Angeles, comparing daunorubicin with either conventionally dosed cytarabine at 200 mg/m^2 continuous infusion to a 500 mg/m^2 i.v. bolus every 12 h during induction did not demonstrate any benefit for this intermediate dose of cytarabine [27].

Several small, uncontrolled studies reported high-remission rates when high doses of cytarabine (1.5–3 gm/m^2 every 12 h for 3–6 days) are used for induction therapy compared with historic controls [28–31]. Two large prospective randomized trials have compared

Table 10.3 Dose intensification of daunorubicin.

Reference	Dose of daunorubicin (mg/m^2)	Complete remission rate (%)	Comments
CALGB 9720; Baer [22]	60	46	>60 years of age
CALGB 9621; Kolitz [23]	≥60	78	<60 years of age
SWOG; Hewlett [24]	70	70	<49 years of age
ECOG 1490; Rowe [25]	60	52	>55 years of age
ECOG 1900; Fernandez [20]	90	70	<50 years of age
HOVAN; Lowenberg [21]	90	64	60–65 years of age

standard-dose continuous-infusion cytarabine with high-dose cytarabine [32,33]. SWOG randomized 665 patients to cytarabine 200 mg/m^2 continuous infusion on days 1–7 and daunorubicin 45 mg/m^2 on days 5–7, or cytarabine 2 gm/m^2 i.v. every 12 h on days 1–6 and the same dose of daunorubicin on days 7–9. CR was similar in the two arms and there was no benefit in overall survival at a median follow-up of 51 months. Furthermore, fatal toxicity due to infection or CNS hemorrhage was significantly more frequent in the high-dose arm compared with the standard-dose arm (14% vs. 5% in patients <50 years of age; 20% vs. 12% for patients >50 years of age). Similar results were seen in a large study by Bishop *et al* [33]. In this study, 301 patients aged 15–60 years with newly diagnosed AML were randomized to either high-dose cytarabine at 3 gm/m^2 every 12 h on days 1, 3, 5, and 7 for eight doses or cytarabine at 100 mg/m^2 continuous infusion on days 1–7 in conjunction with daunorubicin and etoposide during remission induction. All patients received the same postremission consolidation therapy. The CR was comparable in both arms (71% in the high-dose arm vs. 74% in the standard-dose arm). Remission duration was prolonged in the high-dose arm compared with the standard-dose arm (45 vs. 12 months, respectively, $P = 0.0005$). The estimated percentage of patients relapse-free 5 years after achieving CR was 49% in the high-dose arm and 24% in the low-dose arm. However, high-dose cytarabine was associated with significantly higher toxicity in induction with a significantly longer duration of leukopenia and thrombocytopenia. This evidence does not support the use of high doses of cytarabine during induction chemotherapy, especially when using intensified doses of cytarabine in the postremission setting has demonstrated 4-year disease-free intervals of 44% and appears to be safer [34].

Double induction and timed-sequential therapy

Further strategies to intensify induction chemotherapy in the hopes of improving the long-term prognosis of patients with AML have included administering two cycles of induction therapy. In this "double induction" strategy, two courses of induction are administered within 20–22 days of each other regardless of the bone marrow status following the first round. An early study by the German AML Cooperative Group randomized patients to a double induction with two cycles of standard-dose cytarabine, daunorubicin, and 6-thioguanine (TAD-TAD) or double induction with TAD followed by high-dose cytarabine and mitoxantrone (TAD-HAM) [35]. No statistical difference was seen between the two groups in terms of CR rate, hypoplastic death rate, or relapse-free survival at 5 years. In a subsequent study by the same group, double induction containing either two courses or one course of high-dose cytarabine plus mitoxantrone (TAD-HAM vs. HAM-HAM) again demonstrated no benefit from intensified dosing in terms of CR, relapse-free survival, or overall survival, regardless of patient age [36]. There was no significant benefit from the more intensive induction on the outcome for any prognostic subgroup, including secondary AML/myelodysplasia, poor-risk cytogenetics group, high white blood cell count, or high lactate dehydrogenase (LDH) level.

Time-sequential therapy is similar to double induction therapy; however, the second course of therapy is given much closer to the first course, again regardless of the degree of aplasia in the marrow. The scientific rationale behind this approach posits that the initial course of chemotherapy can recruit residual leukemia cells into the cell cycle making residual cells more sensitive to cell-cycle specific agents used in the second course. The second course is applied earlier, between days 8 and 10 in order to achieve a greater cell kill [37–40]. Phase II studies have demonstrated the feasibility of this approach, but the results are mixed with some demonstrating improved disease-free survival but others demonstrating no benefit in terms of relapse-free survival or overall survival compared with historic controls [41–45]. In a recent German study, sequential HAM was administered with pegfilgrastim support [36]. Dose intensity of the sequential HAM was 66% of the HAM-HAM used in the double induction trials secondary to prolonged neutropenia in the group who received sequential HAM at 85% dose intensity of the HAM-HAM. Overall, 113 patients received sequential HAM at 66% and 59 patients at 85%. The more intensive induction regimen using two courses of sequential HAM did not result in any change in outcome including CR, early death rate, or overall survival and disease-free survival.

The Acute Leukemia French Association (ALFA) 9000 study compared standard induction to a double induction and a time-sequential induction approach [46]. Importantly, the dose of daunorubicin in the control group was 80 mg/m^2. In this study, there was no difference in the overall CR rate or treatment-related mortality in either the induction or postremission phase of therapy. A subgroup analysis of patients <50 years of age demonstrated that relapse-free survival was significantly improved in younger patients receiving the timed-sequential induction. However, importantly, there was no difference in event-free survival and overall survival among the three randomized arms. From this study, there appears to be no advantage to timed-sequential therapy or a double-induction regimen compared with standard-induction therapy with an intensified dose of daunorubicin.

Addition of other agents to standard therapy

The antimetabolite 6-thioguanine is often added to the standard "3 plus 7" regimen. The regimens that include thioguanine are often abbreviated with the acronym DAT or TAD. A CALGB study randomized 427 patients to receive daunorubicin plus cytarabine with or without 6-thioguanine, and there was no difference in the CR rate, remission duration, or overall survival between the two regimens [47]. In addition, large randomized trials conducted by the Medical Research Council (MRC) found that replacement of 6-thioguanine with etoposide has no significant effect on the rates of CR, remission duration, or overall survival [48]. The addition of etoposide to standard-induction chemotherapy has also been studied by many groups, including the Australian Leukemia Study Group (ALSG). In addition to standard daunorubicin and cytarabine-induction chemotherapy, patients were randomized to receive etoposide at a dose of 75 mg/m^2 administered intravenously on days 1–7 [49]. There was no difference in the overall complete response rate. However, the median remission duration improved from 18 months to 12 months ($P = 0.01$) in the group that received etoposide.

Priming and growth-factor support

The myeloid growth factors granulocyte colony-stimulating factor (G-CSF) [50–52] and granulocyte-macrophage colony-stimulating factor (GM-CSF) [25,53–57] have been extensively studied in AML. Whether administered before, during, or after chemotherapy for AML, these agents reduce the duration of neutropenia and appear to be safe and well tolerated. Despite consistently demonstrating a shorter duration of neutropenia, multiple prospective randomized trials have documented only modest benefits in terms of reduction in the incidence and severity of infections, without substantial gains or impact in CR, overall survival, and disease-free survival rates. An ECOG study by Rowe *et al.* was the only study to demonstrate a survival benefit for the GM-CSF treated group over placebo (median survival of 10.6 vs. 4.8 months, $P = 0.021$). However, some argue that the median survival in the control arm was inferior to that reported in other studies in the same age group [50,58].

Growth factors have also been used during induction to recruit quiescent leukemia cells into the S phase of the cell cycle to increase their susceptibility to chemotherapy with the goal of reducing relapse and resistance. *In vitro* studies demonstrate that co-culturing leukemia cells with GM-CSF or G-CSF results in a higher proportion of cells in S phase and enhances the incorporation of cytarabine into the DNA of leukemia cells, conferring greater cytotoxicity [59–61]. Randomized trials to evaluate this priming strategy have consistently demonstrated an improvement in terms of disease-free or event-free survival in the intermediate-risk group of patients with AML, but no overall survival benefit with this approach [1,46,62].

Monoclonal antibodies

Several classes of monoclonal antibodies have been developed for treatment in patients with AML. The antibodies target many antigens that are expressed on the surface of leukemia cells, which result in leukemic cell death. Early studies using unconjugated monoclonal antibodies directed against CD14, CD15, and CD33 have been utilized. However, even studies using the humanized anti-CD33 monoclonal antibody (HuM195) resulted in only modest response rates with an overall response of <10% [63,64]. A randomized phase III study adding HuM195 to mitoxantrone, etoposide, and cytarabine in patients with relapsed AML has been recently reported with no improvement in CR, disease-free survival, or overall survival rates for patients receiving HuM195 [65]. As a result, attention has been turned to conjugated monoclonal antibodies.

The advantage of a conjugated monoclonal antibody relates to the potential for a more effective therapy directed against the target leukemia cell. Depending upon the specificity of the target, this strategy may result in decreased toxicity with a sparing of damaged to normal stem cells. CD33 has been the antigen targeted in most studies in patients with AML [66]. CD33 is expressed in the majority of myeloid precursor cells but not on normal hematopoietic stem cells. Unfortunately, CD33 is also present on normal, mature hematopoietic cells as well as on liver stellate cells, and therefore the use of anti-CD33 conjugated-antibody therapy may result in toxicity.

The antibody-conjugate drug that has been most intensely studied is calicheamicin. Calicheamicin can be reversibly linked to humanized anti-CD33 antibodies (CMA7676) [67]. When internalized, the calicheamicin generates an active radical species that binds and intercalates DNA, causing double strand breaks leading to apoptosis. Numerous phase II studies using gemtuzumab ozogamicin (Mylotarg®) has demonstrated significant activity in patients with relapsed or refractory $CD33^+$ AML, which has led to the approval of gemtuzumab in patients >60 years old with relapsed AML. The overall response rate of single-agent gemtuzumab is 40%, with 33% of patients achieving a CR and an additional 8% of patients achieving a CRP (complete remission without recovery of platelets) [68].

With the development of gemtuzumab in patients with relapsed AML, it was tested in two feasibility studies in newly diagnosed patients with AML. The MRC tested gemtuzumab with a variety of induction regimens, including DAT (daunorubicin, cytarabine, thioguanine), DA (daunorubicin plus cytarabine), and FLAG-Ida (fludarabine, cytarabine, G-CSF, idarubicin) with gemtuzumab. Gemtuzumab was dosed at $3\,mg/m^2$ during the first cycle but was not dosed in subsequent cycles because of hepatotoxicity and delayed hematopoietic recovery [69]. A remission with the first course was seen in 86% of patients leading to a randomized phase III study (MRC-AML15) in patients <60 years old. The preliminary report of the MRC15 study on 1115 patients showed that the CR for both arms was 83%. However, patients who received gemtuzumab had a higher disease-free survival at 3 years (51% vs. 40%; $P = 0.008$). Overall survival was not improved with gemtuzumab (53% vs. 46%; $P = 0.4$), which may be attributed to the short follow-up.

The combination of gemtuzumab with daunorubicin and Ara-C was also tested as a feasibility study, with the addition of ozogamicin (GO) leading to an 83% CR and a disease-free survival (DFS) of >50%. Preliminary results from the SWOG 0106 revealed that a phase III randomized trial adding gemtuzumab and GO to standard induction chemotherapy failed to improve the CR or overall survival rate [70]. The complete response rate was 66% in the gemtuzumab arm versus 69% in the control arm. There was also no improvement in the disease-free survival with the addition of gemtuzumab.

FLT3 inhibitors

The FMS-like tyrosine kinase 3 (*FLT3*) gene is mutated in approximately 30% of patients with AML [71]. Approximately 20% of patients with AML, particularly younger patients with a normal karyotype and a high circulating absolute blast count, will harbor an *FLT3* internal tandem duplication (ITD). In addition, approximately 5–7% of patients will have a tyrosine kinase domain mutation (most commonly D835Y). Patients with the *FLT3*-ITD have an extremely poor prognosis, higher rates of disease recurrence, and higher resistance to chemotherapy, suggesting that the standard treatment for AML is generally less effective for this patient population [72]. Several agents have been developed that target the *FLT3* tyrosine kinase. These include midastaurin (PKC412; Novartis Pharmaceuticals, Inc.) [73], tandutinib (MLN518/CT53518; Millennium Pharmaceuticals, Inc., Cambridge, MA, USA) [74], and lestaurtinib (CEP701; Cephalon Pharmaceuticals, Inc., Frazer, PA, USA) [75]. Both tandutinib and midastaurin have been successfully combined with induction chemotherapy using a daunorubicin plus cytarabine backbone [76,77]. Currently, midastaurin is being tested in a phase III randomized, placebo-controlled trial to determine whether or not the addition of an FLT3 inhibitor to standard induction consolidation therapy as well as maintenance therapy may improve overall survival for this high-risk subset of patients.

A phase III study using lestaurtinib in patients with relapsed AML was recently reported [78]. All patients had *FLT3*-ITD or TKD. They were treated with combination chemotherapy with or without lestaurtinib. There was no benefit in terms of CR, disease-free survival, or overall survival in this study. However, the prognostic implication of an *FLT3* mutation in the relapsed refractory setting is unclear. Results from the randomized lestaurtinib trial revealed that the CR rate was 26% in the lestaurtinib arm versus 21% in the control arm ($P = 0.35$), with no difference in overall survival (4.73 months vs. 4.57 months) between the two arms.

Alternative strategies

Inhibitors of the DNA methyltransferase (DNMT), azacitidine (Vidaza; Celgene, Summit, NJ, USA), and decitabine (Dacogen, Bloomington, MN) are approved for the treatment of patients with myelodysplastic syndrome [79–81]. The current WHO definition of AML now includes patients with a blast count of between 20% and 29%, as these patients were previously considered as having myelodysplasia [82,83]. There is a limited experience of the use of these agents in patients with AML. Remission rates are typically in the range of 10–20%. Fenaux *et al.* demonstrated an improved median overall survival in patients treated with acacitadine as compared with conventional care approaches, which included supportive care, low-dose cytarabine, and "3 plus 7" [84].

The novel nucleoside analog clofarabine (Genzyme, Cambridge, MA, USA) is currently being studied in older patients with *de novo* AML. Clofarabine inhibits ribonucleotide reductase and DNA polymerase. It is resistant to cleavage by purine nucleoside phosphorylase and to deamination by adenosine deaminase [85]. A CR of 32% was seen in a phase II trial of patients with relapsed or refractory hematologic malignancies [86,87]. Clofarabine has been combined in an effort to modulate cytarabine triphosphate accumulation in subsequent phase I and II trials [88,89]. Clofarabine as a single agent was studied in 112 patients >60 years old who were deemed to be unlikely to benefit from standard conventional chemotherapy. The CR was 38%, and the overall response rate was 46% with a median disease-free survival of approximately 33 weeks [90]. Cloretazine is a sulfonylhydrazine alkylator of O^6-guanosine [91]. Cloretazine has modest activity in patients with relapsed AML, but it may be more active when combined with other agents such as cytarabine [92–94]. A phase II study in elderly patients with AML >60 years old with at least one poor risk factor, revealed a CR of 25% with an overall response rate of 35% [95].

Conclusion

The treatment of AML is an inherently difficult process. The typical approach is the use of combination cytoreductive chemotherapy with an anthracycline such as daunorubicin or idarubicin for 3 days and standard-dose cytarabine for 7 days (Table 10.4). Depending upon the age of the patients selected, approximately 60–80% of younger adults will achieve a complete remission. The three anthracycline-like drugs—daunorubicin, idarubicin, and mitoxantrone—are all probably equally effective. There is little evidence that adding high-dose cytarabine or a third drug such as etoposide or 6-thioguanine provides any significant benefit, but it may result in additional toxicity. Once a patient enters remission, then a risk-adaptive strategy for postremission therapy should be pursued. The addition of novel agents such as FLT3 inhibitors, histone deacetylase inhibitors, or DNA methyltransferase inhibitors to standard therapy remains to be elucidated.

Induction chemotherapy in older patients remains a problematic venture. Only approximately 30% of patients >60 years old ever receive chemotherapy because of significant comorbidity [96]. When compared with younger patients, older adults have more complications and have a higher inherently resistant disease. Nevertheless, approximately 45–50% of older adults are able to achieve complete remission when receiving an induction regimen (Table 10.5). For those patients deemed suitable, standard anthracycline for 3 days plus a standard dose of cytarabine

Table 10.4 Chemotherapy induction regimens for acute myeloid leukemia.

Drugs	Dosing	Comments
Cytarabine plus daunorubicin	Cytarabine: 100 or 200 mg/m^2 per day as a continuous infusion for 7 days Daunorubicin: 60–90 mg/m^2 intravenous push on each of the first 3 days of treatment	"Standard 7 plus 3" induction regimen resulting in approximately 60–80% remission rate and acceptable toxicity in patients <60 years old
Cytarabine (HDAC) plus daunorubicin	Cytarabine: 1–3 g/m^2 twice daily for a total of 12 doses Daunorubicin: 45 mg/m^2 intravenous push for 3 days following cytarabine	Yields a 90% remission rate; however, substantial toxicity precludes postremission therapy in a high proportion of patients
Cytarabine plus idarubicin	Cytarabine: 100 or 200 mg/m^2 daily as a continuous infusion for 7 days Idarubicin: 12 mg/m^2 i.v. push on each of first 3 days of treatment	Has produced a greater remission rate (88 vs. 70%) than cytarabine/daunorubicin in younger patients; appears superior to daunorubicin in patients with hyperleukocytosis; overall survival not clearly superior to "standard" regimen

Overview of common induction therapy regimens for acute myeloid leukemia in younger adults.
HDAC; high-dose cytarabine.

Table 10.5 Select clinical trials in older adults with acute myeloid leukemia.

Study	Year	Median age (years)	Complete remission (%)	Overall survival (months)
ECOG 1490	1995	64	52	7.8
CALGB 8293	1995	69	52	9.6
SWOG 9031	1998	68	45	8.5
HOVON AML 9	1998	68	42	9.5
MRC AML 11	2001	66	55	10%—5 years
CALGB 9720	2002	70	46	10
SWOG 9333	2002	68	43	9
ECOG 3993	2004	68	42	7.5
AMLCG	2009	66	59	16%—4 years

Adapted with permission from Rowe *et al.* 2009 [97].
Induction death ~15–25%.
Disease-free survival ~6–9 months.
AMLCG, Acute Myeloid Leukemia Cooperative Group; CALGB, Cancer and Leukemia Group B; ECOG, Eastern Cooperative Oncology Group; HOVON AML, Hemato-Oncologie voor Volwassenen Nederland Acute Myeloid Leukemia; MRC, Medical Research Council; SWOG, Southwestern Cooperative Oncology Group.

remains a reasonable option, but for patients >70 years old as well as patients with poor-risk cytogenetic features or significant comorbidity, alternative strategies need to be developed. This remains an active area of investigation.

References

1 Cheson BD, Bennett JM, Kopecky KJ, *et al.* Revised recommendations of the International Working Group for diagnosis, standardization of response criteria, treatment outcomes, and reporting standards for therapeutic trials in acute myeloid leukemia. *J Clin Oncol* 2003;21:4642–9.

2 Lowenberg B, Downing JR, Burnett A. Acute myeloid leukemia. *N Engl J Med* 1999;341:1051–62.

3 Sekeres MA, Elson P, Kalaycio ME, *et al.* Time from diagnosis to treatment initiation predicts survival in younger, but not older, acute myeloid leukemia patients. *Blood* 2009;113:28–36.

4 Grund FM, Armitage JO, Burns P. Hydroxyurea in the prevention of the effects of leukostasis in acute leukemia. *Arch Intern Med* 1977;137:1246–7.

5 Weil M, Glidewell OJ, Jacquillat C, *et al.* Daunorubicin in the therapy of acute granulocytic leukemia. *Cancer Res* 1973;33: 921–8.

6 Rai KR, Holland JF, Glidewell OJ, *et al.* Treatment of acute myelocytic leukemia :a study by cancer and leukemia group B. *Blood* 1981;58:1203–12.

7 Yates J, Glidewell O, Wiernik P, *et al.* Cytosine arabinoside with daunorubicin or adriamycin for therapy of acute myelocytic leukemia: a CALGB study. *Blood* 1982;60:454–62.

8 Hansen OP, Pedersen-Bjergaard J, Ellegaard J, *et al.* Aclarubicin plus cytosine arabinoside versus daunorubicin plus cytosine arabinoside in previously untreated patients with acute myeloid leukemia: a Danish national phase III trial. The Danish Society of Hematology Study Group on AML, Denmark. *Leukemia* 1991;5:510–16.

9 Arlin Z, Case DC, Jr., Moore J, *et al.* Randomized multicenter trial of cytosine arabinoside with mitoxantrone or daunorubicin in previously untreated adult patients with acute nonlymphocytic leukemia (ANLL). Lederle Cooperative Group. *Leukemia* 1990;4:177–83.

10 Berman E, Arlin ZA, Gaynor J, *et al.* Comparative trial of cytarabine and thioguanine in combination with amsacrine or daunorubicin in patients with untreated acute nonlymphocytic leukemia: results of the L-16M protocol. *Leukemia* 1989;3: 115–21.

11 Berman E, Heller G, Santorsa J, *et al.* Results of a randomized trial comparing idarubicin and cytosine arabinoside with daunorubicin and cytosine arabinoside in adult patients with newly diagnosed acute myelogenous leukemia. *Blood* 1991; 77:1666–74.

12 Mandelli F, Petti MC, Ardia A, *et al.* A randomized clinical trial comparing idarubicin and cytarabine to daunorubicin and cytarabine in the treatment of acute non-lymphoid leukemia. A multicentric study from the Italian Co-operative Group GIMEMA. *Eur J Cancer* 1991;27:750–5.

13 Vogler WR, Velez-Garcia E, Weiner RS, *et al.* A phase III trial comparing idarubicin and daunorubicin in combination with cytarabine in acute myelogenous leukemia: a Southeastern Cancer Study Group Study. *J Clin Oncol* 1992;10:1103–11.

14 Reiffers J, Huguet F, Stoppa AM, *et al.* A prospective randomized trial of idarubicin vs daunorubicin in combination chemotherapy for acute myelogenous leukemia of the age group 55 to 75. *Leukemia* 1996;10:389–95.

15 Wiernik PH, Banks PL, Case DC, Jr., *et al.* Cytarabine plus idarubicin or daunorubicin as induction and consolidation therapy for previously untreated adult patients with acute myeloid leukemia. *Blood.* 1992;79:313–19.

16 Rowe JM, Neuberg D, Friedenberg W, *et al.* A phase 3 study of three induction regimens and of priming with GM-CSF in older adults with acute myeloid leukemia: a trial by the Eastern Cooperative Oncology Group. *Blood* 2004;103:479–85.

17 A systematic collaborative overview of randomized trials comparing idarubicin with daunorubicin (or other anthracyclines) as induction therapy for acute myeloid leukemia. AML Collaborative Group. *Br J Haematol* 1998;103:100–9.

18 Cassileth PA, Lynch E, Hines JD, *et al.* Varying intensity of postremission therapy in acute myeloid leukemia. *Blood* 1992;79:1924–30.

19 Cassileth PA, Harrington DP, Appelbaum FR, *et al.* Chemotherapy compared with autologous or allogeneic bone marrow transplantation in the management of acute myeloid leukemia in first remission. *N Engl J Med* 1998;339:1649–56.

20 Fernandez HF, Sun Z, Yao X, *et al.* Anthracycline dose intensification in acute myeloid leukemia. *N Engl J Med* 2009; 361:1249–59.

21 Lowenberg B, Ossenkoppele GJ, van Putten W, *et al.* High-dose daunorubicin in older patients with acute myeloid leukemia. *N Engl J Med* 2009;361:1235–48.

22 Baer MR, George SL, Dodge RK, *et al.* Phase 3 study of the multidrug resistance modulator PSC-833 in previously untreated patients 60 years of age and older with acute myeloid leukemia: Cancer and Leukemia Group B Study 9720. *Blood* 2002;100:1224–32.

23 Kolitz JE, George SL, Dodge RK, *et al.* Dose escalation studies of cytarabine, daunorubicin, and etoposide with and without multidrug resistance modulation with PSC-833 in untreated adults with acute myeloid leukemia younger than 60 years: final induction results of Cancer and Leukemia Group B Study 9621. *J Clin Oncol* 2004;22:4290–301.

24 Hewlett J, Kopecky KJ, Head D, *et al.* A prospective evaluation of the roles of allogeneic marrow transplantation and low-dose monthly maintenance chemotherapy in the treatment of adult acute myelogenous leukemia (AML): a Southwest Oncology Group study. *Leukemia* 1995;9:562–9.

25 Rowe JM, Andersen JW, Mazza JJ, *et al.* A randomized placebo-controlled phase III study of granulocyte-macrophage colony-stimulating factor in adult patients (>55 to 70 years of age) with acute myelogenous leukemia: a study of the Eastern Cooperative Oncology Group (E1490). *Blood* 1995;86:457–62.

26 Dillman RO, Davis RB, Green MR, *et al.* A comparative study of two different doses of cytarabine for acute myeloid leukemia: a phase III trial of Cancer and Leukemia Group B. *Blood* 1991;78:2520–6.

27 Schiller G, Gajewski J, Nimer S, *et al.* A randomized study of intermediate versus conventional-dose cytarabine as intensive induction for acute myelogenous leukemia. *Br J Haematol* 1992;81:170–7.

28 Hines JD, Mazza JJ, Oken MM, *et al.* High-dose cytosine arabinoside and mAMSA induction and consolidation in patients

with previously untreated de novo acute nonlymphocytic leukemia: Phase I Pilot Study for the Eastern Cooperative Oncology Group. *Semin Oncol* 1985;12(2 Suppl.3):117–19.

29 Curtis JE, Messner HA, Minden MD, Minkin S, McCulloch EA. High-dose cytosine arabinoside in the treatment of acute myelogenous leukemia: contributions to outcome of clinical and laboratory attributes. *J Clin Oncol* 1987;5:532–43.

30 Phillips GL, Reece DE, Shepherd JD, *et al.* High-dose cytarabine and daunorubicin induction and postremission chemotherapy for the treatment of acute myelogenous leukemia in adults. *Blood* 1991;77:1429–35.

31 Forman SJ, Nademanee AP, O'Donnell MR, *et al.* High-dose cytosine arabinoside and daunomycin as primary therapy for adults with acute nonlymphoblastic leukemia: a pilot study. *Semin Oncol* 1985;12(2 Suppl.3):114–16.

32 Weick JK, Kopecky KJ, Appelbaum FR, *et al.* A randomized investigation of high-dose versus standard-dose cytosine arabinoside with daunorubicin in patients with previously untreated acute myeloid leukemia: a Southwest Oncology Group study. *Blood* 1996;88:2841–51.

33 Bishop JF, Matthews JP, Young GA, *et al.* A randomized study of high-dose cytarabine in induction in acute myeloid leukemia. *Blood* 1996;87:1710–17.

34 Mayer RJ, Davis RB, Schiffer CA, *et al.* Intensive postremission chemotherapy in adults with acute myeloid leukemia. Cancer and Leukemia Group B. *N Engl J Med* 1994;331:896–903.

35 Buchner T, Hiddemann W, Wormann B, *et al.* Double induction strategy for acute myeloid leukemia: the effect of high-dose cytarabine with mitoxantrone instead of standard-dose cytarabine with daunorubicin and 6-thioguanine: a randomized trial by the German AML Cooperative Group. *Blood* 1999;93:4116–24.

36 Braess J, Spiekermann K, Staib P, *et al.* Dose-dense induction with sequential high-dose cytarabine and mitoxantone (S-HAM) and pegfilgrastim results in a high efficacy and a short duration of critical neutropenia in de novo acute myeloid leukemia: a pilot study of the AMLCG. *Blood* 2009;113:3903–10.

37 Lampkin BC, Nagao T, Mauer AM. Synchronization and recruitment in acute leukemia. *J Clin Invest* 1971;50:2204–14.

38 Karp JE, Burke PJ. Enhancement of drug cytotoxicity by recruitment of leukemic myeloblasts with humoral stimulation. *Cancer Res* 1976;36:3600–3.

39 Karp JE, Donehower RC, Dole GB, Burke PJ. Correlation of drug-perturbed marrow cell growth kinetics and intracellular 1-B-D-arabinofuranosylcytosine metabolism with clinical response in adult acute myelogenous leukemia. *Blood* 1987;69:1134–40.

40 Lampkin BC, McWilliams NB, Mauer AM, Flessa HC, Hake DA, Fisher V. Manipulation of the mitotic cycle in the treatment of acute myelogenous leukemia. *Br J Haematol* 1976;32:29–40.

41 Burke PJ, Karp JE, Geller RB, Vaughan WP. Cures of leukemia with aggressive postremission treatment: an update of timed sequential therapy (Ac-D-Ac). *leukemia.* 1989;3:692–4.

42 Archimbaud E, Leblond V, Fenaux P, *et al.* Timed sequential chemotherapy for advanced acute myeloid leukemia. *Hematol Cell Ther* 1996;38:161–7.

43 Kalaycio M, Advani A, Pohlman B, *et al.* Timed sequential induction chemotherapy and risk-adapted postremission therapy for acute myelogenous leukemia. *Am J Hematol* 2008;83:831–4.

44 He XY, Pohlman B, Lichtin A, Rybicki L, Kalaycio M. Timed-sequential chemotherapy with concomitant granulocyte colony-stimulating factor for newly diagnosed de novo acute myelogenous leukemia. *Leukemia* 2003;17:1078–84.

45 He XY, Elson P, Pohlman B, *et al.* Timed sequential chemotherapy with concomitant granulocyte colony-stimulating factor for high-risk acute myelogenous leukemia: a single arm clinical trial. *BMC Cancer* 2002;2:12.

46 Gardin C, Turlure P, Fagot T, *et al.* Postremission treatment of elderly patients with acute myeloid leukemia in first complete remission after intensive induction chemotherapy: results of the multicenter randomized Acute Leukemia French Association (ALFA) 9803 trial. *Blood* 2007;109:5129–35.

47 Preisler H, Davis RB, Kirshner J, *et al.* Comparison of three remission induction regimens and two postinduction strategies for the treatment of acute nonlymphocytic leukemia: a Cancer and Leukemia Group B study. *Blood* 1987;69:1441–9.

48 Goldstone AH, Burnett AK, Wheatley K, Smith AG, Hutchinson RM, Clark RE. Attempts to improve treatment outcomes in acute myeloid leukemia (AML) in older patients: the results of the United Kingdom Medical Research Council AML11 trial. *Blood* 2001;98:1302–11.

49 Bishop JF, Lowenthal RM, Joshua D, *et al.* Etoposide in acute nonlymphocytic leukemia. Australian Leukemia Study Group. *Blood* 1990;75:27–32.

50 Stone RM, Berg DT, George SL, *et al.* Granulocyte-macrophage colony-stimulating factor after initial chemotherapy for elderly patients with primary acute myelogenous leukemia. Cancer and Leukemia Group B. *N Engl J Med* 1995;332:1671–7.

51 Lowenberg B, Boogaerts MA, Daenen SM, *et al.* Value of different modalities of granulocyte-macrophage colony-stimulating factor applied during or after induction therapy of acute myeloid leukemia. *J Clin Oncol* 1997;15:3496–506.

52 Zittoun R, Suciu S, Mandelli F, *et al.* Granulocyte-macrophage colony-stimulating factor associated with induction treatment of acute myelogenous leukemia: a randomized trial by the European Organization for Research and Treatment of Cancer Leukemia Cooperative Group. *J Clin Oncol* 1996;14:2150–9.

53 Latagliata R, Breccia M, Fazi P, *et al.* Liposomal daunorubicin versus standard daunorubicin: long term follow-up of the GIMEMA GSI 103 AMLE randomized trial in patients older than 60 years with acute myelogenous leukemia. *Br J Haematol* 2008;143:681–9.

54 Freund M, Diedrich H, Ganser A, *et al.* Treatment of relapsed or refractory adult acute lymphocytic leukemia. *Cancer* 1992;69:709–16.

55 Godwin JE, Kopecky KJ, Head DR, *et al.* A double-blind placebo-controlled trial of granulocyte colony-stimulating factor in elderly patients with previously untreated acute myeloid leukemia: a Southwest oncology group study (9031). *Blood* 1998;91:3607–15.

56 Dombret H, Chastang C, Fenaux P, *et al.* A controlled study of recombinant human granulocyte colony-stimulating factor in elderly patients after treatment for acute myelogenous leukemia. AML Cooperative Study Group. *N Engl J Med.* 1995;332:1678–83.

57 Bradstock K, Matthews J, Young G, *et al.* Effects of glycosylated recombinant human granulocyte colony-stimulating factor

after high-dose cytarabine-based induction chemotherapy for adult acute myeloid leukemia. *Leukemia* 2001;15:1331–8.
58 Lowenberg B, Suciu S, Archimbaud E, *et al.* Use of recombinant GM-CSF during and after remission induction chemotherapy in patients aged 61 years and older with acute myeloid leukemia: final report of AML-11, a phase III randomized study of the Leukemia Cooperative Group of European Organization for the Research and Treatment of Cancer and the Dutch Belgian Hemato-Oncology Cooperative Group. *Blood* 1997; 90:2952–61.
59 Cannistra SA, Groshek P, Griffin JD. Granulocyte-macrophage colony-stimulating factor enhances the cytotoxic effects of cytosine arabinoside in acute myeloblastic leukemia and in the myeloid blast crisis phase of chronic myeloid leukemia. *Leukemia* 1989;3:328–34.
60 Hiddemann W, Kiehl M, Zuhlsdorf M, *et al.* Granulocyte-macrophage colony-stimulating factor and interleukin-3 enhance the incorporation of cytosine arabinoside into the DNA of leukemic blasts and the cytotoxic effect on clonogenic cells from patients with acute myeloid leukemia. *Semin Oncol* 1992;19(2 Suppl.4):31–7.
61 Kantarjian HM, Giles F, Gattermann N, *et al.* Nilotinib (formerly AMN107), a highly selective BCR-ABL tyrosine kinase inhibitor, is effective in patients with Philadelphia chromosome-positive chronic myelogenous leukemia in chronic phase following imatinib resistance and intolerance. *Blood* 2007 15;110:3540–6.
62 Hiddemann W, Kern W, Heinecke A, Sauerland C, Buchner T. Priming with G-CSF in acute myeloid leukemia: preliminary data of the AMLCG. *Ann Hematol* 2004;83(Suppl.1):S53–4.
63 Caron P, Dumont L, Scheinberg D. Supersaturating infusional humanized antiCD33 monoclonal antibody HuM195 in myelogenous leukemia. *Clin Cancer Res* 1998;4:1421–8.
64 Feldman E, Kalaycio M, Weiner G, *et al.* Treatment of relapsed or refractory acute myeloid leukemia with humanized antiCD33 monoclonal antibody HuM195. *Leukemia* 2003;17:314–18.
65 Feldman EJ, Brandwein J, Stone R, *et al.* Phase III randomized multicenter study of a humanized antiCD33 monoclonal antibody, lintuzumab, in combination with chemotherapy, versus chemotherapy alone in patients with refractory or first-relapsed acute myeloid leukemia. *J Clin Oncol* 2005;23:4110–16.
66 Sievers EL. Targeted therapy of acute myeloid leukemia with monoclonal antibodies and immunoconjugates. *Cancer Chemother Pharmacol* 2000;46(Suppl.):S18–22.
67 Sievers EL, Appelbaum FR, Spielberger RT, *et al.* Selective ablation of acute myeloid leukemia using antibody-targeted chemotherapy: a phase I study of an antiCD33 calicheamicin immunoconjugate. *Blood* 1999;93:3678–84.
68 Sievers EL, Larson RA, Stadtmauer EA, *et al.* Efficacy and safety of gemtuzumab ozogamicin in patients with CD33-positive acute myeloid leukemia in first relapse. *J Clin Oncol* 2001;19: 3244–54.
69 Kell WJ, Burnett AK, Chopra R, *et al.* A feasibility study of simultaneous administration of gemtuzumab ozogamicin with intensive chemotherapy in induction and consolidation in younger patients with acute myeloid leukemia. *Blood* 2003;102: 4277–83.
70 Petersdorf S, Kopecky KJ, Stuart R, *et al.* Preliminary Results of Southwest Oncology Group Study S0106: An International Intergroup phase 3 randomized trial comparing the addition of gemtuzumab ozogamicin to standard induction therapy versus standard induction therapy followed by a second randomization to post-consolidation gemtuzumab ozogamicin versus no additional therapy for previously untreated acute myeloid leukemia *Blood* 2009;114:326a.
71 Gilliland DG, Griffin JD. The roles of *FLT3* in hematopoiesis and leukemia. *Blood* 2002;100:1532–42.
72 Frohling S, Schlenk RF, Breitruck J, *et al.* Prognostic significance of activating *FLT3* mutations in younger adults (16 to 60 years) with acute myeloid leukemia and normal cytogenetics: a study of the AML Study Group Ulm. *Blood* 2002;100:4372–80.
73 Stone RM, DeAngelo DJ, Klimek V, *et al.* Patients with acute myeloid leukemia and an activating mutation in *FLT3* respond to a small-molecule FLT3 tyrosine kinase inhibitor, PKC412. *Blood* 2005;105:54–60.
74 DeAngelo DJ, Stone RM, Heaney ML, *et al.* Phase 1 clinical results with tandutinib (MLN518), a novel FLT3 antagonist, in patients with acute myelogenous leukemia or high-risk myelodysplastic syndrome: safety, pharmacokinetics, and pharmacodynamics. *Blood* 2006;108:3674–81.
75 Smith BD, Levis M, Beran M, *et al.* Single-agent CEP-701, a novel FLT3 inhibitor, shows biologic and clinical activity in patients with relapsed or refractory acute myeloid leukemia. *Blood* 2004;103:3669–76.
76 Deangelo DJ, Amrein PC, Kovacsovics T, *et al.* Phase 1/2 study of tandutinib (mln518) plus standard induction chemotherapy in newly diagnosed acute myelogenous leukemia (AML). *Blood* 2006;108:51a.
77 Stone RM, Fischer T, Paquette RL, *et al.* A Phase 1b study of midostaurin (pkc412) in combination with daunorubicin and cytarabine induction and high-dose cytarabine consolidation in patients under age 61 with newly diagnosed de novo acute myeloid leukemia: overall survival of patients whose blasts have *FLT3* mutations is similar to those with wild-type FLT3. *Blood* 2009;114:263a.
78 Levis M, Ravandi F, Wang Y, *et al.* Results from a randomized trial of salvage chemotherapy followed by lestaurtinib for *FLT3* mutant AML patients in first relapse. *Blood* 2009;114:325a.
79 Kantarjian H, Issa JP, Rosenfeld CS, *et al.* Decitabine improves patient outcomes in myelodysplastic syndromes: results of a phase III randomized study. *Cancer* 2006;106:1794–803.
80 Silverman LR, Demakos EP, Peterson BL, *et al.* Randomized controlled trial of azacitidine in patients with the myelodysplastic syndrome: a study of the cancer and leukemia group B. *J Clin Oncol* 2002;20:2429–40.
81 Kantarjian H, Oki Y, Garcia-Manero G, *et al.* Results of a randomized study of 3 schedules of low-dose decitabine in higher-risk myelodysplastic syndrome and chronic myelomonocytic leukemia. *Blood* 2007;109:52–7.
82 Harris NL, Jaffe ES, Diebold J, *et al.* World Health Organization classification of neoplastic diseases of the hematopoietic and lymphoid tissues: report of the Clinical Advisory Committee meeting-Airlie House, Virginia, November 1997. *J Clin Oncol* 1999;17:3835–49.
83 Vardiman JW, Harris NL, Brunning RD. The World Health Organization (WHO) classification of the myeloid neoplasms. *Blood* 2002;100:2292–302.
84 Fenaux P, Mufti GJ, Hellstrom-Lindberg E, *et al.* Efficacy of azacitidine compared with that of conventional care regimens in the treatment of higher-risk myelodysplastic syndromes: a

randomized, open-label, phase III study. *Lancet Oncol* 2009;10: 223–32.

85 Jeha S, Gandhi V, Chan KW, *et al.* Clofarabine, a novel nucleoside analog, is active in pediatric patients with advanced leukemia. *Blood* 2004;103:784–9.

86 Kantarjian H, Gandhi V, Cortes J, *et al.* Phase 2 clinical and pharmacologic study of clofarabine in patients with refractory or relapsed acute leukemia. *Blood* 2003;102:2379–86.

87 Kantarjian HM, Gandhi V, Kozuch P, *et al.* Phase I clinical and pharmacology study of clofarabine in patients with solid and hematologic cancers. *J Clin Oncol* 2003;21:1167–73.

88 Faderl S, Gandhi V, O'Brien S, *et al.* Results of a phase 1–2 study of clofarabine in combination with cytarabine (ara-C) in relapsed and refractory acute leukemias. *Blood* 2005;105: 940–7.

89 Faderl S, Verstovsek S, Cortes J, *et al.* Clofarabine and cytarabine combination as induction therapy for acute myeloid leukemia (AML) in patients 50 years of age or older. *Blood* 2006;108: 45–51.

90 Kantarjian HM, Erba HP, Claxton D, *et al.* Phase II study of clofarabine monotherapy in previously untreated older adults with acute myeloid leukemia and unfavorable prognostic factors. *J Clin Oncol* 2009;28:549–555.

91 Giles F, Thomas D, Garcia-Manero G, *et al.* A Phase I and pharmacokinetic study of VNP40101M, a novel sulfonylhydrazine alkylating agent, in patients with refractory leukemia. *Clin Cancer Res* 2004;10:2908–17.

92 Giles F, Verstovsek S, Faderl S, *et al.* A phase II study of cloretazine (VNP40101M), a novel sulfonylhydrazine alkylating agent, in patients with very high risk relapsed acute myeloid leukemia. *Leuk Res* 2006;30:1591–5.

93 Giles F, Verstovsek S, Thomas D, *et al.* Phase I study of cloretazine (VNP40101M), a novel sulfonylhydrazine alkylating agent, combined with cytarabine in patients with refractory leukemia. *Clin Cancer Res* 2005;11:7817–24.

94 Giles F, Vey N, Deangelo D, *et al.* Phase 3 randomized, placebo-controlled, double-blind study of high-dose continuous infusion cytarabine alone or with laromustine (VNP40101M) in patients with acute myeloid leukemia in first relapse. *Blood* 2009;114:4027–33.

95 Schiller G, O'Brien S, Pigneux A, *et al.* Single agent laromustine (VNP40101M), a novel alkylating agent, has significant activity in older patients with previously untreated poor-risk acute myeloid leukemia. *J Clin Oncol* 2010;28:815–21.

96 Menzin J, Lang K, Earle CC, Kerney D, Mallick R. The outcomes and costs of acute myeloid leukemia among the elderly. *Arch Intern Med* 2002;162:1597–603.

97 Rowe JM. Optimal induction and post-remission therapy for AML in first remission. *Hematology Am Soc Hematol Educ Program* 2009:396–405. Review.

Chapter 11
Salvage Therapy for Acute Myeloid Leukemia: Current Strategies and Emerging Therapies

Keith W. Pratz and Judith E. Karp
Sidney Kimmel Comprehensive Cancer Center, Johns Hopkins University, Baltimore, Maryland, USA

Introduction

Acute myeloid leukemia (AML) requires salvage therapy in >60% of patients under the age of 60 and in 80–85% of patients over the age of 60. The only known curative therapy in this setting is allogeneic bone marrow transplant. The outcome of bone marrow transplant is dependant on achieving a remission prior to transplant, but at this time there is no standard approach. For many patients, age or comorbidities precludes bone marrow transplant, thus leaving chemotherapy as the only option for therapy. For patients who achieve a complete remission (CR) with induction chemotherapy but relapse at a later date, a second CR can be achieved in only about 40% of the patients.

Salvage chemotherapy for patients whose first remission lasted >6 months typically includes regimens of similar character to induction therapy. Cytarabine given alone in high dose or in combination with anthracyclines can achieve a second remission in some patients with long initial remissions and/or favorable cytogenetics. For the majority (those with shorter remissions or who are refractory to induction therapy), however, there is no "standard therapy," although a variety of combinations have been studied in this setting with limited favorable results (Table 11.1). For those patients who are eligible for clinical trials, investigational therapy can be recommended as the best option. In this chapter we will review selected emerging conventional cytotoxic chemotherapy, targeted immunotherapy, signal-transduction inhibitors and epigenetic therapies in relapsed and refractory AML. The focus will be discussion of the biologic targets of these therapies and how the investigational agents are being incorporated into clinical regimens.

Leukemias: Principles and Practice of Therapy, 1st edition. Edited by S. Faderl and H. Kantarjian.

Cell cycle-directed therapies

Conventional chemotherapeutics represent a classic subset of cell cycle-directed therapies. Both cytarabine and anthracycline are only effective on cells undergoing active mitoses. Care must be taken when a schedule of therapy is designed to take into account this knowledge, as many new targeted therapies may arrest cells in G1 phase. Specific clinical examples of this phenomenon have been illustrated in the use of epidermal growth factor receptor (EGFR) inhibitors in lung cancer and the multiple negative trials of these agents when used in combination with conventional cell cycle-specific agents [5–8]. Leukemia therapies can take advantage of cell-cycle synchronization by delaying some crucial component of the therapy until the remaining cells are recruited into the cell cycle by the use of continuous or daily infusion over several days targeting the largest fraction of malignant cells possible. Below are selected examples of agents directed against cell-cycle targets that show promise in improving therapy, not just at the time of relapse, but potentially improving induction therapy.

Flavopiridol

Flavopiridol is a synthetic flavone derivative originally isolated from the stem bark of the Indian tree *Dysoxylum binectariferum* [9], which is a potent inhibitor of multiple cyclin-dependant kinases (CDKs) [10, 11]. Flavopiridol is a potent inducer of apoptosis in cell lines derived from B- and T-cell lymphomas, AML, and multiple myeloma [12]. Apoptosis occurs at flavopiridol concentrations of 100–1000 nM and appears to be independent of both p53 and net Bcl-2/Bax expression in the majority of these cell lines [13]. In primary chronic lymphocytic leukemia (CLL) samples, flavopiridol-induced apoptosis is mediated by activation of caspase-3 independently of p53 status or any drug-induced effects on Bcl-2 expression [14].

Table 11.1 Conventional reinduction chemotherapy regimens.

Regimen	Population	Overall response rate (%)	Complete remission (%)	Overall survival
Mitoxantrone days 1–6, etoposide days 1–6, cytarabine days 1–6 [1]	Relapsed and refractory	66	66	36 weeks
Fludarabine days 1–5, cytarabine days 1–5, idarubacin days 1–3, G-CSF daily until recovery [2]	Relapsed and refractory	52	52	13 weeks
Gemtuzumab [3]	Relapsed and refractory	28	13	5.4 months
High-dose cytarabine [4]	Relapsed and refractory	32	32	8.0 months

G-CSF, granulocyte colony-stimulating factor.

Flavopiridol-induced cytotoxicity is followed by recruitment into cell cycle and synchronization of residual A549 cells surviving a 24-h drug exposure [15]. These data suggest flavopiridol may have activity against both cycling and non-cycling cells, and that such activity is cytotoxic as well as cytostatic [11].

Flavopiridol induces cell-cycle arrest at the G1/S and G2/M checkpoints by blocking serine-threonine CDKs through the following two mechanisms: (i) non-cell-cycle dependent binding to the ATP-binding site in the CDK [16] and (ii) cell-cycle dependent interface with the phosphorylation of CDK1, 2, and 4 [10,17]. CDK inhibition occurs when flavopiridol concentration is between 40 and 200 nM, whereas higher concentrations may lead to depletions of cyclin D1 [18]. Flavopiridol at concentrations between 50 and 100 nM decreases the production of vascular-endothelial growth factor (VEGF), which is a growth and survival factor for diverse tumor types, by decreasing the stability of VEGF mRNA in response to a hypoxic stimulus [19]. This activity is also noted to be present *in vivo* with correlative data from a flavopiridol trial indicating reduced circulating VEGF levels in some leukemia patients [20].

Clinically, flavopiridol has been combined with cytarabine and mitoxantrone in a time-sequential manner in a phase II study of patients with poor-risk AML [21]. This study noted a CR in 12 of 15 newly diagnosed secondary leukemia patients, 18 of 24 patients with relapsed leukemia after short remission, and 2 of 13 primary refractory patients. Unfortunately, however, there were no remissions in 10 multiply refractory patients. The 2-year survival of patients achieving a CR was 40%, and for newly diagnosed patients the 2-year survival was 50%. This regimen continues to be studied in patients >50 years of age as a first-line therapy for newly diagnosed patients as flavopiridol is yet to be approved for clinical use.

Clofarabine

Clofarabine is a novel deoxyadenosine analog that is resistant to deamination by adenosine deaminase and has been found clinically to have activity in both AML and acute lymphoblastic leukemia (ALL). Clofarabine's major cytotoxic activity is in inhibition of ribonucleotide reductase and incorporation into DNA, leading to inhibition of DNA polymerase [22–24]. Additionally, mitochondrial membrane polarization and disruption resulting in apoptosis has been reported [25]. Studied in combination with cytarabine, clofarabine was found to be active in relapsed and refractory AML, yielding an overall response rate (ORR) of 38% [26]. In a study of induction therapy for patients with newly diagnosed AML >50 years of age, the ORR was found to be 60% with a median overall survival of 10.3 months [27].

Clofarabine was studied in combination with cyclophosphamide in a time-sequential manner in relapsed and refractory leukemias. This phase I study found modest ORR in AML (3/12) and ALL (4/6) but did demonstrate changes in circulating leukemia cells indicative of DNA damage (via γH2AX), as expected by the combination of a classic alkylating agent along with a potent inhibitor of DNA polymerase [28].

Cloretazine (VNP40101M)

Cloretazine is a novel sulfonylhydralazine alkylating agent with activity in leukemia cell lines with resistance to BCNU, cyclophosphamide, and melphalan. In contrast to BCNU, cloretazine does not generate a hydroxyethylating, vinylating, or aminoethylating species, and alkylation is relatively specific to the O^6 position of guanine [29, 30]. Owing to this relative specificity, cloretazine produces more cross-links and fewer DNA single-strand nicks compared with BCNU in *in vitro* studies [29]. Cloretazine is a pro-drug that is activated intracellularly into two active compounds, 90CE and 101MDCE [31]. 90CE is responsible for selective DNA-synthesis inhibition, whereas 101MDCE causes rapid and non-selective inhibition of DNA, RNA, and protein synthesis. Both 90CE and 101MDCE lead to phosphorylation of histone H2AX, but with distinct kinetics. In animal studies, cloretazine was shown to distribute across the blood–brain barrier [32]. When used in combination with the ribonucleotide-reductase inhibitor, hydroxyurea, in patients >60 years of age with untreated high-risk myelodysplastic syndromes (MDS) or AML, cloretazine resulted in an ORR of 32%, with 28% of patients achieving a CR [33]. The median overall survival was 94 days, and for those achieving a CR, the median survival lengthened to 147 days [34]. In combination with 3 days of cytarabine, similar ORRs were seen (27%) in patients with refractory leukemia [35].

SNS-595

SNS-595 is a novel napthyridine analog which is a first-in-class chemotherapeutic that causes double-stranded DNA breaks in a replication-dependent manner, leading to irreversible G2 arrest and apoptosis [36]. It may also impede net topoisomerase II function through a unique mechanism [37]. In a phase I clinical trial in leukemia, the ORR was reported as 21% (14/67) with four patients achieving a CR and one patient achieving a CRi (complete remission, incomplete platelet recovery). This was a two-arm study comparing dosing on days 1, 8, and 15 with dosing on days 1, 4, 8, and 11. Four of the patients with a CR were on the day 1, 8, and 15 schedule, and correlative assessment of DNA damage through analysis of γH2AX indicated increased levels of DNA damage in responders versus non-responders (3.8- vs. 1.7-fold increase in γH2AX levels). As with all G2-arresting topoisomerase II inhibitors, the dose-limiting toxicity was mucositis. SNS-595 was found to act synergistically with cytarabine in reducing bone marrow cellularity and circulating neutrophils [36]. Taking into account this knowledge, a phase Ib dose-escalation study of SNS-595 in combination with cytarabine in patients with relapsed and refractory AML is ongoing.

Signal transduction-directed therapies

Aberrations in normal signal-transduction pathways represent an emerging target in many malignancies. Chronic myeloid leukemia (CML) with its prototypical aberrant activation of the ABL kinase illustrates the utility of therapy directed against one such aberrant pathway. Several other examples of aberrant signaling cascades exist in leukemia including FLT3, C-Kit, IGF-1R, and VEGF-2 (KDR) and represent important emerging targets in AML. It has been noted that these aberrations can appear in the leukemia stem-cell compartment [38] and may play an important component of intrinsic resistance to conventional chemotherapy. Likewise, ligands involved in these pathways, such as the FLT-ligand, VEGF, and IGF-1, can feed an autocrine loop of malignant clone stimulation [39–41].

FLT3 inhibition

Lestaurtinib (CEP-701)

This indolocarbazole derivative was initially introduced as an inhibitor of TrkA for possible use in prostate cancer [42] but was recognized subsequently as an FLT3 inhibitor [43]. In a phase II study, elderly patients with AML not fit for conventional chemotherapy were treated with lestaurtinib as monotherapy [44]. The results showed partial responses in 8 of 27 patients. The response rate among *FLT3* mutants was three out of five patients. All eight of the responders had plasma levels of drugs sufficient to inhibit FLT3 phosphorylation to levels below 15% of baseline activity.

Drawing on the results of the pre-clinical studies combining lestaurtinib with chemotherapy, the Cephalon 204 trial began accruing patients in 2003. Patients with AML were eligible for this trial if they were in first relapse and they harbored an *FLT3* mutation. The trial was stratified according to the duration of first remission: patients whose first remission lasted <6 months received mitoxantrone, etoposide, and cytarabine [1], while those whose first remission lasted >6 months were treated with high-dose cytarabine [45]. Patients were randomized to receive lestaurtinib at a dosage of 80 mg twice per day beginning after chemotherapy is complete and continuing for up to 16 weeks. The efficacy of target inhibition was determined through the application of a surrogate assay—the plasma inhibitory activity (PIA) assay for FLT3 [46]. The preliminary results from the first 44 patients enrolled on this trial demonstrated 12 remissions in the lestaurtinib arm versus six remissions in the control arm (55% vs. 27%) [47]. Based on these encouraging findings, the Cephalon 204 trial has been expanded to a pivotal trial with a target accrual of 220 patients.

Midostaurin (PKC412)

Midostaurin is an indolocarbazole derivative, originally developed as a protein kinase C inhibitor, which is also under development as an FLT3 inhibitor. Midostaurin was clinically evaluated in a phase II trial for patients with relapsed or refractory AML harboring an *FLT3* mutation [48]. Of 20 patients treated at a dosage of 75 mg three times daily, 14 displayed at least hematologic improvement, with one CR. Midostaurin, an indolocarbazole derivative like lestaurtinib, is tightly bound to alpha-one acid glycoprotein (AAG). Furthermore, midostaurin is converted in the liver into two metabolites, CGP62221 and CGP52421 [48]. CGP52421, by virtue of it being less selective (hence more "multi-targeted") and less bound to AAG than either the parent drug or the other metabolite, and present at much higher levels in plasma, is likely the active compound in patients [43]. Responses in this trial likewise correlated very well with the degree of FLT3 inhibition achieved as determined by the PIA assay [46].

Midostaurin was next evaluated in combination with induction therapy in newly diagnosed patients <60 years of age using a conventional cytarabine and daunorubicin ("7 plus 3") regimen followed by high-dose cytarabine consolidation. In general, midostaurin doses that were well tolerated when used as monotherapy (100 mg orally twice daily) were intolerable (because of nausea) when given concomitantly or following chemotherapy [49]. Midostaurin dosage was subsequently dropped to 50 mg twice daily, and preliminary results reported in 19 patients noted six of six patients with an *FLT3* mutation achieved a CR. By comparison, of the 13 patients with wild-type FLT3, only eight achieved a CR. Based on the results of this pilot trial, a pivotal trial of midostaurin, at a dosage of 50 mg twice daily following induction chemotherapy, is currently planned for patients with newly diagnosed AML.

VEGF-directed therapies

Bevacizumab

An emerging target in a variety of tumor types, including hematologic malignancies, is VEGF. VEGF acts as an autocrine stimulus for both hematologic stem cells and leukemic blast cells. The VEGF-receptor KDR is also noted to be overexpressed in some patients with newly diagnosed AML. Investigations have also shown that, in leukemia patients with high blast counts, there is an inverse correlation with VEGF level and duration of CR and survival [50]. With this knowledge, a phase II study of the humanized anti-VEGF antibody bevacizumab was undertaken in patients with refractory or relapsed AML in combination with cytarabine (2gm/m^2 given as a 72-h continuous infusion on days 1–3) and mitoxantrone (40mg/m^2 on day 4) [51]. Bevacizumab was administered in a time-sequential manner at 10mg/kg on day 8. Forty-eight patients, including patients with primary and multiply refractory AML, were treated with an ORR of 48% (23/48) and a CR rate of 33% (16/48). The toxicity data were notable for decreased ejection fraction in three patients and a cerebrovascular bleed in two patients. The median survival for the entire population was 8.4 months, with the median survival of 16.2 months for those achieving a CR.

Sorafenib

Sorafenib is a biaryl urea that was originally developed as an inhibitor of B-RAF. Subsequent *in vitro* studies have shown it to be a multitargeted tyrosine kinase inhibitor, with activity not only against RAF kinase but also against the VEGF receptors, wild-type and ITD-mutated *FLT3*, the PDGF receptors, and RET kinase [52]. The drug has been studied extensively *in vitro* against human leukemia cell lines in general [53, 54] and against *FLT3* mutant lines in particular [55–57]. To date, there are no published *in vitro* studies in which sorafenib was combined with conventional leukemia chemotherapy. However, it has been studied in combination with bortezomib and vorinostat (SAHA) and was found to be synergistic in both cases in CML-derived cell lines [58, 59]. Sorafenib has been studied in a single agent phase I clinical trial in AML [60]. This two-arm study looked at a 5-day-per-week dosing versus a dosing of 14 days out of 21. Preliminary results showed responses in 6 out of 10 patients receiving a full cycle of therapy. Laboratory correlates in responding patients indicated inhibition of FLT3 phosphorylation in three of three patients studied. Most of the responding patients in this study were those carrying the *FLT3*-ITD, which is consistent with data from our laboratory indicating that sorafenib is unable to inhibit point mutant or wild-type *FLT3* at clinically achievable levels (unpublished observations, Pratz and Levis, John Hopkins University, Baltimore, MD). To date, there have been no reported studies of sorafenib combined with chemotherapy for patients with leukemia. However, a phase I trial in which patients with AML are treated with cytarabine, an anthracycline, and sorafenib has recently begun accruing patients at the M.D. Anderson Cancer Center (Andreeff, M.D. Anderson Cancer Center, Houston, TX).

Protein metabolism-directed therapies

Bortezomib

The 26S proteasome is the predominant location for intracellular protein degradation through ubiquitin conjugation. This system is responsible for intracellular protein homeostasis including degradation of cyclin-dependant kinases, kinase inhibitors, transcription factors, and regulatory proteins such as IκB. Bortezomib is a dipeptide boronic acid derivative and is a potent, reversible inhibitor of the 26S proteasome inhibitor. It is the first drug approved targeting the ubiquitin–proteasome pathway. Bortezomib is particularly clinically effective in multiple myeloma by the induction of accumulation of misfolded proteins in the endoplasmic reticulum and induction of proapoptotic signals as part of an unfolded protein response [61]. Preclinical studies of leukemia stem cells indicted sensitivity to proteasome inhibition through an NF-κB pathway [62]. A phase I study of bortezomib used in combination with idarubicin and cytarabine in relapsed AML or newly diagnosed AML in patients >60 years of age was performed recently [63]. The results demonstrated a CR in 19/31 (61%) and a CRi in 3/31 patients. Specifically in patients with relapsed disease, the CR rate was 6/9 with one additional CRi. The overall survival for the study was 12.4 months, and for those achieving a CR/CRi was 15.4 months.

17-AAG

17-Allylamino-demethoxygeldanamycin (17-AAG) is a heat-shock protein 90 (HSP 90) inhibitor that is in clinical development as a novel therapy of multiple malignancies. HSP 90 is an abundant chaperone protein that mediates stress-induced survival, and in particular stress-induced survival related to nucleoside analogs such as cytarabine as used in hematologic malignances [64]. One mechanism of cytarabine resistance is through the activation of checkpoint kinase 1 (Chk1). Chk1 is a client protein of HSP 90 and *in vitro* inhibition of HSP 90 sensitizes cells to nucleoside cytotoxcity [65]. 17-AAG has been studied as a single agent in solid tumors and is currently under study in combination with cytarabine in leukemia. 17-AAG and a closely related orally available compound 17-dimethylamino-ethylamino–17-demethoxygeldanamycin (17-DMAG) have also been found to have antiangiogenic properties related to direct effects on endothelial cells [66]. 17-DMAG in preclinical *in vitro* studies was noted to be three- to fivefold more potent than 17-AAG in cytotoxicity assays, and in a phase I trial in refractory leukemia the ORR was reported to be 17% (4/24), with a CRi reported in three patients [67]. Given twice weekly, DMAG was well tolerated with dose-limited toxicities reported primarily as cardiac related events (non-ST segment myocardial infarction [NSTEMI] and troponin elevations).

Epigenetic therapies

Epigenetic changes are not found in the specific DNA sequence but rather are changes involving modifications of the DNA to change gene-expression patterns. Alterations in chromatin through acetylation have been found to play a role in malignant transformation by alteration of gene expression. Likewise, elevated levels of DNA methylation have been found in acute leukemias, suggesting DNA methyltransferase (DNMT) overexpression/overactivity may be an important feature of some leukemias. Below are selected therapies under development that aim to correct the epigenetic changes that are found in many cases of leukemia.

DNA methyltransferase inhibitors

DNA methylation is found primarily in areas of palindromic CpG dinucleotide sequences, and aberrant methylation in promoter areas of tumor-suppressor genes has been described in many tumor types [68]. DNA methylation in a promoter area typically silences gene expression and DNMA is responsible for maintenance of methylation through cell division. 5-Azacitidine and decitabine are closely related compounds that both inhibit DNMT by incorporation into DNA as cytosine analogs, and which inactivate DNMT through irreversible bonds leading to subsequent DNMT pool depletion. This depletion does not allow for transmission of the methylation patterns to daughter chromatids.

5-Azacitidine given as a single agent in refractory AML resulted in complete responses in 27% (5/18) of patients, with a median survival of 266 days for those who responded [69]. In a randomized trial for high-risk MDS, 5-azacitidine documented a 60% ORR with a CR rate of 7% when compared with supportive care [70]. Importantly, the transformation rate to AML was significantly lower in the 5-azacitidine arm ($P < 0.001$).

Decitabine is also a DNMT inhibitor with similar characteristics to 5-azacitidine. Decitabine as a single agent in poor-prognosis elderly patients with AML was found to have a response rate of 33% (4/12) with three complete responses [71]. In a phase I study of decitabine in combination with valproic acid, a histone deacetylase (HDAC) inhibitor, in previously treated and untreated AML produced a CR rate of 16% (4/25) [72]. Re-expression of the estrogen receptor was associated with clinical response, suggesting epigenetic changes may have played a role in therapeutic efficacy.

Histone deacetylase inhibitors

Histone modification by acetylation, methylation, or phosphorylation plays a role in gene expression by determining DNA availability to transcription factors. Histone acetylation/deacetylation is performed by two enzymes, histone acetyltransferase and HDAC. Several agents have been found to be active inhibitors of HDAC, including valproic acid, sodium phenylbutyrate, SAHA, and MS-275. As delineated in Table 11.2, each has been found to have some degree of antitumor activity and documentation of increased histone acetylation. Combinations of the diverse HDAC inhibitors with DNMT1 inhibitors are under study, with evidence of clinical responses and molecular evidence for epigenetic modifications in both MDS and MDS-related AML.

Immune-targeted therapies

The use of biologic pharmaceuticals in malignancies can take advantage of specific tumor-based targets through the use of monoclonal antibodies, either alone or conjugated with radioactive or chemical cytotoxics. The clinical utility of rituximab in $CD20^+$ malignancies illustrates this approach. Several other cell-surface markers are of clinical utility in leukemia including CD33, CD45, and CXCR4 specific therapies, which are discussed below. Other approaches, including the therapeutic vaccination with protein derived from human leukemia cells, are under development in attempts to elicit tumor-specific immune reactions similar to the graft-versus-tumor effect seen in allogeneic bone marrow transplantation.

Table 11.2 Selected histone deacetylase inhibitors in trial in acute myeloid leukemia.

Compound	Population	Overall response rate	Complete remission	Comment
Sodium phenylbuterate [73]	MDS or AML	15% (4/27)	0	Increased fetal hemoglobin in 52% of evaluated patients
Valproic acid [74]	AML or MDS	16%	1% (1/75)	Low-risk MDS (blast count >5%) ORR 52%
MS-275 [75]	AML relapsed or refractory	31% (12/39)	0	No classical responders but evidence of histone hyperacetylation in marrow CD34 cells
SAHA [76]	AML or MDS	10% (4/41)	5% (2/41)	Two CRs able to undergo BMT
Combinations				
Phenylbutyrate and 5-azacytadine [77]	High-grade MDS or AML unfit for induction	38% (11/29)	14% (4/29)	6/12 responders underwent demethylation of p15 promoter while non-responders did not
Valproic acid and decitabine [78]	AML: relapsed or >60 years of age	22% (12/54)	19% (10/54)	Median survival of responders 15.3 months
MS-275 and 5-azacytadine [79]	AML and MDS	44% (12/27)	7% (2/27)	Histone hyperacetylation seen in 95% of patients

AML, acute myeloid leukemia; BMT, bone marrow transplant; MDS, myelodysplastic syndrome.

Anti-CD33 constructs

Gemtuzumab ozogamicin is a humanized antibody to CD33 conjugated to the highly toxic anthracycline calicheamicin. Used alone in patients with AML aged >60 years at first relapse, the CR rate was 28% [3], but myelosuppression and hepatic dysfunction limit its use clinically. Current studies combining low-dose gemtuzumab ozogamicin with conventional chemotherapy are ongoing in pediatric and adult populations.

Lintuzumab is a humanized monoclonal antibody to CD33 with a murine complementarity-determining region, and in study alone and in combination with cytarabine in relapsed patients no significant activity was demonstrated. Work with the addition of an α-emitting radioisotope actinium-225 via chelation to anti-CD33 (M195) may allow for increased target cytotoxicity as the decay of actinium-225 yields four high-energy α particles each capable of killing a cell [80]. Recent work on preventing the bioaccumulation of the decay particles in the renal tubules by oral chelation has significantly lowered the secondary renal damage of the primary therapy.

^{131}I-anti-CD45

Radiolabeled murine antibody to CD45 was studied in combination with conventional preparative therapy for myeloablative bone marrow transplant in an attempt to concentrate the effects of radiotherapy in the malignant leukemia clone but lessen the burden of total body irradiation. This strategy was able to deliver higher estimated radiation doses to the marrow and spleen, and a phase II study of ^{131}I-anti-CD45 incorporating into a busulfan/cyclophosphamide preparative regimen for myeloablative bone marrow transplant demonstrated decreased transplant-related and overall survival ($P = 0.09$) [81].

Tumor vaccines

The immunogenicity of malignant clones is implied by the observation of graft-versus-tumor effect in allogeneic bone marrow transplant. Exploitation of this effect outside the transplant setting could potentially lead to marked changes in therapeutic oncology. The roll of T cells in graft versus leukemia is clear and work is under way to select and expand *ex vivo* tumor specific T cells in patients with myeloma. Immunospecific targets of leukemia include Wilms tumor 1 (WT1) protein [82], proteinase 3-derived peptide (PR3) [83], and CD168 (RHAMM)-derived epitope R3 [84]. Ideally, these therapies would be incorporated into treatment during the first complete remission with the goal of decreasing relapse rates.

Conclusion

Relapsed AML is a disease with limited treatment options. For those with known allogeneic bone marrow transplant donors, allogeneic bone marrow transplant at the time of first relapse should be considered the first therapeutic option. Unfortunately, most patients will not have this option, and salvage chemotherapy is necessary. To date, there is no standard salvage therapy except for those with

Table 11.3 Selected emerging therapeutic targets and targeted agents in acute myeloid leukemia.

Target	Compound	Mechanism
PARP	ABT-888	PARP inhibition leads to enhanced cytotoxicity through impaired DNA damage repair. Used in combination with cytotoxics
Pim	ABT-869 [85], quercetagetin [86]	Decreased expression or direct inhibition
Src/Lyn	siRNA or PP2 [87]	Small inhibitory RNA of Lyn proto-oncogene or tyrosine kinase inhibitor or Src family kinases
mTor	Rapamycin [88], temsirolimus, RAD001	Direct inhibition of mTor and interruption of AKT signaling
PI3-kinase	BAG956 [89]	Tyrosine kinase inhibition
Mdm2	Nutlin-3 [90]	Induction of p53 mediated apoptosis by blocking Mdm2 binding to p53
IGF-1R	NVP-AEW541 [39]	Direct tyrosine kinase inhibition
DNA ds breaks	SNS-595 [36]	Replication-dependent DNA damage

long first remissions or favorable cytogenetic changes where high-dose cytarabine can be considered. For all others, experimental therapy, if available, should be considered with the intent of achieving a second remission, which, in turn, allows for transition to the only known curative therapy in this setting—allogeneic bone marrow transplant. We have discussed only a few treatment strategies directed toward selected critical growth and survival pathways. Several emerging molecularly directed therapies are under development (Table 11.3).

Experimental therapies cover a broad range of targets spanning areas from conventional cytotoxic chemotherapies to epigenetic modification to immunotherapeutic modalities. In order to improve the prognosis of this group, continued work on exploring new treatment modalities, and enrollment of patients into these trials, is paramount. Ultimately, as we discover new strategies that can overcome net drug resistance in the setting of relapsed or refractory AML, we will be able to incorporate these new strategies upfront, and hopefully improve the overall survival of all patients with AML by eradicating it first time round.

References

1 Amadori S, Arcese W, Isacchi G, *et al*. Mitoxantrone, etoposide, and intermediate-dose cytarabine: an effective and tolerable regimen for the treatment of refractory acute myeloid leukemia. *J Clin Oncol* 1991;9:1210–14.

2 Pastore D, Specchia G, Carluccio P, *et al*. FLAG-IDA in the treatment of refractory/relapsed acute myeloid leukemia: single-center experience. *Ann Hematol* 2003;82:231–5.

3 Larson RA, Boogaerts M, Estey E, *et al*. Antibody-targeted chemotherapy of older patients with acute myeloid leukemia in first relapse using Mylotarg (gemtuzumab ozogamicin). *Leukemia* 2002;16:1627–36.

4 Karanes C, Kopecky KJ, Head DR, *et al*. A phase III comparison of high dose ARA-C (HIDAC) versus HIDAC plus mitoxantrone in the treatment of first relapsed or refractory acute myeloid leukemia: Southwest Oncology Group Study. *Leukemia Res* 1999;23:787–94.

5 Gatzemeier U, Pluzanska A, Szczesna A, *et al*. Phase III study of erlotinib in combination with cisplatin and gemcitabine in advanced non-small-cell lung cancer: the Tarceva Lung Cancer Investigation Trial. *J Clin Oncol* 2007;25:1545–52.

6 Herbst RS, Prager D, Hermann R, *et al*. TRIBUTE: A phase III trial of erlotinib hydrochloride (OSI-774) combined with carboplatin and paclitaxel chemotherapy in advanced non-small-cell lung cancer. *J Clin Oncol* 2005;23:5892–9.

7 Giaccone G, Herbst RS, Manegold C, *et al*. Gefitinib in combination with gemcitabine and cisplatin in advanced non-small-cell lung cancer: a phase III trial–INTACT 1. *J Clin Oncol* 2004;22: 777–84.

8 Herbst RS, Giaccone G, Schiller JH, *et al*. Gefitinib in combination with paclitaxel and carboplatin in advanced non-small-cell lung cancer: a phase III trial–INTACT 2. *J Clin Oncol* 2004;22: 785–94.

9 Senderowicz AM, Sausville EA. Preclinical and clinical development of cyclin-dependent kinase modulators. *J Natl Cancer Inst* 2000;92:376–87.

10 Kaur G, Stetler-Stevenson M, Sebers S, *et al*. Growth inhibition with reversible cell cycle arrest of carcinoma cells by flavone L86-8275. *J Natl Cancer Inst* 1992;84:1736–40.

11 Bible KC, Kaufmann SH. Flavopiridol: a cytotoxic flavone that induces cell death in noncycling A549 human lung carcinoma cells. *Cancer Res* 1996;56:4856–61.

12 Konig A, Schwartz GK, Mohammad RM, Al-Katib A, Gabrilove JL. The novel cyclin-dependent kinase inhibitor flavopiridol downregulates Bcl-2 and induces growth arrest and apoptosis in chronic B-cell leukemia lines. *Blood* 1997;90:4307–12.

13 Parker BW, Kaur G, Nieves-Neira W, *et al*. Early induction of apoptosis in hematopoietic cell lines after exposure to flavopiridol. *Blood* 1998;91:458–65.

14 Byrd JC, Shinn C, Waselenko JK, *et al*. Flavopiridol induces apoptosis in chronic lymphocytic leukemia cells via activation

of caspase-3 without evidence of bcl-2 modulation or dependence on functional p53. *Blood* 1998;92:3804–16.

15 Bible KC, Kaufmann SH. Cytotoxic synergy between flavopiridol (NSC 649890, L86–8275) and various antineoplastic agents: the importance of sequence of administration. *Cancer Res* 1997; 57:3375–80.

16 Carlson BA, Dubay MM, Sausville EA, Brizuela L, Worland PJ. Flavopiridol induces G1 arrest with inhibition of cyclin-dependent kinase (CDK) 2 and CDK4 in human breast carcinoma cells. *Cancer Res* 1996;56:2973–8.

17 Losiewicz MD, Carlson BA, Kaur G, Sausville EA, Worland PJ. Potent inhibition of CDC2 kinase activity by the flavonoid L86–8275. *Biochem Biophys Res Commun* 1994;201:589–95.

18 Carlson B, Lahusen T, Singh S, *et al.* Down-regulation of cyclin D1 by transcriptional repression in MCF-7 human breast carcinoma cells induced by flavopiridol. *Cancer Res* 1999;59: 4634–41.

19 Melillo G, Sausville EA, Cloud K, Lahusen T, Varesio L, Senderowicz AM. Flavopiridol, a protein kinase inhibitor, down-regulates hypoxic induction of vascular endothelial growth factor expression in human monocytes. *Cancer Res* 1999; 59:5433–7.

20 Karp JE, Passaniti A, Gojo I, *et al.* Phase I and pharmacokinetic study of flavopiridol followed by 1-beta-D-arabinofuranosylcytosine and mitoxantrone in relapsed and refractory adult acute leukemias. *Clin Cancer Res* 2005;11: 8403–12.

21 Karp JE, Smith BD, Levis MJ, *et al.* Sequential flavopiridol, cytosine arabinoside, and mitoxantrone: a phase II trial in adults with poor-risk acute myelogenous leukemia. *Clin Cancer Res* 2007;13:4467–73.

22 Parker WB, Shaddix SC, Chang CH, *et al.* Effects of 2-chloro-9-(2-deoxy-2-fluoro-beta-D-arabinofuranosyl)adenine on K562 cellular metabolism and the inhibition of human ribonucleotide reductase and DNA polymerases by its 5′-triphosphate. *Cancer Res* 1991;51:2386–94.

23 Xie KC, Plunkett W. Deoxynucleotide pool depletion and sustained inhibition of ribonucleotide reductase and DNA synthesis after treatment of human lymphoblastoid cells with 2-chloro-9-(2-deoxy-2-fluoro-beta-D-arabinofuranosyl) adenine. *Cancer Res* 1996;56:3030–7.

24 Xie C, Plunkett W. Metabolism and actions of 2-chloro-9-(2-deoxy-2-fluoro-beta-D-arabinofuranosyl)-adenine in human lymphoblastoid cells. *Cancer Res* 1995;55:2847–52.

25 Genini D, Adachi S, Chao Q, *et al.* Deoxyadenosine analogs induce programmed cell death in chronic lymphocytic leukemia cells by damaging the DNA and by directly affecting the mitochondria. *Blood* 2000;96:3537–43.

26 Faderl S, Gandhi V, O'Brien S, *et al.* Results of a phase 1–2 study of clofarabine in combination with cytarabine (ara-C) in relapsed and refractory acute leukemias. *Blood* 2005;105: 940–7.

27 Faderl S, Verstovsek S, Cortes J, *et al.* Clofarabine and cytarabine combination as induction therapy for acute myeloid leukemia (AML) in patients 50 years of age or older. *Blood* 2006; 108:45–51.

28 Karp JE, Ricklis RM, Balakrishnan K, *et al.* A phase 1 clinical-laboratory study of clofarabine followed by cyclophosphamide for adults with refractory acute leukemias. *Blood* 2007;110: 1762–9.

29 Penketh PG, Shyam K, Sartorelli AC. Comparison of DNA lesions produced by tumor-inhibitory 1,2-bis(sulfonyl)hydrazines and chloroethylnitrosoureas. *Biochem Pharmacol* 2000;59: 283–91.

30 Briscoe WT, Duarte SP. Preferential alkylation by 1,3-bis(2-chloroethyl)–1-nitrosourea (BCNU) of guanines with guanines as neighboring bases in DNA. *Biochem Pharmacol* 1988;37: 1061–6.

31 Ishiguro K, Seow HA, Penketh PG, Shyam K, Sartorelli AC. Mode of action of the chloroethylating and carbamoylating moieties of the prodrug cloretazine. *Mol Cancer Ther* 2006;5: 969–76.

32 Finch RA, Shyam K, Penketh PG, Sartorelli AC. 1,2-Bis(methylsulfonyl)–1-(2-chloroethyl)–2-(methylamino) carbonylhydrazine (101M): a novel sulfonylhydrazine prodrug with broad-spectrum antineoplastic activity. *Cancer Res* 2001; 61:3033–8.

33 Giles F, Verstovsek S, Faderl S, *et al.* A phase II study of cloretazine (VNP40101M), a novel sulfonylhydrazine alkylating agent, in patients with very high risk relapsed acute myeloid leukemia. *Leukemia Res* 2006;30:1591–5.

34 Giles F, Rizzieri D, Karp J, *et al.* Cloretazine (VNP40101M), a novel sulfonylhydrazine alkylating agent, in patients age 60 years or older with previously untreated acute myeloid leukemia. *J Clin Oncol* 2007;25:25–31.

35 Giles F, Verstovsek S, Thomas D, *et al.* Phase I study of cloretazine (VNP40101M), a novel sulfonylhydrazine alkylating agent, combined with cytarabine in patients with refractory leukemia. *Clin Cancer Res* 2005;11:7817–24.

36 Arbitrario J, Kumer J, Howlett A, Silverman J. SNS-595 a novel s phase active cytotoxic acts synergistically with cytarabine to reduce bone marrow cellularity and circulating neutrophils. *Blood* (ASH Annual Meeting Abstracts) 2006;108:2321.

37 Lancet J, Kantarjian H, Ravandi F, *et al.* SNS-595 demonstrates clinical responses in a phase 1 study in acute leukemia. *Blood* (ASH Annual Meeting Abstracts) 2007;110:442.

38 Levis M, Murphy KM, Pham R, *et al.* Internal tandem duplications of the *FLT3* gene are present in leukemia stem cells. *Blood* 2005;106:673–80.

39 Tazzari PL, Tabellini G, Bortul R, *et al.* The insulin-like growth factor-I receptor kinase inhibitor NVP-AEW541 induces apoptosis in acute myeloid leukemia cells exhibiting autocrine insulin-like growth factor-I secretion. *Leukemia* 2007; 21:886–96.

40 Zheng R, Levis M, Piloto O, *et al.* *FLT3* ligand causes autocrine signaling in acute myeloid leukemia cells. *Blood* 2004;103: 267–74.

41 Fiedler W, Graeven U, Ergun S, *et al.* Vascular endothelial growth factor, a possible paracrine growth factor in human acute myeloid leukemia. *Blood* 1997;89:1870–5.

42 George DJ, Dionne CA, Jani J, *et al.* Sustained *in vivo* regression of Dunning H rat prostate cancers treated with combinations of androgen ablation and Trk tyrosine kinase inhibitors, CEP-751 (KT-6587) or CEP-701 (KT-5555). *Cancer Res* 1999;59: 2395–401.

43 Levis M, Allebach J, Tse KF, *et al.* A FLT3-targeted tyrosine kinase inhibitor is cytotoxic to leukemia cells *in vitro* and *in vivo*. *Blood* 2002;99:3885–91.

44 Knapper S, Burnett AK, Littlewood T, *et al.* A phase 2 trial of the *FLT3* inhibitor lestaurtinib (CEP701) as first-line treatment

for older patients with acute myeloid leukemia not considered fit for intensive chemotherapy. *Blood* 2006;108:3262–70.

45 Mayer RJ, Davis RB, Schiffer CA, *et al.* Intensive postremission chemotherapy in adults with acute myeloid leukemia. Cancer and Leukemia Group B. *N Engl J Med* 1994;331:896–903.

46 Levis M, Brown P, Smith BD, *et al.* Plasma inhibitory activity (PIA): a pharmacodynamic assay reveals insights into the basis for cytotoxic response to *FLT3* inhibitors. *Blood* 2006;108: 3477–83.

47 Levis M, Smith BD, Beran M, *et al.* A randomized, open-label study of lestaurtinib (CEP-701), an oral *flt3* inhibitor, administered in sequence with chemotherapy in patients with relapsed AML harboring *FLT3* activating mutations: clinical response correlates with successful *FLT3* inhibition. *Blood* 2005;106:121a.

48 Stone RM, DeAngelo DJ, Klimek V, *et al.* Patients with acute myeloid leukemia and an activating mutation in *FLT3* respond to a small-molecule *FLT3* tyrosine kinase inhibitor, PKC412. *Blood* 2005;105:54–60.

49 Stone RM, Fischer T, Paquette R, *et al.* Phase IB Study of PKC412, an oral *FLT3* kinase inhibitor, in sequential and simultaneous combinations with daunorubicin and cytarabine (DA) induction and high-dose cytarabine consolidation in newly diagnosed patients with AML. *Blood* 2005;106:121a.

50 Aguayo A, Estey E, Kantarjian H, *et al.* Cellular vascular endothelial growth factor is a predictor of outcome in patients with acute myeloid leukemia. *Blood* 1999;94:3717–21.

51 Karp JE, Gojo I, Pili R, *et al.* Targeting vascular endothelial growth factor for relapsed and refractory adult acute myelogenous leukemias: therapy with sequential 1-beta-d-arabinofuranosylcytosine, mitoxantrone, and bevacizumab. *Clin Cancer Res* 2004;10:3577–85.

52 Wilhelm SM, Carter C, Tang L, *et al.* BAY 43–9006 exhibits broad spectrum oral antitumor activity and targets the RAF/MEK/ERK pathway and receptor tyrosine kinases involved in tumor progression and angiogenesis. *Cancer Res* 2004;64:7099–109.

53 Rahmani M, Davis EM, Bauer C, Dent P, Grant S. Apoptosis induced by the kinase inhibitor BAY 43–9006 in human leukemia cells involves down-regulation of Mcl-1 through inhibition of translation. *J Biol Chem* 2005;280:35217–27.

54 Rosato RR, Almenara JA, Coe S, Grant S. The multikinase inhibitor sorafenib potentiates TRAIL lethality in human leukemia cells in association with Mcl-1 and cFLIPL down-regulation. *Cancer Res* 2007;67:9490–500.

55 Lierman E, Lahortiga I, Van Miegroet H, Mentens N, Marynen P, Cools J. The ability of sorafenib to inhibit oncogenic PDGFRbeta and *FLT3* mutants and overcome resistance to other small molecule inhibitors. *Haematologica* 2007;92:27–34.

56 Kancha RK, Grundler R, Peschel C, Duyster J. Sensitivity toward sorafenib and sunitinib varies between different activating and drug-resistant *FLT3-ITD* mutations. *Exp Hematol* 2007;35:1522–6.

57 Auclair D, Miller D, Yatsula V, *et al.* Antitumor activity of sorafenib in *FLT3*-driven leukemic cells. *Leukemia* 2007;21:439–45.

58 Yu C, Friday BB, Lai JP, *et al.* Cytotoxic synergy between the multikinase inhibitor sorafenib and the proteasome inhibitor bortezomib *in vitro*: induction of apoptosis through Akt and c-Jun NH2-terminal kinase pathways. *Mol Cancer Ther* 2006;5: 2378–87.

59 Dasmahapatra G, Yerram N, Dai Y, Dent P, Grant S. Synergistic interactions between vorinostat and sorafenib in chronic myelogenous leukemia cells involve Mcl-1 and p21CIP1 down-regulation. *Clin Cancer Res* 2007;13:4280–90.

60 Quintas-Cardama A, Kantarjian H, Andreef M, *et al.* Phase I trial of intermittent administration of sorafenib (BAY 43–9006) for patients (pts) with refractory/relapsed acute myelogenous leukemia (AML). *J Clin Oncol* 2007;25:7018.

61 Obeng EA, Carlson LM, Gutman DM, Harrington WJ, Jr., Lee KP, Boise LH. Proteasome inhibitors induce a terminal unfolded protein response in multiple myeloma cells. *Blood* 2006;107: 4907–16.

62 Guzman ML, Neering SJ, Upchurch D, *et al.* Nuclear factor-kappaB is constitutively activated in primitive human acute myelogenous leukemia cells. *Blood* 2001;98:2301–7.

63 Attar EC, De Angelo DJ, Supko JG, *et al.* Phase I and pharmacokinetic study of bortezomib in combination with idarubicin and cytarabine in patients with acute myelogenous leukemia. *Clin Cancer Res* 2008;14:1446–54.

64 Mesa RA, Loegering D, Powell HL, *et al.* Heat shock protein 90 inhibition sensitizes acute myelogenous leukemia cells to cytarabine. *Blood* 2005;106:318–27.

65 Arlander SJ, Eapen AK, Vroman BT, McDonald RJ, Toft DO, Karnitz LM. Hsp90 inhibition depletes Chk1 and sensitizes tumor cells to replication stress. *J Biol Chem* 2003;278:52572–7.

66 Kaur G, Belotti D, Burger AM, *et al.* Antiangiogenic properties of 17-(dimethylaminoethylamino)-17-demethoxygeldanamycin: an orally bioavailable heat shock protein 90 modulator. *Clin Cancer Res* 2004;10:4813–21.

67 Lancet J, Baer MR, Gojo I, *et al.* Phase 1, pharmacokinetic (PK) and pharmacodynamic (PD) study of intravenous alvespimycin (KOS-1022) in patients with refractory hematological malignancies. *Blood* (ASH Annual Meeting Abstracts) 2006;108:1961.

68 Jones PA, Baylin SB. The fundamental role of epigenetic events in cancer. *Nat Rev Genet* 2002;3:415–28.

69 Levi JA, Wiernik PH. A comparative clinical trial of 5-azacytidine and guanazole in previously treated adults with acute nonlymphocytic leukemia. *Cancer* 1976;38:36–41.

70 Silverman LR, Demakos EP, Peterson BL, *et al.* Randomized controlled trial of azacitidine in patients with the myelodysplastic syndrome: a study of the Cancer and Leukemia Group B. *J Clin Oncol* 2002;20:2429–40.

71 Petti MC, Mandelli F, Zagonel V, *et al.* Pilot study of 5-aza-2′-deoxycytidine (Decitabine) in the treatment of poor prognosis acute myelogenous leukemia patients: preliminary results. *Leukemia* 1993;7(Suppl.1):36–41.

72 Blum W, Klisovic RB, Hackanson B, *et al.* Phase I study of decitabine alone or in combination with valproic acid in acute myeloid leukemia. *J Clin Oncol* 2007;25:3884–91.

73 Gore SD, Weng LJ, Zhai S, *et al.* Impact of the putative differentiating agent sodium phenylbutyrate on myelodysplastic syndromes and acute myeloid leukemia. *Clin Cancer Res* 2001; 7:2330–9.

74 Kuendgen A, Knipp S, Fox F, *et al.* Results of a phase 2 study of valproic acid alone or in combination with all-trans retinoic acid in 75 patients with myelodysplastic syndrome and relapsed or refractory acute myeloid leukemia. *Ann Hematol* 2005;84(Suppl.1):61–6.

75 Gojo I, Jiemjit A, Trepel JB, *et al.* Phase 1 and pharmacologic study of MS-275, a histone deacetylase inhibitor, in adults with refractory and relapsed acute leukemias. *Blood* 2007;109: 2781–90.

76 Garcia-Manero G, Yang H, Bueso-Ramos C, *et al.* Phase 1 study of the histone deacetylase inhibitor vorinostat (suberoylanilide hydroxamic acid [SAHA]) in patients with advanced leukemias and myelodysplastic syndromes. *Blood* 2008;111:1060–6.
77 Gore SD, Baylin S, Sugar E, *et al.* Combined DNA methyltransferase and histone deacetylase inhibition in the treatment of myeloid neoplasms. *Cancer Res* 2006;66:6361–9.
78 Garcia-Manero G, Kantarjian HM, Sanchez-Gonzalez B, *et al.* Phase 1/2 study of the combination of 5-aza-2′-deoxycytidine with valproic acid in patients with leukemia. *Blood* 2006;108: 3271–9.
79 Gore SD, Jiemjit A, Silverman LB, *et al.* Combined methyltransferase/histone deacetylase inhibition with 5-azacitidine and MS-275 in patients with MDS, CMMoL and AML: clinical response, histone acetylation and DNA damage. *Blood* (ASH Annual Meeting Abstracts) 2006;108:517.
80 McDevitt MR, Ma D, Lai LT, *et al.* Tumor therapy with targeted atomic nanogenerators. *Science* 2001;294:1537–40.
81 Pagel JM, Appelbaum FR, Eary JF, *et al.* 131I-antiCD45 antibody plus busulfan and cyclophosphamide before allogeneic hematopoietic cell transplantation for treatment of acute myeloid leukemia in first remission. *Blood* 2006;107:2184–91.
82 Maslak PG, Krug L, Chanel S, *et al.* Pilot study of a Wilms tumor protein (WT1) heteroclitic peptide vaccine in patients with myeloid and thoracic neoplasms. *Blood* (ASH Annual Meeting Abstracts) 2007;110:903.
83 Hewitt RE, Melenhorst JJ, Price DA, *et al.* Widening the applicability of human neutrophil elastase and proteinase 3 peptide vaccines by elucidating immunogenic non-HLA-A2 MHC Class I restricted epitopes. *Blood* (ASH Annual Meeting Abstracts) 2006;108:3708.
84 Schmitt M, Schmitt A, Rojewski MT, *et al.* RHAMM-R3 peptide vaccination in patients with acute myeloid leukemia, myelodysplastic syndrome, and multiple myeloma elicits immunologic and clinical responses. *Blood* 2008;111:1357–65.
85 Shankar DB, Li J, Tapang P, *et al.* ABT-869, a multitargeted receptor tyrosine kinase inhibitor: inhibition of FLT3 phosphorylation and signaling in acute myeloid leukemia. *Blood* 2007;109:3400–8.
86 Holder S, Zemskova M, Zhang C, *et al.* Characterization of a potent and selective small-molecule inhibitor of the PIM1 kinase. *Mol Cancer Ther* 2007;6:163–72.
87 Dos Santos C, Demur C, Bardet V, Prade-Houdellier N, Payrastre B, Recher C. A critical role for Lyn in acute myeloid leukemia. *Blood* 2008;111:2269–79.
88 Zeng Z, Sarbassov dos D, Samudio IJ, *et al.* Rapamycin derivatives reduce mTORC2 signaling and inhibit AKT activation in AML. *Blood* 2007;109:3509–12.
89 Weisberg E, Banerji L, Wright RD, *et al.* Potentiation of antileukemic therapies by the dual PI3K/PDK-1 inhibitor, BAG956: effects on *BCR–ABL-* and mutant *FLT3*-expressing cells. *Blood* 2008;111:3723–34.
90 Kojima K, Konopleva M, McQueen T, O'Brien S, Plunkett W, Andreeff M. Mdm2 inhibitor Nutlin-3a induces p53-mediated apoptosis by transcription-dependent and transcription-independent mechanisms and may overcome Atm-mediated resistance to fludarabine in chronic lymphocytic leukemia. *Blood* 2006;108:993–1000.

Chapter 12
Hematopoietic Stem-cell Transplantation for Acute Myelogenous Leukemia

Gheath Alatrash and Marcos de Lima
University of Texas M. D. Anderson Cancer Center, Houston, Texas, USA

Introduction

Hematopoietic stem-cell transplant (HSCT) is a major weapon in the armamentarium of therapies used to treat patients with acute myeloid leukemia (AML), providing the possibility of cure of this disease. Although much progress has been made in tissue matching, development of less-toxic preparative regimens, as well as the treatment and prophylaxis of graft-versus-host disease (GVHD), controversy remains about the use and timing of allogeneic or autologous HSCT to treat AML. This chapter discusses the role of this treatment modality, and reviews some of the challenges that have yet to be solved.

Pre-transplant regimens

Prior to the infusion of stem cells, preparative (or conditioning) regimens are administered to the patient to achieve two major goals in the allogeneic setting: leukemia control and immunosuppression, the latter to prevent graft rejection. These regimens can be in the form of chemotherapy, biotherapy, and/or radiation therapy (total body irradiation [TBI]).

Preparative regimens can be divided into three broad categories: myeloablative, non-myeloablative, and reduced intensity conditioning (RIC) regimens. Myeloablative regimens result in the complete eradication of bone marrow function, therefore necessitating autologous or allogeneic stem cells for reconstitution of hematopoiesis. Non-myeloablative regimens do not require stem-cell support, result in neutrophil recovery within 28 days without stem-cell infusion, and frequently show mixed chimerism (coexistence of donor and recipient-derived hematopoiesis) early after transplantation. While decreasing transplant-related mortality (TRM) and morbidity, non-myeloablative regimens may not completely eradicate the malignant clone, thereby depending to a greater extent on the immunologic graft-versus-leukemia (GVL) effect to fully eliminate disease. RIC induces less myelosuppression compared with myeloablative regimens, but cannot be safely administered without stem-cell support.

Allogeneic transplantation

The first reports of antileukemia effects of allogeneic HSCT were noted in murine models in the late 1950s [1] and in humans in the 1960s [2]. Responses using these therapies were noted early on, but were limited by toxicity and GVHD [2]. The pioneering experience of the Seattle group was subsequently reported by Thomas *et al.* in 1977, describing a series of patients with refractory acute leukemia that achieved up to 20% prolonged remissions following HSCT [3].

Graft-versus-leukemia effect and graft-versus-host disease

GVL and GVHD are induced by similar immune mechanisms, primarily mediated by T lymphocytes. The observed remissions following donor lymphocyte infusions (DLI) in patients with relapsed AML, the presence of leukemia-specific lymphocytes in the donor graft, and the reduced incidence of GVHD and higher relapse rates following graft-lymphocyte depletion highlight the importance of T lymphocytes in GVL and GVHD. Donor lymphocytes, if capable of recognizing recipient tumor antigens, lead to GVL effects and disease eradication [4] while causing GVHD if an immunologic response is mounted against normal tissue. In human leukocyte antigen (HLA)-matched donor-recipient sibling pairs, mismatches in minor histocompatibility antigens appear to mediate most of the GVHD, while in the context of unrelated donor transplants, mismatches in loci other than HLA-A, -B, -C, DRB1 and DQB1 also contribute to triggering GVHD. A balance between these two immunologic phenomena determines the success of the transplant. Unfortunately, manipulation of the graft to reduce GVHD by graft T-lymphocyte depletion is often associated with higher post-transplant relapse rates and graft

Leukemias: Principles and Practice of Therapy, 1st edition. Edited by S. Faderl and H. Kantarjian.

rejection. Conditioning regimen-induced inflammation and tissue damage are important components of the "cascade" that leads to the development of GVHD. This has provided the rationale for reducing the intensity of the conditioning regimen to decrease acute GVHD. The trade-off is that RIC regimens may not adequately decrease the disease burden prior to administration of the graft, and may be associated with higher rates of disease relapse.

Unlike low-grade lymphomas, which are highly sensitivity to the GVL effect, AML is considered to be of intermediate sensitivity, hence emphasizing the critical role of the preparative regimen in determining the HSCT outcome. Accordingly, the likelihood of success after non-myeloablative regimens is highly dependent upon the disease stage and biology. Patients with rapidly progressive AML are less likely to benefit from non-myeloablative preparative regimens, especially when accounting for the delayed time for the GVL effect to develop. In such cases, early immunosuppression withdrawal or DLI may hasten the antileukemia immunity or sufficiently delay disease progression until the GVL is achieved.

Stem-cell source

The source of stem cells also impacts transplant outcomes. At this time, there are three possible sources: bone marrow, peripheral blood, and cord blood. The exact cell dose required for stable long-term engraftment is yet to be determined; however, bone marrow nucleated cell dose of $2–3 \times 10^8$/kg is generally preferred. Additionally, a $CD34^+$ cell dose $\geq 3.0 \times 10^6$/kg was associated with improved hematopoietic recovery, TRM, and 5-year survival in some studies [5,6]. Higher cell doses, however, may lead to an increased risk of extensive chronic GVHD following allogeneic HSCT [7].

Steady-state peripheral blood contains few hematopoietic progenitors, but hematopoietic stem cells can be "mobilized" to the peripheral circulation with granulocyte colony stimulating factor (G-CSF). Treatment of donors (or patients) with hematopoietic growth factors improves the yield of peripheral blood stem cell to levels that routinely exceed bone marrow harvest [8,9]. Autologous peripheral-blood stem cells (PBSCs) are frequently procured after standard-dose chemotherapy and G-CSF. In the allogeneic setting, recipient hematologic recovery is faster, but GVHD rates tend to be higher, likely due to the high lymphocyte content of the graft. Cord blood contains a high concentration of hematopoietic stem cells with a high proliferative potential. Procurement of cord blood causes no discomfort to the donor and bypasses the delay encountered with donor medical clearance and stem-cell collection from peripheral blood or bone marrow. In addition, cord blood is more tolerant of histocompatibility mismatches compared with bone marrow and peripheral blood (ie, lower GVHD rates). On the other hand, the relatively small number of hematopoietic progenitors is associated with delayed engraftment and higher mortality rates in adults. Cell doses above 2×10^7 total nucleated cells/kg are generally associated with improved outcomes.

Myeloablative preparative regimens

The number of myeloablative allo-SCT (allogeneic stem-cell transplant) performed for AML has steadily increased over the past 5 years (Figure 12.1). Cyclophosphamide-TBI (CyTBI) and busulfan-cyclophosphamide (BuCy) or busulfan-fludarabine (BuFlu) are commonly used combinations in myeloablative preparative regimens. CyTBI for

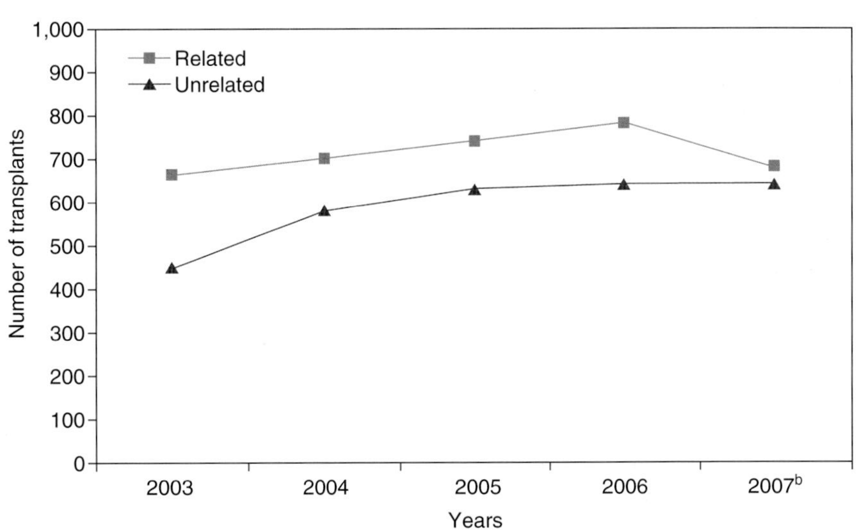

Figure 12.1 Estimated annual numbers of myeloablative hematopoietic cell transplants for acute myeloid leukemia (AML) registered with Center for International Blood and Marrow Transplant Research (CIBMTR) 2003–2007. This figure estimates the total number of hematocrit cell transplants (HCTs) performed in the USA based on the actual numbers of HCTs registered with the CIBMTR and the percent of data collected. We estimate the CIBMTR collects data on about 90% of unrelated donor HCTs and 65% of related donor HCTs performed in the USA. From the Center for International Blood and Marrow Transplant Research, with permission.

patients with AML and acute lymphoblastic leukemia (ALL) was initially proposed in the 1970s by Thomas *et al.* [10]. In subsequent studies, Santos *et al.* [11] successfully substituted oral busulfan (16 mg/kg) for TBI in combination with cyclophosphamide (120 mg/kg) (BuCy2). One of the major limitations of oral busulfan is its unpredictable absorption, which can lead to subtherapeutic or high toxic plasma levels, requiring careful monitoring of drug levels and dose adjustments [12]. This limitation has been overcome by the development of an intravenous formulation by Andersson *et al.* [13,14], with an equivalence ratio of 0.8 mg of intravenous to 1 mg oral busulfan.

The substitution of the nucleoside analog fludarabine for cyclophosphamide in combination with busulfan may increase the safety while maintaining equivalent efficacy [15]. This owes in part to bypassing the shared glutathione-S-transferase conjugation metabolism pathway of busulfan and acrolein (a cyclophosphamide metabolite) and the increase of alkylator-induced cell killing effected by fludarabine DNA-repair inhibition. When cyclophosphamide is avoided, total daily busulfan dose can be delivered in a single administration (130 mg/m^2), allowing a fourfold higher peak area under curve (AUC) (median daily AUC = 4871 μmoles/min) compared with AUC achieved with every 6-hour dosing and possibly providing a better therapeutic index against AML. Additionally, a reduction in acute GVHD rates may also occur with this combination [16,17]. The most commonly used myeloablative regimens for related and unrelated donor transplants (as reported to the Center for International Blood and Marrow Transplant—CIBMTR) are listed in Tables 12.1 and 12.2, respectively.

Comparison of myeloablative preparative regimen

Randomized trials investigating the optimal preparative regimen for patients with AML are scarce; nevertheless, there have been a few trials that shed light into this controversial topic. Two studies have demonstrated superior-

Table 12.1 Most commonly used preparative regimens for related donor myeloablative hematopoietic cell transplants for acute myeloid leukemia in the USA from 2003 to 2007, registered with the Center for International Blood and Marrow Transplant Research.

Conditioning regimen	Year of transplant				
	2003 (% of transplants)	2004 (% of transplants)	2005 (% of transplants)	2006 (% of transplants)	2007 (% of transplants)
Cy + TBI ± other	123 (32)	132 (32)	119 (26)	155 (32)	107 (24)
TBI + other	14 (4)	18 (4)	28 (6)	29 (6)	17 (4)
Bu + Cy ± other	195 (51)	186 (45)	196 (43)	182 (37)	184 (42)
Cy ± other	1 (<1)	3 (1)	5 (1)	4 (1)	3 (1)
Cy + Irr (no TBI) ± other	0	2 (<1)	2 (<1)	0	1 (<1)
Other	48 (13)	70 (17)	100 (22)	116 (24)	125 (29)
Missing	47	43	32	19	5

Bu, busulfan; Cy, cyclophosphamide; Irr, irradiation; TBI, total body irradiation.

Table 12.2 Most commonly used preparative regimens for unrelated donor myeloablative hematopoietic cell transplants for acute myeloid leukemia in the USA from 2003 to 2007, registered with the Center for International Blood and Marrow Transplant Research.

Conditioning regimen	Year of transplant				
	2003 (% of transplants)	2004 (% of transplants)	2005 (% of transplants)	2006 (% of transplants)	2007 (% of transplants)
Cy + TBI ± other	192 (48)	250 (49)	213 (38)	192 (34)	176 (31)
TBI + other	10 (3)	22 (4)	23 (4)	27 (5)	29 (5)
Bu + Cy ± other	127 (32)	161 (31)	185 (33)	183 (32)	161 (28)
Cy ± other	3 (1)	0	1 (<1)	1 (<1)	2 (<1)
Cy + Irr (no TBI) ± other	0	0	0	0	1 (<1)
Other	67 (17)	82 (16)	139 (25)	169 (29)	203 (35)
Missing	7	3	5	5	4

Bu, busulfan; Cy, cyclophosphamide; Irr, irradiation; TBI, total body irradiation.

ity of CyTBI in comparison to BuCy. In the first trial, a heterogeneous group of patients with AML, lymphoid malignancies, and chronic myeloid leukemia (CML) receiving allo-SCT were given either CyTBI or BuCy. Improved efficacy and lower rate of long-term complications were noted in those receiving CyTBI [18]. In a second trial in younger patients with AML in first complete remission (CR1), CyTBI and allo-SCT produced better disease-free survival (DFS) and overall survival (OS) compared with BuCy [19]. One of the major criticisms of these trials is the lack of busulfan blood-level measurements, because approximately 10–20% of patients will have subtherapeutic levels and another 10–20% will have potentially toxic levels of the drug. In a long-term follow-up analysis of these two trials, as well as two additional trials in CML [20,21], Socie *et al.* [22] reported comparable OS and DFS for patients with CML regardless of the preparative regimen, and a 10% statistically insignificant difference in OS and DFS in patients with AML (10-year actuarial survival of 51% and 63% with BuCy and Cy-TBI, respectively). Finally, in a clinical trial conducted by the Southwest Oncology Group in which etoposide/TBI was compared with BuCy for the treatment of patients with AML not in first remission, similar DFS and OS rates were found in both groups [23].

Oral busulfan guided by blood-level monitoring or use of the i.v. formulation minimizes over or underdosing of the drug, which can make significant differences in improving efficacy and decreasing drug-related toxicity. Similarly, improvements in TBI delivery have decreased radiation-related toxicities. Unfortunately, the answer to the critical question of which preparative regimen to use in AML remains to be answered and is dependent on the transplant center and investigator preference.

Transplants for acute myeloid leukemia in complete remission 1

Numerous studies have demonstrated that, although allogeneic transplants are associated with lower relapse rates, they commonly increase the rates of non-relapse mortality in patients who achieved a complete remission (CR), thereby attenuating the benefits of HSCT. Nonetheless, the development of less toxic preparative regimens and advancements in post-transplant supportive care have reduced the risks of HSCT, and, in so doing, have led to improved transplant outcomes in patients with AML in CR1. Unfortunately, there are no recent large randomized trials comparing allogeneic HSCT (which have improved TRM rates) with chemotherapy, and the literature reflects the practice of the mid-to-late 1990s.

Clinical trials comparing chemotherapy with HSCT frequently involve "genetic randomization," which groups patients based on donor availability, irrespective of whether or not the patient receives the HSCT. Nevertheless, non-transplanted patients who are analyzed in the transplant group have, in general, higher relapse rates, while higher rates of TRM are documented in patients who receive HSCT. Interestingly, the Medical Research Council (MRC) AML 10 study confirmed similar survival among patients in the donor group, regardless of whether or not they received a transplant [24].

Cornelissen *et al.* [25] evaluated the outcome of patients entered into three consecutive studies according to a donor-versus-no donor comparison. Of 2287 patients entered, 1032 patients (45%) were eligible for allo-SCT. Only 326 patients had an available HLA-identical sibling donor, of whom 268 received allo-SCT. Cumulative incidence of relapse was 32% versus 59%, favoring patients in the allo-SCT group ($P < 0.001$). DFS was significantly better in the donor group (48% ± 3% versus 37% ± 2% in the no-donor group; $P < 0.001$) at the expense of a higher TRM (21% vs. 4%, $P < 0.001$). Risk-group analysis demonstrated better DFS and OS for younger patients (<40 years) and those without a favorable cytogenetic profile receiving allo-SCT.

Postremission consolidation therapy administered prior to HSCT may also influence the results of clinical trials. Two retrospective studies have investigated the role of postremission consolidation for patients in CR1 receiving HSCT. In a study that compared 146 patients receiving no consolidation with patients receiving standard-dose (<1 g/m^2; $n = 244$) and high-dose (1–3 g/m^2; $n = 249$) cytarabine (Ara-C) prior to autologous HSCT (auto-SCT), 5-year relapse rates, leukemia-free survival (LFS), and OS all favored those who received consolidation [26]. The number of consolidation cycles (one vs. two) and cytarabine dose did not significantly affect transplantation outcome. This effect was not present in another retrospective analysis that enrolled patients receiving HLA-identical sibling transplants. There were no significant differences in OS or LFS noted when comparing subgroups that received no consolidation chemotherapy with standard-dose or high-dose cytarabine consolidation [27].

Patient selection

Determining the ideal transplant candidate in CR1 is critical in interpreting the results of HSCT and in designing future trials in transplantation. As leukemia relapse rates tend to be lower following HSCT, the major limitation to applying HSCT to patients with leukemia in CR1 becomes TRM. Younger patients have good outcomes with high-dose Ara-C, and the risk of allo-SCT may be considered prohibitive if the non-relapse mortality (NRM) is ≥20%. Standard prognostic factors (Table 12.3), including cytogenetics, appear to predict outcomes for HSCT analogous to what is observed with chemotherapy. Nevertheless, there remains disagreement as to which cytogenetic risk group benefits the most from HSCT [24,28].

Table 12.3 Variables that influence outcomes of allogeneic hematopoietic stem-cell transplant for acute myeloid leukemia.

Disease status at time of HSCT
Donor type
Stem-cell source
Karyotype and molecular markers
CR1 duration
Disease "bulk"
Bone marrow blasts
Presence of peripheral blood blasts
Recipient age
Clinical comorbidities

CR1, first complete remission; HSCT, hematopoietic stem-cell transplant.

Numerous studies have shown that patients without a favorable cytogenetic profile (ie, poor and intermediate-risk cytogenetics) benefit the most from HSCT [24,25,29]. A recent study by Schlenk *et al.* demonstrated that, in addition to cytogenetic risk stratification, molecular genetic markers in patients with AML with normal cytogenetics are prognosticators for outcomes following HSCT [30]. Specifically, they studied partial tandem duplications (PTDs) of the mixed lineage leukemia gene (*MLL*), internal tandem duplication (ITDs) or mutations of the tyrosine kinase domain (TKD) of the FMS-related tyrosine kinase 3 gene (*FLT3*), and mutations in the nucleophosmin gene (*NPM1*), the CCAAT/enhancer binding protein α gene (*CEBPA*), and the neuroblastoma RAS viral oncogene homolog gene (*NRAS*). Results demonstrated that allo-SCT was associated with improved relapse-free survival (RFS) in all molecular subgroups, except in those with mutations in NPM1 without *FLT3*-ITD. More studies, however, need to be conducted to further clarify the role of molecular genetic testing in selecting patients for HSCT.

Autologous transplantation

Autologous HSCT for AML remains controversial. Randomized studies have indicated results that were not superior to treatment with chemotherapy alone. Autologous HSCT may provide an alternative form of consolidation for patients lacking an allogeneic donor. TRM and morbidity are usually low (<10%) but have higher relapse rates when compared with allogeneic HSCT [31].

In the European Organisation for Research and Treatment of Cancer (EORTC) Leukemia Group and the Gruppo Italiano Malattie Ematologiche dell'Adulto (GIMEMA) AML 10 trial [29], patients ≤46 years of age were assigned to receive allogeneic or auto-SCT based on donor availability. The 4-year DFS, relapse rates, and OS favored patients in the allo-SCT group, especially younger patients (15–35 years) and those with poor-risk cytogenetics. This latter finding contradicts results of the UK MRC AML 10, where a survival advantage was found only for patients with intermediate-risk disease [24]. In the EORTC GIMEMA AML 13 trial [32], 61 patients aged 61–70 years in CR1 were evaluated for auto-SCT, but only 35 received the transplant and no benefits were noted.

The Bordeaux Grenoble Marseille Toulouse (BGMT) intergroup performed an intent-to-treat analysis [33] based on donor availability investigating the outcomes of HSCT as consolidation for 472 younger patients with AML in CR1. Allo-SCT was used in 171 patients (donor group = 182 patients) while auto-SCT was done in 62% of patients in the no-donor group ($n = 290$). OS at 10 years was 51% and 43% for the donor and no-donor groups, respectively. Independent prognostic factors for survival included initial white blood cell (WBC) count, French–American–British (FAB) subtypes, cytogenetic risk, and number of induction courses. Allo-SCT was associated with a survival advantage for an intermediate-risk group only, as defined by a normal karyotype or an absence of favorable or unfavorable risk cytogenetic abnormalities [32,34].

Since HLA-compatible family donors (HLA-identical sibling or a one-antigen mismatch relative) are available in <35% of the cases in the USA and Europe, and in view of the lengthy process involved in procuring unrelated donor stem cells, auto-SCT has been proposed in such instances. Unfortunately, patients with poor-risk cytogenetics do not appear to benefit significantly from auto-SCT, and it is unclear if auto-SCT is better than high-dose Ara-C-based chemotherapy. If auto-SCT is pursued, stem cells are preferably obtained from peripheral blood upon recovery from consolidation chemotherapy (usually following G-CSF mobilization) with the caveat that patients with AML are often poor mobilizers of stem cells because of AML-related changes in bone marrow stroma and normal stem cells. Additionally, since leukemia stem cells may contaminate the graft, purging techniques have been developed to rid the graft of residual leukemia [35]. *Ex vivo* purging agents affect normal and leukemic stem cells, thereby leading to delayed engraftment [10]. Although purging techniques have not been tested in randomized trials, some data suggest possible benefits for purging autologous grafts. Miller *et al.* [36] investigated the role of purging in 294 patients who received either a 4-hydroperoxycyclophosphamide (4HC)-purged ($n = 211$) or unpurged ($n = 83$) autograft for AML in CR1 ($n = 209$) or second remission ($n = 85$). Post-transplant neutropenia was significantly prolonged following purging (median 40 days; range 10–200 days) versus unpurged autografts (median 29 days; range 9–97 days). Patients receiving 4HC-purged transplants had lower risks of treatment failure than those receiving unpurged transplants (relative risk 0.69; $P = 0.12$ in the first year post transplant; relative risk 0.28; $P < 0.0001$ thereafter). Three-year probabilities of LFS for purged and unpurged autografts were 56% and 31%, respectively, for patients in CR1, and 39% and 10%, respectively, for those in second remission (CR2).

Although auto-SCT is sometimes reserved for elderly patients who may not be able to tolerate the TRM associated with allo-SCT, it did not significantly improve DFS or OS in a large, prospective multicenter trial [32]. Thirty-five of 61 patients aged 61–70 years with good performance status received auto-SCT after first consolidation. Following a median follow-up time of 5 years, the median LFS and OS were 1.1 and 1.6 years, respectively. Successful engraftment was seen in all patients, but delayed platelet recovery was common (median 120 days for platelets $>20 \times 10^9/L$). No benefits were noted in patients who received auto-SCT compared with those who received a second consolidation with standard chemotherapy.

Transplantation for acute myeloid leukemia in primary induction failure or beyond complete remission 1

The duration, karyotype, and age of CR1 are important predictors of outcome after AML recurrence. Short CR1 (ie, ≤6 months) or failure to achieve a CR1 are associated with a likelihood of a CR of <10–20%. Auto-SCT (if cells were harvested while the patient was in CR) for relapsed patients has yielded poor results. Therefore, allo-SCT is considered the treatment of choice for AML in primary induction failure or beyond CR1. This recommendation, however, is derived from the dismal results seen with salvage chemotherapy, and not from randomized trials. Outcomes of allo- and auto-SCT are significantly better if performed in CR2 in contrast to performing these procedures during induction failure, active relapse, or remissions beyond CR2. To some extent, these observations are the result of a selection bias, given that patients in CR2 may be in a better prognostic category compared with those who failed induction or did not enter CR after salvage therapy. In addition, few studies have addressed the influence of covariate variables such as the duration of CR1 or cytogenetics on outcomes of allo-SCT for relapsed disease.

Armistead *et al.* [37] performed a retrospective analysis using a cohort of patients with relapsed AML treated at the M. D. Anderson Cancer Center (MDACC) between 1995 and 2004. The goal was to describe the results of first-salvage therapy for relapsed or refractory disease. The median age was 59 years, and 59% of the patients had poor-risk cytogenetics. Of the 490 patients analyzed, 113 were in CR2 and 377 did not achieve a second CR2. Allo-SCT was associated with a statistically significant survival benefit in both subgroups. In the CR2 group, 2-year OS was 45% versus 20%, favoring the transplanted group ($P = 0.005$). Similarly, for the relapsed refractory group, 2-year OS in the transplant cohort was 13% versus 0% for the non-transplanted patients ($P < 0.001$). Superior survival was demonstrated for allo-SCT patient who were <50 years of age, regardless of cytogenics or remission status. A slight survival benefit was observed for transplanted patients who were ≥50 years of age who failed to achieve CR2, but no survival advantage was seen for patients ≥50 years of age who achieved a CR2. Additionally, a second subgroup analysis in patients ≥50 years of age demonstrated transplant benefit only for patients with a short CR1 (CR1 <36 weeks: 2.7 months vs. 2.5 months, $P = 0.05$) [1]. It is expected (but not proven) that reductions in TRM for the cohort of patients >50 years of age will lead to superior results than those discussed here.

The risks and benefits of administering salvage chemotherapy to achieve CR2 prior to transplant must be taken into consideration. Although patients in CR2 have better outcomes than those transplanted with active disease, the likelihood of entering CR2 is directly related to CR1 duration. For example, CR1 duration <6 months is associated with a low likelihood of response to salvage chemotherapy, which can often lead to complications such as fungal pneumonia and organ toxicity that may prevent an allo-SCT. On the other hand, disease tempo and bulk may dictate an intervention before allo-SCT may be contemplated. Furthermore, the association of aging, shorter remission duration, and disease refractoriness only adds to this therapeutic dilemma. Thus, the issue of salvage chemotherapy before allo-SCT is not solved at this point, although salvage chemotherapy is frequently offered prior to allo-SCT unless the relapse is very indolent in nature and a donor is promptly available.

Therapy following transplant failure

The majority of patients who fail HSCT have a poor prognosis and limited options for therapy. Donor lymphocyte infusion (DLI) in AML may be considered following failure of HSCT. DLI enhances the antileukemia effects by normalizing the T-cell receptor (TCR) repertoire following HSCT and expanding the antileukemic cell population. Although DLIs have been administered to patients with AML, ALL, and myelodysplastic syndromes (MDS), the most significant success with DLI has been documented in patients with relapsed CML [4]. In a retrospective analysis of 399 patients with AML in CR1 following HSCT (171 patients received DLI), the estimated survival at 2 years was 21% ± 3% for patients receiving DLI (vs. 9% ± 2% for patients not receiving DLI). Age <37 years ($P = 0.008$), relapse occurring more than 5 months after HSCT ($P < 0.0001$), and use of DLI ($P = 0.04$) were associated with better outcomes. Additionally, 2-year survival was 56% ± 10%, if DLI was performed in remission or with favorable karyotype and 15% ± 3% if DLI was given with active disease or in aplasia [38]. If DLI is to be used, we recommend association with salvage chemotherapy.

The role of performing a second HSCT after failure of the initial HSCT is also controversial. Oran *et al.* [39] reported results of second allo-SCT (HSCT2) in 18 patients with AML/MDS who relapsed following an initial allo-SCT (HSCT1). HSCT2 performed as initial salvage or as consolidation therapy elicited a median survival of 25.3 months (vs. 2.4 months) when compared with all other salvage approaches, such as DLI or chemotherapy alone ($P = 0.0001$). The largest benefit was noted in patients in CR at HSCT1. In addition to the factors that influence the outcomes of the HSCT1, such as disease status at the time of HSCT, duration of CR after transplant, and performance status, one must take into account the presence of infections and GVHD. Given the extremely poor outcomes when HSCT2 is performed with active disease, our current recommendation is to attempt remission induction prior to proceeding to a second allo-SCT, unless the relapse is detected very early and is indolent in nature.

Aging and allogeneic transplantation for acute myeloid leukemia

The median age of patients with AML at diagnosis is 67 years. Surveillance Epidemiology and End Results (SEER) data show that the 5-year relative survival rates (1998–2003) for patients <65 years of age was 25–35% and 2–6% for patients >65 years of age [40]. Unfortunately, patient-, disease-, and donor-related factors limit the use of allo-SCT in elderly patients. For example, age-associated comorbid conditions can affect tolerance to preparative regimes. The biology of AML in the elderly, which tends to be resistant to chemotherapy compared with AML in younger patients, also worsens allo-SCT outcomes. Elevated levels of pro-inflammatory cytokines such as IL-6 and TNF-α have been noted in elderly individuals, indicating an altered immune response that may interfere with outcomes of allo-SCT or other immunotherapeutic approaches. GVHD rates are higher in elderly individuals and may be, in part, attributed to enhanced allostimulatory activities of antigen-presenting cells [41]. Furthermore, the diversity in the naive T-cell repertoire decreases after the seventh decade of life, a problem that is compounded by a decreased ability of the thymus to rebuild a diverse T-cell repertoire. These defects in T-cell generation can limit the antileukemia activities of T cells post allo-SCT [42]. Stem-cell homing and engraftment may also be affected by aging [43]. Despite these obstacles, the preparative regimen can ablate disease and the transplanted graft may reshape host immunity, thereby allowing elderly individuals to receive allo-SCT, which is now routinely performed in multiple institutions around the world for patients in the sixth and seventh decades of life.

Several indices have been developed to help select patients who may benefit from allo-SCT. The Charlson Comorbidity Index (CCI) accounts for chronic comorbid conditions and decades of life >50 years, and was shown to be a good prognosticator of post-transplant outcomes in retrospective analyses [44,45]. Sorror *et al.* [46,47] reported a more sensitive predictive index than the CCI by using pre-transplant laboratory data to better define previously identified comorbidities and assigning different prognostic values to comorbidities. Prospective evaluation of comorbidity indices is ongoing as a tool for selection of preparative regimen intensity and criteria for enrollment in clinical trials.

As allo-SCT TRM is decreasing substantially with improved tissue matching, GVHD therapy, and post-HSCT supportive care, we consider all adult patients ≤75 years of age in CR1 without good-risk cytogenetics candidates for allo-SCT if a sibling or a molecularly matched-unrelated donor (HLA-A, -B, -C, -DRB1, -DQB1) is available. Recent studies demonstrate similar outcomes for patients in CR1 with use of related or unrelated donors. At the MDACC, the ablative busulfan-fludarabine preparative regimen is used in patients ≤60–65 years, while fludarabine-melphalan or fludarabine-reduced dose busulfan are administered to patients >60–65 years of age or to frail patients prior to HSCT (Figure 12.2).

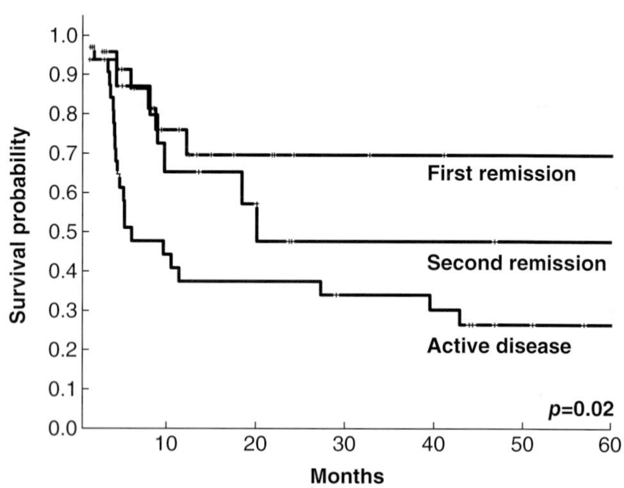

Figure 12.2 Survival probability by pre-transplant disease status (median follow-up is 22 months) in a cohort of 74 patients age ≥55 years with AML ($n = 60$) or MDS ($n = 14$) treated at the M. D. Anderson Cancer Center and who received the preparative regimen consisting of i.v. fludarabine 40 mg/m^2 and i.v. busulfan 130 mg/m^2 given once daily over 3 h on pre-transplant days 6–3.

Reduced-intensity conditioning and preparative regimen intensity

The rate of TRM increases as a function of preparative regimen intensity and in relation to patient age. RIC regimens have been developed in order to extend allo-SCT benefits to older patients and those who may not be ideal candidates for full-dose preparative regimens. Since AML is considered of intermediate sensitivity to the GVL effect, the intensity of the chemotherapy or radiation used in the preparative regimen is critical to the success of the transplant. As may be expected, non-relapse mortality and dose intensity are somewhat correlated [48,49]. Commonly used RIC regimens include fludarabine combined with either low-dose TBI [50], cyclophosphamide [51], busulfan [52], melphalan [53], or other drugs [54].

In a comparison of fludarabine and melphalan versus the non-myeloablative combination of fludarabine, Ara-C, and idarubicin in patients with AML/MDS, melphalan produced better disease control (relapse rate after idarubicin and melphalan was 61% and 30%, respectively) at the expense of higher NRM. The melphalan group comprised patients with refractory and relapsed disease, while the idarubicin cohort had patients with better prognosis and more patients in CR at time of transplantation (44% vs. 16% for idarubicin and melphalan, respectively) [48]. The melphalan regimen has been used extensively at the MDACC and has induced durable disease control in a significant fraction of treated patients. In a study of 112 patients, most of whom had high-risk AML/MDS, approximately 70% of patients transplanted in CR were alive in remission after a median of 29 months [55]. TRM was significantly higher among older patients with relapsed disease compared with patients in CR.

Use of low-dose TBI in non-myeloablative regimens has led to improved TRM rates, possibly at the cost of higher relapse rates (although no direct comparisons of regimens is available). Feinstein *et al.* [56] used either low-dose TBI (2 Gy total body irradiation; $n = 10$) or 2 Gy TBI and 90 mg/m^2 of fludarabine ($n = 8$) in patients with AML in CR1 receiving HLA-identical sibling transplants. Day + 100 NRM was 0%, and 1-year estimated NRM, OS, and PFS were 17%, 54%, and 42%, respectively.

The European Group for Blood and Marrow Transplantation conducted a retrospective analysis to determine clinical outcomes as a function of regimen intensity. Patients with AML >50 years of age who received HLA-identical sibling HSCT after RIC regimens, which consisted of fludarabine and busulfan or low-dose TBI, were eligible. Patients were compared with those who received busulfan-based ablative regimens, with more than 8 mg/kg of the drug or ≥10 Gy TBI-based regimens. Remission rates, LFS, and GVHD incidence was similar in both groups. Those who received RIC regimens experienced less TRM in exchange for a statistically significant higher probability of relapse [57].

Similar results were also obtained by Alyea *et al.* [58], who compared 71 patients who received non-myeloablative conditioning with fludarabine (30 mg/m^2 per day for 4 days) and intravenous busulfan (0.8 mg/kg per day for 4 days) to 81 patients who received myeloablative conditioning using CyTBI. Although patients in the non-myeloablative groups had higher-risk characteristics, OS was improved at 1 year (51% vs. 39%) and at 2 years (39% vs. 29%; $P = 0.056$). PFS (2 years, 27% vs. 25%; $P = 0.24$), and the incidences of grades 2–4 acute GVHD were similar (28% vs. 27%) in the groups. In the non-myeloablative group, the NRM rate was lower (32% vs. 50%; $P = 0.01$), while the relapse rate was higher (46% vs. 30%; $P = 0.052$).

Monoclonal antibodies have also shown efficacy when used in the preparative regimens in AML. Gemtuzumab ozogamicin (Mylotarg™), an anti-CD33 antibody conjugated to calicheamycin, was studied in a phase I/II trial at the MDACC at 2 or 4 mg/m^2 added to the melphalan regimen (melphalan 140 mg/m^2); the dose of 2 mg/m^2 was the most efficacious and least toxic. A group of 52 patients (49 with refractory and/or relapsed disease; median age 53 years) received allo-SCT using this regimen and achieved a longer event-free survival (EFS) when compared with historic controls [59].

Alemtuzumab, an anti-CD52 monoclonal antibody, produces significant recipient, as well as graft, T-cell depletion, thereby leading to a lower incidence of acute and chronic GVHD [60,61]. Unfortunately, this may be associated with higher relapse rates. Antithymocyte globulin (ATG) is frequently employed with the same intent. To date, there are no studies comparing these two approaches. At the MDACC, we use ATG in the context of mismatched-related or unrelated donor transplants.

The development of less toxic myeloablative regimens and improvements in supportive care has enabled patients aged 55–65 years to reap the potential benefits of the lower relapse rates and better disease control observed following myeloablative SCT [62]. Targeted oral and intravenous busulfan-based preparative regimens illustrate this trend [16,63]. In the absence of randomized trials, we recommend that patients with AML receive the highest dose intensity allowed by performance status and comorbid conditions. It is unclear if patients of any age in CR1 should be treated with regimens of lesser intensity in order to minimize TRM, or if this approach should be dictated by age and comorbidities (we support the latter option). These controversies indicate that older patients with AML should be enrolled on clinical trials whenever possible.

Treatment of patients with AML in the sixth decade of life or older is mostly synonymous to treatment of refractory and/or relapsed disease. In order to extend the benefits of allo-SCT to this group of patients, transplants for patients not in CR will have to be increasingly performed.

Schmid *et al.* [64] treated 103 patients with refractory AML with a sequential regimen that consisted of chemotherapy (fludarabine, cytarabine, and amsacrine), followed 4 days later by RIC (4Gy TBI, cyclophosphamide, and ATG), and subsequent related (40%) and unrelated (60%) donor allo-SCT. OS at 1, 2, and 4 years were 54%, 40%, and 32%, respectively; LFS at same time points were 47%, 37%, and 30%, respectively. This approach demonstrates the importance of coordinating chemotherapy and HSCT strategies, and in this case capitalizing on disease control produced by chemotherapy. This strategy of bridging patients to allo-SCT deserves investigation with a variety of drugs, such as hypomethylating agents, FLT3 inhibitors, clofarabine, and others. Additionally, since in refractory patients allo-SCT is usually associated with high but short-lived CRs, maintenance chemotherapy following HSCT may prove to be beneficial. We are currently investigating low-dose 5-azacitadine in this context as a maintenance of remission after allo-SCT.

Patient selection and results of transplantation

As the feasibility and efficacy of allo-SCT for selected patients >50–55 years has been clearly established [65,66], a major question is applicability of these data, mostly derived from phase II studies, to the general population of patients with AML. To address this question, Estey *et al.* [67] prospectively assessed the feasibility of RIC-SCT in 259 patients ≥50 years of age with AML, with or without unfavorable cytogenetics, who received induction chemotherapy at the MDACC from 2001 to 2003. The intent was to consolidate CR1 with a RIC-SCT. Ninety-nine patients entered CR and RIC-SCT was performed in 14 patients, with the majors deterrents to transplant being disease relapse and patient performance status. There was a significant advantage in RFS and OS in patients who received RIC-SCT in CR. The small number of patients who received RIC-SCT in CR reflects the selection bias that is built in the transplant literature. However, the long-term disease control, which approximates 60% for patients in the seventh decade of life, is significantly better than the results achieved with chemotherapy, emphasizing that every effort should be made to extend the option of allo-SCT to patients >60 years of age.

Haploidentical and cord blood transplants

Older patients are less likely to have healthy matched family donors, while availability of unrelated donors is related to ethnicity. Haploidentical donors (sharing at least one HLA haplotype) and unrelated cord blood (UCB) provide a source of hematopoietic stem cells for patients who do not have a readily available matched donor or in patients with highly aggressive disease that does not allow adequate time for the donor search process. Several minority groups, such as African Americans and Hispanics, have a low probability of having an unrelated donor identified. In such cases, haploidentical or UCB transplants may be especially valuable. One of the major limitations of haploidentical transplants is the poor immune recovery that is frequently seen because of the need for extensive *in vivo* or *in vitro* T-cell depletion. UCB transplants are limited by the relatively low number of stem cells when used for the treatment of large adults. On the other hand, cord blood grafts have been shown to cause less GVHD, permitting more donor-recipient HLA mismatches and therefore significantly increasing the donor pool. Although long-term remissions ranging between 20% and 50% have been reported with haploidentical and UCB transplant [68,69], results using these forms of SCT for AML in relapse have been poor. At this time, there are no prospective studies comparing haploidentical with UCB transplants.

In a trial that included 49 patients with a median age of 48 years, diagnosed with various hematologic malignancies and bone marrow failure syndromes (59% AML/MDS), Rizzieri *et al.* [70] showed the feasibility of combining non-myeloablative conditioning and haploidentical SCT. Successful engraftment was seen in 94% of patients and severe GVHD was seen in 8% of patients, the TRM was 10.2%, while 1-year OS was 31%. Similarly, UCB transplantation has been used successfully after reduced-intensity preparative regimens. Uchida *et al.* [71] reported a retrospective analysis of their experience with 70 patients (40% AML), median age of 61 years. NRM rate was 53%, while 2-year OS and progression-free survival (PFS) were both 23%.

Young adults and pediatric patients of lower weight benefit the most from UCB transplantation. Transplants for older adults (a subgroup that usually receive graft low-cell doses) are still complicated by higher rates of morbidity and mortality, and should be performed within a clinical trial whenever possible.

Future directions

While GVL and GVHD are mediated by similar immunologic mechanisms, separating these processes maximizing GVL and reducing GVHD remains a major area of research that can significantly change the field of transplant. Identifying leukemia-associated antigens (LAA) and distinct cytotoxic T-lymphocyte (CTL) populations is critical to the development of leukemia-targeted immunotherapy. Although most of these studies are preclinical, a few have entered clinical trials. PR1-vaccine is an HLA-A201-restricted vaccine that targets leukemia cells that express the neutral serine proteases proteinase-3 (P3) and neutrophil elastase (NE), both shown to be aberrantly expressed in myeloid leukemia [72,73]. Additionally, improved outcomes following IFN-α2b and HSCT have been shown in patients with CML who demonstrated PR1-specific CTL [74,75]. A phase I/II study has been conducted evaluating PR1-vaccine in 66 patients with myeloid leukemia (42 AML; 13 CML; 11 MDS). PR1-specific immune response was observed in 35/44 (57%) of the evaluable patients, positively correlating with clinical responses in 10 of the 25 immune responders ($P = 0.04$). A trend toward longer EFS was noted in patients with PR1 vaccine-induced immune response (8.7 months vs. 4.1 months in immune non-responders). PR1 vaccine is currently in a phase III randomized multicenter international trial.

Promising results were also reported using Wilms tumor peptide (WT1) vaccine in patients with AML. Wilms tumor gene encodes a zinc finger transcription factor that has been linked to leukemogenesis [76]. Increased frequency of WT1-specific T cells in patients with AML and MDS were documented following vaccination with WT1 peptide and correlated with clinical response [77]. A phase II trial of 16 HLA-A2$^+$ patients with AML and one patient with MDS who received up to 18 vaccinations (a median of eight) of WT1 peptide demonstrated evidence of antileukemia activity in six patients and one patient achieved CR for 12 months [78].

Conclusion

With HSCT comes the possibility of cure for a large number of patients with AML. Recent advances in conditioning regimens and supportive care have extended this therapeutic modality to a variety of patients, including the elderly. Despite progress in molecular risk classification, the ideal candidate and the optimal timing of HSCT in CR1, especially for the intermediate-risk patient, are yet to be identified. Disease recurrence and transplant-related toxicity, including GVHD, continue to pose major obstacles to HSCT. Identification of the mechanisms that lead to GVHD or GVL, and the delineation of the pathways involved in these processes, will enable us to maximize the latter while minimizing the former.

References

1 Barnes DW, Loutit JF. Treatment of murine leukaemia with X-rays and homologous bone marrow. II. *Br J Haematol* 1957;3: 241–52.

2 Mathe G, Amiel JL, Schwarzenberg L, *et al.* Successful allogenic bone marrow transplantation in man: chimerism, induced specific tolerance and possible antileukemic effects. *Blood.* 1965;25: 179–96.

3 Thomas ED, Buckner CD, Banaji M, *et al.* One hundred patients with acute leukemia treated by chemotherapy, total body irradiation, and allogeneic marrow transplantation. *Blood* 1977;49: 511–33.

4 Kolb HJ, Schattenberg A, Goldman JM, *et al.* Graft-versus-leukemia effect of donor lymphocyte transfusions in marrow grafted patients. *Blood* 1995;86:2041–50.

5 Bahceci E, Read EJ, Leitman S, *et al.* CD34+ cell dose predicts relapse and survival after T-cell-depleted HLA-identical haematopoietic stem cell transplantation (HSCT) for haematological malignancies. *Br J Haematol* 2000;108:408–14.

6 Bittencourt H, Rocha V, Chevret S, *et al.* Association of CD34 cell dose with hematopoietic recovery, infections, and other outcomes after HLA-identical sibling bone marrow transplantation. *Blood* 2002;99:2726–33.

7 Zaucha JM, Gooley T, Bensinger WI, *et al.* CD34 cell dose in granulocyte colony-stimulating factor-mobilized peripheral blood mononuclear cell grafts affects engraftment kinetics and development of extensive chronic graft-versus-host disease after human leukocyte antigen-identical sibling transplantation. *Blood* 2001;98:3221–7.

8 Siena S, Bregni M, Brando B, Ravagnani F, Bonadonna G, Gianni AM. Circulation of CD34+ hematopoietic stem cells in the peripheral blood of high-dose cyclophosphamide-treated patients: enhancement by intravenous recombinant human granulocyte-macrophage colony-stimulating factor. *Blood* 1989; 74:1905–14.

9 Socinski MA, Cannistra SA, Elias A, Antman KH, Schnipper L, Griffin JD. Granulocyte-macrophage colony stimulating factor expands the circulating haemopoietic progenitor cell compartment in man. *Lancet* 1988;1:1194–8.

10 Smith BD, Jones RJ, Lee SM, *et al.* Autologous bone marrow transplantation with 4-hydroperoxycyclophosphamide purging for acute myeloid leukaemia beyond first remission: a 10-year experience. *Br J Haematol* 2002;117:907–913.

11 Santos GW, Sensenbrenner LL, Anderson PN, *et al.* HL-A-identical marrow transplants in aplastic anemia, acute leukemia, and lymphosarcoma employing cyclophosphamide. *Transplant Proc* 1976;8:607–10.

12 Slattery JT, Sanders JE, Buckner CD, *et al.* Graft-rejection and toxicity following bone marrow transplantation in relation to busulfan pharmacokinetics. *Bone Marrow Transplant* 1995;16: 31–42.

13 Andersson BS, Madden T, Tran HT, *et al.* Acute safety and pharmacokinetics of intravenous busulfan when used with oral busulfan and cyclophosphamide as pretransplantation conditioning therapy :a phase I study. *Biol Blood Marrow Transplant* 2000;6:548–54.

14 Andersson BS, Thall PF, Madden T, *et al.* Busulfan systemic exposure relative to regimen-related toxicity and acute graft-versus-host disease: defining a therapeutic window for i.v. BuCy2 in chronic myelogenous leukemia. *Biol Blood Marrow Transplant* 2002;8:477–85.

15 Russell JA, Tran HT, Quinlan D, *et al.* Once-daily intravenous busulfan given with fludarabine as conditioning for allogeneic stem cell transplantation: study of pharmacokinetics and early clinical outcomes. *Biol Blood Marrow Transplant* 2002;8:468–76.

16 de Lima M, Couriel D, Thall PF, *et al.* Once-daily intravenous busulfan and fludarabine: clinical and pharmacokinetic results of a myeloablative, reduced-toxicity conditioning regimen for allogeneic stem cell transplantation in AML and MDS. *Blood* 2004;104:857–64.

17 Madden T, de Lima M, Thapar N, *et al.* Pharmacokinetics of once-daily IV busulfan as part of pretransplantation preparative regimens: a comparison with an every 6-hour dosing schedule. *Biol Blood Marrow Transplant* 2007;13:56–64.

18 Ringden O, Remberger M, Ruutu T, *et al.* Increased risk of chronic graft-versus-host disease, obstructive bronchiolitis, and alopecia with busulfan versus total body irradiation: long-term results of a randomized trial in allogeneic marrow recipients with leukemia. Nordic Bone Marrow Transplantation Group. *Blood* 1999;93:2196–201.

19 Blaise D, Maraninchi D, Michallet M, *et al.* Long-term follow-up of a randomized trial comparing the combination of cyclophosphamide with total body irradiation or busulfan as conditioning regimen for patients receiving HLA-identical marrow grafts for acute myeloblastic leukemia in first complete remission. *Blood* 2001;97:3669–71.

20 Clift RA, Buckner CD, Thomas ED, *et al.* Marrow transplantation for chronic myeloid leukemia: a randomized study comparing cyclophosphamide and total body irradiation with busulfan and cyclophosphamide. *Blood* 1994;84:2036–43.

21 Devergie A, Blaise D, Attal M, *et al.* Allogeneic bone marrow transplantation for chronic myeloid leukemia in first chronic phase: a randomized trial of busulfan-cytoxan versus cytoxan-total body irradiation as preparative regimen: a report from the French Society of Bone Marrow Graft (SFGM). *Blood* 1995; 85:2263–8.

22 Socie G, Clift RA, Blaise D, *et al.* Busulfan plus cyclophosphamide compared with total-body irradiation plus cyclophosphamide before marrow transplantation for myeloid leukemia: long-term follow-up of 4 randomized studies. *Blood* 2001;98: 3569–74.

23 Blume KG, Kopecky KJ, Henslee-Downey JP, *et al.* A prospective randomized comparison of total body irradiation-etoposide versus busulfan-cyclophosphamide as preparatory regimens for bone marrow transplantation in patients with leukemia who were not in first remission: a Southwest Oncology Group study. *Blood* 1993;81:2187–93.

24 Burnett AK, Wheatley K, Goldstone AH, *et al.* The value of allogeneic bone marrow transplant in patients with acute myeloid leukaemia at differing risk of relapse: results of the UK MRC AML 10 trial. *Br J Haematol* 2002;118:385–400.

25 Cornelissen JJ, van Putten WL, Verdonck LF, *et al.* Results of a HOVON/SAKK donor versus no-donor analysis of myeloablative HLA-identical sibling stem cell transplantation in first remission acute myeloid leukemia in young and middle-aged adults: benefits for whom? *Blood* 2007;109:3658–66.

26 Tallman MS, Perez WS, Lazarus HM, *et al.* Pretransplantation consolidation chemotherapy decreases leukemia relapse after autologous blood and bone marrow transplants for acute myelogenous leukemia in first remission. *Biol Blood Marrow Transplant* 2006;12:204–16.

27 Tallman MS, Rowlings PA, Milone G, *et al.* Effect of postremission chemotherapy before human leukocyte antigen-identical sibling transplantation for acute myelogenous leukemia in first complete remission. *Blood* 2000;96:1254–8.

28 Slovak ML, Kopecky KJ, Cassileth PA, *et al.* Karyotypic analysis predicts outcome of preremission and postremission therapy in adult acute myeloid leukemia: a Southwest Oncology Group/Eastern Cooperative Oncology Group Study. *Blood* 2000;96: 4075–83.

29 Suciu S, Mandelli F, de Witte T, *et al.* Allogeneic compared with autologous stem cell transplantation in the treatment of patients younger than 46 years with acute myeloid leukemia (AML) in first complete remission (CR1): an intention-to-treat analysis of the EORTC/GIMEMAAML-10 trial. *Blood* 2003;102: 1232–40.

30 Schlenk RF, Dohner K, Krauter J, *et al.* Mutations and treatment outcome in cytogenetically normal acute myeloid leukemia. *N Engl J Med* 2008;358:1909–18.

31 Lazarus HM, Perez WS, Klein JP, *et al.* Autotransplantation versus HLA-matched unrelated donor transplantation for acute myeloid leukaemia: a retrospective analysis from the Center for International Blood and Marrow Transplant Research. *Br J Haematol* 2006;132:755–69.

32 Thomas X, Suciu S, Rio B, *et al.* Autologous stem cell transplantation after complete remission and first consolidation in acute myeloid leukemia patients aged 61–70 years: results of the prospective EORTC-GIMEMA AML-13 study. *Haematologica* 2007; 92:389–96.

33 Jourdan E, Boiron JM, Dastugue N, *et al.* Early allogeneic stem-cell transplantation for young adults with acute myeloblastic leukemia in first complete remission: an intent-to-treat long-term analysis of the BGMT experience. *J Clin Oncol* 2005;23: 7676–84.

34 Dastugue N, Payen C, Lafage-Pochitaloff M, *et al.* Prognostic significance of karyotype in de novo adult acute myeloid leukemia. The BGMT group. *Leukemia* 1995;9:1491–8.

35 de Lima M, Shpall EJ. Ex-vivo purging of hematopoietic progenitor cells. *Curr Hematol Rep* 2004;3:257–64.

36 Miller CB, Rowlings PA, Zhang MJ, *et al.* The effect of graft purging with 4-hydroperoxycyclophosphamide in autologous bone marrow transplantation for acute myelogenous leukemia. *Exp Hematol* 2001;29:1336–46.

37 Armistead PM, de Lima M, Pierce S, *et al.* Identifying relapsed AML patients most likely to benefit from allogeneic stem cell transplant: a statistical subgroup analysis. *Blood* (ASH Annual Meeting Abstracts) 2007;110:329.

38 Schmid C, Labopin M, Nagler A, *et al.* Donor lymphocyte infusion in the treatment of first hematological relapse after allogeneic stem-cell transplantation in adults with acute myeloid leukemia: a retrospective risk factors analysis and comparison with other strategies by the EBMT Acute Leukemia Working Party. *J Clin Oncol* 2007;25:4938–45.

39 Oran B, Giralt S, Couriel D, *et al.* Treatment of AML and MDS relapsing after reduced-intensity conditioning and allogeneic hematopoietic stem cell transplantation. *Leukemia* 2007;21: 2540–4.

40 SEER: Surveillance, Epidemiology and End Results. Accessed: April 2008.

41 Ordemann R, Hutchinson R, Friedman J, *et al.* Enhanced allostimulatory activity of host antigen-presenting cells in old mice intensifies acute graft-versus-host disease. *J Clin Invest* 2002; 109:1249–56.

42 Goronzy JJ, Weyand CM. T cell development and receptor diversity during aging. *Curr Opin Immunol* 2005;17:468–75.

43 Liang Y, Van Zant G, Szilvassy SJ. Effects of aging on the homing and engraftment of murine hematopoietic stem and progenitor cells. *Blood* 2005;106:1479–87.

44 Charlson ME, Pompei P, Ales KL, MacKenzie CR. A new method of classifying prognostic comorbidity in longitudinal

studies: development and validation. *J Chronic Dis* 1987;40: 373–83.

45 Diaconescu R, Flowers CR, Storer B, *et al.* Morbidity and mortality with nonmyeloablative compared with myeloablative conditioning before hematopoietic cell transplantation from HLA-matched related donors. *Blood* 2004;104:1550–8.

46 Sorror ML, Maris MB, Storb R, *et al.* Hematopoietic cell transplantation (HCT)-specific comorbidity index: a new tool for risk assessment before allogeneic HCT. *Blood* 2005;106: 2912–19.

47 Sorror ML, Giralt S, Sandmaier BM, *et al.* Hematopoietic cell transplantation specific comorbidity index as an outcome predictor for patients with acute myeloid leukemia in first remission: combined FHCRC and MDACC experiences. *Blood* 2007; 110:4606–13.

48 de Lima M, Anagnostopoulos A, Munsell M, *et al.* Nonablative versus reduced-intensity conditioning regimens in the treatment of acute myeloid leukemia and high-risk myelodysplastic syndrome: dose is relevant for long-term disease control after allogeneic hematopoietic stem cell transplantation. *Blood* 2004; 104:865–72.

49 Clift RA, Buckner CD, Appelbaum FR, Sullivan KM, Storb R, Thomas ED. Long-term follow-up of a randomized trial of two irradiation regimens for patients receiving allogeneic marrow transplants during first remission of acute myeloid leukemia. *Blood* 1998;92:1455–6.

50 Baron F, Maris MB, Sandmaier BM, *et al.* Graft-versus-tumor effects after allogeneic hematopoietic cell transplantation with nonmyeloablative conditioning. *J Clin Oncol* 2005;23: 1993–2003.

51 Childs R, Clave E, Contentin N, *et al.* Engraftment kinetics after nonmyeloablative allogeneic peripheral blood stem cell transplantation: full donor T-cell chimerism precedes alloimmune responses. *Blood* 1999;94:3234–41.

52 Slavin S, Nagler A, Naparstek E, *et al.* Nonmyeloablative stem cell transplantation and cell therapy as an alternative to conventional bone marrow transplantation with lethal cytoreduction for the treatment of malignant and nonmalignant hematologic diseases. *Blood* 1998;91:756–63.

53 Giralt S, Estey E, Albitar M, *et al.* Engraftment of allogeneic hematopoietic progenitor cells with purine analog-containing chemotherapy: harnessing graft-versus-leukemia without myeloablative therapy. *Blood* 1997;89:4531–6.

54 de Lima M, Giralt S. Allogeneic transplantation for the elderly patient with acute myelogenous leukemia or myelodysplastic syndrome. *Semin Hematol* 2006;43:107–17.

55 Oran B, Giralt S, Saliba R, *et al.* Allogeneic hematopoietic stem cell transplantation for the treatment of high-risk acute myelogenous leukemia and myelodysplastic syndrome using reduced-intensity conditioning with fludarabine and melphalan. *Biol Blood Marrow Transplant* 2007;13:454–62.

56 Feinstein LC, Sandmaier BM, Hegenbart U, *et al.* Nonmyeloablative allografting from human leucocyte antigen-identical sibling donors for treatment of acute myeloid leukaemia in first complete remission. *Br J Haematol* 2003;120: 281–8.

57 Aoudjhane M, Labopin M, Gorin NC, *et al.* Comparative outcome of reduced intensity and myeloablative conditioning regimen in HLA identical sibling allogeneic haematopoietic stem cell transplantation for patients older than 50 years of age with acute myeloblastic leukaemia: a retrospective survey from the Acute Leukemia Working Party (ALWP) of the European group for Blood and Marrow Transplantation (EBMT). *Leukemia* 2005;19:2304–12.

58 Alyea EP, Kim HT, Ho V, *et al.* Comparative outcome of nonmyeloablative and myeloablative allogeneic hematopoietic cell transplantation for patients older than 50 years of age. *Blood* 2005;105:1810–14.

59 de Lima M, Giralt S, Caldera Z. Results of a phase I/II study of gemtuzumab ozogamicin added to fludarabine (F), melphalan (M) and allogeneic hematopoietic stem cell transplantation (HSCT) for relapsed myeloid leukemias. *Blood* (ASH Annual Meeting Abstracts) 2004;104:865–72.

60 Chakraverty R, Peggs K, Chopra R, *et al.* Limiting transplantation-related mortality following unrelated donor stem cell transplantation by using a nonmyeloablative conditioning regimen. *Blood* 2002;99:1071–8.

61 van Besien K, Artz A, Smith S, *et al.* Fludarabine, melphalan, and alemtuzumab conditioning in adults with standard-risk advanced acute myeloid leukemia and myelodysplastic syndrome. *J Clin Oncol* 2005;23:5728–38.

62 Wallen H, Gooley TA, Deeg HJ, *et al.* Ablative allogeneic hematopoietic cell transplantation in adults 60 years of age and older. *J Clin Oncol* 2005;23:3439–46.

63 Shimoni A, Kroger N, Zabelina T, *et al.* Hematopoietic stem-cell transplantation from unrelated donors in elderly patients (age >55 years) with hematologic malignancies: older age is no longer a contraindication when using reduced intensity conditioning. *Leukemia* 2005;19:7–12.

64 Schmid C, Schleuning M, Schwerdtfeger R, *et al.* Long-term survival in refractory acute myeloid leukemia after sequential treatment with chemotherapy and reduced-intensity conditioning for allogeneic stem cell transplantation. *Blood* 2006;108: 1092–9.

65 Lioure B, Delaunay J, Blaise D, *et al.* Allogeneic stem cell transplantation (SCT) with non myeloablative conditioning regimen (NST) following intensive consolidation may be equivalent to conventional alloSCT and superior to autoSCT for patients over 50 with acute myeloid leukemia (AML) in 1st CR: first results of the AML 2001 trial. *Blood* 2006;108:319.

66 Niederwieser D, Cornelissen J, Al-Ali HK, *et al.* Hematopoietic cell transplantation after a low-dose, total-body irradiation based regimen in elderly patients with AML: a multicenter, multinational, prospective HOVON/SAKK/OSHO Study. *Blood* (ASH Annual Meeting Abstracts) 2006;108:321.

67 Estey E, de Lima M, Tibes R, *et al.* Prospective feasibility analysis of reduced-intensity conditioning (RIC) regimens for hematopoietic stem cell transplantation (HSCT) in elderly patients with acute myeloid leukemia (AML) and high-risk myelodysplastic syndrome (MDS). *Blood* 2007;109:1395–400.

68 Aversa F, Terenzi A, Tabilio A, *et al.* Full haplotype-mismatched hematopoietic stem-cell transplantation: a phase II study in patients with acute leukemia at high risk of relapse. *J Clin Oncol* 2005;23:3447–54.

69 Rocha V, Labopin M, Sanz G, *et al.* Transplants of umbilical-cord blood or bone marrow from unrelated donors in adults with acute leukemia. *N Engl J Med* 2004;351:2276–85.

70 Rizzieri DA, Koh LP, Long GD, *et al.* Partially matched, nonmyeloablative allogeneic transplantation: clinical outcomes and immune reconstitution. *J Clin Oncol* 2007;25:690–7.

71 Uchida N, Wake A, Takagi S, *et al.* Umbilical cord blood transplantation after reduced-intensity conditioning for elderly patients with hematologic diseases. *Biol Blood Marrow Transplant* 2008;14:583–90.

72 Yong AS, Rezvani K, Savani BN, *et al.* High PR3 or ELA2 expression by CD34+ cells in advanced-phase chronic myeloid leukemia is associated with improved outcome following allogeneic stem cell transplantation and may improve PR1 peptide-driven graft-versus-leukemia effects. *Blood* 2007;110: 770–5.

73 Dengler R, Munstermann U, al-Batran S, *et al.* Immunocytochemical and flow cytometric detection of proteinase 3 (myeloblastin) in normal and leukaemic myeloid cells. *Br J Haematol* 1995;89:250–7.

74 Molldrem JJ, Lee PP, Wang C, Champlin RE, Davis MM. A PR1-human leukocyte antigen-A2 tetramer can be used to isolate low-frequency cytotoxic T lymphocytes from healthy donors that selectively lyse chronic myelogenous leukemia. *Cancer Res* 1999;59:2675–81.

75 Molldrem JJ, Lee PP, Wang C, *et al.* Evidence that specific T lymphocytes may participate in the elimination of chronic myelogenous leukemia. *Nat Med* 2000;6:1018–23.

76 Tsuboi A, Oka Y, Ogawa H, *et al.* Constitutive expression of the Wilms' tumor gene *WT1* inhibits the differentiation of myeloid progenitor cells but promotes their proliferation in response to granulocyte-colony stimulating factor (G-CSF). *Leuk Res* 1999;23:499–505.

77 Oka Y, Tsuboi A, Taguchi T, *et al.* Induction of *WT1* (Wilms' tumor gene)-specific cytotoxic T lymphocytes by *WT1* peptide vaccine and the resultant cancer regression. *Proc Natl Acad Sci U S A* 2004;101:13885–90.

78 Scheibenbogen C, Letsch A, Thiel E, *et al.* CD8 T-cell responses to Wilms tumor gene product *WT1* and proteinase 3 in patients with acute myeloid leukemia. *Blood.* 2002;100:2132–7.

Part 4
Acute Promyelocytic Leukemia

Chapter 13
The Pathophysiology of Acute Promyelocytic Leukemia

Francesco Lo-Coco and Syed Khizer Hasan
University Tor Vergata, Rome, Italy

Introduction

Acute promyelocytic leukemia (APL) is a distinct subset of acute myeloid leukemia (AML) associated with unique features and requiring specific management. The disease was initially recognized in 1957 by Hillestad, who described three patients with a rapidly fatal acute leukemia characterized by abundant number of abnormal promyelocytes infiltrating the marrow and a severe hemorrhagic syndrome [1]. In the following decades, APL has become a well-recognized entity, characterized as the M3 subtype of AML within the French–American–British (FAB) morphologic classification and accounting for approximately 10% of AML cases [2].

Clinically, APL is associated with a bleeding diathesis due to excessive fibrinolysis, which worsens during initial administration of chemotherapy. Most patients present with a low white blood cell (WBC) count, but 10–30% have a WBC count >10,000/μL, with increased risk of serious and potentially fatal hemorrhages into the central nervous system and lungs. The disease is initiated by a malignant transformation of an immature myeloid cell followed by a block in differentiation at the promyelocyte stage. The promyelocytes and blasts in >95% of APL cases harbor a balanced, reciprocal translocation involving the long arms of chromosomes 15 and 17, which is often the only cytogenetic abnormality present [3,4].

In spite of being an infrequent disease, APL represents one of the most successful examples of translational research in medicine. Over the past two decades, considerable progress has been made in the treatment of this leukemia, such that it has been converted nowadays into the most frequently curable adult leukemia [5,6]. Moreover, the APL model provides an extraordinary opportunity to investigate key mechanisms of leukemogenesis and a paradigm for innovative treatments including differentiation therapy and the use of chromatin remodeling agents and antibody-directed therapy.

Leukemias: Principles and Practice of Therapy, 1st edition. Edited by S. Faderl and H. Kantarjian.

Molecular architecture of the t(15;17)

In 1977, Rowley *et al.* [7], from the University of Chicago, reported on the consistent occurrence of a chromosomal translocation t(15;17)(q22;q21) in APL. This aberration was subsequently found to be uniquely associated to, and therefore pathognomonic of, the disease. Upon cloning the translocation in the late 1980s, it was shown that chromosome breakpoints lie within the *RARA* locus on chromosome 17 and the *PML* locus on chromosome 15, resulting in the fusion of the two genes [8,9]. Based on the location of breakpoints within the *PML* locus, the *PML–RARA* transcript isoforms bcr1, bcr2, and bcr3 may be formed. The bcr1, bcr2, and bcr3 transcripts derive from PML breakpoints in intron 6, exon 6, and intron 3, and are referred to as long (L) isoform, variable (V) isoform, and short (S) isoform, respectively [4]. Breakpoints in *RARA* invariably occur in all patients in intron 2. *PML–RARA* L isoform accounts for approximately 55% of APL cases, while the S and V isoforms are detected in approximately 35% and 8% of patients, respectively. The *PML–RARA* fusion is detectable by fluorescence *in situ* hybridization (FISH) or reverse-transcriptase polymerase chain reaction (RT-PCR) in >95% of APLs morphologically defined by FAB criteria, while in the remaining cases, several variant rearrangements have been described that constantly involve *RAR* and partner genes other than *PML* [4] (described in more detail below).

Structure and function of PML and RARα

The human *PML* gene comprises nine exons, with exons 7 to 9 having potential to generate, by alternative splicing, a number of C-terminally divergent PML isoforms [10]. The exact functions of these isoforms are not clear at present. PML belongs to a family of proteins containing a distinctive C_3HC_4 zinc-binding domain referred to as RING (really interesting new gene) finger. Similarly to other members of this family, such as BRCA1, PML acts as a tumor suppressor and has been implicated in the

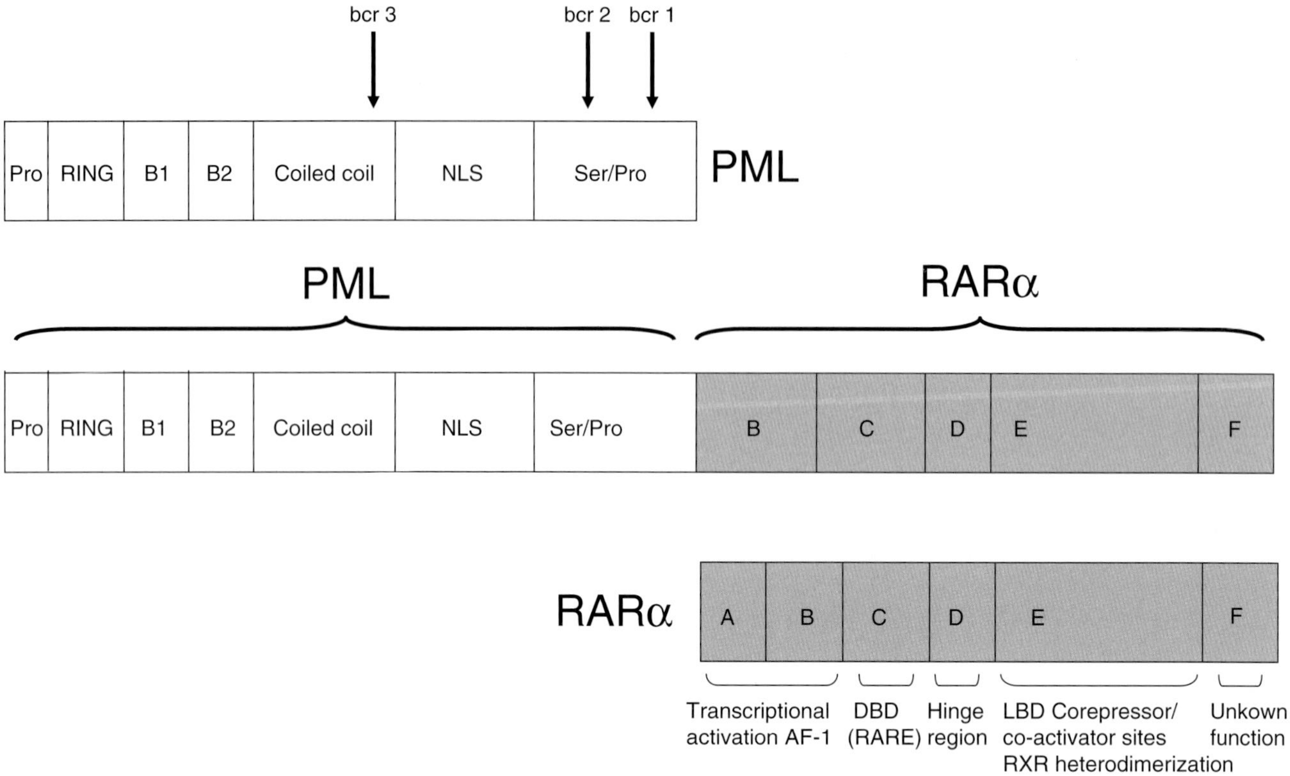

Figure 13.1 Schematic representation of PML–RARα fusion protein. PML regions labeled as RING, B1, and B2 represents cysteine-histidine rich domains, coiled-coil region; nuclear localization signal (NLS) and an acidic C-terminal Ser/Pro-rich domain, positions of three breakpoint cluster regions indicated by arrows (upper panel), A-F; RARα functional domains. DBD-DNA binding domain; LBD, ligand binding domain (lower panel); RARE, retinoic acid receptor element. In the fusion protein (middle panel), RING finger, B boxes, and the coiled-coil regions are consistently retained, whereas the C-terminal portion of PML varies depending on alternative splicing of the *PML* exons. RARA is fused through B to F domain.

control of genomic stability [11]. PML controls p53-dependent apoptosis, growth suppression, and cellular senescence in response to ionizing radiation and oncogenic transformation [12]. In the nucleus, PML co-localizes with other proteins such as p53, pRb, Daxx, and CBP [12,13] and organizes into a multiprotein complex termed "PML nuclear bodies" through its ability to form homomultimers. The PML protein has a modular structure with several domains (Figure 13.1). These include the following: a cysteine-rich region (aa 57–222) composed of three zinc finger-like structures. The first is a Zn^{2+}-binding motif, RING finger. The following two are called B-box zinc fingers (aa 140–161 and aa 189–222). RING-finger /B-box proteins often are linked to a coiled-coil (CC) domain and comprise a subfamily of RING proteins (RBCC for RING-B-box coiled coil). In addition to the RBCC motif, a nuclear localization signal (NLS), which is required for biologic activity of proteins, and an acidic Ser-Pro-rich region of unknown function is present within the C-terminal portion of PML. The RING-finger/B-box region is involved in localization of PML into nuclear bodies (NB). The CC motif mediates oligomerization of PML-RARα and its interaction with wild-type PML [8–10,14,15].

RARα is a member of the retinoic acid (RA) nuclear receptor family, serving as a ligand-inducible transcription factor by binding through its DNA-binding domain "C" to specific retinoic acid response elements (RAREs), which are located in the promoters of many genes including those of RARα, RARβ, and RARγ. The RARE are composed of hexanucleotide direct repeats with a variable number of spacer nucleotides between the repeated motifs. As shown in Figure 13.1, RARα contains two domains, AF-1 (A/B domain) and AF-2 (E domain), which can cooperate to activate transcription. The RA-RARα pathway indeed plays an important role in the control of myeloid cell differentiation. In the absence of ligand, RARα forms heterodimers with the retinoid X receptor (RXR) through its ligand binding domain "E" and recruits a co-repressor complex containing histone deacetylase (HDAC) activities that induces chromatin condensation and transcriptional repression [16].

Retinoids, natural or synthetic derivatives of vitamin A, are necessary dietary constituents that exert profound effects on development, cell proliferation, and differentiation in normal cells and various cancer cells by regulating the expression of specific genes. RARs (α, β, and γ) are activated by both all-trans-retinoic acid (ATRA, also called tretinoin, which is an acid form of vitamin A) and 9-cis-RA, whereas RXRs (α, β, and γ) are activated by 9-cis-RA only. Physiologic concentrations of RA (1×10^{-9} M) are able to release the nuclear co-repressors complex from the RARα-RXR and recruit co-activators with histone acetyltransferase activities (HAT). This results in hyperacetylation of histones at RARE sites, chromatin remodeling, and transcriptional activation of RARα target genes [17–19].

Both PML and RARαmoiety of the PML–RARα fusion protein have functional domains from each of the two native proteins. The N-terminal proline-rich domain, together with the RBCC motifs of PML, is fused to domains B–F of RARα [16].

Biologic effects of PML-RARα

The t(15;17) translocation results into two fusion gene products, *PML–RARA* and *RARA–PML*, on the $15q^+$ and $17q^-$ derivatives, respectively. Whereas *PML–RARA* is invariably expressed in all patients, the reciprocal *RARA–PML* fusion is detectable only in ~70% of cases [4,20,21], suggesting that the former hybrid is the one contributing a major role in disease pathogenesis.

Both *in vivo* studies in transgenic animals and *in vitro* analysis in hematopoietic cells have demonstrated that the PML–RARα fusion protein contributes to the leukemic phenotype by inhibiting differentiation and promoting survival of hematopoietic precursors. In PML–RARα fusion proteins, oligomerization of RARα through the CC domain of PML is responsible for the oncogenic activity [22]. As a consequence of heterodimerization through the RING finger domain of wild-type PML with PML-RARα, wild-type PML becomes de-localized into microspeckled nuclear particles. This variation in subcellular distribution of PML in APL bearing the PML-RARα rearrangement is clinically relevant as it allows rapid diagnosis through immunostaining techniques [21,23]. The PML-RARα protein alters the intranuclear distribution of PML and other nuclear body-associated proteins, and is a stronger transcriptional repressor than RARα. This results from its increased affinity for the SMRT (silencing mediator for retinoid and thyroid hormone receptors) and nuclear receptor co-repressors (N-CoR) [24,25].

The co-repressors N-CoR and SMRT are part of a multiprotein complex that includes HDACs. In the absence of ligand, both wild-type RARα and PML-RARα repress transcription by increasing the recruitment of co-repressors and HDAC complexes to the promoter region of RA target genes, resulting in deacetylation of histones. Deacetylated histones alter the conformation of chromatin and its accessibility to the transcriptional machinery, resulting in transcriptional silencing [19,26]. Pharmacologic doses of RA are able to release the interaction between HDACs and co-repressors, favoring the recruitment of coactivators, leading to active transcription on the DNA of target genes. In turn, these molecular events overcome the maturation arrest of leukemic promyelocytes resulting in *in vivo* differentiation of blasts and clinical remission.

Variant RARα translocations

In the vast majority of FAB defined M3 cases, the classical t(15;17) is detected [27]; however, a series of variant chromosomal aberrations have been reported, including t(11;17)(q23;q21), t(5;17)(q35;q12–21), t(11;17)(q13;q21), and der(17), whereby *RARA* is fused to the *PLZF*, *NPM*, *NuMA*, and *STAT5b* genes, respectively [28–31]. In common with *PML–RARA*-associated APL, patients with fusion genes involving *NPM* and *NuMA* appear to be sensitive to ATRA. In contrast, APL associated with a *PLZF-RARA* rearrangement is characterized by lack of a differentiation response to retinoids, and patients harboring this variant translocation treated with ATRA alone have a poor prognosis [32]. At pharmacologic levels of ATRA, the co-repressor complex is released from the retinoid receptor moiety of PML–RARα, NPM–RARα, PLZF–RARα, and presumably NuMA–RARα fusion proteins; however, the PLZF moiety of the PLZF–RARα fusion protein contains a BTB/POZ repression domain that binds the N-CoR and SMRT co-repressors in a retinoid-independent manner so that transcriptional repression is not relieved by ATRA. This latter phenomenon has been proposed to account for the lack of response to ATRA that characterizes cases of APL with the t(11;17) (q23;q21) chromosomal aberration.

Molecular basis for response to all-trans-retinoic acid and arsenic trioxide

PML-RARα in its basal state interacts with N-CoR and SMRT co-repressors that mediate transcriptional silencing. Transcriptional activation by PML-RARα in response to pharmacologic doses of ATRA (10^{-6}–10^{-7}) occurs via a conformational shift, which releases these co-repressors and instead recruits co-activator proteins. This co-regulator exchange model (replacement of co-repressors by co-activators) is supported by recent transcriptome and proteome analyses [33] with modulation of a large number of genes involved in the initiation/promotion of granulocytic differentiation, such as the upregulation of granulopoiesis-associated transcription factors *C/EBPs*, cytokines/cytokine receptors, as well as their corresponding post-receptor signal transduction molecules. Furthermore, ATRA induces the degradation of the PML-RARα chimeric protein by triggering caspase-mediated cleavage [34]. Further studies on the pathways involved in PML-RARα catabolism led to the discovery of a ubiquitin/proteasome-mediated degradation of PML-RARα and RARα, which was dependent on the binding of 26S proteasome regulatory subunit 1 (SUG-1) in the AF-2 transactivation domain of RARα [35,36]. Indeed, a number of components of the proteasome pathway appear to be necessary for the degradation of PML-RARα can be significantly enhanced upon ATRA [37].

Arsenic trioxide (ATO) exerts dose-dependent effects on APL cells [38]. At high concentration ($1–2 \times 10^{-6}$ M), ATO induces apoptosis, mainly through activating the mitochondria-mediated intrinsic apoptotic pathway. At low concentrations ($0.25–0.5 \times 10^{-6}$ M), and with a longer treatment course, ATO tends to promote differentiation of APL cells. Several mechanisms have been implicated in the action of arsenic in APL. One of the most intensively studied mechanisms is the induction of reactive oxygen species (ROS) in cells treated with arsenic [39,40]. ROS species include hydrogen peroxide and superoxide, which could be scavenged by systems that include glutathione, glutathione-S-transferase, catalase, and *N*-acetylcysteine (NAC). These systems can decrease arsenic-induced cell death [41,42]. ROS production can induce phosphorylation and activate Jun N-terminal kinase (JNK), which in turn triggers apoptosis [43,44].

Other biologic features of APL and their impact on therapy

In addition to PML-RARα, other biologic features of APL account for its unique phenotype and provide potential targets for tailored treatment. As with their surface markers, APL cells are characterized by a virtually absent or minimally expressed gp-170, for example the main effector of the multidrug resistance phenotype that is found in a high proportion of AML. Immunophenotypic studies have also shown that APL is featured by a distinctive antigen profile that includes strong positivity for CD33, expression of CD13 and CD117, infrequent expression of HLA-DR and CD34, and lack of CD7, CD11a, CD11b, CD14, and CD18 [45,46]. In addition, leukemic promyelocytes frequently show aberrant expression of the T-cell-associated antigen CD2 and low or negative CD34 expression [46,47]. A negative impact on outcome has been suggested for CD2 and CD56 expression, although studies in large series of patients receiving modern ATRA plus chemotherapy regimens have not confirmed these associations [6,47]. CD33 is detected in virtually 100% of APL cases at high density and homogeneity. This may account, together with lack of gp-170 expression, for the optimal therapeutic response observed with the anti-CD33 monoclonal antibody (MoAb) gemtuzumab ozogamicin, a compound that may induce molecular remission even if used as single agent and/or in advanced disease [48,49]. The cytotoxic agent of gemtuzumab ozogamicin is N-acetyl gamma calicheamicin dimethyl hydrazide, a derivative of gamma calicheamicin [50]. Binding of gemtuzumab ozogamicin to the CD33 antigen is followed by endocytosis, cleavage of the covalent link between the MoAb and calicheamicin in lysosomes by acid hydrolysis, and release of calicheamicin. Glutathion reduction produces a reactive intermediate of calicheamicin, which in turn causes DNA double-strand breaks [51–56]. Gemtuzumab ozogamicin allows delivery of an anthracycline-like compound (calicheamicin) directly to leukemia blasts. Although at present only a few reports have been published on gemtuzumab ozogamicin treatment for APL, it is presumable that its use in this leukemic subset will be expanded in the near future and most investigators believe that APL represents an ideal target disease for gemtuzumab ozogamicin.

The FLT3 receptor is involved in the proliferation and differentiation of hematopoietic stem cells. Following binding to its ligand, the FLT3 receptor activates several intracellular signaling pathways that ultimately lead to cell proliferation. FLT3 receptor internal tandem duplications (ITD) in the juxtamembrane domain and point mutations in the tyrosine kinase II domain have been reported to occur in up to 45% of APL cases. This suggests that targeted therapies using FLT3 inhibitors may prove effective in APL. Both ITD and mutations in the tyrosine kinase II domain have been correlated with a higher WBC count at presentation, and ITD mutations have been more frequently detected in cases harboring the S-type *PML–RARA* [57,58]. Expression profile studies in patients with mutated *FLT3* have shown increased expression of genes involved in cell growth, cell-cycle control, and cell adhesion and migration, suggesting a role of these alterations in the pathogenesis of the disease and its clinical manifestations [57,59]. Concerning their prognostic significance, a presumed negative impact of mutations on treatment outcome has not been confirmed in the large clinical studies with modern ATRA and chemotherapy reported by the GIMEMA (Gruppo Italiano Malattie Ematologiche dell'Adulto) and MRC (Medical Research Council) groups [57,58]. Although FLT3 inhibitors have been successfully used in APL mouse models [60], because of the availability of several other effective agents, no clinical trials have been conducted so far in patients.

Conclusions and future perspectives

Elucidation of the pathophysiology of APL by the identification of the specific PML-RARα oncoprotein and of its biochemical functions has provided relevant information to unravel key mechanisms of leukemogenesis. In particular, recruitment of the co-repressor complex by a fusion protein leading to transcription inhibition and maturation arrest represents a frequent finding in AML pathogenesis and provides a rationale for transcription therapeutic targeting. Moreover, molecular insights into APL have proved extremely useful to improve rapid and specific diagnosis of this leukemia and to sensitively monitor minimal residual disease. Tailored treatment with ATRA and chemotherapy results in the cure of nearly 80% of patients with APL, and attempts to substitute cytotoxic therapy with combinatorial ATRA plus ATO are currently under way. In spite of this progress, the therapeutic benefit achieved in APL through targeted therapy has not yet been translated into other leukemic subsets, which remain essentially unresponsive to differentiating agents. Further studies on the mechanisms underlying the maturation block of AML, and unravelling relevant pathways for therapeutic targeting, are warranted to improve treatment results in the other AML subsets.

References

1 Hillestad LK. Acute promyelocytic leukemia. *Acta Med Scand* 1957;159:189–94.

2 Bennett JM, Catovsky D, Daniel MT, *et al.* Proposed revised criteria for the classification of acute myeloid leukemia. A report of the French-American-British Cooperative Group. *Ann Intern Med* 1985;103:620–5.

3 Melnick A, Licht JD. Deconstructing a disease: RARalpha, its fusion partners, and their roles in the pathogenesis of acute promyelocytic leukemia. *Blood* 1999;93:3167–215.

4 Grimwade D. The pathogenesis of acute promyelocytic leukemia: evaluation of the role of molecular diagnosis and monitoring in the management of the disease. *Br J Haematol* 1999; 106:591–613.

5 Tallman MS, Nabhan C, Feusner JH, Rowe JM. Acute promyelocytic leukemia: evolving therapeutic strategies. *Blood* 2002; 99:759–67.

6 Sanz MA, Tallman MS, Lo-Coco F. Tricks of the trade for the appropriate management of newly diagnosed acute promyelocytic leukemia. *Blood* 2005;105:3019–25.

7 Rowley JD, Golomb HM, Dougherty C. 15/17 translocation, a consistent chromosomal change in acute promyelocytic leukemia. *Lancet* 1977;1:549–50.

8 de Thé H, Chomienne C, Lanotte M, Degos L, Dejean A. The t(15;17) translocation of acute promyelocytic leukemia fuses the retinoic acid receptor alpha gene to a novel transcribed locus. *Nature* 1990;347:558–61.

9 Kakizuka A, Miller WH, Jr., Umesono K, *et al.* Chromosomal translocation t(15;17) in human acute promyelocytic leukemia fuses RAR alpha with a novel putative transcription factor, PML. *Cell* 1991;66:663–74.

10 Fagioli M, Alcalay M, Pandolfi PP, *et al.* Alternative splicing of PML transcripts predicts coexpression of several carboxy-terminally different protein isoforms. *Oncogene* 1992;7: 1083–91.

11 Salomoni P, Pandolfi PP. p53 De-ubiquitination: at the edge between life and death. *Nat Cell Biol* 2002;4:E152–3.

12 Gurrieri C, Capodieci P, Bernardi R, *et al.* Loss of the tumor suppressor PML in human cancers of multiple histologic origins. *J Natl Cancer Inst* 2004;96:269–79.

13 Jensen K, Shiels C, Freemont PS. PML protein isoforms and the RBCC/TRIM motif. *Oncogene* 2001;20:7223–33.

14 Goddard AD, Borrow J, Freemont PS, Solomon E. Characterization of a zinc finger gene disrupted by the t(15;17) in acute promyelocytic leukemia. *Science* 1991;254:1371–4.

15 de Thé H, Lavau C, Marchio A, *et al.* The PML–RAR alpha fusion mRNA generated by the t(15;17) translocation in acute promyelocytic leukemia encodes a functionally altered RAR. *Cell* 1991;66:675–84.

16 Mistry AR, Pedersen EW, Solomon E, Grimwade D. The molecular pathogenesis of acute promyelocytic leukemia: implications for the clinical management of the disease. *Blood Rev* 2003;17:71–97.

17 Chambon P. A decade of molecular biology of retinoic acid receptors. *FASEB J* 1996;10:940–54.

18 Mangelsdorf DJ, Evans RM. The RXR heterodimers and orphan receptors. *Cell* 1995;83:841–50.

19 Minucci S, Ozato K. Retinoid receptors in transcriptional regulation. *Curr Opin Genet Dev* 1996;6:567–74.

20 Alcalay M, Zangrilli D, Fagioli M, *et al.* Expression pattern of the *RARalpha–PML* fusion gene in acute promyelocytic leukemia. *Proc Natl Acad Sci U S A* 1992;89:4840–4.

21 Grimwade D, Howe K, Langabeer S, *et al.* Establishing the presence of the t(15;17) in suspected acute promyelocytic leukemia: cytogenetic, molecular and PML immunofluorescence assessment of patients entered into the M.R.C. ATRA trial. M.R.C. Adult Leukemia Working Party. *Br J Haematol* 1996;94: 557–73.

22 Wang ZY, Chen Z. Acute promyelocytic leukemia: from highly fatal to highly curable. *Blood* 2008;111:2505–15.

23 Falini B, Flenghi L, Fagioli M, *et al.* Immunocytochemical diagnosis of acute promyelocytic leukemia (M3) with the monoclonal antibody PG-M3 (antiPML). *Blood* 1997;90:4046–53.

24 Lin RJ, Evans RM. Acquisition of oncogenic potential by RAR chimeras in acute promyelocytic leukemia through formation of homodimers. *Mol Cell* 2000;5:821–30.

25 Minucci S, Maccarana M, Cioce M, *et al.* Oligomerization of RAR and AML1 transcription factors as a novel mechanism of oncogenic activation. *Mol Cell* 2000;5:811–20.

26 Grignani F, De Matteis S, Nervi C, *et al.* Fusion proteins of the retinoic acid receptor- recruit histone deacetylase in promyelocytic. *Nature* 1998;391:815–18.

27 Larson RA, Kondo K, Vardiman JW, *et al.* Evidence for a 15;17 translocation in every patient with acute promyelocytic leukemia. *Am J Med* 1984;76:827–841.

28 Arnould C, Philippe C, Bourdon V, *et al.* The signal transducer and activator of transcription *STAT5b* gene is a new partner of retinoic acid receptor alpha in acute promyelocytic-like leukemia. *Hum Mol Genet* 1999 8:1741–9.

29 Chen Z, Brand NJ, Chen A, *et al.* Fusion between a novel Kruppel-like zinc finger gene and the retinoic acid receptor-alpha locus due to a variant t(11;17) translocation associated with acute promyelocytic leukemia. *EMBO J* 1993;12:1161–7.

30 Redner RL, Rush EA, Faas S, Rudert WA, Corey SJ. The t(5;17) variant of acute promyelocytic leukemia expresses a nucleophosmin-retinoic acid receptor fusion. *Blood* 1996;87: 882–6.

31 Wells RA, Catzavelos C, Kamel-Reid S. Fusion of retinoic acid receptor alpha to NuMA, the nuclear mitotic apparatus protein, by a variant translocation in acute promyelocytic leukemia. *Nat Genet* 1997;17:109–13.

32 Licht JD, Chomienne C, Goy A, *et al.* Clinical and molecular characterization of a rare syndrome of acute promyelocytic leukemia associated with translocation (11;17). *Blood* 1995; 85:1083–94.

33 Zheng PZ, Wang KK, Zhang QY, *et al.* Systems analysis of transcriptome and proteome in retinoic acid/arsenic trioxide-induced cell differentiation/apoptosis of promyelocytic leukemia. *Proc Natl Acad Sci U S A* 2005;102:7653–8.

34 Nervi C, Ferrara FF, Fanelli M, *et al.* Caspases mediate retinoic acid-induced degradation of the acute promyelocytic leukemia PML/RARalpha fusion protein. *Blood* 1998;92:2244–51.

35 Brown D, Kogan S, Lagasse E, *et al.* A *PMLRARalpha* transgene initiates murine acute promyelocytic leukemia. *Proc Natl Acad Sci U S A* 1997;94:2551–6.

36 vom Baur E, Zechel C, Heery D, *et al.* Differential ligand-dependent interactions between the AF-2 activating domain of nuclear receptors and the putative transcriptional intermediary factors mSUG1 and TIF1. *EMBO J* 1996;15:110–24.

37 Zhu J, Gianni M, Kopf E, *et al.* Retinoic acid induces proteosome-dependent degradation of retinoic acid receptor α (RARα) and oncogenic RARα fusion proteins. *Proc Natl Acad Sci U S A* 1999;96;14807–12.

38 Chen GQ, Shi XG, Tang W, *et al.* Use of arsenic trioxide (As2O3) in the treatment of acute promyelocytic leukemia (APL): I. As2O3 exerts dose-dependent dual effects on APL cells. *Blood* 1997;89:3345–53.

39 Hei TK, Filipic M. Role of oxidative damage in the genotoxicity of arsenic. *Free Radic Biol Med* 2004;37:574–81.

40 Hei TK, Liu SX, Waldren C. Mutagenicity of arsenic in mammalian cells: role of reactive oxygen species. *Proc Natl Acad Sci U S A* 1998;95:8103–7.

41 Chou WC, Jie C, Kenedy AA, *et al.* Role of NADPH oxidase in arsenic-induced reactive oxygen species formation and cytotoxicity in myeloid leukemia cells. *Proc Natl Acad Sci U S A* 2004;101:4578–83.

42 Zhou L, Jing Y, Styblo M, Chen Z, Waxman S. Glutathione-S-transferase pi inhibits As2O3-induced apoptosis in lymphoma cells: involvement of hydrogen peroxide catabolism. *Blood* 2005;105:1198–203.

43 Davison K, Mann KK, Waxman S, Miller WH, Jr. JNK activation is a mediator of arsenic trioxide-induced apoptosis in acute promyelocytic leukemia cells. *Blood* 2004;103:3496–502.

44 Huang C, Ma WY, Li J, Dong Z. Arsenic induces apoptosis through a c-Jun NH2-terminal kinase-dependent, p53-independent pathway. *Cancer Res* 1999;59:3053–8.

45 Paietta E. Expression of cell-surface antigens in acute promyelocytic leukemia. *Best Pract Res Clin Haematol* 2003;16:369–85.

46 Paietta E, Goloubeva O, Neuberg D, *et al.* A surrogate marker profile for *PML/RAR alpha* expressing acute promyelocytic leukemia and the association of immunophenotypic markers with morphologic and molecular subtypes. *Cytometry B Clin Cytom* 2004;59:1–9.

47 Albano F, Mestice A, Pannunzio A, *et al.* The biological characteristics of CD34+ CD2+ adult acute promyelocytic leukemia and the CD34 CD2 hypergranular (M3) and microgranular (M3v) phenotypes. *Haematologica* 2006;91:311–16.

48 Lo-Coco F, Cimino G, Breccia M, *et al.* Gemtuzumab ozogamicin (Mylotarg) as a single agent for molecularly relapsed acute promyelocytic leukemia. *Blood* 2004;104:1995–1999.

49 Gale RE, Hills R, Pizzey AR, *et al.* Relationship between *FLT3* mutation status, biologic characteristics, and response to targeted therapy in acute promyelocytic leukemia. *Blood* 2005; 106:3768–76.

50 Sievers E, Larson R, Stadmauer E, *et al.* Efficacy and safety of gemtuzumabozogamicin in patients with CD33-positive acute myeloid leukemia in first relapse. *J Clin Oncol* 2001;19: 3244–54.

51 Wellhausen SR, Peiper SC. CD33: biochemical and biological characterization and evaluation of clinical relevance. *J Biol Regul Homeost Agents* 2002;16:139–43.

52 Dedon PC, Salzberg AA, Xu J. Exclusive production of bistranded DNA damage by calicheamicin. *Biochemistry* 1993; 32:3617–22.

53 LaMarr WA, Yu L, Nicolaou KC, Dedon PC. Supercoiling affects the accessibility of glutathione to DNA-bound molecules: positive supercoiling inhibits calicheamicin-induced DNA damage. *Proc Natl Acad Sci U S A* 1998;95:102–7.

54 Yu L, Goldberg IH, Dedon PC. Enediyne-mediated DNA damage in nuclei is modulated at the level of the nucleosome. *J Biol Chem* 1994;269:4144–51.

55 Kumar RA, Ikemoto N, Patel DJ . Solution structure of the calicheamicin gamma 1I–DNA complex. *J Mol Biol* 1997;265: 187–201.

56 Zein N, Sinha AM, McGahren WJ, *et al.* Calicheamicin gamma 1I: an antitumor antibiotic that cleaves double-stranded DNA site specifically. *Science* 1988;240:1198–201.

57 Noguera NI, Breccia M, Divona M, *et al.* Alterations of the *FLT3* gene in acute promyelocytic leukemia: association with diagnostic characteristics and analysis of clinical outcome in patients treated with the Italian AIDA protocol. *Leukemia* 2002; 16:2185–9.

58 Marasca R, Maffei R, Zucchini P, *et al.* Gene expression profiling of acute promyelocytic leukemia identifies two subtypes mainly associated with *FLT3* mutational status. *Leukemia* 2006; 20:103–14.

59 Kelly LM, Kutok JL, Williams IR, *et al.* *PML/RARalpha* and *FLT3*-ITD induce an APL-like disease in a mouse model. *Proc Natl Acad Sci U S A* 2002;99:8283–8.

60 Kelly LM, Kutok JL, Williams IR, *et al.* *PML/RARalpha* and *FLT3*-ITD induce an APL-like disease in a mouse model. *Proc Natl Acad Sci U S A* 2002;99:8283–8.

Chapter 14
Acute Promyelocytic Leukemia: Manifestations and Therapy

Sylvain Thépot, Lionel Ades, and Pierre Fenaux
Service d'hématologie clinique, Hôpital Avicenne (Assistance Publique—Hôpitaux de Paris) and Paris 13 University, Bobigny, France

Introduction

First described in 1957 by Hillestad as a peculiar form of acute myeloid leukemia (AML) associated with morphologic characteristics of blast cells and a fatal evolution due to bleeding events [1], acute promyelocytic leukemia (APL) was later correlated in 1977 with a specific cytogenetic translocation, t(15;17) [2], which was shown in 1991 to fuse the *PML* and the *RARA* genes [3]. APL is probably the acute leukemia subtype that has benefited most from therapeutic progress over the last 20 years, a large majority of the patients being now cured using a combination of all-trans-retinoic acid (ATRA) and anthracycline-based chemotherapy, while arsenic derivatives occupy a growing place in the therapeutic armamentum by being the reference treatment of relapse and playing an increasing role in first-line treatment.

Clinical and biologic characteristics of acute promyelocytic leukemia

Clinical findings

The occurrence of APL is a relatively rare: the number of newly diagnosed cases per year is less than one case per million, representing <10% of all AML [4]. Its incidence seems to depend partly on ethnic and environmental factors, and previous exposures are increasingly incriminated (up to 15% of the cases in recent series), especially breast carcinoma treated by topoisomerase 2 inhibitors (anthracyclines, mitoxantrone, and, less often, VP-16) [5]. Contrary to other subsets of AML, the incidence increases with age until it reaches a plateau and decreases after the age of 55 [6].

Patients generally present with bleeding or, less often, other signs of bone marrow failure (fever, anemia) and pancytopenia on peripheral blood count. Bleeding is often severe, caused by the combination of thrombocytopenia (secondary to bone marrow failure) and coagulopathy (see below). It can include cutaneous purpura, often suggestive of the diagnosis in the presence of pancytopenia if extensive, and is associated with bleeding at injection sites (or, for example, at the site of marrow aspirate). The most severe form of bleeding is central nervous system (CNS) bleeding, which can be a presenting factor. Severe pulmonary bleeding can also develop. Organomegaly is rarely found at diagnosis, except sometimes in hyperleukocytic forms, while involvement of other organs at diagnosis (especially in the CNS and skin) is also rare.

Diagnosis is almost always suggested by the characteristic morphology of the leukemic population in bone marrow aspiration (M3 or M3v in the World Health Organization [WHO] classification), the presence of severe coagulopathy combining disseminated intravascular coagulopathy (DIC), fibrinolysis, and non-specific proteolysis, and is confirmed by the presence of t(15;17) translocation and of *PML–RARA* fusion gene by molecular analysis.

Blood and bone marrow examination in acute promyelocytic leukemia

As said above, the blood count is generally characterized by pancytopenia, with leukopenia being found in about 70% of the cases, and blast cells inconstantly seen in the blood. Leukocytosis (>10 g/L) is found in only about 25% of the cases, white blood cell (WBC) count being rarely >100 g/L. On bone marrow examination, the blast morphology in APL is characterized by cell nuclear shape, often kidney-shaped or bi-lobed, cytoplasm completely occupied by densely packed or even coalescent granules. In some cells the cytoplasm is filled with fine dust-like granules. At least a proportion of promyelocytic blasts contain several Auer rods, generally in bundles ("faggot cells"). Myeloperoxidase (MPO) is always strongly positive in all blast cells. Flow cytometry has been described

Leukemias: Principles and Practice of Therapy, 1st edition. Edited by S. Faderl and H. Kantarjian.

as $CD34^{-/+}$ heterogeneous, $CD117^{-/+}$ dim, $HLADR^{-/+}$ dim, $CD11b^{-}$, low levels of CD15, and frequent coexpression of the T-lineage marker CD2 with myeloid markers $CD13^{+}$ (heterogeneous) and $CD33^{+}$ (homogeneous) [7].

An atypical form (called an M3 variant or hypogranular form), usually associated with peripheral hyperleukocytosis, is observed in 10–20% of cases and is characterized by paucity or absence of granules, but a prominently bilobed nuclear shape. Careful examination often finds a few cells with several Auer rods.

Cytogenetic and molecular biology

A specific t(15;17)(q22;q12) translocation characterizes APL and is observed in >95% of the cases, leading to fusion of the retinoic acid receptor (*RAR*) gene on chromosome 17q12 to the promyelocytic leukemia (*PML*) gene on chromosome 15q22, and to a fusion mRNA and chimeric protein PML–RAR, with three different breakpoints at the mRNA level (Bcr1, 2, and 3).

Molecular analysis is mandatory to confirm the presence of the specific *PML–RAR* fusion and characterize its isoform, especially for subsequent molecular monitoring of minimal residual disease (MRD) during treatment.

Three very rare other different gene rearrangements can be observed, fusing (very rarely) RAR to promyelocytic leukemia zinc finger (*PLZF*, located in 11q23), or (quite exceptionally) *RAR* to nucleophosmin (*NPM*, located in 5q35), or nuclear matrix associated (*NuMA*, located in 11q13) genes.

Confirmation of genetic diagnosis should be performed on leukemia cells from bone marrow. Fluorescence *in situ* hybridization (FISH) analysis, which can be useful in case of conventional cytogenetic failure, is also preferably performed in bone marrow samples, as is real-time polymerase chain reaction (RT-PCR) analysis of *PML–RARA*, although the fusion transcript is usually readily detectable in peripheral blood (PB).

FLT3 internal tandem duplications (ITDs) are seen in one-third of the cases and are generally associated with a higher WBC count at presentation so that they do not add important independent prognostic information to WBC count, and, currently, *FLT3*-ITDs do not influence management [8,9].

Coagulopathy

In APL, patients can develop a fatal hemorrhage during diagnostic evaluation, even before beginning antileukemic therapy or during the first days of induction. It has been published that as many as 3% of patients with APL might die of hemorrhage before the onset of therapy [10]. The coagulation/bleeding syndrome at the onset of APL is a complex disorder that combines DIC, fibrinolysis, and a more general proteolysis. DIC involves the rapid consumption of coagulation factors and platelets and an intravascular clotting activation. Biologic clotting tests reveal hypofibrinogenemia, increased fibrinogen-fibrin degradation products (FDP), and prolonged prothrombin and thrombin times. When cytotoxic chemotherapy was the only treatment available, coagulation parameters usually worsened when it was initiated, resulting in severe hemorrhagic complications while, in contrast, ATRA rapidly improves the hemostatic laboratory parameters and bleeding complications and should therefore be started as soon as the diagnosis of APL is suspected upon morphologic examination, without waiting for genetic confirmation of diagnosis.

Prognostic factors in acute promyelocytic leukemia

Pretreatment factors associated with a higher risk of relapse include high WBC counts, M3v morphology, presence of the short Bcr3 transcript, CD2 and CD34 expression, *FLT3*-ITD, and slow and incomplete *in vitro* differentiation of blasts with ATRA [11–16].

With the exception of the last, these parameters are, in fact, generally correlated to high WBC counts. The Sanz score is a predictive model for relapse risk based on patient leukocyte and platelet counts at diagnosis that distinguishes three groups: low-risk patients with a WBC count <10 g/L and a platelet count >40 g/L; intermediate-risk patients with a WBC count <10 g/L and a platelet count <40 g/L; and high-risk patients with a WBC count >10 g/L [17]. In fact, for therapeutic purposes, low and intermediate-risk groups are often combined, individualizing the high-risk group characterized by a WBC count >10 g/L that carries a greater risk of early death and relapse. However, some therapeutic improvements in APL have particularly benefited patients with high WBC counts, and their prognosis now appears almost identical to that of patients with lower WBC counts in very recent experiences [18].

The major prognostic factor of relapse during or after treatment is the amount of fusion PML–RARα mRNA transcripts, determined by RT-PCR in bone marrow cells, increasingly using a quantitative method [19–23]. However, kinetics of the disappearance of the PML-RARα transcript depend on the sensitivity of the RT-PCR method used. Persistent positivity after consolidation treatment or, later on, switch to positivity in patients who were negative using low-sensitivity methods (sensitivity of 10^{-3} to 10^{-4}) indicates probable relapse in the following few weeks or months. On the other hand, very sensitive quantitative methods require interpretation based on the detection limit, and require repeated examinations to assess the increase, stability, or decrease of the abnormal signal during follow-up.

First-line treatment of acute promyelocytic leukemia

Background: ATRA combined with anthracycline-based chemotherapy in the treatment of newly diagnosed APL

Before the advent of ATRA, APL was treated exclusively by conventional chemotherapy using anthracycline with or without cytarabine. With this chemotherapy and intensive platelet support during induction treatment, complete remission (CR) rates of 70–80% were obtained, and about 40% of the patients who achieved CR could be cured of their disease with consolidation chemotherapy—more than other types of AML [24].

ATRA can differentiate APL blasts both *in vitro* and *in vivo*. With ATRA treatment alone, 85–90% of newly diagnosed APL cases can obtain CR through differentiation of APL blasts into mature granulocyte [24–28]. In addition, ATRA rapidly improves the biologic signs of APL coagulopathy. However, in some cases, ATRA can also lead to major blood hyperleukocytosis and potentially fatal "ATRA syndrome" (subsequently renamed "leukocyte-activation syndrome" [LAS], as it can also be observed with arsenic derivatives). Furthermore, almost all patients relapse unless they receive consolidation chemotherapy. Those findings rapidly lead clinical groups to combine ATRA and classical anthracycline-Ara-C chemotherapy in the treatment of newly diagnosed APL, in order to reduce the incidence and severity of ATRA syndrome and the incidence of relapse. Many trials, including two randomized trials performed in the 1990s (European APL 91 trial and a US intergroup trial) clearly showed that ATRA followed by two or three anthracycline-Ara-C chemotherapy cycles could reduce the incidence of relapse from 50% with chemotherapy alone to about 25%, while slightly increasing the CR rate from 80% to about 90% [29,30].

This, however, means that about 10% of the patients still did not achieve CR and about 25% relapsed with a regimen (combining ATRA and several courses of anthracycline-Ara-C courses) that was associated with important myelosuppression, and there was also a mortality rate of about 5% in CR (up to 15–20% in elderly patients). Failure to achieve CR owed mainly to bleeding (principally in the CNS), infection, or LAS rather than leukemic failure, which is extremely rare (about 1 in 500 in confirmed cases of APL).

Optimization of first-line APL treatment in the late 1990s and early 2000s

The following years were therefore used to improve results obtained with this ATRA and anthracycline-based chemotherapy "backbone." Many experiences have reported that early addition of chemotherapy to ATRA, optimal prevention and treatment of LAS, intensive treatment of coagulopathy, and maintenance treatment could further reduce early mortality and the incidence of relapse, while reduction of the intensity of chemotherapy (by the possible avoidance of Ara-C in most cases) has reduced treatment toxicity. Finally, the most recent years have been characterized by introduction of arsenic derivatives in the first-line treatment of APL by several groups.

With those improvements, reported CR rates are now closer to 95% than 90%, relapse rates have dropped to <10% (although they remain a little higher in patients with high WBC counts), and mortality in CR has also diminished, giving the hope that APL may now be cured in the vast majority of cases.

Role of early addition of chemotherapy to ATRA

It was clearly shown that treatment with ATRA combined with intensive chemotherapy gave better results than intensive chemotherapy alone in newly diagnosed APL and that ATRA should be started immediately after APL diagnosis wass suspected; however, whether chemotherapy should be administered after or concomitantly with ATRA remained uncertain.

Results of a trial randomizing ATRA followed by chemotherapy and ATRA with early addition of chemotherapy (on day 3 of ATRA treatment) in APL with WBC counts <10 g/L showed similar CR rates but a strong trend for few relapses (21.6% vs. 13.2% at 10 years, $P = 0.09$) in patients who had early addition of chemotherapy. Early addition of chemotherapy also reduced the incidence of LAS, one of the persisting causes of failure to achieve CR in APL [31]. In patients with a WBC count >10 g/L, rapid addition of chemotherapy to ATRA appears particularly recommended to avoid the risk of severe LAS [18].

Prophylaxis and treatment of the leukocyte differentiation or activation syndrome and other side-effects of ATRA

The LAS was first described with ATRA [32] but is also seen with arsenic derivatives. Its pathophysiology remains uncertain, but probably includes the release of various cytokines by differentiating leukocytes: induction of interleukin 1 α (IL1-α) and G-CSF secretion by APL cells under ATRA treatment may contribute to hyperleukocytosis *in vivo*, while the secretion of IL1-α, IL6, tumor necrosis factor α (TNF-α), and IL8—which are involved in leukocyte activation and adherence, and are implicated in the development of acute respiratory distress syndrome (ARDS)—could play a pathogenetic role in LAS [33,34]. More recently, it has been shown that ATRA induces aggregation of NB4 cells (an APL cell line). This process was mediated by the adhesion molecules lymphocyte function associated antigen 1 (LFA-1) and intercellular adhesion molecule 2 (ICAM-2), and was reversed by addition of methylprednisolone [35]. These findings suggest that modification of the adhesive properties of APL cells by ATRA could play a role in LAS.

Diagnosis of this syndrome should be suspected clinically in the presence of one of the following symptoms and signs: dyspnea, unexplained fever, weight gain, peripheral edema, unexplained hypotension, acute renal failure, or congestive heart failure, but particularly by a chest radiograph demonstrating interstitial pulmonary infiltrates or pleuropericardial effusion. Those symptoms are not pathognomonic of the syndrome, as they could in this context be due to bacteremia, sepsis, fungal infection, or congestive heart failure. Incidence of LAS ranges from 10% to 15% in different series [36,37]. Symptoms generally occur around 7 and 11 days after drug onset and are generally, but not always, preceded by an increase of WBC. In some cases, LAS occurs very early but can also occur at the time of recovery from aplasia in patients treated with ATRA who received early intensive chemotherapy. LAS is fatal in 5–15% of cases. In addition, its occurrence is associated with an increased risk of subsequent relapse [38]. As said above, in our experience (APL 93 trial), early addition of chemotherapy to ATRA in newly diagnosed APL with low WBC counts significantly reduced the incidence of ATRA syndrome [39].

In APL presenting with high WBC counts, very early addition of chemotherapy to ATRA (on day 1 or 2 of ATRA treatment) is recommended by most teams to prevent a risk of severe LAS.

Specific treatment with dexamethasone at a dosage of 10 mg twice daily by intravenous injection should be started promptly at the very earliest symptom or sign of LAS [40]. Temporary discontinuation of ATRA or arsenic trioxide (ATO) is indicated only in case of severe LAS (ie, patients developing renal failure or requiring admission to the intensive care unit owing to respiratory distress). Otherwise, these differentiating agents can generally be maintained unless progression to overt syndrome or lack of response to dexamethasone is observed. If a favorable response is obtained, dexamethasone should be maintained until complete disappearance of symptoms, and then ATRA or ATO should be resumed.

While this pre-emptive therapy with dexamethasone currently represents a standard approach to treat patients developing LAS, there is no evidence that prophylactic corticosteroids are useful to reduce rates of morbidity and mortality associated with this syndrome. Nevertheless, in uncontrolled studies, very low mortality or morbidity due to LAS was reported following ATRA treatment when corticosteroids were administered prophylactically in patients presenting with a WBC count >5–10×10^9/L, particularly in our experience [18].

Other side-effects of ATRA include dryness of lips and mucosae that are usual but reversible with symptomatic treatment. Increases in transaminases and triglycerides are common, but they have never required treatment discontinuation in our experience. Headache, caused by intracranial hypertension, is generally moderate in adults but may be severe in children and associated with signs of pseudotumor cerebri [41].

Lower ATRA doses (25 mg/m^2 per day) reduce this side-effect in children and seem as effective as conventional doses of 45 mg/m^2 per day in inducing CR. Isolated fever frequently develops in the absence of other signs of ATRA syndrome (or infection) and is reversible within 48 h of ATRA discontinuation.

A few other side-effects, including bone marrow necrosis, hypercalcemia, erythema nodosum, marked basophilia, severe myositis, Sweet syndrome, Fournier gangrene (necrotizing fasciitis of the penis and scrotum), thrombocytosis, and necrotizing vasculitis have rarely been reported with ATRA treatment [42–51].

Optimal treatment of coagulopathy

Intracerebral and pulmonary bleeding are not only the most frequent causes of death early during induction therapy but they can also occur before the diagnosis of APL has been made and therapy started. To prevent them, supportive measures should be instituted immediately after a diagnosis of APL is suspected. ATRA should be started before the diagnosis is confirmed in order to minimize the risk of severe bleeding [52].

Supportive care consists of an extremely large transfusion of platelets in order to maintain a platelet count >50 g/L whenever possible. Fresh frozen plasma and fibrinogen are advocated in case of a fibrinogen level <150 mg/dL. Platelet and fibrinogen monitoring is required once a day or more.

Central venous catheterization, lumbar puncture, and other invasive procedures (eg, bronchoscopy) should be avoided at this stage of the treatment.

The benefit of heparin, tranexamic acid, or another anticoagulant or antifibrinolytic therapy in attenuating the hemorrhagic syndrome is unclear.

Role of maintenance treatment

Two randomized studies, the APL 93 and the US intergroup trials, showed that maintenance treatment with continuous low-dose chemotherapy (in the APL 93 trial), with ATRA (in the US and APL 93 trials), or with both (in the APL 93 trial) significantly decreased the incidence of relapse in comparison to cases with no maintenance treatment at all, with an additional effect on relapse of the two modalities in newly diagnosed APL [53,54].

Patients with a high WBC count particularly seemed to benefit from maintenance in the APL 93 trial: in patients with a WBC count >5 g/L, the relapse rate dropped from 64.5% with no maintenance to 20.5% with combined ATRA and chemotherapy maintenance. Interestingly, the effect of the low-dose chemotherapy component of maintenance treatment seemed even more important than that of maintenance ATRA. Long-term results in APL 93 also showed significantly more relapse in patients who discontinued maintenance treatment before 1 year (for reasons other than relapse) compared with patients who received longer maintenance.

Role of Ara-C

Classical consolidation chemotherapy cycles combining an anthracycline and Ara-C are associated with a mortality rate of about 5% in younger adults, which can, however, reach 15–20% in elderly patients. Further improvement in the outcome of APL would require a reduction of this mortality in CR, especially through a reduction of the intensity of consolidation chemotherapy. Owing to this perspective, a major attempt has been made to avoid using Ara-C during consolidation chemotherapy courses.

Before the era of ATRA, a few studies had suggested that chemotherapy with an anthracycline alone, especially idarubicin, provided it was given at relatively high dose, gave similar results as anthracycline-Ara-C regimens.

Since the advent of ATRA, the Spanish PETHEMA group have gained the most experience of chemotherapy with ATRA and anthracycline alone in patients with APL, with two successive trials (LPA 96 and 99 trials) [55,56]. The induction regimen consists of ATRA and idarubicin ($12\,mg/m^2 \times 4$) followed by three consolidation courses with idarubicin or mitoxantrone (with ATRA in patients at intermediate- or high-risk of relapse) and a 2-year maintenance therapy combining low-dose 6-mercaptopurine and methotraxane chemotherapy and ATRA. The consolidation chemotherapy courses with an anthracycline alone could be generally administered in outpatients and are associated with low morbidity and no mortality. Five-year cumulative incidence of relapse (CIR) and disease-free survival were 11% and 84%, respectively. Nevertheless, in patients with a WBC count >10 g/L and a WBC count >50 g/L, the 5-year cumulative incidence of relapse was 23% and 34%, respectively.

In order to confirm these results in a randomized trial, the APL 2000 trial (conducted by the European APL group) randomized, in patients aged ≤60 years with a WBC count of <10 g/L, the best treatment group from the APL 93 trial (ATRA with early introduction of anthracycline-Ara-C chemotherapy [Ara-C group]) followed by a group with two consolidation anthracycline-Ara-C courses and maintenance combining continuous chemotherapy and intermittent ATRA to the same regimen, but without Ara-C (no Ara-C group). In the Ara-C and the no Ara-C group, the CR rate was 99% versus 94% ($P = 0.066$), the 2-year CIR was 4.7% versus 15.9% ($P = 0.011$) and overall survival (OS) was 97.9% versus 89.6% ($P = 0.0066$). These results suggested that, in patients with a WBC <10 g/L (ie, at low risk of relapse), an anthracycline alone for chemotherapy instead of the classical anthracycline–Ara-C combination could lead to an increased risk of relapse. Discrepancies between our results and those of the PETHEMA group studies could be due to the higher cumulative dose of anthracycline administered in the Spanish studies or to a superiority of idarubicin (used in Spanish trial) over daunorubicin (used in European and US intergroup trials) in APL. Thus, substituting idarubicin for daunorubicin during induction and consolidation treatment could improve long-term results in APL. Finally, using ATRA during consolidation courses, as in LPA 99 trial, may have had a positive impact on the risk of relapse.

To better understand these discrepancies, a joint analysis was performed in younger patients included in the Spanish PETHEMA LPA 99 trial (without Ara-C) and the APL 2000 trial (with Ara-C). In low and intermediate-risk patients, the CR rates, 2-year CIR, event-free survival (EFS), and OS were not significantly different in the LPA 99 and the APL 2000 trials. In high-risk patients, the CR rate was significantly better for those included in the APL 2000 trial, and the CIR was significantly lower than in patients treated in the LPA 99 trial [57].

This analysis suggests that, in patients with a WBC count <10 g/L, the current PETHEMA approach is not associated with more relapses than a classic ATRA plus daunorubicin plus Ara-C regimen, while also being clearly less myelosuppressive. It also strongly suggests that, if one uses an anthracycline alone, daunorubicin should not be substituted for idarubicin, as it may be less effective in APL. In patients with high WBC counts, the APL 2000 results yielded better EFS and OS and a strong trend for fewer relapses than the PETHEMA results, suggesting a beneficial role for Ara-C, possibly at high dose, in this subset of patients [58]. The Italian GIMEMA group and German group results, although they were not randomized, also strongly support a role for Ara-C in reducing the relapse rate in cases of APL with a WBC count >10 g/L [59,60]. In the ongoing Spanish PETHEMA LPA 2005 trial, which now includes Ara-C during consolidation in patients with high WBC counts, a great reduction in the risk of relapse has been observed in this subset of patients [61]. As shown below, it is currently being investigated whether arsenic derivatives could be substituted for Ara-C in this situation.

Role of arsenic derivatives

The most commonly used arsenic derivative for the treatment of APL is ATO, which is the treatment of choice for patients with relapsing APL. It is not particularly associated with the toxicities commonly observed with other anthracycline-based chemotherapies, especially myelosuppression (see Treatment of relapses section). Owing to this, investigators from China, Iran, and India, as well as Western countries, are assessing the role of ATO in newly diagnosed APL in three approaches: (i) ATO used in addition to ATRA and anthracycline-based chemotherapies, particularly in cases with an increased risk of relapse (mainly patients with high WBC counts); (ii) ATO used as a possible replacement for some of the chemotherapies administered; and (iii) ATO used to completely avoid any concomitant chemotherapy [62–64].

Using the first approach, a Chinese trial randomized patients with newly diagnosed APL for induction between ATRA alone, ATO alone, and the combination of both. Patients who achieved CR then received anthracycline-based consolidation chemotherapy. The CR rate was the same in the three treatment arms, but decrease of the fusion transcript was faster and, more importantly, the incidence of relapse was significantly lower in patients treated with the ATRA–ATO combination upfront [62]. A US intergroup trial randomly evaluated the benefit of two additional courses of ATO as the first postremission therapy in a standard treatment based on ATRA and anthracycline–Ara-C chemotherapy. Three-year EFS was 77% in the ATO arm compared with 59% in the standard arm, and 3-year overall survival (OS) was 86% in the ATO arm compared with 77% in the standard arm. The benefit of the addition of two courses of ATO consolidation following remission induction was particularly important in patients presenting with high WBC counts (Powell, Comprehensive Cancer Center, Wake Forest University, Winston-Salem, NC, presented at ASCO 2007, no full paper as yet).

For investigating the second approach, ATO was used alone or with limited ATRA and chemotherapy. In a trial in India, patients received ATO as a single agent for induction and one consolidation course of 28 days, followed by maintenance courses of 10 days per month over 6 months. The CR rate was 86%, and the disease-free survival and OS were 87% and 86%, respectively [64].

Similar results, although with a higher relapse rate (40% vs. 15%), were observed in an Iranian trial that used the same approach of induction and one consolidation course of ATO alone, but without maintenance treatment. The M. D. Anderson group also reported on 44 patients who received ATO and ATRA for induction (associated with gemtuzumab ozogamycin in high-risk patients) with an 89% CR rate (all with molecular CR) [65]. In low- and intermediate-risk patients, the CR rate was 96%. Very few relapses (exclusively in high-risk patients) were seen with ATRA–ATO maintenance.

These reports are impressive, as they constitute the first demonstration that a leukemia can be cured without any chemotherapy. On the other hand, the experiences using ATO as a single agent during induction treatment of APL generally reported relatively high incidences of sometimes-fatal LAS. The risk may even be higher if ATRA is combined with ATO upfront. This complication could be avoided by early introduction of chemotherapy or gemtuzumab ozogamicin , as reported by the M. D. Anderson group [65]. However, given the very high CR rates obtained with ATRA anthracycline-based chemotherapy, now about 95% in most trials, we feel that induction protocols without chemotherapy—with ATO alone or with ATO combined to ATRA—need to be validated in large multicenter trials before they can be recommended outside of specialized centers.

Central nervous system prophylaxis

The CNS is the commonest site of extramedullary disease in APL [66]. In the European and PETHEMA group experience, 10 of the 169 relapses observed were extramedullary, mainly in the CNS ($n = 9$), and, less often, the skin ($n = 1$). In eight of the cases, the marrow was also involved by the relapse, with the presence of blasts in seven but only molecular relapse in one. Patients with extramedullary relapse in the CNS were characterized by younger age, higher WBC count, and treatment without high-dose Ara-C [67]. Prognosis was poor with a median survival of 13 months. Because the majority of CNS relapses occur in patients presenting with hyperleukocytosis, some groups, including ours, therefore include CNS prophylaxis for patients presenting with high WBC counts, using intrathecal methotraxane plus Ara-C and/or systemic high-dose Ara-C, although the benefit of this policy has not been established in prospective studies. Intrathecal therapy, in addition, should not be performed during induction treatment owing to the risk of bleeding, but started only during consolidation treatment.

In patients without hyperleukocytosis, in whom the risk of extramedullary relapse in the CNS is extremely low, there is a general consensus to avoid CNS prophylaxis. Finally, preliminary findings suggest that ATO may cross the blood–brain barrier, further supporting its wider use during consolidation first-line treatment of APL [68].

Molecular and cytogenetic evaluation

The molecular status at the end of induction has no predictive value on patient outcome even using low-sensitivity methods (ie, with detection threshold between 10^{-3} and 10^{-4}) [69]. After consolidation treatment, molecular evaluation of MRD performed on bone marrow cells using low-sensitivity methods is well correlated to the risk of relapse. Patients with persistent MRD at the end of consolidation using such low-sensitivity methods should be considered for further treatment instead of only maintenance [70] remission as well as molecular relapse have recently been incorporated in response criteria in APL [71]. During maintenance and follow-up in patients with undetectable MRD, conversion to MRD positivity is associated with generally rapid hematologic relapse [72], leading more and more groups to treat those patients without waiting for marrow relapse [73].

Patients at higher risk of relapse, such as patients with a WBC count >10 g/L at diagnosis, should be closely monitored—at least five or six times per year during the first year and then every 3 months during the second and third year. The monitoring of patients at low risk of relapse is nowadays a question of debate. Finally, quantitative RT-PCR techniques (RQ-PCR) are increasingly being used in APL, and efforts are being made to reach consensus technical approaches [21]. The kinetics of evolution of the fusion transcript may sometimes give more adequate and/or rapid information than the positive versus negative information provided by RQ-PCR. However, the clinical advantage of RQ-PCR over classic techniques needs to be more firmly determined.

Treatment of relapsing acute promyelocytic leukemia

Induction treatment

Arsenic derivatives

Arsenic derivatives, especially ATO, currently constitute the reference induction treatment of APL in first relapse (or subsequent relapses in patients who have not previously received arsenic derivatives).

ATO induces 80–90% of second hematologic CR, in most cases associated to molecular CR after two cycles (contrary to that achieved with ATRA alone) [74]. ATO may act on APL cells in several ways, including induction of differentiation and/or apoptosis, growth inhibition, and angiogenesis inhibition. Like ATRA, ATO triggers the degradation of the PML–RARα fusion protein, but contrary to ATRA, ATO targets the PML part rather than the RARα part of this fusion protein. The safety profile of ATO compares favorably with the safety profile of intensive salvage chemotherapy, particularly as it lacks profound cytopenia and cardiac failure [75]. Treatment with ATO is associated with electrolyte abnormalities and prolongation of the QT interval, both of which require careful monitoring. Maintenance of serum potassium >4.0 mmol/L and serum magnesium >0.82 mmol/L, well above the lower limit of normal, is mandatory to avoid the risk of cardiac arrhythmias, the most severe being torsades de pointe. Medications that may cause prolonged QTc intervals have to be stopped. If the QTc interval is prolonged for longer than 500 ms, ATO should be discontinued. ATO also carries the risk of LAS; however, this is generally less important in relapse than in newly diagnosed patients. However, if a major increase in WBC counts is seen, preventive and therapeutic measures could be rapidly taken, as for first-line treatment.

Other induction treatments of relapse

Even before the ATO era, relatively high rates of second CR could be obtained with intensive anthracycline-based chemotherapy or, in patients who had not received ATRA within a few months of relapse, with ATRA chemotherapy combinations. This treatment was, however, associated with major toxicity, and poorer results of subsequent allogeneic stem-cell transplantation (SCT) [76].

Preliminary results indicate that gemtuzumab ozogamicin might be a promising agent in patients with APL, particularly in case of molecular relapse [77]. The M. D. Anderson group also reported interesting results with gemtuzumab ozogamicin in consolidation with ATO and ATRA after ATO induction in first relapse [65].

Tamibarotène (Am80) is a new synthetic retinoid approximately 10 times more potent than ATRA as an *in vitro* differentiation inducer. This drug is potentially capable of overcoming resistance to ATRA because of its hypermetabolism. In a Japanese study, Am80 produced 58% CR in patients who had relapsed from CR induced by ATRA. However, because all those patients had discontinued ATRA for at least 18 months, it is unclear whether Am80 was superior to ATRA in this situation, and whether it would be able to overcome resistance to ATRA [78].

Finally, it is unclear, with the probable exception of gemtuzumab ozogamicin, if those approaches can be effective in patients who have already received ATO, especially in first relapse.

Consolidation/maintenance treatment

At least two, and sometimes three, cycles of ATO (ie, at least one induction course and one or two consolidation courses for 5 days per week over 5 weeks) are generally required to achieve molecular remission in relapsing APL. Once this has been obtained, consolidation with autologous or allogeneic SCT is strongly recommended to obtain sustained second CR [75]. Because it is associated with few relapses (if stem cells are collected after molecular CR has been achieved) and low toxicity, autologous SCT is increasingly advocated at the expense of allogeneic SCT. Reaching molecular CR may, however, sometimes require consolidation chemotherapy or gemtuzumab ozogamicin before stem-cell collection in addition to ATO [79]. If molecular CR cannot be obtained, and probably also in younger patients (<30 years), allogeneic SCT is preferred to autologous SCT. In patients who can be neither allo- nor autografted, maintenance treatment should use variable combinations of ATRA, ATO, anthracyclines with or without Ara-C, gemtuzumab ozogamicin, and maintenance with 6-mercaptopurine and methotrexate, depending on what the patient received before relapse.

The improvement in the treatment of relapsing APL is stressed by the results of our group, with a 2-year survival of 77% in patients with relapsing APL salvaged by ATO (and consolidated by allogeneic SCT, autologous SCT, or various maintenance regimens), as compared with 51% in a similar population treated before the arsenic era [76].

Treatment in elderly patients and in children

Acute promyelocytic leukemia in the elderly

As mentioned above, APL is relatively uncommon in older patients, as only 20% of APL are aged >60 years.

Elderly patients with APL are more likely to present with low-risk features than younger patients [80]. In our experience (APL 93 trial), the CR rate was 94% for those <60 years of age compared with 85% for those >70 years of age [81], the difference exclusively due to a higher incidence of early deaths in older patients, as those patients, like younger ones, had no case of resistant leukemia. The relapse rate was not higher in elderly patients compared with younger adults, but the mortality rate in CR was 19% in patients >70 years of age, mainly due to sepsis secondary to neutropenia [81]. Reducing the intensity of consolidation therapy in elderly patients is therefore of utmost importance. The PETHEMA group reported, with their regimen devoid of Ara-C, a 6-year CIR of 8.5% in elderly patients consolidated without Ara-C, with <8.2% mortality in CR [80].

The intensity of consolidation chemotherapy can probably be even further decreased by using ATO during consolidation courses. On the other hand, as said above for all patients, caution must be exercised during induction treatment if one is to use ATO with or without ATRA without chemotherapy because of the risk of severe LAS, particularly in this fragile population [65].

Acute promyelocytic leukemia in children

The occurrence of APL in children is also rare. Compared with the disease in adults, APL in childhood more frequently presents with hyperleukocytosis (approximately 40% in children vs. 20–25% in adults) [82]. The therapeutic strategy for children has generally been similar to that used for adults, combining ATRA and chemotherapy [82,83–85]. Owing to the frequent occurrence of headaches, and even clinical features of pseudointracranial hypertension, however, reduced doses of ATRA (ie, $25\,mg/m^2$ per day) are often used either systematically or only if those symptoms occur (and we would favor this latter approach in order to maximize the quantity of ATRA administered) [86].

Some attempts have been made to reduce the cumulative dose of anthracyclines in children because of their potential long-term cardiac toxicity. However, preliminary analysis of the US Intergroup study of children treated with ATRA and reduced dose intensity of anthracycline-based chemotherapy has not been encouraging [87]. Although ATO also appears to be effective in pediatric APL [88], there is only very limited experience of this agent in children with newly diagnosed APL, possibly because of the concerns of pediatricians about using a drug with potential long-term side-effects [89].

Conclusion

With protocols combining ATRA and idarubicin, intensive supportive care during induction treatment (especially platelet transfusions), and prolonged maintenance, >95% of cases of APL with WBC counts $<10{,}000/mm^3$ reach CR and <10% relapse. Patients with higher WBC counts have an early death risk of around 10%, which, however, can be further reduced by rapid introduction of chemotherapy and particularly intensive platelet support. In those patients, Ara-C or possibly ATO (in addition to maintenance) should be added to idarubicin in order to reduce the relapse rate (probably to ≤10%). ATO, which remains the gold standard for relapse, can be administered during first-line treatment in addition to chemotherapy in order to reduce the relapse risk (in patients with high WBC counts) or, to some extent, be substituted for chemotherapy (in elderly or frail patients), mainly during the consolidation period. On the other hand, we feel that its place during first-line induction treatment has to be further validated in multicenter trials, particularly because of the risk of LAS. Finally, owing to the drug armamentum we have, allogeneic or autologous SCT are now generally restricted to the consolidation treatment of first relapse.

References

1 Hillestad LK. Acute promyelocytic leukemia. *Acta Med Scand* 1957;159:189–94.

2 Rowley J, Golomb HM, Dougherty C. 15/17 translocation, a consistent chromosomal change in acute promyelocytic leukemia. *Lancet* 1977;1:549–50.

3 de Thé H, Lavau C, Marchio A, Chomienne C, Degos L, Dejean A. The PML–RARA fusion mRNA generated by the t(15,17) translocation in PML. *Cell* 1991;66:675–84.

4 Ribeiro R, Rego R. Management of APL in developing countries: epidemiology, challenges and opportunities for international collaboration. *Hematology Am Soc Hematol Educ Program* 2006;162–8.

5 Beaumont M, Sanz M, Carli PM, *et al*. Therapy related acute promyelocytic leukemia. A report on 106 cases. *J Clin Oncol* 2003;21:2123–37.

6 Vickers M, Jackson G, Taylor P. The incidence of acute promyelocytic leukemia appears constant over most of a human lifespan, implying only one rate limiting mutation. *Leukemia* 2000;14:722–6.

7 Orfao A, Ortuño F, de Santiago M, Lopez A, San Miguel JF. Immunophenotyping of acute leukemias and myelodysplastic syndromes. *Cytometry* 2004;58A:62–71.

8 Callens C, Chevret S, Cayuela JM, *et al*. Prognostic implication of *FLT3* and *Ras* gene mutations in patients with acute promyelocytic leukemia (APL): a retrospective study from the European APL Group. *Leukemia* 2005;19:1153–60.

9 Gale RE, Hills R, Pizzey AR, *et al*. Relationship between *FLT3* mutation status, biologic characteristics, and response to tar-

geted therapy in acute promyelocytic leukemia. *Blood* 2005; 106:3768–76.

10 De la Serna J, Montesinos P, Vellenga E, *et al.* Causes and prognostic factors of remission induction failure in patients with acute promyelocytic leukemia treated with all-trans retinoic acid and idarubicin. *Blood* 2008;111:3395–402.

11 Asou N, Adachi K, Tamura J, *et al.* Analysis of prognostic factors in newly diagnosed acute promyelocytic leukemia treated with all-trans retinoic acid and chemotherapy. Japan Adult Leukemia Study Group. *J Clin Oncol* 1998;16:78–85.

12 Claxton DF, Reading CL, Nagarajan L, *et al.* Correlation of CD2 expression with *PML* gene breakpoints in patients with acute promyelocytic leukemia. *Blood* 1992;80:582–6.

13 Paietta E, Andersen J, Gallagher R, *et al.* The immunophenotype of acute promyelocytic leukemia (APL): an ECOG study. *Leukemia* 1994;8:1108–12.

14 Guglielmi C, Martelli MP, Diverio D, *et al.* Immunophenotype of adult and childhood acute promyelocytic leukemia correlation with morphology, type of *PML* gene breakpoint and clinical outcome, a cooperative Italian study on 196 cases. *Br J Haematol* 1998;102:1035–41.

15 Murray CK, Estey E, Paietta E, *et al.* CD56 expression in acute promyelocytic leukemia: a possible indicator of poor treatment outcome? *J Clin Oncol* 1999;17:293–7.

16 Cassinat B, Chevret S, Zassadowski F, *et al.* *In vitro* all-trans retinoic acid sensitivity of acute promyelocytic leukemia blasts: a novel indicator of poor patient outcome. *Blood* 2001;98:2862–4.

17 Sanz MA, Lo Coco F, Martin G, *et al.* Definition of relapse risk and role of non anthracycline drugs for consolidation in patients with acute promyelocytic leukemia: a joint study of the PETHEMA and GIMEMA cooperative groups. *Blood* 2000;96: 1247–53.

18 Kelaidi C, Chevret S, De Botton S, *et al.* Improved outcome of acute promyelocytic leukemia with high WBC counts over the last 15 years: the European APL group experience. J *Clin Oncol* 2009;27:2668–76.

19 Jurcic JG, Nimer SD, Scheinberg DA, de Blasio T, Warrell RP, Jr., Miller WH, Jr. Prognostic significance of minimal residual disease detection and PML/RAR- isoformtype: long-term follow-up in acute promyelocytic leukemia. *Blood* 2001;98: 2651–6.

20 Diverio D, Rossi V, Avvisati G, *et al.* Early detection of relapse by prospective reverse transcriptase-polymerase chain reaction analysis of the *PML/RARalpha* fusion gene in patients with acute promyelocytic leukemia enrolled in the GIMEMA-AIEOP multicenter "AIDA" trial. GIMEMA AIEOP Multicenter "AIDA" Trial. *Blood* 1998;92:784–9.

21 Cassinat B, Zassadowski F, Balitrand N, *et al.* Quantitation of minimal residual disease in acute promyelocytic leukemia patients with t(15;17) translocation using real-time RTPCR. *Leukemia* 2000;14:324.

22 Visani G, Buonamici S, Malagola M, *et al.* Pulsed ATRA as single therapy restores longterm remission PML-RARalpha-positive acute promyelocytic leukemia patient real time quantification of minimal residual disease. A pilot study. *Leukemia* 2000; 15:1696–700.

23 Gallagher RE, Yeap BY, Bi W, *et al.* Quantitative real-time RT-PCR analysis of PML-RAR alpha mRNA in acute promyelocytic leukemia: assessment of prognostic significance in adult patients from intergroup protocol 0129. *Blood* 2003;101:2521–8.

24 Bernard J, Weil M, Boiron M, Jacquillat C, Flandrin G, Gemon MF. Acute promyelocytic leukemia: results of treatment by daunorubicin. *Blood* 1973;41:489–96.

25 Castaigne S, Chomienne C, Daniel MT, *et al.* All-trans retinoic acid as a differentiation therapy for acute promyelocytic leukemia. I. Clinical results. *Blood* 1990;76:1704–9.

26 Degos L, Chomienne C, Daniel MT, *et al.* Treatment of first relapse in acute promyelocytic leukemia with all-trans retinoic acid. *Lancet* 1990;336:1440–1.

27 Chen ZX, Xue YQ, Zhang R, *et al.* A clinical and experimental study on all-trans retinoic acid-treated acute promyelocytic leukemia patients. *Blood* 1991;78:1413–1.9

28 Warrell RP, Jr., Frankel SR, Miller WH, Jr., *et al.* Differentiation therapy of acute promyelocytic leukemia with tretinoin (all-trans-retinoic acid). *N Engl J Med* 1991;324:1385–93.

29 Fenaux P, Le Deley MC, Castaigne S, *et al.* Effect of all transretinoic acid in newly diagnosed acute promyelocytic leukemia. Results of a multicenter randomized trial. European APL 91 Group. *Blood* 1993;82:3241–9.

30 Tallman MS, Andersen JW, Schiffer CA, *et al.* All-transretinoic acid in acute promyelocytic leukemia. *N Engl J Med* 1997; 337:1021–8.

31 Fenaux P, Chastang C, Chevret S, *et al.* A randomized comparison of all transretinoic acid (ATRA) followed by chemotherapy and ATRA plus chemotherapy and the role of maintenance therapy in newly diagnosed acute promyelocytic leukemia. The European APL Group. *Blood* 1999;94:1192–200.

32 Frankel SR, Eardley A, Lauwers G, Weiss M, Warrell RP, Jr. The "retinoic acid syndrome" in acute promyelocytic leukemia. *Ann Intern Med* 1992;117:292–6.

33 Dubois C, Schlageter MH, de Gentile A, *et al.* Modulation of IL-8, IL-1 beta, and G-CSF secretion by all-trans retinoic acid in acute promyelocytic leukemia. *Leukemia* 1994;8:1750–7.

34 Dubois C, Schlageter MH, de Gentile A, *et al.* Hematopoietic growth factor expression and ATRA sensitivity in acute promyelocytic blast cells. *Blood* 1994;83:3264–70.

35 Larson RS, Brown DC, Sklar LA. Retinoic acid induces aggregation of the acute promyelocytic leukemia cell line NB-4 by utilization of LFA-1 and ICAM-2. *Blood* 1997;90: 2747–56.

36 Kanamaru A, Takemoto Y, Tanimoto M, *et al.* All-trans retinoic acid for the treatment of newly diagnosed acute promyelocytic leukemia. Japan Adult Leukemia Study Group. *Blood* 1995;85: 1202–6.

37 Vahdat L, Maslak P, Miller WH, Jr. Early mortality and the retinoic acid syndrome in acute promyelocytic leukemia: impact of leukocytosis, low-dose chemotherapy, PMN/RAR-alpha isoform, and CD13 expression in patients treated with all-trans retinoic acid. *Blood* 1994;84:3843–9.

38 de Botton S, Dombret H, Sanz M, *et al.* Incidence, clinical features, and outcome of all trans-retinoic acid syndrome in 413 cases of newly diagnosed acute promyelocytic leukemia. The European APL Group. *Blood* 1998;92:2712–18.

39 de Botton S, Coitteux V, Chevret S, *et al.* Early onset chemotherapy can reduce the incidence of ATRA syndrome in newly diagnosed acute promyelocytic leukemia (APL). Results of a randomized study. *Blood* 2001;98:766a.

40 Tallman MS, Andersen JW, Schiffer CA, *et al.* All-transretinoic acid in acute promyelocytic leukemia. *N Engl J Med* 1997; 337:1021–8.

41 Mahmoud HH, Hurwitz CA, Roberts WM, Santana VM, Ribeiro RC, Krance RA. Tretinoin toxicity in children with acute promyelocytic leukemia. *Lancet* 1993;342:1394–5.
42 Hakimian D, Tallman MS, Zugerman C, Caro WA. Erythema nodosum associated with all-trans-retinoic acid in the treatment of acute promyelocytic leukemia. *Leukemia* 1993;7: 758–9.
43 Koike T, Tatewaki W, Aoki A, *et al*. Brief report: severe symptoms of hyperhistaminemia after the treatment of acute promyelocytic leukemia with tretinoin (all-trans-retinoic acid). *N Engl J Med* 1992;327:385–7.
44 Iwakiri R, Inokuchi K, Dan K, Nomura T. Marked basophilia in acute promyelocytic leukemia treated with all-trans retinoic acid: molecular analysis of the cell origin of the basophils. *Br J Haematol* 1994;86:870–2.
45 Miranda N, Oliveira P, Frade MJ, Melo J, Marques MS, Parreira A. Myositis with tretinoin. *Lancet* 1994;344:1096.
46 Tomas JF, Escudero A, Fernandez-Ranada JM. All-trans retinoic acid treatment and Sweet syndrome. *Leukemia* 1994;8:1596.
47 Arun B, Berberian B, Azumi N, Frankel SR, Luksenburg H, Freter C. Sweet's syndrome during treatment with all-trans retinoic acid in a patient with acute promyelocytic leukemia. *Leuk Lymphoma* 1998;31:613–15.
48 Levy V, Jaffarbey J, Aouad K, Zittoun R. Fournier's gangrene during induction treatment of acute promyelocytic leukemia, a case report. *Ann Hematol* 1998;76:91–2.
49 Mori A, Tamura S, Katsuno T, *et al*. Scrotal ulcer occurring in patients with acute promyelocytic leukemia during treatment with all-trans retinoic acid. *Oncol Rep* 1999;6:55–8.
50 Kentos A, LeMoine F, Crenier L, *et al*. All-trans retinoic acid induced thrombocytosis in a patient with acute promyelocytic leukemia. *Br J Haematol* 1997;97:685.
51 Paydas S, Sahin B, Zorludemir S, Hazar B. All trans retinoic acid as the possible cause of necrotizing vasculitis. *Leuk Res* 1998;22:655–7.
52 Tapiovaara H, Matikainen S, Hurme M, Vaheri A. Induction of differentiation of promyelocytic NB4 cells by retinoic acid is associated with rapid increase in urokinase activity subsequently downregulated by production of inhibitors. *Blood* 1994;83:1883–91.
53 Tallman MS, Andersen JW, Schiffer CA, *et al*. All-transretinoic acid in acute promyelocytic leukemia. *N Engl J Med* 1997; 337:1021–8.
54 Fenaux P, Chastang C, Chevret S, *et al*. A randomized comparison of all transretinoic acid (ATRA) followed by chemotherapy and ATRA plus chemotherapy and the role of maintenance therapy in newly diagnosed acute promyelocytic leukemia. The European APL Group. *Blood* 1999;94:1192–200.
55 Sanz MA, Lo-Coco F. Definition of relapse risk and role of nonanthracycline drugs for consolidation in patients with acute promyelocytic leukemia: a joint study of the PETHEMA and GIMEMA cooperative groups. *Blood* 2000;96:1247–53.
56 Sanz A, Martin G, Gonzalez M, *et al*. Risk-adapted treatment of acute promyelocytic leukemia with all-trans-retinoic acid and anthracycline monochemotherapy: a multicenter study by the PETHEMA group. *Blood* 2004;103:1237.
57 Lo-Coco F, Vignetti M, Avvisatti G, *et al*. Front-line treatment of acute promyelocytic leukemia with AIDA induction followed by risk-adapted consolidation: results of the AIDA-2000 trial of the Italian GIMEMA group. *Blood* 2004;104(Suppl.1):392.
58 Lengfelder E, Reichert A, Schoch C, *et al*. Double induction strategy including high dose cytarabine in combination with all-trans retinoic acid: effects in patients with newly diagnosed acute promyelocytic leukemia. German AML Cooperative Group. *Leukemia* 2000;14:1362–70.
59 Adès L, Sanz MA, Chevret S. Treatment of newly diagnosed acute promyelocytic leukemia (APL): a comparison of French-Belgian-Swiss and PETHEMA results. *Blood* 2008;111:1078–84.
60 Adès L, Chevret S, Raffoux E, *et al*. Is cytarabine useful in the treatment of acute promyelocytic leukemia? Results of a randomized trial from the European Acute Promyelocytic Leukemia Group. *J Clin Oncol* 2006;24:5703–10.
61 Sanz M, Montesinos P, Rayón C, *et al*. Risk-adapted treatment of acute promyelocytic leukemia based on all-*trans* retinoic acid and anthracycline with addition of cytarabine in consolidation therapy for high-risk patients: further improvements in treatment outcome. *Blood* 2010;115:5137–46.
62 Shen ZX, Shi ZZ, Fang J, *et al*. All-trans retinoic acid/As2O3 combination yields a high quality remission and survival in newly diagnosed acute promyelocytic leukemia. *Proc Natl Acad Sci U S A* 2004;101:5328–35.
63 Ghavamzadeh A, Alimoghaddam K, Ghaffari SH, *et al*. Treatment of acute promyelocytic leukemia without ATRA and/or chemotherapy. *Ann Oncol* 2006;17:131–4.
64 Mathews V, George B, Lakshmi KM, *et al*. Single-agent arsenic trioxide in the treatment of newly diagnosed acute promyelocytic leukemia: durable remissions with minimal toxicity. *Blood* 2006;107:2627–32.
65 Estey E, Garcia-Manero G, Ferrajoli A, *et al*. Use of all-trans retinoic acid plus arsenic trioxide as an alternative to chemotherapy in untreated acute promyelocytic leukemia. *Blood* 2006; 107:3469–73.
66 Evans GD, Grimwade DJ. Extramedullary disease in acute promyelocytic leukemia. *Leuk Lymphoma* 1999;33:219–29.
67 de Botton S, Sanz MA, Chevret S, *et al*. Extramedullary relapse in acute promyelocytic leukemia treated with all-trans retinoic acid and chemotherapy. *Leukemia* 2005;20:35–41.
68 Wing-Yan Au, *et al*. Determinants of cerebrospinal fluid arsenic concentration in patients with acute promyelocytic leukemia on oral arsenic trioxide therapy. *Blood* 2008;112:3587–90.
69 Santamaria C, Chillon MC, Fernandez C, *et al*. Relapse-risk stratification in acute promyelocytic leukemia patients by PML-RAR transcript quantification. *Haematologica* 2007;92:316–23.
70 Grimwade D, Lo Coco F. Acute promyelocytic leukemia: a model for the role of molecular diagnosis and residual disease monitoring in directing treatment approach in acute myeloid leukemia. *Leukemia* 2002;16:1959–73.
71 Cheson BD. International Working Group for diagnosis, standardization of response criteria, treatment outcomes, and reporting standards for therapeutic trials in acute myeloid leukemia. *J Clin Oncol* 2003;21:4642–9.
72 Diverio D, Rossi V, Avvisati G, *et al*. Early detection of relapse by prospective reverse transcriptase-polymerase chain reaction analysis of the *PML/RARa* fusion gene in patients with acute promyelocytic leukemia enrolled in the GIMEMA-AIEOP multicenter "AIDA" trial. *Blood* 1998:92; 784–9.
73 Gallagher RE, Yeap BY, Bi W, *et al*. Quantitative real-time RT-PCR analysis of PML-RAR alpha mRNA in acute promyelocytic leukemia: assessment of prognostic significance in adult patients from intergroup protocol 0129. *Blood* 2003;101:2521–8.

74 Niu C, Yan H, Yu T, *et al.* Studies on treatment of acute promyelocytic leukemia experience with arsenic trioxide: remission induction, follow-up, and molecular monitoring in 11 newly diagnosed and 47 relapsed acute promyelocytic leukemia patients. *Blood* 1999;94:3315–24.

75 Sanz MA, Fenaux P, Lo Coco F. On behalf of the European APL Group of Experts. Arsenic trioxide in the current treatment of acute promyelocytic leukemia. A review of current evidence. *Haematologica* 2005;90:1231–5.

76 Thomas X, Pigneux A, Raffoux E, Huguet F, Caillot D, Fenaux P. Superiority of an arsenic trioxide-based regimen over a historic control combining all-trans retinoic acid plus intensive chemotherapy in the treatment of relapsed acute promyelocytic leukemia. *Haematologica* 2006;91:996–7.

77 Lo-Coco F, Cimino G, Breccia M, *et al.* Gemtuzumab ozogamicin (Mylotarg) as a single agent for molecularly relapsed acute promyelocytic leukemia. *Blood* 2004;104:1995–9.

78 Tobita T, Takeshita A, Kitamura K, *et al.* Treatment with a new synthetic retinoid, AM80, of acute promyelocytic leukemia relapsed from complete remission induced by all-trans retinoic acid. *Blood* 1997;90:967–73.

79 Douer D, Hu W, Giralt S, *et al.* Arsenic trioxide (trisenox) therapy for acute promyelocytic leukemia in the setting of hematopoietic stem cell transplantation. *Oncologist* 2003;8:132–40.

80 Sanz MA, Vellenga E, Rayón C, *et al.* All-trans retinoic acid and anthracycline monochemotherapy for the treatment of elderly patients with acute promyelocytic leukemia. *Blood* 2004;104: 3490–3.

81 Adès L, Chevret S, de Botton S, *et al.* Outcome of acute promyelocytic leukemia treated with all trans retinoic acid and chemotherapy in elderly patients: the European group experience. *Leukemia* 2005;19:230–3.

82 de Botton S, Coiteux V, Chevret S, *et al.* Outcome of childhood acute promyelocytic leukemia with all-trans-retinoic acid and chemotherapy. *J Clin Oncol* 2004;22:1404–12.

83 Testi AM, Biondi A, Lo Coco F, *et al.* GIMEMA-AIEOPAIDA protocol for the treatment of newly diagnosed acute promyelocytic leukemia (APL) in children. *Blood* 2005;106:447–53.

84 Ortega JJ, Madero L, Martín G, *et al.* PETHEMA Group Treatment with all-trans retinoic acid and anthracycline monochemotherapy for children with acute promyelocytic leukemia: a multicenter study by the PETHEMA Group. *J Clin Oncol* 2005;23:7632–40.

85 Mann G, Reinhardt D, Ritter J, *et al.* Treatment with all-trans retinoic acid in acute promyelocytic leukemia reduces early deaths in children. *Ann Hematol* 2001;80:417–22.

86 Castaigne S, Lefebvre P, Chomienne C, *et al.* Effectiveness and pharmacokinetics of low-dose all-trans retinoic acid (25 mg/ m^2) in acute promyelocytic leukemia. *Blood* 1993;82:3560.

87 Powell BL, Moser B, Stock W, *et al.* Effect of consolidation with arsenic trioxide (As2O3) on event-free survival (EFS) and overall survival (OS) among patients with newly diagnosed acute promyelocytic leukemia (APL): North American Intergroup Protocol C9710 [Abstract] *J Clin Oncol* 2007;25 (Suppl.18):2.

88 Fox E, Razzouk BI, Widemann BC, *et al.* Phase 1 trial and pharmacokinetic study of arsenic trioxide in children and adolescents with refractory or relapsed acute leukemia, including acute promyelocytic leukemia or lymphoma. *Blood* 2008;111: 566–73.

89 George B, Mathews V, Poonkuzhali B, *et al.* Treatment of children with newly diagnosed acute promyelocytic leukemia with arsenic trioxide: a single center experience. *Leukemia* 2004;18: 1587–90.

Part 5
Acute Lymphoblastic Leukemia

Chapter 15
Acute Lymphoblastic Leukemia: Presentation, Diagnosis and Classification

Sandeep Gurbuxani and John Anastasi
University of Chicago, Chicago, Illinois, USA

Introduction

Acute lymphoblastic leukemia (ALL) is a neoplasm of precursor B- or precursor T-lymphoid cells. The development of leukemia is a consequence of genetic or molecular lesions affecting these progenitors that permit them to evade normal control mechanisms that regulate their proliferation and differentiation. These genetic and molecular abnormalities result in a differentiation arrest, abnormal proliferation, and resistance to apoptosis, and subsequently cause an accumulation of leukemic cells, typically in the bone marrow or occasionally in extramedullary sites such as the thymus. In the bone marrow, crowding-out of normal hematopoiesis in turn leads to anemia, infection, and bleeding, and to the associated signs and symptoms common at presentation.

Epidemiology

Considered primarily to be a cancer of childhood, the peak incidence of ALL is between the ages of 1 and 4 years [1], and approximately 61% of acute leukemias are diagnosed in patients <20 years of age [1]. This first peak is followed by a progressive decline in incidence during adolescence and early adulthood. A second, much smaller peak begins to emerge in the fifth decade of life, with the highest incidence for this second peak being 1.9473/100,000 reached in those aged ≥85 years. The overall age adjusted incidence of ALL has increased progressively from 0.9287/100,000 in 1975 to 1.5333/100,000 in 2005 [1]. The reason for this increase is not entirely clear, but appears to be due in part to an increased incidence of ALL in patients <45 years of age.

There are conflicting, frequently isolated, reports of possible risk factors for the development of ALL. These include parental tobacco or alcohol use, exposure to pesticides or solvents, and cigarette smoking. However, only ionizing radiation has been significantly linked to an increased risk of developing ALL [2]. In addition, a very small minority of cases (<5%) are associated with inherited, predisposing syndromes such as Down syndrome, Bloom syndrome, ataxia telangiectasia, and Nijmegen breakage syndrome [3]. In the vast majority of cases, no underlying predisposing factors have been found.

An infective etiology has been proposed by two different groups and continues to be an area of investigation. The underlying basis for these hypotheses is the increased prevalence of ALL in industrialized, urban, affluent societies as well as an occasional clustering of cases, particularly in new urban developments. Greaves has attempted to explain the increased prevalence of ALL in affluent societies by the "delayed infection" theory. According to this hypothesis, susceptible individuals acquire a preleukemic clone prenatally. Expansion of the clone is held in check in an affluent, hygienic environment as younger infants are protected from common infections and the associated stimulation of lymphoid cells. Exposure to an, as yet, unidentified infective agent in later life results in abnormal, excessive lymphoid proliferation, which triggers the development of overt leukemia [4]. The second, parallel "population mixing" hypothesis is proposed by Kinlen [5]. This hypothesis was proposed to explain the clustering of leukemia cases. According to this hypothesis, ALL clusters occur when a previously unexposed community is exposed to infectious agents brought into the community by a large influx of new residents, as might happen during urbanization of rural communities.

Presentation

The presentation is usually acute, with non-specific symptoms and signs that are a consequence of either bone marrow failure and blood cytopenias or organ infiltration. Pallor, lethargy, malaise (anemia), fever, infection (neutropenia), spontaneous bruising, purpura, bleeding gums, and menorrhagia (thrombocytopenia) are all consequences of a bone marrow packed with leukemic blasts that is incapable of producing normal hematopoietic forms. Splenomegaly, hepatomegaly, lymphadenopathy, mediastinal mass, tender bones, and meningeal syndrome

Leukemias: Principles and Practice of Therapy, 1st edition. Edited by S. Faderl and H. Kantarjian.

(headache, nausea, vomiting, blurring of vision, and double vision) are manifestations of organ infiltration.

Diagnosis

Diagnosis and appropriate classification of ALL requires integration of all available data including information from flow cytometry, cytogenetic studies, and molecular studies. Evaluation of morphology should be performed on the peripheral blood, bone core biopsy, and bone marrow aspirate. To the greatest extent possible, all findings (including immunophenotype, karyotype, and genetic features) should be a part of a single, integrated report. Parameters such as LDH and uric acid levels, while not essential for diagnosis, provide crucial information about the tumor burden and are an integral part of the laboratory work-up of a newly diagnosed leukemia. At the outset, it needs to be emphasized that the term acute lymphoblastic leukemia and acute lymphoblastic lymphoma indicate identical biologic entities. The term "lymphoma" is preferred when the presentation is primarily nodal or extramedullary with a relatively lower percentage of blasts in the bone marrow (arbitrarily defined as <25%). Finally, while the most recent World Health Organization (WHO) classification [6] uses the term "B-lymphoblastic leukemia/lymphoma" rather than "precursor B-lymphoblastic leukemia/lymphoma," the entity is still considered a neoplasm of progenitor B cells that does not include Burkitt lymphoma/leukemia, which is a malignant neoplasm of mature B cells.

Initial laboratory evaluation

A complete blood count (CBC) and a morphologic evaluation of the peripheral blood smear is the starting point for the laboratory diagnosis of any hematologic malignancy. An abnormality in at least one of the CBC parameters is detected in >90% of patients with ALL at diagnosis. A normochromic, normocytic anemia with reticulocytopenia is the most common abnormality, and >75% of patients will present with a hemoglobin concentration of <9g/dL. Thrombocytopenia is frequent, and approximately 70% will present with platelet counts of $<100 \times 10^9/L$ [7]. Neutropenia is almost always present. Approximately 50% of patients present with an initial white blood count (WBC) of $<10 \times 10^9/L$, another 40% with counts between 10 and $100 \times 10^9/L$, and only 10% present with a WBC $>100 \times 10^9/L$ [8]. Blasts account for a variable proportion of the cells in the peripheral blood and can range from being undetectable to numerous, accounting for the entire leukocyte population. Occasionally, a leukoerythroblastic picture with circulating nucleated red cells and immature granulocytes may be present. An uncommon extreme manifestation of this is the situation where left-shifted granulocytic elements, including numerous myelocytes and myeloblasts, predominate with only rare circulating lymphoblasts. This can complicate the diagnosis from the peripheral blood. It therefore has to be emphasized that a bone marrow examination is absolutely critical for the morphologic diagnosis of a clinically suspected acute leukemia presenting with a low WBC and only a few circulating blasts. Eosinophilia as a presentation of ALL is extremely uncommon. However, when present, it is likely indicative of a specific chromosomal abnormality—t(5;14)(q31;q32), described in greater detail below. Amongst the non-hematologic parameters, lactate dehydrogenase levels are frequently elevated, and almost 50% of patients will have levels between 300 and 1000IU/L at the time of presentation [7]. The LDH level usually correlates with the WBC and blast count, and is an indicator of tumor burden.

Morphology

Peripheral blood smear, bone marrow aspirate smear, and touch imprints

Morphology is best appreciated on Romanowsky-based stains such as a Giemsa or Wright–Giemsa stain of the peripheral blood smear (Figure 15.1 a and b), bone

Figure 15.1 (a-n) Illustrations depicting various aspects of acute lymphoblastic leukemia (ALL). (a) Peripheral blood smear illustrates ALL with a marked lymphoblastosis. Some patients, however, can present with a leukopenia, and some with few or no circulating blasts. Higher magnification of the smear showing lymphoblasts compared with a single small lymphocyte (center top). (c) A hypercellular bone packed with blasts. (d) The bone marrow aspirate typically shows sheets of lymphoblasts with few residual normal hematopoietic elements, but hypocellular presentation does occur. (e-i) Cytologic variants of lymphoblasts. (e) Typical lymphoblast with smudgy nuclear chromatin, inconspicuous nucleoli and scant cytoplasm. (f) Large lymphoblast with prominent nucleoli and more abundant cytoplasm. (g) Smaller lymphoblast with more condensed chromatin ("lymphocyte-like"); (h) "Hand-mirror" cell. (i) Lymphoblast with faint azurophilic granules (arrow), and scant vacuolization. (j) A Burkitt cell is shown for comparison. Note the more condensed nuclear chromatin, the deep coloration of the cytoplasm, and the prominent vacuolization in the Burkitt cell compared with the lymphoblast. (k) Lymphoblasts are illustrated in a cytospin preparation of cerebral spinal fluid from a patient with leukemic meningitis. (l) A bone marrow biopsy at presentation illustrating marrow necrosis and "ghost" cells. (m) Bone marrow aspirate after recovery from chemotherapy illustrating hematogones (arrow) associated with numerous small lymphocytes. Hematogones can be difficult to distinguish from lymphoblasts cytologically, but can be recognized by flow cytometry. In a flow histogram (n) showing CD20 (ordinate) and CD10 (abscissa) expression on $CD19^+$ cells, hematogones show a spectrum of CD10 and C20 staining, illustrating a reduction of CD10 as CD20 becomes expressed on maturing lymphoid cells (arrows). In the histogram, in addition to the hematogones, there is a small, distinct population of $CD20^-$ cells with bright CD10 (bottom right gate) representing a small population of residual neoplastic lymphoblasts.

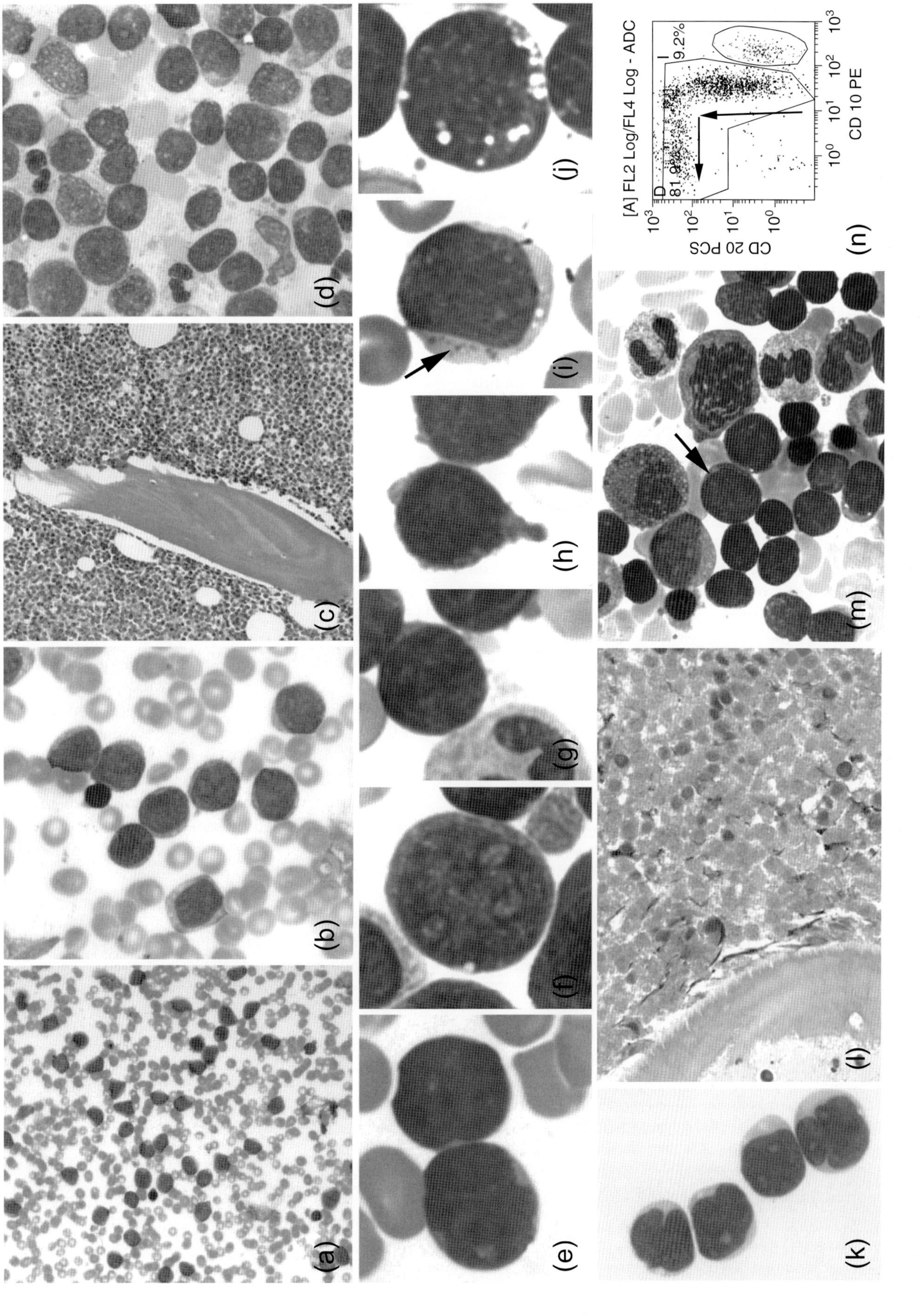

(a)
(b)
(c)
(d)
(e)
(f)
(g)
(h)
(i)
(j)
(k)
(l)
(m)
(n)
[A] FL2 Log/FL4 Log - ADC
D
I
81.9%
9.2%
CD 20 PCS
CD 10 PE

marrow aspirate smear and touch imprints, or cytospin specimens (Figure 15.1 d and k). B-lymphoblasts are morphologically indistinguishable from T-lymphoblasts and this distinction requires evaluation of antigen expression by flow cytometry or immunohistochemistry. The lymphoblasts vary from small cells with a high nuclear–cytoplasmic ratio and scant cytoplasm to larger cells with more abundant, bluish-gray cytoplasm (Figure 15.1 e and f). The nuclei are usually round and the chromatin is variably described as "smudged" or uniformly condensed, and rarely as fine as in myeloblasts. The nucleoli are usually inconspicuous, but can sometimes be more prominent. Occasionally, the blasts can be small with more condensed chromatin (Figure 15.1g). These "lymphocyte-like" blasts can cause difficulty in diagnosis, particularly in distinguishing the cells from those of mature B-cell malignancies in adults. Another variant that is frequently discussed in the context of ALL morphology includes blasts with a "hand mirror" appearance (Figure 15.1h). The "hand-mirror" variant is generally considered an artifact of preparation and, together with the other morphologic variants, has little biologic significance.

Blasts with coarse azurophilic granules (Figure 15.1i) can be seen in a subset of blasts in 5–8% of children presenting with ALL. This morphologic feature is seen even more infrequently in adult ALL. When present, the blasts can be distinguished from myeloblasts since the granules are negative for the myeloperoxidase reaction. An association has been reported between lymphoblasts with granular cytoplasm and either the presence of the Philadelphia chromosome [9] or ALL in the setting of Down syndrome [10]. In the latter situation, the granules comprise accumulations of mitochondria. Another morphologic finding that can sometimes pose a diagnostic challenge is the presence of cytoplasmic vacuoles in the lymphoblasts. Cytoplasmic vacuolation in >10% of the blasts can be seen in as many as 28% of childhood ALL cases, and can cause one to consider a leukemic presentation of Burkitt lymphoma, which is characterized by vacuolated cells (Figure 15.1j) [11]. In most cases, the distinction from a leukemic presentation of Burkitt lymphoma can be made on other morphologic features, such as the smaller cell size, lack of deep-blue cytoplasm, and less coarse chromatin in ALL blasts. However, even when morphology is somewhat confounding, the distinction can be made by immunophenotyping of the malignant cells to demonstrate the expression of TdT and absence of surface immunoglobulin in ALL. Very frequently, these vacuoles stain positively with the periodic acid-Schiff (PAS) reaction and therefore represent glycogen deposits [12].

Bone marrow biopsy and tissue sections

Trephine biopsy sections usually show hypercellular bone marrow (Figure 15.1c). On the hematoxylin and eosin (H&E)-stained section the marrow appears to be packed with a relatively uniform population of blasts. These blasts are small to intermediate in size and have round to oval nuclei. Less frequently, the blasts can have a more variable morphology with indented, clefted, convoluted, and variably sized nuclei. The chromatin is typically described as being finely dispersed. The nucleoli are usually inconspicuous, but can be more prominent in some cases. Mitotic activity is readily appreciated. Residual hematopoiesis is markedly reduced and, in most cases, comprises a few megakaryocytes and small erythroid islands. Partial and focal involvement by ALL is rare at the time of presentation. Less commonly, the bone marrow can be normocellular or even hypocellular. Hypocellular or aplastic presentation of ALL is seen in 1–2% of children. This is characterized by a younger age at presentation (<10 years), female sex, and the prevalence of fever associated with an underlying infection [13]. Making the diagnosis of ALL from hypocellular bone marrow can be particularly challenging since the biopsy has to be frequently interpreted with little ancillary information available because of the lack of cells in a bone marrow aspirate. It is notable that the hypocellular phase is frequently followed by partial recovery and finally overt leukemia within 6 months of initial presentation [13]. Bone marrow necrosis at the time of diagnosis can be seen in up to 1% of cases of childhood ALL (Figure 15.1i) [14]. This can also pose a diagnostic challenge when the necrosis is extensive and no viable material is available for characterization. It needs to be emphasized that a necrotic bone marrow is usually indicative of an underlying malignancy—the most frequent in children being ALL. Therefore, when dealing with a biopsy showing necrosis that is not interpretable, a repeat biopsy from a different site should be attempted, which usually provides appropriate material for a definitive diagnosis. Some degree of reticulin fibrosis has been documented in up to 64% of adult patients with ALL [15] and in 70% of childhood cases at the time of diagnosis [16]. Increased fibrosis is more frequently associated with precursor B-than precursor T-ALL. Furthermore, 8–10% show marked fibrosis, making aspiration impossible. The diagnosis and immunophenotyping of the leukemia is, out of necessity, based on the interpretation of the biopsy and the immunohistochemistry performed on the biopsy sections.

Extramedullary (lymphomatous) presentation of ALL is seen more frequently with T-ALL than with B-ALL. This can be in the form of a mediastinal mass, lymphadenopathy, and organ enlargement. Less frequently, infiltration can be seen in other organs such as the kidney, skin, testis, central nervous system (CNS), and breast. Whenever there is concern of a lymphoblastic process, a careful review of the peripheral blood and an evaluation of the bone marrow is imperative. The morphology of the lymphoblasts in tissue sections is similar to that described in the bone core biopsy. Lymph node involvement is usually diffuse, but can be paracortical with sparing of the follicles.

Cytochemistry

The use of cytochemistry is currently limited to the use of the myeloperoxidase reaction to make a rapid and quick distinction from most cases of acute myeloid leukemia (AML). Lymphoblasts, by definition, are negative for myeloperoxidase. Sudan Black B is also negative. Similarly, while one continues to find the description of block-like positivity with the PAS stain corresponding to the glycogen deposits, this stain is also no longer performed in most laboratories. Focal, punctuate, or a Golgi zone pattern of the non-specific esterase (NSE) reaction is sometimes observed. When present, this is distinctively different from the diffuse and homogeneous positivity seen in monocytic cells.

Immunophenotype

Extensive immunophenotypic characterization is a prerequisite for the appropriate classification of ALL. When adequate material is available, immunophenotyping should be performed using multicolor flow cytometry so that multiple antigens can be examined simultaneously on the surface of the lymphoblasts. This is crucial since no single antigen is specific for any one lineage. Equally importantly, aberrant antigen expression on the malignant blasts provides a footprint that can be followed to monitor residual disease post therapy. When adequate material is not available, as might happen when the bone marrow is fibrotic, by necessity immunophenotyping has to be performed by immunohistochemistry on the bone core biopsy. Even here multiple antibodies directed against multiple antigens should be used to assign a lineage with certainty and exclude the possibility of an AML or a neoplasm of ambiguous lineage.

B-ALL

By definition, B-ALLs express one or more of the B-cell antigens CD19, CD79a, and CD22 by flow cytometry. They also express Pax5 and CD79a, which can be evaluated from paraffin-imbedded tissue sections. However, while Pax5 is considered to be the most reliable marker for B-lineage commitment by immunohistochemistry, expression of this antigen has been reported in 36–100% of AML with t(8;21) [17]. Similarly, CD79a expression is absent in up to 20% of B-ALLs and can be seen in 10% of T-ALLs, further underscoring the importance of using more than one antigen to assign a lineage to a blast population. While CD20 is another reliable B-cell marker that can be detected by flow cytometry or immunohistochemistry, it is expressed on mature cells and frequently lacking or expressed only dimly on lymphoblasts. Cytoplasmic immunoglobulin μ chains are expressed in about 20% of B-ALL cases. Surface immunoglobulin is usually not expressed. However, the expression of surface immunoglobulin does not preclude the diagnosis of B-ALL provided other criteria for the diagnosis are met and the malignant cells show no rearrangements of the *c-myc* gene. Surface immunoglobulin-positive ALL cases are quite rare. Other antigens that are not lineage specific but are variably expressed in B-ALL are CD10, TdT, CD34, HLADR, and CD45. Myeloid antigens such as CD13 and CD33 have been reported with variable frequency. The expression of these antigens does not preclude the diagnosis of B-ALL. Furthermore, in the recent WHO classification scheme, these antigens are no longer part of the algorithm used to diagnose mixed lineage leukemia. On the other hand, the expression of MPO by cytochemical reaction or by flow immunophenotyping does exclude the diagnosis of B-ALL. When MPO positivity is detected with the expression of multiple B-lineage antigens, including CD19, a diagnosis of acute leukemia of ambiguous lineage has to be rendered. Similarly, when in addition to B-lineage markers there is expression of multiple monocytic markers (at least two) such as NSE, CD11c, CD14, CD64, and lysozyme, the finding should be used to make the diagnosis of acute leukemia of ambiguous lineage rather than B-ALL.

In as much as the maturation of the B-lymphoblasts corresponds to normal B-cell maturation, an attempt has been made to classify B-ALL based on the antigen expression profile. Thus, the most immature B-ALL, also referred to as "early" precursor B- or "Pro-B"-ALL, is characterized by the expression of CD19, CD79a, cyCD22, and TdT. The intermediate stage of maturation is characterized by the expression of the common ALL antigen (CALLA or CD10) in addition to the above mentioned B-cell antigens. This stage has been referred to as "common" precursor B-ALL. Finally, the most mature B-ALL, also referred to as "Pre-B"-ALL, is characterized by cytoplasmic immunoglobulin μ chain expression and a variable expression of CD10. All of these can have variable expressions of CD34 and HLADR.

T-ALL

Cytoplasmic CD3 (cCD3) is by far the most reliable marker for assigning T-lineage to the lymphoblasts. The antibody used for the detection of T-ALL has to be specific for the epsilon chain. Polyclonal CD3 antibodies used for immunohistochemistry frequently stain the CD3 zeta chain and are not T-cell specific. Other T-cell antigens that are expressed more variably include CD1a, CD2, surface CD3 (sCD3), CD4, CD5, CD7, and CD8. CD10 expression can be seen in up to 20% of the cases and CD79a is expressed in 10% of T-ALL. Similar to the B-ALLs, expression of the myeloid associated markers, CD13 and CD33, is not uncommon and does not in any manner impact the diagnosis of T-ALL. CD117 is expressed only rarely and appears to be associated with *FLT3* mutations. Expression of MPO by cytochemistry or by antigen expression, or the expression of at least two monocytic antigens including NSE, CD11c, CD14, CD64, or lysozyme, precludes the diagnosis of T-ALL and indicates an ambiguous lineage leukemia.

Similar to B-ALL, T-ALL has been classified according to the stage of maturation. The most immature of the T-ALLs are called pro-T-ALL (or immature thymocyte stage) and are characterized by the expression of cCD3, CD7, and variable expression of CD34. These T-ALLs lack CD2 and CD1a expression. Pre-T-ALL is more mature and expresses CD2 along with cCD3 and CD7 and continues to be negative for the expression of CD1a. The intermediate stage of maturation is the cortical T-ALL (or common thymocyte stage), characterized by the expression of cCD3, CD7, CD2, CD1a, and double positivity for CD4 and CD8. These leukemias almost invariably lack the expression of CD34. Finally, the most mature T-ALL is "medullary" T-ALL (or mature thymocyte stage), which no longer expresses CD1a and is positive for the expression of either CD4 or CD8.

Differential diagnoses

Considerations for differential diagnoses depend, at least in part, on the patient's age [18]. In pediatric patients with a high WBC (20–30 × 10^9/L), the possibility of pertussis must be excluded. The lymphoid cells in pertussis are morphologically mature with clumped chromatin, but they can be deceptive. The immunophenotype of these cells is a mixture of $CD4^+$ and $CD8^+$ mature T-cells that are TdT^-. In the bone marrow, hematogones (normal immature lymphoid precursors) can be increased in children and require careful morphologic and immunophenotypic evaluation to distinguish them from leukemic blasts. Morphologically, hematogones usually have round nuclei, smooth chromatin and an invariable absence of nucleoli (Figure 15.1m). Immunophenotypically, hematogones show a distinct pattern of maturation with reduction of CD10 as the cells mature and become $CD20^+$. The flow immunophenotypic pattern is particularly helpful in distinguishing hematogones from residual lymphoblasts during recovery from therapy (Figure 15.1n). Small, round blue cell tumors seen in the pediatric age group can histologically mimic ALL. However, these tumors can be easily distinguished by immunohistochemical staining. In older patients, chronic lymphocytic leukemia (CLL) and leukemic manifestations of lymphoma, particularly the blastoid variant of mantle cell lymphoma, can present with overlapping morphology. However, these entities can be distinguished from ALL by their distinct mature immunophenotype. Entities that can present in all age groups that morphologically mimic ALL include AML (particularly AML with minimal differentiation), chronic myeloid leukemia (CML) presenting in blast crisis, and mixed lineage leukemia. The distinction from ALL requires appropriate and comprehensive morphologic and immunophenotypic analysis as well as molecular and/or cytogenetic correlation.

Cytogenetic and molecular characterization

Leukemogenesis in ALL follows the general theme of tumor development characterized by multiple cooperating genetic lesions. The overall consequence of these lesions is the acquisition of a capacity to proliferate independently of the normal environmental cues and homeostatic controls, to resist signals for cell death, and to inhibit differentiation. In as much as these genetic lesions frequently involve transcription factors involved in the ontogenic cascade of B- or T-cell development, each of the lesions is likely characterized by a distinct gene expression profile, biology, and response to therapy [19]. While the biology of ALL associated with specific genetic lesions does not vary between adult and pediatric cases, the frequency with which these genetic lesions occur does vary with age [20] and, at least in part, contributes to the differences in treatment outcome between younger and older patients (Figure 15.2). In recognition of the significance of cytogenetic abnormalities in ALL, the most recent WHO classification includes multiple subtypes of B-ALL characterized by recurrent cytogenetic abnormalities (Table 15.1) [6]. While not entirely exhaustive and somewhat arbitrary, the inclusion of non-random cytogenetic abnormalities as defining features of a diagnostic entity reflects a paradigm shift in the work-up and classification of ALL. The currently included entities are associated with distinctive clinical phenotype and biologic behavior as reflected by response to specific therapeutic regimens. Even when the cytogenetic abnormality noted is not one of the specific entities defined in the WHO classification, it is recommended that this information be included in the synoptic diagnosis to facilitate data collection for future analyses. It is expected that, as we accumulate more information about the significance of various molecular lesions in ALL, the list of entities defined by these lesions will continue to increase. A brief discussion of the molecular abnormalities including the ones that are used to define unique entities in the WHO classification is included. The interested reader is referred to two excellent recent reviews that discuss this area in greater detail [20,21].

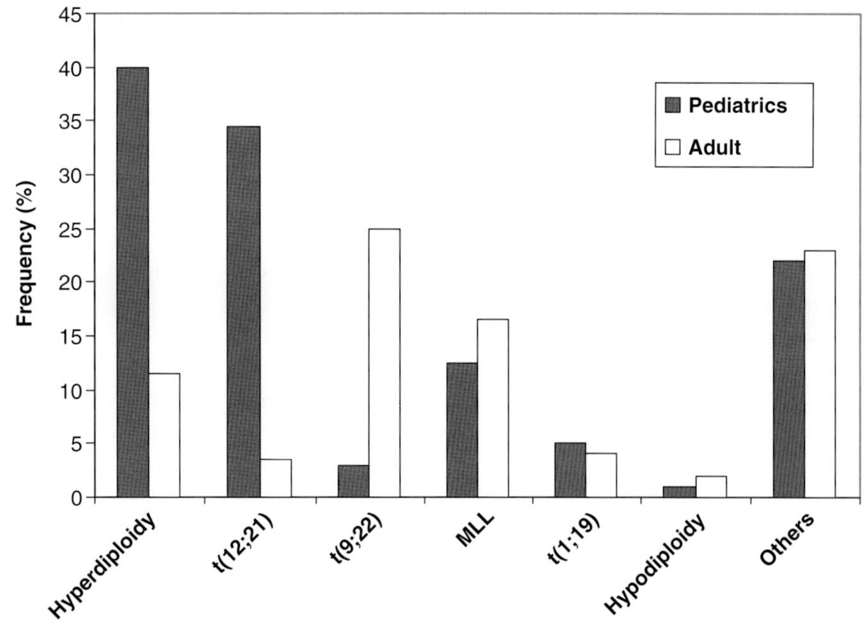

Figure 15.2 Comparison of the frequencies of various cytogenetic abnormalities in B-acute lymphoblastic leukemia in pediatric and adult cases.

Table 15.1 World Health Organization classification of precursor lymphoid neoplasms.

1. B-lymphoblastic leukemia/lymphoma, not otherwise specified
2. B-lymphoblastic leukemia/lymphoma with recurrent cytogenetic abnormalities
B-ALL/LBL with t(9;22)(q34;q11.2)
B-ALL/LBL with t(v;11q23); *MLL* rearranged
B-ALL/LBL with t(12;21)(p13;q22)
B-ALL/LBL with hyperploidy
B-ALL/LBL with hypoploidy
B-ALL/LBL with t(5;14)(q31;q32)
B-ALL with t(1;19)(q23;p13.3)
3. T-lymphoblastic leukemia/lymphoma

Cytogenetic and molecular lesions in B-ALL

The frequency of the various genetic lesions varies depending on age group. This difference is particularly striking for B-ALL (Figure 15.2), with a prominent skewing of the distribution of favorable cytogenetic abnormalities such as t(12;21) and hyperdiploid ALL in the pediatric group. Salient features of the entities included in the WHO classification are discussed.

B-lymphoblastic leukemia/lymphoma with t(9;22)(q34;q11.2); *BCR–ABL1*

This cytogenetic abnormality is seen in up to 25% of adult ALL and 2–4% of childhood ALL. The t(9;22) results in the fusion of *BCR* on 22q11.2 to *ABL1* on 9q34 locus. The resultant chimeric protein is the constitutively active ABL1 tyrosine kinase implicated in excessive proliferation of cells and leukemogenesis. The breakpoints in the *BCR* gene are somewhat variable. In the majority of childhood ALL associated with the t(9;22), the breakpoint is in the minor breakpoint region of *BCR* (exons 1–2) and results in the production of a 190-kD p190 protein. In adults, about half the patients have the breakpoint in the major breakpoint cluster region spanning exons 12–16, and this results in the formation of the 210-kD p210 protein. The remaining adult patients have the p190 fusion protein like the pediatric patients. There are no unique morphologic features associated with the t(9;22) cases or with the different break points of the *BCR* gene. However, most children with Ph^+ ALL present with a higher WBC, a $CD19^+$, $CD10^+$, TdT^+ immunophenotype, and frequent coexpression of myeloid antigens, commonly CD13 and CD33. CD25 coexpression is strongly associated with Ph^+ ALL, at least in adults [22]. CD117 is typically not expressed and only rarely is t(9;22) seen in T-lymphoblastic leukemia. Patients with t(9;22) ALL have a poor prognosis.

B-lymphoblastic leukemia/lymphoma with t(v;11q23); *MLL* rearranged

This is the most frequent cytogenetic abnormality observed in infant ALL where the translocation may occur *in utero*. Translocations involving the 11q23 locus result in the fusion of the N-terminal portion of the *MLL* (mixed lineage leukemia) gene with the C-terminal portion of one of more than 50 translocation partners. In its non-mutated state, the *MLL* gene is a methyl transferase involved in the regulation of expression of the

HOX family and methylation of histone H3 lysine residue 4 (H3K4). The chimeric protein that results from the translocations no longer has the capacity to act as a methyltransferase, is associated with enhanced transcriptional activity, and causes disruption in the normal expression of *HOX* genes [23]. Typically, patients with *MLL* rearrangements present with very high white cell counts, often >100,000/mL, and frequently have CNS involvement. However, there are no distinguishing morphologic features. B-lymphoblastic leukemia with MLL translocations, particularly t(4;11), are $CD19^+$, $CD10^-$, $CD24^-$, with frequent coexpression of the myeloid antigen CD15. If MPO and/or multiple monocytic markers are present, the leukemia should be classified as "ambiguous" or of mixed phenotype with t(v;11q23).

B-lymphoblastic leukemia with t(12;21) (p13;q22); *ETV6–RUNX1* (*TEL–AML1*)

This is one of the most common cytogenetic abnormalities observed in lymphoblastic leukemia and is reported in up to 25% of the children presenting with B-ALL. The translocation is usually cryptic and the detection rate by standard karyotype analyses is <0.05% [24]. The use of fluorescence *in situ* hybridization (FISH) and molecular techniques are required to detect the mutation in the majority of the cases. The translocation results in the fusion of the 5′ portion of the *ETV6* (also known as *TEL*) gene on chromosome 12p13 to the almost entire coding region of the *RUNX1* (also known as *AML1*, *CBFα*) on chromosome 21q22. The resultant chimeric protein retains the protein–protein interaction domain of the ETV6 protein and the DNA-binding transcriptional regulatory sequence of RUNX1 [25]. The normal RUNX1 protein binds DNA at the core-enhanced sequence and recruits other transcription factors and co-activators with resultant changes in the chromatin structure that are permissive to enhanced transcription of target genes. The chimeric protein produced as a consequence of the t(12;21) instead recruits histone deacetylases that result in chromatin closure and inhibition of crucial transcription programs essential for maturation of hematopoietic stem cells [26]. The translocation occurs early in life and can be frequently detected in retrospective studies performed from blood spots taken at birth. Thus, it appears that the translocation is essential, but not sufficient for leukemic transformation [27]. There are no unique morphologic features associated with the translocation. The immunophenotype of B-ALL with t(12;21) is $CD19^+$, $CD10^+$, and $CD34^+$. CD9, CD20, and CD66c are expressed only rarely. Expression of myeloid antigen CD13 is common but has no prognostic or diagnostic implication.

B-lymphoblastic leukemia with hyperdiploidy

Hyperdiploidy, as defined by the presence of >50 and usually <66 chromosomes, is present in up to 25% of childhood ALL. The karyotype is not seen in infants and is infrequent in adult ALL. ALL with hyperdiploidy is usually not associated with balanced translocations. While hyperdiploidy can involve any chromosome, there appears to be a distinct, non-random sequential pattern of gain of specific chromosomes as the modal number of chromosome increases [28]. Additions of chromosomes 21, 6, X, 14, 4, 17, and 19 occur most frequently. While, in general, this karyotype has been associated with a favorable outcome, whether this is dependent on the modal chromosome number or the gain of specific chromosomes remains a matter of controversy and continued investigation [29,30]. Some investigators believe cases with trisomy of both chromosomes 4 and 10 have a superior prognosis. Hyperdiploid B-ALL can be detected by standard karyotyping, FISH, or flow cytometric measurement of DNA index. There are no unique morphologic features that distinguish hyperdiploid ALL from other types of ALL. The blasts are $CD19^+$ and $CD10^+$, with most cases being $CD34^+$ as well. CD45 expression is usually not seen. It needs to be emphasized that the T-ALL cases that are hyperdiploid usually present near tetraploid karyotypes and are biologically distinct from hyperdiploid B-ALL.

B-lymphoblastic leukemia with hypodiploidy

By definition, hypodiploid B-ALL includes leukemias where blasts have a chromosome number <46. However, a stricter definition of a chromosome number <45 probably defines the clinical, biologic entity more accurately [31,32]. There are no distinct morphologic features associated with this karyotype. The immunophenotype is typically $CD19^+$, $CD10^+$. Structural abnormalities may be seen in the remaining chromosomes, but there are none that are characteristically associated. Patients with <44 chromosomes have significantly poorer survival when compared with patients with 44 chromosomes. Finally, within the group of patients with 44 chromosomes, monosomy 7, the presence of a dicentric chromosome, or both is associated with a poorer event-free survival (EFS) [32]. Doubling of the hypodiploid clone is not uncommon, but has no prognostic implication.

B-lymphoblastic leukemia with t(1;19) (q23;p13.3); TCF3–PBX1 (E2A–PBX1)

This leukemia is found in both adults and children and accounts for 5–6% of B-ALL. The translocation results in the fusion of the transactivation domain of the TCF3 (E2A) protein on chromosome 19 to the HOX protein PBX1 on chromosome 1. The resultant haplo-insufficiency of TCF3 protein and the chimeric HOX protein likely contribute to leukemogenesis [21]. There are no unique morphologic features. The immunophenotype of the blasts is $CD19^+$, $CD10^+$, and cytoplasmic μ heavy chain-positive ("Pre-B"-ALL). In addition, the t(1;19) associated leukemias show a bright expression of CD9 and usually lack CD34 expression. However, it needs to be pointed out that not all B-ALLs expressing cytoplasmic μ will be associated with a t(1;19). Initially associated with a poor prognosis, B-ALLs with t(1;19) have an excellent outcome with currently used chemotherapy regimens.

An alternative translocation involving the *TCF3* gene and the *HLF* gene on chromosome 17 has been reported. The translocation is extremely uncommon, is associated with an extremely poor prognosis, and is not biologically related to the t(1;19) leukemias in spite of the involvement of *TCF3* in both translocations. Similarly, a variant t(1;19), seen rarely in hyperdiploid ALL, does not involve either the *TCF3* or the *PBX1* gene and is also not biologically related to t(1;19) B-ALL as defined by the WHO.

B-lymphoblastic leukemia with t(5;14) (q31;q32); *IL3–IGH*

This is an extremely uncommon disease. However, the unique presentation merits its description as a specific entity in the WHO classification. The t(5;14) results in the fusion of the *IL3* gene on chromosome 5 with the *IGH* gene on chromosome 14 [33], which results in constitutive overexpression of IL3. The high IL3 levels in turn drive proliferation of eosinophils. The t(5;14) leukemias therefore present with variable eosinophilia that can be so impressive as to obscure the blast population. The diagnosis of ALL can be established in the presence of eosinophilia and the demonstration of the cytogenetic abnormality even when the bone marrow blast percentage is relatively low. The eosinophils are reactive and not related to the leukemic clone. The blasts themselves have no distinct morphology. The immunophenotype is $CD19^+$, $CD10^+$. There are too few cases with t(5;14) reported in the literature to draw definitive conclusions about the prognostic impact of this translocation. The development of eosinophilia without obvious blasts after treatment can sometimes herald overt relapse.

Cytogenetic and molecular lesions in T-ALL

The genetic lesions associated with T-ALL are a myriad of abnormalities, and in the current WHO classification they are not recognized as unique entities. They do provide insight into the underlying molecular pathogenesis in T-ALL and may be associated with prognostic significance. Overall, 50–70% of T-ALL cases have an abnormal karyotype, which commonly involves translocations of the different T-cell receptor (TCR) loci on 14q11.2, 7q35 or 7p14–15. The translocations involve a growing list of partner genes including *bHLH* genes (*MYC, SCL* [*TAL1*], and *LYL1*), *LMO* genes (*LMO1* and *LMO2*), and *HOX* genes (*HOX11, HOX11L2*) [21]. When rearranged close to the enhancer with the *TCR* genes, some of these partner regulatory genes become active and produce protein products that bind inappropriately to promoters or enhancers of downstream targets. For example, *TAL1* is activated owing to the t(1;14) translocation, and subsequently activates a number of genes that are typically quiescent in T-cell precursors. The *HOX* genes, which are developmental genes with homologs in mouse embryogenesis, likewise transactivate downstream targets. In addition to activating proto-ongogenes, translocations in T-ALL produce fusion genes, and the *MLL–ELL*, seen in about 2% of adult and pediatric cases, is an interesting example. It occurs with the t(11;19) and produces a fusion protein that alters self-renewal and growth. Another significant genetic defect reported in >50% of T-ALLs are activating mutations of *NOTCH1*. These are seen not infrequently in conjunction with some of the other abnormalities. How these mutations promote leukemogenesis is a matter of intense investigation. However, inhibition of γ secretase, required for activity of the mutant *NOTCH1* is being investigated as therapeutic target for treating ALL.

Conclusion

Advances in the molecular characterization of B- and T-cell ALL have led to the identification of a growing number of molecular subtypes that hold great potential for understanding the molecular pathogenesis of the disease and discovering possible targets for future therapies. The initial diagnosis of ALL is still based on careful evaluation of blood, bone marrow, and tissue biopsy specimens, and through appropriate immunophenotypic analysis of the leukemic cells. Only through the precise pathologic diagnosis, careful genetic analysis, and skilled clinical management of patients with ALL, will future progress be realized.

References

1 Ries LAG, Melbert D, Krapcho M, *et al.* SEER Cancer Statistics Review, 1975–2005. Bethesda, MD: National Cancer Institute, 2008.

2 Belson M, Kingsley B, Holmes A. Risk factors for acute leukemia in children: a review. *Environ Health Perspect* 2007;115:138–45.

3 Pui CH, Robison LL, Look AT. Acute lymphoblastic leukemia. *Lancet* 2008;371:1030–43.

4 Greaves MF, Alexander FE. An infectious etiology for common acute lymphoblastic leukemia in childhood? *Leukemia* 1993;7:349–60.

5 Kinlen L. Evidence for an infective cause of childhood leukemia: comparison of a Scottish new town with nuclear reprocessing sites in Britain. *Lancet* 1988;2:1323–7.

6 Swerdlow SH, Campo E, Harris NL, *et al.* (eds). *WHO Classification of Tumors of the Hematopoietic and Lymphoid Tissue.* IARC Press: Lyon, 2008.

7 Pui CH, Dodge RK, Dahl GV, *et al*. Serum lactic dehydrogenase level has prognostic value in childhood acute lymphoblastic leukemia. *Blood* 1985;66:778–82.

8 Moricke A, Reiter A, Zimmermann M, *et al*. Risk-adjusted therapy of acute lymphoblastic leukemia can decrease treatment burden and improve survival: treatment results of 2169 unselected pediatric and adolescent patients enrolled in the trial ALL-BFM 95. *Blood* 2008;111:4477–89.

9 Fulcher JW, Allred TJ, Kulharya A, *et al*. Granular acute lymphoblastic leukemia in adults: report of a case and review of the literature. *South Med J* 2006;99:894–7.

10 Hodson D, Gatward G, Erber W. Azurophilic granules in acute lymphoblastic leukemia resulting from abundant mitochondria. *Br J Haematol* 2004;125:265.

11 Lilleyman JS, Hann IM, Stevens RF, Richards SM, Eden OB. Blast cell vacuoles in childhood lymphoblastic leukemia. *Br J Haematol* 1988;70:183–6.

12 Lilleyman JS, Britton JA, Anderson LM, Richards SM, Bailey CC, Chessells JM. Periodic acid Schiff reaction in childhood lymphoblastic leukemia. The Medical Research Council Working Party on Childhood Leukemia. *J Clin Pathol* 1994;47: 689–92.

13 Matloub YH, Brunning RD, Arthur DC, Ramsay NK. Severe aplastic anemia preceding acute lymphoblastic leukemia. *Cancer* 1993;71:264–8.

14 Macfarlane SD, Tauro GP. Acute lymphocytic leukemia in children presenting with bone marrow necrosis. *Am J Hematol* 1986;22:341–6.

15 Thomas X, Le QH, Danaïla C, Lhéritier V, Ffrench M. Bone marrow biopsy in adult acute lymphoblastic leukemia: morphological characteristics and contribution to the study of prognostic factors. *Leuk Res* 2002;26:909–18.

16 Wallis JP, Reid MM. Bone marrow fibrosis in childhood acute lymphoblastic leukemia. *J Clin Pathol* 1989;42:1253–4.

17 Feldman AL, Dogan A. Diagnostic uses of Pax5 immunohistochemistry. *Adv Anat Pathol* 2007;14:323–34.

18 Kebriaei P, Anastasi J, Larson RA. Acute lymphoblastic leukemia: diagnosis and classification. *Best Pract Res Clin Haematol* 2002;15:597–621.

19 Yeoh EJ, Ross ME, Shurtleff SA, *et al*. Classification, subtype discovery, and prediction of outcome in pediatric acute lymphoblastic leukemia by gene expression profiling. *Cancer Cell* 2002;1:133–43.

20 Pui CH, Relling MV, Downing JR. Acute lymphoblastic leukemia. *N Engl J Med* 2004;350:1535–48.

21 Armstrong SA, Look AT. Molecular genetics of acute lymphoblastic leukemia. *J Clin Oncol* 2005;23:6306–15.

22 Paietta E, Racevskis J, Neuberg D, Rowe JM, Goldstone AH, Wiernik PH. Expression of CD25 (interleukin-2 receptor alpha chain) in adult acute lymphoblastic leukemia predicts for the presence of BCR/ABL fusion transcripts: results of a preliminary laboratory analysis of ECOG/MRC Intergroup Study E2993. Eastern Cooperative Oncology Group/Medical Research Council. *Leukemia* 1997;11:1887–90.

23 Krivtsov AV, Armstrong SA. MLL translocations, histone modifications and leukemia stem-cell development. *Nat Rev Cancer* 2007;7:823–33.

24 Raimondi SC. Current status of cytogenetic research in childhood acute lymphoblastic leukemia. *Blood* 1993;81:2237–51.

25 Golub TR, Barker GF, Bohlander SK, *et al*. Fusion of the *TEL* gene on 12p13 to the *AML1* gene on 21q22 in acute lymphoblastic leukemia. *Proc Natl Acad Sci U S A* 1995;92: 4917–21.

26 Perry C, Eldor A, Soreq H. *Runx1/AML1* in leukemia: disrupted association with diverse protein partners. *Leuk Res* 2002;26: 221–8.

27 Greaves MF, Wiemels J. Origins of chromosome translocations in childhood leukemia. *Nat Rev Cancer* 2003;3:639–49.

28 Heerema NA, Raimondi SC, Anderson JR, *et al*. Specific extra chromosomes occur in a modal number dependent pattern in pediatric acute lymphoblastic leukemia. *Genes Chromosomes Cancer* 2007;46:684–93.

29 Arico M, Valsecchi MG, Rizzari C, *et al*. Long-term results of the AIEOP-ALL-95 Trial for Childhood Acute Lymphoblastic Leukemia: insight on the prognostic value of DNA index in the framework of Berlin-Frankfurt-Muenster based chemotherapy. *J Clin Oncol* 2008;26:283–9.

30 Sutcliffe MJ, Shuster JJ, Sather HN, *et al*. High concordance from independent studies by the Children's Cancer Group (CCG) and Pediatric Oncology Group (POG) associating favorable prognosis with combined trisomies 4, 10, and 17 in children with NCI standard-risk B-precursor acute lymphoblastic leukemia: a Children's Oncology Group (COG) initiative. *Leukemia* 2005;19:734–40.

31 Harrison CJ, Moorman AV, Broadfield ZJ, *et al*. Three distinct subgroups of hypodiploidy in acute lymphoblastic leukemia. *Br J Haematol* 2004;125:552–9.

32 Nachman JB, Heerema NA, Sather H, *et al*. Outcome of treatment in children with hypodiploid acute lymphoblastic leukemia. *Blood* 2007;110:1112–15.

33 Grimaldi JC, Meeker TC. The t(5;14) chromosomal translocation in a case of acute lymphocytic leukemia joins the *Interleukin-3* gene to the immunoglobulin heavy chain gene. *Blood* 1989;73:2081–5.

Chapter 16
Induction Therapy in Adult Acute Lymphoblastic Leukemia

Xavier Thomas
Leukemia Unit, Department of Hematology, Edouard Herriot Hospital, Hospices Civils de Lyon, Lyon, France

Introduction

Acute lymphoblastic leukemia (ALL) is a malignant neoplasm of lymphocyte-precursor cells. ALL is characterized by aberrations in proliferation and differentiation of leukemic lymphoblasts, leading to failure of normal immune response and a decreased production of normal hematopoiesis responsible for anemia, thrombocytopenia, and neutropenia. Both T-cell and B-cell precursors can be involved in the malignant process. ALL is a heterogeneous disease with distinct morphologic, cytogenetic, and molecular groupings, some of which have important clinical implications. The French–American–British (FAB) classification, which recognized three subtypes of ALL, was based strictly on morphology and cytochemistry [1], whereas the current World Health Organization (WHO) classification also incorporates immunophenotyping and cytogenetics [2]. ALL represents <1% of adult cancers, while it represents 25% of all childhood cancers. Principles of induction therapy of adult ALL are therefore based on those initially developed for children. Treatment is often tailored to specific disease entities. Remission induction regimens classically involve cyclical combination chemotherapy, usually including prednisolone, vincristine, and an anthracycline with or without L-asparaginase, cytosine arabinoside, and cyclophosphamide.

Historical considerations

First chemotherapies

The era of chemotherapy began in the 1940s with the first uses of nitrogen mustards and antifolate drugs. Folate analogs—first aminopterin and then amethopterin (methotrexate)—became the first drugs to successfully induce remission in children with ALL by blocking the function of folate-requiring enzymes [3,4]. Methotrexate was also the first drug for which pharmacokinetic analysis was routinely used to monitor drug clearance and identify patients at risk of severe toxicity [5]. The therapeutic value of corticosteroids was discovered in 1949, of which prednisone became the most widely used. Their capacity to cause lymphocyte death was exploited promptly in the clinical treatment of acute leukemias [6]. Other antileukemic drugs came to clinical trials in the1950s and the 1960s, such as 6-mercaptopurine [7] and vinca alkaloids [8]. The kinetics of tumor growth were analyzed and *in vivo* assays for quantifying cytotoxicity were created [9]. Inhibitors of DNA synthesis, such as cytosine arabinoside (Ara-C) [10], proved most effective against rapidly dividing cells, while drugs that physically damaged DNA, such as alkylating agents, were cell-cycle non-specific.

Combination chemotherapy

In 1965, a combination of methotrexate, vincristine, 6-mercaptopurine, and prednisone—which together were referred to as the POMP regimen—was shown to induce long-term remissions in children with ALL [11]. Cytotoxicity was shown as a direct function of dose, suggesting the use of high-dose chemotherapy, and the effectiveness of combination chemotherapy was demonstrated in preventing drug resistance. Other effective molecules, including anthracyclines and epidophyllotoxins, emerged during the period 1970–1990 [12,13]. Through these approaches, the cure of ALL in children evolved from an anecdotal wonder to a quantifiable reality. Methods of dealing with complications of leukemia, such as meningeal leukemia, were developed [14]. Supportive care concomitantly improved. Blood transfusion technology advanced rapidly. Platelet transfusions became available [15]. Advances in the control of infections have been a major factor in the improved outcome of leukemia therapy. The recombinant hematopoietic growth factors (HGFs) were introduced during the mid-1980s. These factors were used for their ability to stimulate normal hematopoiesis and thereby reduce the toxicity of conventional cytotoxic therapies. Although giving less spectacular results than those seen in children, these therapeutic

Leukemias: Principles and Practice of Therapy, 1st edition. Edited by S. Faderl and H. Kantarjian.

strategies have been applied to adults with ALL, leading to an improved response rate and survival over the past two decades.

Targeted therapy

Signaling networks that regulate cellular activities were explored, and many of them were found to be altered in malignant cells. This leads to the era of targeted therapy with the aim to repair these molecular defects. Innovations in technology increased the success of finding inhibitors of specific targets. The new targets included growth factors, signaling molecules, cell-cycle proteins, modulators of apoptosis, and molecules that promoted angiogenesis [16]. One of the landmark events in the revolution of targeted therapies has been the development of imatinib mesylate, a potent inhibitor of the Bcr–Abl kinase, the fusion protein product of translocation t(9;22) that is involved in the pathogenesis of Philadelphia chromosome-positive ALL [17].

Antileukemic drugs used in induction schedules

Corticosteroids

The adrenocorticosteroids most commonly used are prednisone and its soluble analog, prednisolone. These drugs are usually given daily in dosages ranging from $40\,mg/m^2$ to $80\,mg/m^2$. Their mechanisms of action probably involve the activation of nucleases leading to DNA fragmentation [18]. Dexamethasone has a higher antileukemic activity and is administered at dosage of $6\,mg/m^2$ to $10\,mg/m^2$ [19]. It may provide greater control of central nervous system (CNS) leukemia [20], but can increase susceptibility to severe infections [21]. Prednisolone given at intervals less frequent than daily [22] or steroids given at higher doses have also been used without significantly improved complete remission (CR) rates [23].

Vinca alkaloids

A single intravenous dosage of 2 mg/week has become the consensus mode for vincristine administration. More frequent injections [24] and continuous infusions [25] not only increase the biologic effects of vincristine, but also the toxicity with peripheral neuropathy or paralytic ileus. Other vinca alkaloids (vinblastine, vindesine) have been used in ALL with equal activity compared with vincristine [26], but with less neurotoxicity.

Anthracyclines and non-anthracycline DNA intercalators

Anthracyclines (daunorubicin, adriamycin) induce a 25–50% CR in patients with ALL. Anthracyclines in combination add to the effectiveness of induction regimens [27]. The application of dose-intensive anthracyclines during induction therapy may contribute to an improvement of CR rate [28]. The relative value of newer anthracyclines (rubidazone and idarubicin) in comparison to daunorubicin has not yet been established [29,30]. However, idarubicin may circumvent P-glycoprotein-mediated drug resistance. Its breakdown product idarubidazol may also be found in the CNS, suggesting its use in the treatment or prophylaxis of CNS leukemia.

Two non-anthracycline DNA intercalators, 4′-[9-acridinylamino]methansulfon-m-anisidide and mitoxantrone, have proved to be effective in ALL therapy. 4′-[9-Acridinylamino]methansulfon-m-anisidide is not cross-resistant with anthracyclines and is generally used in salvage combination chemotherapy at doses ranging from 90 to $120\,mg/m^2$. Mitoxantrone, a synthetic anthraquinone, is generally given at $10\,mg/m^2$/day for 5 days, but in combination with high-dose cytarabine it is given for 3 or 4 days only.

Alkylating agents

The alkylating agents are directly descended from the sulfur mustard used in the trenches during the World War I. They interact with DNA, which makes them cytotoxic and cell-cycle phase non-specific. General mechanisms of resistance include drug deactivation by conjugation with glutathione and increased repair of alkylated bases by a number of specific repair systems. Cyclophosphamide is the most commonly used alkylating agent for ALL. It is effective in T-cell ALL and may act synergistically with cytarabine [31]. In B-cell lineage ALL, cyclophosphamide is used in moderate to high doses [32,33]. At $200\,mg/m^2$ for 5 days in combination with prednisolone, it can induce tumor-mass reduction in mature B-ALL as the initial phase of treatment [34]. Ifosfamide is another alkylating agent with remission induction potential comparable to cyclophosphamide [35].

L-Asparaginase

L-Asparaginase may be given at various doses and schedules, but higher doses increase its CR induction potential [36]. Caution is required to avoid life-threatening anaphylactoid reactions and coagulation disturbances. Preparations from different origins (*Erwinia carotovora* or *Escherichia coli*) are available. These preparations show differences in terms of half-life, which has consequences for dose schedules. At the same dose level, *Erwinia carotovora* has been associated with less toxicity but also with inferior efficacy [37]. A polyethylene glycol (PEG) encapsulated L-asparaginase has been explored as part of multi-drug induction therapy. Higher CR rates and more rapid response have been described with PEG-asparaginase [38]. A dose level of $1000\,IU/m^2$ may yield sufficient asparaginase activity for at least 14 days. PEG-asparaginase did not show higher toxicity compared with native *Escherichia coli* asparaginase [39].

Folic acid antimetabolites

Methotrexate, a less toxic analog of ametopterin, is currently the most widely used antifolate. The terminal elimination half-life is about 8–10h but may be prolonged considerably in patients with impaired renal function or a third-space compartment. The major toxicities are myelosuppression, renal toxicity, and mucositis. High-dose methotrexate provides effective antileukemic drug concentrations and has the potential to overcome mechanisms of resistance against methotrexate. Higher doses (>100 mg/m^2) are typically used with a rescue dose of reduced folate, N5-formyl-tetrahydrofolate (calcium folinate, leucovorin), with the dose administered determined by the methotrexate concentration at 24h. Methotrexate is also used as intrathecal therapy, both for CNS prophylaxis and in the treatment of established meningeal leukemia.

Nucleoside analogs

Ara-C is a potent inhibitor of a number of DNA polymerases involved in DNA replication and repair, resulting in termination of strand elongation [40]. High-dose Ara-C (2–3 g/m^2) has been used extensively in ALL and may be particularly useful in T-cell ALL [41]. It is more active when administered every 12h by injection or by continuous infusion. High-dose Ara-C yields cytotoxic drug levels in the cerebrospinal fluid and has also been used for remission induction in CNS leukemia [42]. Fludarabine is a newer purine analog that exerts synergistic activity with cytarabine. Regimens including fludarabine and high-dose Ara-C followed by granulocyte colony-stimulating factor (G-CSF) or in combination with additional idarubicin have shown promising activity [43].

Epidophyllotoxines

Podophyllotoxin is a natural product extracted from the roots of *Podophyllum peltatum* and *Podophyllum emodi*. Two derivatives, etoposide (VP16) and tenoposide (VM26), are used increasingly in combination, particularly with Ara-C. They induce DNA strand breaks, resulting in a block in the cell cycle in late S or G_2 [44]. Resistance is mainly due to two mechanisms: increased expression of the *MDR1* gene resulting in increased P-glycoprotein, increased efflux of drug from the cell, and decreased activity of topoisomerase II.

Tyrosine kinase inhibitors

The most promising current approach using targeted therapy with signal transduction inhibitors is the use of imatinib mesylate (STI571, Gleevec; Novartis, Basel, Switzerland) to treat Philadelphia chromosome-positive (Ph^+) ALL. Abl kinase blockade by imatinib mesylate has proven remarkably active. However, the benefit is seen only when Bcr–Abl inhibitors are combined with chemotherapy, either concomitantly or sequentially. Imatinib mesylate is a member of the 2-phenylaminopyrimidine class of small molecules that has a high affinity and selectivity for Abl. Protein kinases contain within their catalytic domain a nucleotide-binding pocket and an activation loop that controls activity [45]. Imatinib, which binds to the Abl nucleotide-binding pocket, recognizes and stabilizes a distinct, inactive conformation of the activation loop of Abl and precludes adenosine triphosphate (ATP) binding. This prevents Bcr–Abl from phosphorylating tyrosine residues of substrate proteins, thereby interrupting Bcr–Abl signal transduction pathways. Imatinib mesylate is a Bcr–Abl tyrosine kinase inhibitor that has shown equal activity against p210 and p190 disease [17,46]. Various mechanisms of resistance have been documented [47]. Imatinib resistance may occur on the basis of clonal selection of cells that reactivate Bcr–Abl despite continuation of imatinib therapy. The reactivation may be accompanied by genomic amplification, overexpression of Bcr–Abl, or spontaneous mutations of the tyrosine kinase domain of Bcr–Abl, resulting in insensibility to imatinib. The emergence of resistance to imatinib mesylate reinforces the need for additional strategies. A series of substituted 2-(aminopyridyl)- and 2-(aminopyrimidinyl)thiazole-5-carboxamides was identified as potent Src/Abl kinase inhibitors with excellent antiproliferative activity against hematologic cell lines [48]. Dasatinib (BMS-354825, Sprycel; Bristol-Myers Squibb, New York, NY, USA) has demonstrated two-log increased potency relative to imatinib that retains activity against imatinib-resistant *BCR–ABL* mutants [49]. Nilotinib (AMN-107, Tasigna; Novartis) was also found to be significantly more potent than imatinib against Ph^+ ALL [50].

Remission induction

Most therapeutic advances in adult ALL have arisen from the successful adaptation of ALL treatment in children. It has been well demonstrated that induction of remission improves survival and is essential for the chance of cure. Rapid remission induction reduces the likelihood for development of clinical resistance to the drugs. Currently, intensive combination therapy in adult ALL has resulted in CR rates of 80–90% [30,51–66] (Table 16.1). Despite high CR rates, there is still no unanimity among hematologists regarding drugs, doses, or schedules.

Standard treatment

Historically, induction therapy for adult ALL has been built around a "backbone" of vincristine and prednisone. The combination of vincristine and prednisone alone produces CR rates of approximately 35–65% but a median remission duration of only 3–7 months. Intensifying induction therapy by adding an anthracycline was first shown in a randomized Cancer and Leukemia Group B

Table 16.1 Results of induction chemotherapy in adult acute lymphoblastic leukemia.

Reference	Patients	Age (range) (years)	Induction therapy (without CNS prophylaxis)	Complete remission (%)	Death during induction (%)
Larson *et al.* [51]	198	35 (16–83)	CP 1200 mg/m^2 d1, DNR 45 mg/m^2 days 1–3, Vcr 2 mg days 1, 8, 15, 22, Pred 60 mg/m^2 days 1–2L, L-aspa 6000 IU/m^2 days 5, 8, 11, 15, 18, 22	82	8
Thiebaut *et al.* [52]	572	33 (15–60)	RBZ 100 mg/m^2 or DNR 50 mg/m^2 days 1–3, Vcr 1.5 mg/m^2 days 1, 8, 15, 22, CP 600 mg/m^2 days 1, 8, Pred 60 mg/m^2 days 1–22	76	9
Kantarjian *et al.* [53]	203	39 (16–79)	Part 1: CP 300 mg/m^2 every 12 h days 1–3, Adria 50 mg/m^2 day 4, Vcr 2 mg day 4, 11, Dex 40 mg days 1–4, 11–14 Part 2: MTX 200 then 800 mg/m^2 day1, Ara-C 3g/m^2 every 12 h days 2, 3, MetPred 50 mg d 1–3	91	6
Rowe *et al.* [54]	871	30 (14–60)	Phase I: DNR 60 mg/m^2 days 1, 8, 15, 22, Vcr 1.4 mg/m^2 days 1, 8, 15, 22, L-aspa 10,000 IU days 17–28, Pred 60 mg/m^2 days 1–28 Phase II: CP 650 mg/m^2 days 1, 15, 29, Ara-C 75 mg/m^2 days 1–4, 8–11, 15–18, 22–25, 6MP 6 mg/m^2 days 1–28	89	5
Dekker *et al.* [55]	193	33 (15–60)	Phase I: Pred 60 mg/m^2 days 1–28, Vcr 1.5 mg/m^2 days 1, 8, 15, 22, DNR 45 mg/m^2 days 1, 8, 15, 22, L-aspa 5000 IU/m^2 days 15–28 Phase II: CP 650 mg/m^2 days 1, 15, 29, Ara-C 75 mg/m^2 days 4–7, 11–14, 18–21, 25–28	82	ND
Bassan *et al.* [56]	121	35 (ND–ND)	Ida 10 mg/m^2 days 1, 2, Vcr 2 mg days 1, 8, 15, L-aspa 6000 IU/m^2 days 8, 10, 12, 16, 18, Pred 60 mg/m^2 days 1–21, (CP 150 mg/m2 day 3 to day 0; only for T-ALL), G-CSF 5 μg/kg day 3 to recovery	84	ND
Gökbuget *et al.* [57]	1200	35 (15–65)	Phase I: Pred 60 mg/m^2 days 1–29, Vcr 2 mg days 1, 8, 15, 22, DNR 45 mg/m^2 days 1, 8, 15, 22, L-aspa 5000 IU/m^2 days 15, 17, 19, 22, 24, 26, 28 Phase II: CP 1000 mg/m^2 days 29, 43, 57, Ara-C 75 mg/m^2 days 31–34, 38–41, 45–48, 52–55, G-CSF (during phase II)	86	5
Hallbook *et al.* [58]	120	44 (16–82)	HD-Ara-C 3 g/m^2/12h days 1–3, CP 600 mg/m^2 day 1, DNR 30 mg/m^2 days 1–3, Vcr 2 mg day 1, beta 20 mg/m^2 days 1–5	85	5
Takeuchi *et al.* [59]	263	31 (15–59)	Vcr 1.3 mg/m^2 (max. 2 mg) days 1, 8, 15, 22, Adria 30 mg/m^2 days 1, 2, 3, 8, (9, 10)[a], Pred 40 mg/m^2 days 1–10, L-aspa 6000 IU/m^2 days 29–35, CP 600 mg/m^2 days 29, G-CSF 200 μg/m^2 days 12–26	78	6
Linker *et al.* [60]	84	27 (18–59)	DNR 60 mg/m2 days 1–3,(15)[b], Vcr 1.4 mg/m^2 days 1, 8, 15, 22, Pred 60 mg/m^2 days 1–28, L-aspa 6000 IU/m^2 days 17–28	93	ND
Annino *et al.* [61]	794	27 (12–60)	Prephase: Pred 20–60 mg/m^2 day 7 to day 1 Induction: CP 800 mg/m^2 days 1, 2, DNR 40 mg/m^2 days 1, 8, 15, 22, Vcr 2 mg/m^2 days 1, 8, 15, 22, Pred 60 mg/m^2 days 1–14, 40 mg/m^2 days 15–31, L-aspa 6000 IU/m^2 days 22–31	82	7
Kantarjian *et al.* [62]	288	40 (15–92)	Part 1: CP 300 mg/m^2/12 h d1–3, Adria 50 mg/m^2 day 4, Vcr 2 mg days 4, 11, Dex 40 mg days 1–4, 11–14 Part 2: MTX 200 then 800 mg/m^2 day 1, Ara-C 3g/m^2/12 h days 2, 3, MetPred 50 mg days 1–3	92	5

Table 16.1 Continued

Reference	Patients	Age (range) (years)	Induction therapy (without CNS prophylaxis)	Complete remission (%)	Death during induction (%)
Labar *et al.* [63]	340	33 (14–79)	DNR 45 mg/m² days 1, 2, 3, CP 600 mg/m² days 1, 8, Vcr 1.5 mg/m² days 1, 8, 15, 22, Pred 60 mg/m² days 1–22	74	ND
Hunault *et al.* [64]	198	33 (15–59)	Prephase: Pred 40 mg/m² day 3 to day 1 Induction: Pred 40 mg/m² days 1-d21, Vcr 1.5 mg/m² days 1, 8, 15, 22, Ida 5 mg/m² days 1, 8, 15, 22, L-aspa 7500 IU/m² days 10, 13, 16, 19, 22, 25	86	2
Thomas *et al.* [30]	922	33 (15–55)	Ida 9 mg/m² days 1–3, 8, or DNR 30 mg/m² days 1–3, 15, 16, Vcr 1.5 mg/m² days 1, 8, 15, 22, CP 750 mg/m² days 1, 8, Pred 60 mg/m² days 1–7, 15–21	84	5
Ribera *et al.* [65]	222	27 (15–50)	Vcr 2 mg days 1, 8, 15, 22, DNR 30 mg/m² days 1, 8, 15, 22, Pred 60 mg/m² days 1–28, 30 mg/m² days 29–33, 15 mg/m² days 34–38, L-aspa 10,000 IU/m² days 16–20, days 23–27, CP 1000 mg/m² day 36	82	6
Rowe *et al.* [66]	1521	ND (15–59)	Phase I: DNR 60 mg/m² days 1, 8, 15, 22, Vcr 1.4 mg/m² days 1, 8, 15, 22, L-aspa 10,000 IU days 17–28, Pred 60 mg/m² days 1–28 Phase II: CP 650 mg/m² days 1, 15, 29, Ara-C 75 mg/m² days 1–4, 8–11, 15–18, 22–25, 6MP 6 mg/m² days 1–28	91	ND

Adria, adriamycin; Ara-C, cytarabine; beta, betamethasone; CNS, central nervous system; CP, cyclophosphamide; DNR, daunorubicin; G-CSF, granulocyte colony-stimulating factor; HD-Ara-C, high-dose cytarabine; Ida, idarubicin; L-aspa, L-asparaginase; MetPred, methylprednisolone; MTX, methotrexate; 6MP, 6-mercaptopurine; ND, not done; Pred, prednisone or prednisolone; RBZ, rubidazone; Vcr, vincristine.

[a]Except if day 8 bone marrow showed <20% leukemic cells.

[b]If day 14 bone marrow had residual leukemia.

(CALGB) trial to significantly increase the likelihood of achieving a CR from about 50% to 78% [27]. These results were then confirmed by other studies. The anthracyclines used include doxorubicin (adriamycin), daunorubicin, and more recently idarubicin and ribidazone. Daunorubicin has been the most extensively studied because of its availability for the longest period of time, its activity, and its lower gastrointestinal mucosal toxicity. The optimal schedule of anthracyclines is controversial. The two most common schedules are once weekly or daily for 3 days for each course. According to pediatric experience [67], administration over 2 or 3 days is more active through greater myelosuppression. Although there are no randomized studies addressing further intensification of induction therapy, almost all modern treatment regimens add L-asparaginase or cyclophosphamide to induction therapy. Asparaginase does not affect the CR rate but probably improves leukemia-free survival (LFS) and, if not used during induction therapy, it is often included as part of the consolidation treatment [68]. However, the addition of L-asparaginase to vincristine and prednisolone has led to improved CR rates in relapsed pediatric patients with ALL [69]. Cyclophosphamide also does not raise the overall CR rate, but possibly improves the remission quality. Accordingly, standard induction regimens can be labeled as four-drug (vincristine, prednisone, anthracycline, and cyclophosphamide or L-asparaginase) or five-drug (vincristine, prednisone, anthracycline, cyclophosphamide, and L-asparaginase) regimens. No data favor one of these induction regimens over another. A pediatric study showed that the sum of the percentages of three induction drugs (vincristine, L-asparaginase and anthracyclines) delivered were critical in predicting relapse, supporting the concept that dose intensity during induction is important for long-term prognosis [70]. To improve outcome, modifications of these standard treatments have been proposed by adding known chemotherapy drugs, intensifying chemotherapy doses, or incorporating new and "targeted" drugs. Although the addition of other cytotoxic drugs does not increase CR rates substantially, the highest remission rates have been achieved with multidrug induction regimens.

Prephase with corticosteroids

The majority of ALL blast cells are sensitive to steroids. Response to a 7-day pretreatment with prednisolone as measured by the reduction of leukemia cells in the peripheral blood is considered as a significant prognostic factor [61]. Furthermore, a cautious cell reduction phase is recommended for patients with a large leukemic cell burden at diagnosis. Steroid pre-induction phase in combination with urate oxidase has dramatically decreased the frequency of tumor lysis syndrome and, in combination with chemotherapy, the need for hemodialysis in patients with B-cell ALL [33].

Addition of other drugs to induction

High-dose cytarabine

The aim of treatment with high-dose Ara-C (HD-Ara-C) is not only to improve the CR rate but also to increase the quality of remission and to provide efficient prophylaxis of CNS relapse. The addition of HD-Ara-C (1–3 g/m^2, generally for 12 doses) after the standard induction therapy has resulted in CR rates ranging from 67% to 94% [71–75]. This approach does not appear superior to conventional treatment, and it remains uncertain for which subgroups it may be beneficial for LFS. The exception is the hyper-CVAD regimen, which yielded a high CR rate of 91% [53]. The hyper-CVAD regimen follows the principles developed by Murphy *et al.* [76], who developed a short-term dose-intense chemotherapy regimen that consisted of a combination of fractionated cyclophosphamide, followed by vincristine and adriamycin, followed after hematologic recovery by a second cycle with a non-cross-resistant combination of high-dose intravenous methotrexate and cytarabine. Another approach is the upfront administration of HD-Ara-C before standard induction treatment. This yielded, in two preliminary reports, remission rates of 85% [58,77].

High-dose methotrexate

Methotrexate at a dosage of 6 g/m^2 resulted in an 80% CR rate in children with CNS ALL, indicating that systemic application yields cytotoxic levels in the cerebrospinal fluid [78]. Several studies have investigated the efficacy of high-dose methotrexate as induction treatment in combination with other chemotherapeutic agents in adult ALL [79,80].

Intensification of anthracycline doses

Anthracyclines have become a fundamental part for remission induction in adult ALL. Although CR can be achieved without the use of anthracyclines, data support the role of anthracyclines in increasing the CR rate [27] and inducing more rapid reduction of leukemic cells, before the development of drug resistance [81]. In a retrospective analysis, the long-term disease-free survival (DFS) was found to improve when an anthracycline was administered at high doses delivered in short time [82]. Retrospective studies suggested that early dose intensification of daunorubicin would lead to superior leukemia-free survival [83]. Induction therapy was based on a combination of vincristine, prednisone, and daunorubicin, in which daunorubicin was administered daily for 3 consecutive days [84]. High dose was defined as >175 mg/m^2 in induction, and low dose as <175 mg/m^2. The cut-off for dose intensity was 21 mg/m^2/week. Higher dose and dose intensity of daunorubicin given in induction affected long-term DFS. In a subsequent study [83], the median dose was increased by 47%, from 175 mg/m^2 to 257.5 mg/m^2, and the dose intensity was increased by 81%, from 21 mg/m^2/week to 38 mg/m^2/week. The CR rate improved from 79% to 93%, and the rate of resistant cases decreased from 3.5% to 1.6%. However, the dose-limiting toxicity of these schedules was cardiac toxicity [85]. To reduce this risk, the total planned dose of daunorubicin was stopped at 550 mg/m^2 [83]. The preventive use of dexrazoxane also has been suggested. Other studies have not confirmed an improvement in DFS, but have shown fewer relapses [86].

Dexamethasone instead of prednisone

Dexamethasone is five- to six times more cytotoxic than prednisolone in stroma-supported cultures of ALL blasts [19], and has shown a 16-fold higher antileukemic activity in an *in vitro* drug sensitivity assay [87]. The half-life of dexamethasone is also longer in the cerebrospinal fluid (CSF) compared with prednisolone [20]. This was confirmed in a randomized study comparing dexamethasone and prednisolone during induction therapy in childhood ALL, by a lower rate of CNS relapses with dexamethasone [88]. Dexamethasone has therefore progressively replaced prednisone for better antileukemia activity and achievement of higher levels in the CSF [88,89]. However, the extensive use of dexamethasone may increase the risk of severe infections and the risk of bone marrow necrosis [21]. Furthermore, dexamethasone pharmacokinetics depend on concurrent use of particular drugs [90]. Patients with diminished exposure to asparaginase may experience fewer antileukemic effects of dexamethasone by maintaining high clearance of dexamethasone.

Incorporation of novel agents

Pegylated asparaginase

Native asparaginase, because of immunogenicity, can result in anaphylactic reactions or development of neutralizing antibodies with rapid clearance and short plasma half-life of asparaginase [91]. Recently, *E. Coli* asparaginase has been covalently linked to monomethoxy-polyethylene glycol, rendering native asparaginase less immunogenic with a longer plasma half-life, and enabling up to bi-weekly administrations. Limited experience is available in adult ALL. However, randomized studies in children have shown higher CR rates in the PEG-asparaginase group that more rapidly cleared lymphoblasts from early marrow samples and developed antibodies less frequently [92,93]. In adults, the data are still scarce. A high CR rate of 93% was achieved in one study using intensified PEG-asparaginase [38].

Recently, a new enzyme formulation of L-asparaginase (GRASPA®), with a safer and broader range of clinical uses compared with existing forms, has been developed [94]. This formulation (encapsuling L-asparaginase in homologous red blood cells) is able to overcome limitations associated with conventional L-asparaginase, making it satisfactory even for hypersensitive or elderly patients, or patients with neutralizing antibodies.

Liposomal preparations

Liposomal preparations of chemotherapeutic agents change the pharmacologic properties of the active compound, generally resulting in better efficacy with reduced toxicity. Several liposomal agents have been investigated.

Conventional anthracyclines are active against leukemic cells [83], but cardiotoxicity related to cumulative dose limits their use. Encapsuling conventional anthracyclines in liposomes, microscopic vesicles, consisting of concentric lipid membranes, reduced the incidence and severity of cardiomyopathy while preserving antitumor activity. Two preparations containing doxorubicin (doxil; Shering-Plough, Kenilworth, NJ, USA, and evacet; The Liposome Company, Princeton, NJ, USA) and one containing daunorubicin (daunoxome, Gilead Sciences, Foster City, CA, USA) have been undergoing widespread clinical study. The three compounds vary widely in their pharmacology [95]. High doses of liposomal daunorubicin (daunoxome) during ALL remission induction may achieve the same goals with lower rates of cardiotoxicity and mucositis. A daunoxome dosage of 100–125 mg/m^2 per day for 3 days has been shown safe and effective in combination with high-dose cytarabine [96].

Doxil, a pegylated "stealth" liposomal formulation of doxorubicin hydrochloride, avoids uptake by the reticuloendothelial system, thus improving drug delivery to malignant cells while decreasing toxicity. Liposome-encapsulated doxorubicin citrate complex (Myocet; Cephalon Limited, Oxford, UK), another liposomal delivery system for doxorubicin, lacks the polyethylene glycol coating, resulting in much shorter circulation times than those of doxil [97].

Liposomal vincristine has also been studied. Whereas the half-life of free vincristine is only 10 min, that of liposomal vincristine is up to 8 h [98]. Liposomal vincristine is well tolerated with only mild neurotoxicity. Substitution of vincristine for the liposomal preparation in ALL induction protocols is planned.

New cytotoxic drugs under investigation

Nucleoside analogs, which demonstrate additional metabolic properties and mechanisms of actions, are under investigation in adult ALL and could be included in the near future into remission induction regimens [99].

Clofarabine is a second-generation purine analog with activity in acute leukemias and approval for use in children with ALL relapse. It exerts an antiproliferative effect by inhibiting ribonucleotide reductase and by direct DNA incorporation [100].

Fludarabine is a DNA synthesis inhibitor that was also shown to be an effective drug for remission induction in ALL [101]. However, doses required to achieve CR are associated with unacceptable CNS toxicity. In view of its potent antileukemic activity, further evaluation of fludarabine at lower doses may be warranted in combination with other agents. Regimens combining fludarabine with cytarabine and liposomal daunorubicin have already been shown as an effective alternative treatment for patients with ALL who failed first-line therapy [102].

Nelarabine is an inactive pro-drug of guanine arabinoside (ara-G). It is rapidly activated by adenosine deaminase to ara-G, resulting in cytotoxic levels of ara-GTP in circulating leukemia cells. Ara-GTP is accumulated at higher levels in T-lymphoblasts than in B-lymphoblasts [103].

Decitabine is an inhibitor of DNA methyltransferase, preventing methylation of cytosine residues on DNA and leading to hypomethylation of gene promoters, thereby reactivating silenced genes. Interest in the drug was renewed following the discovery of potential synergies between decitabine and chemotherapy, and immunostimulants and histone deacetylase inhibitors [104]. Although experience with this agent is scarce in ALL, understanding epigenetic changes may offer another mechanism, the targeting of which may lead to risk-adapted therapies.

Monoclonal antibodies

Monoclonal antibody (MoAb) therapy in ALL is based on two characteristics: selectivity of the tumor target and different mechanisms of actions compared with traditional cytotoxic chemotherapy. CD20 is expressed in about 35% of patients with ALL with higher expression in Ph$^+$ ALL and mature B-cell ALL. ALL blasts also show high expression of CD19 and CD52.

Rituximab is a chimeric MoAb directed against CD20. Moreover, the presence of CD20 on ALL blasts is associated with a worse outcome [105]. Rituximab plus hyper-CVAD has been reported [106]. When compared with the previous trial with chemotherapy alone, 89% complete responses were observed without additional toxicity. The addition of rituximab in CD20$^+$ patients may therefore have a favorable impact on outcome in mature B-ALL and Ph$^+$ ALL [107].

CD19 is highly expressed in most patients with B-lineage ALL. Several antibodies targeting CD19 have been developed. Most MoAbs targeting the CD19 antigen are conjugated with immunotoxins. Blocked ricin is a toxin that was conjugated with the anti-CD19 MoAb (anti-B4-bR) and showed enhanced cytotoxic activity in lymphoid malignancies [108]. Experience with other conjugates (tyrosine kinase inhibitor genistein, pokeweed antiviral protein immunotoxin) suggested antitumor activity, but experience remains limited. It has been demonstrated that the imatinib-encapsulated CD19 liposomes induced specific and efficient death of Ph^+ ALL cells. This new therapeutic approach might be a useful treatment for Ph^+ ALL, with a higher cytocidal effect than that of free imatinib [109].

CD52 is expressed to a higher degree in T- rather than B-lymphoblasts, and use of the anti-CD52 MoAb alemtuzumab may provide additional benefit to patients with T-cell leukemias [110]. CD52 is detected in 30–50% of ALL blasts. Alemtuzumab is currently being investigated as part of intense induction programs in T-cell ALL.

Central nervous system treatment and prophylaxis

Central nervous system treatment

At the time of diagnosis, CNS involvement is identified in <10% of adults with ALL, mostly in those with T-cell lineage ALL or B-cell mature ALL and who are more likely to have lymph node enlargement, mediastinal mass, and other extramedullary localizations [29,53,111–115]. Most antileukemic agents do not penetrate the blood–brain barrier to a significant extent. Factors that influence CNS drug penetration include the physicochemical properties of the drug, the degree of protein binding of the drug, and the affinity of the drug for carriers facilitating transport into the CNS. No superiority of idarubicin over daunorubicin has been established [30]. However, it is assumed that idarubicin may circumvent P-glycoprotein-mediated drug resistance. After intravenous application, its breakdown product idarubidazol reaches measurable levels in the CNS, although its potential advantages in the treatment of CNS leukemia remain to be established. Systemic high-dose therapy with cytarabine and/or methotrexate has been used mainly to overcome drug resistance and to achieve therapeutic drug levels in the CSF [116]. High-dose cytarabine has been successfully used for remission induction in CNS leukemia [42]. At a dose of $3\,g/m^2$ given every 12h, persistent cytotoxic concentrations of cytarabine can be achieved in the CSF. The elimination half-life of cytarabine in the CSF is eight times greater than in plasma. The effect of high-dose methotrexate on CNS leukemia also may be an important factor. With the use of calcium folinate rescue, high systemic doses of methotrexate can be administered safely and therapeutic CSF methotrexate levels can be achieved despite the limited penetration of methotrexate into the CSF. When administered at a dosage of $6\,g/m^2$, cytotoxic levels have been shown in the CSF [78].

Intrathecal methotrexate is the most commonly used intrathecal agent. The drug can safely be given at a dose of 12.5mg although lower doses (6mg) should be used when administered through an Omaya reservoir. CSF methotrexate concentrations were shown to be highly variable and actually correlated better with patient age than body surface area. However, ventricular CSF methotrexate concentrations following an intrathecal dose are quite variable and approximate only 10% of simultaneously drawn lumbar levels. Neurotoxicity associated with intrathecal methotrexate has been correlated with both the total amount of the drug administered and with elevated methotrexate concentrations in the CNS. It can be given either alone or in conjunction with cytarabine and hydrocortisone. In one trial, three-agent therapy was no more effective than two-agent therapy with methotrexate and hydrocortisone [117]. Intrathecal cytarabine is the second most widely used intrathecal agent and is usually administered at dosages of $30\,mg/m^2$. After intrathecal injection, conversion to the inactive metabolite uracil arabinoside is negligible because of the significantly lower cytidine deaminase activity in the brain and CSF. This is responsible for a prolonged half-life of this agent in CSF versus plasma. Recently, intrathecal depot cytarabine has been used in the treatment of CNS involvement. It has been shown that intrathecal depot cytarabine administered every 2–4 weeks is more effective than intrathecal methotrexate administered twice weekly [118]. Intrathecal depot cytarabine has an advantage over both methotrexate and native cytarabine in its frequency of administration.

The CR rates for patients presenting with CNS involvement do not differ from those observed in patients without CNS disease, with the exeption of a smaller series where the CR rate was significantly lower in patients with CNS disease at diagnosis [114,119]. The management of patients with CNS leukemia has not been standardized. Patients with CNS leukemia at the time of diagnosis generally receive more intensive intrathecal therapy, starting early during induction remission therapy. One suggested regimen is intrathecal chemotherapy twice a week until CR, then weekly for a total of 12 administrations. Concomitant systemic therapy should include agents with good CNS penetration, such as dexamethasone, methotrexate, and cytarabine, with or without cranial irradiation [53,112,120]. In adults, it has been shown that patients who had an isolated CNS leukemia and did not also receive systemic therapy eventually relapsed in the bone marrow [111].

Central nervous system prophylaxis

CNS prophylaxis, including intrathecal chemotherapy, cranial or craniospinal irradiation, and high-dose systemic chemotherapy with agents that can cross the blood–brain barrier, has impoved the long-term prognosis of patients [121]. Early initiation of CNS prophylaxis is important, particularly in high-risk patients [122,123]. In adults, the value of CNS prophylaxis has been established in a randomized trial [124], although no agreement exists about the optimal strategy. Intrathecal chemotherapy is the preferred method for CNS prophylaxis, with generally four intrathecal injections during a 4-week or 5-drug standard induction regimen. In some instances, intrathecal methotrexate has been used alone [122,123], whereas other studies have used a triple intrathecal combination of methotrexate, cytarabine, and hydrocortisone administered simultaneously [30]. Steroids can also be useful. Dexamethasone achieves higher CSF levels and has a longer half-life in the CSF than prednisone [19]. Systemic administration of L-asparaginase can deplete the CSF of L-asparagine for prolonged periods of time [125]. Systemic high-dose treatment alone does not provide sufficient prophylaxis. In high-risk patients, the best prophylaxis has been achieved with high-dose systemic chemotherapy combined with intrathecal chemotherapy [53,113,126]. Results in adults have shown that effective prophylaxis can be achieved without cranial irradiation after the initial phase, but only with intrathecal injections continued throughout maintenance [113]. Although high-dose systemic chemotherapy plus intrathecal chemotherapy has been effective in mature B-cell ALL [127], the combination of cranial irradiation (24 Gy) with intrathecal chemotherapy has also been shown to be of value in this subtype of ALL [34]. A risk-oriented approach should be used to minimize risks and optimize efficacy.

Subset-specific approaches

Increasingly, ALL is recognized as a group of heterogeneous disease entities with unique responses to therapy. Specific approaches are pursued in ALL subsets based on cytogenetic and molecular markers, immunophenotypic features, and age.

Immunologic subtypes

B-cell lineage acute lymphoblastic leukemia

B-cell lineage constitutes about 75% of ALL in adults. Common ALL is the most frequent subtype. In adults, B-precursor ALL has an inferior outcome compared with T-lineage ALL, both in terms of the CR rate and survival duration. Higher doses of anthracyclines given in induction may be associated with improved results [84]. Chemotherapy including high-dose cytarabine appears to be an effective treatment strategy in early pre-B-ALL [128]. This has been confirmed by the higher sensitivity of early pre-B-ALL blast cells compared with other ALL blast cell subgroups in *in vitro* drug resistance tests [129].

T-cell lineage acute lymphoblastic leukemia

T-cell lineage represents about 24% of ALL in adults. In recent trials, results for T-ALL have improved, with CR rates >80%. The combination of cytarabine and cyclophosphamide, when added to conventional drugs, are responsible for this improvement [130]. A lower rate of induction failure has also been reported after introduction of a prephase treatment with cyclophosphamide [131]. As in childhood ALL, the introduction of high-dose methotrexate, high-dose cytarabine, and L-asparaginase into chemotherapy regimens has contributed to a better outcome in T-ALL. CR rates have been shown as inferior for pre/pro-T-ALL compared with thymic or mature T-ALL [132]. This might be in part due to a higher expression of multidrug resistance (MDR) and a higher median age for pre/pro-T-ALL. Higher CNS relapse rates and the presence of mediastinal tumors represent specific treatment problems in T-lineage ALL. Intensive CNS prophylaxis during first-line therapy is therefore mandatory. Mediastinal irradiation has been proposed after initial cell reduction by chemotherapy [132]. However, because of its toxicity, the additional mediastinal irradiation should be restricted to patients with large mediastinal masses at diagnosis or residual tumors after induction therapy.

Philadelphia chromosome-positive acute lymphoblastic leukemia

The Philadelphia chromosome (Ph) (t(9;22) and/or *BCR–ABL* ALL) can be detected in 20–40% of adults with ALL [133]. Historically, chemotherapy regimens induced CR in about 70% of the cases (moderately lower than in Ph^- ALL), but most patients relapsed faster and died as a result of the disease [61,134,135]. Only the hyper-CVAD chemotherapy (fractionated cyclophosphamide, vincristine, doxorubicin, and dexamethasone alternating with cycles of high-dose methotrexate and cytarabine) from the M. D. Anderson Cancer Center reported higher CR rate (91%) with a better outcome [53]. Chemotherapy in elderly patients with Ph^+ ALL was also associated with a very poor prognosis, but, in contrast with younger adults, the presence of the Ph chromosome had less impact on the prognosis because of the poor overall outcome of ALL in the elderly [136].

Following initial studies showing that the use of imatinib mesylate as a single agent in Ph^+ ALL yielded potential responses but was unlikely to be sufficient for long-term disease control, the efficacy of imatinib was explored as front-line treatment combined with chemotherapy, either concurrently or sequentially (Table 16.2) [137–141]. Imatinib was given concurrently at 400 mg/day for the

Table 16.2 Imatinib-based induction chemotherapy regimens for de novo adult Ph⁺ acute lymphoblastic leukemia.

Reference	Induction chemotherapy	Imatinib dosing	Patients	Age (range) (years)	Complete remission (%)
Thomas *et al.* [137]	Cycle 1: CP 300 mg/m² every 12 h days 1–3 Vcr 2 mg day 4, day 11 ADR 50 mg/m² day 4 Dex 40 mg d ays 1–4, d ays 11–14 Cycle 2: HD-MTX 1 g/m² day 1 HD-Ara-C 3 g/m² every 12 h day 2, day 3	400 mg/d days 1–14 (Cycle 2)	39	42 (17–75)	92
Lee *et al.* [139]	Induction: DNR 50 mg/m² per day days 1–3 Vcr 2 mg day 8, day 15, day 22 L-aspa 4000 IU/m² days 17–28 Pred 60 mg/m² days 1–28	600 mg per day days 1–28	20	37 (15–67)	95
Yanada *et al.* [138]	Induction: CP 1200 mg/m² day 1 DNR 60 mg/m² days 1–3 Vcr 1.3 mg/m² day 1, day 8, day 15, day 22 Pred 60 mg/m² days 1–21	600 mg per day days 8–63	80	48 (15–63)	96
Ottmann *et al.* [140]	Prephase: Dex 10 mg/m² days 1–5 CP 200 mg/m² per day days 3–5	600 mg per day days 1–28	28	66 (54–79)	96
Vignetti *et al.* [141]	Prephase: Pred 10–40 mg/m² days 1–7 Induction: Pred 40 mg/m² days 1–45	800 mg per day days 1–45	30	69 (61–83)	100

ADR, adriamycin; CP, cyclophosphamide; CR, complete remission; Dex, dexamethasone; DNR, daunorubicin; HD-Ara-C, high-dose cytarabine; HD-MTX, high-dose methotrexate; L-aspa, L-asparaginase; Pred, prednisone or prednisolone; Vcr, vincristine.

first 14 days with each cycle of the hyper-CVAD regimen [137]. In this study, the CR rate was 96%. There was no unexpected toxicity related to the addition of imatinib. Similarly encouraging data were reported by the Japanese Adult Leukemia Study Group (JALSG), in which imatinib was started after 1 week of induction therapy and then co-administered with chemotherapy during the remainder of a standard induction [138]. The CR rate was 96% (median time to CR: 28 days), and a remarkably high molecular response rate became apparent as early as 2 months after starting the treatment. Transplant candidates had a better chance to receive allogeneic stem-cell transplantation (SCT) with imatinib-combined regimens. Alternating and concurrent imatinib–chemotherapy combinations were compared by the German Multicenter Acute Lymphoblastic Leukemia (GMALL) trial in two sequential patient cohorts [142]. Efficacy analyses based on Bcr–Abl transcript levels showed a clear advantage of the simultaneous over the alternating schedule, with 52% of patients achieving polymerase chain reactivity (PCR) negativity (vs. 19%). Several approaches using imatinib-based induction therapy have been explored for elderly patients. With relatively minimal use of imatinib (600 mg/day for phase II induction), the Group for Research on Adult Acute Lymphoblastic Leukemia (GRAALL) showed higher CR rates compared with historical controls [143]. Similar results were reported by the Italian group using continuous administration of imatinib (800 mg) only combined with prednisone [141]. The GMALL conducted a randomized study comparing induction therapy with single-agent imatinib with standard induction chemotherapy [140]. The response rate was better with single-agent imatinib (96% vs. 50%). Achievement of molecular remission was associated with longer DFS. Unfortunately, imatinib resistance developed rapidly and was quickly followed by disease progression. Disease recurrence was related with a high rate of *ABL* mutations in the tyrosine kinase domain [144]. Despite these encouraging results, data from the United Kingdom Acute Lymphoblastic Leukemia (UKALL) XII/Eastern Cooperative Oncology Group (ECOG) 2993 study, in which imatinib (600 mg) was started with phase II induction, did not provide clear evidence that imatinib alters the outcome of the disease [145].

New strategies using new tyrosine kinase inhibitors are being developed to overcome resistance to imatinib. A recent phase II study combining the hyper-CVAD regimen with dasatinib (50 mg twice a day) for the first 14 days of each cycle showed a CR achievement in 93% of newly diagnosed Ph^+ ALL, with molecular remissions observed even after the first cycle [146]. In a series combining dasatinib (70 mg twice a day) with steroids only, CR was achieved in all cases with a marked clearance of blasts already at day 22 [147]. Nilotinib as monotherapy also appeared to have promising activity and a favorable safety profile [148]. Its use in combination with chemotherapy is currently being tested.

Burkitt cell acute lymphoblastic leukemia

Accounting for 1–3% of all cases of ALL, Burkitt cell ALL is characterized by the morphology of blast cells, the presence of monoclonal surface immunoglobulins, and by chromosomal translocations—t(8;14)(q24;q32), t(2;8)(p12;q24) or t(8;22)(q24;q11)—that lead to rearrangements of the proto-oncogene *c-myc*, located at the band 8q24 [1,149,150]. Additional chromosomal abnormalities are found in 30–40% of the cases, but do not appear to carry prognostic value. Burkitt cell ALL prognosis had long been regarded as uniformly poor, because of frequent CNS involvement and early relapses. Conventional ALL treatments combining vincristine, prednisone, an anthracycline, L-asparaginase, and intrathecal injections of methotrexate only produced a 30–50% CR rate, with most patients subsequently presenting with CNS relapses [32,151–154]. Over the past 15 years, survival has improved in children with the use of aggressive protocols including intensive induction and early CNS treatment. Introduction of fractionated high doses of cyclophosphamide (or ifosfamide), moderate or high-dose methotrexate and cytarabine, and an epidophyllotoxin (VP16 or VM26) in addition to an anthracycline and vincristine yielded improvements in the outcome of the disease. A 1-week phase combining cyclophosphamide, vincristine, and prednisone usually preceded high-dose chemotherapy in order to reduce the risk of tumor lysis syndrome. Concomitantly, the poor outcome of Burkitt cell ALL patients with CNS involvement led to approaches using an intensification of CNS therapy combining high-dose methotrexate (5–8 g/m^2) and more intrathecal injections (with cytarabine, methotrexate, and hydrocortisone), followed by consolidation with etoposide, high-dose cytarabine, and cranial irradiation [155–158]. These approaches, which showed improved results in children, were tried for adults, leading to similar improved results, with CR rates ranging from 38% to 100% (median, 73%) [32,34,53,127,159–165] (Table 16.3). Recently, rituximab has been combined with Burkitt-tailored chemotherapy, with preliminary results showing a high response rate [163–165]. Only occasional cases of human immunodeficiency virus (HIV)-associated Burkitt cell ALL have been reported [32,151,152]. In Burkitt's lymphoma, treatment results were less favorable in HIV-positive than in HIV-negative patients (40% CR rate vs. 65%) [166]. The impact of highly active antiretroviral therapy in combinations with intensive Burkitt protocols has been recently investigated and showed possible applications in patients without symptoms of advanced HIV disease [167].

Acute lymphoblastic leukemia in adolescents

Currently, an 18-year-old patient referred to a pediatric hematologist is treated rather differently from the same patient who happens to be referred to an adult hematologist. Retrospective comparisons demonstrate that adolescents with ALL significantly benefit from pediatric rather than adult chemotherapy regimens [168–172] (Table 16.4). Although no major differences were demonstrated in terms of CR achievement, all pediatric trials report CR at the end of approximately 1 month of multi-agent chemotherapy whereas many adult trials report on the CR rates after 2 months of treatment. Pediatric regimens generally include greater dose densities of many chemotherapeutic agents (such as L-asparaginase, vincristine, corticosteroids, and methotrexate) than adult regimens. Differences in drug and dose intensity may explain the superior results with pediatric regimens. The choice of antileukemic agents may also play a role. In addition, there are cultural differences between care of pediatric and adult patients with ALL, with a pediatricians' tighter adherence to complex treatment protocols. It was determined that the median number of days from the time of initial CR until the time of the first postremission chemotherapy was 2 days in a pediatric study and 7 days in an adult study [169]. It is possible that adolescents and younger adult patients are currently being underdosed with the standard adult ALL regimens. These results have led to new pediatric-inspired therapeutic approaches that might also improve the efficacy of CNS leukemia prophylaxis [173].

Acute lymphoblastic leukemia in the elderly

A number of clinical and laboratory characteristics influence the response to treatment and thus the survival of patients with ALL. Among them, patient age is one of the most important prognostic variables [112,153]. Increasing age is the most adverse factor for the CR rate and is associated with shorter remissions. Very few reports have been published on ALL in the elderly but all confirmed the poor prognosis of the disease in this age group. In patients >60 years old, the remission rate ranges from 31% to 67% (Table 16.5a) [174–183]. This is mainly owing to a high mortality rate, ranging from 15% to 37%. Toxicity is probably not mostly hematologic, since regeneration after chemotherapy is not significantly delayed, but mainly extrahematologic. Comorbidities, interactions with other medications, nutritional status, and adherence to complex

Table 16.3 Induction treatment of adult Burkitt cell acute lymphoblastic leukemia with intensive protocols.

References	Induction therapy	Patients	Complete remission (%)	Early death (%)
Fenaux *et al.* [32]	Prephase: Vcr, CP, Pred, MTX (IT); COPADM1: Vcr, CP, ADR, HD-MTX, MTX (IT), Pred; COPADM2: idem with increased dose of Vcr and CP	9	88	11
Pees *et al.* [160]	Prephase: Pred, CP, MTX (IT), Ara-C (IT), Pred (IT); Course A: Dex, Ifo, MTX, Vcr, Ara-C, Eto, MTX (IT), Ara-C (IT), Pred (IT)	5	60	20
Soussain *et al.* [159]	Prephase: Vcr, CP, Pred, MTX (IT); COPADM1: Vcr, CP, ADR, HD-MTX, MTX (IT), Pred; COPADM2: idem with increased dose of Vcr and CP	24	38	8
Hoelzer *et al.* [34]	Prephase: CP, Pred; Block A: MTX (IT), MTX, CP, VM26, Ara-C, Pred; Block B: MTX (IT), MTX, CP, ADR, Pred	24	63	8
Hoelzer *et al.* [34]	Prephase: CP, Pred; Block A: MTX + Ara-C + Dex (IT), Vcr, MTX, Ifo, VM26, Ara-C, Dex; Block B: MTX + Ara-C + Dex (IT), Vcr, MTX, CP, ADR, Dex	35	74	9
Todeschini *et al.* [161]	Phase A: CP + Vcr + ADR + CNS prophylaxis Phase B: HD-MTX + HD-Ara-C	6	100	0
Thomas *et al.* [127]	CP, Vcr, Dex, HD-MTX, Ara-C, MTX (IT), Ara-C (IT)	26	81	19
Kantarjian *et al.* [53]	CP, Vcr, Dex, HD-MTX, Ara-C, MTX (IT), Ara-C (IT)	11	73	–
Lee *et al.* [162]	Prephase: CP, Pred; Cycle 1: Ifo, MTX, Vcr Ara-C, Eto, Dex, MTX (IT), Ara-C (IT), Pred (IT)	24	73	–
Cabanillas *et al.* [164]	R, CP, Vcr, Dex, HD-MTX, Ara-C, MTX (IT), Ara-C (IT)	20	89	0
Hoelzer *et al.* [165]	Prephase: CP, Pred; Block A: MTX + Ara-C + Dex (IT), R, Vcr, MTX, Ifo, VM26, Ara-C, Dex; Block B: MTX + Ara-C + Dex (IT), R, Vcr, MTX, CP, ADR, Dex	11	91	9
Thomas *et al.* [163]	R, CP, Vcr, Dex, HD-MTX, Ara-C, MTX (IT), Ara-C (IT)	31	86	0

ADR, adriamycin; Ara-C, cytarabine; CNS, central nervous system; CP, cyclophosphamide; Dex, dexamethasone; Eto, etoposide; HD-Ara-C, high-dose cytarabine; HD-MTX, high-dose methotrexate; Ifo, ifosphamide; IT, intrathecal; MTX, methotrexate; Pred, prednisone or prednisolone; Pts, patients; R, rituximab; Vcr, vincristine; VM26, teniposide.

Table 16.4 Induction treatment in adolescents with acute lymphoblastic leukemia: comparison between pediatric and adult trials.

Reference	Type of trial	Induction therapy (trial)	Age range (years)	Patients	Complete remission (%)	5-year DFS (%)
Stock *et al.* [168]	Pediatric	CGC	16–21	196	96	64
	Adult	CALGB		103	93	38
Boissel *et al.* [169]	Pediatric	FRALLE 93	15–20	77	94	67
	Adult	LALA94		100	83	41
DeBont *et al.* [170]	Pediatric	DCOG	15–18	47	98	69
	Adult	HOVON		44	91	34
Testi *et al.* [171]	Pediatric	AIEOP	14–18	150	94	80
	Adult	GIMEMA		95	89	71
Ramanujachar *et al.* [172]	Pediatric	ALL97	15–17	61	98	65
	Adult	UKALLXII		67	94	49

AIEOP, Associazione Italiana Ematologia Oncologia Pediatrica; CALGB, Cancer and Leukemia Group B; CGC, Children's Cancer Group; DCOG, Dutch Childhood Oncology Group; DFS, disease-free survival; FRALLE, French Acute Lymphoblastic Leukemia; GIMEMA, Gruppo Italiano Malattie Ematologiche dell' Adulto; HOVON, Hemato-Oncologie voor Volwassenen Nederland; LALA, Leucémies Aiguës Lymphoblastiques de l'Adulte; UKALL, United Kingdom Acute Lymphoblastic Leukaemia.

Table 16.5 Results of induction therapy in elderly patients with acute lymphoblastic leukemia: (a) retrospective studies using various induction regimens and (b) prospective studies.

(a)

Reference	Patients	Median age (years)	Complete remission (%)	Death during induction (%)
Delannoy *et al.* [174]	18	>59	47	30
Taylor *et al.* [175]	49	>59	31	16
Späth *et al.* [176]	29	>59	42	37
Mandelli *et al.* [177]	80	>60	46	NR
Ferrari *et al.* [178]	49	>60	59	23
Legrand *et al.* [179]	46	>59	43	17
Nagura *et al.* [180]	20	>59	55	NR
Pagano *et al.* [181]	37	>65	67	24
Thomas *et al.* [182]	69	>59	67	27
Houot *et al.* [136][a]	25	>55	76	0
Robak *et al.* [183]	87	>60	45	15

NR, not reported.
[a]Ph$^+$ acute lymphoblastic leukemia.

(b)

Reference	Patients	Median age (years)	Complete remission (%)	Death during induction (%)	Induction therapy
Kantarjian *et al.* [184]	52	>59	65	12	Vcr, Adria, Dex CP, Vcr, Adria, Dex
Bassan *et al.* [185]	22	59	59	18	Ida, Vcr, L-aspa, Pred
Delannoy *et al.* [186]	40	>54	85	7	Vcr, CP, Pred, DNR
Delannoy *et al.* [187]	58	>54	58	12	(Vcr or Vds), CP, Pred, DNR
Offidani *et al.* [188]	15	>60	73	20	Vcr, DXM, Dex

Adria, adriamycin; CP, cyclophosphamide; DEX, dexamethasone; DXM, daunoXome; Ida, idarubicin; L-aspa, L-asparaginase; Pred, prednisone; Vds, vindesine; Vcr, vincristine.

treatment regimens all influence the pharmacokinetic profile in older patients. The volume of distribution of a drug may be less than in younger adults. Hepatic blood flow and renal clearance may be diminished in older patients. Specific drugs may have toxicities that require special attention in older patients: vincristine may cause severe constipation, corticosteroids can exacerbate diabetes, and L-asparaginase can cause cognitive impairment leading to encephalopathy. Intensification of induction therapy must therefore be carefully weighed against the possible disadvantages of toxicity. This may lead to incomplete application of a proposed treatment schedule, which additionally worsens the outcome. Another major reason for the poor outcome in elderly patients with ALL is a higher prevalence of disease refractory to standard chemotherapy programs related to the higher incidence of adverse risk factors, particularly the increasing frequency of Ph$^+$ ALL with age [136]. Studies of prognostic factors showed some differences compared with what was usually found in an overall adult ALL population. CR rates were lower with higher white blood cell (WBC) counts, a worse performance status, and presence of hemorrhage at diagnosis [182].

Elderly patients, therefore, have often been excluded from protocols with curative intent. Palliative chemotherapy approaches have been occasionally recommended to older patients because of poor performance status or the presence of comorbidities. Several studies have addressed the question of whether these treatments, consisting mostly of vincristine and prednisolone, may be preferable in order to maintain quality of life [175,181]. Despite the poor prognosis in this type of leukemia, improvements have, however, been observed with time. This is mainly a result of an improvement in supportive care, but also an improvement of specific therapies against leukemia. "Personalized" treatments have been progressively replaced (at least in all patients with a WHO performance status <3) by therapeutic schedules either similar to those administered to adults <60 years of age or specifically designed for elderly patients [184–188] (Table 16.5b). Although very few clinical trials have focused on induction therapies designed specifically for older patients with ALL, the best results were observed with schedules using lower doses of chemotherapy, prednisone administered on alternate days, and anthracycline administration tailored according to response at day 15 [182]. Advances of supportive care and introduction of growth factors could also be responsible for notable improvements in outcome [189]. On the other hand, the lower toxicity of less intense induction combinations was counterbalanced by a higher relapse rate so that "age-adapted" therapies did not translate into better DFS or overall survival (OS) [182].

Supportive care

Improvements in supportive care have been of significant benefit to the individual with ALL. Although many symptoms may be attribuable to the underlying disease, many are iatrogenic.

Indwelling venous catheters

An important advance in the supportive care has been the evolution of the indwelling central venous catheter (tunneled Hickman and Groshong catheters, and Port-a-cath systems with subcutaneous reservoir), providing access for blood sampling and the administration of blood products, fluids, and antibiotics. However, the increased use of indwelling catheters has been paralleled by an increase in the incidence of Gram-positive infections [190]. Thrombotic complications are also common [191].

Antimicrobial prophylaxis

The incidence of infections in patients with ALL ranged from 30% to 100% during induction. Infection death rates during induction therapy were 0–20% [22,29,41,53,84,192]. Gram-negative bacterial infections occur commonly after induction chemotherapy. The incidence of and morbidity from Gram-negative sepsis have been reduced with the use of prophylactic quinolone antibiotics with and without non-absorbable antibiotics [193]. Infection and death from *Pneumocystis carinii* pneumonia became infrequent during induction after the introduction of prophylactic trimethoprim-sulfamethoxazole. Fungal infections have increased and tend to occur earlier during the course of the disease [194]. Prophylactic approaches using various antifungal agents remain controversial. However, imidazoles have been promising in recent studies [195].

Hematopoietic growth factors

Induction protocols for ALL commonly use schedules in which cytotoxic drugs are administered in divided doses over a prolonged period of time, thus requiring simultaneous administration of HGFs and chemotherapy. The safety of simultaneous administration of HGFs and chemotherapy in adult patients with ALL has been well established in numerous clinical trials [189,196]. Based on these studies, the efficacy of the concurrent administration of G-CSF and granulocyte-macrophage colony-stimulating factor (GM-CSF) was tested in larger, prospective trials and are summarized in Table 16.6. G-CSF markedly ameliorated neutropenia, and more importantly reduced the incidence of febrile neutropenia and documented infections [197,198]. Patients receiving GM-CSF did not have shorter intercycle times or a lower incidence of documented infections than those who did not receive GM-CSF [199]. A reduction of mucositis was the only significant effect observed during induction [200]. In a randomized comparison of G-CSF and GM-CSF administration in ALL during a 28-day induction cycle, HGFs showed a trend for a reduced incidence of severe infections and of days with antibiotics as compared with controls without a growth factor, but overall there was no significant difference between the individual growth factors [201]. Results were heterogeneous in studies using HGFs only after chemotherapy. In one study, there was a non-significant reduction of febrile neutropenia and incidence of documented infections [202]. In another study, patients receiving G-CSF had fewer days in the hospital, a higher CR rate, and fewer deaths during remission induction [51,203]. A time-sequenced administration of HGFs together with remission induction and consolidation was also explored. The aim of this schedule was to generate cell cycle-dependent protection of normal hematopoietic progenitors and to stimulate granulopoiesis. Patients who received HGFs had shorter periods of neutropenia, a lower infection rate, more rapid completion of therapy, shorter hospitalization, and required less intravenous antibiotic and antifungal medications [204–206]. Based on results of randomized studies showing generally fewer severe infections with HGFs as an adjunct in adult ALL, HGF support has been integrated as a routine element of supportive therapy during induction treatment in most current trials.

Symptom control

Nausea and vomiting may be ameliorated to a large extent by antiemetics: prokinetic antiemetics, antiemetics acting on the vomiting center, and 5-hydroxytryptamine antagonists [207]. Anorexia with associated weight loss is usually multifactorial. Although corticosteroids used during induction therapy have an appetite-stimulatory effect, their role is minor. Factors associated with diarrhea include broad-spectrum antibiotics, clostridium difficile-associated colitis, mucositis, infection, and drugs. Special attention to the individual's psychologic need is also required.

Complications during induction

Hyperleukocytosis

Hyperleukocytosis is observed in 10–30% of patients with ALL. However, symptomatic leukostasis is rare [208].

Table 16.6 Use of hematopoietic growth factors during induction chemotherapy in adult acute lymphoblastic leukemia.

Reference	Treatment	HGF	Patients	Results in the group with HGF
Ohno *et al.* [202]	After induction	G-CSF (2 vs. 5 vs. 10 μg/kg)	41	↓neutropenia, ↓ febrile neutropenia, ↓infections after 5 or 10 μg/kg
Ottmann *et al.* [197]	Induction (second phase)	G-CSF Control	37 39	↓neutropenia, ↓infections, ↓prolonged interruptions of chemotherapy
Papamichael *et al.* [199]	Induction (from day 4)	GM-CSF Control	26	No difference
Welte *et al.* [203]	Induction (from day 7)	G-CSF Control	17 17	↓ febrile neutropenia, ↓infections, ↓prolonged interruptions of chemotherapy
Geisller *et al.* [198]	Induction (from day 2)	G-CSF Control	25 26	↓neutropenia, ↓febrile neutropenia, ↓ infections
Bassan *et al.* [205]	Induction (from day 4 vs. day 15)	G-CSF	65	Early > late, ↓neutropenia, ↓infections, ↓antibiotic and antifungal medications
Larson *et al.* [51]	Induction (from day 4)	G-CSF Placebo	102 96	↓neutropenia, ↓thrombocytopenia, ↑CR rate, ↓ death during induction, ↓days in hospital
Ifrah *et al.* [200]	Induction (from day 7)	GM-CSF Placebo	35 29	↓mucositis, ↓days with fever
Weiser *et al.* [206]	Induction (from day 5 vs. day 10)	G-CSF	199	Delayed administration not associated with ↑infections, nor with ↑TRM during consolidation
Holowiecki *et al.* [204]	Induction (time-sequenced)	G-CSF Control	64	↓neutropenia, ↓infections, ↓days in hospital
Thomas *et al.* [201]	Trial 1: Induction (from day 9 or day 17) Trial 2: Induction (from day 4)	GM-CSF G-CSF Control GM-CSF G-CSF Control	41 58 49 26 37 25	↓neutropenia, ↓days in hospital, ↓days with antibiotics, ↓infections with G-CSF; ↑CR rate with GM-CSF; early therapy > late therapy

G-CSF, granulocyte colony-stimulating factor; GM-CSF, granulocyte-macrophage colony-stimulating factor; HGF, hematopoietic growth factor; Pts, patients; TRM, treatment-related mortality.

Historically, leukapheresis has been used in symptomatic patients with a high WBC count (>200 × 10^9/L) [209]. However, the benefits of this procedure remain controversial, and no data have suggested that the response rate and overall outcome were improved [210]. Leukapheresis in adult ALL is not recommended except in rare instances, such as when leukemia occurs during pregnancy. A pre-induction phase with steroids or combining steroids with vincristine or cyclophosphamide is a preferred means for the amelioration of hyperleukocytosis. For mature B-ALL, initial treatment with cyclophosphamide and prednisone for 1 week usually results in lysis of large tumor masses [34].

Hypercalcemia

Severe hypercalcemia has been reported in 4–5% of cases at diagnosis [211]. Paraneoplastic production of parathyroid hormone-related protein is thought to be responsible for hypercalcemia by way of a humoral effect, while osteolytic skeletal localizations and cytokines may be responsible for local osteolytic hypercalcemia [212]. An adequate control of hypercalcemia can be achieved by the combination of hydration, diuretics, biphosphonates, corticosteroids, and calcitonin [213].

Metabolic complications

Metabolic disturbances may arise during the first phase of the induction chemotherapy. In case of hyperleukocytosis, patients are at risk of developing acute tumor lysis syndrome, manifesting by electrolyte abnormalities. This syndrome may lead to oliguric renal failure (tubular precipitation of urate and calcium phosphate crystals), fatal cardiac arrthythmias, and seizures (hypercalcemia). Vigorous intravenous hydration, oral or intravenous allopurinol, and phosphate binders represent the standard therapy for managing this syndrome. Recombinant urate oxidase (rasburicase) has been recently introduced to prevent uric acid formation, and was demonstrated to be a safe and effective alternative to allopurinol [214]. Lactic acidosis is frequently associated and correlated with the severity of acute tumor lysis syndrome [215]. Hemodialysis and hemofiltration with bicarbonate-based replacement fluid is a successful therapy for severe lactic acidosis. However, plasma lactate levels decrease only after the initiation of chemotherapy.

Coagulopathy

Coagulopathy is a common complication of ALL. Disseminated intravascular coagulation (DIC) in adults has been reported in about 35–75% during remission induction therapy [216,217]. Hypofibrinogenemia has been detected in about 40% of patients after initiation of therapy [218]. The best way to treat coagulopathy is to treat the underlying ALL. However, exacerbation of DIC has been observed during induction therapy and could be associated with tumor lysis syndrome. Activated partial thromboplastin times must be kept at levels of about 1.5 times normal with fresh frozen plasma (FFP), platelet counts at about 50×10^9/L with platelet transfusions, and fibrinogen levels over 100 mg/dL with cryoprecipitate.

L-asparaginase can produce depletion of many of the hemostatic, anticoagulant, and fibrinolytic factors such as fibrinogen, factors IX and XI, antithrombin III, proteins C and S, and plasminogen with an associated risk of thrombosis and hemorrhage [219]. Therapy with cryoprecipitate or FFP is usually successful in correcting the hemostatic defect. Furthermore, it is reasonable to temporarily discontinue the administration of L-asparaginase. CNS thrombosis occurs in approximately 4% of cases, usually 2–3 weeks after the initiation of therapy with L-asparaginase [220]. While the risk is greatest during the remission induction phase, it may occur at any stage of therapy.

Mediastinal mass

Compression of great vessels by a bulky mediastinal mass (particularly in T-cell lineage ALL) may lead to a life-threatening superior vena cava syndrome. A mediastinal mass may also be responsible for dyspnea or dysphagia from a tracheal and oesophageal compression. Therapy with steroids, chemotherapy, and/or radiation must be initiated promptly [221].

Evaluation of induction therapy

Assessment of response

Complete response is usually evaluated after 4 weeks and also after 8 weeks, when a second phase of induction is applied. Traditionally, a reduction of blast cells to <5% together with return of marrow cellularity and function to normal levels and the disappearance of all extramedullary manifestations of leukemia infiltration constituted a CR [222]. However, the criteria for response are changing as a result of increasing expectations of therapy and improvements in technology. The criteria have evolved from the disappearance of cytohistologically detectable leukemia cells from the blood and bone marrow to the absence of immunologically distinctive leukemia cells and cytogenetic abnormalities and to the disappearance of leukemia-specific genes and transcripts assessed by PCR or reverse transcriptase (RT)-PCR. Molecular methods or flow cytometry for detection of minimal residual disease (MRD) are therefore increasingly developed to achieve a quantitative measurement of residual blasts with a high sensitivity (10^{-4}–10^{-6}) far below the detection level of conventional morphologic and cytogenetic analyses. In patients with childhood ALL, it has been noted that those in whose remission marrows 10^5 leukemia cells can be detected are more likely to relapse, whereas those with 10^4 cells and below almost always remain in long-lasting remission [223].

Drug resistance or death during induction

Between 15% and 20% of adult patients with ALL will not achieve CR after induction therapy. The number of patients who are refractory to induction chemotherapy is steadily decreasing with the use of more intensive regimens, which, however, lead more frequently to toxic death. <10% die during the induction period. Mortality is age-dependent, increasing from <3% in adolescents to 20–30% in patients >60 years old [224]. The main causes of death are infectious complications.

Prognostic factors

Time to response

The time or the number of chemotherapy courses required to achieve CR is a major prognostic factor. Adults with ALL not responding within 4 or 5 weeks fare poorly [112]. This may be explained by a more resistant blast-cell population. As early blast clearance is an important predictor for survival, response to chemotherapy is now evaluated earlier, after 7 days of prephase therapy with steroids [173] and/or 1 or 2 weeks after start of chemotherapy [225] in order to better define risk groups and risk-adapted continuation therapy.

Minimal residual disease after induction therapy

Detection of MRD is based on the analysis of immunophenotype with multiparameter flow cytometry, quantitative measurement of gene products from gene translocation such as *BCR–ABL*, *E2A–PBX1*, *MLL–AFA*, or *TEL–AML1* by PCR or more recently RT-PCR, and/or quantitative measurement of individual rearrangements of the T-cell receptor or immunoglobulin-heavy chain genes. MRD evaluation after induction therapy shows that most patients with ALL remain MRD⁺ despite CR achievement as defined by conventional morphologic analysis [226,227]. In Ph⁺/*BCR–ABL*⁺ ALL, however, recent trials using a combination of imatinib with chemotherapy as induction therapy report a higher percentage of MRD negativity [137,138]. Efficacy analyses based on Bcr–Abl transcript levels show a clear advantage of the simultaneous over the alternating schedules [142].

References

1 Bennett JM, Catovsky D, Daniel MT, *et al.* The morphological classification of acute lymphoblastic leukemia: Concordance among observers and clinical correlations. *Br J Haematol* 1981;47:553–61.

2 Harris NL, Jaffe ES, Diebold J, *et al.* The World Health Organization classification of neoplasms of the hematopoietic and lymphoid tissues: Report of the Clinical Advisory Committee meeting—Airlie House, Virginia, November 1997. *Hematol J* 1997;1:53–66.

3 Gilman A. The initial clinical trial of nitrogen mustard. *Am J Surg* 1963;105:574–8.

4 Farber S, Diamond LK, Mercer RD, *et al.* Temporary remissions in acute leukemia in children prolonged by folic acid antagonist 4-amethopteroylglutamic acid (aminopterin). *N Engl J Med* 1948;238:787–93.

5 Stoller RG, Hande KR, Jacobs SA, *et al.* Use of plasma pharmacokinetics to predict and prevent methotrexate toxicity. *N Engl J Med* 1977;297:630–4.

6 Pearson OH, Eliel LP, Rawson RW, *et al.* Adrenocorticotrophic hormone- and cortisone-induced regression of lymphoid tumors in man: a preliminary report. *Cancer* 1949;2:943–5.

7 Skipper HE, Thomson JR, Elion GB, *et al.* Observations on the anticancer activity of 6-mercaptopurine. *Cancer Res* 1954;14: 294–8.

8 Johnson IS, Armstrong JG, Gorman M, *et al.* The Vinca alkaloids: a new class of oncolytic agents. *Cancer Res* 1963;23: 1390–427.

9 Skipper HE, Schabel FM Jr, Wilcox WS. Experimental evaluation of potential anticancer agents. XIII. On the criteria and kinetics associated with 'curability' of experimental leukemia. *Cancer Chemother Rep* 1964;35:1–111.

10 Ellison RR, Holland JF, Weil M, *et al.* Arabinosyl cytosine, a useful agent in the treatment of acute leukemia in adults. *Blood* 1968;32:507–23.

11 Frei E III, Karon M, Levin RH, *et al.* The effectiveness of combinations of antileukemic agents in inducing and maintaining remission in children with acute leukemia. *Blood* 1965;26: 642–56.

12 Ross WE, Bradley MO. DNA double-stand breaks in mammalian cells after exposure to intercalating agents. *Biochem Biophys Acta* 1981;654:129–34.

13 Minocha A, Long BH. Inhibition of the DNA catenation activity of type II topoisomerase by VP16–213 and VM26. *Biochem Biophys Res Commun* 1984;122:165–70.

14 Whiteside JA, Phillips F, Dargeon HW, *et al.* Intrathecal aminopterin in neurologic manifestations of acute leukemia. *AMA Arch Intern Med* 1958;101:279–85.

15 Djerassi I. Platelet transfusions and supportive care. A requirement for currently effective chemotherapy. *JAMA* 1972;222: 1172–3.

16 Hanahan D, Weinberg RA. The hallmarks of cancer. *Cell* 2000; 100:57–70.

17 Druker BJ, Talpaz M, Resta DJ, *et al.* Efficacy and safety of a specific inhibitor of the Bcr–Abl tyrosine kinase in chronic myeloid leukemia. *N Engl J Med* 2001;344:1031–7.

18 Distelhorst CW. Glucocorticosteroids induce DNA fragmentation in human lymphoid leukemia cells. *Blood* 19887;2:1305–9.

19 Ito C, Evans WE, McNinch L, *et al.* Comparative cytotoxicity of dexamethasone and prednisolone in childhood acute lymphoblastic leukemia. *J Clin Oncol* 1996;14:2370–6.

20 Balis FM, Lester CM, Chrousos GP, *et al.* Differences in cerebrospinal fluid penetration of corticosteroids: Possible relationship to the prevention of meningeal leukemia. *J Clin Oncol* 1987;5:202–7.

21 Hurwitz CA, Silverman LB, Schorin MA, *et al.* Substituting dexamethasone for prednisone complicates remission induction in children with acute lymphoblastic leukemia. *Cancer* 2000;88:1964–9.

22 Thomas X, Danaïla C, Bach QK, *et al.* Sequential induction chemotherapy with vincristine, daunorubicin, cyclophosphamide, and prednisone in adult acute lymphoblastic leukemia. *Ann Hematol* 1995;70:65–9.

23 Shanbrom E, Miller S. Critical evaluation of massive steroid therapy of acute leukemia. *N Engl J Med* 1962;266:1354–8.

24 Carbone PP, Bono V, Frei EI, *et al.* Clinical studies with vincristine. *Blood* 1963;21:640–7.

25 Weber W, Nagel GA, Nagel-Stuer E, *et al.* Vincristine infusion: A phase I study. *Cancer Chemother Pharmacol* 1979;3:49–55.

26 Vats T, Buchanan G, Mehta P, *et al.* A study of toxicity and comparative therapeutic efficacy of vindesine-prednisone vs. vincristine-prednisone in children with acute lymphoblastic leukemia in relapse: A Pediatric Oncology Group study. *Invest New Drugs* 1992;10:231–4.

27 Gottlieb AJ, Weinberg V, Ellison RR, *et al.* Efficacy of daunorubicin in the therapy of adult acute lymphocytic leukemia: A prospective randomized trial by the Cancer and Leukemia Group B. *Blood* 1984;64:267–74.

28 Bassan R, Lerede T, Rambaldi A, *et al.* Role of anthracyclines in the treatment of adult acute lymphoblastic leukemia. *Acta Haematol* 1996;95:188–92.

29 Fiere D, Lepage E, Sebban C, *et al.* Adult acute lymphoblastic leukemia: A multicentric randomized trial testing bone marrow transplantation as postremission therapy. *J Clin Oncol* 1993;11:1990–2001.

30 Thomas X, Boiron JM, Huguet F, *et al.* Outcome of treatment in adults with acute lymphoblastic leukemia: Analysis of the LALA-94 trial. *J Clin Oncol* 2004;22:4075–86.

31 Lauer SJ, Pinkel D, Buchanan GR, *et al.* Cytosine arabinoside/cyclophosphamide pulses during continuation therapy for childhood acute lymphoblastic leukemia. *Cancer* 1987;60: 2366–71.

32 Fenaux P, Lai JL, Miaux O, *et al.* Burkitt cell acute leukemia (L3 ALL) in adults: A report of 18 cases. *Br J Haematol* 1989; 71:371–6.
33 Patte C, Philip T, Rodary C, *et al.* High survival rate in advanced-stage B-cell lymphomas and leukemias without CNS involvement with a short intensive polychemotherapy: Results from the French Pediatric Oncology Society of a randomized trial of 216 children. *J Clin Oncol* 1991;9:123–32.
34 Hoelzer D, Ludwig WD, Thiel E, *et al.* Improved outcome in adult B-cell acute lymphoblastic leukemia. *Blood* 1996;87: 495–508.
35 Rodriguez V, McCredie KB, Keating MJ, *et al.* Isophosphamide therapy for hematologic malignancies in patients refractory to prior treatment. *Cancer Treat Rep* 1978;62:493–7.
36 Keating MJ, Smith TL, Gehan EA, *et al.* Factors related to length of complete remission in adult acute leukemia. *Cancer* 1980;45:2017–29.
37 Otten J, Suciu S, Lutz P, *et al.* The importance of L-asparaginase (A'ase) in the treatment of acute lymphoblastic leukemia (ALL) in childen: Results of the EORTC 58881 randomized phase III trial showing greater efficiency of Escherichia Coli (E.Coli) as compared to Erwinia (ERW) A'ase. *Blood* 1996;88(Suppl.1):669a.
38 Douer D, Yampolsky H, Cohen LJ, *et al.* Pharmacodynamics and safety of intravenous pegaspargase during remission induction in adults aged 55 years or younger with newly diagnosed acute lymphoblastic leukemia. *Blood* 2007;109: 2744–50.
39 Wetzler M, Sanford BL, Kurtzberg J, *et al.* Effective asparagine depletion with pegylated asparaginase results in improved outcomes in adult acute lymphoblastic leukemia: Cancer and Leukemia Group B Study 9511. *Blood* 2007;109:4164–7.
40 Ross ED, Chen SRS, Cuddy DP. Effects of 1-beta-D-arabinofuranosyl-cytosine on DNA replication intermediates monitored by pH-step alkaline elution. *Cancer Res* 1990;50: 2658–66.
41 Rohatiner AZ, Bassan R, Battista R, *et al.* High dose cytosine arabinoside in the initial treatment of adults with acute lymphoblastic leukemia. *Br J Cancer* 1990;62:454–8.
42 Morra E, Lazzarino M, Brusamolino E, *et al.* The role of systemic high-dose cytarabine in the treatment of central nervous system leukemia: Clinical results in 46 patients. *Cancer* 1993; 72:439–45.
43 Virchis A, Koh M, Rankin P, *et al.* Fludarabine, cytosine arabinoside, granulocyte-colony stimulating factor with or without idarubicin in the treatment of high risk acute leukemia or myelodysplastic syndrome. *Br J Haematol* 2004;124: 26–32.
44 Barlogie B, Drewinko B. Cell cycle stage-dependent induction of G2 arrest by different antitumor agents. *Eur J Cancer* 1978; 14:741–5.
45 Nagar B, Bornmann WG, Pellicena P, *et al.* Crystal structure of the kinase domain of c-Abl in complex with the small molecule inhibitors PD173955 and imatinib (STI-571). *Cancer Res* 2002;62:4236–43.
46 Beran M, Cao X, Estrov Z, *et al.* Selective inhibition of cell proliferation and Bcr–Abl phosphorylation in acute lymphoblastic leukemia cells expressing M, 190,000 Bcr–Abl protein by a tyrosine kinase inhibitor (CGP-57148). *Clin Cancer Res* 1998; 4:1661–72.
47 Daub H, Specht K, Ullrich A. Strategies to overcome resistance to targeted protein kinase inhibitors. *Nature Rev Drug Discov* 2004;3:1001–10.
48 Lombardo LJ, Lee FY, Chen P, *et al.* Discovery of N-(2-chloro-6-methyl-phenyl)–2-(6-(4-(2-hydroxyethyl)-piperazin-1-yl)–2-methylpyrimidin-4-ylamino)thiazole-5-carboxamide (BMS-354825), a dual Src/Abl kinase inhibitor with potent antitumor activity in preclinical assays. *J Med Chem* 2004;47: 6658–61.
49 Shah NP, Tran C, Lee FY, *et al.* Overriding imatinib resistance with a novel ABL kinase inhibitor. *Science* 2004;305:399–401.
50 Verstovsek S, Golemovic M,, Kantarjian H, *et al.* AMN107, a novel aminopyrimidine inhibitor of p190 Bcr–Abl activation and of *in vitro* proliferation of Philadelphia-positive acute lymphoblastic leukemia cells. *Cancer* 2005;104:1230–6.
51 Larson RA, Dodge RK, Linker CA, *et al.* A randomized controlled trial of filgrastim during remission induction and consolidation chemotherapy for adults with acute lymphoblastic leukemia: CALCB study 9111. *Blood* 1998;92:1556–64.
52 Thiebaut A, Vernant JP, Degos L, *et al.* Adult acute lymphocytic Leukemia study testing chemotherapy and autologous and allogeneic transplantation. A follow-up report of the French protocol LALA 87. *Hematol Oncol Clin North Am* 2000;14: 1353–65.
53 Kantarjian HM, O'Brien S, Smith TL, *et al.* Results of treatment with hyper-CVAD, a dose-intensive regimen, in adult acute lymphocytic Leukemia. *J Clin Oncol* 2000;18:547–61.
54 Rowe JM, Richards SM, Burnett AK, *et al.* Favorable results of allogeneic bone marrow transplantation (BMT) for adults with Philadelphia (Ph)-chromosome-negative acute lymphoblastic leukemia (ALL) in first complete remission (CR): Results from the International ALL trial (MRC UKALL XII/ECOG E2993). *Blood* 2001;98(Suppl.1):481a.
55 Dekker AW, van't Veer MB, van der Holt B, *et al.* Postremission treatment with autologous stem cell transplantation (Auto-SCT) or allogeneic stem cell transplantation (Allo-SCT) in adults with acute lymphoblastic leukemia (ALL). A Phase II clinical trial (HOVON 18 ALL). *Blood* 2001;98(Suppl.1):859a.
56 Bassan R, Pogliani E, Casula P, *et al.* Risk-oriented postremission strategies in adult acute lymphoblastic leukemia: prospective confirmation of anthracycline activity in standard-risk class and role of hematopoietic stem cell transplants in high-risk groups. *Hematol J* 2001;2:117–26.
57 Gökbuget N, Arnold R, Büchner T, *et al.* Intensification of induction and consolidation improves only subgroups of adult ALL: Analysis of 1200 patients in GMALL study 05/93. *Blood* 2001;98(Suppl.1):802a.
58 Hallbook H, Simonsson B, Ahlgren T, *et al.* High-dose cytarabine in upfront therapy for adult patients with acute lymphoblastic leukemia. *Br J Haematol* 2002;118:748–54.
59 Takeuchi J, Kyo T, Naito K, *et al.* Induction therapy by frequent administration of doxorubicin with four other drugs, followed by intensive consolidation and maintenance therapy for adult acute lymphoblastic leukemia: the JALSG-ALL93 study. *Leukemia* 2002;16:1259–66.
60 Linker C, Damon L, Ries C, *et al.* Intensified and shortened cyclical chemotherapy for adult acute lymphoblastic leukemia. *J Clin Oncol* 2002;20:2464–71.
61 Annino L, Vegna ML, Camera A, *et al.* Treatment of adult acute lymphoblastic leukemia (ALL): long-term follow-up of

the GIMEMA ALL 0288 randomized study. *Blood* 2002;99: 863–71.

62 Kantarjian H, Thomas D, O'Brien S, *et al.* Long-term follow-up results of hyperfractionated cyclophosphamide, vincristine, doxorubicin, and dexamethasone (Hyper-CVAD), a dose-intenseve regimen, in adult acute lymphocytic leukemia. *Cancer* 2004;101:2788–801.

63 Labar B, Suciu S, Zittoun R, *et al.* Allogeneic stem cell transplantation in acute lymphoblastic leukemia and non Hodgkin's lymphoma for patents < or = 50 years old in first complete remission: results of the EORTC ALL-3 trial. *Haematologica* 2004;89:809–17.

64 Hunault M, Harousseau JL, Delain M, *et al.* Better outcome of adult acute lymphoblastic leukemia after early genoidentical allogeneic bone marrow transplantation (BMT) than after late high-dose therapy and autologous BMT: a GOELAMS trial. *Blood* 2004;104:3028–37.

65 Ribera JM, Oriol A, Bethencourt C, *et al.* Comparison of intensive chemotherapy, allogeneic or autologous stem cell transplantation as post-remission treatment for adult patients with high-risk acute lymphoblastic leukemia. Results of the PETHEMA ALL-93 trial. *Haematologica* 2005;90: 1346–56.

66 Rowe JM, Buck G, Burnett AK, *et al.* Induction therapy for adults with acute lymphoblastic leukemia: results of more than 1500 patients from the international ALL trial MRC UKALL XII/ECOG E2993. *Blood* 2005;106: 3760–7.

67 Shaw PJ, Eden T, Paradisis M. Induction toxicity in childhood acute lymphoblastic leukemia: A comparison of two schedules of daunorubicin administration. *Med Pediatr Oncol* 1995;24: 18–22.

68 Nagura E, Kimura K, Yamada K, *et al.* Nation-wide randomized comparative study of doxrubicin, vincristine and prednisolone combination therapy with and without L-asparaginase for adult acute lymphoblastic leukemia. *Cancer Chemother Pharmacol* 1994;33:359–65.

69 Ertel I, Nesbit M, Hammond D, *et al.* Effective dose of L-asparaginase for induction of remission in previously treated children with acute lymphocytic leukemia: A report from Children's Cancer Study Group. *Cancer Res* 1979;39: 3893–6.

70 Gaynor PS, Steinherz PG, Bleyer WA, *et al.* Association of delivered drug dose and outcome for children with acute lymphoblastic leukemia and unfavorable presenting features. *Med Pediatr Oncol* 1991;19:221–7.

71 Bassan R, Battista R, Rhatiner AZS, *et al.* Treatment of adult acute lymphoblastic leukemia (ALL) over a 16 year period. *Leukemia* 1992;6(Suppl.2):186–90.

72 Cassileth PA, Andersen JW, Bennett JM, *et al.* Adult acute lymphocytic leukemia: the Eastern Cooperative Oncology Group experience. *Leukemia* 1992;6(Suppl.2):178–81.

73 Willemze R, Zijlmans JM, den Ottolander GJ, *et al.* High-dose Ara-C for remission induction and consolidation of previously untreated adults with ALL or lymphoblastic lymphoma. *Ann Hematol* 1995;70:71–4.

74 Kaufmann SH, Karp JE, Burke PJ, *et al.* Addition of etoposide to initial therapy of adult acute lymphoblastic leukemia: a combined clinical and laboratory study. *Leuk Lymphoma* 1996;23:71–83.

75 Wernli M, Abt A, Bargetzi M, *et al.* A new therapeutic strategy in adult acute lymphoblastic leukemia: intensive induction consolidation, early transplant, maintenance-type in relapse only. *Proc Am Soc Clin Oncol* 1997;16:6a.

76 Murphy SB, Bowman WP, Abromowitch M, *et al.* Results of treatment of advanced-stage Burkitt's lymphoma and B cell (sIg+) acute lymphoblastic leukemia with high-dose fractionated cyclophosphamide and coordinated high-dose methotrexate and cytarabine. *J Clin Oncol* 1986;4:1732–9.

77 Weiss M, Maslak P, Feldman E, *et al.* Cytarabine and high-dose mitoxantrone induces rapid complete remission in adult acute lymphoblastic leukemia without the use of vincristine or prednisone. *J Clin Oncol* 1996;14:2480–5.

78 Balis FM, Savitch JL, Bleyer WA, *et al.* Remission induction of meningeal leukemia with high-dose intravenous methotrexate. *J Clin Oncol* 1985;3:485–9.

79 Cuttner J, Mick R, Budman DR, *et al.* Phase III trial of brief intensive treatment of adult acute lymphocytic leukemia comparing daunorubicin and mitoxantrone: a CALGB study. *Leukemia* 1991;5:425–31.

80 Elonen E, Almqvist A, Hänninen A, *et al.* Intensive treatment of acute lymphocytic leukemia in adults: ALL86 protocol. *Haematologica* 1991;76(Suppl.4):133.

81 Sebban C, Browman GP, Lepage E, *et al.* Prognostic value of early response to chemotherapy assessed by the 15 day bone marrow aspiration in adult acute lymphoblastic leukemia: A prospective analysis of 437 cases and its application for designing induction chemotherapy trials. *Leuk Res* 1995;19: 861–8.

82 Bassan R, Lerede T, Rambaldi A, *et al.* The use of anthracyclines in adult acute lymphoblastic leukemia. *Haematologica* 1995;80:280–91.

83 Todeschini G, Tecchio C, Meneghini V, *et al.* Estimated 6-year event-free survival of 55% in 60 consecutive adult acute lymphoblastic leukemia patients treated with an intense phase II protocol on high induction dose of daunorubicin. *Leukemia* 1998;12:144–8.

84 Todeschini G, Meneghini V, Pizzolo G, *et al.* Relationship between daunorubicin dosage delivered during induction therapy and outcome in adult acute lymphoblastic leukemia. *Leukemia* 1994;8:376–81.

85 Nysom K, Holm K, Lipsitz SR, *et al.* Relationship between cumulative anthracycline dose and late cardiotoxicity in childhood acute lymphoblastic leukemia. *J Clin Oncol* 1998;16: 545–50.

86 Larson RA. The US trials in adult acute lymphoblastic leukemia. *Ann Hematol* 2004;83(Suppl.1):S127–8.

87 Kaspers GJ, Veerman AJ, Popp-Snijders C, *et al.* Comparison of the antileukemic activity *in vitro* of dexamethasone and prednisolone in childhood acute lymphoblastic leukemia. *Med Pediatr Oncol* 1996;27:114–21.

88 Jones B, Freeman AI, Shuster JJ, *et al.* Lower incidence of meningeal leukemia when prednisone is replaced by dexamethasone in the treatment of acute lymphocytic leukemia. *Med Pediatr Oncol* 1991;19:269–75.

89 Bostrom BC, Sensel MR, Sather HN, *et al.* Dexamethasone versus prednisone and daily oral versus weekly intravenous mercaptopurine for patients with standard-risk acute lymphoblastic leukemia: A report from the Children's Cancer Group. *Blood* 2003;101:3809–17.

90 Yang L, Panetta JC, Cai X, *et al.* Asparaginase may influence dexamethasone pharmacokinetics in acute lymphoblastic leukemia. *J Clin Oncol* 2008;26:1932–9.

91 Graham ML. Pegasparaginase: A review of clinical studies. *Adv Drug Delivery Rev* 2003;55:1293–302.

92 Abshire TC, Pollock BH, Billett AL, *et al.* Weekly polyethylene glycol conjugated L-asparaginase compared with biweekly dosing produces superior induction remission rates in childhood relapsed acute lymphoblastic leukemia: A Pediatric Oncology Group study. *Blood* 2000;96:1709–15.

93 Avramis VI, Sencer D, Periclou AP, *et al.* A randomized comparison of native Escherichia Coli asparaginase and polyethylene glycol conjugated asparaginase for treatment of children with newly diagnosed standard-risk acute lymphoblastic leukemia: a Children's Cancer Group study. *Blood* 2002;99: 1986–94.

94 Bertrand Y, Thomas X, Godfrin Y. L-asparaginase loaded into erythrocytes (GRASPA): Principle and interests in acute lymphoblastic leukemia. *Ann Hematol* 2008;87(Suppl.1):S5-S6.

95 Muggia FM. Liposomal encapsuled anthracyclines: new therapeutic horizons. *Curr Oncol Rep* 2001;3:156–62.

96 Cortes J, O'Brien S, Estey E, *et al.* Phase I study of liposomal daunorubicin in patients with acute leukemia. *Invest New Drugs* 1999;17:81–7.

97 Allen TM, Martin FJ. Advantages of liposomal delivery systems for anthracyclines. *Semin Oncol* 2003;31:5–15.

98 Krishna R, Webb MS, St Onge G, *et al.* Liposomal and nonliposomal drug pharmacokinetics after administration of liposome-encapsulated vincristine and their contribution to drug tissue distribution properties. *J Pharmacol Exp Ther* 2001;298:1206–12.

99 Faderl S, Gandhi V, Kantarjian H, *et al.* New nucleotide analogs in clinical development. *Cancer Chemother Biol Response Modif* 2002;20:37–58.

100 Jeha S, Gandhi V, Chan KW, *et al.* Clofarabine, a novel nucleoside analog, is active in pediatric patients with advanced leukemia. *Blood* 2004;103:784–9.

101 Warrell RP, Jr., Berman E. Phase I and II study of fludarabine phosphate in leukemia: therapeutic efficacy with delayed central nervous system toxicity. *J Clin Oncol* 1986;4:74–9.

102 Clavio M, Venturino C, Pierri I, *et al.* Combination of liposomal daunorubicin (DaunoXome), fludarabine, and cytarabine (FLAD) in patients with poor-risk acute leukemia. *Ann Hematol* 2004;83:696–703.

103 Lambe CU, Averett DR, Paff MT, *et al.* 2-amino-6-methoxypurine arabinoside: An agent for T-cell malignancies. *Cancer Res* 1995;55:3352–6.

104 Garcia-Manero G, Bueso-Ramos C, Daniel J, *et al.* DNA methylation patterns at relapse in adult acute lymphocytic leukemia. *Clin Cancer Res* 2002;8:1897–903.

105 Thomas DA, Cortes J, O'Brien SM, *et al.* Significance of CD20 positivity in de novo acute lymphocytic leukemia (ALL). *Blood* 2000;96(Suppl.1):109a.

106 Thomas DA, Cortes J, Giles F, *et al.* Update of the modified hyper-CVAD regimen in newly diagnosed adult acute lymphocytic leukemia (ALL). *Blood* 2003;102(Suppl.1):880a.

107 Thomas DA, Cortes J, Faderl S, *et al.* Hyper-CVAD and rituximab therapy in HIV-negative Burkitt (BL) or Burkitt-like (BLL) leukemia/lymphoma and mature B-cell acute lymphocytic leukemia (B-ALL). *J Clin Oncol* 2005;23:567s.

108 Grossbard ML, Freedman AS, Ritz J, *et al.* Serotherapy of B-cell neoplasms with antiB4-blocked ricin: A phase I trial of daily bolus infusion. *Blood* 1992;79:576–85.

109 Harata M, Soda Y, Tani K, *et al.* CD19-targeting liposomes containing imatinib efficiently kill Philadelphia chromosome-positive acute lymphoblastic leukemia cells. *Blood* 2004;104: 1442–9.

110 Tibes R, Keating MJ, Ferrajoli A, *et al.* Activity of alemtuzumab in patients with CD52-positive acute leukemia. *Cancer* 2006; 106:2645–51.

111 Larson RA, Dodge RK, Burns CP, *et al.* A five-drug remission induction regimen with intensive consolidation for adults with acute lymphoblastic leukemia. Cancer and Leukemia Group B study 8811. *Blood* 1995;85:2025–37.

112 Hoelzer D, Thiel E, Löffler H, *et al.* Prognostic factors in a multicenter study for treatment of acute lymphoblastic leukemia in adults. *Blood* 1988;71:123–31.

113 Cortes J, O'Brien SM, Pierce S, *et al.* The value of high-dose systemic chemotherapy and intrathecal therapy for central nervous system prophylaxis in different risk groups of adult acute lymphoblastic leukemia. *Blood* 1995;86:2091–7.

114 Lazarus HM, Richards SM, Chopra M, *et al.* Central nervous system involvement in adult acute lymphoblastic leukemia at diagnosis: results from the international ALL trial MRC UKALL XII/ECOG E2993. *Blood* 2006;108:465–72.

115 Kantarjian HM, Walters RS, Smith TL, *et al.* Identification of risk groups for development of central nervous system leukemia. *Blood* 1988;72:1784–9.

116 Morra E, Lazzarino M, Inverdadi D, *et al.* Systemic high-dose ara-C for the treatment of meningeal leukemia in adult acute lymphoblastic leukemia and non-Hodgkin's lymphoma. *J Clin Oncol* 1986;4:1207–11.

117 Sullivan M, Moon T, Trueworthy R, *et al.* Combination intrathecal therapy for meningeal leukemia: Two versus three drugs. *Blood* 1977;50:471–9.

118 Glantz MJ, Jaeckle KA, Chamberlain MD, *et al.* () A randomized controlled trial comparing intrathecal sustained-release cytarabine (DepoCyt) to intrathecal methotrexate in patients with meningitis from solid tumors. *Clin Cancer Res* 1999;5:3394–402.

119 Petersdorf SH, Kopecky KJ, Head DR, *et al.* Comparison of the L10M consolidation regimen including escalating methotrexate/L-asparaginase for adult acute lymphoblastic leukemia: a Southwest Oncology Group Study. *Leukemia* 2001;15:208–16.

120 Linker CA, Levitt LJ, O'Donnell M, *et al.* Treatment of adult acute lymphoblastic leukemia with intensive cyclical chemotherapy: A follow-up report. *Blood* 1991;78:2814–22.

121 Bleyer WA, Poplack DA. Prophylaxis and treatment of leukemia in the central nervous system and other sanctuaries. *Semin Oncol* 1985;12:131–48.

122 Hussein KK, Dahlberg S, Head D, *et al.* Treatment of acute lymphoblastic leukemia in adults with intensive induction, consolidation, and maintenance chemotherapy. *Blood* 1989;73: 57–63.

123 Schauer P, Arlin ZA, Mertelsmann R, *et al.* Treatment of acute lymphoblastic leukemia in adults: Results of the L-10 and L-10M protocols. *J Clin Oncol* 1983;1:462–70.

124 Omura GA, Moffitt S, Vogler WR, *et al.* Combination chemotherapy of adult acute lymphoblastic leukemia with rand-

omized central nervous system prophylaxis. *Blood* 1980;55: 199–204.

125 Riccardi R, Holcenberg JS, Glaubiger DL, *et al.* L-asparaginase pharmacokinetics and asparaginase levels in cerebrospinal fluid of rhesus monkeys and humans. *Cancer Res* 1981;41: 4554–8.

126 Wiernik PH, Dutcher JP, Paietta E, *et al.* Long-term follow-up of treatment and potential cure of adult acute lymphocytic leukemia with MOAD: A non-anthracycline containing regimen. *Leukemia* 1993;7:1236–41.

127 Thomas DA, Cortes J, O'Brien S, *et al.* Hyper-CVAD program in Burkitt's-type adult acute lymphoblastic leukemia. *J Clin Oncol* 1999;17:2461–70.

128 Ludwig WD, Rieder H, Bartram CR, *et al.* Immunogenotype and genotypic features, clinical characteristics, and treatment outcome of adult pro-B acute lymphoblastic leukemia: Results of the German multicenter trials. *Blood* 1998;92:1898–909.

129 Pieters R, den Boer ML, Durian M, *et al.* Relation between age, immunophenotype and *in vitro* drug resistance in 395 children with acute lymphoblastic leukemia: Implication for treatment of infants. *Leukemia* 1998;12:1344–8.

130 Schiffer CA, Larson RA, Bloomfield CD. Cancer and Leukemia Group B studies in adult acute lymphocytic leukemia. *Leukemia* 1992;6:171–4.

131 Bassan R, Pogliani E, Lerede T, *et al.* Fractionated cyclophosphamide added to the IVAD regimen (idarubicin-vincristine-L-asparaginase-prednisolone) could lower the risk of primary refractory disease in T-lineage but not B-lineage acute lymphoblastic leukemia: First results from a phase II clinical study. *Haematologica* 1999;84:1088–93.

132 Hoelzer D, Arnold R, Freund M, *et al.* Characteristics, outcome and risk factors in adult T-lineage acute lymphoblastic leukemia (ALL). *Blood* 1999;94(Suppl.1):659a.

133 Groupe Français de Cytogénétique Hématologique. Cytogenetic abnormalities in adult acute lymphoblastic leukemia: correlations with hematologic findings and outcome. *Blood* 1996;87:3135–42.

134 Dombret H, Gabert J, Boiron JM, *et al.* Outcome of treatment in adults with Philadelphia chromosome-positive leukemia—results of the prospective multicenter LALA-94 trial. *Blood* 2002;100:2357–66.

135 Westbrook CA, Hooberman AL, Spino C, *et al.* Clinical significance of the *BCR–ABL* fusion gene in adult acute lymphoblastic leukemia: a Cancer and Leukemia Group B Study (8762). *Blood* 1992;80:2983–90.

136 Houot R, Tavernier E, Le QH, *et al.* Philadelphia chromosome-positive acute lymphoblastic leukemia in the elderly: prognostic factors and treatment outcome. *Hematology* 2004;9:369–76.

137 Thomas DA, Faderl S, Cortes J, *et al.* Treatment of Philadelphia chromosome-positive acute lymphoblastic leukemia with hyper-CVAD and imatinib mesylate. *Blood* 2004;103:4396–407.

138 Yanada M, Takeuchi J, Sugiura I, *et al.* High complete remission rate and promising outcome by combination of imatinib and chemotherapy for newly diagnosed *BCR–ABL*-positive acute lymphoblastic leukemia: a phase II study by the Japan Adult Leukemia Study Group. *J Clin Oncol* 2006;24:460–6.

139 Lee KH, Lee JH, Choi SJ, *et al.* Clinical effect of imatinib added to intensive combination chemotherapy for newly diagnosed Philadelphia chromosome-positive acute lymphoblastic leukemia. *Leukemia* 2005;19:1509–16.

140 Ottmann OG, Wassmann B, Pfeifer H, *et al.* Imatinib compared with chemotherapy as front-line treatment of elderly patients with Philadelphia chromosome-positive acute lymphoblastic leukemia (Ph^+ ALL). *Cancer* 2007;109:2068–76.

141 Vignetti M, Fazi P, Cimino G, *et al.* Imatinib plus steroids induces complete remissions and prolonged survival in elderly Philadelphia chromosome-positive patients with acute lymphoblastic leukemia without additional chemotherapy: results of the Gruppo Italiano Malattie Ematologiche dell' Adulto (GIMEMA) LAL0201-B protocol. *Blood* 2007;109: 3676–8.

142 Wassmann B, Pfeifer H, Goekbuget N, *et al.* Alternating versus concurrent schedules of imatinib and chemotherapy as front-line therapy for Philadelphia-positive acute lymphoblastic leukemia (Ph^+ ALL). *Blood* 2006;108:1469–77.

143 Delannoy A, Delabesse E, Lhéritier V, *et al.* Imatinib and methylprednisolone alternated with chemotherapy improve the outcome of elderly patients with Philadelphia-positive acute lymphoblastic leukemia: results of the GRAALL AFR09 study. *Leukemia* 2006;20:1526–32.

144 Pfeifer H, Wassmann B, Pavlova A, *et al.* Kinase domain mutations of Bcr–Abl frequently precede imatinib-based therapy and give rise to relapse in patients with de novo Philadelphia-positive acute lymphoblastic leukemia (Ph^+ ALL). *Blood* 2007; 110:727–34.

145 Fielding AK, Richards SM, Lazarus HM, *et al.* Does imatinib change the outcome in Philadelphia chromosome positive acute lymphoblastic leukemia in adults? Data from the UKALLXII/ECOG2993 study. *Blood* 2007;110:10a.

146 Ravandi F, Thomas D, Kantarjian H, *et al.* Phase II study of combination of the hyperCVAD regimen with dasatinib in patients with Philadelphia chromosome (Ph) or *BCR–ABL* positive acute lymphoblastic leukemia (ALL) and lymphoid blast phase chronic myeloid leukemia (CML-LB). *Blood* 2007; 110:828A.

147 Foa R, Vignetti M, Vitale A, *et al.* Dasatinib as front-line monotherapy for the induction treatment of adult and elderly Ph^+ acute lymphoblastic leukemia (ALL) patients: Interim analysis of the GIMEMA prospective study LAL1205. *Blood* 2007;110:10a.

148 Ottmann OG, Larson RA, Kantarjian HM, *et al.* Nilotinib in patients (pts) with relapsed/refractory Philadelphia chromosome-positive acute lymphoblastic leukemia (Ph^+ ALL) who are resistant or intolerant to imatinib. *Blood* 2007;110:828A.

149 Berger R, Bernheim A. Cytogenetic studies on Burkitt's lymphoma-leukemia. *Cancer Genet Cytogenet* 1982;7:231–44.

150 Dalla-Favera R, Gregni M, Erikson J, *et al.* Human c-myc oncogene is located on the region of chromosome 8 that is translocated in Burkitt's lymphoma cells. *Proc Natl Acad Sci U S A* 1982;79:7824–7.

151 Bernasconi C, Brusamolino E, Pagnucco G, *et al.* Burkitt's lymphoma/leukemia: A clinocopathologic study on 24 adult patients. *leukemia* 1991;5(Suppl.1):90–4.

152 Gill PS, Meyer PR, Pavlova Z, *et al.* B cell acute lymphocytic leukemia in adults. Clinical, morphologic, and immunologic findings. *J Clin Oncol* 1986;4:737–43.

153 Baccarani M, Corbelli G, Amadori S, *et al.* Adolescent and adult acute lymphoblastic leukemia: Prognostic features and outcome of therapy. *Blood* 1982;60:677–84.

154 Lerede T, Bassan R, Rossi A, *et al.* Therapeutic impact of adult-type acute lymphoblastic leukemia regimens in B-cell/L3

acute leukemia and advanced-stage Burkitt's lymphoma. *Haematologica* 1996;81:442–9.
155 Patte C, Michon J, Frappaz D, *et al.* Therapy of Burkitt and other b-cell acute lymphoblastic leukemia and lymphoma: Experience with the LMB protocols of the SFOP (French Paedriatric Oncology Society) in children and adults. *Baillieres Clin Haematol* 1994;7:339–48.
156 Reiter A, Schrappe M, Tiemann M, *et al.* Improved treatment results in childhood B-cell neoplasms with tailored intensification of therapy: A report of the Berlin-Frankfurt-Munster Group Trial NHL-BFM 90. *Blood* 1999;94:3294–306.
157 Patte C, Auperin A, Michon J, *et al.* The Société Française d'Oncologie Pédiatrique LMB89: Highly effective multiagent chemotherapy tailored to the tumor burden and initial response in 561 unselected children with B-cell lymphomas and L3 leukemia. *Blood* 2001;97:3370–9.
158 Mead GM, Sydes MR, Walewski J, *et al.* An international evaluation of CODOX-M and CODOX-M alternating with IVAC in adult Burkitt's lymphoma: Results of United Kingdom Lymphoma Group LY06 study. *Ann Oncol* 2002;13:1264–74.
159 Soussain C, Patte C, Ostronoff M, *et al.* Small noncleaved cell lymphoma and leukemia in adults. A retrospective study of 65 adults treated with the LMB pediatric protocols. *Blood* 1995;85:664–74.
160 Pees HW, Radtke H, Schwamborn J, *et al.* The BFM-protocol for HIV-negative Burkitt's lymphomas and L3 ALL in adult patients: A high chance for cure. *Ann Hematol* 1992;65:201–5.
161 Todeschini G, Tecchio C, Degani D, *et al.* Eighty-one percent event-free survival in advanced Burkitt's lymphoma/leukemia: No differences in outcome between pediatric and adult patients treated with the same intensive pediatric protocol. *Ann Oncol* 1997;8(Suppl.1):77–81.
162 Lee EJ, Petroni GR, Schiffer CA, *et al.* Brief-duration high-intensity chemotherapy for patients with small non-cleaved-cell lymphoma or FAB L3 acute lymphocytic leukemia: Results of Cancer and Leukemia Group B study 9251. *J Clin Oncol* 2001;19:4014–22.
163 Thomas DA, Faderl S, O'Brien S, *et al.* Chemoimmunotherapy with hyper-CVAD plus rituximab for the treatment of adult Burkitt and Burkitt-type lymphoma or acute lymphoblastic leukemia. *Cancer* 2006;106:1569–89.
164 Cabanillas ME, Tomas D, Cortes J, *et al.* Outcome with hyper-CVAD and rituximab in Burkitt (BL) and Burkitt-like (BLL) leukemia/lymphoma. *Proc Am Soc Clin Oncol* 2003;22:574, Abstract 2309.
165 Hoelzer D, Baur KH, Giagounidis A, *et al.* Short intensive chemotherapy with rituximab seems successful in Burkitt NHL, mature B-ALL and other high-grade B-NHL. *Blood* 2003;102:70a.
166 Spina M, Tirelli U, Zagonel V, *et al.* Burkitt's lymphoma in adults with or without human immunodeficiency virus infection: A single-institution clinicopathologic study of 75 patients. *Cancer* 1998;82:766–74.
167 Cortes J, Thomas D, Rios A, *et al.* Hyperfractionated cyclophosphamide, vincristine, doxorubicin, and dexamethasone and highly active antiretroviral therapy for patients with acquired immunodeficiency syndrome-related Burkitt lymphoma/leukemia. *Cancer* 2002;94:1492–9.
168 Stock W, Sather H, Dodge RK, *et al.* Outcome of adolescents and young adults with ALL: A comparison of Children's Cancer Group (CCG) and Cancer and Leukemia Group B (CALGB) regimens. *Blood* 2000;96(Suppl.1):467a.
169 Boissel N, Auclerc MF, Lhéritier V, *et al.* Should adolescents with acute lymphoblastic leukemia be treated as old children or young adults? Comparison of the French FRALLE-93 and LALA-94 trials. *J Clin Oncol* 2003;21:774–80.
170 DeBont JM, van der Holt B, Dekker AW, *et al.* Significant difference in outcome for adolescents with acute lymphoblastic leukemia treated on pediatric vs adult protocols in the Netherlands. *Leukemia* 2004;18:2032–5.
171 Testi AM, Valsecchi MG, Conter V, *et al.* Difference in outcome of adolescents with acute lymphoblastic leukemia (ALL) enrolled in pediatric (AEIOP) and adult (GIMEMA) protocols. *Blood* 2004;104(Suppl.1):1954a.
172 Ramanujachar R, Richards S, Hann I, *et al.* Adolescents with acute lymphoblastic leukemia: Emerging from the shadow of pediatric and adult treatment protocols. *Pediatr Blood Cancer* 2006;47:748–56.
173 Huguet F, Raffoux E, Thomas X, *et al.* Toward a pediatric approach in adults with acute lymphoblastic leukemia (ALL): the GRAALL-2003 study. *Blood* 2006;108(Suppl.1): 48a.
174 Delannoy A, Ferrant A, Bosly A, *et al.* Acute lymphoblastic leukemia in the elderly. *Eur J Haematol* 1990;45:90–3.
175 Taylor PRA, Reid MM, Proctor SJ. Acute lymphoblastic leukemia in the elderly. *Leuk Lymph* 1994;13:373–80.
176 Späth-Schwalbe E, Heil G, Heimpel H. Acute lymphoblastic leukemia in patients over 59 years of age. Experience in a single center over a 10-year period. *Ann Hematol* 1994;69: 291–6.
177 Mandelli F, Annino L, Ferrari A for the GIMEMA Group. ALL in the elderly: the GIMEMA trials. *Ann Hematol* 1995;70 (Suppl.2):41.
178 Ferrari A, Annino L, Crescenzi S, *et al.* Acute lymphoblastic leukemia in the elderly: results of two different treatment approaches in 49 patients during a 25-year period. *Leukemia* 1995;9:1643–7.
179 Legrand O, Marie JP, Marjanovic Z, *et al.* Prognostic factors in elderly acute lymphoblastic leukemia. *Br J Haematol* 1997;97: 596–602.
180 Nagura E, Minami S, Nagata K, *et al.* Analysis of elderly patients, aged 60 year old or older, with acute lymphoblastic leukemia. *Nippon Ronen Igakkai Zasshi* 1999;36:52–8.
181 Pagano L, Mele L, Casorelli I, *et al.* Acute lymphoblastic leukemia in the elderly. A twelve-year retrospective, single center study. *Haematologica* 2000;85:1327–9.
182 Thomas X, Olteanu N, Charrin C, *et al.* Acute lymphoblastic leukemia in the elderly: The Edouard Herriot Hospital experience. *Am J Hematol* 2001;67:73–83.
183 Robak T, Szmigielska-Kaplon A, Wrzesien-Kus A, *et al.* =Acute lymphoblastic leukemia in elderly: the Polish Adult Leukemia Group experience. *Ann Hematol* 2004;83:225–31.
184 Kantarjian HM, O'Brien S, Smith T, *et al.* Acute lymphocytic leukemia in the elderly: characteristics and outcome with the vincristine-adriamycin-dexamethasone (VAD) regimen. *Br J Haematol* 1994;88:94–100.
185 Bassan R, Di Bona E, Lerede T, *et al.* Age-adapted moderate-dose induction and flexible outpatient postremission therapy for elderly patients with acute lymphoblastic leukemia. *Leuk Lymphoma* 1996;22:295–301.

186 Delannoy A, Sebban C, Cony-Makhoul P, *et al.* Age-adapted induction treatment of acute lymphoblastic leukemia in the elderly and assessment of maintenance with interferon combined with chemotherapy. A multicentric prospective study in forty patients. *Leukemia* 1997;11:1429–34.

187 Delannoy A, Cazin B, Thomas X, *et al.* Treatment of acute lymphocytic leukemia in the elderly: an evaluation of vindesine during induction and of interferon alpha given as a single agent after comlete remission. *Leuk Lymphoma* 2002;43: 75–81.

188 Offidani M, Corvatta L, Centurioni R, *et al.* High-dose daunorubicin as liposomal compound (daunoxome) in elderly patients with acute lymphoblastic leukemia. *Hematol J* 2003;4: 47–53.

189 Ottmann OG, Ganser A, Freund M, *et al.* Simultaneous administration of granulocyte colony-stimulating factor (filgrastim) and induction chemotherapy in acute lymphoblastic leukemia. *Ann Hematol* 1993;67:161–7.

190 Mueller BU, Skelton J, Callender DP, *et al.* A prospective randomized trial comparing the infectious and noninfectious complications of externalized catheter versus a subcutaneously implanted device in cancer patients. *J Clin Oncol* 1992; 10:1943–8.

191 Raad II, Luna M, Khalil SA, *et al.* The relatioship between thrombotic and infective complications of central venous catheters. *JAMA* 1994;271:1014–16.

192 Kantarjian HM, Walters RS, Keating MJ, *et al.* Results of the vincristine, doxorubicin, and dexamethasone regimen in adults with standard and high-risk acute lymphocytic leukemia. *J Clin Oncol* 1990;8:994–1004.

193 Arning M, Wolf HH, Aul C, *et al.* Infection prophylaxis in neutropenic patients with acute leukemia—a randomized, comparative study with ofloxacin, ciprofloxacin and co-tromoxazole/colistin. *J Antimicrob Chemother* 1990;26(Suppl.D): 137–42.

194 Büchner T, Roos N. Antifungal treatment strategy in leukemia patients. *Ann Hematol* 1992;65:153–61.

195 Robenshtok E, Gafter-Gvili A, Goldberg E, *et al.* Antifungal prophylaxis in cancer patients after chemotherapy or hematopoietic stem-cell transplantation: systematic review and meta-analysis. *J Clin Oncol* 2007;25:5471–89.

196 Scherrer R, Geissler K, Kyrle PA, *et al.* Granulocyte colony-stimulating factor (G-CSF) as an adjunct to induction chemotherapy in acute lymphoblastic leukemia. A pilot study. *Ann Hematol* 1993;66:283–9.

197 Ottmann OG, Hoelzer D, Gracien E, *et al.* Concomitant granulocyte colony-stimulating factor and induction chemoradiotherapy in adult acute lymphocytic leukemia: A randomized phase III trial. *Blood* 1995;86:444–50.

198 Geissler K, Koller E, Hubmann E, *et al.* Granulocyte colony-stimulating factor as an adjunct to induction chemotherapy for adult acute lymphoblastic leukemia—A randomized phase-III study. *Blood* 1997;90:590–6.

199 Papamichael D, Andrews T, Owen D, *et al.* Intensive chemotherapy for adult acute lymphoblastic leukemia given with or without granulocyte-macrophage colony-stimulating factor. *Ann Hematol* 1996;73:259–63.

200 Ifrah N, Witz F, Jouet JP, *et al.* Intensive short term therapy with granulocyte-macrophage colony-stimulating factor support, similar to therapy for acute myeloblastic leukemia, does not improve overall results for adults with acute lymphoblastic leukemia. *Cancer* 1999;86:1496–505.

201 Thomas X, Boiron JM, Huguet F, *et al.* Efficacy of granulocyte and granulocyte-macrophage colony-stimulating factors in the induction treatment of adult acute lymphoblastic leukemia: a multicenter randomized study. *Hematol J* 2004;5: 384–94.

202 Ohno R, Tomonaga M, Ohshima T, *et al.* A randomized controlled study of granulocyte colony-stimulating factor after intensive induction and consolidation therapy in patients with acute lymphoblastic leukemia. *Int J Hematol* 1993;58:73–81.

203 Welte K, Reiter A, Mempel K, *et al.* A randomized phase-III study of the efficacy of granulocyte colony-stimulating factor in children with high-risk acute lymphoblastic leukemia. *Blood* 1996;87:3143–50.

204 Holowiecki J, Giebel S, Krzemien S, *et al.* G-CSF administered in time-sequenced setting during remission induction and consolidation therapy of adult acute lymphoblastic leukemia has beneficial influence on early recovery and possibly improves long-term outcome: a randomized multicenter study. *Leuk Lymphoma* 2002;43:315–25.

205 Bassan R, Battista R, Viero P, *et al.* Granulocyte colony-stimulating factor (G-CSF, filgrastim) after or during an intensive remission induction therapy for adult acute lymphoblastic leukemia: Effects, role of patient pretreatment characteristics, and costs. *Leuk Lymphoma* 1997;26:153–61.

206 Weiser MA, O'Brien S, Thomas DA, *et al.* Comparison of two different schedules of granulocyte colony-stimulating factor during treatment for acute lymphocytic leukemia with a hyper-CVAD (cyclophosphamide, doxorubicin, vincristine, and dexamethasone) regimen. *Cancer* 2002;94:285–91.

207 Twycross R. Palliative care: anorexia, cachexia, nausea and vomiting. *Medicine* 2000;28:7–12.

208 Porcu P, Cripe LD, Ng EW, *et al.* Hyperleukocytic leukemias and leukostasis: A review of pathophysiology, clinical presentation and management. *Leuk Lymphoma* 2000;39:1–18.

209 Strauss RA, Gloster ES, McCallister JA, *et al.* Acute cytoreduction techniques in the early treatment of hyperleukocytosis associated with childhood hematologic malignancies. *Med Pediatr Oncol* 1985;13:346–51.

210 Maurer HS, Steinherz PG, Gaynon PS, *et al.* The effect of initial management of hyperleukocytosis on early complications and outcome of children with acute lymphoblastic leukemia. *J Clin Oncol* 1988;6:1425–32.

211 Fukasawa H, Kato A, Fijigaki Y, *et al.* Hypercalcemia in a patient with B-cell acute lymphoblastic leukemia: A role of proinflammatory cytokine. *Am J Med Sci* 2001;322:109–12.

212 Esbrit P. Hypercalcemia of malignancy—New insights into an old syndrome. *Clin Lab* 2001;47:67–71.

213 Schmid I, Stachel D, Schon C, *et al.* Pamidronate and calcitonin as therapy of acute cancer-related hypercalcemia in children. *Klin Padiatr* 2001;213:30–4.

214 Goldman SC, Holcenberg JS, Finklestein JZ, *et al.* A randomized comparison between rasburicase and allopurinol in children with lymphoma or leukemia at high risk for tumor lysis. *Blood* 2001;97:2998–3003.

215 Sillos EM, Shenep JL, Burghen GA, *et al.* Lactic acidosis: A metabolic complication of hematologic malignancies: Case report and review of the literature. *Cancer* 2001;92: 2237–46.

216 Sarris AH, Kempin S, Berman E, *et al.* High incidence of disseminated intravascular coagulation during remission induction of adult patients with acute lymphoblastic leukemia. *Blood* 1992;79:1305–10.
217 Higuchi T, Mori H, Niikura H, *et al.* Disseminated intravascular coagulation in acute lymphoblastic leukemia at presentation and in early phase of remission induction therapy. *Ann Hematol* 1998;76:263–9.
218 Solano C, Lopez J, Gomez N, *et al.* Acute lymphoblastic leukemia: Hypofibrinogenemia with a low incidence of clinical complications is often found during induction remission therapy. *Blood* 1992;80:1366–8.
219 Priest JR, Ramsay NK, Bennett AJ, *et al.* The effect of L-asparaginase on antithrombin, plasminogen, and plasma coagulation during therapy for acute lymphoblastic leukemia. *J Pediatr* 1982;100:990–5.
220 Gugliotta L, Mazzucconi MG, Leone G, *et al.* Incidence of thrombotic complications in adult patients with acute lymphoblastic leukemia receiving L-asparaginase during induction therapy: A retrospective study. *Eur J Haematol* 1992;49: 63–6.
221 Lam JC, Chui CH, Jacobsen AS, *et al.* When is a mediastinal mass critical in a child? An analysis of 29 patients. *Pediatr Surg Int* 2004;20:180–4.
222 Cheson BD, Cassileth PA, Head DR, *et al.* Report of the National Cancer Institute-sponsored workshop on definitions of diagnosis and response in acute myeloid leukemia. *J Clin Oncol* 1990;8:813–19.
223 Pui CH, Campana D. New definition of remission in childhood acute lymphoblastic leukemia. *Leukemia* 2000;14: 783–5.
224 Gaynor J, Chapman D, Little C, *et al.* A cause-specific hazard rate analysis of prognostic factors among 199 adults with acute lymphoblastic leukemia: The Memorial Hospital experience since 1969. *J Clin Oncol* 1988;6:1014–30.
225 Thomas X, Huguet F, Delannoy A, *et al.* Early resistance to induction chemotherapy assessed by residual blasts in bone marrow and/or peripheral blood at day 8 is associated with unfavorable outcomes in adult acute lymphoblastic leukemia. In: Torres LS (ed.) *Cancer Drug Resistance Research Perspectives.* Commack, USA: Nova Science Publishers, 2007. pp.107–18.
226 Goulden NJ, Knechtli CJ, Garland RJ, *et al.* Minimal residual disease analysis for the prediction of relapse in children with standard-risk acute lymphoblastic leukemia. *Br J Haematol* 1998;100:235–44.
227 Van Dongen JJ, Seriu T, Panzer-Grümayer ER, *et al.* Prognostic value of minimal residual disease in acute lymphoblastic leukemia in childhood. *Lancet* 1998;352:1731–8.

Chapter 17
Salvage Therapy of Adult Acute Lymphoblastic Leukemia

Nicola Gökbuget and Dieter Hoelzer
Goethe University Hospital, Frankfurt, Germany

Introduction

Treatment results in adult acute lymphoblastic leukemia (ALL) have improved considerably in the past decade with an increase in complete remission (CR) rates to 85–90% and overall survival (OS) rates to 40–50%. Improved chemotherapy and supportive care, the integration of stem-cell transplants (SCT) in front-line therapy, as well as optimized risk stratification were all important developments. Even more impressive is the success of targeted therapies in subgroups of ALL. In the formerly most unfavorable subgroup, Ph/*BCR–ABL*$^+$ (Ph$^+$) ALL, survival now ranges from 40% to 50% after the invention of imatinib in combination with chemotherapy. In mature B-ALL, survival rates increased to >80% with the combination of short intensive chemotherapy and rituximab [1]. Despite all improvements of first-line therapy, the outcome after relapse is extremely poor (<10%). Prevention of relapse is therefore the major aim. However, for further improvement of overall outcome it is also essential to optimize salvage therapy. In contrast to childhood ALL, rational and comprehensive strategies, or even consecutive studies, for treatment optimization have been rarely reported for relapsed adult ALL, which is due in part to fatalities that occur once an adult patient with ALL has relapsed.

Definitions of refractory and relapsed disease, including minimal residual disease response evaluation

For reporting of clinical trials, and also management of patients, it is essential to have clear definitions. First, for outcome and selection of treatment it is important to differentiate whether a patient presents with refractory or relapsed disease. Primary refractory disease, which means that a patient did not achieve a complete remission (CR) after standard induction therapy, is an indicator of resistance to conventional ALL drugs. Relapsed disease is present if a patient has achieved a CR during front-line therapy and then relapsed during, or even after, continuation therapy. A similar classification is possible for salvage therapy, for example refractory relapse (no CR after first-line of salvage therapy) or second or later relapse (CR after first-line of salvage therapy). These differentiations are even relevant for pivotal studies with new drugs, which are in some cases tailored to recruit patients in very specific situations (eg, second relapse, non-response to a certain number of treatment lines).

In addition, nowadays, the molecular definition of refractory and relapsed disease should be considered not only for *de novo* but also for relapsed ALL. In ALL there is the fortunate situation that evaluation of minimal residual disease (MRD) allows refined and standardized response evaluation. Compared with cytology, the most exact and sensitive measurement of response can be performed by the evaluation of MRD [2]. Similarly to achievement of complete hematologic response, measured by cytomorphology, the achievement of response on the MRD level has become an essential prognostic factor and a central part of prospective clinical trials in adult and pediatric ALL. Persistent MRD after induction can be classified as molecular refractory disease, and reappearance of MRD after initial achievement of negative status can be classified as molecular relapse. It has been demonstrated unequivocally that molecular relapse leads to cytologic relapse in the majority of cases [3] and should therefore be treated similarly to clinical relapse.

Treatment principles

Treatment of relapsed ALL follows some general principles that can facilitate the treatment decision considerably. Criteria for decision making are summarized in Table 17.1.

Patients with a higher age have a significantly poorer long-term outcome. This is partly because of a higher incidence of poor prognostic features but predominantly due to a poorer tolerability of chemotherapy, which is

Leukemias: Principles and Practice of Therapy, 1st edition. Edited by S. Faderl and H. Kantarjian.

Table 17.1 Factors influencing decision making for salvage therapy in acute lymphoblastic leukemia.

Immunologic subgroup	T-ALL, B-ALL
Age	Feasibility for SCT
Donor availability	Treatment plan with/without SCT
Status of disease	Refractory disease/early relapse vs. late relapse
Previous therapy	Chemotherapy or SCT Drug combinations
Level of disease	Molecular or clinical relapse
Localization	BM, isolated/combined; CNS, other extramedullary
Surface markers	CD20, CD19, CD22, CD33, CD52
Molecular aberrations	Bcr–Abl, FLT3

ALL, acute lymphoblastic leukemia; BM, bone marrow; CNS, central nervous system; SCT, stem-cell transplant.

associated with higher mortality, higher morbidity, and reduced time and dose intensity of treatment. Furthermore, older patients, even in the presence of high-risk factors, are rarely candidates for SCT in CR1. Older patients are therefore treated with less intensive chemotherapy. If they do not respond adequately to initial treatment or undergo relapse, further treatment options are very limited. Therefore, it is important to consider age, general condition, and comorbidities in order to assess whether a patient with relapsed ALL is a candidate for SCT—including dose-reduced conditioning—at all. In older patients without the option of transplant, a less intensive salvage treatment with the aim to control the disease with as high a quality of life as possible could be considered. On the other hand, in adolescents and young adults, intensive chemotherapy-based salvage regimens developed for pediatric patients with ALL may be considered.

The same applies for donor availability. A donor search should be initiated immediately because remission duration and the resulting time interval for realization of SCT after achievement of second CR is short. The search includes family, matched-unrelated and even alternative donors, such as cord blood or haploidentical donors, since it is unequivocal that SCT offers the only chance of cure in relapsed ALL. If no sibling donor is available and the donor search starts at the time of relapse, it may be realistic to assume that SCT cannot be realized within 3 months and the treatment strategy has to be planned accordingly.

The status of disease, particularly the differentiation between (i) refractory disease or early relapse during the intensive treatment phase, compared with (ii) late relapse after the end of treatment or during maintenance therapy, is important for treatment selection. In the former, experimental or alternative drug combinations have to be considered, whereas in the latter repeated induction therapy may be the most promising option.

In this respect, knowledge of previous treatment cycles is important for the selection of salvage therapy. In patients with relapse after SCT, particularly early after SCT, less intensive treatments may be preferable. In patients with relapse during intensive chemotherapy, it makes no sense to repeat treatment elements that have already been administered. In molecular relapse, continuation of treatment (if available), targeted therapies, or immediate SCT may be considered, whereas in clinical relapse a formal salvage treatment is indicated.

The localization of relapse should be considered for additional treatment elements, for example irradiation, although all relapse localizations unequivocally require systemic treatment.

At first diagnosis and again at relapse, the prerequisite for comprehensive treatment planning is diagnostic classification as a basis for treatment stratification. At relapse the major aim is to define subgroup-specific and targeted approaches. This includes the identification of potential therapeutic targets, for example CD20, CD19, CD33, CD22, CD52, Bcr–Abl, FLT3, etc. This information facilitates decision-making regarding the potential use of antibodies as single drugs or in conjunction with chemotherapy, and/or a selection of targeted drugs such as tyrosine-kinase inhibitors.

Outcome after relapse

Recently, four large study groups have reported retrospective analyses of outcome after relapse from adult ALL. The reports were compiled from the databases of the respective study groups and included patient characteristics, in some cases applied salvage treatments, overall outcome, and prognostic factors. Ph^+ ALL was included in all trials. The results are summarized in Table 17.2.

The French group reported an overall CR rate of 44% in 421 relapsed patients. Risk status at first diagnosis had an impact on the remission rate, with a 52% CR for patients with initial standard risk compared with 37% with high risk. A variety of regimens was administered in this retrospective study, with CR rates ranging between 44% and 62%. The median survival was 6.3 months with 8% OS at 5 years. In this study, the only prognostic factor for survival was transplantation of any type [4].

The Medical Research Council (MRC)/Eastern Cooperative Oncology Group (ECOG) study group performed a retrospective analysis of 609 patients with first

Table 17.2 Retrospective studies on outcome of adult patients with acute lymphblastic leukema in first relapse.

Reference	Thomas *et al.* [7]	Tavernier *et al.* [4]	Fielding *et al.* [5]	Vives *et al.* [6]
Year	1999	2007	2007	2008
n	314	421	609	198
Patient characteristics				
Median age (range) (years)	34 (15–81)	34 (15–55)	n.r.	30 (15–69)
B-lineage (%)	59	68	67	64
CNS involvement (%)	16	15	9	n.r.
Duration of first complete remission (%)	30 (12 months)	16 (2 years)	19 (2 years)	n.r.
Outcome				
Complete remission rate (%)	31	44	44	42
Early death (%)	21	n.r.	n.r.	15
Overall survival				
Probability at 5 years (%)	6	8	7	5
Median (months)	6	6	24	n.r.
Survival after SCT				
Autologous (%)	n.r.	4	15	n.r.
Allogeneic sibling (%)	n.r.	21	23	n.r.
Allogeneic unrelated (%)	n.r.	31	16	n.r.

CNS, central nervous system; SCT, stem-cell transplant.

relapse. The CR rate was 44%; details on treatment regimens were not reported. The median survival was 24 months with an OS of 7% at 5 years. Prognostic factors for survival were age (<35 years of age vs. >35 years of age; 3% vs. 12%), gender (female vs. male; 3% vs. 8%), site of relapse (extramedullary vs. central nervous system [CNS] vs. bone marrow; 14% vs. 0% vs. 6%), and duration of first remission (<2 years of age vs. >2 years of age; 5% vs. 11%). In this study, SCT was scheduled as part of an upfront therapy in all patients with sibling donors. After relapse, the outcome of patients with or without prior SCT showed no difference [5].

The Spanish Programma para el Tratamiento de Hemopatìas Malignas (PETHEMA) reported the outcome of 198 patients with relapse after chemotherapy or SCT. The CR rate with various treatment approaches was 42%. Although 35% of the patients could be transferred to SCT, the OS was only 5%. Age was significantly associated with survival (<30 years of age vs. >30 years of age; 7 vs. 3 months). Also, the duration of first remission was a significant prognostic factor for OS (<1 year vs. >1 year; 0% vs. 11%). However, even the most favorable group of young patients with duration of initial remission >1 year had a survival of only 13% [6].

The M. D. Anderson group reported a cohort of 314 patients with an overall CR rate of 31% after a variety of salvage regimens. The CR rates after different salvage regimens showed a wide range (8–33%). The highest CR rate (60%) was achieved in patients with a duration of first remission being >2 years. The OS at 5 years was 5%. In a multivariate regression model for survival age (< vs. >40 years), presence of peripheral blasts (yes vs. no) and duration of first remission (< vs. >1 year) were significant factors. Patients without any risk factor had a significantly better median survival (48 months) than patients with up to three adverse features. Achievement of CR after salvage therapy compared with failure was an additional favorable prognostic feature, with a 12 versus 5 months median survival, respectively [7].

In another report, the M. D. Anderson group focused specifically on the outcome of 288 patients with relapsed ALL who received a second salvage therapy. One aim of the study was to provide some general comparative data since the Food and Drug Administration (FDA) had registered drugs, for example clofarabine, specifically for this instance. The reponse rate with second salvage therapy was 18% and thus seems to be lower compared with first salvage therapy. The overall median survival was only 3 months. Multivariate analysis identified a number of poor prognostic factors for survival, duration of first remission (< or >3 years), bone marrow blasts (< or >50%), platelet count (< or >50,000/μL), and albumin (< or >3 g/L). The OS rate in this study was not reported, but subgroup analysis for patients with none/one, two, three, or four adverse features showed significant differences regarding CR rate (44%, 25%, 12%, and 9%, respectively) and survival (33%, 14%, 8%, and 0%, respectively). The achievement of CR had a significant impact on survival as well. The type of salvage therapy had a significant effect on the outcome, with more favorable results for salvage therapies based on hyper-CVAD, high-dose cytarabine, or direct allogeneic SCT [8].

Table 17.3 Larger prospective trials on combination regimens for adult acute lymphoblastic leukemia.

Reference	Year	Therapy	Patients (*n*)	Complete remission rate (%)	Overall survival
Giona *et al.* [10]	1997	IDA, HDAC, PRED	61	56	10% (3 years)
Koller *et al.* [9]	1997	HDAC, MITOX	64	38	4.6 months
Koller *et al.* [9]	1997	Hyper-CVAD	66	44	9.7 months
Martino *et al.* [13]	1999	VDS, MITOX, CP, HDAC, PRED, MTX	45	74	5.7 months
Camera *et al.* [11]	2004	IDA, HDAC	135	55	6.4 months, 10% (3 years)
Giebel *et al.* [12]	2006	FLU, HDAC, MITOX	50	50	12% (2 years)

Prospective studies of salvage therapy

In a few larger studies, groups have evaluated prospectively defined salvage regimens (Table 17.3).

The hyper-CVAD regimen, which is now front-line therapy in the M. D. Anderson studies, was originally developed as salvage therapy. It consists of alternating cycles with cyclophosphamide, doxorubicin, vincristine, dexamethasone, and cycles with high-dose cytarabine and high-dose methotrexate. The hyper-CVAD regimen in 66 patients was compared with 63 patients treated with high-dose cytarabine and mitoxantrone, with resulting CR rates of 44% and 38%, respectively. Although this difference is not significant, the hyper-CVAD regimen appears to be better tolerated and is associated with a prolonged survival (42 vs. 20 weeks) [9].

The Italian ALL R-87 study used a combination of high-dose cytarabine, idarubicin, and prednisone. In 61 patients the CR rate was 56% and the OS was 10% after 3 years [10]. The subsequent ALL R-97 protocol again included high-dose cytarabine and idarubicin followed by a consolidation with vindesine, high-dose methotrexate, and dexamethasone. Non-responders were treated with high-dose cytarabine and fludarabine. The CR rate in 135 patients was 55%, with no difference between refractory leukemia (57%) and relapse (55%). The mortality during salvage therapy was 12%. Overall, 50 patients (37%) were transferred to SCT but the relapse rate after transplant was remarkably high (53%). The OS at 3 years was 10% [11].

The Polish group reported the results from a combination of fludarabine, cytarabine, and mitoxantrone (FLAM). The CR rate in 50 patients was 50%, with significantly better results for application as second-line treatment compared with more advanced disease (a 66% vs. 13% CR rate). The early mortality was considerable (33%) in patients >40 years compared with younger patients (8%). The OS at 2 years was 12% [12].

The Spanish group evaluated a salvage therapy with vindesine, mitoxantrone, cyclophosphamide, intermediate-dose cytarabine, prednisolone, and methotrexate, which is a regimen more suited to ALL type. The CR rate was 74% in 45 patients. Sixty-eight percent of patients in CR received subsequent SCT. The median OS was still only 5.7 months. The only prognostic factor for survival was availability of a donor for SCT [13].

A variety of other small studies with different drug combinations has also been reported. Single agents generally yield CR rates of only 10–15% [14–16]. These results clearly underline the fact that single drug treatment is not an option in relapsed ALL and this should include pivotal trials with new drugs.

The repetition of regimens (including vincristine, anthracyclines, and steroids), similar to standard induction treatment, led to CR rates of 61% in early studies. This is the preferred approach for late relapses of ALL.

High-dose cytarabine as single drug or in combinations based on AML-type has been extensively studied in adults with relapsed ALL. From several small pilot studies comprising 90 patients in total, the weighted mean CR rate was 37% [17]. Higher CR rates were achieved with combinations, for example with mitoxantrone (17–80%) [16], idarubicin (46– 64% CR rate) [10,11,18,19], fludarabine (39–83% CR rate) [20,21,22–24], mitoxantrone, and VP16 (17–23% CR rate) [25,26] or amsacrine (40% CR) [27]. Because high-dose cytarabine is increasingly administered during front-line treatment, its efficacy during relapse treatment may be impaired. Median remission duration or survival was only reported by a few groups, but did not exceed 5 months and 16%, respectively.

High-dose methotrexate, followed by rescue with folinic acid and combined with asparaginase, led to response rates of 22–79% in early studies [14]. This combination is no longer administered in relapses of ALL, but is incorporated into several regimens for *de novo* ALL.

Overall, it is questionable whether these data are still valid, since all the above-mentioned drugs are generally also used in upfront treatment of adult ALL. Thus, earlier trials may overestimate response rates to salvage therapy. No relevant conclusion can be made regarding the most effective salvage therapies owing to the variability regarding treatment regimens, pretreatments, study size, patient characteristics, number of participating centers, and prior drug exposure. Despite favorable response rates in some trials, overall outcome after relapse is extremely poor, particularly in early relapse. One reason might be the low realization rate of SCT in second CR, another might be that treatment is, in many cases, too short and inconsequent. In patients with late relapse, a modified induction is often successful, whereas in patients with early relapse during intensive chemotherapy, new, experimental, or more intensive regimens are considered. Prospective treatment optimization trials for relapsed ALL are urgently required.

Stem-cell transplant after relapse

It is generally agreed that SCT after achievement of second CR is the treatment of choice in relapsed ALL. This was underlined by an evidence-based review stating an advantage for SCT over chemotherapy in second remission [28]. However, it has to be considered that patients with transplants always represent a selected group of individuals surviving at least as long as the donor search is performed and being in sufficiently good condition to qualify for SCT.

For allogeneic SCT from sibling donors, the European Group for Blood and Marrow Transplant (EBMT) and the International Bone Marrow Transplant Registry (IBMTR) reported a survival rate of 29–34% in second remission and 15–18% in more advanced disease [29,30]. Similarly, survival after matched-unrelated SCT was 28% in second remission and 11% in advanced disease, particularly low because of a higher transplant-related mortality in heavily pretreated patients [30]. Results are quite similar in a pooled literature analysis (Table 17.4).

It is very questionable whether direct SCT without additional chemotherapy is an adequate treatment of relapse. Salvage chemotherapy before SCT should be attempted in order to achieve at least a good partial remission and to reduce tumor load before SCT. As a final option, direct SCT or SCT in aplasia may be attempted. Survival after SCT as a direct treatment of relapse was 18% [8] and 8% [4] in two studies. Compared with acute myeloid leukemia (AML), the reduction of tumor load before SCT appears to be more important in ALL. In a prospective trial on early SCT after salvage therapy with high-dose etoposide and cyclophosphamide in refractory acute leukemia, the CR rates were similar for AML and ALL (54% vs. 67%), but event-free survival was significantly lower for ALL (52% for AML vs. 14% at 5 years) [31].

In the MRC UK study, 120 patients (20%) were able to receive an SCT after relapse, either autologous (n = 13), matched unrelated (n = 65), or matched related (n = 42). The survival rates were 15%, 16%, and 23%, respectively (Table 17.2). The outcome was significantly better compared with that of chemotherapy (4% OS), excluding those who died within the estimated realization time of SCT (100 days) in a landmark analysis. Survival rates were 15% for autograft, 16% for unrelated, and 23% for sibling transplantation after 2 years [5].

The French group identified transplantation in second CR as favorable prognostic factor for OS. Survival after SCT was 25%, with a slightly better outcome for matched-unrelated versus sibling SCT (31% vs. 21%, respectively). The results for SCT were significantly better if performed in second CR compared with failure or immediate SCT at relapse (OS 33% vs. 12% vs. 8%), partly due to a significantly lower transplant-related mortality (23% vs. 79% vs. 65%). The relapse probability was highest for SCT at relapse (54% vs. 41% vs. 78%) [4].

Table 17.4 Results of stem-cell transplant in relapsed/refractory acute lymphoblastic leukemia (pooled from published studies).

Type of SCT	Stage	n	TRM (%)	Relapse rate (%)	LFS (%)
Allogeneic sibling	≥CR2	1019	29	48	34
	Rel/Refr	216	47	75	18
Allogeneic MUD	≥CR2	231	8	75	27
	Rel/Refr[a]	47	64	31	5
Autologous	≥CR2	258	18	70	24

CR, complete remission; LFS, leukemia-free survival; MUD, matched unrelated; Refr, refractory; Rel, relapsed; SCT, stem-cell transplant; TRM, transplant associated mortality.

[a]One trial, Cornellissen *et al.* [32]

For all chemotherapy regimens, the duration of second remission is usually short (maximum 6 months) and the only curative chance for adult patients with relapsed or resistant ALL is SCT. The major aim of relapse treatment is the induction of a second remission with sufficient duration to prepare for SCT. Thus all attempts—including experimental drugs—should be made to obtain a second remission and to transfer patients to SCT. The results of SCT may be improved by optimized conditioning regimens and, moreover, consequent follow-up with additional therapeutic interventions after SCT.

Management of specific situations

Treatment and prevention of extramedullary relapse

A small proportion of relapses in adult ALL are located extramedullary, for example in the CNS or testes. In contrast to childhood ALL, the outcome of extramedullary relapse in adult ALL, either isolated or combined, is not different from bone marrow relapse [4,5]. The reason is probably that, in the majority of extramedullary relapses, bone marrow involvement can be detected by MRD evaluation [33–35]. Out of 64 pediatric patients with ALL with extramedullary relapse, 46 had MRD $> 10^{-4}$, 11 had MRD $> 10^{-4}$, and for seven patients, no MRD was detected. The presence of MRD is an unfavourable prognostic factor [36].

If only local treatment is performed, for example intrathecal therapy, the extramedullary relapse is usually followed by bone marrow relapse. It is therefore recommendable to always consider ALL relapse as a systemic disease and to combine, if necessary, local approaches such as intrathecal therapy in CNS relapse with systemic treatment. MRD evaluation may help with the decision on intensity of treatment, for example in CNS relapse, where additional neurotoxicity could be avoided in patients without MRD in the bone marrow. The risk of cumulative toxicities, particularly if several CNS toxic treatments are combined, should be evaluated carefully.

On the other hand, in patients with bone marrow relapse, the need for CNS prophylaxis should not be forgotten. Although not evaluated systematically, patients after relapse should receive intrathecal therapy for CNS prophylaxis.

Treatment of relapse in Ph/Bcr–Abl$^+$ acute lymphoblastic leukemia

Treatment of Ph/Bcr–Abl$^+$ ALL has been revolutionized by the use of targeted therapies with tyrosine-kinase (TK) inhibitors. At relapse, treatment decisions depend on prior treatment, including applied TK inhibitors, and the presence of mutations associated with resistance to TK inhibitors. The topic is discussed in Chapter 18.

Relapse after stem-cell transplantation

Data on relapse after SCT are very scarce. In an early report from the EBMT that included 76 patients with ALL (adults and children), 42% achieved a CR with subsequent chemotherapy. The median survival was 14 months [37] and only one of nine patients with second transplant achieved long-term survival. No homogeneous series has been reported but two major problems are evident, which are toxicity, particularly in early relapses after SCT, and a high relapse rate [16,38]. Nevertheless, relapse after SCT should be treated as analogous to relapse after chemotherapy.

In the meantime, more experience with second transplants has been accumulated, and for younger patients particularly a second transplant, preferably from an alternative donor, is a realistic option. Decision-making depends, however, on a number of individual factors—time to relapse, general condition, history of or presence of graft-versus-host-disease (GVHD), and many others. Immunomodulation is another option, for example through the withdrawal of GVHD prophylaxis or donor–lymphocyte infusion, although these are less effective in ALL than in other leukemias. The early detection of relapse, already on the molecular level, may be more promising for these approaches.

Minimal residual disease monitoring after relapse and stem-cell transplant

As in front-line therapy, MRD analysis can also be employed to assess responses to salvage therapies. The ultimate goal is to achieve not only a complete hematologic remission, but also a good molecular remission. In pediatric patients with ALL, the MRD level after salvage treatment [39] was predictive for survival. Furthermore, the MRD level was predictive for the outcome of subsequent SCT [40–42]. Because all patients receiving transplant after relapse are at high risk, the follow-up of MRD may help to identify patients who could benefit from additional treatment measures such as immunologic treatments, for example the reduction of GVHD prohylaxis and/or the application of donor lymphocytes are promising approaches for preventing overt relapse. In Ph$^+$ ALL, post-transplant treatment with imatinib—either upfront or after detection of MRD—appears to be a very successful approach.

Prognostic factors for outcome of relapse

A number of prognostic factors for the achievement of CR and OS after relapse have been reported (see above). Overall, with an extremely poor OS after relapse, the value of prognostic factors can be questioned and the majority are not helpful for the evaluation and design of salvage therapies. There are, however, four relevant factors.

Duration of first remission

The most significant predictive factor for treatment response in relapsed patients is the duration of first remission. The term has been defined in different ways, for example relapse before or after 1 year, before or after 18 months, before or after 2 years, and relapse during or after treatment. The difference in outcome may be in part due to different pathogenetic mechanisms of early and late relapse. Early relapse, including molecular, identifies patients with resistance to standard chemotherapy. Although a variety of resistance mechanisms are underlying, the risk for non-response to further chemotherapy approaches is high. In late relapse it may well be that a quiescent leukemic clone, present as MRD at a non-detectable level, acquires additional mutations that then lead to relapse. Consequently, in early relapse, innovative approaches with alternative mechanisms of action should be attempted, whereas in late relapse the chance to achieve remission with repeated induction chemotherapy is rather good.

Age

Older age is associated with a higher mortality during salvage treatment and the lack of SCT as a therapeutic option. Both factors are relevant for the evaluation of CR and OS. In the majority of trials for salvage therapy in adult ALL, older patients are not included at all.

Achievement of complete remission

The achievement of CR after relapse, namely rapid achievement of CR already at the first salvage attempt, is a significant prognostic factor for OS. This means that achievement of CR is a surrogate marker for clinical endpoint. Nowadays, molecular CR assessed by measurement of MRD provides a more standardized and refined approach to assess achievement of CR.

Treatment lines

Consequently, the chance to achieve a CR decreases with the number of applied treatment approaches, not only because of cumulative toxicity, but also as a result of the selection of more resistant leukemia cell clones. This fact has to be considered for the evaluation of new drugs, which are often tested in patients with a number of prior treatment lines. Therefore, the potential benefit of these drugs in front-line therapy may be underestimated.

In addition, in pediatric ALL, the outcome after extramedullary relapse is significantly better than for bone marrow relapse. Based on the duration of first remission, relapse localistion (bone marrow involvement vs. extramedullary only), and achievement of molecular CR (negative MRD status), pediatric study groups have established a risk-adapted treatment of relapsed ALL with intensive chemotherapy for low-risk patients and STC in high-risk patients. CR rates varied between 60% and 91% and survival varied between 10% and 35% for early relapses. For late relapses, CR rates ranged between 81% and 96% and survival ranged between 33% and 71% [43].

New drugs

Fortunately, a number of new drugs are available that may be either integrated in prospective trials for innovative salvage therapies or that are still in clinical testing before registration [44–46]. Treatment with new drugs is an option, particularly in patients with early relapse and as a second approach to salvage therapy, since access to new drugs usually needs some logistic preparation—first salvage treatment should not be postponed for organisational reasons.

The design of phase I and II trials with new drugs for ALL has to be discussed carefully with the regulatory authorities. Monotherapies in selected situations, for example second relapse, do not reflect the clinical needs and do not offer the patients an optimal chance to benefit from a new treatment. Also, randomized studies at relapse of ALL are generally unrealistic because of the small patient number, the biologic diversity, and the fact that no standard treatment is defined that could be compared. In contrast to oncology trials, comparison with best supportive care is no option, partly for ethical reasons as patients with acute leukemia have an extremely short survival with this approach. Furthermore, for quicker assessments of the benefits of new drugs, surrogate markers for efficacy evaluation are essential. Long-term follow-up endpoints such as OS are not very suitable since they depend too much on covariates, for example the realization of SCT. Fortunately, achievement of CR and also molecular CR, defined as MRD-based response evaluation, are ideal surrogate markers because they are strongly correlated to clinical outcome.

Nucleoside analogs or related drugs

Nelarabine is a water-soluble prodrug of arabinosylguanine. It inhibits DNA synthesis and leads to DNA fragmentation, and is specifically active in T-ALL. Pivotal studies in pediatric ALL demonstrated a CR rate of 48% in patients with one prior induction and 23% with two or more prior inductions. In combined CNS and bone marrow relapse, the CR rate was 21% [47]. In adult T-ALL, the response rates were slightly inferior at 27% versus 21% in patients with one compared with more prior inductions. One-year survival was 36% and 29%, respectively

[48]. Whereas bone marrow toxicity is limited, nelarabine can potentially lead to severe neurotoxicities. At present, the integration into front-line therapy is assessed as well as the design of combination regimens.

Clofarabine is a deoxyadenosine analog with several pharmacologic advantages compared with fludarabine or cladribine. It shows activity in myeloid and lymphoid malignancies with no lineage specificity [49]. When tested in relapsed/refractory pediatric ALL, it resulted in a CR rate of 20%. It was tested in different combination regimens; the combination with cyclophosphamide and VP16 yielded a CR/CRp (CR without platelet recovery) rate of 64% in pediatric patients with ALL [50]. The dose-limiting toxicity was veno-occlusive disease (VOD). Therefore, patients with pre-existing liver toxicity and patients with prior SCT were no longer included. So far there is little experience with single-drug clofarabine or combination regimens in adult ALL, but further testing is certainly of interest.

Forodesine hydrochloride is not a cytostatic drug but an inhibitor of purine nucleoside phosphorylase. Finally, similar to nelarabine, it leads to accumulation of deoxyguanosine and thereby to inhibition of DNA synthesis [51]. Activity has been demonstrated in T- and B-ALL, and there may be a specific activity in relapse after SCT [52]. The drug has a very favorable safety profile and may have a role in maintenance therapy, particularly because of its available oral formulation.

Liposomal drugs

PEG-asparaginase is *Escheria coli* L-asparaginase conjugated to polyethylene glycol. Compared with native *E. coli* asparaginase it has the advantage of longer activity—approximately 10 days after one application of 2000–2500 U/m^2. Furthermore, it seems to be less immunogenic. This is an advantage because, during long-term use, a lower proportion of patients may suffer from silent inactivation or clinical hypersensitivity. In adult patients, the German Multicenter Study Group for Adult ALL (GMALL) has used doses of 1000–2000 U/m^2 with acceptable toxicity and favorable interim results for efficacy [53]. Asparaginase encapsulated into erythrocytes is another new formulation of *E.coli* asparaginase with similar advantages [54]. Both drugs could contribute to improved efficacy of salvage regimens based on typical ALL induction.

Liposomal daunorubicin and doxorubicin are pegylated formulations of the respective conventional drugs. Data obtained in ALL so far show no clear advantage compared with conventional preparations of the drug [55]. Recently, a study with liposomal daunorubicin in combination with high-dose cytarabine yielded in 25 patients with relapsed ALL, including one-third Ph$^+$ ALL, a CR rate of 80%. Of note is that 39% of the patients showed an overexpression of MDR related proteins. The survival at 1 year was 39% [56].

Liposomal vincristine has, similarly to other liposomal drugs, a prolonged half-life. Side-effects are similar to conventional vincristine. In 36 patients with refractory/relapsed ALL, a response rate of 19% has been observed, which is a favorable result for monotherapy. The CR rate was 29% if liposomal vincristine was administered as the first salvage attempt [57]. Future application of liposomal vincristine should certainly be as part of a combination regimen.

Liposomal cytarabine is a cytarabine preparation for intrathecal application. After one application cytotoxicity is maintained for 14 days and the drug achieves a more even distribution in the cerebrospinal fluid [58]. It is also a highly active drug in CNS relapse of ALL, but because of the potential cumulative toxicity combination with systemic high-dose therapy it must be evaluated carefully.

Monoclonal antibodies

Rituximab is the monoclonal antibody for which most experience in ALL has been accumulated so far. If not already used in front-line therapy, as in several trials for mature B-ALL/Burkitt lymphoma or B-ALL, it may be combined with any relapse therapy in order to increase efficacy.

Alemtuzumab is potentially useful for the treatment of relapsed ALL since CD52 is expressed on the majority of ALL blasts, B- or T-lineage. Activity in ALL has been demonstrated in single cases.

Epratuzumab is an antibody to CD22 that is present in most cases of B-ALL. Experience so far is mainly available in non-Hodgkin lymphoma, but a trial in relapsed pediatric ALL is ongoing [59].

Gemtuzumab ozogamicin is an antibody to CD33 that is expressed in a subset of patients with ALL, particularly immature, early subtypes such as pro-B-ALL and early T-ALL. Single-drug activity has been demonstrated but prospective trials are so far missing [60].

Molecular therapies

Dasatinib and nilotinib are second-generation TK inhibitors that may be used for the treatment of relapsed Ph/Bcr–Abl$^+$ ALL, either as single drugs or in combination with chemotherapy.

FLT3 inhibitors are an option in patients with ALL with *FLT3* mutations, as they are observed particulary in immature subtypes of ALL, such as pro-B-ALL.

A number of other treatment approaches is currently under investigation in ALL including histone deacetylase inhibitors, DNA methylase inhibitors, mTOR inhibitors, farnesyl transferase inhibitors, CDK inhibitors, γ-secretase inhibitors, or proteasome inhibitors [61]. These studies are still in the early phases, but after proof-of-principle many of these drugs will be suitable partners for combination regimens.

Summary and conclusions

The overall outcome of adult patients with relapsed ALL is extremely poor. With a variety of salvage therapies, CR rates of 30–80% are achieved. The most important prognostic factor for the achievement of CR is the duration of first remission. Achievement of CR after salvage treatment and realization of SCT is the most relevant factor for survival.

Although a large number of different salvage regimens have been evaluated, there is no standard approach to therapy of relapsed ALL. Treatment must be selected rationally, based on factors such as age, subtype, availability of targeted therapies, stage of disease, and many others. In older patients without the option of transplant, a palliative approach appears to be justified. In patients with late relapse the basis of treatment is a repeated induction therapy. In early relapse, new drugs with preferable alternative mechanisms of action are of interest. MRD evaluation is a new method not only to identify patients with upcoming relapse earlier but to improve the outcome of salvage therapy by application at a lower level of tumor load. MRD evaluation may also serve as sensitive method for evaluation of salvage regimens. Achievement of CR and achievement of molecular CR, defined as negative MRD status, are factors correlated to clinical outcome and therefore are surrogate markers for clinical trials.

It is generally agreed that SCT after achievement of CR is the treatment of choice in relapsed ALL. Survival rates of around 30% are achieved for matched-unrelated or sibling SCT in second CR. In many studies, the realisation rate of SCT in relapsed patients is still low, probably owing to logistics. Furthermore, increased treatment-related mortality and relapse rate has to be expected.

Prospective trials are needed, not only for the evaluation of new drugs, but also for academic treatment optimization trials. This includes optimization of combination chemotherapy with induction and subsequent consolidations, realization of SCT by optimized logistics, optimized SCT, and post-SCT procedures. SCT in second CR is the preferred treatment in patients with relapsed ALL but it has to be demonstrated that it can contribute to an improved overall outcome of ALL after relapse.

The major challenges are slightly different for early and late relapse. In early relapse, new targeted and subgroup-adjusted treatments with alternative mechanisms of action are most promising. Since remission duration is short logistics for SCT realization have to be optimized. In late relapse response rates are favorable but a comprehensive strategy including procedures for failure patients, measurement of MRD, consolidation therapies, improved realization of SCT, and optimized SCT procedures, including post-transplant strategies for relapse prophylaxis, is needed.

References

1 Gökbuget N, Hoelzer D. Treatment of adult acute lymphoblastic leukemia. *Sem Hematol* 2009;46:64–75.

2 Szczepanski T. Why and how to quantify minimal residual disease in acute lymphoblastic leukemia? *Leukemia* 2007;21: 622–6.

3 Raff T, Gökbuget N, Luschen S, *et al.* Molecular relapse in adult standard-risk ALL patients detected by prospective MRD monitoring during and after maintenance treatment: data from the GMALL 06/99 and 07/03 trials. *Blood* 2007;109:910–15.

4 Tavernier E, Boiron JM, Huguet F, *et al.* Outcome of treatment after first relapse in adults with acute lymphoblastic leukemia initially treated by the LALA-94 trial. *Leukemia* 2007;21: 1907–14.

5 Fielding AK, Richards SM, Chopra R, *et al.* Outcome of 609 adults after relapse of acute lymphoblastic leukemia (ALL); an MRC UKALL12/ECOG 2993 study. *Blood* 2007;109:944–50.

6 Oriol A, Vives S, Hernández-Rivas JM, *et al.* Outcome after relapse of acute lymphoblastic leukemia in adult patients included in four consecutive risk-adapted trials by the PETHEMA Study Group. *Haematologica* 2010;95:589–96.

7 Thomas DA, Kantarjian H, Smith TL, *et al.* Primary refractory and relapsed adult acute lymphoblastic leukemia: characteristics, treatment results, and prognosis with salvage therapy. *Cancer* 1999;86:1216–30.

8 O'Brien S, Thomas D, Ravandi F, *et al.* Outcome of adults with acute lymphocytic leukemia after second salvage therapy. *Cancer* 2008;113:3186–91.

9 Koller CA, Kantarjian HM, Thomas D, *et al.* The hyper-CVAD regimen improves outcome in relapsed acute lymphoblastic leukemia. *Leukemia* 1997;11:2039–44.

10 Giona F, Annino L, Rondelli R, *et al.* Treatment of adults with acute lymphoblastic leukemia in first bone marrow relapse. *Br J Haematol* 1997;97:896–903.

11 Camera A, Annino L, Chiurazzi F, *et al.* GIMEMA ALL—Rescue 97: a salvage strategy for primary refractory or relapsed adult acute lymphoblastic leukemia. *Haematologica* 2004;89:145–53.

12 Giebel S, Krawczyk-Kulis M, Adamczyk-Cioch M, *et al.* Fludarabine, cytarabine, and mitoxantrone (FLAM) for the treatment of relapsed and refractory adult acute lymphoblastic leukemia. A phase study by the Polish Adult Leukemia Group (PALG). *Ann Hematol* 2006;85:717–22.

13 Martino R, Bellido M, Brunet S, *et al.* Intensive salvage chemotherapy for primary refractory or first relapsed adult acute lymphoblastic leukemia: results of a prospective trial. *Haematologica* 1999;84:505–10.

14 Welborn JL. Impact of reinduction regimens for relapsed and refractory acute lymphoblastic leukemia in adults. *Am J Hematol* 1994;45:341–344.

15 Bassan R, Lerede T, Barbui T. Strategies for the treatment of recurrent acute lymphoblastic leukemia in adults. *Haematologica* 1996;81:20–36.
16 Garcia-Manero G, Thomas DA. Salvage therapy for refractory or relapsed acute lymphocytic leukemia. *Hematol Oncol Clin North Am* 2001;15:163–205.
17 Hoelzer D. High-dose chemotherapy in adult acute lymphoblastic leukemia. *Semin Hematol* 1991;28(Suppl.4):84–9.
18 Arcese W, Meloni G, Giona F, *et al.* Idarubicin plus ARA-C followed by allogeneic or autologous bone marrow transplantation in advanced acute lymphoblastic leukemia in adults. *Bone Marrow Transplant* 1991;2:38a.
19 Freund M, Heil G, Arnold R, *et al.* Treatment of relapsed ALL—studies of the German ALL Cooperative Group. *Ann Hematol* 1997;74:A15.
20 Montillo M, Tedeschi A, Discepoli G, *et al.* Fludarabine and cytosine arabinoside + G-CSF in the treatment of relapsed acute lymphoblastic leukemia: preliminary results. *Blood* 1994; 94:622a.
21 Visani G, Tosi P, Zinzani PL, *et al.* FLAG (fludarabine, cytarabine, G-CSF) as a second line therapy for acute lymphoblastic leukemia with myeloid antigen expression: *in vitro* and *in vivo* effects. *Eur J Haematol* 1996;56:308–12.
22 Montillo M, Tedeschi A, Centuriono R, Leoni P. Treatment of relapsed adult acute lymphoblastic leukemia with fludarabine and cytosine arabinoside followed by granulocyte colony-stimulating factor (FLAG-GCSF). *Leuk Lymphoma* 1997;25: 579–82.
23 Specchia G, Pastore D, Carluccio P, *et al.* FLAG-IDA in the treatment of relapsed/refractory adult acute lymphoblastic leukemia. *Ann Hematol* 2005;84:792–5.
24 Yavuz S, Paydas S, Disel U, Sahin B. IDA-FLAG regimen for the therapy of primary refractory and relapse acute leukemia: a single-center experience. *Am J Ther* 2006;13:389–93.
25 Mazza JJ, Leong T, Rowe JM, Wiernik PH, Cassileth PA. Treatment of adult patients with acute lymphocytic leukemia in relapse. *Leuk Lymphoma* 1996;20:317–19.
26 Rosen PJ, Rankin C, Head DR, *et al.* A phase II study of high dose ARA-C and mitoxantrone for treatment of relapsed or refractory adult acute lymphoblastic leukemia. *Leuk Res* 2000; 24:183–7.
27 Reman O, Buzyn A, Lhéritier V, *et al.* Rescue therapy combining intermediate-dose cytarabine with amsacrine and etoposide in relapsed adult acute lymphoblastic leukemia. *Hematol J* 2004; 5:123–9.
28 Hahn T, Wall D, Camitta B, *et al.* The role of cytotoxic therapy with hematopoietic stem cell transplantation in the therapy of acute lymphoblastic leukemia in adults: an evidence-based review. *Biol Blood Marrow Transplant* 2006;12:1–30.
29 Loberiza F. Summary Slides 2003—part III. IMBTR/ABMTR Newsletter 2006;10:6–9.
30 Chaidos A, Kanfer E, Apperley JF. Risk assessment in haemotopoietic stem cell transplantation: disease and disease stage. *Best Pract Res Clin Haematol* 2007;20:125–54.
31 Johny A, Song KW, Nantel SH *et al.* Early stem cell transplantation for refractory acute leukemia after salvage therapy with high-dose etoposide and cyclophosphamide. *Biol.Blood.Marrow. Transplant.* 2006;12:480–489.
32 Cornelissen JJ, Carston M, Kollman C, *et al.* Unrelated marrow transplantation for adult patients with poor-risk acute lymphoblastic leukemia: strong graft-versus-leukemia effect and risk factors determining outcome. *Blood* 2001;97:1572–7.
33 Goulden N, Langlands K, Steward C, *et al.* PCR assessment of bone marrow status in 'isolated' extramedullary relapse of childhood B-precursor acute lymphoblastic leukemia. *Br J Haematol* 1994;87:282–5.
34 O'Reilly J, Meyer B, Baker D, *et al.* Correlation of bone marrow minimal residual disease and apparent isolated extramedullary relapse in childhood acute lymphoblastic leukemia. *Leukemia* 1995;15:624–7.
35 Neale GAM, Pui C-H, Mahmoud HH, *et al.* Molecular evidence for minimal residual bone marrow disease in children with 'isolated' extra-medullary relapse of T-cell acute lymphoblastic leukemia. *Leukemia* 1994;8:768–75.
36 Hagedorn N, Acquaviva C, Fronkova E, *et al.* Submicroscopic bone marrow involvement in isolated extramedullary relapses in childhood acute lymphoblastic leukemia: a more precise definition of "isolated" and its possible clinical implications, a collaborative study of the Resistant Disease Committee of the International BFM study group. *Blood* 2007;110:4022–9.
37 Frassoni F, Barrett AJ, Granena A, *et al.* Relapse after allogeneic bone marrow transplantation for acute leukemia: a survey by the E.B.M.T. of 117 cases. *Br J Haematol* 1988;70:317–20.
38 Kumar L. Leukemia: management of relapse after allogeneic bone marrow transplantation. *J Clin Oncol* 1994;12:1710–17.
39 Eckert C, Biondi A, Seeger K, *et al.* Prognostic value of minimal residual disease in relapsed childhood acute lymphoblastic leukemia. *Lancet* 2001;358:1239–41.
40 Knechtli CJC, Goulden NJ, Hancock JP, *et al.* Minimal residual disease status before allogeneic bone marrow transplantation is an important determinant of successful outcome for children and adolescents with acute lymphoblastic leukemia. *Blood* 1998;92:4072–9.
41 Bader P, Hancock J, Kreyenberg H, *et al.* Minimal residual disease (MRD) status prior to allogeneic stem cell transplantation is a powerful predictor for post-transplant outcome in children with ALL. *Leukemia* 2002;16:1668–72.
42 Goulden N, Bader P, van der Velden V, *et al.* Minimal residual disease prior to stem cell transplant for childhood acute lymphoblastic leukemia. *Br J Haematol* 2003;122:24–9.
43 Bailey LC, Lange BJ, Rheingold SR, Bunin NJ. Bone-marrow relapse in pediatric acute lymphoblastic leukemia. *Lancet Oncol* 2008;9:873–83.
44 Pui CH, Jeha S. New therapeutic strategies for the treatment of acute lymphoblastic leukemia. *Nat Rev Drug Discov* 2007;6: 149–65.
45 Thomas X. Emerging drugs for adult acute lymphoblastic leukemia. *Expert Opin Emerg Drugs* 2005;10:591–617.
46 Gökbuget N, Hoelzer D. Treatment of adult acute lymphoblastic leukemia. *Hematology Am Soc Hematol Educ Program* 2006;133–141.
47 Berg SL, Blaney SM, Devidas M, *et al.* Phase II study of nelarabine (compound 506U78) in children and young adults with refractory T-cell malignancies:a report from the Children's Oncology Group. *J Clin Oncol* 2005;23:3376–82.
48 Deangelo DJ, Yu D, Johnson JL, *et al.* Nelarabine induces complete remissions in adults with relapsed or refractory T-lineage acute lymphoblastic leukemia or lymphoblastic lymphoma: cancer and leukemia group B study 19801. *Blood* 2007. [Epub ahead of print.]

49 Jeha S, Gandhi V, Chan KW, *et al.* Clofarabine, a novel nucleoside analog, is active in pediatric patients with advanced leukemia. *Blood* 2004;103:784–9.

50 Hijiya N, Gaynon PS, Fernandez M, *et al.* Durable remissions observed in a Phase I/II study of clofarabine in combination with etoposide and cyclophosphamide in pediatric patients with refractory or relapsed acute leukemia. *Blood* (ASH Annual Meeting Abstracts) 2008;112:2925.

51 Gandhi V, Kilpatrick JM, Plunkett W, *et al.* A proof-of-principle pharmacokinetic, pharmacodynamic, and clinical study with purine nucleoside phosphorylase inhibitor immucillin-H (BCX-1777, forodesine). *Blood* 2005;106:4253–60.

52 Stelljes M, Kienast J, Berning B, *et al.* Forodesine in patients with refractory/relapsed T-ALL can induce prolonged stable remission with minimal toxicity before and after allogeneic hematopoietic stem cell transplantation. *Blood* 2006;108:5340.

53 Gökbuget N, Baumann A, Beck J, *et al.* PEG-asparaginase in adult acute lymphoblastic leukemia (ALL): efficacy and feasibility analysis with increasing dose levels. *Blood* (ASH Annual Meeting Abstracts) 2008;112:302.

54 Bertrand Y, Thomas X, Baruchel A, *et al.* GRASPALL 2005.01 Clinical Study: L-Asparaginase loaded into red blood cells is effective at depleting serum asparagine in children and adults with relapsed acute lymphoblastic leukemia (ALL). *Blood* (ASH Annual Meeting Abstracts) 2008;112:306.

55 Offidani M, Corvatta L, Malerba L, *et al.* Comparison of two regimens for the treatment of elderly patients with acute lymphoblastic leukemia (ALL). *Leuk Lymphoma* 2005;46:233–8.

56 Candoni A, Michelutti A, Simeone E, *et al.* Efficacy of liposomal daunorubicin and cytarabine as reinduction chemotherapy in relapsed acute lymphoblastic leukemia despite expression of multidrug resistance-related proteins. *Eur J Haematol* 2006;77: 293–9.

57 Thomas DA, Kantarjian HM, Stock W, *et al.* Phase 1 multicenter study of vincristine sulfate liposomes injection and dexamethasone in adults with relapsed or refractory acute lymphoblastic leukemia. *Cancer* 2009;115:5490–8.

58 Benesch M, Urban C. Liposomal cytarabine for leukemic and lymphomatous meningitis: recent developments. *Expert Opin Pharmacother* 2008;9:301–9.

59 Raetz EA, Cairo MS, Borowitz MJ, *et al.* Chemoimmunotherapy reinduction with epratuzumab in children with acute lymphoblastic leukemia in marrow relapse: a Children's Oncology Group Pilot Study. *J Clin Oncol* 2008;26:3756–62.

60 Chevallier P, Mahe B, Garand R, *et al.* Combination of chemotherapy and gemtuzumab ozogamicin in adult Philadelphia positive acute lymphoblastic leukemia patient harboring CD33 expression. *Int J Hematol* 2008;88:209–11.

61 Crazzolara R, Bendall L. Emerging treatments in acute lymphoblastic leukemia. *Curr Cancer Drug Targets* 2009;9:19–31.

Chapter 18
Philadelphia Chromosome-positive Acute Lymphoblastic Leukemia: Current Treatment Status and Perspectives

Olga Sala-Torra and Jerald P. Radich
Fred Hutchinson Cancer Research Center, Seattle, Washington, USA

Introduction

Philadelphia chromosome-positive acute lymphoblastic leukemia (Ph^+ ALL) accounts for approximately 25–30% of ALL diagnosed in adults, but <5% of ALL diagnosed in pediatric patients. The Philadelphia chromosome is a well-characterized recurrent chromosomal abnormality that confers adverse prognosis to ALL. Although 70–90% of cases of Ph^+ ALL achieve complete remission (CR) with conventional chemotherapy regimes, long-term survival does not surpass 20%, reflecting a high rate of relapse and failure of salvage regimens. Thus, patients diagnosed with Ph^+ ALL are considered to be candidates for hematopoietic stem-cell transplant (HSCT) if a suitable donor is available.

The initial treatment of Ph^+ ALL has been dramatically changed by the introduction of Abl tyrosine kinase inhibitors (TKI). Used as a single agent, or in combination with chemotherapy, CR is common although, even with combination approaches, relapse is the rule. A more complete understanding of the biology of the Ph chromosome is needed in order to cure patients who cannot receive an HSCT.

The molecular biology of the philadelphia chromosome

The Ph is the shortened chromosome 22 that results from the reciprocal translocation of the long arms of chromosomes 9 and 221—t (9; 22). While chromosome 9 breaks almost invariably in the 5′ region of Abl, the breakpoint in chromosome 22 varies, with predilection for two different sites in the *BCR* gene, the major (M-*BCR*) and the minor (m-*BCR*) breakpoint cluster regions. This produces the two common Bcr–Abl fusion variants, p210 and p190, with different molecular weights determined by the different amount of *BCR* that they include [1–4]. The Ph is the hallmark of chronic myeloid leukemia (CML), and it is also the most common recurrent cytogenetic abnormality in adult ALL. The larger 210 kD fusion protein (p210 variant) is almost invariably found in CML, but it is also present in 10–50% of Ph^+ ALL. It occurs in <10% of pediatric Ph^+ ALL, and its prevalence increases with age to 40% in patients >50 years old [5,6]. Inversely, the p190 kD Bcr–Abl protein is found in the majority of pediatric Ph^+ ALL, in two-thirds to one-half of adult Ph^+ ALL, and only rarely in patients with CML. A small percentage of patients with Ph^+ ALL present with both p210 and p190 isoforms, a result of the alternative splicing of the *BCR* exons contributing to Bcr–Abl [7].

Several diagnostic approaches can detect the presence of the Ph. Conventional cytogenetics detect the Ph directly, with known limitations of sensitivity (1–5%) and the fact that in ~20–30% of cases, the bone marrow samples prove inadequate for metaphase preparations [8,9]. In addition, conventional cytogenetics fail to detect cryptic translocations that may occur in a small percentage of Ph^+ ALL cases. Fluorescence *in situ* hybridization (FISH) allows the analysis of interphase cells with a sensitivity down to 0.5–5%, depending on the probe used and the laboratory using it [10]. Reverse-transcriptase polymerase chain reaction (RT-PCR) detects the chimeric mRNA arising from the *BCR–ABL* genomic recombination and is the most sensitive of the diagnostic techniques (it can detect one $Bcr–Abl^+$-containing cell in a background of 100,000–1,000,000 normal cells). RT-PCR can discriminate between p190 and p210 Bcr–Abl by using oligonucleotide primers with sequences specific to the Bcr fragments involved in each isoform [2,11,12]. Limitations of this technique include the risk of false-positives resulting from contamination, and the risk of false-negatives owing to the exquisite susceptibility of RNA to degradation [13].

Abl is a non-receptor tyrosine kinase localized both in the nucleus and the cytoplasm [14]. However, in the Bcr–Abl fusion protein, Abl is constitutively activated through

Leukemias: Principles and Practice of Therapy, 1st edition. Edited by S. Faderl and H. Kantarjian.

the formation of Bcr–Abl homotetramers (mediated by the Bcr coiled-coil domain included in the fusion protein) [15]. Bcr–Abl is kept in the cytoplasm [16,17], and when forcedly entrapped in the nucleus after treatment with the TKI imatinib and leptomycin B, it induces apoptosis [18]. Bcr–Abl phosphorylates itself and multiple signaling proteins [19], activating pathways that are usually regulated by receptor tyrosine kinases and annulling the cytokine-dependence of the cell for functions such as proliferation or apoptosis. The expression of p190 or p210 Bcr–Abl fusion forms is sufficient to cause leukemia in animal models [20–24], but how both isoforms interfere with the specific cellular pathways ultimately determining cell transformation, and how these pathways differ in each myeloid and lymphoid environment, is not completely understood.

Among the pathways activated by Bcr–Abl are the JAK–STAT, Ras–Raf–MEK–ERK, PI3K–AKT, c-Myc, SAPK–JNK, and NF-κB pathways. The JAK–STAT pathway is involved in cell proliferation and inhibition of apoptosis, and Bcr–Abl$^+$ cells (both p190 and p210) constitutively present phosphorylation of multiple STAT proteins, STAT5 among them [25]. STAT5 phosphorylation results in the activation of gene expression, such as the antiapoptotic protein Bcl-xL [26]. Recent studies in animal models suggest that STAT5A/b is required for lymphoid transformation by Bcr–Abl [27,28], and that deletion of Bcl-xL is not enough to reverse leukemia [29]. In addition, constitutive phosphorylation of Stat6 is only present in p190$^+$ cells, and may be important in determining the preference of p190 for lymphoid transformation [25]. Finally, JAK2 is involved in the induction of the transcription factor c-Myc [30], required for Bcr–Abl transformation [31].

The Ras–Raf–MEK–ERK and PI3K–AKT pathways are also involved in inhibition of apoptosis and regulation of cell-cycle progression, and activation of Ras and AKT are required for Bcr–Abl transformation of hematopoietic cells [32–34]. Autophosphorylation of Tyr177, in the Grb2-binding motif in *BCR*, is essential for Bcr binding to Grb2, which mediates phosphorylation and complex formation with Gab2 and is linked to Ras activation [35,36]. Mutation of Tyr177 or deletion of Gab2 results in decreased activation of PI3K–AKT and Ras–ERK pathways, with decreased cell proliferation and migration [36]. *BCR–ABL* mutated on the Y177 site does not induce myeloproliferative disease, and mice transplanted with marrow transduced with this mutant die from B and T leukemias after a long latency [37]. Similarly, Gab2–/– mice myeloid progenitors transduced with *BCR–ABL* are resistant to transformation, and the transformation of lymphoid progenitors is decreased owing to increased apoptosis [36]. Y177 site and Gab2 also seem to be involved in the constitutive activation of PI3K pathway in Bcr–Abl$^+$ cells [36], which results in AKT phosphorylation and can increase in β-catenin stability [38]. Phosphorylation of downstream targets of AKT, such as Bad and mTOr, promote cell survival [39]. The transcription NF-κB, which inhibits apoptosis, is also activated by Bcr–Abl in a kinase-dependent manner [40].

Bcr–Abl$^+$ leukemias are characterized by a high degree of genomic instability that is induced by this oncogenic protein, as demonstrated by the increased frequency of DNA insertions and deletions present in Bcr–Abl pre-leukemic mice [41]. Bcr–Abl increases polymerase-β expression [42], downregulates DNA-repair enzymes (DNA-PKcs) [43], and deregulates RAD51 [44] and BRCA-1 [45], all of which can cause increased mutations.

Ph$^+$ ALL typically presents a pre-B phenotype, reflecting an arrest in B-cell maturation, and aberrant coexpression of some myeloid cell-surface markers and myeloid specific genes [46]. Ph$^+$ ALL often presents aberrant splicing of key genes in lymphoid development, such as *BTK* and *SLP-65*, and deleterious mutations of *IKZF1*, a gene that encodes the zinc-finger transcription factor Ikaros [46–50]. The aberrant splicing of SLP-65 and Btk in B-cell precursors results in shorter transcripts that halt lymphoid maturation [51]. Bcr–Abl lymphoblastic leukemia cells can express high levels of an alternative splice variant of SLP-65 that introduces additional exons with an early termination codon. Treatment with Abl kinase inhibitors restores the normal SLP-65 variant in some of these cells, which also progress to a more differentiated phenotype [47]. Btk deficiency defines the X-linked agammaglobulinemia syndrome, characterized by a differentiation block of B-cell precursors at the pre-B state. Similar to SLP-65, mutants that lack the Btk kinase domain have been identified in pre-B Ph$^+$ ALL [49]. These truncated forms may act as a link between Bcr–Abl and wild-type Btk, facilitating Btk phosphorylation by Bcr–Abl that activates downstream cell-survival signals [52]. Finally, the deletion of exons 3–6 of *IKZF1*, perhaps as a result of an aberrant Rag-mediated recombination [50], results in a dominant negative form of Ikaros that lacks the DNA-binding domain. This mutated form, denominated IK6, halts B-cell differentiation and contributes to the expression of some myeloid specific genes [46]. It has been suggested that overexpression of IK6 may contribute to resistance to tyrosine kinase inhibitors [53].

A common additional mutation in patients with Ph$^+$ ALL is the deletion of 9p21, compromising the *INK4A–ARF* gene that has been detected in up to 30% of adult and pediatric patients in some cohorts [54–56]. The activation of $p14^{ARF}$ induces cell-cycle arrest and apoptosis through p53 activation, and Arf-null BCR–ABL$^+$ cells induce more severe leukemia in irradiated mice recipients, and with reduced latency when compared with Arf$^+$ *BCR–ABL* transformed cells. Additionally, Arf-null p210 or p190$^+$ mice leukemias are resistant to Abl kinase inhibitors *in vivo* [56].

Another particularity of Ph+ ALL is the dependence of Bcr–Abl transformation on Src kinases that do not appear to be required for the induction of CML [57], at least in the murine model. Bcr–Abl activates Src kinases in a kinase-independent manner, as the inhibition of Bcr–Abl by imatinib does not decrease Src activation [58]. At the same time, the specific inhibition of Src kinases (without inhibition of Bcr–Abl) induces apoptosis in leukemia cells and extends survival in mice with Ph+ ALL, confirming the role of Src kinases in the Bcr–Abl transformation of lymphoid cells [58]. CML progression to lymphoid blast crisis may also depend on Src kinases [58] as lymphoid blast crisis cells are also extremely dependent on Lyn for survival, to a higher extent than myeloid blast crisis CML cells, suggesting a lineage-specific signaling pathway or mechanism [59]. Src kinases activate β-catenin in an *in vitro* model, and the specific inhibition of Src kinases in BCR–ABL+ leukemic cells inhibits this activation, suggesting that Src inhibition may impact the leukemia stem cells [60].

Are p190 and p210 BCR–ABL different?

The presence of p190 in Ph+ ALL, and p210 in Ph+ ALL and lymphoid blast crisis CML (CML-LBC), suggests that both fusion proteins can transform normal lymphoblasts into malignant lymphoblasts. However, several lines of data indicate that p190 and p210 diseases may be subtly different. First, p190 and p210 differ in their *in vitro* kinase activity, with p190 exhibiting higher kinase activity than p210 [61,62]. Additionally, despite both proteins transforming murine IL-3-dependent cell lines from myeloid (32D cl3) and lymphoid (Ba/F3) lineage, p190 transformation of Ba/F3 resulted in a higher proliferation rate [61].

p190 and p210 Bcr–Abl also produce different effects in murine models. While p190 transgenic mice develop a rapidly progressive pre-B leukemia [22,23], p210 transgenic mice develop B, T, and myeloid diseases with more chronic features and experience a longer median survival [21]. In the murine transplant model, mice transplanted with bone marrow transduced with p190 or p210 Bcr–Abl and treated with 5-FU (which enriches the marrow for myeloid precursors) developed a myeloproliferative disease, arising from a pluripotential cell resembling CML, that transformed to acute leukemia similar to blast crisis [20,61]. However, when the transduced marrow was not enriched for myeloid progenitors, differences between diseases were displayed, with p210 generating a CML-like disease originating in a pluripotential cell in 50% of the animals, while p190 produced a B-cell leukemia arising from a lineage-committed progenitor with shorter latency in most of the animals and rapid death [61].

Studies of human Ph+ ALL are inconsistent in regards to the effect of p190 versus p210 Bcr–Abl and outcome. Several studies have shown no difference in prognosis at the time of diagnosis [5,9,63], while others have demonstrated a worse prognosis with p190 disease, especially in the context of detection in the setting of minimal residual disease (MRD) [64–66].

Lineage restriction of the Philadelphia chromosome

How is Ph+ ALL different from lymphoid blast crisis CML? Attempts to address this question initially focused on studies aiming to discover the nature of the cell in which each disease originates. As CML is a hematopoietic stem cell disease, the Ph should be found in myeloid and lymphoid cells in CML-LBC. On the other hand, if Ph+ ALL is lineage restricted, one should find the Ph only in lymphoid cells. However, original studies in patients did not yield such a clear-cut distinction and data showing lymphoid restriction or multilineage involvement in both p190 and p210 Ph+ ALL cases have been published [67–76], with some suggestion that myeloid involvement in Ph+ ALL had a relatively favorable prognosis [67,70,73].

Recent functional studies have shed some light on the issue. Three different studies conclude that the leukemia stem cell (LSC) in Ph+ ALL is a primitive cell lymphoid that is restricted, as it will not originate from myeloid or erythroid colonies, although the studies differ on the characterization of this LSC [77–79]. First, Cobaleda *et al.* described that only the $CD34^+$ $CD38^-$ fraction of patients with p190+ ALL was able to engraft in non-obese diabetic/severe combined immune-deficient (NOD/SCID) mice and reconstitute the marrow with a leukemia of an identical phenotype as the donor, without reconstituting myeloid colonies in culture [78]. Second, Hotfilder *et al.* [79] showed that the $CD34^+$ $CD19^-$ cells were the most undifferentiated leukemia progenitors in pediatric patients with Ph+ ALL, but they did not differentiate into myeloid colonies. Finally, Castor *et al.* [77] detected p210 in undifferentiated ($CD34^+$ $CD38^-$, and $CD34^+$ $CD38^-$ $CD19^-$) fractions as well as in myeloid and lymphoid fractions of the bone marrow of five patients with p210 Ph+ ALL, but they could not detect p190 in the $CD34^+$ $CD38^-$ $CD19^-$ or myeloid fractions of four patients with p190 Ph+ ALL. Surprisingly, despite the detection of p210 in a multipotent hematopoietic stem cell (HSC), only $CD19^+$ cells reconstituted NOD/SCID mice with leukemia, defining LSC in this disease also as a B-cell-committed precursor.

Treatment

The Ph has historically been the worst prognostic indicator in ALL, and complex chemotherapy regimens have not made the Ph relinquish this grim title. The Ph occurs in an age-dependent manner, as the incidence rises with age from <5% in pediatric patients [80,81] to around 40% or higher in patients >40 years [82]. The Ph is usually associated with additional negative prognosis factors such as a high white blood cell (WBC) count and blast count [5,83]. In the elderly population, the prognosis of any category of ALL is poor, and in this setting the Ph does not add an additional prognostic burden [84].

Conventional chemotherapy

The rates of CR in adults with Ph⁺ ALL with conventional chemotherapy range from 60% to 90% [5,6,63,82,83, 85–94]—somewhat inferior to CR rates achieved in patients with Ph-ALL. The gradual intensification of chemotherapy regimens over time has increased CR rates, but this has not translated into a higher overall survival (OS) [87,91,94] and, as a consequence, most adult patients with Ph⁺ ALL treated with chemotherapy alone will relapse. The long-term survival of patients with Ph⁺ ALL treated with chemotherapy alone ranges from 0% to 20% [6,9,63,83,87,91,95–97]. In older patients, CR rates are only around 50% [98], and long-term survival is <10% [99]. Once patients with Ph⁺ ALL relapse, long-term survival following salvage chemotherapy is quite rare, with a 5-year OS after relapse of only 3–6% [100–102].

Overall, pediatric ALL is the showcase for demonstrating the curative potential of intense chemotherapy, with disease-free survival (DFS) rates of >80%. However, pediatric patients with Ph⁺ ALL have a DFS and an OS of <50% [81,103–112], despite achieving CR rates of 80–100%. In this age group, initial WBC count, age [107], and response to a round of steroids pre-chemotherapy [104] enable the subclassification of patients according to prognosis. Patients <10 years of age with Ph⁺ ALL who present with a WBC count at diagnosis of <50,000/μL, have a 5-year DFS rate of 49% compared with 20% for those >10 years old and presenting with a WBC count >50,000/μL. Similarly, all patients with Ph⁺ ALL who have a good response to prednisone pulse prior to chemotherapy and who receive intrathecal methotrexate had a 4-year event-free survival (EFS) of 52%, compared with only a 30% CR rate and a 10% 4-year EFS in the poor prednisone responders group. The percentage of patients with Ph⁺ ALL who have a poor response to prednisone is over twofold higher than that of unselected patients with ALL [104,107].

Hematopoietic stem cell transplantation

Given the low frequency of Ph⁺ ALL, most clinical data regarding the efficacy of HSCT are derived from relatively small retrospective studies, and thus may be associated with inherent biases regarding patient selection and time from diagnosis to transplantation, for example. Despite these caveats, allogeneic HSCT from a matched-related donor is widely regarded as the treatment of choice for adults and children with Ph⁺ ALL in first CR (CR1) [113]. However, not all patients in remission will have access to this treatment because of lack of a donors, age, or comorbidities that limit eligibility for HSCT. Moreover, the aggressive nature of Ph⁺ ALL often results in a rapid relapse prior to transplant. Thus, it has been estimated that only ~30–50% of patients diagnosed with Ph⁺ ALL eventually undergo allogeneic transplant in CR1 [6,107,114–117]. Transplant results for the "pre-TKI" era are shown in Table 18.1.

The first substantial evidence that allogeneic HSCT improved survival in adult patients with Ph⁺ ALL was from International Bone Marrow Transplant Registry (IBMTR) data of 67 transplants from matched siblings, reporting a 31% DFS at 2 years, with similar outcomes in patients transplanted in first remission and after relapse [118]. Other reports have shown a worse outcome for patients transplanted in relapse [119–121]. Esperou *et al.* [122] reviewed the outcomes of 121 patients with Ph⁺ ALL who received an allogeneic transplant on three French prospective trials, and showed that the only independent factor associated with survival was disease status at transplant (CR1 vs. >CR1).

Recent prospective studies confirm the survival advantage for patients with an allogeneic donor in first remission. The intention-to-treat analysis of 103 adult patients with Ph⁺ ALL in the French Leucémies Aiguës Lymphoblastiques de l'Adulte (LALA)-94 study concluded that a matched HSCT from a related or unrelated donor in CR1 was the first treatment choice because an allogeneic donor was a prognostic factor for both survival and remission duration [6]. Similarly, the United Kingdom Acute Lymphoblastic Leukemia (UKALL) XI/Eastern Cooperative Oncology Group (ECOG) 2993 international study of 267 adult patients with Ph⁺ ALL demonstrated a 10% better 5-year OS for patients with a matched-related donor available compared with those without one ($P = 0.4$) [114]. Finally, in a retrospective review of pediatric patients, Arico *et al.* [107] described that those undergoing a matched-related HSCT in CR1 had a lower risk of death or adverse events (relative risk = 0.3), and of death from any cause (relative risk = 0.4) than patients treated with chemotherapy alone. Pediatric patients with Ph⁺ ALL in CR2/3 at the time of transplant achieved a long-term survival of 17%, while those transplanted in relapse had only a 5% survival at 2 years [129].

Compared with matched-related HSCT, unrelated transplants are generally associated with a greater risk of treatment-related mortality, principally from graft-versus-host disease (GVHD), but lower relapse rates attributed to the graft-versus-leukemia (GVL) effect. These competing risks make matched-unrelated donor transplants similar in outcome to matched-related transplants [6,130]. In the circumstances where patients have excessive transplant-related mortality, or in advanced disease where the GVL effect cannot intercede, the benefits of an unrelated transplant are not so clear [107,129].

Given the widening pool of unrelated donors, the role of autologous transplantation in ALL is shrinking. Relapse

Table 18.1 Outcome with allogeneic stem cell transplant for patients with Philadelphia chromosome-positive acute lymphoblastic leukemia pre-tyrosine kinase inhibitors.

Reference	Year	N	Age (range) (years)	Status (*n*)	Donor (*n*)	TRM (years)	Probability of relapse (years)	OS % (years)	DFS % (years)
Barrett [118]	1992	67	28 (5–49)	CR1 (33)	MRD	42 (2)	34 (2)	NA	38 (2)
				>CR1 (22)	MRD	40 (2)	32 (2)	NA	41 (2)
				PIF (12)	MRD	42 (2)	57 (2)	NA	25 (2)
Chao [119]	1995	38	NA	CR1 (17) >CR1 (21)	MRD MRD	NA NA	NA NA	NA NA	46 (2) 28 (2)
Dunlop [125]	1996	11	27 (3–37)	CR1 (5)/>CR1 (6)	MRD	NA	63 (3)		22 (3)
Sierra [123]	1997	18	25 (2–51)	CR1 (7)/>CR1 (11)	MUD	NA	22[e]	NA	49 (2)
Kroger [120]	1998	19	29 (2–60)	CR1 (15)/>CR1 (4)	MRD (13)/ MUD (6)	NA	NA	38 (5) [1]	34 (5)[a]
Marks (p) [124]	1998	15	8 (3–19)	CR1 (9)/>CR1 (6)	MUD[g]	NA	40	44 (2)	37 (2)
Snyder [126]	1999	23	30 (6–44)	CR1 (23)	MRD	30[e]	12% (3)	65 (3)	65 (3)
Arico (p) [107]	2000	38	8 (0–20)	CR1 (38)	MRD	8	24	72 (5)	65 (5)
Dombret[c] [6]	2002	60	NA	CR1	MRD (46)/ MUD (14)	24[e] (2)	50 (3)	37 (3)	NA
Lee [121]	2003	23	36 (15–44)	CR1 (14)/CR2 (9)	MRD	28[e]	40 (2)		43.5 (2)
Esperou [122]	2003	121	35 (1–53)	CR1 (76)	MRD (59)/ MUD (15)/ Oher (2)	NA	37 (2)	50 (2)	NA
				>CR1 (45)	MRD (29)/ MUD (16)	NA	62 (2)	17 (2)	NA
Goldstone [114]	2003	87	<50	CR1 (80)/>CR1 (7)	MRD (57) MUD (30)	35[d] 57[d]	37 (5) 25 (5)	42 (5) 36 (5)	41 (5) 32 (5)
Sharathkumar (p) [116]	2004	11	9 (2–16)	CR1	MRD (4) MUD (7)	NA NA	NA NA	NA NA	75 (4)[f] 36 (4)
Thomas[b] [115]	2004	75	NR	CR1	MRD (65)/ MUD (10)	22 (5)	58 (5)	36 (3)	34 (3)
Satwani (p) [127]	2007	9	12 (2–13)	CR1	MRD	NA	NA	NA	66.7 (5)
Chim [128]	2007	25	NR	CR1 (18)/>CR 1 (7)	MRD (19)/ MUD (6)	19.5 (15)	55 (15)	41 (15)	33 (15)

CR, complete remission; DFS, disease-free survival; MRD, matched-related donor; MUD, matched-unrelated donor; N, number of patients transplanted; OS, overall survival; (p), pediatric study; PIF, primary induction failure; Ref., reference number; TRM, transplant related mortality; Y, years.

[a]For patients in first complete remission.

[b]Intention to treat analysis: outcome variables reported for all patients eligible for allogeneic hematopoietic stem-cell transplant (HSCT) in complete remission. Actual number of patients who underwent HSCT in first complete remission: 43 (MRD) and 8 (MUD).

[c]Update on LALA-94 reported by Dombret.

[d]Rate of death in remission.

[e]Death other than for leukemia.

[f]Estimated from the published curves.

[g]Includes four patients mismatched at one or two HLA loci. All 15 patients had a T-cell depleted HSCT.

rates following autologous transplant are similar to chemotherapy [107,115,120,125]. Although the re-infusion of leukemia cells during autologous transplant may account for some proportion of the relapse risk, more likely is that relapse mainly occurs owing to the lack of a GVL effect. The relapse-free survival advantage in recipients of an allogeneic transplant who develop acute [122] or chronic [66,121] GVHD and the description of patients converting to PCR⁻ after developing GVHD [121] are clues to the immunologic effect achieved by an allogeneic graft. Cornelissen [129] suggested that Ph^+ ALL was particularly sensitive to the GVL effect as the presence of this translocation was an independent favorable prognosis factor for DFS and relapse in a study of patients with high-risk ALL undergoing unrelated HSCT.

The molecular detection of the Bcr–Abl fusion mRNA by PCR has been shown to be an effective method for monitoring disease [117,121]. Bcr–Abl levels before transplantation are prognostic in adult and pediatric patients undergoing HSCT, with patients who are in remission morphologically and molecularly enjoying the best outcome, whereas patients who are molecularly positive for Bcr–Abl, although still in conventional remission, suffer a relatively higher relapse rate [6,131,132]. Patients in whom Bcr–Abl is detected after transplant have an approximately fivefold relative risk of relapse compared with patients without Bcr–Abl. The risk is higher for those patients expressing the p190 Bcr–Abl variant (~10-fold relative risk of relapse), whereas little risk is conveyed by the presence of the p210 variant post transplant [64,66].

Despite the significant progress made, there is not enough evidence regarding the use of alternative sources of stem cells [133] (haploidentical donors [134] or umbilical cord blood stem cells [135,136]), or non-myeloablative conditioning [137,138] in Ph^+ ALL to recommend the use of these approaches outside clinical trials.

Tyrosine kinase inhibitors

Imatinib mesylate, 2-phenylamino pirimidine, binds the Abl–ATP site in a competitive manner, stabilizing Abl in its inactive conformation and inhibiting its tyrosine kinase activity. Initial clinical trials with imatinib as monotherapy were conducted in patients with relapsed or refractory Ph^+ ALL [139–142]. Responses were seen in 60–70% of patients, with 20% achieving CR, and 10% achieving complete cytogenetic responses (CCyR). Unfortunately, these responses were short-lived and patients relapsed within a few weeks, although in some cases it allowed long enough time to proceed to HSCT [142].

The low toxicity profile of imatinib, together with published data suggesting synergy with chemotherapy drugs *in vitro* [143–145], encouraged its addition to conventional chemotherapy ALL regimens. A summary of published studies incorporating imatinib at different stages of Ph^+ ALL treatment is shown in Table 18.2. The addition of imatinib to induction and consolidation chemotherapy regimens for Ph^+ ALL resulted in CR rates of ~90% or higher in newly diagnosed patients [146–155,158,159]. Wassmann *et al.* [153] compared two sequential patient cohorts; the first received imatinib concomitant with induction chemotherapy, and the second received alternate consolidation chemotherapy–imatinib cycles after chemotherapy induction. There were no statistically significant differences in OS and DFS between the two cohorts, though a higher rate of Bcr–Abl negativity was achieved in the cohort receiving imatinib and chemotherapy concurrently.

Complete molecular responses are reported in 20–70% of the studies. A high percentage (≥65%) of patients in CR1 maintained remission long enough to undergo HSCT, compared with historic rates for regimens without imatinib (~20–50%) [6]. So far, studies have suggested that treatment with imatinib prior to HSCT does not affect transplant outcomes [142,148,149,153].

Imatinib has improved the outcome of elderly patients with Ph^+ ALL, a subpopulation with a historically very poor prognosis and who are not generally candidates for HSCT. Induction with imatinib alone resulted in higher CR rates than chemotherapy induction, with no mortality in a randomized study conducted by the GMALL group [150]. However, there were no differences in OS at 24 months between the two groups. A second study showed imatinib and steroid induction therapy, with no additional chemotherapy, achieved a similar OS to the imatinib arm in the German Multicenter Acute Lymphoblastic Leukemia (GMALL) article [156]. A third study in older patients with Ph^+ ALL incorporated imatinib in consolidation and maintenance chemotherapy regimens after induction chemotherapy, resulting in significantly higher DFS and OS than historic cohorts [147]. On the opposite side of the age continuum, ongoing pediatric studies report that the incorporation of imatinib to chemotherapy and administered post HSCT improves early EFS compared with historic cohorts [160].

The incidence of central nervous system (CNS) involvement in Ph^+ ALL is around 17% [161]. In patients treated with imatinib as a single agent, CNS relapses have been described with relative frequency [162,163], and imatinib cerebrospinal fluid levels have been measured to only ~1.5% of those in serum [162,163]. These data reflects the limited distribution of imatinib into the CNS as a consequence of imatinib being a substrate for P-glycoprotein [164,165], which results in CNS subtherapeutic levels of imatinib. Consequently, CNS prophylactic chemotherapy remains a critical aspect of the treatment of Ph^+ ALL.

Clinical trials have also addressed the use of imatinib after HSCT to treat MRD, as the detection of Bcr–Abl after HSCT predicts the probability of relapse [64]. Imatinib therapy after the detection of MRD post HSCT reverts approximately 50% of these patients to PCR negativity

Table 18.2 Outcome with imatinib ± chemotherapy and hematopoietic stem-cell transplant for patients with Philadelphia chromosome-positive acute lymphoblastic leukemia.

Study	Year	Tmt. phase with imatinib	Cht	N	Age (range) (years)	CR (%)	Mol CR (%)	% patients who undergo SCT CR1 (allo)	OS (%) (months)	DFS (%) (months)
Champagne (COG)[b] [139]	2004	Salvage	N	10	NR (3–20)	70	NA	NA	50 (15)	NA
Wassmann [157]	2004	Salvage	N	68	48 (17–76)	30	15	NA	22.6 (18)	22.8 (6)
Lee [149]	2005	Consolidation and salvage	Y	29	36 (18–55)	96	24	86 (100)	78 (36)	78 (36)
Lee [148]	2005	Induction, consolidation, and maintenance	Y	20	37 (15–67)	95	71 (at the time of HSCT)	75	50 (30)	50 (27)
Delannoy (GRAALL AFR09) [147]	2006	Consolidation/ salvage and maintenance	Y	30	65.8 (58–78)	90 (after salvage therapy)		NA	66 (12)	58 (12)
Rea (GRAALL) [151]	2006	Salvage	Y	31 (includes 13 patients with CML LBC)	45 (10–70)	90	8	NA	50 (13.5)	50 (9.5)
Wassmann [153]	2006	Consolidation and maintenance	Y	47	46 (21–65)	NA[a]	19 (prior to C1)*	85 (90)	36 (24)	52 (24)
		Induction, consolidation, and maintenance	Y	45	41 (19–63)	96	52 (prior to C1)*	80 (97)	43 (24)	61 (24)
Yanada (JALGS ALL202) [155]	2006	Induction, consolidation, and maintenance	Y	80	48 (15–63)	96	71.3	55 (100)	58 (24)	50.5 (24)
de Labarthe (GRAAPH-2003) [146]	2007	Induction, consolidation, and maintenance	Y	45	45 (16–59)	96	38 (after consolidation and DIV for poor early responders)	65 (79)	65 (18)	51 (18)
Thomas [152]	2007	Induction and consolidation	Y	54	51 (17–84)	93	52	30 (100)	55 (36)	66 (36)
Ottmann [150]	2007	Induction and consolidation	Y[c]	28	66 (54–79)	96**	37	NA	57 (24)	29.5 (18)
		Consolidation	Y	27	68 (58–78)	50**	50	NA	41 (24)	34.6 (18)
Vignetti [156]	2007	Induction	N[d]	30	69 (61–83)	100	4	NA	74 (12)	48 (12)

Cht, chemotherapy; CR, complete remission; CRI, first complete remission; DIV, vincristine and dexamethasone regime; HSCT, hematopoietic stem-cell transplant; Mol CR, molecular complete remission; N, number of patients transplanted; OS, oversall survival; Tmt, treatment.

*$P = 0.01$.

**$P = 0.0001$.

[a]Patients in CR when entering the study.

[b]Phase 1 study in pediatric patients.

[c]This arm included imatinib monotheray as induction therapy.

[d]Induction therapy with Imatinib plus steroids.

within 1.5 months, and they maintain this status while on imatinib. Conversely, patients who fail to achieve PCR negativity shortly after initiating imatinib have a 90% relapse rate at 3 months. The response to imatinib pre-transplant predicts the molecular response to imatinib post-MRD detection after transplant [166]. Imatinib has also been administered prophylactically in patients with Ph^+ ALL and advanced-phase CML undergoing HSCT. Patients were able to start imatinib at a median of 27 days after transplant without serious adverse effects, and the results suggested a therapeutic effect in regards to molecular response compared with historical controls [167].

Resistance to imatinib

Resistance to imatinib can be primary (no response or poor initial response) or secondary (manifesting after an initial response). Both are observed in a substantial fraction of patients with Ph^+ ALL. Multiple mechanisms of resistance to imatinib have been described: Bcr–Abl kinase-domain point mutations [168], overexpression of Bcr–Abl mRNA, genomic amplification of Bcr–Abl [168], increased imatinib efflux through P-glycoprotein mechanisms, and activation of Bcr–Abl-independent pathways such as Src kinases [169].

Secondary resistance is generally related to the emergence of a leukemic clone bearing a point mutation in the Abl kinase domain. These mutations may affect the transformation potency of Bcr–Abl, and confer a proliferation advantage even in the absence of imatinib [170] in addition to interfering with the binding of imatinib to the Abl ATP-binding site. While mutations have been described in different sites in the Abl molecule, those affecting the P-loop region (destabilizing the inactive conformation of Abl to which imatinib binds) and the *T315I* (which affects the hydrogen bond between Abl and imatinib) are significant, conferring the worst prognosis. Mutations in Ph^+ ALL and lymphoid blast crisis are detected in up to 80% of patients with imatinib resistance [95,171]. Most of these mutations are overcome, albeit briefly, by newly developed TKI, with the exception of the *T315I* that is detected in ~10% of patients with imatinib resitance [95].

The median time from initiating imatinib to developing resistance is only approximately 3 months, which suggests that clones bearing the mutation must be present at the initiation of therapy, and thereafter selected by the use of imatinib [172]. In an analysis of 48 patients >55 years of age with Ph^+ ALL [95], 40% harbored mutations in the Abl KD at the onset of imatinib therapy. That same mutation was found at relapse in 90% of the cases, suggesting outgrowth of the mutated clone under the selective pressure of imatinib. However, the initial clinical and molecular response to imatinib was not affected by the Abl mutation status, despite the mutations conferring imatinib resistance *in vitro*. Still, all but two patients harboring mutations at diagnosis eventually relapsed in contrast to 50% of patients with unmutated Abl, and patients with a *T315I* mutation had a shorter time to progression.

Second-generation Abl inhibitors

Dasatinib is an orally available TKI now licensed for resistant or advanced-phase CML. Like imatinib, it inhibits a broad spectrum of tyrosine kinases, including Abl and the Src family of kinases. Unlike imatinib, it can bind Abl in its active and inactive conformations [173], blocking Abl with a 300-fold higher potency than imatinib [174]; it is not a substrate for drug-efflux pumps (P-glycoprotein); and it can cross the blood–brain barrier [175]. Shah *et al.* [173] showed that dasatinib is active against wild-type Abl and against most of the mutant forms that confer resistance to imatinib, with the exception of the *T315I* mutation. The resistance displayed by *T315I* has been confirmed in clinical studies [176,177]. Phase I [176] and II [177] clinical studies have been conducted in patients with imatinib-intolerant or imatinib-resistant Ph^+ ALL. The phase II study (with 36 cases of Ph^+ ALL) reported a 42% major hematologic response (MHR), 67% of whom showed a sustained response with an 8-month follow-up, and 58% of whom displayed major cytogenetic responses (MCyR). Except for *T315I* mutations, responses are seen similarly between cases with and without Abl mutations. Unfortunately, treatment with dasatinib has been shown to select for new *BCR–ABL* mutations that inhibit dasatinib activity [178–181].

Nilotinib is a designed offspring of imatinib, and is a relatively selective inhibitor of Abl. Nilotinib has a greater potency than imatinib against wild-type *BCR–ABL* and most of its mutants except for the *T315I* mutation [174]. The phase I dose-escalation study included 13 patients with Ph^+ ALL who were resistant to imatinib. One of 10 patients enrolled with relapsed ALL had a partial hematologic response, and one of three patients who enrolled with persistent molecular disease after imatinib achieved a complete molecular remission [182]. The phase II clinical trial reported a 24% CR rate and 68% disease progression in a series of 41 patients [183]. Nevertheless, the results of these trials seem poor, but the fact that they are obtained with nilotinib monotherapy in patients with resistant disease encourages future trials in combination with chemotherapy.

A few other Abl inhibitors have not yet reached clinical trials. The first one is the dual Abl-Lyn/Lck inhibitor INNO-406 (NS-187). It inhibits Bcr–Abl with a higher potency and specificity than imatinib, and selectively inhibits the phosphorylation of Src kinases Lyn and Lck [184]. This profile may prove clinically relevant, as Lyn has been associated with imatinib resistance [169,184,185]. INNO-406 is also effective in inhibiting most of the mutated forms of Abl tested, but is still ineffective against *T315I* mutation in *in vitro* and *in vivo* experiments [186,187]. This compound, like imatinib, is a substrate for

P-glycoprotein [188]. The second compound is SKI-606, yet another potent Abl-Src inhibitor that is effective in inhibiting CML cell proliferation and inducing cell death [189]. Unlike imatinib, it preserves PDGF and Kit kinases [190], which may give it some advantage regarding toxicities. It is active against a number of Abl point mutations, but shows only partial activity against E255K, and no activity against *T315I* [190]. Finally, ON012380 has the peculiarity of inhibiting Bcr–Abl by binding in a different site to the ATP-binding pocket. It induces cell death in Ph$^+$ CML cells, including those with the *T315I*-resistant isoform in mouse models, and it acts synergistically with imatinib [191].

Other targeted therapies

Because different kinases share similar structures for the ATP-binding pocket, a variety of kinase inhibitors are being screened to see whether they include Abl inhibition as one of their "off" targets. As an example, MK-0457 (VX-680) was initially developed as an aurora kinase inhibitor [192] but it binds with a high affinity to both Abl wild type and the *T315I* mutant, potently inhibiting their kinase activity [193,194], and it is active in patients with *BCR–ABL T315I* leukemias [195]. In a different category is FTY720, as it is an immunomodulator currently in phase III trials in solid-organ transplant and multiple sclerosis. It induces the activation of PP2A (a phosphatase with reduced activity in CML) that results in apoptosis in CML and Ph$^+$ ALL cell lines, regardless of their sensitivity to TKIs, at a dose that does not affect normal hematopoietic progenitors [196].

Other promising therapies in the pipeline are histone deacetylase inhibitors that induce apoptosis of *BCR–ABL*$^+$ cells. These inhibitors have a synergistic effect with TKIs, and may overcome resistant *BCR–ABL* mutations including *T315I* [197–200]. MEK1/2 inhibitors also show synergy with dasatinib, although they do not overcome the resistance of *T315I* mutations [201,202].

Conclusion

Despite the advent of combination chemotherapy and TKIs, most patients with Ph$^+$ ALL will succumb to the disease. Allogeneic transplantation is still the treatment of choice, preferably in first remission. Molecular monitoring may be helpful in patients before and after transplantation, as outcomes are better for those patients transplanted in molecular remission, and post-transplant treatment or intervention for molecular relapse may be efficacious. Hopefully, the advances in drug development, new treatment design (*in vitro* data suggest that combination therapy with multiple kinase inhibitors may be able to reduce the frequency of primary resistance [203]), monitoring, and low-intensity transplantation will afford a brighter future for the care of patients with Ph$^+$ ALL.

References

1 Hermans A, Heisterkamp N, von Linden M, *et al*. Unique fusion of *BCR* and *C-ABL* genes in Philadelphia chromosome positive acute lymphoblastic leukemia. *Cell* 1987;51:33–40.

2 Hooberman AL, Carrino JJ, Leibowitz D, *et al*. Unexpected heterogeneity of Bcr–Abl fusion mRNA detected by polymerase chain reaction in Philadelphia chromosome-positive acute lymphoblastic leukemia. *Proc Natl Acad Sci U S A* 1989;86: 4259–63.

3 Kurzrock R, Shtalrid M, Gutterman JU, *et al*. Molecular analysis of chromosome 22 breakpoints in adult Philadelphia-positive acute lymphoblastic leukemia. *Br J Haematol* 1987;67: 55–9.

4 Rubin CM, Carrino JJ, Dickler MN, Leibowitz D, Smith SD, Westbrook CA. Heterogeneity of genomic fusion of *BCR* and *ABL* in Philadelphia chromosome-positive acute lymphoblastic leukemia. *Proc Natl Acad Sci U S A* 1988;85:2795–9.

5 Gleissner B, Gokbuget N, Bartram CR, *et al*. Leading prognostic relevance of the Bcr–Abl translocation in adult acute B-lineage lymphoblastic leukemia: a prospective study of the German Multicenter Trial Group and confirmed polymerase chain reaction analysis. *Blood* 2002;99:1536–43.

6 Dombret H, Gabert J, Boiron JM, *et al*. Outcome of treatment in adults with Philadelphia chromosome-positive acute lymphoblastic leukemia–results of the prospective multicenter LALA-94 trial. *Blood* 2002;100:2357–66.

7 van Rhee F, Hochhaus A, Lin F, Melo JV, Goldman JM, Cross NC. p190 Bcr–Abl mRNA is expressed at low levels in p210-positive chronic myeloid and acute lymphoblastic leukemias. *Blood* 1996;87:5213–17.

8 Kantarjian H, Talpaz M, Estey E, Ku S, Kurzrock R. What is the contribution of molecular studies to the diagnosis of *BCR–ABL*-positive disease in adult acute leukemia? *Am J Med* 1994;96:133–8.

9 Moorman AV, Harrison CJ, Buck GA, *et al*. Karyotype is an independent prognostic factor in adult acute lymphoblastic leukemia (ALL): analysis of cytogenetic data from patients treated on the Medical Research Council (MRC) UKALLXII/ Eastern Cooperative Oncology Group (ECOG) 2993 trial. *Blood* 2007;109:3189–97.

10 Nashed AL, Rao KW, Gulley ML. Clinical applications of Bcr–Abl molecular testing in acute leukemia. *J Mol Diagn* 2003;5:63–72.

11 Gehly GB, Bryant EM, Lee AM, Kidd PG, Thomas ED. Chimeric Bcr–Abl messenger RNA as a marker for minimal residual disease in patients transplanted for Philadelphia chromosome-positive acute lymphoblastic leukemia. *Blood* 1991;78:458–65.

12 Maurer J, Kinzel H, Nentwig T, Thiel E. Molecular diagnosis of the Philadelphia chromosome in chronic myelogenous and acute lymphoblastic leukemias by PCR. *Dis Markers* 1990;8: 211–18.

13 Gleissner B, Rieder H, Thiel E, *et al*. Prospective Bcr–Abl analysis by polymerase chain reaction (RT-PCR) in adult acute B-lineage lymphoblastic leukemia: reliability of RT-nested-

PCR and comparison to cytogenetic data. *Leukemia* 2001;15: 1834–40.

14 Taagepera S, McDonald D, Loeb JE, *et al*. Nuclear-cytoplasmic shuttling of C-ABL tyrosine kinase. *Proc Natl Acad Sci U S A* 1998;95:7457–62.

15 McWhirter JR, Galasso DL, Wang JY. A coiled-coil oligomerization domain of Bcr is essential for the transforming function of Bcr–Abl oncoproteins. *Mol Cell Biol* 1993;13:7587–95.

16 McWhirter JR, Wang JY. Activation of tyrosinase kinase and microfilament-binding functions of C-Abl by Bcr sequences in Bcr–Abl fusion proteins. *Mol Cell Biol* 1991;11:1553–65.

17 McWhirter JR, Wang JY. An actin-binding function contributes to transformation by the Bcr–Abl oncoprotein of Philadelphia chromosome-positive human leukemias. *Embo J* 1993;12: 1533–46.

18 Vigneri P, Wang JY. Induction of apoptosis in chronic myelogenous leukemia cells through nuclear entrapment of Bcr–Abl tyrosine kinase. *Nat Med* 2001;7:228–34.

19 Goss VL, Lee KA, Moritz A, *et al*. A common phosphotyrosine signature for the Bcr–Abl kinase. *Blood* 2006;107:4888–97.

20 Pear WS, Miller JP, Xu L, *et al*. Efficient and rapid induction of a chronic myelogenous leukemia-like myeloproliferative disease in mice receiving P210 Bcr–Abl-transduced bone marrow. *Blood* 1998;92:3780–92.

21 Voncken JW, Kaartinen V, Pattengale PK, Germeraad WT, Groffen J, Heisterkamp N. BCR/ABL P210 and P190 cause distinct leukemia in transgenic mice. *Blood* 1995;86:4603–11.

22 Heisterkamp N, Jenster G, ten Hoeve J, Zovich D, Pattengale PK, Groffen J. Acute leukemia in bcr/abl transgenic mice. *Nature* 1990;344:251–3.

23 Voncken JW, Morris C, Pattengale P, *et al*. Clonal development and karyotype evolution during leukemogenesis of *BCR–ABL* transgenic mice. *Blood* 1992;79:1029–36.

24 Huettner CS, Zhang P, Van Etten RA, Tenen DG. Reversibility of acute B-cell leukemia induced by *BCR–ABL1*. *Nat Genet* 2000;24:57–60.

25 Ilaria RL, Jr., Van Etten RA. P210 and P190 (*BCR–ABL*) induce the tyrosine phosphorylation and DNA binding activity of multiple specific STAT family members. *J Biol Chem* 1996; 271:31704–10.

26 Horita M, Andreu EJ, Benito A, *et al*. Blockade of the Bcr–Abl kinase activity induces apoptosis of chronic myelogenous leukemia cells by suppressing signal transducer and activator of transcription 5-dependent expression of Bcl-xL. *J Exp Med* 2000;191:977–84.

27 Hoelbl A, Kovacic B, Kerenyi MA, *et al*. Clarifying the role of Stat5 in lymphoid development and Abelson-induced transformation. *Blood* 2006;107:4898–906.

28 Sexl V, Piekorz R, Moriggl R, *et al*. Stat5a/b contribute to interleukin 7-induced B-cell precursor expansion, but *ABL*- and *BCR–ABL*-induced transformation are independent of stat5. *Blood* 2000;96:2277–83.

29 Harb JG, Chyla BI, Huettner CS. Loss of Bcl-x in Ph+ B-ALL increases cellular proliferation and does not inhibit leukemogenesis. *Blood* 2008;111:3760–9.

30 Xie S, Lin H, Sun T, Arlinghaus RB. Jak2 is involved in c-Myc induction by *BCR–ABL*. *Oncogene* 2002;21:7137–46.

31 Sawyers CL, Callahan W, Witte ON. Dominant negative MYC blocks transformation by *ABL* oncogenes. *Cell* 1992;70: 901–10.

32 Sawyers CL, McLaughlin J, Witte ON. Genetic requirement for Ras in the transformation of fibroblasts and hematopoietic cells by the *BCR–ABL* oncogene. *J Exp Med* 1995;181:307–13.

33 Skorski T, Bellacosa A, Nieborowska-Skorska M, *et al*. Transformation of hematopoietic cells by *BCR–ABL* requires activation of a PI-3k/Akt-dependent pathway. *Embo J* 1997; 16:6151–61.

34 Skorski T, Kanakaraj P, Nieborowska-Skorska M, *et al*. Phosphatidylinositol-3 kinase activity is regulated by Bcr–Abl and is required for the growth of Philadelphia chromosome-positive cells. *Blood* 1995;86:726–36.

35 Puil L, Liu J, Gish G, *et al*. Bcr–Abl oncoproteins bind directly to activators of the Ras signaling pathway. *Embo J* 1994; 13:764–73.

36 Sattler M, Mohi MG, Pride YB, *et al*. Critical role for Gab2 in transformation by *BCR–ABL*. *Cancer Cell* 2002;1:479–92.

37 Million RP, Van Etten RA. The Grb2 binding site is required for the induction of chronic myeloid leukemia-like disease in mice by the Bcr–Abl tyrosine kinase. *Blood* 2000;96:664–70.

38 Fukumoto S, Hsieh CM, Maemura K, *et al*. Akt participation in the Wnt signaling pathway through Dishevelled. *J Biol Chem* 2001;276:17479–83.

39 Neshat MS, Raitano AB, Wang HG, Reed JC, Sawyers CL. The survival function of the *BCR–ABL* oncogene is mediated by Bad-dependent and -independent pathways: roles for phosphatidylinositol 3-kinase and Raf. *Mol Cell Biol* 2000;20: 1179–86.

40 Reuther JY, Reuther GW, Cortez D, Pendergast AM, Baldwin AS, Jr. A requirement for NF-kappaB activation in *BCR–ABL*-mediated transformation. *Genes Dev* 1998;12:968–81.

41 Brain JM, Goodyer N, Laneuville P. Measurement of genomic instability in preleukemic P190 *BCR–ABL* transgenic mice using inter-simple sequence repeat polymerase chain reaction. *Cancer Res* 2003;63:4895–8.

42 Canitrot Y, Lautier D, Laurent G, *et al*. Mutator phenotype of *BCR–ABL* transfected Ba/F3 cell lines and its association with enhanced expression of DNA polymerase beta. *Oncogene* 1999; 18:2676–80.

43 Deutsch E, Dugray A, AbdulKarim B, *et al*. Bcr–Abl down-regulates the DNA repair protein DNA-PKcs. *Blood* 2001; 97:2084–90.

44 Slupianek A, Schmutte C, Tombline G, *et al*. Bcr–Abl regulates mammalian RecA homologs, resulting in drug resistance. *Mol Cell* 2001;8:795–806.

45 Deutsch E, Jarrousse S, Buet D, *et al*. Down-regulation of BRCA1 in *BCR–ABL*-expressing hematopoietic cells. *Blood* 2003;101:4583–8.

46 Klein F, Feldhahn N, Herzog S, *et al*. *BCR–ABL1* induces aberrant splicing of IKAROS and lineage infidelity in pre-B lymphoblastic leukemia cells. *Oncogene* 2006;25:1118–24.

47 Klein F, Feldhahn N, Harder L, *et al*. The Bcr–Abl1 kinase bypasses selection for the expression of a pre-B cell receptor in pre-B acute lymphoblastic leukemia cells. *J Exp Med* 2004; 199:673–85.

48 Jumaa H, Bossaller L, Portugal K, *et al*. Deficiency of the adaptor SLP-65 in pre-B-cell acute lymphoblastic leukemia. *Nature* 2003;423:452–6.

49 Feldhahn N, Rio P, Soh BN, *et al*. Deficiency of Bruton's tyrosine kinase in B cell precursor leukemia cells. *Proc Natl Acad Sci U S A* 2005;102:13266–71.

50 Mullighan CG, Miller CB, Radtke I, *et al*. *BCR–ABL1* lymphoblastic leukemia is characterized by the deletion of Ikaros. *Nature* 2008;453:110–14.
51 Jumaa H, Mitterer M, Reth M, Nielsen PJ. The absence of SLP65 and Btk blocks B cell development at the pre-B cell receptor-positive stage. *Eur J Immunol* 2001;31:2164–9.
52 Feldhahn N, Klein F, Mooster JL, *et al*. Mimicry of a constitutively active pre-B cell receptor in acute lymphoblastic leukemia cells. *J Exp Med* 2005;201:1837–52.
53 Iacobucci I, Lonetti A, Messa F, *et al*. Expression of spliced oncogenic Ikaros isoforms in Philadelphia-positive acute lymphoblastic leukemia patients treated with tyrosine kinase inhibitors: implications for a new mechanism of resistance. *Blood* 2008;112:3847–55.
54 Heerema NA, Harbott J, Galimberti S, *et al*. Secondary cytogenetic aberrations in childhood Philadelphia chromosome positive acute lymphoblastic leukemia are nonrandom and may be associated with outcome. *Leukemia* 2004;18:693–702.
55 Primo D, Tabernero MD, Perez JJ, *et al*. Genetic heterogeneity of *BCR–ABL+* adult B-cell precursor acute lymphoblastic leukemia: impact on the clinical, biological and immunophenotypical disease characteristics. *Leukemia* 2005;19:713–20.
56 Williams RT, Roussel MF, Sherr CJ. *Arf* gene loss enhances oncogenicity and limits imatinib response in mouse models of *BCR–ABL*-induced acute lymphoblastic leukemia. *Proc Natl Acad Sci U S A* 2006;103:6688–93.
57 Hu Y, Liu Y, Pelletier S, *et al*. Requirement of Src kinases Lyn, Hck and Fgr for *BCR–ABL1*-induced B-lymphoblastic leukemia but not chronic myeloid leukemia. *Nat Genet* 2004;36: 453–61.
58 Hu Y, Swerdlow S, Duffy TM, Weinmann R, Lee FY, Li S. Targeting multiple kinase pathways in leukemic progenitors and stem cells is essential for improved treatment of Ph+ leukemia in mice. *Proc Natl Acad Sci U S A* 2006;103:16870–5.
59 Ptasznik A, Nakata Y, Kalota A, Emerson SG, Gewirtz AM. Short interfering RNA (siRNA) targeting the Lyn kinase induces apoptosis in primary, and drug-resistant, *BCR–ABL1(+)* leukemia cells. *Nat Med* 2004;10:1187–9.
60 Li S, Li D. Stem cell and kinase activity-independent pathway in resistance of leukemia to Bcr–Abl kinase inhibitors. *J Cell Mol Med* 2007;11:1251–62.
61 Li S, Ilaria RL, Jr., Million RP, Daley GQ, Van Etten RA. The P190, P210, and P230 forms of the *BCR–ABL* oncogene induce a similar chronic myeloid leukemia-like syndrome in mice but have different lymphoid leukemogenic activity. *J Exp Med* 1999;189:1399–412.
62 Lugo TG, Pendergast AM, Muller AJ, Witte ON. Tyrosine kinase activity and transformation potency of *BCR–ABL* oncogene products. *Science* 1990;247:1079–82.
63 Secker-Walker LM, Craig JM, Hawkins JM, Hoffbrand AV. Philadelphia positive acute lymphoblastic leukemia in adults:age distribution, BCR breakpoint and prognostic significance. *Leukemia* 1991;5:196–9.
64 Radich J, Gehly G, Lee A, *et al*. Detection of Bcr–Abl transcripts in Philadelphia chromosome-positive acute lymphoblastic leukemia after marrow transplantation. *Blood* 1997;89:2602–9.
65 Cimino G, Pane F, Elia L, *et al*. The role of Bcr–Abl isoforms in the presentation and outcome of patients with Philadelphia-positive acute lymphoblastic leukemia: a seven-year update of the GIMEMA 0496 trial. *Haematologica* 2006;91:377–80.
66 Stirewalt DL, Guthrie KA, Beppu L, *et al*. Predictors of relapse and overall survival in Philadelphia chromosome-positive acute lymphoblastic leukemia after transplantation. *Biol Blood Marrow Transplant* 2003;9:206–12.
67 Anastasi J, Feng J, Dickstein JI, *et al*. Lineage involvement by *BCR–ABL* in Ph+ lymphoblastic leukemias: chronic myelogenous leukemia presenting in lymphoid blast vs Ph+ acute lymphoblastic leukemia. *Leukemia* 1996;10:795–802.
68 Craig JM, Hawkins JM, Yamada T, Ganeshaguru K, Mehta AB, Secker-Walker LM. First intron and M-bcr breakpoints are restricted to the lymphoid lineage in Philadelphia positive acute lymphoblastic leukemia. *Leukemia* 1990;4:678–81.
69 Estrov Z, Talpaz M, Kantarjian HM, Zipf TF, McClain KL, Kurzrock R. Heterogeneity in lineage derivation of Philadelphia-positive acute lymphoblastic leukemia expressing p190 *BCR–ABL* or p210 *BCR–ABL*: determination by analysis of individual colonies with the polymerase chain reaction. *Cancer Res* 1993;53:3289–93.
70 Haferlach T, Winkemann M, Ramm-Petersen L, *et al*. New insights into the biology of Philadelphia-chromosome-positive acute lymphoblastic leukemia using a combination of May-Grunwald-Giemsa staining and fluorescence in situ hybridization techniques at the single cell level. *Br J Haematol* 1997; 99:452–9.
71 Schenk TM, Keyhani A, Bottcher S, *et al*. Multilineage involvement of Philadelphia chromosome positive acute lymphoblastic leukemia. *Leukemia* 1998;12:666–74.
72 Secker-Walker LM, Cooke HM, Browett PJ, *et al*. Variable Philadelphia breakpoints and potential lineage restriction of bcr rearrangement in acute lymphoblastic leukemia. *Blood* 1988;72:784–91.
73 Secker-Walker LM, Craig JM. Prognostic implications of breakpoint and lineage heterogeneity in Philadelphia-positive acute lymphoblastic leukemia: a review. *Leukemia* 1993;7: 147–51.
74 Kasprzyk A, Harrison CJ, Secker-Walker LM. Investigation of clonal involvement of myeloid cells in Philadelphia-positive and high hyperdiploid acute lymphoblastic leukemia. *Leukemia* 1999;13:2000–6.
75 Pajor L, Vass JA, Kereskai L, *et al*. The existence of lymphoid lineage restricted Philadelphia chromosome-positive acute lymphoblastic leukemia with heterogeneous *BCR–ABL* rearrangement. *Leukemia* 2000;14:1122–6.
76 Cuneo A, Bigoni R, Grazia Roberti M, Castoldi G. Lineage involvement and prognosis in Ph chromosome positive acute lymphoblastic leukemia. *Br J Haematol* 1998;101:394–6.
77 Castor A, Nilsson L, Astrand-Grundstrom I, *et al*. Distinct patterns of hematopoietic stem cell involvement in acute lymphoblastic leukemia. *Nat Med* 2005;11:630–7.
78 Cobaleda C, Gutierrez-Cianca N, Perez-Losada J, *et al*. A primitive hematopoietic cell is the target for the leukemic transformation in human philadelphia-positive acute lymphoblastic leukemia. *Blood* 2000;95:1007–13.
79 Hotfilder M, Rottgers S, Rosemann A, *et al*. Leukemic stem cells in childhood high-risk ALL/t(9;22) and t(4;11) are present in primitive lymphoid-restricted CD34+CD19- cells. *Cancer Res* 2005;65:1442–9.
80 Pui CH, Crist WM, Look AT. Biology and clinical significance of cytogenetic abnormalities in childhood acute lymphoblastic leukemia. *Blood* 1990;76:1449–63.

81 Schlieben S, Borkhardt A, Reinisch I, *et al*. Incidence and clinical outcome of children with *BCR–ABL*-positive acute lymphoblastic leukemia (ALL). A prospective RT-PCR study based on 673 patients enrolled in the German pediatric multicenter therapy trials ALL-BFM-90 and CoALL-05–92. *Leukemia* 1996;10:957–63.

82 Cytogenetic abnormalities in adult acute lymphoblastic leukemia: correlations with hematologic findings outcome. A Collaborative Study of the Group Francais de Cytogenetique Hematologique. *Blood* 1996;87:3135–42.

83 Pullarkat V SM, Kopecky KJ, Forman SJ, Appelbaum FR. Impact of cytogenetics on the outcome of adult acute lymphoblastic leukemia: results of Southwest Oncology Group 9400 study. *Blood* 2008;111:2563–72.

84 Thomas X, Olteanu N, Charrin C, Lheritier V, Magaud JP, Fiere D. Acute lymphoblastic leukemia in the elderly: The Edouard Herriot Hospital experience. *Am J Hematol* 2001;67:73–83.

85 Gotz G, Weh HJ, Walter TA, *et al*. Clinical and prognostic significance of the Philadelphia chromosome in adult patients with acute lymphoblastic leukemia. *Ann Hematol* 1992;64: 97–100.

86 Westbrook CA, Hooberman AL, Spino C, *et al*. Clinical significance of the *BCR–ABL* fusion gene in adult acute lymphoblastic leukemia: a Cancer and Leukemia Group B Study (8762). *Blood* 1992;80:2983–90.

87 Larson RA, Dodge RK, Burns CP, *et al*. A five-drug remission induction regimen with intensive consolidation for adults with acute lymphoblastic leukemia: cancer and leukemia group B study 8811. *Blood* 1995;85:2025–37.

88 Chim CS, Kwong YL, Chu YC, Chan CH, Chan YT, Liang R. Improved treatment outcome in adult acute lymphoblastic leukemia using the intensive German protocol, a preliminary report. *Hematol Oncol* 1997;15:19–26.

89 Secker-Walker LM, Prentice HG, Durrant J, Richards S, Hall E, Harrison G. Cytogenetics adds independent prognostic information in adults with acute lymphoblastic leukemia on MRC trial UKALL XA. MRC Adult Leukemia Working Party. *Br J Haematol* 1997;96:601–10.

90 Wetzler M, Dodge RK, Mrozek K, *et al*. Prospective karyotype analysis in adult acute lymphoblastic leukemia: the cancer and leukemia Group B experience. *Blood* 1999;93:3983–93.

91 Faderl S, Kantarjian HM, Thomas DA, *et al*. Outcome of Philadelphia chromosome-positive adult acute lymphoblastic leukemia. *Leuk Lymphoma* 2000;36:263–73.

92 Thomas X, Danaila C, Le QH, *et al*. Long-term follow-up of patients with newly diagnosed adult acute lymphoblastic leukemia: a single institution experience of 378 consecutive patients over a 21-year period. *Leukemia* 2001;15:1811–22.

93 Annino L, Vegna ML, Camera A, *et al*. Treatment of adult acute lymphoblastic leukemia (ALL): long-term follow-up of the GIMEMA ALL 0288 randomized study. *Blood* 2002;99: 863–71.

94 Kantarjian HM, O'Brien S, Smith TL, *et al*. Results of treatment with hyper-CVAD, a dose-intensive regimen, in adult acute lymphocytic leukemia. *J Clin Oncol* 2000;18:547–61.

95 Pfeifer H, Wassmann B, Pavlova A, *et al*. Kinase domain mutations of *BCR–ABL* frequently precede imatinib-based therapy and give rise to relapse in patients with de novo Philadelphia-positive acute lymphoblastic leukemia (Ph+ ALL). *Blood* 2007;110:727–34.

96 Faderl S, Jeha S, Kantarjian HM. The biology and therapy of adult acute lymphoblastic leukemia. *Cancer* 2003;98: 1337–54.

97 Radich JP. Philadelphia chromosome-positive acute lymphocytic leukemia. *Hematol Oncol Clin North Am* 2001;15: 21–36.

98 Brandwein JM, Gupta V, Wells RA, *et al*. Treatment of elderly patients with acute lymphoblastic leukemia–evidence for a benefit of imatinib in *BCR–ABL* positive patients. *Leuk Res* 2005;29:1381–6.

99 Larson RA. Management of acute lymphoblastic leukemia in older patients. *Semin Hematol* 2006;43:126–33.

100 Fielding AK, Richards SM, Chopra R, *et al*. Outcome of 609 adults after relapse of acute lymphoblastic leukemia (ALL); an MRC UKALL12/ECOG 2993 study. *Blood* 2007;109:944–50.

101 Tavernier E, Boiron JM, Huguet F, *et al*. Outcome of treatment after first relapse in adults with acute lymphoblastic leukemia initially treated by the LALA-94 trial. *Leukemia* 2007;21: 1907–14.

102 Camera A, Annino L, Chiurazzi F, *et al*. GIMEMA ALL – Rescue 97:a salvage strategy for primary refractory or relapsed adult acute lymphoblastic leukemia. *Haematologica* 2004;89: 145–53.

103 Uckun FM, Nachman JB, Sather HN, *et al*. Clinical significance of Philadelphia chromosome positive pediatric acute lymphoblastic leukemia in the context of contemporary intensive therapies:a report from the Children's Cancer Group. *Cancer* 1998;83:2030–9.

104 Schrappe M, Arico M, Harbott J, *et al*. Philadelphia chromosome-positive (Ph+) childhood acute lymphoblastic leukemia: good initial steroid response allows early prediction of a favorable treatment outcome. *Blood* 1998;92:2730–41.

105 Roy A, Bradburn M, Moorman AV, *et al*. Early response to induction is predictive of survival in childhood Philadelphia chromosome positive acute lymphoblastic leukemia: results of the Medical Research Council ALL 97 trial. *Br J Haematol* 2005;129:35–44.

106 Ribeiro RC, Broniscer A, Rivera GK, *et al*. Philadelphia chromosome-positive acute lymphoblastic leukemia in children: durable responses to chemotherapy associated with low initial white blood cell counts. *Leukemia* 1997;11:1493–6.

107 Arico M, Valsecchi MG, Camitta B, *et al*. Outcome of treatment in children with Philadelphia chromosome-positive acute lymphoblastic leukemia. *N Engl J Med* 2000;342:998–1006.

108 Pui CH, Sandlund JT, Pei D, *et al*. Improved outcome for children with acute lymphoblastic leukemia: results of Total Therapy Study XIIIB at St Jude Children's Research Hospital. *Blood* 2004;104:2690–6.

109 Arico M, Valsecchi MG, Conter V, *et al*. Improved outcome in high-risk childhood acute lymphoblastic leukemia defined by prednisone-poor response treated with double Berlin-Frankfurt-Muenster protocol II. *Blood* 2002;100:420–6.

110 Silverman LB, Gelber RD, Dalton VK, *et al*. Improved outcome for children with acute lymphoblastic leukemia: results of Dana-Farber Consortium Protocol 91–01. *Blood* 2001;97: 1211–18.

111 Forestier E, Johansson B, Gustafsson G, *et al*. Prognostic impact of karyotypic findings in childhood acute lymphoblastic leukemia: a Nordic series comparing two treatment periods. For the Nordic Society of Pediatric Hematology and Oncology

(NOPHO) Leukemia Cytogenetic Study Group. *Br J Haematol* 2000;110:147–53.

112 Hann I, Vora A, Harrison G, *et al.* Determinants of outcome after intensified therapy of childhood lymphoblastic leukemia: results from Medical Research Council United Kingdom acute lymphoblastic leukemia XI protocol. *Br J Haematol* 2001;113:103–14.

113 Fielding AK, Goldstone AH. Allogeneic hematopoietic stem cell transplant in Philadelphia-positive acute lymphoblastic leukemia. *Bone Marrow Transplant* 2008;41:447–53.

114 Goldstone AH, Chopra R, Buck G, *et al.* The Outcome of 267 Philadelphia Positive Adults in the International UKALL12/ECOG E2993 Study. Final Analysis and the Role of Allogeneic Transplant in Those under 50 years. *Blood* 2003;102: 268a.

115 Thomas X, Boiron JM, Huguet F, *et al.* Outcome of treatment in adults with acute lymphoblastic leukemia: analysis of the LALA-94 trial. *J Clin Oncol* 2004;22:4075–86.

116 Sharathkumar A, Saunders EF, Dror Y, *et al.* Allogeneic bone marrow transplantation vs chemotherapy for children with Philadelphia chromosome-positive acute lymphoblastic leukemia. *Bone Marrow Transplant* 2004;33:39–45.

117 Mitterbauer G, Nemeth P, Wacha S, *et al.* Quantification of minimal residual disease in patients with *BCR–ABL*-positive acute lymphoblastic leukemia using quantitative competitive polymerase chain reaction. *Br J Haematol* 1999;106:634–43.

118 Barrett AJ, Horowitz MM, Ash RC, *et al.* Bone marrow transplantation for Philadelphia chromosome-positive acute lymphoblastic leukemia. *Blood* 1992;79:3067–70.

119 Chao NJ, Blume KG, Forman SJ, Snyder DS. Long-term follow-up of allogeneic bone marrow recipients for Philadelphia chromosome-positive acute lymphoblastic leukemia. *Blood* 1995;85:3353–4.

120 Kroger N, Kruger W, Wacker-Backhaus G, *et al.* Intensified conditioning regimen in bone marrow transplantation for Philadelphia chromosome-positive acute lymphoblastic leukemia. *Bone Marrow Transplant* 1998;22:1029–33.

121 Lee S, Kim DW, Cho B, *et al.* Risk factors for adults with Philadelphia-chromosome-positive acute lymphoblastic leukemia in remission treated with allogeneic bone marrow transplantation:the potential of real-time quantitative reverse-transcription polymerase chain reaction. *Br J Haematol* 2003; 120:145–53.

122 Esperou H, Boiron JM, Cayuela JM, *et al.* A potential graft-versus-leukemia effect after allogeneic hematopoietic stem cell transplantation for patients with Philadelphia chromosome-positive acute lymphoblastic leukemia: results from the French Bone Marrow Transplantation Society. *Bone Marrow Transplant* 2003;31:909–18.

123 Sierra J, Radich J, Hansen JA, *et al.* Marrow transplants from unrelated donors for treatment of Philadelphia chromosome-positive acute lymphoblastic leukemia. *Blood* 1997;90: 1410–14.

124 Marks DI, Bird JM, Cornish JM, *et al.* Unrelated donor bone marrow transplantation for children and adolescents with Philadelphia-positive acute lymphoblastic leukemia. *J Clin Oncol* 1998;16:931–6.

125 Dunlop LC, Powles R, Singhal S, *et al.* Bone marrow transplantation for Philadelphia chromosome-positive acute lymphoblastic leukemia. *Bone Marrow Transplant* 1996;17:365–9.

126 Snyder DS, Nademanee AP, O'Donnell MR, *et al.* Long-term follow-up of 23 patients with Philadelphia chromosome-positive acute lymphoblastic leukemia treated with allogeneic bone marrow transplant in first complete remission. *Leukemia* 1999;13:2053–8.

127 Satwani P, Sather H, Ozkaynak F, *et al.* Allogeneic bone marrow transplantation in first remission for children with ultra-high-risk features of acute lymphoblastic leukemia: A children's oncology group study report. *Biol Blood Marrow Transplant* 2007;13:218–27.

128 Chim CS, Lie AK, Liang R, Au WY, Kwong YL. Long-term results of allogeneic bone marrow transplantation for 108 adult patients with acute lymphoblastic leukemia: favorable outcome with BMT at first remission and HLA-matched unrelated donor. *Bone Marrow Transplant* 2007;40:339–47.

129 Cornelissen JJ, Carston M, Kollman C, *et al.* Unrelated marrow transplantation for adult patients with poor-risk acute lymphoblastic leukemia: strong graft-versus-leukemia effect and risk factors determining outcome. *Blood* 2001;97:1572–7.

130 Kiehl MG, Kraut L, Schwerdtfeger R, *et al.* Outcome of allogeneic hematopoietic stem-cell transplantation in adult patients with acute lymphoblastic leukemia: no difference in related compared with unrelated transplant in first complete remission. *J Clin Oncol* 2004;22:2816–25.

131 Krejci O, van der Velden VH, Bader P, *et al.* Level of minimal residual disease prior to hematopoietic stem cell transplantation predicts prognosis in pediatric patients with acute lymphoblastic leukemia:a report of the Pre-BMT MRD Study Group. *Bone Marrow Transplant* 2003;32:849–51.

132 Goulden N, Bader P, Van Der Velden V, *et al.* Minimal residual disease prior to stem cell transplant for childhood acute lymphoblastic leukemia. *Br J Haematol* 2003;122:24–9.

133 Marks DI, Aversa F, Lazarus HM. Alternative donor transplants for adult acute lymphoblastic leukemia:a comparison of the three major options. *Bone Marrow Transplant* 2006;38: 467–75.

134 Ciceri F, Labopin M, Aversa F, *et al.* A survey of fully-haploidentical hematopoietic stem cells transplantation in adults with high-risk acute leukemia: a risk factor analysis of outcomes for patients transplanted in remission. *Blood* 2008; 112:3574–81.

135 Eapen M, Rubinstein P, Zhang MJ, *et al.* Outcomes of transplantation of unrelated donor umbilical cord blood and bone marrow in children with acute leukemia: a comparison study. *Lancet* 2007;369:1947–54.

136 Laughlin MJ, Eapen M, Rubinstein P, *et al.* Outcomes after transplantation of cord blood or bone marrow from unrelated donors in adults with leukemia. *N Engl J Med* 2004;351:2265–75.

137 Arnold R, Massenkeil G, Bornhauser M, *et al.* Nonmyeloablative stem cell transplantation in adults with high-risk ALL may be effective in early but not in advanced disease. *Leukemia* 2002; 16:2423–8.

138 Martino R, Giralt S, Caballero MD, *et al.* Allogeneic hematopoietic stem cell transplantation with reduced-intensity conditioning in acute lymphoblastic leukemia: a feasibility study. *Haematologica* 2003;88:555–60.

139 Champagne MA, Capdeville R, Krailo M, *et al.* Imatinib mesylate (STI571) for treatment of children with Philadelphia chromosome-positive leukemia: results from a Children's Oncology Group phase 1 study. *Blood* 2004;104:2655–60.

140 Druker BJ, Sawyers CL, Kantarjian H, *et al.* Activity of a specific inhibitor of the Bcr–Abl tyrosine kinase in the blast crisis of chronic myeloid leukemia and acute lymphoblastic leukemia with the Philadelphia chromosome. *N Engl J Med* 2001; 344:1038–42.

141 Ottmann OG, Druker BJ, Sawyers CL, *et al.* A phase 2 study of imatinib in patients with relapsed or refractory Philadelphia chromosome-positive acute lymphoid leukemias. *Blood* 2002; 100:1965–71.

142 Wassmann B, Pfeifer H, Scheuring U, *et al.* Therapy with imatinib mesylate (Glivec) preceding allogeneic stem cell transplantation (SCT) in relapsed or refractory Philadelphia-positive acute lymphoblastic leukemia (Ph+ALL). *Leukemia* 2002;16: 2358–65.

143 Kano Y, Akutsu M, Tsunoda S, *et al. In vitro* cytotoxic effects of a tyrosine kinase inhibitor STI571 in combination with commonly used antileukemic agents. *Blood* 2001;97:1999–2007.

144 Thiesing JT, Ohno-Jones S, Kolibaba KS, Druker BJ. Efficacy of STI571, an abl tyrosine kinase inhibitor, in conjunction with other antileukemic agents against *BCR–ABL*-positive cells. *Blood* 2000;96:3195–9.

145 Topaly J, Zeller WJ, Fruehauf S. Synergistic activity of the new ABL-specific tyrosine kinase inhibitor STI571 and chemotherapeutic drugs on *BCR–ABL*-positive chronic myelogenous leukemia cells. *Leukemia* 2001;15:342–7.

146 de Labarthe A, Rousselot P, Huguet-Rigal F, *et al.* Imatinib combined with induction or consolidation chemotherapy in patients with de novo Philadelphia chromosome-positive acute lymphoblastic leukemia: results of the GRAAPH-2003 study. *Blood* 2007;109:1408–13.

147 Delannoy A, Delabesse E, Lhéritier V, *et al.* Imatinib and methylprednisolone alternated with chemotherapy improve the outcome of elderly patients with Philadelphia-positive acute lymphoblastic leukemia:results of the GRAALL AFR09 study. *Leukemia* 2006;20:1526–32.

148 Lee KH, Lee JH, Choi SJ, *et al.* Clinical effect of imatinib added to intensive combination chemotherapy for newly diagnosed Philadelphia chromosome-positive acute lymphoblastic leukemia. *Leukemia* 2005;19:1509–16.

149 Lee S, Kim YJ, Min CK, *et al.* The effect of first-line imatinib interim therapy on the outcome of allogeneic stem cell transplantation in adults with newly diagnosed Philadelphia chromosome-positive acute lymphoblastic leukemia. *Blood* 2005;105:3449–57.

150 Ottmann OG, Wassmann B, Pfeifer H, *et al.* Imatinib compared with chemotherapy as front-line treatment of elderly patients with Philadelphia chromosome-positive acute lymphoblastic leukemia (Ph + ALL). *Cancer* 2007;109:2068–76.

151 Rea D, Legros L, Raffoux E, *et al.* High-dose imatinib mesylate combined with vincristine and dexamethasone (DIV regimen) as induction therapy in patients with resistant Philadelphia-positive acute lymphoblastic leukemia and lymphoid blast crisis of chronic myeloid leukemia. *Leukemia* 2006;20:400–3.

152 Thomas DA, Kantarjian HM, Ravandi F, *et al.* Long-term follow-up after frontline therapy with the hyper-CVAD and imatinib mesylate Regimes in adults with philadelphia (Ph) positive acute lymphoblastic leukemia (ALL). *Blood* 2007;110, Abstract 4.

153 Wassmann B, Pfeifer H, Goekbuget N, *et al.* Alternating versus concurrent schedules of imatinib and chemotherapy as front-line therapy for Philadelphia-positive acute lymphoblastic leukemia (Ph+ ALL). *Blood* 2006;108:1469–77.

154 Yanada M, Takeuchi J, Sugiura I, *et al.* Karyotype at diagnosis is the major prognostic factor predicting relapse-free survival for patients with Philadelphia chromosome-positive acute lymphoblastic leukemia treated with imatinib-combined chemotherapy. *Haematologica* 2008;93:287–90.

155 Yanada M, Takeuchi J, Sugiura I, *et al.* High complete remission rate and promising outcome by combination of imatinib and chemotherapy for newly diagnosed *BCR–ABL*-positive acute lymphoblastic leukemia: a phase II study by the Japan Adult Leukemia Study Group. *J Clin Oncol* 2006;24:460–6.

156 Vignetti M, Fazi P, Cimino G, *et al.* Imatinib plus steroids induces complete remissions and prolonged survival in elderly Philadelphia chromosome-positive patients with acute lymphoblastic leukemia without additional chemotherapy: results of the Gruppo Italiano Malattie Ematologiche dell'Adulto (GIMEMA) LAL0201-B protocol. *Blood* 2007;109: 3676–8.

157 Wassmann B, Pfeifer H, Scheuring UJ, *et al.* Early prediction of response in patients with relapsed or refractory Philadelphia chromosome-positive acute lymphoblastic leukemia (Ph+ALL) treated with imatinib. *Blood* 2004;103:1495–8.

158 Thomas DA, Faderl S, Cortes J, *et al.* Treatment of Philadelphia chromosome-positive acute lymphocytic leukemia with hyper-CVAD and imatinib mesylate. *Blood* 2004; 103:4396–407.

159 Towatari M, Yanada M, Usui N, *et al.* Combination of intensive chemotherapy and imatinib can rapidly induce high-quality complete remission for a majority of patients with newly diagnosed *BCR–ABL*-positive acute lymphoblastic leukemia. *Blood* 2004;104:3507–12.

160 Schultz KR, Bowman WP, Aledo A, *et al.* Improved early event free survival (EFS) in children with philadelphia chromosome positive (Ph+) acute lymphoblastic leukemia (ALL) with imatinib in combination with high dose chemotherapy: Children's Oncology Group (COG) Study AALL0031. *Blood* 2007;110.

161 Lazarus HM, Richards SM, Chopra R, *et al.* Central nervous system involvement in adult acute lymphoblastic leukemia at diagnosis: results from the international ALL trial MRC UKALL XII/ECOG E2993. *Blood* 2006;108:465–72.

162 Pfeifer H, Wassmann B, Hofmann WK, *et al.* Risk and prognosis of central nervous system leukemia in patients with Philadelphia chromosome-positive acute leukemias treated with imatinib mesylate. *Clin Cancer Res* 2003;9:4674–81.

163 Leis JF, Stepan DE, Curtin PT, *et al.* Central nervous system failure in patients with chronic myelogenous leukemia lymphoid blast crisis and Philadelphia chromosome positive acute lymphoblastic leukemia treated with imatinib (STI-571). *Leuk Lymphoma* 2004;45:695–8.

164 Dai H, Marbach P, Lemaire M, Hayes M, Elmquist WF. Distribution of STI-571 to the brain is limited by P-glycoprotein-mediated efflux. *J Pharmacol Exp Ther* 2003;304:1085–92.

165 Hamada A, Miyano H, Watanabe H, Saito H. Interaction of imatinib mesilate with human P-glycoprotein. *J Pharmacol Exp Ther* 2003;307:824–8.

166 Wassmann B, Pfeifer H, Stadler M, *et al.* Early molecular response to posttransplantation imatinib determines outcome in MRD+ Philadelphia-positive acute lymphoblastic leukemia (Ph+ ALL). *Blood* 2005;106:458–63.

167 Carpenter PA, Snyder DS, Flowers ME, *et al.* Prophylactic administration of imatinib after hematopoietic cell transplantation for high-risk Philadelphia chromosome-positive leukemia. *Blood* 2007;109:2791–3.

168 Gorre ME, Mohammed M, Ellwood K, *et al.* Clinical resistance to STI-571 cancer therapy caused by *BCR–ABL* gene mutation or amplification. *Science* 2001;293:876–80.

169 Donato NJ, Wu JY, Stapley J, *et al.* Bcr–Abl independence and LYN kinase overexpression in chronic myelogenous leukemia cells selected for resistance to STI571. *Blood* 2003;101: 690–8.

170 Griswold IJ, MacPartlin M, Bumm T, *et al.* Kinase domain mutants of *BCR–ABL* exhibit altered transformation potency, kinase activity, and substrate utilization, irrespective of sensitivity to imatinib. *Mol Cell Biol* 2006;26:6082–93.

171 Soverini S, Colarossi S, Gnani A, *et al.* Contribution of Abl kinase domain mutations to imatinib resistance in different subsets of Philadelphia-positive patients: by the GIMEMA Working Party on Chronic Myeloid Leukemia. *Clin Cancer Res* 2006;12:7374–9.

172 Hofmann WK, Komor M, Wassmann B, *et al.* Presence of the *BCR–ABL* mutation Glu255Lys prior to STI571 (imatinib) treatment in patients with Ph+ acute lymphoblastic leukemia. *Blood* 2003;102:659–61.

173 Shah NP, Tran C, Lee FY, Chen P, Norris D, Sawyers CL. Overriding imatinib resistance with a novel ABL kinase inhibitor. *Science* 2004;305:399–401.

174 O'Hare T, Walters DK, Stoffregen EP, *et al.* *In vitro* activity of Bcr–Abl inhibitors AMN107 and BMS-354825 against clinically relevant imatinib-resistant Abl kinase domain mutants. *Cancer Res* 2005;65:4500–5.

175 Porkka K, Koskenvesa P, Lundan T, *et al.* Dasatinib crosses the blood–brain barrier and is an efficient therapy for central nervous system Philadelphia chromosome-positive leukemia. *Blood* 2008;112:1005–12.

176 Talpaz M, Shah NP, Kantarjian H, *et al.* Dasatinib in imatinib-resistant Philadelphia chromosome-positive leukemias. *N Engl J Med* 2006;354:2531–41.

177 Ottmann O, Dombret H, Martinelli G, *et al.* Dasatinib induces rapid hematologic and cytogenetic responses in adult patients with Philadelphia chromosome positive acute lymphoblastic leukemia with resistance or intolerance to imatinib:interim results of a phase 2 study. *Blood* 2007;110: 2309–15.

178 Burgess MR, Skaggs BJ, Shah NP, Lee FY, Sawyers CL. Comparative analysis of two clinically active Bcr–Abl kinase inhibitors reveals the role of conformation-specific binding in resistance. *Proc Natl Acad Sci U S A* 2005;102:3395–400.

179 Soverini S, Martinelli G, Colarossi S, *et al.* Second-line treatment with dasatinib in patients resistant to imatinib can select novel inhibitor-specific *BCR–ABL* mutants in Ph+ ALL. *Lancet Oncol* 2007;8:273–4.

180 Soverini S, Colarossi S, Gnani A, *et al.* Resistance to dasatinib in Philadelphia-positive leukemia patients and the presence or the selection of mutations at residues 315 and 317 in the Bcr–Abl kinase domain. *Haematologica* 2007;92:401–4.

181 Shah NP, Skaggs BJ, Branford S, *et al.* Sequential Abl kinase inhibitor therapy selects for compound drug-resistant *BCR–ABL* mutations with altered oncogenic potency. *J Clin Invest* 2007;117:2562–9.

182 Kantarjian H, Giles F, Wunderle L, *et al.* Nilotinib in imatinib-resistant CML and Philadelphia chromosome-positive ALL. *N Engl J Med* 2006;354:2542–51.

183 Ottmann OG, Larson RA, Kantarjian HM, *et al.* Nilotinib in patients with relapsed/refractory philadelphia chromosome-positive acute lymphoblastic leukemia who are resistant or intolerant to imatinib. *Blood* 2007;110:2815.

184 Deguchi Y, Kimura S, Ashihara E, *et al.* Comparison of imatinib, dasatinib, nilotinib and INNO-406 in imatinib-resistant cell lines. *Leuk Res* 2008;32:980–3.

185 Dai Y, Rahmani M, Corey SJ, Dent P, Grant S. A Bcr–Abl-independent, Lyn-dependent form of imatinib mesylate (STI-571) resistance is associated with altered expression of Bcl-2. *J Biol Chem* 2004;279:34227–39.

186 Kimura S, Naito H, Segawa H, *et al.* NS-187, a potent and selective dual Bcr–Abl/Lyn tyrosine kinase inhibitor, is a novel agent for imatinib-resistant leukemia. *Blood* 2005;106: 3948–54.

187 Naito H, Kimura S, Nakaya Y, *et al.* *In vivo* antiproliferative effect of NS-187, a dual Bcr–Abl/Lyn tyrosine kinase inhibitor, on leukemic cells harboring Abl kinase domain mutations. *Leuk Res* 2006;30:1443–6.

188 Yokota A, Kimura S, Masuda S, *et al.* INNO-406, a novel Bcr–Abl/Lyn dual tyrosine kinase inhibitor, suppresses the growth of Ph+ leukemia cells in the central nervous system, and cyclosporine A augments its *in vivo* activity. *Blood* 2007;109: 306–14.

189 Golas JM, Arndt K, Etienne C, *et al.* SKI-606, a 4-anilino-3-quinolinecarbonitrile dual inhibitor of Src and Abl kinases, is a potent antiproliferative agent against chronic myelogenous leukemia cells in culture and causes regression of K562 xenografts in nude mice. *Cancer Res* 2003;63:375–81.

190 Puttini M, Coluccia AM, Boschelli F, *et al.* *In vitro* and *in vivo* activity of SKI-606, a novel Src-Abl inhibitor, against imatinib-resistant *BCR–ABL+* neoplastic cells. *Cancer Res* 2006;66: 11314–22.

191 Gumireddy K, Baker SJ, Cosenza SC, *et al.* A non-ATP-competitive inhibitor of Bcr–Abl overrides imatinib resistance. *Proc Natl Acad Sci U S A* 2005;102:1992–7.

192 Harrington EA, Bebbington D, Moore J, *et al.* VX-680, a potent and selective small-molecule inhibitor of the Aurora kinases, suppresses tumor growth *in vivo*. *Nat Med* 2004;10:262–7.

193 Carter TA, Wodicka LM, Shah NP, *et al.* Inhibition of drug-resistant mutants of Abl, KIT, and EGF receptor kinases. *Proc Natl Acad Sci U S A* 2005;102:11011–16.

194 Young MA, Shah NP, Chao LH, *et al.* Structure of the kinase domain of an imatinib-resistant Abl mutant in complex with the Aurora kinase inhibitor VX-680. *Cancer Res* 2006;66: 1007–14.

195 Giles FJ, Cortes J, Jones D, Bergstrom D, Kantarjian H, Freedman SJ. MK-0457, a novel kinase inhibitor, is active in patients with chronic myeloid leukemia or acute lymphocytic leukemia with the *T315I BCR–ABL* mutation. *Blood* 2007;109: 500–2.

196 Neviani P, Santhanam R, Oaks JJ, *et al.* FTY720, a new alternative for treating blast crisis chronic myelogenous leukemia and Philadelphia chromosome-positive acute lymphocytic leukemia. *J Clin Invest* 2007;117:2408–21.

197 Fiskus W, Pranpat M, Balasis M, *et al.* Cotreatment with vorinostat (suberoylanilide hydroxamic acid) enhances activity of

dasatinib (BMS-354825) against imatinib mesylate-sensitive or imatinib mesylate-resistant chronic myelogenous leukemia cells. *Clin Cancer Res* 2006;12:5869–78.

198 Fiskus W, Pranpat M, Bali P, *et al*. Combined effects of novel tyrosine kinase inhibitor AMN107 and histone deacetylase inhibitor LBH589 against Bcr–Abl-expressing human leukemia cells. *Blood* 2006;108:645–52.

199 Nimmanapalli R, Fuino L, Bali P, *et al*. Histone deacetylase inhibitor LAQ824 both lowers expression and promotes proteasomal degradation of Bcr–Abl and induces apoptosis of imatinib mesylate-sensitive or -refractory chronic myelogenous leukemia-blast crisis cells. *Cancer Res* 2003;63:5126–35.

200 Nimmanapalli R, Fuino L, Stobaugh C, Richon V, Bhalla K. Cotreatment with the histone deacetylase inhibitor suberoylanilide hydroxamic acid (SAHA) enhances imatinib-induced apoptosis of *Bcr–Abl*-positive human acute leukemia cells. *Blood* 2003;101:3236–9.

201 Nguyen TK, Rahmani M, Harada H, Dent P, Grant S. MEK1/2 inhibitors sensitize *BCR–ABL+* human leukemia cells to the dual Abl/Src inhibitor BMS-354/825. *Blood* 2007;109: 4006–15.

202 Yu C, Krystal G, Varticovksi L, *et al*. Pharmacologic mitogen-activated protein/extracellular signal-regulated kinase kinase/mitogen-activated protein kinase inhibitors interact synergistically with STI571 to induce apoptosis in Bcr/Abl-expressing human leukemia cells. *Cancer Res* 2002;62:188–99.

203 Azam M, Nardi V, Shakespeare WC, *et al*. Activity of dual SRC-Abl inhibitors highlights the role of Bcr–Abl kinase dynamics in drug resistance. *Proc Natl Acad Sci U S A* 2006;103:9244–9.

Chapter 19
Acute Lymphoblastic Leukemia in Adolescents and Young Adults

Michael E. Rytting
M. D. Anderson Cancer Center, Houston, Texas, USA

Introduction

Acute lymphoblastic leukemia (ALL) in adolescents and young adults is a rare and challenging clinical problem. Even defining the age of the patients to fill the adolescent and young adult (AYA) group is problematic. Whereas age between 15 and 30 years is the currently accepted age range, the boundaries for this age group are not absolute, but rather fit well with the 5-year divisions of the population used by the Surveillance, Epidemiology, and End Results (SEER) program to describe cancer incidence and mortality. As an example, current national pediatric ALL trials allow enrollment of young adults up to the age of 30. Nevertheless, some trials at adult institutions, including the M. D. Anderson Cancer Center (MDACC), enrol older patients with ALL, even up to the age of 55. What constitutes a "young adult" probably is in the eye of the beholder or of the person writing the protocol.

Incidence of acute lymphoblastic leukemia in adolescents and young adults

The rarity of ALL in the young adult population is reflected in the above-mentioned SEER data. For the years 2001–2005, the incidence of ALL in the USA was 1.6 cases per 100,000 people. For the population aged between 15 and 29 years, ALL accounts for about 6% of all invasive cancer diagnoses [1]. The incidence of leukemia is lowest in 15–29-year-old patients because of a decrease in incidence of ALL and a low incidence of other leukemias compared with older age groups [2]. In absolute numbers, each year there are approximately 540 patients diagnosed with ALL in the US population who are aged 15–29 years.

Leukemias: Principles and Practice of Therapy, 1st edition. Edited by S. Faderl and H. Kantarjian.

Therapeutic approach to adolescents and young adults with acute lymphoblastic leukemia

In clinical practice, AYA patients, particularly the younger adolescents, may be seen by either pediatric or adult oncologists. This has led, as would be expected, to comparisons of outcomes for adolescents treated on pediatric or adult services. For patients up to age 21, several published studies report that pediatric-type therapy results in superior overall survival (OS) and event-free survival (EFS) when compared with adult therapies [3,4].

One must remain cognisant of the fact that no such comparisons exist for patients >21 years old. Applying pediatric therapy to this group of patients, while perhaps appealing, is experimental and should be performed in the setting of a clinical trial. So far, the toxicities reported appear to be acceptable. In fact, some studies of induction show remarkably few grade III–IV toxicities in adults treated with pediatric therapy [5,6]. At MDACC, approximately 30 adults >21 years old have been enrolled on pediatric protocols—although toxicities have been acceptable and manageable, approximately 20% have had grade III–IV adverse events not including expected hematologic toxicities. The role of pediatric protocols in young adults is not clear at this point, and whether they will be successful requires more time and a longer follow-up to establish.

Various different factors between adult trials and pediatric trials contribute to the several disparities found in comparable patient populations: (i) Familiarity with the disease must be considered. ALL is the most common malignancy in pediatric patients, and most pediatric oncologists are very familiar with the care of these patients, which provides pediatric oncologists with a tremendous advantage. On the other hand, ALL is far from common in adults, and thus adult oncologists may not focus on such a rare disease. This is particularly important in ALL, where patient management and therapy are very complex. (ii) Pediatric patients with cancer are frequently treated at academic medical centers. A much larger percentage of adult patients with leukemia are treated in community settings. Protocol therapy is strongly emphasized in pediatric leukemia clinics—although the adolescent population may not be as rigorously entered on national therapies as previously thought—and trials are audited strictly. Young adults >21 years old are poorly enrolled on trials; enrollment of these patients on national studies, fortunately, is now being emphasized. Therapy provided by dedicated adult leukemia services should obviate the effects of these differences. (iii) Patients seen in a pediatric office are, in general, more compliant. Pediatric patients and young adults who visit pediatric offices with their parents generally have strong support systems and frequently have no choice but to take their medicines and keep their appointments. This is an essential facet in following complex, onerous regimens that may easily last for 3 years. (iv) Finally, there are biologic differences in young adult ALL when compared with much younger patients, including far fewer cases of TEL–AML translocations and hyperdiploid leukemia, more cases of Philadelphia chromosome-positive ALL, higher presenting white blood cell (WBC) counts, and an increased proportion of T-cell ALL.

Adolescent patients with ALL who are seen on a pediatric leukemia service have several tested, effective regimens to choose from. In addition, they are eligible for ongoing national protocols. The current Children's Oncology Group protocol, open for patients up to age 30, is based on augmented Berlin–Frankfurt–Muenster (BFM) therapy. Results for the standard arm in this trial, augmented BFM with a single delayed-intensification phase, were recently published [7]. The trial achieved an 81% 6-year EFS and an 89% 6-year OS for patients who responded rapidly to therapy, with little difference found between age groups. Rapid responders were those patients who achieved <25% blasts in the marrow by day 7 of therapy and were in morphologic remission by day 28 of induction. The arm of the trial that was chosen as the most efficacious uses a single delayed-intensification phase and augmented therapy with increased intensity of vincristine, asparaginase, and methotrexate. This therapy, with slight modification, is given to adolescents and other patients with high-risk ALL at the MDACC pediatric clinic if the family does not wish to participate in a national experimental trial. Other options with known excellent outcomes for adolescents include the Dana Farber Cancer Institute (DFCI) high-risk ALL regimen and BFM therapy employing high-dose methotrexate. DFCI protocols employ intensive asparaginase treatment. An analysis of the subset of patients aged 15–18 years treated on two consecutive DFCI trials shows a 78% EFS for these patients. The DFCI 95-01 protocol uses cranial radiation therapy in all patients >15 years old [8]. For adolescent patients with T-ALL, the Pediatric Oncology Group (POG) 9404 regimen has produced excellent results as well. This trial again used intensive asparaginase and high-dose methotrexate. An interesting finding in many recent trials of therapy for high-risk ALL in adolescents is that patients with T-ALL do as well as their pre-B-cell ALL counterparts [9–11]. Ongoing national experimental protocols for adolescents with ALL include a high-risk protocol based on an augmented BFM backbone and a very high-risk protocol for those patients with very high-risk features such as hypodiploidy, primary refractory disease, or *MLL* gene rearrangements with a slow response to therapy.

Adolescents who are seen in adult clinics are usually placed on adult ALL regimens such as the hyper-CVAD regimen. Hyper-CVAD alternates courses of fractionated cyclophosphamide, vincristine, corticosteroids, and adriamycin with courses of intermediate-dose methotrexate and high-dose cytarabine. Intrathecal therapy is included, with the frequency determined by the risk for central nervous system (CNS) disease and cerebrospinal fluid (CSF) status at the first lumbar puncture. This regimen has at least a 95% complete remission rate and does not employ craniospinal radiation except in cases of cranial nerve palsy. The CNS relapse rate is <5%. The published 5-year EFS for hyper-CVAD is 38%, but this includes all patients [12]. A similar complete remission rate was achieved by using intensified therapy for ALL [13]. This protocol uses relatively high doses of anthracyclines as well as large doses of cytarabine and methotrexate. The therapy is short compared with that used for pediatric regimens, and there is no prolonged maintenance phase. For patients with pre-B-ALL treated with this regimen, the 5-year EFS is estimated at 52% for all patients. It was not successful in cases of high WBC count or in cases of *MLL* gene rearrangement. An analysis of patients <30 years old treated with this regimen was not presented. The Cancer and Leukemia Group B (CALGB) 8811 study demonstrated a 5-year EFS of 69% for adults <30 years old with pre-B-ALL [14]. The results of a larger Medical Research Council (MRC)/Eastern Cooperative Oncology Group (ECOG) trial were not as encouraging [15]. In this trial, chemotherapy consisted of a four-drug induction followed by a second phase of induction using cyclophosphamide and cytarabine. This initial therapy is very similar to pediatric ALL treatment, while later therapy varied moderately from the pediatric schema. For patients aged 15–19 years treated on the ECOG trial, the 5-year OS was 44%. Interestingly, the OS for patients aged 20–29 was practically the same as for the teenagers at 45%.

Disease-specific therapy

Adult strategies for ALL are now moving forward at a rapid pace and stratification into different subtypes is now being attempted. Adult patients with pre-B-ALL who express CD20 have been enrolled on treatment with rituximab and hyper-CVAD. Comparing the outcome of non-T-CD20$^+$ ALL with historic experience, the addition of rituximab improved disease-free survival (DFS) rates (62% vs. 28%, $P = 0.005$) in patients <30 years old. The impact on OS was not significant and no improvement in DFS was demonstrated in older patients [16]. The addition of rituximab to standard therapy for ALL in teenagers and young adults may therefore be an attractive option and requires further study. Many adult groups have, by now, adopted the incorporation of tyrosine kinase inhibitors (TKIs) into therapy for Philadelphia chromosome-positive ALL [17,18]. Adult studies show that if testing for the Philadelphia chromosome is done rapidly, imatinib can be added at the onset of therapy and is well tolerated. In a long-term follow-up of hyper-CVAD with imatinib with a median age of 51 years (range 17–84 years), 93% of the patients achieved complete morphologic remission and 52% achieved a molecular response as determined by nested polymerase chain reaction (PCR) testing [18]. Compared with hyper-CVAD alone, DFS and OS rates at 3 years remain significantly superior (66% vs. 14% and 55% vs. 15%, respectively; $P < 0.001$). The second-generation TKI, dasatinib, is now being tested in combination with hyper-CVAD in adult patients with Philadelphia chromosome-positive ALL, but it is still too early to determine clear results. Young adults with T-ALL may be assigned to hyper-CVAD combined with nelarabine. This is similar to the Childrens' Oncology Group (COG) strategy for T-ALL that incorporates nelarabine into augmented BFM therapy with high-dose methotrexate. The value of the addition of nelarabine to current therapy is not yet known.

Central nervous sytem therapy

All strategies employ some form of therapy to protect the CNS from relapse or to actively treat CNS leukemia. But how much CNS directed therapy is enough and who should receive such therapy? Recently, some groups using BFM-based therapy have questioned whether cranial radiation is essential to maintain high cure rates [11,19]. The BFM group found that the moderate-risk group of patients with pre-B-ALL did not require radiation treatment [20]. The moderate-risk group included teenage patients with pre-B-ALL with a good response to steroids. The Children's Cancer Group (CCG) trial with augmented BFM therapy radiated all slow early responders, although the radiation dose was small and did not include the spine [7]. Cranial radiation is given to all teenage patients on other consortium trials [21]. On the other hand, the therapeutic approach at some research hospitals does not include CNS radiation even for patients with overt CNS leukemia at diagnosis. The hyper-CVAD regimen employs intensified intrathecal treatment for overt CNS leukemia and only employs radiation for patients with cranial nerve palsies. The CNS relapse rate is low for hyper-CVAD, perhaps owing to the use of high-dose cytarabine. It seems very possible, depending on the chemotherapeutic regimen, to achieve an acceptable cure rate for ALL in teenagers and young adults without the use of cranial radiation.

The number of lumbar punctures that are needed is debatable and probably depends on the systemic chemotherapy regimen chosen. Intrathecal treatments range from eight in hyper-CVAD to >25 in patients treated for slow early response using some pediatric protocols. The required number is most likely somewhere in between. Currently, young adults with pre-B-ALL treated at MDACC receive 15 lumbar punctures in the context of augmented BFM therapy and pegylated asparaginase. Another variable in the approach to CNS prophylaxis is the effect of traumatic lumbar puncture with possible introduction of leukemic blasts into the CNS. Studies report a worsened outcome for patients with ALL who have an initial traumatic lumbar puncture [22,23]. Such traumatic punctures are bound to increase as the AYA population becomes more obese. It has been suggested that obese patients should delay the first lumbar puncture until the circulating blasts are cleared, thus decreasing the chance of CNS contamination.

Information is now beginning to accrue for young adults treated on pediatric-based therapy. One of the foremost concerns, toxicity, appears to be acceptable [5,6,24]. As noted above, treatments based on intensive asparaginase have been well tolerated, and the standard four- or five-drug induction accompanied by intrathecal treatments have also worked well, with excellent complete remission rates at the end of induction. It remains to be seen which single regimen produces the best EFS and OS. Early results, however, at least suggest that an age-unrestricted approach to ALL, at least in patients <30 years old, should be pursued [6,25]. One advantage so far is that the pediatric regimens generally require decreased inpatient stays compared with some adult treatments. Also, it is not known whether agents such as TKIs, rituximab, or nelarabine may be safely and effectively added to a pediatric regimen that is then used in the young adult population. These investigations will probably be undertaken in the near future.

Stem-cell transplantation

Pediatric strategies now recommend transplantation for very high-risk patients with pre-B-ALL. This group of patients includes those with any of the following: induction failure based on morphology or persistent minimal residual disease (MRD); Philadelphia chromosome; *MLL* gene rearrangement with slow response to therapy; and hypodiploidy with ≤44 chromosomes or a DNA index <0.81 in leukemic blasts. If there is a matched-related donor or a single antigen mismatched-related donor, excluding HLA-DR, then pediatric protocol patients in remission may proceed to transplant after initial chemotherapy. These protocols allow enrollment up to the age of 30. It remains to be seen whether stem-cell transplantation will improve leukemia-free survival (LFS) in the AYA patients enrolled on this study.

What is the role of bone marrow transplant in adolescents and young adults with ALL? The EFS in adult patients with ALL transplanted in first remission is generally in the range of 30–40%, with much poorer results in adults in second CR or later [26–30]. EFS is sometimes not presented for different adult age groups, and, in some studies, age did not influence survival. Others have found that there is improved LFS in adults <30 years old compared with older adults with ALL transplanted in first CR [31,32]. While these studies indicate that LFS after transplant might be superior to LFS after chemotherapy, this is a conclusion that others have not confirmed [33,34]. In studies of high-risk adult ALL, those patients who have an initial high WBC count are Philadelphia chromosome positive, are slow responders to therapy or resistant to primary induction, or have *MLL* rearrangements in general demonstrate a very poor outcome with chemotherapy; in this setting, transplant in first remission should be strongly considered. Interestingly, as opposed to children, hypodiploidy is not frequently mentioned as a high-risk feature for adults with ALL. With the use of pediatric protocols in the young adult population being so new, there is no information comparing the efficacy of the new chemotherapeutic strategies with stem-cell transplantation in this population. As more information is gathered, it may very well be necessary to build transplant options into new protocols for the high-risk young adult patient with ALL.

Relapsed and refractory acute lymphoblastic leukemia

The therapy of relapsed ALL in young adults centers around marrow transplant. Chemotherapy in this setting, even in the first remission, is over two years and is unlikely to provide a cure [32]. If there is an acceptable donor and a second remission can be achieved, then moving to transplant as soon as possible is generally the accepted standard procedure. The difficulties lie in locating a compatible donor and inducing a second remission. Even in patients that do go to transplant after a first relapse, maintaining remission is very difficult. For CNS relapse the data are sparse [35,36]. Intensive intrathecal therapy combined with systemic treatment can successfully generate a remission but long-term survival is poor. The hyper-CVAD regimen augmented with increased doses of vincristine, asparaginase, and decadron has an approximate 45% success rate in inducing a second remission—this is a viable option for the young adult who has relapses on a pediatric regimen as well [37]. Alternatively, patients who have relapsed after hyper-CVAD may respond to induction regimens based on pediatric regimens.

Conclusions

Treatment for AYA patients is at a crossroads between pediatric and adult disciplines. This has resulted in fragmentation of the patient population between adult and pediatric groups. Nevertheless, being at a crossroads may prove to be a boon, not just for young adult patients, but for patients with ALL on each end of the age spectrum. The middle ground of AYA patients has the potential to bring adult and pediatric experiences together, providing impetus for testing new ideas in the younger and in the older populations with ALL. A prime example of a recent addition to pediatric ALL therapy, which was initially studied in adult patients with ALL, is the incorporation of TKIs as early as possible in the treatment of Philadelphia chromosome-positive acute leukemia. Testing of second-generation and later TKIs in the AYA population, if successful, will lend strong support for moving such drugs to the forefront in treating Philadelphia chromosome-positive ALL in children. As another example, rituximab, if it proves beneficial in young adults with ALL, may well be worth testing in high-risk pediatric patients with $CD20^+$ non-T-ALL. For adult patients with leukemia, the current interest in pediatric-type chemotherapy regimens may result in improvements in survival with fewer inpatient days. In addition, the pediatric focus on late effects, particularly cognitive function, is clearly also applicable to adult patients. In the future, the treatment of AYA patients with ALL will hopefully continue to borrow from both adult and pediatric experiences. This will probably be the case for MRD, as both adult and pediatric groups are studying how to use it in treating ALL. As in pediatric studies, transplant might be considered for adolescents and young adults with ALL and persistent MRD. Another area for exploration is epigenetic therapy. Already, groups have shown that hypermethylation of DNA portends a poor outcome in adolescents with ALL. Indeed, accumulated epigenetic modifications that occur over time might explain the steady worsening in outcome in ALL that follows increasing age.

References

1 Ries LAG, Melbert D, Krapcho M, *et al. SEER Cancer Statistics Review, 1975–2005*. National Cancer Institute, 2008.

2 Mattano L, Jr., Nachman J, Ross J, *et al. Leukemias: Cancer Epidemiology in Older Adolescents and Young Adults 15 to 29 Years of Age, Including SEER Incidence and Survival: 1975–2000*. National Cancer Institute, 2006. pp. 39–51.

3 Boissel N, Auclerc MF, Lhéritier V, *et al*. Should adolescents with acute lymphoblastic leukemia be treated as old children or young adults? Comparison of the French FRALLE and LALA-94 trials. *J Clin Oncol* 2003;21:774–80.

4 Stock W, Sather H, Dodge RK, *et al*. Outcome of adolescents and young adults with ALL: a comparison of Children's Cancer

Group (CCG) and Cancer and Leukemia Group B (CALGB) regimens. *Blood* 2000;96:467a.

5 Douer D, Yampolsky H, Cohen LF, *et al.* Pharmacodynamics and safety of intravenous pegaspargase during remission induction in adults aged 55 years or younger with newly diagnosed acute lymphoblastic leukemia. *Blood* 2007;109:2744–50.

6 Ribera JM, Oriol A, Sanz MA, *et al.* Comparison of the results of the treatment of adolescents and young adults with standard-risk acute lymphoblastic leukemia with the Program Espanol de Tratamiento en Hematologia pediatric-based protocol ALL-96. *J Clin Oncol* 2008;26:1843–9.

7 Seibel NL, Steinherz PG, Sather HN, *et al.* Early postinduction intensification therapy improves survival for children and adolescents with high-risk acute lymphoblastic leukemia: a report from the Children's Oncology Group. *Blood* 2008;111:2548–55.

8 Loh ML, Goldwasser MA, Silverman LB, *et al.* Prospective analysis of TEL/AML1-positive patients treated on Dana-Farber Cancer Institute consortium protocol 95–01. *Blood* 2006; 107:4508–13.

9 Goldberg JM, Silverman LB, Levy DE, *et al.* Childhood T-cell acute lymphoblastic leukemia: the Dana-Farber Cancer Institute acute lymphoblastic leukemia consortium experience. *J Clin Oncol* 2003;21:3616–22.

10 Hann IM, Richards SM, Eden OB, *et al.* Analysis of the immunosphenotype of children treated on the Medical Research Council United Kingdom Acute Lymphoblastic Leukemia Trial XI (MRC UKALLXI). Medical Research Council Leukemia Working Party. *Leukemia* 1998;12:1249–55.

11 Kamps WA, Bokkerink JPM, Hakvoort-Cammel FGAJ, *et al.* BFM-oriented treatment for children with acute lymphoblastic leukemia without cranial irradiation and treatment reduction for standard risk patients: results of DCLSG protocol ALL-8 (1991–1996). *Leukemia* 2002;16.1099–111

12 Kantarjian H, Thomas D, O'Brien S, *et al.* Long-term follow-up results of hyperfractionated cyclophosphamide, vincresitine, doxorubicin, and dexamethasone (hyper-CVAD), a dose-intensive regimen, in adult acute lymphocytic leukemia. *Cancer* 2004;101:2788–801.

13 Linker C, Damon L, Ries C, *et al.* Intensified and shortened cyclical chemotherapy for adult acute lymphoblastic leukemia. *J Clin Oncol* 2002;20:2464–71.

14 Larson R, Dodge R, Burns P, *et al.* A five-drug remission induction regimen with intensive consolidation for adults with acute lymphoblastic leukemia: Cancer and Leukemia Group B Study 8811. *Blood* 1995;85:2025–37.

15 Rowe J, Buck G, Burnett A, *et al.* Induction therapy for adults with acute lymphoblastic leukemia: results of more than 1500 patients from the International ALL Trial: MRC UKALL XII/ECOG E2993. *Blood* 2005;106:3760–7.

16 Thomas D, Kantarjian H, Faderl S, *et al.* Update of the modified hyper-CVAD regimen with or without rituximab as frontline therapy of adults with acute lymphocytic leukemia (ALL or lymphoblastic lymphoma (LL). *Blood* 2007;110, Abstract 2824.

17 Thomas DA. Philadelphia chromosome-positive acute lymphocytic leukemia: a new era of challenges. *Am Soc Hematol Educ Prog* 2007;435–443.

18 Thomas DA, Kantarjian HM, Ravandi F, *et al.* Long-term follow-up after frontline therapy with the Hyper-CVAD and imatinib mesylate regimen in adults with Philadelphia (Ph) positive acute lymphoblastic leukemia (ALL). *Blood* 2007;110:10a.

19 Conter V, Arico M, Valsecchi MG, *et al.* Extended intrathecal methotrexate may replace cranial irradiation for prevention of cns relapse in children with intermediate-risk acute lymphoblastic leukemia treated with Berlin-Frankfurt-Munster-based intensive chemotherapy. The Associazione Italiana di Ematologia ed Oncologia Pediatrica. *J Clin Oncol* 1995;13: 2480–2.

20 Moricke A, Reiter A, Zimmerman M, *et al.* Risk-adjusted therapy of acute lymphoblastic *leukemia* can decrease treatment burden and improve survival: treatment results of 2169 unselected pediatric and adolescent patients enrolled in the trial ALL-BFM 95. *Blood* 2008;111:4477–89.

21 Barry E, DeAngelo D, Newberg D, *et al.* Favorable outcome for adolescents with acute lymphoblastic leukemia treated on Dan-Farber Cancer Institute acute lymphoblastic leukemia consortium protocols *J Clin Oncol* 2007;25:813–20.

22 Gajjar A, Harrison PL, Sandlund JT *et al.* Traumatic lumbar puncture at diagnosis adversely affects outcome in childhood acute lymphoblastic leukemia. *Blood* 2000;96:3381–4.

23 Burger B, Zimmermann M, Mann G, *et al.* Diagnostic cerbrospinal fluid examination in children with acute lymphoblastic leukemia: significance of low leukocyte counts with blasts or traumatic lumbar puncture. *J Clin Oncol* 2003;21:184–8.

24 DeAngelo D. The treatment of adolescents and young adults with acute lymphoblastic leukemia. *Am So Hematol Educ Prog* 2005;123–130.

25 Huguet F, Raffoux E, Thomas X, *et al.* Toward a pediatric approach in adults with acute lymphoblastic leukemia (ALL): the GRAALL-2003 study. *Blood* 2006;108, Abstract 147.

26 Hallbook H, Haggulund H, Stockelberg D, *et al.* Autologous and allogeneic stem cell transplantation in adult ALL: the Swedish Adult ALL Group Experience. *Bone Marrow Transplant* 2005;35:1141–8.

27 Chim CS, Lie, AK, Liang R, *et al.* Long-term results of allogeneic bone marrow transplantation for 108 adult patients with acute lymphoblastic leukemia: favorable outcome with BMT at first remission and HLA-matched unrelated donor. *Bone Marrow Transplant* 2007;40:339–47.

28 Cornelissen JJ Carston M, Kollman C, *et al.* Unrelated marrow transplantation for adult patients with poor-risk acute lymphoblastic leukemia: strong graft-versus-leukemia effect and risk factors determining outcome. *Blood* 2001;99:2270–1.

29 Kiehl MG, Kraut L, Schwerdtfeger R, *et al.* Outcome of allogeneic hematopoietic stem cell transplantation in adult patients with acute lymphoblastic leukemia: no difference in related compared with unrelated transplant in first complete remission. *J Clin Oncol* 2004;22:2816–25.

30 Fielding AK, Richards SM, Chopra R, *et al.* Outcome of 609 adults after relapse of acute lymphoblastic leukemia (ALL); an MRC UKALL12/ECOG 2993 study. *Blood* 2007;109:944–50.

31 Goldstone AH, Richards SM, Lazarus HM, *et al.* In adults with standard-risk acute lymphoblastic leukemia, the greatest benefit is achieved from a matched sibling allogeneic transplantation in first complete remission, and an autologous transplantation is less effective than conventional consolidation/maintenance chemotherapy in all patients: final results of the international ALL trial (MRC UKALL XII/ECOGE2993). *Blood* 2008;111:1827–33.

32 Oh H, Gale RP, Zhang MJ, *et al.* Chemotherapy vs. HLA-identical sibling bone marrow transplants for adults with acute

lymphoblastic leukemia in first remission. *Bone Marrow Transplant* 1998;22:253–7.

33 Zhang MJ, Hoelzer D, Horowitz MM, *et al*. Long-term Follow-up of adults with acute lymphoblastic leukemia in first remission treated with chemotherapy or bone marrow transplantation. The Acute Lymphoblastic Leukemia Working Committee. *Ann Intern Med* 1995;123:428–31.

34 Ribera JM, Oriol A, Bethencourt C, *et al*. Comparison of intensive chemotherapy, allogeneic or autologous stem cell transplantation as post-remission treatment of adult patients with high-risk acute lymphoblastic leukemia. Results of the PETHEMA ALL-93 trial. *J Hematol* 2005;90:1346–56.

35 Sancho JM, Ribera JM, Oriol A, *et al*. Central nervous system recurrence in adult patients with acute lymphoblastic leucemia: frequency and prognosis in 467 patients without cranial irradiation for prophylaxis. *Cancer* 2006;106:2540–6.

36 Surapaneni UR, Cortes JE, Thomas D, *et al*. Central nervous system relapse in adults with acute lymphoblastic leukemia. *Cancer* 2002;94:773–9.

37 Faderl S, Thomas DA, Ravandi F, *et al*. Intensification of Hyper-CVAD with L-Asparaginase, vincristine, and dexamethasone ("augmented Hyper-CVAD") has activity in adult patients with relapsed/refractory acute lymphoblastic leukemia (ALL). *Blood* 2007;110, Abstract 4324.

Chapter 20
The Role of Hematopoietic Stem-cell Transplantation in Adults with Acute Lymphoblastic Leukemia

Partow Kebriaei
University of Texas M. D. Anderson Cancer Center, Houston, Texas, USA

Abstract

Adult patients with acute lymphoblastic leukemia (ALL) can now achieve complete remission (CR) rates of 80–90%. However, only 25–50% of these patients achieve long-term disease-free survival (DFS). Current research efforts are focused on innovative postremission strategies with the goal of improving DFS and overall survival (OS). The identification of different prognostic groups based on the biology of the malignant clone and well-characterized prognostic factors allow for risk-adapted therapy. Multiple randomized trials have demonstrated that allogeneic hematopoietic stem-cell transplantation (SCT) improves the outcome of patients with high-risk ALL. Furthermore, recent trials suggest that patients with standard-risk ALL may also benefit from allogeneic SCT. In this chapter, we will define the different disease risk groups, the clinical outcomes of major transplant trials for ALL, and the therapeutic factors that affect the outcome following SCT.

General principles of acute lymphoblastic leukemia therapy

Treatment for adult ALL is modeled on the therapy developed for childhood ALL, and consists of remission induction, consolidation, maintenance therapy, and CNS prophylaxis using a risk-stratified approach. Selecting therapy based on patient- and disease-specific prognostic factors has led to a significant improvement in outcomes for childhood ALL [1], and the more recent adoption of this approach for adults has had a similar favorable impact [2–4]. Hematopoietic SCT is considered the optimal form of consolidation in a select group of patients.

Leukemias: Principles and Practice of Therapy, 1st edition. Edited by S. Faderl and H. Kantarjian.

Prognostic factors and risk assessment

Several classic evaluations of prognostic features in adult ALL have been made and have led to five widely accepted prognostic features: age, white blood cell (WBC) count, leukemic cell immunophenotype, cytogenetic subtype, and time to achieve CR [5–7] (Table 20.1). The presence of any of these features portends a high risk for relapse following standard ALL therapy, and the remaining patients are considered as standard risk. Up to 75% of adults with ALL are considered to be poor-risk patients with an expected DFS rate of 25%, and 25% of adults with ALL constitute standard-risk patients with a projected DFS rate of >50% [8]. However, recent advances in ALL biology and therapy are changing the risk assignment of some of these features.

Age, WBC count, and treatment response during induction therapy remain classic prognostic features. Age is a continuous variable, with OS decreasing with increasing age; OS ranges from 34% to 57% for patients <30 years old compared with only 15–17% for patients >50 years old [9–13]. A high WBC count is also a continuous variable; generally, a WBC count >30,000/μL or 50,000/μL for B-lineage ALL and >100,000/uL for T-lineage ALL predict for poor prognosis [9,12–14]. Of note, while an increased WBC count holds prognostic significance independently as a measure of tumor burden, a high WBC count may also be associated with increased risk of complications during induction therapy, increased risk of central nervous system (CNS) relapse, and poor-risk cytogenetic subgroups (eg, t(4;11) and t(9;22)). Finally, the achievement of CR and time to CR after induction therapy carries significant prognostic implications, with patients who require >4 weeks to achieve a CR having a lower likelihood of being cured [5,13]. The emergence of minimal residual disease (MRD) monitoring provides an even more accurate assessment of disease response. In contrast to children, decrease in MRD burden occurs more slowly in adults [15–17]. In general, the presence of MRD, defined as 10^{-4} leukemic cells, at any time after the start of consolidation therapy is associated with an increased relapse

Table 20.1 Prognostic factors in adult acute lymphoblastic leukemia.

Characteristic	High-risk factor(s)	Standard-risk factor(s)
Patient-related		
Age	>50 years	<35 years
Performance status	Poor	Good
Gender	Male	
Race	Black	
Plasma albumin levels	Low	Normal
Treatment-related		
Late response	Time to CR >4 weeks Persistence of blasts in PB at day 7 and BM at day 14	Time to CR <4 weeks Timely clearance of blasts
Response to steroids	Delayed, incomplete	Fast, complete
Dose intensity	Decreased	
Pharmacodynamics	Non-therapeutic levels of 6-MP, MTX	Therapeutic levels of drugs
Disease-related		
Leukocytosis	>30 × 10^9/L (B-lineage) >100 × 10^9/L (T-lineage)	<30 × 10^9/L
Cytogenetics	t(9;22), t(4;11)	t(12;21), hyperdiploid
Immunophenotype	Early and mature T-ALL, pro-B-ALL (null type)	Cortical T-ALL
Other characteristics		
P-glcyoprotein	Greater expression	
p53	Aberrant expression	
$p15^{INK4b}$	Greater methylation	
Glutathione	High levels	
Caspase 2 and 3	High levels	

From Faderl *et al.* (2003), with permission.
ALL, acute lymphoblastic leukemia; BM, bone marrow; CR, complete remission; MTX, methotrexate; PB, peripheral blood; 6-MP, 6-mercaptopurine.

risk, and the predictive value increases at later time points [16]. The German Multicenter Adult ALL Study Group (GMALL) prospectively analyzed post-consolidation samples of 105 patients who had completed 1 year of chemotherapy and were in molecular remission; 27% of patients subsequently had molecular relapse, with 61% of these patients developing overt relapse at a median of 9.5 months. However, MRD evaluation has certain limitations, and in contrast to childhood ALL protocols, MRD positivity is not yet universally accepted as an independent prognostic factor in all adult regimens. The predictive value of MRD depends on the technical quality of the assay and the frequency of monitoring. Furthermore, there is not yet consensus on standard methodology to measure MRD.

Specific recurring cytogenetic abnormalities portend significant prognosis. The presence of the Philadelphia chromosome and t(4;11)(q21;q23) have been associated with inferior survival in multiple large series [18,33]. Additionally, the presence of the t(8;14)(q24.1;q32) complex karyotype, defined as more than five chromosomal abnormalities, or low hypodiploidy/near triploidy were noted to have poor survival in a more recent analysis of patients treated on the Medical Research Council (MRC) United Kingdom Acute Lymphoblastic Leukemia (UKALL) XII/Eastern Cooperative Oncology Group (ECOG) 2993 trial [19]; in contrast, the presence of hyperdiploidy or del(9p) indicated a good prognosis [19]. Of note, the t(8;14) associated with a mature B-ALL phenotype has a poor prognosis when treated with standard

ALL regimens. However, modified ALL regimens, incorporating CD20-targeted therapy, suggest better survival for this group. Similarly, while the Philadelphia chromosome has traditionally been considered a marker of high-risk disease, the outcome for this subset of patients may greatly change with the incorporation of tyrosine kinase inhibitors into classic ALL therapy. Reports from studies incorporating imatinib into their regimens show a greater proportion of patients achieving CR and MRD negativity, and thus suggest a better prognosis [20–25].

Finally, patients with T-lineage ALL formerly had inferior CR rates in comparison with precursor-B-ALL. However, modification of the standard ALL therapy to include cytarabine, cyclophosphamide, and CNS prophylaxis in T-lineage ALL regimens now result in uniformly better outcomes for these patients as compared with their B-lineage ALL counterparts, with CR rates up to 80% and leukemia-free survival (LFS) >50% [10,26].

Hematopoietic stem-cell transplantation in first complete remission

Reviews of a number of small, phase II trials in high-risk adult patients with ALL who have undergone allogeneic SCT in CR1 suggest a higher DFS when compared with historical controls based on conventional chemotherapy, ranging broadly from 21% to 71% [27–32]. These findings were then investigated in several multicenter randomized, prospective studies (Table 20.2). To minimize patient selection bias, these trials employed a "genetic" randomization method, offering allogeneic SCT in CR1 to all patients with a sibling donor, and chemotherapy versus autologous SCT [9,14,35–37,38], chemotherapy only [39], or autologous SCT only [40] to patients without a donor. Results were then analyzed using "intent-to-treat" methods that compared patients with and without donors.

The multicenter French study group Leucémies Aiguës Lymphoblastiques de l'Adulte completed two large studies between 1986 and 1991 (LALA-87) [14] and between 1994 and 2002 (LALA-94) [35]. Using an intent-to-treat analysis, a significant DFS and OS benefit was observed for allogeneic SCT in high-risk patients in both trials. High risk was defined as having one or more of the following factors: presence of the Philadelphia chromosome, null ALL, age >35 years, WBC count $>30 \times 10^9/L$, or time to CR >4 weeks. The international MRC UKALL XII/ECOG E2993 trial also noted significantly improved survival (53% vs. 45%) for patients who received an allogeneic SCT in CR1 as compared with chemotherapy or autologous SCT [36]. However, in contrast to the LALA study, this advantage was confined to the standard-risk patient subset (OS 63% vs. 51%) because of the high treatment-related mortality (TRM) observed in the high-risk group (39%) as compared with the standard-risk group (20%). Of note, high risk in this study was defined as age >35 years or a high WBC count (>30,000 for B-lineage or >100,000 for T-ALL); Philadelphia chromosome-positive patients were excluded in this analysis. The international MRC UKALL XII/ECOG E2993 trial also noted significantly improved survival (53% vs. 45%) for patients who receive an allogeneic SCT in CRI as compared with chemotherapy or autologous SCT [40]. However, in contrast to the LALA study, this advantage was confined to the standard-risk patient subset (OS 62% vs. 52%) because of the high treatment-related mortality (TRM) observed in the high-risk group (36%) compared with the standard-risk group.

Table 20.2 Selected prospective trials in adult acute lymphoblastic leukemia.

Study	Year	N	Median age (range)	SCT	Complete remission rate (%)	Early death (%)	Survival (%) (years)
CALGB 8811 [7]	1995	197	32 (16–80)	–	85	9	50 (3)
CALGB 9111 [11]	1998	198	35 (16–83)	Ph$^+$	82	8	40 (3)
LALA 87 [14]	2000	572	33 (15–60)	D	76	9	27 (10)
GMALL 05/93 [26]	2001	1163	35 (15–65)	R	83	n.r.	35 (5)
JALSG-ALL93 [9]	2002	263	31 (15–59)	D	78	6	33 (6)
GIMEMA 0288 [13]	2002	767	28 (12–60)	–	82	11	27 (9)
M. D. Anderson [12]	2004	288	40 (15–92)	Ph$^+$	92	5	38 (5)
EORTC ALL-3 [38]	2004	340	33 (14–79)	D	74	n.r.	36 (6)
LALA 94 [35]	2004	922	33 (15–55)	R	84	5	36 (5)
MRC XII/ECOG E 2993 [36]	2008	1913	31 (15–65)	D	91	n.r.	39 (5)
Pethema ALL-93 [37]	2005	222	27 (15–50)	HR	82	6	34 (5)

CALGB, Cancer and Leukemia Group B; D, prospective hematopoietic stem-cell transplant in all patients with donor; ECOG, Eastern Cooperative Oncology Group; EORTC, European Organisation for Research and Treatment of Cancer; GIMEMA, Gruppo Italiano Malattie Ematologiche dell'Adulto; GMALL, German Multicenter Acute Lymphoblastic Leukemia; HR, prospective hematopoietic stem-cell transplant in high-risk patients only; JALSG-ALL, Japanese Adult Leukemia Study Group—Acute Lymphoblastic Leukemia; LALA, Leucémies Aiguës Lymphoblastiques de l'Adulte; MRC, Medical Research Council; n.r., not reported; Ph$^+$, hematopoietic stem-cell transplant in Philadelphia-positive acute lymphoblastic leukemia; R, hematopoietic stem-cell transplant according to prospective risk model.

In contrast to these three studies, no survival advantage was noted for allogeneic SCT in CR1 in three other multicenter, prospective studies [9,37,38]. In the European Organisation for Research and Treatment of Cancer (EORTC) ALL-3 trial, although the donor group had a lower relapse rate (38% vs. 56%, $P = 0.001$), they had also had a higher cumulative incidence of death in CR (23% vs. 7%, $P = 0.0004$), resulting in similar survival rates (41% vs. 39%) [38]. Finally, no survival advantage has ever been shown for autologous SCT as compared with chemotherapy for patients who do not have a matched-related donor [14,35–37,38].

Unfortunately, less than 30% of patients will have a matched sibling donor, and a matched-unrelated donor (MUD) transplant may be considered. Historically, these transplants have been associated with a higher risk of graft rejection, graft-versus-host disease (GVHD), and infection. However, more precise human leukocyte antigen (HLA) matching of the donor and recipient through the use of high-resolution allele-based typing for class 1 and 2 HLA molecules has allowed the selection of better-matched donors; this has resulted in a progressive improvement in the incidence of severe GVHD and survival in patients undergoing MUD transplantation [41]. Currently, outcomes are similar for patients in CR1 receiving a MUD versus matched sibling SCT, with DFS rates ranging from 40% to 45% [42,43].

Hematopoietic stem-cell transplantation beyond first complete remission

Unfortunately, 60–70% of patients who achieve a CR eventually relapse. A second CR can often be achieved, but these are typically transient, short-lived responses. Allogeneic SCT remains the most effective modality for achieving durable remissions for patients in, or beyond, CR2. The outcome of 609 adults with relapsed ALL, all of whom were previously treated on the MRC UKALL 12/ECOG 2993 study, was investigated [44]. The survival at 5 years after relapse was 7%. Factors predicting a good outcome after salvage therapy were young age and long duration of first remission. When survival was evaluated based on treatment strategy, survival following SCT ranged from 15% to 23% depending on donor type (15% for autograft, 16% for MUD, 23% for MRD), and was significantly better than chemotherapy at only 4% ($P < 0.00005$) [44]. Similar long-term LFS rates of 14–43% have been reported from other small series for patients receiving SCT in CR2 [29,31,45]. As expected, the primary cause of treatment failure is relapse (>50%).

Hematopoietic stem-cell transplantation for primary refractory acute lymphoblastic leukemia

Most current induction regimens obtain a CR in 80–90% of newly diagnosed patients. Early deaths account for some of the induction failures, but, in most studies, 5–10% of patients have disease that is resistant to the remission induction regimen. These patients often have poor prognostic factors at presentation, and additional attempts at induction chemotherapy may be unsuccessful. Several studies suggest that patients with a human leukocyte antigen (HLA)-identical sibling can benefit if they proceed directly to allogeneic transplantation without undergoing a second attempt at induction therapy [46–48]. In the largest of these studies, approximately 35% of these patients with primary refractory disease became long-term disease-free survivors [48]. In a retrospective review of patients with primary refractory or relapsed ALL, the records of 314 adults were reviewed for disease outcome at M. D. Anderson Cancer Center between 1980 and 1997. Allogeneic SCT was performed in 29 patients (13 in salvage and 16 in CR2). The rates for durable CR post transplant were comparable between the two groups—5/13 (38%) in the salvage group and 5/16 (31%) in the remission group. Although patient numbers are small and a variety of transplant conditioning regimens were used, these results corroborate the findings of earlier studies and suggest that allogeneic transplant should be considered for these patients with an otherwise dismal chance of long-term survival [49].

Philadelphia chromosome-positive acute lymphoblastic leukemia

Historically, patients with Ph^+ ALL have been difficult to treat with long-term DFS rates of 10–20% [6]. Allogeneic transplantation from a related or unrelated donor has been the standard form of consolidation, with 27–65% long-term survival for patients receiving SCT in CR1 [32,50,51]. Beyond CR1, SCT is curative in only a small fraction of patients, with DFS ranging between 5% and 17% [52].

The recent development of potent inhibitors of the tyrosine kinase activity of the *BCR–ABL* fusion product resulting from the Ph chromosome translocation has revolutionized therapy for Ph-associated leukemias [53]. Imatinib mesylate has demonstrated significant activity in patients with chronic myeloid leukemia (CML) [54] and Ph^+ ALL [55], although the response duration in Ph^+ ALL has been limited, with a median time to progression and median OS of 2.2 and 4.9 months, respectively [55]. However, synergistic effects have been observed *in vitro* when imatinib has been combined with commonly used chemotherapy agents [56]. As a result, a number of studies have investigated the benefit of concurrent or sequential administration of imatinib with chemotherapy [20–25]. Results from these single insitution [20,25] and multicenter trials [21–24] suggest that the incorporation of imatinib into standard ALL therapy results in improved remission induction rates of 95% with 50–70% of patients achieving molecular negativity. Furthermore, more patients are able to receive SCT in CR1, resulting in improved OS rates of 43–78% with 1–3 years of follow-up.

One exception to these general findings is the data from the Ph+ arm of the UKALL XII/ECOG 2993 study that found no improvement in the rate of patients eligible to receive SCT in CR1 (58% vs. 62% in the pre-imatinib era), or in the 3-year OS rates (23% vs. 26% in the pre-imatinib era) for patients treated with and without imatinib [51]. One explanation for this discrepancy may be the dose scheduling of imatinib; here, most patients began imatinib after induction therapy. Of note, thus far there does not appear to be a survival difference between patients who receive an allogeneic SCT for consolidation versus those who do not [20,23], albeit with short follow-up for the non-transplanted patients. Whether consolidation with SCT in CR1 will remain the standard of care for patients with Ph+ ALL will depend on the durability of the remission inductions, which is currently under investigation.

Factors influencing transplant outcome

The relation between donor and recipient, the chemotherapy preparative regimen, the source of stem cells, and GVHD prophylaxis regimen all impact on transplant outcome. Although there is currently no role for alternative donor transplants (haploidentical, cord blood) in CR1 [57], they may be reasonable options for patients with more advanced disease, since disease control beyond CR1 is limited with chemotherapy. Transplants using haploidentical donors are most successful if undertaken in CR and can result in event-free survival rates up to 25%; however, graft rejection, severe GVHD, and infection are limiting complications [58]. Cord blood transplantation is still in the early stages of development. This graft source has the potential advantage of the most readily available cell source, but is limited by the small stem cell numbers in each cord unit. Investigations are under way to advance this field, including *ex vivo* umbilical cord blood (UCB) unit expansion and the use of double UCB grafts in the setting of reduced-intensity conditioning—the latter appears to provide greater antileukemic benefit [59].

In contrast to other hematologic malignancies, total body irradiation (TBI) remains the standard backbone for myeloablative ALL transplant preparative regimens. The most widely used regimen remains the combination of TBI and cyclophosphamide, although a retrospective analysis of registry data from the Center for International Blood and Marrow Transplant Research (CIBMTR) suggests that the combination of TBI and etoposide may afford better survival for patients in CR2 when compared with cyclophosphamide and TBI [60]. Non-radiation-containing regimens, most commonly busulfan and cyclophosphamide, have been investigated in the hope of decreasing radiation-related complications, with no significant differences noted in the outcome [61]. Novel preparative regimens incorporating disease-directed monoclonal antibodies, both radiolabelled [34,62] and non-radiolabelled [63,64] are under investigation. The use of rituximab in the transplant preparative regimen seemed to lower the incidence of acute GVHD in a phase II study from M. D. Anderson [63]; a randomized study investigating this issue is currently ongoing.

As illustrated in the MRC UKALL XII/ECOG 2993 study, the TRM rate begins to obscure the survival advantage for older patients. Since the incidence of ALL increases in adults >50 years old, transplant approaches with reduced TRM are needed. Non-myeloablative transplant regimens use less-intense chemotherapy combinations, which still provide adequate immunosuppression to allow for successful donor stem-cell engraftment. The major benefit of this approach is a lower risk of drug toxicity and TRM, which is most relevant to older or debilitated patients unable to tolerate ablative preparative regimens; disease control occurs through the immune graft versus leukemia (GVL) effect. GVL is operative in ALL [65], but to a lesser degree than in other hematologic malignancies [66]. Martino *et al.* [67] published the largest series of non-myeloablative SCT in ALL. He analyzed the results of 27 patients, with a median age of 55 years. The incidence of TRM was 23%, OS 31%, and disease progression 49% at 2 years. The incidence of disease relapse was 33% in patients transplanted in CR compared with 60% in those with overt disease [67]. In this study, and others, a higher relapse rate was observed for patients transplanted with overt disease. However, in older patients in CR1 this strategy appears favorable, but it must be validated in multicenter, prospective studies.

Finally, the effect of bone marrow versus peripheral blood stem cells (PBSC) as the source of stem cells in SCT has been evaluated. Allogeneic PBSC result in faster engraftment, but may be associated with an increased rate of chronic GVHD [68]. A multicenter prospective study is currently ongoing to help define the role of PBSC in allogeneic SCT. In this study, adult patients with leukemia requiring MUD HSCT will be randomized to bone marrow or PBSC donors. The results of this trial are eagerly anticipated.

Immunomodulation post transplant

Allogeneic SCT is associated with a potent GVL effect mediated by donor immunocompetent cells, including T-cell and normal karyotype (NK) cells [69–72]. The presence of a GVL effect is based primarily on observations of lower relapse rates in patients who develop GVHD [30,71,73]. A GVL effect that is associated with the presence of GVHD has been described in ALL, acute myeloid leukemia (AML), and CML; interestingly, this effect appears most potent in ALL [74]. Donor-lymphocyte infusion (DLI) has been widely used to augment GVL effects in patients with residual or recurrent malignancy following SCT. However, in contrast to CML and AML, where DLI often results in a CR in patients with relapsed disease following allogeneic transplant, DLI does not appear to be effective for relapsed ALL following SCT [75,76]. The reasons for this observation are likely multifactorial. First, the target antigens for the GVL response are unknown. Second, it is difficult to generate a T-cell response to lymphoblasts. Finally, ALL cells do not express co-stimulatory molecules and are poor stimulators of T-cell reactivity. Still, small studies using granulocyte colony-stimulating factor (G-CSF) mobilized PBSC as the source of DLI (which may have more T cells and NK cells) [77] or the addition of IL-2 to the DLI in efforts to augment the immune response to the DLI [77] presented better results, suggesting that immunomodulatory therapies may be further developed as a treatment modality for ALL.

Long-term complications of allogeneic stem-cell transplant

Socie *et al.* [78] analyzed the characteristics of 6691 patients listed in the IBMTR who underwent allogeneic SCT for AML, ALL, CML, or aplastic anemia between January 1980 and December 1993. The median duration of follow-up was 80 months. Mortality rates in this cohort were compared with those of an age-, sex-, and nationality-matched general population. All patients were free from disease 2 years post transplant, with 89% survival at 5 years. Mortality rates remained significantly higher than the general population throughout the study among patients who underwent transplantation for ALL or CML, and through the ninth year for patients who had AML. Specifically, for patients with ALL the relative mortality rate was 20.1 2 years after transplantation, 25.9 5 years after transplantation, and 15.4 10 years after transplantation. Not surprisingly, recurrent leukemia was the chief cause of death for patients who underwent SCT for leukemia and GVHD among those in either disease category, followed by infection, new cancer, and organ failure. Older age was associated with an increased risk of relapse in the ALL group, with 48% relapse observed in ALL compared with 11% relapses in the overall group. Chronic GVHD was the second leading cause of death overall, with 23% observed in the ALL cohort.

A low incidence of secondary cancer was reported overall (6%), with a slightly higher rate observed in the ALL group (10%) [78]. However, with longer follow-up time the incidence of secondary cancers was reported to be up to 12.8% ± 2.6% at 15 years by the European Group for Blood and Marrow Transplantation (EBMT) [79]. The most frequent malignant diseases were neoplasms of the skin, oral cavity, uterus (including cervix), thyroid gland, breast, and glial tissue. Older patient age and treatment of GVHD with cyclosporine were significant risk factors for new malignant neoplasms after SCT in multivariate analysis [79]. The risk for specifically secondary breast cancer among cancer survivors was recently reported in a study by Friedman *et al.* [80]. In a multivariable analysis, increased risk was associated with longer time from transplantation (hazard ratio [HR] for 20+ years after transplantation = 10.8), use of TBI (HR = 4.0), and younger age at transplantation (HR = 9.5 for HSCT <18 years). The hazard for death associated with breast cancer was 2.5 (95% confidence interval: 1.1–5.8) [80].

Quality of life and psychosocial functioning are major issues following allogeneic SCT. Broers *et al.* [81] evaluated the quality of life in a prospective study of 125 consecutive patients who underwent SCT between 1987 and 1992. Patients were evaluated with questionnaires measuring quality of life, functional limitations, psychologic distress, anxiety, depression, and self-esteem. Questionnaires were answered prior to the SCT, 1 month after discharge, and 6 months, 1 year, and 3 years after SCT. Nearly 90% of patients reported a good-to-excellent quality of life at 3 years. Changes in quality of life and psychologic distress could be explained entirely by changes in functional limitations and somatic symptoms. The minority of patients who reported a worse quality of life reported experiencing continued serious functional limitations. One such limitation is the late neurotoxic effects of SCT on cognitive functioning. Harder *et al.* [84] investigated this phenomenon in a consecutively treated cohort of long-term adult SCT survivors. Forty patients were included, 87.5% had undergone allogeneic transplantation. All received TBI up to 12 Gy. Assessment took place 22–82 months after SCT. Mild to moderate cognitive impairment was found in 24 patients (60%). Compared with healthy population norms, selective attention and executive function, information processing speed, verbal learning, and verbal and visual memory were most likely to be affected [82]. Therefore, cognitive functioning should be used as an outcome parameter in SCT studies, and emphasis should be placed on interventions that help patients cope with their physical limitations.

Conclusion

In conclusion, allogeneic SCT has been demonstrated to have a major therapeutic benefit for selected patients with high-risk ALL. However, much work remains to be done to improve survival for patients with this challenging disease. Results of trials of novel strategies are eagerly awaited, including the incorporation of molecularly targeted chemotherapy, targeted immunotherapy using monoclonal antibodies or adoptive cellular therapy, and novel non-myeloablative preparative regimens with promise to decrease TRM and improve survival.

References

1 Pui CH, Evans WE. Acute lymphoblastic leukemia. *N Engl J Med* 1998;339:605–15.

2 Linker C, Damon L, Ries C, Navarro W. Intensified and shortened cyclical chemotherapy for adult acute lymphoblastic leukemia. *J Clin Oncol* 2002;20:2464–71.

3 Larson RA. Recent clinical trials in acute lymphocytic leukemia by the Cancer and Leukemia Group B. *Hematol Oncol Clin North Am* 2000;14:1367–79.

4 Kantarjian HM, O'Brien S, Smith TL, *et al.* Results of treatment with hyper-CVAD, a dose-intensive regimen, in adult acute lymphocytic leukemia. *J Clin Oncol* 2000;18:547–61.

5 Hoelzer D. Which factors influence the different outcome of therapy in adults and children with ALL? *Bone Marrow Transplant.* 1989;4(Suppl.1):98–100.

6 Faderl S, Garcia-Manero G, Thomas DA, Kantarjian HM. Philadelphia chromosome-positive acute lymphoblastic leukemia- current concepts and future perspectives. *Rev Clin Exp Hematol* 2002;6:142–60; discussion 200–2.

7 Larson RA, Dodge RK, Burns CP, *et al.* A five-drug remission induction regimen with intensive consolidation for adults with acute lymphoblastic leukemia: cancer and leukemia group B study 8811. *Blood* 1995;85:2025–37.

8 Gokbuget N, Hoelzer D. Treatment of adult acute lymphoblastic leukemia. *Am Soc Hematol* 2006:133–41.

9 Takeuchi J, Kyo T, Naito K, *et al.* Induction therapy by frequent administration of doxorubicin with four other drugs, followed by intensive consolidation and maintenance therapy for adult acute lymphoblastic leukemia: the JALSG-ALL93 study. *Leukemia* 2002;16:1259–66.

10 Rowe JM, Buck G, Burnett AK, *et al.* Induction therapy for adults with acute lymphoblastic leukemia: results of more than 1500 patients from the international ALL trial: MRC UKALL XII/ECOG E2993. *Blood* 2005;106:3760–7.

11 Larson RA, Dodge RK, Linker CA, *et al.* A randomized controlled trial of filgrastim during remission induction and consolidation chemotherapy for adults with acute lymphoblastic leukemia: CALGB study 9111. *Blood* 1998;92:1556–64.

12 Kantarjian H, Thomas D, O'Brien S, *et al.* Long-term follow-up results of hyperfractionated cyclophosphamide, vincristine, doxorubicin, and dexamethasone (Hyper-CVAD), a dose-intensive regimen, in adult acute lymphocytic leukemia. *Cancer* 2004;101:2788–801.

13 Annino L, Vegna ML, Camera A, *et al.* Treatment of adult acute lymphoblastic leukemia (ALL): long-term follow-up of the GIMEMA ALL 0288 randomized study. *Blood* 2002;99:863–71.

14 Thiebaut A, Vernant JP, Degos L, *et al.* Adult acute lymphocytic leukemia study testing chemotherapy and autologous and allogeneic transplantation. A follow-up report of the French protocol LALA 87. *Hematol Oncol Clin North Am* 2000;14:1353–66.

15 Coustan-Smith E, Behm FG, Sanchez J, *et al.* Immunological detection of minimal residual disease in children with acute lymphoblastic leukemia. *Lancet* 1998;351:550–4.

16 Bruggemann M, Raff T, Flohr T, *et al.* Clinical significance of minimal residual disease quantification in adult patients with standard-risk acute lymphoblastic leukemia. *Blood* 2006;107:1116–23.

17 Mortuza FY, Papaioannou M, Moreira IM, *et al.* Minimal residual disease tests provide an independent predictor of clinical outcome in adult acute lymphoblastic leukemia. *J Clin Oncol* 2002;20:1094–104.

18 Faderl S, Kantarjian HM, Talpaz M, Estrov Z. Clinical significance of cytogenetic abnormalities in adult acute lymphoblastic leukemia. *Blood* 1998;91:3995–4019.

19 Moorman AV, Harrison CJ, Buck GA, *et al.* Karyotype is an independent prognostic factor in adult acute lymphoblastic leukemia (ALL): Analysis of cytogenetic data from patients treated on the Medical Research Council (MRC) UKALLXII/Eastern Cooperative Oncology Group (ECOG) 2993 Trial. *Blood* 2007;109:3189–97.

20 Thomas DA, Faderl S, Cortes J, *et al.* Treatment of Philadelphia chromosome-positive acute lymphocytic leukemia with hyper-CVAD and imatinib mesylate. *Blood* 2004;103:4396–407.

21 Towatari M, Yanada M, Usui N, *et al.* Combination of intensive chemotherapy and imatinib can rapidly induce high-quality complete remission for a majority of patients with newly diagnosed *BCR–ABL*-positive acute lymphoblastic leukemia. *Blood* 2004;104:3507–12.

22 Wassmann B, Pfeifer H, Goekbuget N, *et al.* Alternating versus concurrent schedules of imatinib and chemotherapy as front-line therapy for Philadelphia-positive acute lymphoblastic leukemia (Ph+ ALL). *Blood* 2006;108:1469–77.

23 Yanada M, Takeuchi J, Sugiura I, *et al.* High complete remission rate and promising outcome by combination of imatinib and chemotherapy for newly diagnosed *BCR–ABL*-positive acute lymphoblastic leukemia: a phase II study by the Japan Adult Leukemia Study Group. *J Clin Oncol* 2006;24:460–6.

24 de Labarthe A, Rousselot P, Huguet-Rigal F, *et al.* Imatinib combined with induction or consolidation chemotherapy in patients with de novo Philadelphia chromosome-positive acute lymphoblastic leukemia: results of the GRAAPH-2003 study. *Blood* 2007;109:1408–13.

25 Lee S, Kim YJ, Min CK, *et al.* The effect of first-line imatinib interim therapy on the outcome of allogeneic stem cell transplantation in adults with newly diagnosed Philadelphia chromosome-positive acute lymphoblastic leukemia. *Blood* 2005;105:3449–57.

26 Gokbuget N, Arnold R, Buechner T, *et al.* Intensification of induction and consolidation improves only subgroups of adult ALL: Analysis of 1200 patients in the GMALL study 05/93. *Am Soc Hematol* 2001;98:Abstract 3338.

27 Blaise D, Gaspard MH, Stoppa AM, *et al.* Allogeneic or autologous bone marrow transplantation for acute lymphoblastic leukemia in first complete remission. *Bone Marrow Transplant* 1990;5:7–12.

28 Wingard JR, Piantadosi S, Santos GW, *et al.* Allogeneic bone marrow transplantation for patients with high-risk acute lymphoblastic leukemia. *J Clin Oncol* 1990;8:820–30.

29 Chao NJ, Forman SJ, Schmidt GM, *et al.* Allogeneic bone marrow transplantation for high-risk acute lymphoblastic leukemia during first complete remission. *Blood* 1991;78:1923–7.

30 Doney K, Fisher LD, Appelbaum FR, *et al.* Treatment of adult acute lymphoblastic leukemia with allogeneic bone marrow transplantation. Multivariate analysis of factors affecting acute graft-versus-host disease, relapse, and relapse-free survival. *Bone Marrow Transplant* 1991;7:453–9.

31 Sutton L, Kuentz M, Cordonnier C, *et al.* Allogeneic bone marrow transplantation for adult acute lymphoblastic leuke-

mia in first complete remission: factors predictive of transplant-related mortality and influence of total body irradiation modalities. *Bone Marrow Transplant* 1993;12:583–9.

32 De Witte T, Awwad B, Boezeman J, *et al*. Role of allogenic bone marrow transplantation in adolescent or adult patients with acute lymphoblastic leukemia or lymphoblastic lymphoma in first remission. *Bone Marrow Transplant* 1994;14:767–74.

33 Wetzler M, Dodge RK, Mrozek K, *et al*. Prospective karyotype analysis in adult acute lymphoblastic leukemia: the cancer and leukemia Group B experience. *Blood* 1999;93:3983–93.

34 Matthews DC, Appelbaum FR, Eary JF, *et al*. Phase I study of (131)I-antiCD45 antibody plus cyclophosphamide and total body irradiation for advanced acute leukemia and myelodysplastic syndrome. *Blood* 1999;94:1237–47.

35 Thomas X, Boiron JM, Huguet F, *et al*. Outcome of treatment in adults with acute lymphoblastic leukemia: analysis of the LALA-94 trial. *J Clin Oncol* 2004;22:4075–86.

36 Goldstone AH, Richards SM, Lazarus HM, *et al*. In adults with standard-risk acute lymphoblastic leukemia, the greatest benefit is achieved from a matched sibling allogeneic transplantation in first complete remission, and an autologous transplantation is less effective than conventional consolidation/maintenance chemotherapy in all patients: final results of the International ALL Trial (MRC UKALL XII/ECOG E2993). *Blood* 2008;111:1827–33.

37 Ribera JM, Oriol A, Bethencourt C, *et al*. Comparison of intensive chemotherapy, allogeneic or autologous stem cell transplantation as post-remission treatment for adult patients with high-risk acute lymphoblastic leukemia. Results of the PETHEMA ALL-93 trial. *Haematologica* 2005;90:1346–56.

38 Labar B, Suciu S, Zittoun R, *et al*. Allogeneic stem cell transplantation in acute lymphoblastic leukemia and non-Hodgkin's lymphoma for patients <or = 50 years old in first complete remission: results of the EORTC ALL-3 trial. *Haematologica* 2004;89:809–17.

39 Gupta V, Yi QL, Brandwein J, *et al*. The role of allogeneic bone marrow transplantation in adult patients below the age of 55 years with acute lymphoblastic leukemia in first complete remission: a donor vs no donor comparison. *Bone Marrow Transplant* 2004;33:397–404.

40 Hunault M, Harousseau JL, Delain M, *et al*. Better outcome of adult acute lymphoblastic leukemia after early genoidentical allogeneic bone marrow transplantation (BMT) than after late high-dose therapy and autologous BMT: a GOELAMS trial. *Blood* 2004;104:3028–37.

41 Petersdorf EW, Hansen JA, Martin PJ, *et al*. Major-histocompatibility-complex class I alleles and antigens in hematopoietic-cell transplantation. *N Engl J Med* 2001;345:1794–800.

42 Kiehl MG, Kraut L, Schwerdtfeger R, *et al*. Outcome of allogeneic hematopoietic stem-cell transplantation in adult patients with acute lymphoblastic leukemia: no difference in related compared with unrelated transplant in first complete remission. *J Clin Oncol* 2004;22:2816–25.

43 Doney K, Hagglund H, Leisenring W, Chauncey T, Appelbaum FR, Storb R. Predictive factors for outcome of allogeneic hematopoietic cell transplantation for adult acute lymphoblastic leukemia. *Biol Blood Marrow Transplant* 2003;9:472–81.

44 Fielding AK, Richards SM, Chopra R, *et al*. Outcome of 609 adults after relapse of acute lymphoblastic leukemia (ALL); an MRC UKALL12/ECOG 2993 study. *Blood* 2007;109:944–50.

45 Greinix HT, Reiter E, Keil F, *et al*. Leukemia-free survival and mortality in patients with refractory or relapsed acute leukemia given marrow transplants from sibling and unrelated donors. *Bone Marrow Transplant* 1998;21:673–8.

46 Martino R, Bellido M, Brunet S, *et al*. Intensive salvage chemotherapy for primary refractory or first relapsed adult acute lymphoblastic leukemia: results of a prospective trial. *Haematologica* 1999;84:505–10.

47 Forman SJ, Schmidt GM, Nademanee AP, *et al*. Allogeneic bone marrow transplantation as therapy for primary induction failure for patients with acute leukemia. *J Clin Oncol* 1991;9:1570–4.

48 Biggs JC, Horowitz MM, Gale RP, *et al*. Bone marrow transplants may cure patients with acute leukemia never achieving remission with chemotherapy. *Blood* 1992;80:1090–3.

49 Thomas DA, Kantarjian H, Smith TL, *et al*. Primary refractory and relapsed adult acute lymphoblastic leukemia: characteristics, treatment results, and prognosis with salvage therapy. *Cancer* 1999;86:1216–30.

50 Snyder DS, Nademanee AP, O'Donnell MR, *et al*. Long-term follow-up of 23 patients with Philadelphia chromosome-positive acute lymphoblastic leukemia treated with allogeneic bone marrow transplant in first complete remission. *Leukemia* 1999;13:2053–8.

51 Fielding AK, Rowe JM, Richards SM, *et al*. Prospective outcome data on 267 unselected adult patients with Philadelphia chromosome-positive acute lymphoblastic leukemia confirms superiority of allogeneic transplantation over chemotherapy in the pre-imatinib era: results from the International ALL Trial MRC UKALLXII/ECOG-2993. *Blood* 2009;113:4489–96.

52 Cornelissen JJ, Carston M, Kollman C, *et al*. Unrelated marrow transplantation for adult patients with poor-risk acute lymphoblastic leukemia: strong graft-versus-leukemia effect and risk factors determining outcome. *Blood* 2001;97:1572–7.

53 Druker BJ, Tamura S, Buchdunger E, *et al*. Effects of a selective inhibitor of the Abl tyrosine kinase on the growth of *BCR–ABL* positive cells. *Nat Med* 1996;2:561–6.

54 Druker BJ, Sawyers CL, Kantarjian H, *et al*. Activity of a specific inhibitor of the Bcr–Abl tyrosine kinase in the blast crisis of chronic myeloid leukemia and acute lymphoblastic leukemia with the Philadelphia chromosome. *N Engl J Med* 2001;344:1038–42.

55 Ottmann OG, Druker BJ, Sawyers CL, *et al*. A phase 2 study of imatinib in patients with relapsed or refractory Philadelphia chromosome-positive acute lymphoid leukemias. *Blood* 2002;100:1965–71.

56 Kano Y, Akutsu M, Tsunoda S, *et al*. *In vitro* cytotoxic effects of a tyrosine kinase inhibitor STI571 in combination with commonly used antileukemic agents. *Blood* 2001;97:1999–2007.

57 Hahn T, Wall D, Camitta B, *et al*. The role of cytotoxic therapy with hematopoietic stem cell transplantation in the therapy of acute lymphoblastic leukemia in adults: an evidence-based review. *Biol Blood Marrow Transplant* 2006;12:1–30.

58 Marks DI, Aversa F, Lazarus HM. Alternative donor transplants for adult acute lymphoblastic leukemia: a comparison of the three major options. *Bone Marrow Transplant* 2006;38:467–75.

59 Verneris MR, Brunstein C, Defor TE, Barker J, Weisdorf DJ. *Risk of relapse after umbilical cord blood transplantation in patients with acute leukemia: Marked reduction in recipients of two units.* International Umbilical Cord Transplantation Symposium: Los Angeles, CA, 2006.
60 Marks DI, Forman SJ, Blume KG, *et al.* A comparison of cyclophosphamide and total body irradiation with etoposide and total body irradiation as conditioning regimens for patients undergoing sibling allografting for acute lymphoblastic leukemia in first or second complete remission. *Biol Blood Marrow Transplant* 2006;12:438–53.
61 Blume KG, Kopecky KJ, Henslee-Downey JP, *et al.* A prospective randomized comparison of total body irradiation-etoposide versus busulfan-cyclophosphamide as preparatory regimens for bone marrow transplantation in patients with leukemia who were not in first remission: a Southwest Oncology Group study. *Blood* 1993;81:2187–93.
62 Buchmann I, Bunjes D, Kotzerke J, *et al.* Myeloablative radioimmunotherapy with Re-188-antiCD66-antibody for conditioning of high-risk leukemia patients prior to stem cell transplantation: biodistribution, biokinetics and immediate toxicities. *Cancer Biother Radiopharm* 2002;17:151–63.
63 Kebriaei P, Saliba RM, Ma C, *et al.* Allogeneic hematopoietic stem cell transplantation after rituximab-containing myeloablative preparative regimen for acute lymphoblastic leukemia. *Bone Marrow Transplant* 2006;38:203–9.
64 Novitzky N, Thomas V, Hale G, Waldmann H. Ex vivo depletion of T cells from bone marrow grafts with CAMPATH-1 in acute leukemia: graft-versus-host disease and graft-versus-leukemia effect. *Transplantation* 1999;67:620–6.
65 Sanchez-Garcia J, Serrano J, Gomez P, *et al.* The impact of acute and chronic graft-versus-host disease on normal and malignant B-lymphoid precursors after allogeneic stem cell transplantation for B-lineage acute lymphoblastic leukemia. *Haematologica* 2006;91:340–7.
66 Niederwieser D, Gentilini C, Hegenbart U, *et al.* Allogeneic hematopoietic cell transplantation (HCT) following reduced-intensity conditioning in patients with acute leukemias. *Crit Rev Oncol Hematol* 2005;56:275–81.
67 Martino R, Giralt S, Caballero MD, *et al.* Allogeneic hematopoietic stem cell transplantation with reduced-intensity conditioning in acute lymphoblastic leukemia: a feasibility study. *Haematologica* 2003;88:555–60.
68 Champlin RE, Schmitz N, Horowitz MM, *et al.* Blood stem cells compared with bone marrow as a source of hematopoietic cells for allogeneic transplantation. IBMTR Histocompatibility and Stem Cell Sources Working Committee and the European Group for Blood and Marrow Transplantation (EBMT). *Blood* 2000;95:3702–9.
69 Bortin MM, Truitt RL, Rimm AA, Bach FH. Graft-versus-leukemia reactivity induced by alloimmunisation without augmentation of graft-versus-host reactivity. *Nature* 1979;281: 490–1.
70 Barrett AJ, Malkovska V. Graft-versus-leukemia: understanding and using the alloimmune response to treat haematological malignancies. *Br J Haematol* 1996;93:754–61.
71 Horowitz MM, Gale RP, Sondel PM, *et al.* Graft-versus-leukemia reactions after bone marrow transplantation. *Blood* 1990;75:555–62.
72 Appelbaum FR. Hematopoietic cell transplantation as immunotherapy. *Nature* 2001;411:385–9.
73 Sullivan KM, Weiden PL, Storb R, *et al.* Influence of acute and chronic graft-versus-host disease on relapse and survival after bone marrow transplantation from HLA-identical siblings as treatment of acute and chronic leukemia. *Blood* 1989;73: 1720–8.
74 Appelbaum FR. Graft versus leukemia (GVL) in the therapy of acute lymphoblastic leukemia (ALL). *Leukemia* 1997;11 (Suppl.4):S15–17.
75 Collins RH, Jr., Shpilberg O, Drobyski WR, *et al.* Donor leukocyte infusions in 140 patients with relapsed malignancy after allogeneic bone marrow transplantation. *J Clin Oncol* 1997;15: 433–44.
76 Kolb HJ, Schattenberg A, Goldman JM, *et al.* Graft-versus-leukemia effect of donor lymphocyte transfusions in marrow grafted patients. *Blood* 1995;86:2041–50.
77 Slavin S, Naparstek E, Nagler A, *et al.* Allogeneic cell therapy with donor peripheral blood cells and recombinant human interleukin-2 to treat leukemia relapse after allogeneic bone marrow transplantation. *Blood* 1996;87:2195–204.
78 Socie G, Stone JV, Wingard JR, *et al.* Long-term survival and late deaths after allogeneic bone marrow transplantation. Late Effects Working Committee of the International Bone Marrow Transplant Registry. *N Engl J Med* 1999;341:14–21.
79 Kolb HJ, Socie G, Duell T, *et al.* Malignant neoplasms in long-term survivors of bone marrow transplantation. Late Effects Working Party of the European Cooperative Group for Blood and Marrow Transplantation and the European Late Effect Project Group. *Ann Intern Med* 1999;131:738–44.
80 Friedman DL, Rovo A, Leisenring W, *et al.* Increased risk of breast cancer among survivors of allogeneic hematopoietic cell transplantation: a report from the FHCRC and the EBMT-Late Effect Working Party. *Blood* 2008;111:939–44.
81 Broers S, Kaptein AA, Le Cessie S, Fibbe W, Hengeveld MW. Psychological functioning and quality of life following bone marrow transplantation: a 3-year follow-up study. *J Psychosom Res* 2000;48:11–21.
82 Harder H, Cornelissen JJ, Van Gool AR, Duivenvoorden HJ, Eijkenboom WM, van den Bent MJ. Cognitive functioning and quality of life in long-term adult survivors of bone marrow transplantation. *Cancer* 2002;95:183–92.

Part 6
Chronic Myeloid Leukemia

Chapter 21
Pathophysiology of Chronic Myeloid Leukemia

Agnes S. M. Yong[1] *and Junia V. Melo*[2]
[1]National Heart, Lung, and Blood Institute, National Institutes of Health, Bethesda, Maryland, USA
[2]Institute of Medical and Veterinary Science, Adelaide, Australia

Introduction

Chronic myeloid leukemia (CML) was the first human cancer to be associated with a consistent chromosomal abnormality [1]—the Philadelphia (Ph) chromosome (22q–), generated by a reciprocal translocation between chromosomes 9 and 22 [2]. The Ph chromosome contains the hallmark *BCR–ABL* hybrid gene, which encodes a tyrosine kinase with excessive activity compared with the product of its normal *ABL* counterpart [3]. *BCR–ABL*$^+$ bone marrow transplanted into mice caused a CML-like disease, suggesting that the presence of the *BCR–ABL* gene is sufficient to cause CML [4]. The Bcr–Abl oncoprotein is responsible for most of the clinical features of CML, as confirmed by the resolution of the malignant phenotype when this enzyme is blocked by the tyrosine kinase inhibitor (TKI) imatinib *in vitro* [5] as well as *in vivo* [6,7].

The molecular biology of chronic myeloid leukemia

The reciprocal t(9;22)(q34;q11) translocation in CML is initiated in the multipotent hematopoietic progenitor. However, the trigger for its formation is unknown in the majority of patients. Ionizing radiation is the only confirmed risk factor for CML from epidemiologic studies of atomic bomb survivors [8,9] and patients receiving radiotherapy [10], as well as from *in vitro* studies [11]. Furthermore, the topographic arrangement of chromosomes 9 and 22 during a critical period of the cell cycle favors the juxtaposition of the partner *ABL* and *BCR* genes that may predispose to *BCR–ABL* formation [12,13].

The breakpoints within the *ABL* gene occur in a 5′ segment that extends over 300 kB, typically within intronic sequences [14]. The most common breakpoints form between the two alternative first exons of *ABL*, 1b and 1a, resulting in a *BCR–ABL* fusion gene containing exon 1a alone or in combination with exon 1b, or containing neither of the alternative first exons. Splicing of the hybrid *BCR–ABL* transcript yields an mRNA that consists of *BCR* exons directly fused to *ABL* exon a2. The *BCR* breakpoint in 95% of patients with CML and one-third of all patients with acute lymphoblastic leukemia (ALL) occurs within a 5.8-kB region known as the major breakpoint cluster region (Bcr), which consists of five exons, e12 to e16 (formerly b1 to b5). The majority of *BCR* breakpoints form within introns downstream of exons 13 or 14 (previously b2 and b3, respectively). Hybrid *BCR–ABL* mRNA transcripts e13a2 or e14a2 consist of an 8.5-kB sequence that encodes the 210 kD Bcr–Abl fusion protein (Figure 21.1).

In the majority of patients with Ph$^+$ ALL, the minority of patients with CML, and rarely in patients with acute myeloid leukemia (AML), the *BCR* breakpoint occurs upstream of the major Bcr in the intronic area known as the minor Bcr. This produces a hybrid *BCR–ABL* mRNA of 7 kB, which consists of the fusion of *BCR* exon e1 with *ABL* exon a2 and encodes a 190-kD Bcr–Abl fusion protein. Rarely, other breakpoints in the *BCR* gene have been reported, including the micro-Bcr between exons e19 and e20, transcribing an e19a2 *BCR–ABL* fusion transcript that is translated into a 230 kD oncoprotein, associated in many cases with chronic neutrophilic leukemia [14,15].

Although a functional *BCR–ABL* gene generates the leukemic phenotype, *BCR–ABL* transcripts are found in healthy individuals by using sensitive techniques that can detect one *BCR–ABL* transcript in 10^8 cells [16,17], suggesting that *BCR–ABL* alone may not be sufficient to effect malignant transformation in some individuals. The presence of *BCR–ABL* without manifestation of disease may be interpreted as a result of (i) the hybrid gene encoding a truncated, non-functional fusion protein; (ii) the fusion gene being formed in a cell incapable of self-renewal or clonal expansion; or (iii) the cells that bear this abnormality being recognized by the immune system and destroyed prior to further proliferation. The report that individuals who express the human leukocyte antigen (HLA)-B8 with or without HLA-A3 may be protected

Leukemias: Principles and Practice of Therapy, 1st edition. Edited by S. Faderl and H. Kantarjian.

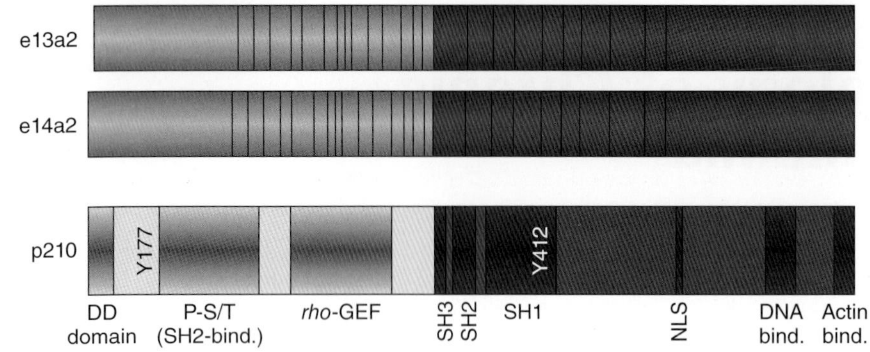

Figure 21.1 Schematic representation of the commonest forms of the *BCR–ABL* oncogene product of the t(9;22)(q34;q11) translocation in CML, transcribing mRNA with e13a2 or e14a2 junctions. The encoded p210 kD Bcr–Abl oncoprotein contains functional domains from the amino-terminus of Bcr (dimerization [DD], Src homology [SH2]-binding [SH2-bind] and the *rho* GTP-GDP exchange factor domains [*rho*-GEF]) and the carboxy-terminus of Abl (only the SH3, SH2, and SH1 regions and the DNA- and actin-binding domains [DNA bind., Actin bind.] are shown). Tyrosine 177 in the Bcr and tyrosine 412 in the Abl regions are important for docking of adaptor proteins and for Bcr–Abl autophosphorylation, respectively.

against the development of CML appears to support the latter hypothesis [18]. Conversely, *BCR–ABL* may require a cooperating genetic lesion in some individuals prior to the initiation of CML [15]. A multistep pathogenesis of CML is suggested by the demonstration of clonality in Ph^- Epstein–Barr virus-transformed B-cell lines derived from a patient with Ph^+ CML [19]. The finding of clonal chromosomal abnormalities in Ph^- bone marrow cells of patients who have a complete cytogenetic remission with imatinib treatment appears to support this [20,21].

The *BCR* gene is ubiquitously expressed, with the highest mRNA levels found in brain and hematopoeitic cells [22]. The normal 160 kD Bcr protein is expressed mainly in early myeloid progenitors [22] and has several structural motifs that are retained in the Bcr–Abl chimeric protein (Figure 21.1). The first N-terminal *BCR* exon is critically significant for leukemogenesis as its encoded sequence is present in all known Bcr–Abl fusion proteins. This region contains the oligomerization domain, a serine/threonine kinase, whose known substrates are Bcr and Bap-1 (a member of the 14-3-3 family of proteins) and two serine-rich boxes containing Src homology (SH2)-binding domains [22]. The coiled-coil oligomerization domain is essential for the dimerization of Bcr–Abl and the subsequent activation of its kinase activity. It also enhances the F-actin binding capacity of Bcr–Abl and may be responsible for its cytoplasmic localization [23]. The binding of SH2 domains, which are highly conserved non-catalytic regions of approximately 100 amino acids, to SH2-binding sites (which consist of three to five amino acids including a phosphotyrosine) is important in the assembly of signal-transduction complexes. The SH2 regions of Abl bind to the SH2-binding domains of Bcr–Abl via phosphorylated serines and threonines, and this interaction is essential for the oncogenic activation of Bcr–Abl. Phosphorylation of Bcr–Abl on tyrosine 177 forms a binding site for Grb-2, which is an adaptor molecule involved in the activation of the Ras signal transduction pathway [24]. The central *Rho*-guanidine exchange factor (GEF) domain stimulates the exchange of guanidine triphosphate (GTP) for guanidine diphosphate (GDP) on Rho proteins, which subsequently coordinate diverse functions including actin cytoskeletal, transcriptional, and cell-cycle regulation [25].

The *ABL* gene is also ubiquitously expressed and is the human homolog of the *v-abl* oncogene in the Abelson murine leukemia virus that targets early B-cells [26,27]. Abl, the encoded non-receptor tyrosine kinase, is a 145 kD protein with two isoforms arising from alternative splicing of the first exon [3]. Several structural domains in the normal Abl are also retained in the Bcr–Abl chimeric protein. These include the SH1 domain, which has tyrosine kinase function, the SH2 domain that binds phosphotyrosine-containing consensus sites, and the SH3 domain that binds to proline-rich consensus sequences in proteins such as Crk and Crkl. In contrast to Src, Abl contains actin- and DNA-binding domains. Although Abl is mainly found in the nucleus of most cells and is able to shuttle between the nucleus and cytoplasm, in hematopoietic cells a significant fraction is localized to the cytoplasm and associates with F-actin [28,29]. The many cellular functions of Abl include cell-cycle inhibition, response to genotoxic stress, and signal transduction from growth factor receptors and integrins [15].

The activity of normal Abl is tightly regulated, as shown by its inability to transform fibroblasts or hematopoietic cells when overexpressed [29]. Autoinhibition of Abl is maintained by its SH2 and SH3 domains, which are bound to the kinase domain distal from the active site [30,31]. This inactive conformation is stabilized by the interaction of the N-terminal myristoyl group with a hydrophobic groove at the base of the kinase domain, which induces a sharp bend of the C-terminal helix of the kinase. Thus, the N-terminal cap region of Abl is crucial for its autoregulation. Activation of Abl also results from mutations in the linker between the SH2 and SH1 domains, or mutations or positional changes in the SH3 domain [15].

Transcription of the *BCR–ABL* hybrid gene is under the control of the *BCR* promoter. The fusion of N-terminal Bcr sequences to the Abl sequence deregulates the tyrosine kinase through a series of events involving the combination of (i) Bcr–Abl dimerization effected by the Bcr coiled-coil oligomerization domain, (ii) transphosphorylation of a regulatory tyrosine in the kinase activation loop in the Abl portion of the oncoprotein (Figure 21.1, tyrosine 412), and (iii) phosphorylation of tyrosine 245 in the SH2-kinase domain linker. The latter disrupts the interaction with the SH3 domain and results in full activation of the kinase [15]. The TKI imatinib binds to the inactive form of the kinase. Thus, mutations that impair the conserved autoregulatory mechanism and, as a consequence, favor the active conformation lead to resistance to imatinib. Dasatinib, a newer TKI that has entered clinical practice, has the ability to bind both active and inactive kinase forms and is effective in imatinib-resistant cells [32].

Pathogenetic consequences of Bcr–Abl

The constitutive activation of the Bcr–Abl tyrosine kinase results in several abnormalities that characterize the CML cell: (i) altered cell adhesion; (ii) activation and perturbation of several downstream signal transduction pathways; (iii) inhibition of apoptosis; and (iv) induction of proteasomal degradation of key proteins. Biologic pathways impacted by Bcr–Abl include the activation of Ras, MAPK, JAK-STAT, PI3K, and Myc pathways, the molecular details of which are extensively reviewed elsewhere [15]. The myriad downstream effects of Bcr–Abl tyrosine kinase is augmented by its primary cytoplasmic location, which permits it to perturb cellular processes through its actions on multiple substrates [28,33].

In its usual role as a cytoplasmic oncoprotein, Bcr–Abl is a potent inhibitor of apoptosis [34]. The enforced nuclear localization of kinase active Bcr–Abl using leptomycin-B to block its nuclear export is proapoptotic [35,36]. The antiapoptotic effect of Bcr–Abl is also independent of its tyrosine kinase activity [37]. Thus, cells that escape the effects of TKIs, such as primitive quiescent stem cells [38,39], may be sustained in an antiapoptotic state owing to alternative mechanisms and may retain the ability to undergo further transformation, resulting in subsequent disease progression.

The transforming potential of Bcr–Abl is enhanced by its ability to induce the proteasomal degradation of diverse proteins. Among these are the Abl interactor proteins, which antagonise the oncogenic activity of Abl [40], and the DNA-dependent protein kinase catalytic subunit (DNA-PKcs) component of the DNA-dependent protein kinase complex that is downregulated in cells from patients with CML [41]. Downregulation of the cyclin-dependent kinase inhibitor p27 by Bcr–Abl by way of both PI3K-dependent and independent mechanisms also involves proteasomal degradation [42]. The p53/Mdm2 pathway induces cell-cycle arrest or apoptosis in response to genotoxic stress. Although mutations in the *p53* gene are rare in CML, Mdm2, a key regulator of p53 function, has been shown to be upregulated by Bcr–Abl [43]. In addition to inhibiting *p53* transcription, Mdm2 binds to the p53 protein and targets it to proteasomal degradation. Bcr–Abl maintains a high Mdm2 level by stabilizing it against proteasomal degradation [43], thus inhibiting apoptosis. Overexpression of Mdm2 may also further compromise the genomic stability of Bcr–Abl$^+$ cells and result in progressive DNA damage.

The clinical evolution of chronic myeloid leukemia

The median age of patients with CML at diagnosis is around 60 years, with <10% diagnosed under the age of 20 [44]. CML is a triphasic disease that typically presents in chronic phase (CP), when the disease generally responds well to treatment. Prior to the advent of imatinib, CP lasted 4–5 years before terminating in the usually fatal acute phase, blast crisis (BC), which is highly resistant to standard chemotherapy (Table 21.1). BC is usually preceded by a poorly defined intermediate stage—"accelerated phase"— that is less responsive to therapy than the CP [44]. Compared with previous drug therapy, patients on imatinib have higher rates of Ph chromosome elimination in all stages of CML [46–48], better overall survival [49,50], and a decreased incidence of BC [51]. The

Table 21.1 Criteria for accelerated phase and blast crisis in chronic myeloid leukemia [45].

Accelerated phase[a]
1. Persistent or increasing WBC count (>10 × 10^9/L)
2. Persistent or increasing splenomegaly
3. Persistent thrombocytosis (>1000 × 10^9/L)
4. Persistent thrombocytopenia (<100 × 10^9/L) unrelated to therapy
5. Clonal cytogenetic evolution not present at the time of diagnosis
6. ≥20% basophils in peripheral blood
7. 10–19% blasts in peripheral blood or bone marrow
Blast crisis
1. ≥20% blasts in peripheral blood or bone marrow
2. Extramedullary blast proliferation

WBC, white blood cell.

[a]Criteria 1–5 are more associated with a transition between the chronic phase and accelerated phase; criteria 6–7 usually indicate the transition between accelerated phase and blast crisis.

only curative treatment for CML is an allogeneic stem-cell transplantation (allo SCT), which is applicable to only a minority of patients. However, allo SCT is second-line therapy in the majority of patients diagnosed in the imatinib era in affluent countries [52,53], although it is first-line therapy in many middle- and low-income countries for prevailing economic reasons [54]. Increasingly, patients with low-risk CML are reported to have a much better survival with imatinib treatment, although this treatment can not yet be considered a "cure" [51,55]. The threat of progression to BC, which was inevitable with previous therapy such as interferon-α and/or hydroxyurea, seems to be transmuted with imatinib [51]. In patients with a good response to imatinib, *BCR–ABL* transcripts continue to decline steadily after several years' follow-up [56]. However, *BCR–ABL* transcripts [50] and Bcr–Abl$^+$ CD34$^+$ progenitors [57] are still found in a substantial proportion of imatinib-responders, and these residual leukemia cells retain the potential of blastic transformation. Patients in the CP who are in molecular remission on imatinib, without detectable *BCR–ABL* transcripts for as long as 45 consecutive months, were still susceptible to disease relapse upon discontinuation of the drug [58,59]. The emergence of resistance to imatinib, owing to various mechanisms such as mutations of the kinase domain preventing proper binding of the drug [60] or amplification of *BCR–ABL* [61], has led to the development of more efficacious second-generation TKIs, of which dasatinib and nilotinib are preeminent [32]. Furthermore, as quiescent leukemic stem cells in CML are unaffected by imatinib [38,57], dasatinib [39], or nilotinib [62], new therapeutic strategies that target them are being explored [63].

Disease heterogeneity

A highly intriguing feature in patients with CML is the clinical heterogeneity of the duration of disease between transformation from CP to BC, which may be as short as a few months or as long as 20 years [64,65]. The Sokal and Hasford (Euro) clinical scores were devised to prognosticate patients from diagnosis and subsequently individualize therapy [66,67]. Although markers of clonal evolution, such as additional chromosomal abnormalities represented predominantly by iso17q and double Ph chromosomes, are identified *ab initio* in some patients [68–70], in the majority the features of disease heterogeneity remain a mystery. Deletions adjacent to the translocation breakpoint on the derivative 9q$^+$ chromosome, which are detectable from diagnosis, were originally associated with an adverse prognosis in CML [71–74]. However, recent analyses suggest that imatinib treatment may abrogate this deleterious effect [75,76].

Biologic features, such as the effects of autocrine growth-factor regulation of CML progenitors via interleukin-3 and granulocyte colony-stimulating factor (G-CSF), also vary between different CP patients at diagnosis [77–79]. The differential encoding of mRNA transcripts (e13a2 vs. e14a2) and cognate p210 fusion proteins, arising from *BCR–ABL* hybrid genes formed by different breakpoints in *BCR*, have no prognostic significance [15]. Telomere lengths, which are already shorter in CML cells than in normal cells, are further shortened in CP patients with early disease progression [80–82], suggesting a correlation with disease evolution.

Although a functional *BCR–ABL* gene is essential to initiate CML, additional factors may shape its biologic behavior. CML stem cells exhibit a hierarchy of transplantable leukemic cells [83] analogous to those seen in AML, where different functional subsets of leukemic stem cells with varying self-renewal and differentiation capacity exist [84,85]. Gene expression profiling of CD34$^+$ progenitor cells from patients with CP-CML reveals a differential dominance of varying subsets of CD34$^+$ progenitors that are present from diagnosis [86]. The combination of lower CD7 expression and higher elastase or proteinase 3 expression in CD34$^+$ progenitors is highly predictive of longer survival [86]. Interestingly, both elastase and proteinase 3 can elicit cytotoxic T-lymphocyte (CTL) responses that selectively lyse CML cells [87,88]. However, high expression of both these proteins is inversely correlated to the presence of proteinase 3- or elastase-associated peptide-specific native CTLs in patients with CML [89], most probably resulting from a tolerance mechanism where high avidity specific CTLs are deleted by the patient's immune system [90]. Thus, the better prognosis conferred by a higher expression of proteinase 3 and elastase may be due to identification of patients with CML who have more differentiated leukemic progenitors. Furthermore, CD7, a surface marker on immature myeloid progenitors [91], is associated with early disease progression and poor prognosis in CML-CP [92,93], as in AML and myelodysplastic syndrome [94,95]. A larger population of CD34$^+$ CD7$^+$ progenitor cells, which may be more poorly differentiated, may be more likely to harbor cells that have the ability to transform to BC [96]. Some of these cells may have a greater self-renewal capacity and higher risk of random mutation. The finding that CP patients who progress more rapidly to BC have a higher expression of one of the stem-cell renewal regulators, the polycomb group gene *BMI1*, at diagnosis seems to support this view [97].

Pathobiology of transformation from chronic phase to blast crisis

The transformation from CP to BC appears to be the consequence of a multistep pathogenetic progression involving differentiation arrest, genomic instability, telomere shortening, and loss of tumor-suppressor functions [98]. CML progenitor cells continue to express *BCR–ABL* upon progression to BC, with amplification of both mRNA and protein [99]. CML progenitors in BC still retain dependence on Bcr–Abl but, in clinical practice, rapidly develop resistance to TKIs [52,53], which may be related to their increased Bcr–Abl expression [99].

Although CML is initiated in the multipotent hematopoietic stem cell, recent data suggest that a committed granulocyte-macrophage progenitor (GMP) is responsible for myeloid blastic transformation [100,101]. The reduction in the incidence of BC in patients with good clinical responses to imatinib therapy [51] and mathematic modeling of disease kinetics appear to support this [102,103]. The acquisition of stem-cell characteristics by GMP in BC appears to occur through activation of nuclear β-catenin [100], although a direct molecular connection between Bcr–Abl and the Wnt-β-catenin pathway is yet to be unraveled. Furthermore, other genes associated with stem-cell renewal, such as *BMI1*, are also elevated in advanced-phase CML and, when overexpressed in CP, correlated with a more rapid disease progression to BC [97]. The presence of these proteins associated with self-renewal in BC cells characterizes and identifies their stem cell-like phenotype, but does not specify the trigger behind the transformation from CP to BC.

Differentiation arrest

In BC, undifferentiated leukemic blast cells accumulate in a background of mature myeloid progenitors and granulocytes. In the majority of patients with CML, the number of blasts in the peripheral blood rises steadily, usually over years, with the accelerated phase bridging the transition between CP and BC. This observation implies a differentiation arrest that may be instigated by several critical steps involving major genes that are crucial to hematopoietic differentiation, such as CEBPα—a transcription factor and a key regulator of myeloid differentiation that activates G-CSF receptor transcription [104,105]. In BC cells, Bcr–Abl inhibits the translation of CEBPα by inducing hnRNP E2, a poly(rC) binding protein that interacts with CEBPα mRNA [106]. Inactivating mutations in *CEBPA* are found in a minority of patients with AML [107] and confer a favorable prognosis [108]. However, similar *CEBPA* mutations are not associated with CML-BC [109].

Transformation to lymphoid BC appears to have a similar molecular pathogenesis as Ph^+ ALL, involving deletions of *IKZF1*, which are not found in CP-CML [110]. *IKZF1* encodes the transcription factor Ikaros, an essential component of normal lymphoid development.

Genomic instability

Both failure of genome surveillance and DNA repair deficiencies are present in CML, resulting in an overall genomic instability. This state predisposes CML cells to acquiring mutations, which subsequently drive blastic transformation. DNA damage sensors, such as ataxia telangiectasia and RAD3-related (ATR) nuclear protein kinases, are inhibited, resulting in inappropriate DNA replication despite DNA damage [98]. Double-stranded DNA break repair, by either non-homologous end-joining (NHEJ) or homologous recombination (HR), is defective in CML. A major effector of NHEJ, DNA PKcs, which is dependent on the proteasomal pathway for degradation, is downregulated in cells from patients with CML [41]. Bcr–Abl also upregulates the transcription of RAD51 and activates this DNA repair protein, with a net result of compromising the fidelity of HR DNA repair [98].

Loss of tumor-suppressor function

The dominance of the Bcr–Abl tyrosine kinase activity tends to eclipse other factors, such as the downregulation of tumor-suppressor functions in the pathobiology of CML. PP2A (protein phosphatase 2A) antagonises Bcr–Abl, and its inactivation is found in BC. Bcr–Abl inhibits PP2A indirectly by upregulating SET, the physiologic phosphoprotein inhibitor of PP2A [111]. The activation of PP2A by an immunomodulating drug, FTY720 (fingolimod), antagonizes Bcr–Abl activity and suppresses leukemogenesis in mice [112]. Fingolimod also suppresses Bcr–Abl in TKI-resistant CML cells, and is a promising therapeutic agent.

Challenges for the future

Although the majority of patients with CP-CML are effectively treated with TKIs, a significant proportion, particularly those in advanced-phase disease, acquire drug resistance (see Chapter 23) and are candidates for investigative treatments. Some of the prevailing questions facing clinician-scientists include "How could we eliminate CML cells not targeted in imatinib-responders"? "Can we cure CML without allo-SCT?" "Is the development of further targeted therapy the answer to managing resistance to TKIs?" and "How can we improve the outcome of BC"?

Targeting quiescent and primitive stem cells

The majority of patients with CML who have a complete cytogenetic response following imatinib therapy still harbor $Bcr–Abl^+$ progenitors [50,56,57]. Primitive and non-cycling (quiescent) CML progenitors are resistant to TKIs [38,39,62] through a variety of biologic mechanisms [113,114]. Stimulating quiescent cells to enter the cell cycle with G-CSF reduces the overall non-cycling cell population *in vitro* [115,116] but does not impact disease outcome in clinical practice [117]. Recently, a farnesyl transferase inhibitor, BMS-214662, was found to kill quiescent CML progenitors and BC-CML cells *in vitro*, and its effect was enhanced when combined with either imatinib or dasatinib [63], making it a promising agent for clinical development.

Immunotherapy using peptide vaccines directed against leukemia-specific or leukemia-associated antigens is another promising treatment modality [118]. In addition to Bcr–Abl, proteins such as WT1 (Wilms tumor 1), proteinase 3, and PRAME (preferentially expressed antigen of melanoma) are overexpressed in CML progenitors, and immunogenic peptides from these, which can elicit CTL responses that specifically kill CML cells [87,119,120], are entering clinical trials. WT1 and PR1-peptide vaccines in patients with CML have promising results [121–123] and the potential to target primitive CML progenitors [124]. The limitation of T-cell immunotherapy is the HLA-restricted nature of CTLs, with the majority of peptides being restricted to HLA-A*0201, which is more prevalent in Caucasian populations.

Advanced phase and blast crisis chronic myeloid leukemia

Despite the progress in CML therapy, advanced-phase disease, particularly BC, still confers a grim outlook. Even allo-SCT, the only "curative" treatment in CML, offers <20% overall survival for patients with BC [125], mainly because of relapse and refractory disease. Responses to TKIs in BC patients are usually short-lived. The potential in new drug discovery lies with exploration of the various non-tyrosine kinase associated pathways affected by Bcr–Abl, as recently shown with protein phosphatase [112,126], as well as maximizing immunotherapeutic options in the context of allo SCT [89], or as adjunct treatment with other pharmacologic agents. Ensuring that patients have the opportunity to undertake investigational treatment in clinical trials would further expedite our understanding of this disease.

References

1 Nowell PC, Hungerford DA. A minute chromosome in human chronic granulocytic leukemia. *Science* 1960;132:1497.

2 Rowley JD. Letter: A new consistent chromosomal abnormality in chronic myelogenous leukemia identified by quinacrine fluorescence and Giemsa staining. *Nature* 1973;243:290–3.

3 Deininger MW, Goldman JM, Melo JV. The molecular biology of chronic myeloid leukemia. *Blood* 2000;96:3343–56.

4 Daley GQ, Van Etten RA, Baltimore D. Induction of chronic myelogenous leukemia in mice by the P210 *BCR–ABL* gene of the Philadelphia chromosome. *Science* 1990;247:824–30.

5 Druker BJ, Tamura S, Buchdunger E, *et al*. Effects of a selective inhibitor of the Abl tyrosine kinase on the growth of *BCR–ABL* positive cells. *Nat Med* 1996;2:561–6.

6 Deininger MW, Goldman JM, Lydon N, Melo JV. The tyrosine kinase inhibitor CGP57148B selectively inhibits the growth of *BCR–ABL*-positive cells. *Blood* 1997;90:3691–8.

7 Druker BJ, Talpaz M, Resta DJ, *et al*. Efficacy and safety of a specific inhibitor of the Bcr–Abl tyrosine kinase in chronic myeloid leukemia. *N Engl J Med* 2001;344:1031–7.

8 Brill AB, Tomonaga M, Heyssel RM. Leukemia in man following exposure to ionizing radiation. A summary of the findings in Hiroshima and Nagasaki, and a comparison with other human experience. *Ann Intern Med* 1962;56:590–609.

9 Heyssel R, Brill AB, Woodbury LA, *et al*. Leukemia in Hiroshima atomic bomb survivors. *Blood* 1960;15:313–31.

10 Brown WM, Doll R. Mortality from cancer and other causes after radiotherapy for ankylosing spondylitis. *Br Med J* 1965; 5474:1327–32.

11 Deininger MW, Bose S, Gora-Tybor J, Yan XH, Goldman JM, Melo JV. Selective induction of leukemia-associated fusion genes by high-dose ionizing radiation. *Cancer Res* 1998;58: 421–5.

12 Neves H, Ramos C, da Silva MG, Parreira A, Parreira L. The nuclear topography of *ABL*, *BCR*, *PML*, and *RARalpha* genes: evidence for gene proximity in specific phases of the cell cycle and stages of hematopoietic differentiation. *Blood* 1999;93: 1197–207.

13 Anastasi J, Moinuddin R, Daugherty C. The juxtaposition of *ABL* with *BCR* and risk for fusion may come at the time of *BCR* replication in late S-phase. *Blood* 1999;94:1137–8.

14 Melo JV. The diversity of Bcr–Abl fusion proteins and their relationship to leukemia phenotype. *Blood* 1996;88:2375–84.

15 Melo JV, Deininger MW. Biology of chronic myelogenous leukemia–signaling pathways of initiation and transformation. *Hematol Oncol Clin North Am* 2004;18:545–68.

16 Bose S, Deininger M, Gora-Tybor J, Goldman JM, Melo JV. The presence of typical and atypical *BCR–ABL* fusion genes in leukocytes of normal individuals: biologic significance and implications for the assessment of minimal residual disease. *Blood* 1998;92:3362–7.

17 Biernaux C, Loos M, Sels A, Huez G, Stryckmans P. Detection of major *BCR–ABL* gene expression at a very low level in blood cells of some healthy individuals. *Blood* 1995;86:3118–22.

18 Posthuma EF, Falkenburg JH, Apperley JF, *et al*. HLA-B8 and HLA-A3 coexpressed with HLA-B8 are associated with a reduced risk of the development of chronic myeloid leukemia. The Chronic Leukemia Working Party of the EBMT. *Blood* 1999;93:3863–5.

19 Fialkow PJ, Martin PJ, Najfeld V, Penfold GK, Jacobson RJ, Hansen JA. Evidence for a multistep pathogenesis of chronic myelogenous leukemia. *Blood* 1981;58:158–63.

20 Jabbour E, Kantarjian HM, Abruzzo LV, *et al*. Chromosomal abnormalities in Philadelphia chromosome negative metaphases appearing during imatinib mesylate therapy in patients with newly diagnosed chronic myeloid leukemia in chronic phase. *Blood* 2007;110:2991–5.

21 Deininger MW, Cortes J, Paquette R, *et al*. The prognosis for patients with chronic myeloid leukemia who have clonal cytogenetic abnormalities in philadelphia chromosome-negative cells. *Cancer* 2007;110:1509–19.

22 Laurent E, Talpaz M, Kantarjian H, Kurzrock R. The *BCR* gene and philadelphia chromosome-positive leukemogenesis. *Cancer Res* 2001;61:2343–55.

23 McWhirter JR, Galasso DL, Wang JY. A coiled-coil oligomerization domain of Bcr is essential for the transforming function of Bcr–Abl oncoproteins. *Mol Cell Biol* 1993;13:7587–95.

24 Pendergast AM, Quilliam LA, Cripe LD, *et al*. *BCR–ABL*-induced oncogenesis is mediated by direct interaction with the SH2 domain of the GRB-2 adaptor protein. *Cell* 1993;75: 175–85.

25 Coleman ML, Marshall CJ, Olson MF. RAS and RHO GTPases in G1-phase cell-cycle regulation. *Nat Rev Mol Cell Biol* 2004;5: 355–66.

26 Rosenberg NE, Clark DR, Witte ON. Abelson murine leukemia virus mutants deficient in kinase activity and lymphoid cell transformation. *J Virol* 1980;36:766–74.

27 Whitlock CA, Ziegler SF, Treiman LJ, Stafford JI, Witte ON. Differentiation of cloned populations of immature B cells after transformation with Abelson murine leukemia virus. *Cell* 1983;32:903–11.

28 Wetzler M, Talpaz M, Van Etten RA, Hirsh-Ginsberg C, Beran M, Kurzrock R. Subcellular localization of Bcr, Abl, and Bcr–Abl proteins in normal and leukemic cells and correlation of expression with myeloid differentiation. *J Clin Invest* 1993; 92:1925–39.

29 Van Etten RA. Cycling, stressed-out and nervous: cellular functions of c-Abl. *Trends Cell Biol* 1999;9:179–86.

30 Nagar B, Hantschel O, Young MA, *et al.* Structural basis for the autoinhibition of c-Abl tyrosine kinase. *Cell* 2003;112: 859–71.

31 Hantschel O, Nagar B, Guettler S, *et al.* A myristoyl/phosphotyrosine switch regulates c-Abl. *Cell* 2003;112:845–57.

32 Weisberg E, Manley PW, Cowan-Jacob SW, Hochhaus A, Griffin JD. Second generation inhibitors of Bcr–Abl for the treatment of imatinib-resistant chronic myeloid leukemia. *Nat Rev Cancer* 2007;7:345–56.

33 Van Etten RA, Jackson P, Baltimore D. The mouse type IV *C-ABL* gene product is a nuclear protein, and activation of transforming ability is associated with cytoplasmic localization. *Cell* 1989;58:669–78.

34 Wang JY. Regulation of cell death by the Abl tyrosine kinase. *Oncogene* 2000;19:5643–50.

35 Vigneri P, Wang JY. Induction of apoptosis in chronic myelogenous leukemia cells through nuclear entrapment of Bcr–Abl tyrosine kinase. *Nat Med* 2001;7:228–34.

36 Aloisi A, Di Gregorio S, Stagno F, *et al.* Bcr–Abl nuclear entrapment kills human CML cells: ex vivo study on 35 patients with the combination of imatinib mesylate and leptomycin B. *Blood* 2006;107:1591–8.

37 Bueno-da-Silva AE, Brumatti G, Russo FO, Green DR, Amarante-Mendes GP. Bcr–Abl-mediated resistance to apoptosis is independent of constant tyrosine-kinase activity. *Cell Death Differ* 2003;10:592–8.

38 Graham SM, Jorgensen HG, Allan E, *et al.* Primitive, quiescent, Philadelphia-positive stem cells from patients with chronic myeloid leukemia are insensitive to STI571 *in vitro*. *Blood* 2002; 99:319–25.

39 Copland M, Hamilton A, Elrick LJ, *et al.* Dasatinib (BMS-354825) targets an earlier progenitor population than imatinib in primary CML but does not eliminate the quiescent fraction. *Blood* 2006;107:4532–9.

40 Dai Z, Quackenbush RC, Courtney KD, *et al.* Oncogenic Abl and Src tyrosine kinases elicit the ubiquitin-dependent degradation of target proteins through a Ras-independent pathway. *Genes Dev* 1998;12:1415–24.

41 Deutsch E, Dugray A, AbdulKarim B, *et al.* Bcr–Abl down-regulates the DNA repair protein DNA-PKcs. *Blood* 2001;97: 2084–90.

42 Jonuleit T, van der Kuip H, Miething C, *et al.* Bcr–Abl kinase down-regulates cyclin-dependent kinase inhibitor p27 in human and murine cell lines. *Blood* 2000;96:1933–9.

43 Goetz AW, van der Kuip H, Maya R, Oren M, Aulitzky WE. Requirement for Mdm2 in the survival effects of Bcr–Abl and interleukin 3 in hematopoietic cells. *Cancer Res* 2001;61: 7635–41.

44 Cortes J. Natural history and staging of chronic myelogenous leukemia. *Hematol Oncol Clin North Am* 2004;18:569–84.

45 Vardiman JW, Melo JV, Baccarani M, Thiele J. Chronic myelogenous leukemia, *BCR–ABL1* positive. In: Swerdlow SH, Campo E, Harris NL, *et al.* (eds). *WHO Classification of Tumors of Haematopoietic and Lymphoid Tissues*. IARC Press: Lyon, 2008. pp. 32–7.

46 O'Brien SG, Guilhot F, Larson RA, *et al.* Imatinib compared with interferon and low-dose cytarabine for newly diagnosed chronic-phase chronic myeloid leukemia. *N Engl J Med* 2003;348:994–1004.

47 Talpaz M, Silver RT, Druker BJ, *et al.* Imatinib induces durable hematologic and cytogenetic responses in patients with accelerated phase chronic myeloid leukemia: results of a phase 2 study. *Blood* 2002;99:1928–37.

48 Kantarjian HM, Cortes J, O'Brien S, *et al.* Imatinib mesylate (STI571) therapy for Philadelphia chromosome-positive chronic myelogenous leukemia in blast phase. *Blood* 2002;99: 3547–53.

49 Kantarjian HM, Cortes JE, O'Brien S, *et al.* Long-term survival benefit and improved complete cytogenetic and molecular response rates with imatinib mesylate in Philadelphia chromosome-positive chronic-phase chronic myeloid leukemia after failure of interferon-{alpha}. *Blood* 2004;104: 1979–88.

50 Hughes TP, Kaeda J, Branford S, *et al.* Frequency of major molecular responses to imatinib or interferon alfa plus cytarabine in newly diagnosed chronic myeloid leukemia. *N Engl J Med* 2003;349:1423–32.

51 Druker BJ, Guilhot F, O'Brien SG, *et al.* Five-year follow-up of patients receiving imatinib for chronic myeloid leukemia. *N Engl J Med* 2006;355:2408–17.

52 Baccarani M, Saglio G, Goldman J, *et al.* Evolving concepts in the management of chronic myeloid leukemia: recommendations from an expert panel on behalf of the European leukemiaNet. *Blood* 2006;108:1809–20.

53 Goldman JM. How I treat chronic myeloid leukemia in the imatinib era. *Blood* 2007;110:2828–37.

54 Gratwohl A, Baldomero H, Schwendener A, Gratwohl M, Urbano-Ispizua A, Frauendorfer K. Hematopoietic stem cell transplants for chronic myeloid leukemia in Europe–impact of cost considerations. *Leukemia* 2007;21:383–6.

55 Hehlmann R, Berger U, Pfirrmann M, *et al.* Drug treatment is superior to allografting as first-line therapy in chronic myeloid leukemia. *Blood* 2007;109:4686–92.

56 Branford S, Seymour JF, Grigg A, *et al.* Bcr–Abl messenger RNA levels continue to decline in patients with chronic phase chronic myeloid leukemia treated with imatinib for more than 5 years and approximately half of all first-line treated patients have stable undetectable Bcr–Abl using strict sensitivity criteria. *Clin Cancer Res* 2007;13:7080–5.

57 Bhatia R, Holtz M, Niu N, *et al.* Persistence of malignant hematopoietic progenitors in chronic myelogenous leukemia patients in complete cytogenetic remission following imatinib mesylate treatment. *Blood* 2003;101:4701–7.

58 Cortes J, O'Brien S, Kantarjian H. Discontinuation of imatinib therapy after achieving a molecular response. *Blood* 2004;104: 2204–5.

59 Rousselot P, Huguet F, Rea D, *et al*. Imatinib mesylate discontinuation in patients with chronic myelogenous leukemia in complete molecular remission for more than 2 years. *Blood* 2007;109:58–60.

60 Shah N, Nicoll J, Nagar B, *et al*. Multiple Bcr–Abl kinase domain mutations confer polyclonal resistance to the tyrosine kinase inhibitor imatinib (STI571) in chronic phase and blast crisis chronic myeloid leukemia. *Cancer Cell* 2002;2:117–25.

61 Gorre ME, Mohammed M, Ellwood K, *et al*. Clinical resistance to STI-571 cancer therapy caused by *BCR–ABL* gene mutation or amplification. *Science* 2001;293:876–80.

62 Jorgensen HG, Allan EK, Jordanides NE, Mountford JC, Holyoake TL. Nilotinib exerts equipotent antiproliferative effects to imatinib and does not induce apoptosis in CD34+ CML cells. *Blood* 2007;109:4016–19.

63 Copland M, Pellicano F, Richmond L, *et al*. BMS-214662 potently induces apoptosis of chronic myeloid leukemia stem and progenitor cells and synergises with tyrosine kinase inhibitors. *Blood* 2008;111:2843–53.

64 Cortes J, Kantarjian HM, Giralt S, Talpaz M. Natural history and staging of chronic myelogenous leukemia. *Baillieres Clin Haematol* 1997;10:277–90.

65 Kantarjian HM, O'Brien S, Cortes JE, *et al*. Complete cytogenetic and molecular responses to interferon-alpha-based therapy for chronic myelogenous leukemia are associated with excellent long-term prognosis. *Cancer* 2003;97: 1033–41.

66 Sokal JE, Cox EB, Baccarani M, *et al*. Prognostic discrimination in "good-risk" chronic granulocytic leukemia. *Blood* 1984;63: 789–99.

67 Hasford J, Pfirrmann M, Hehlmann R, *et al*. A new prognostic score for survival of patients with chronic myeloid leukemia treated with interferon alfa. Writing Committee for the Collaborative CML Prognostic Factors Project Group. *J Natl Cancer Inst* 1998;90:850–8.

68 O'Brien S, Thall PF, Siciliano MJ. Cytogenetics of chronic myelogenous leukemia. *Baillieres Clin Haematol* 1997;10: 259–76.

69 Sokal JE, Gomez GA, Baccarani M, *et al*. Prognostic significance of additional cytogenetic abnormalities at diagnosis of Philadelphia chromosome-positive chronic granulocytic leukemia. *Blood* 1988;72:294–8.

70 Kantarjian HM, Smith TL, McCredie KB, *et al*. Chronic myelogenous leukemia: a multivariate analysis of the associations of patient characteristics and therapy with survival. *Blood* 1985;66:1326–35.

71 Huntly BJ, Reid AG, Bench AJ, *et al*. Deletions of the derivative chromosome 9 occur at the time of the Philadelphia translocation and provide a powerful and independent prognostic indicator in chronic myeloid leukemia. *Blood* 2001;98:1732–8.

72 Sinclair PB, Nacheva EP, Leversha M, *et al*. Large deletions at the t(9;22) breakpoint are common and may identify a poor-prognosis subgroup of patients with chronic myeloid leukemia. *Blood* 2000;95:738–43.

73 Huntly BJ, Bench A, Green AR. Double jeopardy from a single translocation: deletions of the derivative chromosome 9 in chronic myeloid leukemia. *Blood* 2003;102:1160–8.

74 Huntly BJ, Guilhot F, Reid AG, *et al*. Imatinib improves but may not fully reverse the poor prognosis of patients with CML with derivative chromosome 9 deletions. *Blood* 2003;102: 2205–12.

75 Quintas-Cardama A, Kantarjian H, Talpaz M, *et al*. Imatinib mesylate therapy may overcome the poor prognostic significance of deletions of derivative chromosome 9 in patients with chronic myelogenous leukemia. *Blood* 2005;105: 2281–6.

76 Kreil S, Pfirrmann M, Haferlach C, *et al*. Heterogeneous prognostic impact of derivative chromosome 9 deletions in chronic myelogenous leukemia. *Blood* 2007;110:1283–90.

77 Jiang X, Lopez A, Holyoake T, Eaves A, Eaves C. Autocrine production and action of IL-3 and granulocyte colony-stimulating factor in chronic myeloid leukemia. *Proc Natl Acad Sci U S A* 1999;96:12804–9.

78 Holyoake TL, Jiang X, Jorgensen HG, *et al*. Primitive quiescent leukemic cells from patients with chronic myeloid leukemia spontaneously initiate factor-independent growth *in vitro* in association with up-regulation of expression of interleukin-3. *Blood* 2001;97:720–8.

79 Jiang X, Fujisaki T, Nicolini F, *et al*. Autonomous multi-lineage differentiation *in vitro* of primitive CD34+ cells from patients with chronic myeloid leukemia. *Leukemia* 2000;14:1112–21.

80 Boultwood J, Peniket A, Watkins F, *et al*. Telomere length shortening in chronic myelogenous leukemia is associated with reduced time to accelerated phase. *Blood* 2000;96: 358–61.

81 Brummendorf TH, Holyoake TL, Rufer N, *et al*. Prognostic implications of differences in telomere length between normal and malignant cells from patients with chronic myeloid leukemia measured by flow cytometry. *Blood* 2000;95:1883–90.

82 Drummond M, Lennard A, Brummendorf T, Holyoake T. Telomere shortening correlates with prognostic score at diagnosis and proceeds rapidly during progression of chronic myeloid leukemia. *Leuk Lymphoma* 2004;45:1775–81.

83 Eisterer W, Jiang X, Christ O, *et al*. Different subsets of primary chronic myeloid leukemia stem cells engraft immunodeficient mice and produce a model of the human disease. *Leukemia* 2005;19:435–41.

84 Bonnet D, Dick JE. Human acute myeloid leukemia is organized as a hierarchy that originates from a primitive hematopoietic cell. *Nat Med* 1997;3:730–7.

85 Hope KJ, Jin L, Dick JE. Acute myeloid leukemia originates from a hierarchy of leukemic stem cell classes that differ in self-renewal capacity. *Nat Immunol* 2004;5:738–43.

86 Yong AS, Szydlo RM, Goldman JM, Apperley JF, Melo JV. Molecular profiling of CD34+ cells identifies low expression of CD7, along with high expression of proteinase 3 or elastase, as predictors of longer survival in patients with CML. *Blood* 2006;107:205–12.

87 Molldrem JJ, Clave E, Jiang YZ, *et al*. Cytotoxic T lymphocytes specific for a nonpolymorphic proteinase 3 peptide preferentially inhibit chronic myeloid leukemia colony-forming units. *Blood* 1997;90:2529–34.

88 Fujiwara H, El Ouriaghli F, Grube M, *et al*. Identification and *in vitro* expansion of CD4+ and CD8+ T cells specific for human neutrophil elastase. *Blood* 2004;103:3076–83.

89 Yong AS, Rezvani K, Savani BN, *et al*. High PR3 or ELA2 expression by CD34+ cells in advanced phase chronic myeloid leukemia is associated with improved outcome following

allogeneic stem cell transplantation and may improve PR1 peptide driven graft-versus-leukemia effects. *Blood* 2007;110: 770–5.
90 Molldrem JJ, Lee PP, Kant S, *et al.* Chronic myelogenous leukemia shapes host immunity by selective deletion of high-avidity leukemia-specific T cells. *J Clin Invest* 2003;111: 639–47.
91 Chabannon C, Wood P, Torok-Storb B. Expression of CD7 on normal human myeloid progenitors. *J Immunol* 1992;149: 2110–13.
92 Martin-Henao GA, Quiroga R, Sureda A, Garcia J. CD7 expression on CD34+ cells from chronic myeloid leukemia in chronic phase. *Am J Hematol* 1999;61:178–86.
93 Normann AP, Egeland T, Madshus IH, Heim S, Tjonnfjord GE. CD7 expression by CD34+ cells in CML patients, of prognostic significance? *Eur J Haematol* 2003;71:266–75.
94 Ogata K, Nakamura K, Yokose N, *et al.* Clinical significance of phenotypic features of blasts in patients with myelodysplastic syndrome. *Blood* 2002;100:3887–96.
95 Ogata K, Yokose N, Shioi Y, *et al.* Reappraisal of the clinical significance of CD7 expression in association with cytogenetics in de novo acute myeloid leukemia. *Br J Haematol* 2001; 115:612–15.
96 Kosugi N, Tojo A, Shinzaki H, Nagamura-Inoue T, Asano S. The preferential expression of CD7 and CD34 in myeloid blast crisis in chronic myeloid leukemia. *Blood* 2000;95: 2188–9.
97 Mohty M, Yong AS, Szydlo RM, Apperley JF, Melo JV. The polycomb group *BMI-1* gene is a molecular marker for predicting prognosis of chronic myeloid leukemia. *Blood* 2007; 110:380–3.
98 Melo JV, Barnes DJ. Chronic myeloid leukemia as a model of disease evolution in human cancer. *Nat Rev Cancer* 2007;7: 441–53.
99 Barnes DJ, Palaiologou D, Panousopoulou E, *et al.* Bcr–Abl expression levels determine the rate of development of resistance to imatinib mesylate in chronic myeloid leukemia. *Cancer Res* 2005;65:8912–19.
100 Jamieson CH, Ailles LE, Dylla SJ, *et al.* Granulocyte-macrophage progenitors as candidate leukemic stem cells in blast-crisis CML. *N Engl J Med* 2004;351:657–67.
101 Savona M, Talpaz M. Getting to the stem of chronic myeloid leukemia. *Nat Rev Cancer* 2008;8:341–50.
102 Michor F. Chronic myeloid leukemia blast crisis arises from progenitors. *Stem Cells* 2007;25:1114–18.
103 Michor F, Hughes TP, Iwasa Y, *et al.* Dynamics of chronic myeloid leukemia. *Nature* 2005;435:1267–70.
104 Smith LT, Hohaus S, Gonzalez DA, Dziennis SE, Tenen DG. PU.1 (Spi-1) and C/EBP alpha regulate the granulocyte colony-stimulating factor receptor promoter in myeloid cells. *Blood* 1996;88:1234–47.
105 Zhang DE, Zhang P, Wang ND, Hetherington CJ, Darlington GJ, Tenen DG. Absence of granulocyte colony-stimulating factor signaling and neutrophil development in CCAAT enhancer binding protein alpha-deficient mice. *Proc Natl Acad Sci U S A* 1997;94:569–74.
106 Perrotti D, Cesi V, Trotta R, *et al.* Bcr–Abl suppresses C/EBPalpha expression through inhibitory action of hnRNP E2. *Nat Genet* 2002;30:48–58.
107 Pabst T, Mueller BU, Zhang P, *et al.* Dominant-negative mutations of *CEBPA*, encoding CCAAT/enhancer binding protein-alpha (C/EBPalpha), in acute myeloid leukemia. *Nat Genet* 2001;27:263–70.
108 Frohling S, Schlenk RF, Stolze I, *et al.* *CEBPA* mutations in younger adults with acute myeloid leukemia and normal cytogenetics: prognostic relevance and analysis of cooperating mutations. *J Clin Oncol* 2004;22:624–33.
109 Pabst T, Stillner E, Neuberg D, *et al.* Mutations of the myeloid transcription factor CEBPA are not associated with the blast crisis of chronic myeloid leukemia. *Br J Haematol* 2006;133: 400–2.
110 Mullighan CG, Miller CB, Radtke I, *et al.* *BCR–ABL1* lymphoblastic leukemia is characterized by the deletion of Ikaros. *Nature* 2008;453:110–14.
111 Neviani P, Santhanam R, Trotta R, *et al.* The tumor suppressor PP2A is functionally inactivated in blast crisis CML through the inhibitory activity of the BCR/ABL-regulated SET protein. *Cancer Cell* 2005;8:355–68.
112 Neviani P, Santhanam R, Oaks JJ, *et al.* FTY720, a new alternative for treating blast crisis chronic myelogenous leukemia and Philadelphia chromosome-positive acute lymphocytic leukemia. *J Clin Invest* 2007;117:2408–21.
113 Holtz MS, Forman SJ, Bhatia R. Nonproliferating CML CD34+ progenitors are resistant to apoptosis induced by a wide range of proapoptotic stimuli. *Leukemia* 2005;19:1034–41.
114 Jiang X, Zhao Y, Smith C, *et al.* Chronic myeloid leukemia stem cells possess multiple unique features of resistance to Bcr–Abl targeted therapies. *Leukemia* 2007;21:926–35.
115 Jorgensen HG, Copland M, Allan EK, *et al.* Intermittent exposure of primitive quiescent chronic myeloid leukemia cells to granulocyte-colony stimulating factor in vitro promotes their elimination by imatinib mesylate. *Clin Cancer Res* 2006;12: 626–33.
116 Holtz M, Forman SJ, Bhatia R. Growth factor stimulation reduces residual quiescent chronic myelogenous leukemia progenitors remaining after imatinib treatment. *Cancer Res* 2007;67:1113–20.
117 Heaney N, Drummond M, Kaeda J, *et al.* A Phase 3 pilot study of continuous imatinib versus pulsed imatinib with or without G-CSF in patients with chronic phase CML who have achieved a complete cytogenetic response to imatinib. *Blood* 2007;110: 313a.
118 Barrett AJ, Rezvani K. Translational mini-review series on vaccines: peptide vaccines for myeloid leukaemias. *Clin Exp Immunol* 2007;148:189–98.
119 Oka Y, Elisseeva OA, Tsuboi A, *et al.* Human cytotoxic T-lymphocyte responses specific for peptides of the wild-type Wilms' tumor gene (*WT1*) product. *Immunogenetics* 2000;51: 99–107.
120 Grunebach F, Mirakaj V, Mirakaj V, Muller MR, Brummendorf T, Brossart P. Bcr–Abl is not an immunodominant antigen in chronic myelogenous leukemia. *Cancer Res* 2006;66:5892–900.
121 Oka Y, Tsuboi A, Taguchi T, *et al.* Induction of *WT1* (Wilms' tumor gene)-specific cytotoxic T lymphocytes by *WT1* peptide vaccine and the resultant cancer regression. *Proc Natl Acad Sci U S A* 2004;101:13885–90.
122 Qazilbash MH, Wieder ED, Thall PF, *et al.* PR1 peptide vaccine-induced immune response is associated with better

event-free survival in patients with myeloid leukemia. *Blood* 2007;110:90a.

123 Rezvani K, Yong AS, Mielke S, *et al.* Leukemia-associated antigen-specific T-cell responses following combined PR1 and WT1 peptide vaccination in patients with myeloid malignancies. *Blood* 2008;111:236–42.

124 Yong AS, Keyvanfar K, Eniafe R, *et al.* Hematopoietic stem cells and primitive progenitors express leukemia-associated antigens that may be targets for graft-versus-leukemia effect or for vaccine-based immunotherapy in chronic myeloid leukemia. *Blood* 2006;108:2125.

125 Barrett J. Allogeneic stem cell transplantation for chronic myeloid leukemia. *Semin Hematol* 2003;40:59–71.

126 Perrotti D, Neviani P. From mRNA metabolism to cancer therapy: chronic myelogenous leukemia shows the way. *Clin Cancer Res* 2007;13:1638–42.

Chapter 22
Therapy of Newly Diagnosed and Chronic-phase Chronic Myeloid Leukemia

Andreas Hochhaus
Universitätsklinikum Jena, Abteilung Hämatologie und Internistische Onkologie, Jena, Germany

Introduction

Chronic myeloid leukemia (CML), which accounts for 15% of adult leukemias, can occur at any age. The incidence of the disease increases with age, with the median age at diagnosis is between 55 and 60 years. The annual incidence of CML is approximately 1–2 per 100,000 people, and slightly more men than women are affected [1,2]. Most patients are diagnosed in chronic phase (CP), which is characterized by <10% blasts in the peripheral blood and bone marrow, with mild to no symptoms and a high likelihood of treatment response [3,4]. Accelerated phase (AP) is a transition phase with resistance to initial therapy accompanied by aquiration of multiple cytogenetic abnormalities. Blast crisis (BC), with >30% of blasts in the peripheral blood and/or bone marrow, may arise directly from CP or after AP CML [1,4].

Although a relatively rare disease, CML has captured attention as a model for the role of targeted therapies in the treatment of human malignancies. Prior to the introduction of targeted therapies, busulfan, hydroxyurea, and interferon alpha (IFN-α)-based therapies or allogeneic hematopoietic stem-cell transplantation (SCT) were offered to most patients, with SCT being the recommended initial treatment for younger patients with matched donors. Treatment with IFN was started in the 1980s and was the first drug treatment that was able to induce complete cytogenetic responses (CCyR). While allogeneic SCT is potentially curative, its utility is limited by donor availability and considerable morbidity, which precludes its use in most patients ≥65 years old.

The introduction of the tyrosine kinase inhibitor (TKI) imatinib mesylate revolutionized the treatment paradigm for CML [5]. Imatinib is a selective inhibitor of BCR–ABL, the oncogenic gene product associated with the Philadelphia (Ph) chromosome, the hallmark of CML. The Ph chromosome results from the reciprocal chromosomal translocation, t(9;22)(q34;q11) [6,7]. The high cytogenetic and molecular response rates of imatinib [8–11], its long-term efficacy in preventing disease progression [12], and its notably superior tolerability over IFN [11] led to the approval of the drug in the USA, the European Union, and Japan in 2001. Imatinib is acknowledged as the standard of care for patients with newly diagnosed CML [12–14] and is also approved for Ph^+ acute lymphoblastic leukemia, hypereosinophilic syndrome and chronic eosinophilic leukemia, aggressive systemic mastocytosis; myelodysplastic syndrome/myeloproliferative disease (MDS/MPD) with translocation involving 5q33, dermatofibrosarcoma protuberans, and Kit^+ gastrointestinal stromal tumor. The success of imatinib as an agent designed to target a specific oncogenic event has broad implications for the field of cancer therapy.

Chronic myeloid leukemia pathophysiology

Chronic myeloid leukemia is a clonal neoplasm originating from a single hematopoietic stem cell. It is the first hematologic malignancy consistently associated with a chromosomal abnormality. CML is characterized by a translocation event involving the fusion of the Abelson oncogene (ABL) located on chromosome 9q34 with the breakpoint cluster region (BCR) on chromosome 22q11.2, resulting in the cytoplasmic fusion protein BCR–ABL [7].

The functional consequences of the formation of the BCR–ABL fusion protein include constitutive activation of the ABL kinase, enhanced binding of ABL to the cytoskeleton, and loss of ABL binding capacity to DNA. The activation of signal-transduction pathways is associated with increased proliferation, genetic instability, impaired adhesion, and suppression of apoptosis.

Various translocation breakpoints result in different isoforms of BCR–ABL associated with specific leukemia

Leukemias: Principles and Practice of Therapy, 1st edition. Edited by S. Faderl and H. Kantarjian.

phenotypes [7,15]. The predominant isoform of BCR–ABL is a 210 kDa protein that is found in >90% of patients with CML. In the rare group of patients with the smaller 190 kDa BCR–ABL isoform, a common characteristic is monocytosis and a low neutrophil-to-monocyte ratio. The larger 230 kDa BCR–ABL protein appears to disrupt granulocytic differentiation and is classified as chronic neutrophilic leukemia. The correlation between phenotype and genotype is, however, rather loose.

Use of tyrosine kinase inhibitors for the treatment of chronic myeloid leukemia

The identification of BCR–ABL as the defining leukemogenic event in CML revolutionized the treatment of the disease. Animal models revealed that constitutive BCR–ABL kinase activity leads to development of leukemia [16,17]. These, and other, preclinical findings supported the central role of BCR–ABL in the pathophysiology of CML, and prompted the search for drugs targeting this tyrosine kinase. With the understanding that the formation of BCR–ABL is a crucial event in the development of the disease, CML serves as a model for the potential utility of molecularly targeted drugs in hematologic malignancies and other cancers.

While it is clear that BCR–ABL is necessary for leukemic transformation, the cooperation of other oncogenes may be required for CML progression. Actually, BCR–ABL can be detected at very low levels in healthy human subjects [18,19]. The fact that these individuals do not show evidence of CML suggests that other molecular events must occur before CML can develop. The TKIs currently available for CML treatment demonstrate different response profiles: imatinib targets BCR–ABL, ABL, the ABL-related gene (ARG) product, KIT, the platelet-derived growth factor receptors alpha and beta (PDGFRα and β), and c-fms [20,21]. Dasatinib targets a number of kinases including ABL, BCR–ABL, EPHA2, KIT, PDGFR, and SRC family members, while nilotinib targets *BCR–ABL, ABL*, ARG, KIT, and PDGFR [21]. In addition to BCR–ABL, other defining molecular events underlying CML development are under investigation and may reveal new therapeutic targets for the disease.

Imatinib

Imatinib is the standard of care for first-line treatment of CML-CP because of its high long-term response rates and favorable tolerability profile compared with previous standard therapies, allogeneic SCT, and IFN. As an effective inhibitor of BCR–ABL, imatinib targets a key initiation event in the development of CML [22,23]. In colony-forming assays of the peripheral blood or bone marrow from patients with CML, there was a 92–98% decrease in the number of BCR–ABL positive colonies formed but no inhibition of normal colony formation [23]. Imatinib also inhibited proliferation in hematopoietic cell lines positive for BCR–ABL but had no effect on BCR–ABL$^-$ cell lines [24]. The activity of imatinib in these cell-culture studies provided the rationale for clinical studies.

After the safety of the drug was established in phase I studies [22], a phase II study of imatinib was initiated in 532 IFN-resistant or refractory patients with late-phase CML-CP [25]. Imatinib was associated with high response rates in this study, with major cytogenetic response (MCyR) in 67%, CCyR in 57%, and complete hematologic response (CHR) in 96%. Imatinib was well tolerated and also appeared to confer survival benefits, with a 6-year progression-free survival (PFS) rate and an overall survival (OS) rate of 61% and 76%, respectively. Serious grade 3/4 adverse events (AE) were uncommon, occurring in <5% of patients. At the 6-year cut-off, 255 (56%) patients discontinued the study, 8% discontinued treatment owing to AE.

The superiority of imatinib over IFN was established in the International Randomized Study of Interferon versus STI571 (IRIS) study [10,11]. In this phase III study, 1106 treatment-naïve patients with CML-CP were randomized to either imatinib at 400 mg daily (n = 553) or IFN plus cytarabine (n = 553). At 18 months, an MCyR was achieved in 87% of patients initially treated with imatinib, compared with 35% of IFN-treated patients (P < 0.001). Most imatinib-treated patients experienced CCyR (76.2% vs. 14.5% with IFN, P < 0.001). Major molecular responses (MMRs), defined as at least a 3-log decrease in BCR–ABL transcripts compared with a standardized baseline, were more common with imatinib, occurring in 39% of imatinib-treated patients versus 2% of IFN-treated patients (P < 0.001). Rates of MMR were higher in patients with CCyR; 57% for imatinib versus 24% for IFN (P = 0.003).

After 6 years of imatinib therapy, long-term response rates remained high [26]. Of the 456 patients who achieved CCyR on imatinib therapy, 325 (71%) were still on study treatment and maintained CCyR at 6 years. From year 1 to 6, the annual event rate (loss of CHR, loss of MCyR, progression to AP/BC, or death) on imatinib decreased over time from 3.3%, 7.5%, 4.8%, 1.7%, 0.8%, to 0.4%. There is a downward trend in risk of disease progression on imatinib, with a 0.4% event rate and no transformations to AP/BC between years 5 and 6. Approximately 83% of patients were event-free, and 93% were free of progression to AP or BC at 6 years. The estimated 6-year survival rate for all patients who received imatinib as initial therapy was 88%. When only CML-related deaths were considered, the estimated survival was 95%. Achievement of any cytogenetic response within 6 months was a prognostic factor for freedom from progression. Six-year PFS occurred in 97% of patients achieving CCyR within 6 months, compared with 80% of patients without a CCyR at this early time point ($P < 0.001$).

The IRIS study showed that, in addition to its efficacy advantages, imatinib is better tolerated than high-dose IFN [26]. Grade 3/4 AE, including fatigue, depression, myalgias, arthralgias, neutropenia, and thrombocytopenia, were more common in the IFN arm. The most common grade 3/4 AE among patients treated with imatinib were neutropenia (14%), thrombocytopenia (8%), anemia (3%), and elevated liver enzymes (5%). The AE frequency decreased over time, occurring mostly in years 1 and 2, with rates decreasing to <2% after year 4. Follow-up at 6 years on therapy revealed that imatinib has a favorable long-term safety profile. No new serious AE were identified between years 5 and 6. Furthermore, first-line treatment with imatinib did not affect later success on salvage therapies (IFN, allogeneic SCT), further emphasizing the low risk of imatinib use in the front-line setting [27,28].

The survival benefits of imatinib could not be determined in the IRIS study because of patient crossover, but were confirmed by historic comparison studies [29,30] (Figure 22.1). A retrospective comparison of newly diagnosed patients with CML treated with imatinib ($n = 279$) or IFN ($n = 650$) at the M. D. Anderson Cancer Center (MDACC) in Houston, TX, demonstrated improved response and survival for imatinib-treated patients [29]. CCyR rates were 87% for imatinib-treated patients versus 28% for IFN-treated patients ($P < 0.001$). Survival correlated with cytogenetic response for both imatinib and IFN, suggesting that the survival benefits of imatinib are a result of the high-cytogenetic response rates induced by this drug. The estimated 5-year survival rate was significantly higher (88%) for imatinib-treated patients, compared with 63% for patients on IFN ($P = 0.001$). The benefits of imatinib were seen in all prognostic risk groups. Another retrospective study examining outcomes from the imatinib arm of the IRIS trial and the IFN/cytarabine arm of the CML91 trial were in concordance with the MDACC study [30]. The safety, response, and survival advantages of imatinib over IFN has led to broad acceptance of imatinib as the drug of choice for initial therapy of CML.

Assessing imatinib response and resistance

The National Comprehensive Cancer Network (NCCN) and European LeukemiaNet (ELN) have recommended a similar monitoring schedule for patients treated with imatinib (Table 22.1) [12–14]. When a patient initiates treatment with a TKI, bone marrow cytogenetics should be measured every 6 months until CCyR, then every 1–3 years as long as the MMR is stable. BCR–ABL transcript levels should be monitored at least every 3 months and then every 3–6 months once CCyR is reached [31]. To assess MMR, major guidelines recommend that BCR–ABL transcript levels should be determined every 3–6 months using real-time reverse transcriptase-polymerase chain reaction (RT-PCR) and expressed according to an international scale (IS) [32]. In the case of rising BCR–ABL levels, transcript testing may be performed more frequently and BCR–ABL mutation analysis considered.

Definitions of imatinib response are provided in Table 22.2. Poor risk factors associated with decreased response to therapy include high Sokal risk [33], additional chromosome aberrations in Ph^+ cells at diagnosis, less than CCyR at 12 months, any increase in transcript levels of BCR–ABL, or other chromosomal aberrations at any time [12,13]. Importantly, these poor risk factors appear to differ among CML therapies. This has been shown in the

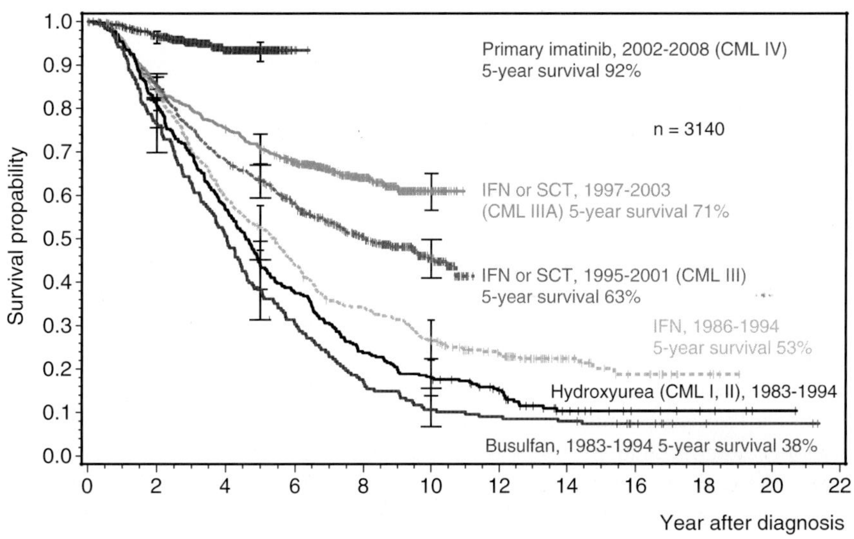

Figure 22.1 Outcome of patients with CML diagnosed and treated between 1983 and 2008 in consecutive prospective randomized trials in Germany.

Table 22.1 Monitoring the response to imatinib [12–14,31].

Cytogenetics	At diagnosis At 3 months At 6 months Every 6 months until a CCyR has been achieved and confirmed, then every 12 months if regular molecular monitoring cannot be assured Always in case of failure (primary or secondary resistance) and in case of unexplained anemia, leukopenia, or thrombocytopenia Every 3 months, until an MMR has been achieved and confirmed, then at least every 6 months
Molecular (mutational analysis)	In case of suboptimal response or failure. It is always required before switching to other TKIs or other therapies.

Testing plasma level of imatinib may help in case of suboptimal response, failure, excess toxicity, or low compliance. It is recommended in case of simultaneous treatment with agents metabolized by the P450 cytochrome isoenzymes CYP3A4 and CYP3A5.
CCyR, complete cytogenetic response; MMR, major molecular response; TKI, tyrosine kinase inhibitors.

Table 22.2 Definitions of unsatisfactory response to imatinib, adapted from [13].

Time on imatinib (months)	Response	
	Failure	Suboptimal
3	No CHR	No CyR
6	No CyR	<PCyR ($Ph^+ \geq 35\%$)
12	<PCyR	<CCyR ($Ph^+ \geq 5\%$)
18	<CCyR	No MMR
Any	Loss of CHR Loss of CCyR Mutations with virtual intensitivity to imatinib Clonal evolution	Loss of MMR Other BCR–ABL mutation associated with diminished response.

CHR, complete hematologic response; CCyR, complete cytogenetic response; CyR, cytogenetic response; MMR, major molecular response; PCyR, partial cytogenetic response.

5-year follow-up of the IRIS study, where 97% of patients with a CCyR within 12 months after starting imatinib did not progress by 60 months, irrespective of the Sokal score at the time of diagnosis. Patients with high Sokal risk had a lower rate of CCyR (69%) than patients with low or intermediate risk (89% and 82%, respectively). However, the risk of relapse in patients after having achieved a CCyR was not associated with the Sokal score. With IFN treatment, the Sokal and Hasford [34] scores are important indicators of response even among patients in CCyR. The 2009 ELN recommendations include updates to the response criteria. Changes include the following: no CHR at 3 months is considered a failure; no CyR at 3 months is considered a suboptimal response; and clonal evolution arising at any time is considered a failure (Table 22.2) [13].

Factors affecting imatinib concentration in target cells

The importance of imatinib plasma concentration was raised by the report that mean through plasma levels (C_{min}) of imatinib were higher in the patients who achieved CCyR and MMR [35]. A plasma level of 1002 ng/mL was considered the threshold. Confirmatory data came from the IRIS study, where the C_{min} plasma level at day 29 was higher in patients achieving a CCyR and was significantly related to a better molecular response and longer event-free survival, but with more side-effects [36]. However, the results of individual imatinib blood level tests may not be a true reflection of long-term imatinib blood levels, and thus may not necessarily affect the course of therapy.

Other reports have demonstrated that multidrug resistance (MDR)-associated ATP-binding cassette transporters affect the intracellular concentration of imatinib [37–39]. MDR transporters are also overexpressed in hematopoietic stem cells and can contribute to the resistance to imatinib. The clinical relevance of the expression and functional activity of the transporters is still unclear. Instead, more focus is being placed on the human organic cation transporter 1 (hOCT-1), which has been reported to be a key determinant of the response to imatinib [40,41].

Effect on leukemic stem cells

Studies on Ph^+ stem cells are difficult to perform and should be interpreted with caution. Quiescent Ph^+ stem cells are resistant to imatinib, either prior to treatment or in patients in CCyR or CMR. The existence of quiescent and persisting stem cells has fostered controversial hypotheses on the curability of CML with TKI and is still a major threat regarding the long-term outcome of therapy, despite the decreasing rate of failure over time, while patients receive imatinib.

High-dose imatinib

Based on IRIS, the recommended starting dose of imatinib is 400 mg once daily. However, higher doses are currently being investigated in previously treated, slowly responding patients, patients with loss of response, and in treatment-naïve CML populations. High-dose imatinib has also shown high cytogenetic and molecular response rates in patients with newly diagnosed CML-CP. In a cohort of 114 newly diagnosed patients treated with 800 mg/day imatinib, high-dose imatinib was associated with improved CCyR ($P = 0.0005$), MMR ($P = 0.00001$), and CMR ($P = 0.001$) compared with a historical control group receiving standard-dose imatinib [42]. A phase II dose-escalation study in imatinib-naïve patients, who were started on 600 mg/day and increased to 800 mg/day if response criteria were not met, further demonstrated CCyR and MMR rates that exceeded those of the IRIS study [43].

These promising results prompted the initiation of several prospective randomized trials evaluating high-dose imatinib in newly diagnosed patients. The randomized phase III "Tyrosine Kinase Inhibitor Optimization and Selectivity (TOPS)" trial is evaluating 400 mg versus 800 mg imatinib in patients with newly diagnosed, previously untreated CML-CP. The primary endpoint of the trial is MMR rate at 12 months. Preliminary results from this study show that CCyR was significantly better at 6 months with 800 mg (45% 400 mg vs. 57% 800 mg; $P = 0.0146$), but there was no statistical difference in CCyR at 12 months (66% 400 mg versus 70% 800 mg). MMR rates were higher with 800 mg at 3 and 6 months compared with 400 mg (12% vs. 3% at 3 months; $P = 0.0011$, and 34% vs. 17% at 6 months; $P = 0.0002$), although no difference in MMR rate at 12 months was observed (46% vs. 40%, $P = 0.20$). Treatment discontinuation as a result of side-effects was higher in the 800 mg cohort [44]. The ELN also performed a randomized study of standard (400 mg) versus high-dose (800 mg) imatinib as front-line therapy in patients with high Sokal-risk CML-CP, where CCyR at 12 months was the primary endpoint [45]. There was no difference in the CCyR rate at 12 months in the intention-to-treat analysis. CCyR correlated with the mean daily dose, where the rate of CCyR was 86% among patients receiving a median daily imatinib dose of 600–800 mg, compared with 66% for patients receiving a median daily dose <600 mg ($P = 0.013$). High-dose imatinib was associated with higher rates of AE, including grade 3/4 anemia, neutropenia, and thrombocytopenia, rash (5.7% vs. 2.5%), diarrhea (4.1% vs. 1.3%), myalgia (3.5% vs. 0.6%), superficial edema (3.2% vs. 0%), and dyspnea (2.5% vs. 0%).

Combination with other agents

Imatinib-based combinations may increase the efficacy of imatinib and decrease the risk of resistance [46–50]. The first interim analysis of the French Spirit Study, wherein 636 patients were assigned to receive either imatinib 400 mg or 600 mg or imatinib 400 mg with either pegylated IFN-α 2a or with low-dose Ara-C, reported the best response in the imatinib plus IFN arm, with a 12-month CCyR of 71% versus 57% for imatinib 400 mg alone, and a 12-month MMR rate of 61% versus 40% for imatinib 400 alone, although 46% of the patients discontinued IFN during the first year of therapy [50]. The efficacy and tolerability of IFN maintenance therapy after experimental imatinib–IFN induction has been explored in an attempt to avoid the need for lifelong imatinib therapy. In 20 patients with CML-CP, this approach resulted in improved or continuous molecular remissions in 17 patients (85%) [51].

Second-generation tyrosine kinase inhibitors

Possibly the most promising future developments in CML therapy will be the use of second-generation TKIs, such as nilotinib or dasatinib, in the front-line setting. Nilotinib (800 mg/day) treatment is being assessed in newly diagnosed patients with CML-CP in several ongoing studies. In a study being conducted at the MDACC, CCyR was achieved in 97% of patients within 6 months of therapy, and 50% of patients achieved an MMR by 6 months of therapy. Both CCyR and MMR were maintained for 12 months [52]. In another study, the Gruppo Italiano Malattie Ematogiche dell'Adulto (GIMEMA) Working Party reported a 97% CCyR rate on nilotinib by 6 months, and an MMR rate of 75% [53]. Dasatinib has also been evaluated as front-line therapy in a phase II study being conducted at MDACC. At 6 months, the rate of CCyR was 94% and MMR was 36% [54].

Treatment discontinuation and interruption

The optimal duration of imatinib treatment is yet to be identified. Discontinuation is an appealing and logical consequence of successful treatment, but the number of patients who achieve a stable CMR is still small. Early discontinuation of imatinib treatment, despite previous achievement of CMR, is associated with loss of CMR in the majority of patients. In a study of patients with CML who discontinued imatinib after >2 years of undetectable residual disease, about 50% experienced molecular relapse with a detectable BCR–ABL transcript within 6 months [55,56]. Molecular response was regained in most patients after reintroduction of imatinib.

Allogeneic stem-cell transplantation

The assessment of the long-term outcome of allogeneic SCT from HLA-identical siblings is still based on the data collected by the international registries between 1978 and 1997 [57–60]. These results encompassed a 15–20 year period with survival rates of about 50%. The transplantation risk score proposed by the European Group for Blood and Marrow Transplant (EBMT) in 1998 [58] has not undergone any substantial modification. The EBMT report [60] on patients who were submitted to a reduced-intensity conditioning procedure between 1994 and 2002 shows a 3-year OS of 70% for the patients with an EBMT risk score of 0–2. A report from the EBMT analyzed the outcomes of patients transplanted in three different time cohorts (1980–1990, 1991–1999, and 2000–2003) [59]. For the patients with an EBMT score of 0–1, transplant-related mortality was reduced from 31% in the earlier cohort to 17% in the most recent cohort. Of 80 patients who were enrolled in a prospective study of imatinib-based treatment in Germany after 2002, 5-year OS was 88% [61]. Thus, today, the early outcome of allogeneic SCT is certainly superior to that of a decade ago. However, more data are needed to determine if leukemia-free survival, quality of life, and long-term OS will likewise be improved. Prior treatment with imatinib does not affect the outcome of allogeneic SCT [62–64].

Prognostic factors

Imatinib base-line prognostic factors

The prognostic classification that was proposed by Sokal *et al.* [33], and the later proposal published by Hasford *et al.* [34], have been confirmed to apply to the outcome of imatinib treatment (Table 22.3). In the IRIS study, the CCyR rate at 12 months was 78%, 68%, and 51%; for Sokal low-, intermediate- and high-risk patients [11], the MMR rate among CCyRs was 66%, 45%, and 38%, respectively [10]; and the 6-year OS, PFS, and event-free survival (EFS) were 94%, 97%, and 91% for low-risk patients, 87%, 92%, and 81% for intermediate-risk patients, and 76%, 83%, and 64% for high-risk patients, all differences being significant ($P \leq 0.002$) [26]. Once CCyR was achieved, the outcome was not significantly affected by the pretreatment score, with a reported PFS for patients in CCyR of 99%, 95%, and 95% ($P = 0.20$). The detection of a deletion of the long arm of chromosome 9, found in 10–15% of patients, has not been confirmed as a significant prognostic factor for any efficacy endpoints [65,66]. Variant translocations occur in 4–8% of patients, and were not found to be prognostically significant in imatinib-treated patients [67,68]. The prognostic value of the gene expression profile of Ph^+ cells remains undetermined [69].

Imatinib first-line response-related prognostic factors

For the few patients who fail to achieve a CHR after 3 months of imatinib therapy, the probability of achieving a CCyR is very small ($P = 0.0003$), and the OS and PFS are significantly shorter (60% and 56%, respectively, $P = 0.003$ and 0.002, respectively) [70]. After 6 months, the patients without any cytogenetic response had a significantly lower chance of achieving a subsequent CCyR and MMR (25% and 12%) [71], and the patients who achieved a CCyR or partial cytogenetic response (PCyR) had a significantly better 5-year PFS, EFS, and OS [26]. After 12

Table 22.3 Calculation of relative risk.

Sokal *et al.* 1984 [33]	Exponential 0.0116 × (age − 43.4) + 0.0345 × (spleen − 7.51) + 0.188 × (platelet count/700)^2 − 0.563) + 0.0887 × (blast cells − 2.10).
Hasford *et al.* 1998 [34]	0.666 when age ≥50 + (0.042 × spleen) + 1.0956 when platelet count >1500 × 10^9L + (0.0584 × blast cells) + 0.20399 when basophils >3% + (0.0413 × eosinophils) × 100

The relative risk according to Sokal *et al.* was defined based on patients treated with conventional chemotherapy; it is calculated as exponential of the total: low <0.8; intermediate 0.8–1.2; high >1.2. The relative risk according to Hasford *et al.* was defined based on patients treated with IFN-based regimes. It is calculated as total ×1000; low ≤780; intermediate 781–1480; high >1480. Age is in years. Spleen is in cm below costal margin, maximum distance. Blast cells, eosinophils and basophils are in percent of peripheral blood differential.

months, a CCyR yielded superior results compared with a PCyR for the 5-year PFS and OS. After 18 months of imatinib therapy, the PFS and the OS of patients in CCyR were superior to those with PCyR (99% vs. 87%, 98% vs. 76%) [9,26,71]. The exact value of molecular response is more difficult to assess. The first analysis of the IRIS study indicated that achieving an MMR at 12 months predicted a better PFS [10], but in the most recent update it was reported that a MMR predicted a better 6-year EFS (98% vs. 88%, $P = 0.01$) at 18 months but not at 12 months (94% vs. 93%) [72]. Any loss of CHR or CCyR predicts a shorter PFS ($P \leq 0.001$) and a shorter OS ($P \leq 0.04$) [70]. The prognostic value of the loss of MMR is controversial, but all reports point out that a rise in the level of transcripts should raise the level of attention and suspicion for relapse [31,71].

The prognostic value of other chromosome abnormalities in Ph^- cells at diagnosis [73] is not clear [74]. An evolution toward acute myeloid leukemia or MDS has been reported in <10% of cases, mainly with a loss of chromosome 7.

Response definitions

Based on the degree of hematologic, cytogenetic, and molecular responses, and on the time when these responses are achieved, the overall response to imatinib can be defined as optimal, suboptimal, and failure. The response is optimal when, based on current knowledge and expectation, results predicts normal survival. Suboptimal response means that the patient may still have a substantial long-term benefit from continuing a specific treatment, but the chances of an optimal outcome are reduced. Failure means that continuing a specific treatment is no longer appropriate and a favorable outcome is unlikely. A patient who fails should receive a different treatment, even investigational, whenever available and applicable. The relevance of these definitions—optimal, suboptimal, and failure—is modulated by the coexistence of warning prognostic factors. "Warnings" may negatively affect the response to that therapy, and require more stringent and careful monitoring. An optimal responder must be in CHR and have at least minor CyR (Ph^+ ≤65%) by 3 months, at least PCyR (Ph^+ ≤35%) by 6 months, CCyR by 12 months, MMR by 18 months, and must remain in CCyR and MMR (Table 22.2).

Treatment recommendations

Hydroxyurea may still be used, but only for a short period of time until BCR–ABL positivity is confirmed or in a patient who cannot take a TKI and is not eligible for allogeneic SCT. IFN is still an option in case of pregnancy, and in some (mainly low-risk) patients who cannot take a TKI and are not eligible for allogeneic SCT. Apart from these exceptions, the standard initial treatment of CML-CP is imatinib at a dosage of 400 mg daily. In case of imatinib intolerance, the second-generation inhibitors dasatinib and nilotinib are available. In the case of a suboptimal response to imatinib, such as a transitory condition, there is no solid, confirmed evidence that a change in treatment will improve the eventual outcome, but there are at least three other possible options, namely an increase of imatinib dose or changing to dasatinib or nilotinib. In case of imatinib failure, drug therapy should be changed to dasatinib or nilotinib. Allogeneic SCT is recommended in cases of AP, blast phase, or T315I mutation and for patients who do not show optimal responses to second-line TKIs [13].

Conclusions

As the first neoplasm for which knowledge of genotype led to a rationally designed therapy, CML serves as a model for the promise of molecularly targeted therapy in cancer. Imatinib has revolutionized the treatment of CML, providing effective and safe long-term therapy. It is not clear whether imatinib is able to eradicate the malignant CML clone. Maintenance therapy with immunomodulators, such as IFN, may also play a role in inducing sustained responses to TKI.

Many outstanding issues remain in the field of CML therapy. These include the role of molecular testing in routine patient monitoring, the preferred second-line treatment regimen in patients with imatinib failure, the role of nilotinib and dasatinib as first-line CML therapy, and the future use of novel treatment approaches and combination therapies in both newly diagnosed and treated patients. Results from ongoing studies initiated to address these issues are eagerly anticipated.

Acknowledgments and disclosures

Andreas Hochhaus was supported by the German José Carreras Foundation (H 03/01), Novartis, and Bristol Myers Squibb.

References

1 Hehlmann R, Hochhaus A, Baccarani M. Chronic myeloid leukemia. *Lancet* 2007:370;342–50.
2 Parkin DM, Pisani P, Ferlay J. Estimates of the worldwide incidence of eighteen major cancers in 1985. *Int J Cancer* 1985;54: 594–606.
3 Vardiman JW, Harris NL, Brunning RD. The world health organization (WHO) classification of the myeloid neoplasms. *Blood* 2002;100:2292–302.
4 Tefferi A, Thiele J, Orazi A, *et al.* Proposals and rationale for revision of the world health organization diagnostic criteria for

polycythemia vera, essential thrombocythemia, and primary myelofibrosis: Recommendations from an ad hoc international expert panel. *Blood* 2007;110:1092–7.
5 Druker BJ, Talpaz M, Resta DJ, *et al.* Efficacy and safety of a specific inhibitor of the BCR–ABL tyrosine kinase in chronic myeloid leukemia. *N Engl J Med* 2001;344:1031–7.
6 Rowley JD. A new consistent chromosomal abnormality in chronic myelogenous leukemia identified by quinacrine fluorescence and giemsa staining. *Nature* 1973;243:290–3.
7 Melo JV, Deininger MW. Biology of chronic myelogenous leukemia–signaling pathways of initiation and transformation. *Hematol Oncol Clin North Am* 2004;18:545–68.
8 Kantarjian H, Sawyers C, Hochhaus A, *et al.* Hematologic and cytogenetic responses to imatinib mesylate in chronic myelogenous leukemia. *N Engl J Med* 2002;346:645–52.
9 Druker BJ, Guilhot F, O'Brien SG, *et al.* Five-year follow-up of patients receiving imatinib for chronic myeloid leukemia. *N Engl J Med* 2006;355:2408–17.
10 Hughes TP, Kaeda J, Branford S, *et al.* Frequency of major molecular responses to imatinib or interferon alfa plus cytarabine in newly diagnosed chronic myeloid leukemia. *N Engl J Med* 2003;349:1423–32.
11 O'Brien SG, Guilhot F, Larson RA, *et al.* Imatinib compared with interferon and low-dose cytarabine for newly diagnosed chronic-phase chronic myeloid leukemia. *N Engl J Med* 2003; 348:994–1004.
12 Baccarani M, Saglio G, Goldman J, *et al.* Evolving concepts in the management of chronic myeloid leukemia: Recommendations from an expert panel on behalf of the European LeukemiaNet. *Blood* 2006;108:1809–20.
13 Baccarani M, Cortes JE, Pane F, *et al.* Chronic myeloid leukemia. an update of concepts and management. Recommendations of European LeukemiaNet. *J Clin Oncol* 2009;27:6041–51.
14 NCCN Clinical Practice Guidelines in Oncology: Chronic Myelogenous Leukemia. v.2.2010. http://www.nccn.org/professionals/physician_gls/PDF/cml.pdf (accessed October 2009).
15 Melo JV. The diversity of BCR–ABL fusion proteins and their relationship to leukemia phenotype. *Blood* 1996;88:2375–84.
16 Daley GQ, Van Etten RA, Baltimore D. Induction of chronic myelogenous leukemia in mice by the P210 *BCR–ABL* gene of the Philadelphia chromosome. *Science* 1990;247:824–30.
17 Pear WS, Miller JP, Xu L, *et al.* Efficient and rapid induction of a chronic myelogenous leukemia-like myeloproliferative disease in mice receiving P210 bcr/abl-transduced bone marrow. *Blood* 1998;92:3780–92.
18 Biernaux C, Loos M, Sels A, Huez G, Stryckmans P. Detection of major *BCR–ABL* gene expression at a very low level in blood cells of some healthy individuals. *Blood* 1995;86:3118–22.
19 Bose S, Deininger M, Gora-Tybor J, Goldman JM, Melo JV. The presence of typical and atypical *BCR–ABL* fusion genes in leukocytes of normal individuals: Biologic significance and implications for the assessment of minimal residual disease. *Blood* 1998;92:3362–7.
20 Buchdunger E, Zimmermann J, Mett H, *et al.* Inhibition of the abl protein-tyrosine kinase *in vitro* and *in vivo* by a 2-phenylaminopyrimidine derivative. *Cancer Res* 1996;56:100–4.
21 Hantschel O, Rix U, Superti-Furga G. Target spectrum of the BCR–ABL inhibitors imatinib, nilotinib and dasatinib. *Leuk Lymphoma* 2008;49:615–19.
22 Druker BJ, Sawyers CL, Kantarjian H, *et al.* Activity of a specific inhibitor of the BCR–ABL tyrosine kinase in the blast crisis of chronic myeloid leukemia and acute lymphoblastic leukemia with the Philadelphia chromosome. *N Engl J Med* 2001;344: 1038–42.
23 Druker BJ, Tamura S, Buchdunger E, *et al.* Effects of a selective inhibitor of the abl tyrosine kinase on the growth of *BCR–ABL* positive cells. *Nat Med* 1996;2:561–6.
24 Deininger MW, Goldman JM, Lydon N, Melo JV. The tyrosine kinase inhibitor CGP57148B selectively inhibits the growth of *BCR–ABL*-positive cells. *Blood* 1997;90:3691–8.
25 Hochhaus A, Druker B, Sawyers C, *et al.* Favorable long-term follow-up results over 6 years for response, survival, and safety with imatinib mesylate therapy in chronic-phase chronic myeloid leukemia after failure of interferon-alpha treatment. *Blood* 2008;111:1039–43.
26 Hochhaus A, O'Brien SG, Guilhot F, *et al.* Six-year follow-up of patients receiving imatinib for the first-line treatment of chronic myeloid leukemia. *Leukemia* 2009. [Epub ahead of print.]
27 Deininger M, Schleuning M, Greinix H, *et al.* The effect of prior exposure to imatinib on transplant-related mortality. *Haematologica* 2006;91:452–9.
28 Hess G, Bunjes D, Siegert W, *et al.* Sustained complete molecular remissions after treatment with imatinib-mesylate in patients with failure after allogeneic stem cell transplantation for chronic myelogenous leukemia: Results of a prospective phase II open-label multicenter study. *J Clin Oncol* 2005;23: 7583–93.
29 Kantarjian HM, Talpaz M, O'Brien S, *et al.* Survival benefit with imatinib mesylate versus interferon-alpha-based regimens in newly diagnosed chronic-phase chronic myelogenous leukemia. *Blood* 2006;108:1835–40.
30 Roy L, Guilhot J, Krahnke T, *et al.* Survival advantage from imatinib compared with the combination interferon-alpha plus cytarabine in chronic-phase chronic myelogenous leukemia: Historical comparison between two phase 3 trials. *Blood* 2006; 108:1478–84.
31 Hughes T, Deininger M, Hochhaus A, *et al.* Monitoring CML patients responding to treatment with tyrosine kinase inhibitors: Review and recommendations for harmonizing current methodology for detecting BCR–ABL transcripts and kinase domain mutations and for expressing results. *Blood* 2006;108: 28–37.
32 Branford S, Fletcher L, Cross NCP, *et al.* Desirable performance characteristics for BCR–ABL measurement on an international reporting scale to allow consistent interpretation of individual patient response and comparison of response rates between clinical trials. *Blood* 2008;112:3330–7.
33 Sokal JE, Cox EB, Baccarani M, *et al.* Prognostic discrimination in "good-risk" chronic granulocytic leukemia. *Blood* 1984;63: 789–99.
34 Hasford J, Pfirmann M, Hehlmann R, *et al.* A new prognostic score for survival of patients with chronic myeloid leukemia treated with interferon alfa. *J Natl Cancer Inst* 1998;90:850–8.
35 Picard S, Titier K, Etienne G, *et al.* Through imatinib plasma levels are associated with both cytogenetic and molecular responses to standard-dose imatinib in chronic myeloid leukemia. *Blood* 2007;109:3496–9.
36 Larson RA, Druker BJ, Guilhot F, *et al.* Imatinib pharmacokinetics and its correlation with response and safety in chronic-

phase chronic myeloid leukemia: a subanalysis of the IRIS study. *Blood* 2008;111:4022–8.

37 Nakanishi T, Shiozawa K, Hassel BA, *et al.* Complex interaction of BCRP/ABCG2 and imatinib in BCR–ABL-expressing cells: BCRP-mediated resistance to imatinib is attenuated by imatinib-induced reduction of BCRP expression. *Blood* 2006;108:678–84.

38 Brendel C, Scharenberg C, Dohse M, *et al.* Imatinib mesylate and nilotinib (AMN107) exhibit high–affinity interaction with ABCG2 on primitive hematopoietic stem cells. *Leukemia* 2007; 21:1267–75.

39 Dulucq S, Bouchet S, Tuecq B, *et al.* Multidrug resistance gene (MDR1) polymorphisms are associated with major molecular responses to standard-dose imatinib in chronic myeloid leukemia. *Blood* 2008;112:2024–7.

40 Jordanides NE, Jorgensen HG, Holyoake TL, *et al.* Functional ABCG2 is overexpressed on primary CML CD34+ cells and inhibited by imatinib mesylate. *Blood* 2006;108:1370–3.

41 White DL, Saunders VA, Dang P, *et al.* OCT-1-mediated influx is a kay determinant of the intracellular uptake of imatinib but not nilotinib (AMN107): reduced OCT-1 activity is the cause of low *in vitro* sensitivity to imatinib. *Blood* 2006;108:697–704.

42 Kantarjian H, Talpaz M, O'Brien S, *et al.* High-dose imatinib mesylate therapy in newly diagnosed Philadelphia chromosome-positive chronic phase chronic myeloid leukemia. *Blood* 2004; 103:2873–8.

43 Hughes T, Branford S, Reynolds J, *et al.* Higher dose imatinib (600 mg/day) with selective intensification in newly diagnosed CML patients in chronic phase: Cytogenetic response rates at 12 months are superior to IRIS. *Blood* 2004;104, Abstract 1001.

44 Cortes J, Baccarani M, Guilhot F, *et al.* A phase III, randomized, open-label study of 400 mg versus 800 mg of imatinib mesylate (IM) in patients (pts) with newly diagnosed, previously untreated chronic myeloid leukemia in chronic phase (CML-CP) using molecular endpoints: 1-year results of TOPS (tyrosine kinase inhibitor optimization and selectivity) study. *Blood* 2008;112:130–1.

45 Baccarani M, Castagnetti F, Simonsson B, *et al.* Cytogenetic and molecular response to imatinib in high risk (Sokal) chronic myeloid leukemia (CML): Results of an European LeukemiaNet prospective study comparing 400 mg and 800 mg front-line. *Blood* 2008;112:75.

46 Cortes J, Quintas-Cardama A, Garcia-Manero G, *et al.* Phase 1 study of tipifarnib in combination with imatinib for patients with chronic myelogenous leukemia in chronic phase after imatinib failure. *Cancer* 2007;110:2000–6.

47 Cortes J, Jabbour E, Daley GQ, *et al.* Phase 1 study of lonafarnib (SCH 66336) and imatinib mesylate in patients with chronic myeloid leukemia who have failed prior single-agent therapy with imatinib. *Cancer* 2007;110:1295–302.

48 Singh N, Kumar L, Kochupillae V, *et al.* To assess the response and toxicity of imatinib mesylate and low-dose cytarabine in imatinib non-responder chronic myeloid leukemia, chronic phase (CML-CP) patients: A pilot study. *J Clin Oncol* 2007;25:680s.

49 Hochhaus A, Neubauer A, Mueller MC, *et al.* Safety and efficacy of a combination of imatinib and pegylated interferon 2a (pegasys) in newly diagnosed patients with chronic myelogenous leukemia: A phase II cohort study. *Blood* 2007;110:311a.

50 Guilhot F, Mahon FX, Guilhot J, *et al.* Randomized comparison of imatinib versus imatinib combination therapies in newly diagnosed chronic myeloid leukemia (CML) patients in chronic phase (CP): first results of the phase III (SPIRIT) trial from the French CML Group (FI LMC). *Blood* 2008;112:74.

51 Hochhaus A, Neubauer A, Mueller MC, *et al.* Sustained molecular responses with interferon 2a maintenance therapy after imatinib plus IFN induction treatment for chronic phase chronic myelogenous leukemia. *Blood* 2007;110:16–17a.

52 Cortes J, O'Brien S, Jones D, *et al.* Efficacy of nilotinib (formerly AMN107) in patients (pts) with newly diagnosed, previously untreated philadelphia chromosome (ph)-positive chronic myelogenous leukemia in early chronic phase (CML-CP). *Blood* 2008;112:170.

53 Rosti G, Castagnetti F, Poerio A, *et al.* High and early rates of cytogenetic and molecular response with nilotinib 800 mg daily as first line treatment of ph-positive chronic myeloid leukemia in chronic phase: Results of a phase 2 trial of the GIMEMA CML working party. *Blood* 2008;112:73–4.

54 Cortes J, O'Brien S, Borthakur G, *et al.* Efficacy of dasatinib in patients (pts) with previously untreated chronic myelogenous leukemia (CML) in early chronic phase (CML-CP). *Blood* 2008;112:74.

55 Rousselot P, Huguet F, Rea D, *et al.* Imatinib mesylate discontinuation in patients with chronic myelogenous leukemia in complete molecular remission for more than 2 years. *Blood* 2007;109:58–60.

56 Mahon FX, Huguet F, Guilhot F, *et al.* Is it possible to stop imatinib in patients with chronic myeloid leukemia? an update from a French pilot study and first results from the multicentre study. *Blood* 2008;112:76.

57 Gratwohl A, Brand R, Apperley J, *et al.* Allogeneic hematopoietic stem cell transplantation for chronic myeloid leukemia in Europe 2006: transplant activity, long-term data and current results. An analysis by the chronic leukemia working party of the European group for blood and marrow transplantation (EBMT). *Haematologica* 2006;91:513–21.

58 Gratwohl A, Hermans J, Goldman JM, *et al.* Risk assessement for patients whith chronic myeloid leukemia before allogenic *Blood* or marrow transplantation: Chronic Leukemia Working Party of the European Group for Blood and Marrow Transplatation. *Lancet* 1998;352:1087–92.

59 Passweg JR, Walker I, Sobocinski KA, *et al.* Validation and extention of the EBMT risk score for patients with chronic myeloid leukemia receiving allogeneic hematopoietic stem cell transplants. *Br J Haematol* 2004;125:613–20.

60 Crawley C, Szydlo R, Lalancette M, *et al.* Outcome of reduced-intensity transplantation for chronic myeloid leukemia: an analysis of prognostic factors from the chronic leukemia working party of the EBMT. *Blood* 2005;106:2969–76.

61 Saussele S, Lauseker M, Gratwohl A, *et al.* Allogeneic hematopoietic stem cell transplantation (HSCT) in the imatinib-era: high survival rate following allogeneic HSCT after imatinib failure: results of the German CML study IV. *Blood* 2008;112:171.

62 Deininger M, Schleuning M, Greinix H, *et al.* The effect of prior exposure to imatinib on transplant-related mortality. *Haematologica* 2006;91:452–9.

63 Oehler VG, Gooley T, Snyder DS, *et al.* The effects of imatinib mesylate treatment before allogeneic tranplantation for chronic myeloid leukemia. *Blood* 2007;109:1782–9.

64 Lee SJ, Kukreja M, Wang T, *et al.* Impact of prior imatinib mesylate on the outcome of hematopoietic cell transplantation for chronic myeloid leukemia. *Blood* 2008;112:3500–7.

65 Kim DHD, Popradi G, Sriharsha L, *et al.* No significance of derivative chromosome 9 deletion on the clearance kinetics of BCR–ABL fusion transcripts, cytogenetic or molecular response, loss of response, or treatment failure to imatinib mesylate therapy for chronic myeloid leukemia. *Cancer* 2008;113: 772–81.
66 Castagnetti F, Testoni N, Marzocchi G, *et al.* Deletions of the derivative chromosome 9 do not influence response to imatinib mesylate in early chronic phase chronic myeloid leukemia patients: a GIMEMA CML Working Party analysis. *J Clin Oncol* 2010;28:2748–54.
67 Richebourg S, Eclache V, Perot C, *et al.* Mechanisms of genesis of variant translocation in chronic myeloid leukemia are not correlated with ABL1 or BCR deletion status or response to imatinib therapy. *Cancer Gen Cytogen* 2008;182:95–102.
68 Batty N, Kantarjian H, Borthakur G, *et al.* Patients with chronic myeloid leukemia with variant Philadelphia chromosome (Ph) translocations have a similar outcome as those with classic Ph when treated with imatinib or 2nd generation TKI. *Blood* 2008; 112:1108.
69 Radich JP, Dai H, Mao M, *et al.* Gene expression changes associated with progression and response in chronic myeloid leukemia. *Proc Natl Acad Science* 2006;103:2794–9.
70 Marin D, Milojkovic D, Olavarria E, *et al.* European leukemiaNet criteria for failure or suboptimal response reliably identify patients with CML in early chronic phase treated with imatinib whose eventual outcome is poor. *Blood* 2008;112:4437–44.
71 de Lavallade H, Apperley JF, Khorashad JS, *et al.* Imatinib for newly diagnosed patients with chronic myeloid leukemia: incidence of sustained responses in an intention-to-treat analysis. *J Clin Oncol* 2008;26:3358–63.
72 Hughes T, Hochhaus A, Branford S, *et al.* Reduction of BCR–ABL transcript levels at 6, 12, and 18 months (mo) correlates with long-term outcomes on imatinib (IM) at 72 mo: an analysis from the international randomized study of interferon versus STI571 (IRIS) in patients (pts) with chronic phase chronic myeloid leukemia (CML-CP). *Blood* 2008;112:129–30.
73 Zaccaria A, Valenti AM, Donti E, *et al.* Persistence of chromosomal abnormalities additional to the philadelphia chromosome after Philadelphia chromosome disappearance during imatinib therapy for chronic myeloid leukemia. *Haematologica* 2007;92:564–5.
74 Deininger MWN, Cortes J, Paquette R, *et al.* The prognosis for patients with chronic myeloid leukemia who have clonal cytogenetic abnormalities in Philadelphia chromosome-negative cells. *Cancer* 2007;110:1509–19.

Chapter 23
Therapy of Advanced-stage and Resistant Chronic Myeloid Leukemia

Devendra K. Hiwase and Timothy P. Hughes
Institute of Medical and Veterinary Science, Adelaide, Australia

Introduction

Chronic myeloid leukemia (CML) is characterized by the t(9;22) chromosome, which produces the constitutively active Bcr–Abl oncoprotein. The Bcr–Abl chimeric oncoprotein leads to enhanced cellular proliferation, resistance to apoptosis, and altered cell adhesion. Imatinib binds to the ATP-binding pocket of the Bcr–Abl kinase domain, blocks phosphorylation of downstream proteins, and induces apoptosis in CML cells. Five-year follow-up of the IRIS study (International Randomized Study of Interferon and STI571) demonstrated the effectiveness of imatinib as front-line therapy for patients in CML-chronic phase (CP). At 60 months, estimated major cytogenetic response (MCyR) and complete cytogenetic response (CCyR) were achieved in 92% and 87% of patients, respectively. Estimated overall survival (OS) and progression-free survival (PFS, progression to accelerated and blast crisis phase) was 89% and 93%, respectively [1].

The response to imatinib in patients with newly diagnosed CML-CP varies considerably in both the speed and depth of response (degree of reduction of leukemic burden). Landmark analysis of the IRIS study demonstrated that patients who achieved major molecular response (MMR, ≥3 log reduction in Bcr–Abl transcripts from the standardized baseline) by 12 months have a 100% PFS at 60 months (disease progression was defined by any of the following events: death, accelerated-phase or blast-crisis CML, loss of complete hematologic response, or loss of major cytogenetic response). This compares favourably with patients who achieved CCyR or MCyR by 12 months [1]. This demonstrates that the risk of developing progressive disease is related to the depth of early molecular response achieved. Hence, it is important to closely monitor patients on imatinib and identify patients who are not responding well. Recently, an expert panel on behalf of European LeukemiaNet proposed guidelines for monitoring response (Table 23.1) [2].

Leukemias: Principles and Practice of Therapy, 1st edition. Edited by S. Faderl and H. Kantarjian.

How to monitor newly diagnosed patients with chronic-phase chronic myeloid leukemia receiving imatinib as a first-line therapy

Patients who are on imatinib should be monitored with complete blood counts (CBC) every 2 weeks until complete hematologic response (CHR) is achieved, and then three-monthly CBCs unless indicated otherwise. Real-time quantitative polymerase chain reaction (RQ-PCR) for Bcr–Abl transcripts should be conducted every 3 months. Bone marrow cytogenetics should be undertaken at 6 months, 12 months, and then every 12 months. Bone marrow cytogenetic examination should also be repeated if there is a progressive rise in Bcr–Abl transcripts.

Imatinib resistance

Imatinib failure could be due to imatinib resistance, poor compliance, toxicity leading to dose interruption, and drug interaction. imatinib resistance can be divided into two broad categories, primary and secondary. Primary resistance to imatinib is defined as an inability to achieve a landmark response, whereas secondary resistance is defined as loss of an established response [3]. imatinib resistance can be further subdivided into hematologic, cytogenetic, and molecular resistance. Failure to achieve CHR (normalization of peripheral blood counts, the differential leukocyte counts, and spleen size) by 3 months despite therapeutic dose of imatinib is quite rare (2–4%) in newly diagnosed patients with CML-CP [1]. A more commonly encountered problem is cytogenetic resistance (15–25% of patients), which includes failure to achieve any cytogenetic response after 6 months of treatment, MCyR (<35% of Ph$^+$ chromosome) at 12 months, and CCyR at 18 months [1].

Table 23.1 Operational definition of suboptimal response, failure of response, and warning signs in previously untreated patients with chronic-phase chronic myeloid leukemia [2].

Time point after starting imatinib	Definition of failure	Definition of suboptimal response	Warning signs
At diagnosis	NA	NA	High risk, del9q+, ACAs∞ in Ph+ cells
3 month0073	No HR (stable disease or disease progression)	Less than CHR	NA
6 months	Less than CHR, no CyR[a]	Less than PcyR[b]	NA
12 months	Less than PcyR[a]	Less than CcyR[c]	Less than MMR[d]
18 months	Less than CcyR[c]	Less than MMR	NA
Anytime	Loss of CH, Loss of CCyR[#] Mutation	ACA in Ph+ cells Loss of MMR[$] Mutation	Any rise in transcript level, OCA

Adapted from Baccarani M, Saglio G, Goldman J, *et al.* Evolving concepts in the management of chronic myeloid leukemia: recommendations from an expert panel on behalf of the European LeukemiaNet. *Blood* 2006;108:1809–20.
Failure: means that continuing imatinib treatment at the current dose is no longer appropriate for these patients, who would likely benefit more from other treatment.
Suboptimal response: means that patients may still achieve a substantial benefit from continuing imatinib, but that the long-term outcome of the treatment would not likely be as favorable as switching to another treatment.
Warning signs: factors which are considered as strong cautionary indicators that standard-dose imatinib treatment may not be the best choice for these patients.
ACA, additional chromosomal abnormalities; CCyR, complete cytogenic response; CHR, complete hematologic response; HR, hematologic response; MMR, major molecular response; NA, not applicable; OCA, other chromosomal abnormalities; PCyr, partial cytogenic response.
[a]No CyR: >95% Ph+ chromosomes.
[b]35% of Ph+ chromosomes.
[c]No Ph+ chromosome.
[d]0.1% on the International Scale.

Factors that can predict primary imatinib resistance

Data from correlative studies suggest that primary resistance is linked to the inability of the drug to effectively inhibit Bcr–Abl kinase. $IC50^{imatinib}$ is defined as the concentration of imatinib needed *in vitro* to inhibit phosphorylation of Crkl (a surrogate marker of Bcr–Abl kinase activity) by 50%. We have demonstrated that 47% of patients with low *in vitro* $IC50^{imatinib}$ (<0.6 μM imatinib) achieved MMR by 12 months compared with 23% of patients with high $IC50^{imatinib}$ [4]. This was further strengthened by *in vivo* kinase inhibition within the first 28 days, which predicted the molecular response at 24 months. All patients who achieved ≥50% kinase inhibition within the first month achieved MMR by 24 months compared with only 50% patients who had <50% kinase inhibition [5]. Patients treated with a high dose of imatinib (600–800 mg daily) achieved an earlier cytogenetic response compared with standard-dose imatinib [6]. Similarly, some patients resistant to standard-dose imatinib were rescued by high-dose imatinib [7]. Therefore, primary imatinib resistance is most likely due to inadequate inhibition of Bcr–Abl kinase activity.

Inadequate *in vivo* Bcr–Abl kinase inhibition can be multifactorial, and early detection of these patients is crucial to optimize the therapy. imatinib plasma concentration is determined by drug absorption and metabolism, as well as actual dose received. Subanalysis of the IRIS study demonstrated that, at 12 months, CCyR was achieved in 73%, 71%, and 59% of patients with trough plasma imatinib of >1170 ng/mL, ≥647–1170 ng/mL, and <647 ng/mL, respectively [8]. Moreover, CCyR was more durable in patients with high-plasma trough imatinib level (13% vs. 24% of patients lost CCyR) compared with patients with low-plasma trough imatinib level [8].

While plasma concentration of imatinib is important, the most relevant indication of kinase inhibition achieved may be the level of intracellular imatinib. For maximum Bcr–Abl kinase inhibition, higher intracellular tyrosine kinase inhibitors (TKI) concentration is also crucial. We have demonstrated that the variation in *in vitro* $IC50^{imatinib}$ is predominantly due to a variation in intracellular imatinib cellular uptake and retention (IUR). Wang *et al.* [9] initially reported that imatinib is actively transported into cells by human organic cation transporter (hOCT1). Patients with high OCT-1 activity have low $IC50^{imatinib}$, presumably because at a given imatinib concentration they achieve higher intracellular drug concentrations [10]. Our group also demonstrated that low OCT-1 activity is the major determinant of a suboptimal response to imatinib. In our study, 85% of patients with high OCT-1 activity achieved MMR by 24 months versus 45% with low OCT-1 activity [11]. Clark and colleagues [12] have recently reported that patients with high OCT-1 mRNA expression prior to treatment had a higher response compared with patients with low OCT-1 mRNA expression.

Sokal score at diagnosis also predicts the response—49%, 67%, and 76% of patients with high-, intermediate- and low-risk Sokal scores achieved CCyR at 12 months [13]. The probability of primary imatinib resistance also depends on the duration of disease prior to starting imatinib and response to previous treatment. MCyR and CCyR were achieved in 67% and 57% of patients in late CP who failed interferon therapy [14] compared with 92% and 87% of patients with newly diagnosed CML-CP [1]. imatinib failure is also more common in advanced phase patients—76% of patients in accelerated phase (AP) and 84% of patients in blast crisis (BC) failed to achieve MCyR [15,16].

As multiple mechanisms may contribute to primary resistance, the best management will be to identify patients who may be susceptible to imatinib resistance and tailor the treatment accordingly. Patients with low OCT-1 activity and high $IC50^{imatinib}$ may benefit from higher-dose imatinib or second-generation TKIs (dasatinib or nilotinib) that are not predominantly dependent on OCT-1 for their cellular transport [10,17]. However, these predictive assays need to be prospectively validated before they can be applied clinically.

Risk factors and mechanisms of secondary resistance

Secondary resistance frequently evolves from primary resistance, hence primary resistance should be considered as an important risk factor for secondary resistance. Other risk factors for secondary resistance are disease phase and duration of chronic phase prior to imatinib. After 60 months, 16% of patients with early CML-CP developed secondary resistance or disease progression [1]. At 48 months, 26% of patients in late CP previously treated with interferon-α developed secondary resistance or progressive disease. The secondary resistance rate was significantly higher in AP (73%) and BC patients (95%) with CML [3].

Resistance to imatinib could theoretically be either due to a failure to maintain kinase inhibition or the capacity of resistant CML cells to propagate and survive despite kinase inhibition. In most cases, there is reactivation of Bcr–Abl kinase activity within leukemic cells despite the presence of imatinib. Point mutation in the Bcr–Abl kinase domain is the most common cause (50–60% of cases) of acquired imatinib resistance [18–23]. Mutations that cause imatinib resistance are usually those that lead to a Bcr–Abl protein with a functional Abl tyrosine kinase domain but impaired drug binding. More than 90 mutations have been identified in association with resistance, and they are located throughout the kinase domain, including the ATP binding loop (P loop), imatinib binding sites, activation loop (A loop), catalytic domain, and the carboxy terminal. However, 15 common mutations account for >90% of all mutations (Figure 23.1). These common mutations include *T315I*, *Y253F/H*, *E255D/K/R/V*, *M351T*, *G250A/E*, *F359C/L/V*, and *H396P/R* [24].

Other proposed mechanisms of acquired imatinib resistance include overexpression and amplification of the *BCR–ABL* gene [18,19], activation of Bcr-Abl independent pathways such as members of the Src kinase family [25], binding of imatinib to serum alpha 1 acid glycoprotein [26], and increased drug efflux through the multidrug resistance protein [9,27].

Therapy for imatinib-resistant patients with chronic-phase chronic myeloid leukemia

Approximately 30% of patients with CML who are receiving imatinib as a first-line therapy will discontinue treatment within 5 years because of resistance or intolerance. As Bcr–Abl signaling is usually reactivated at the time of resistance, it remains the critical target for therapy.

High-dose imatinib for resistant patients

High-dose imatinib (300–400 mg twice daily) achieved CHR, McyR, and CCyR in 45%, 56%, and 18% of evaluable patients with CML-CP who were resistant to lower doses (300–400 mg daily) [7]. These findings were supported by another study in which high-dose imatinib induced CHR, MCyR, CcyR, and MMR in 82%, 33%, 16%, and 4% of patients resistant to standard-dose imatinib [28]. Thus, some patients resistant to lower doses of imatinib can be rescued by a high dose.

Nilotinib trials in imatinib-resistant/intolerant patients with chronic-phase chronic myeloid leukemia

Nilotinib, a phenylaminopyrimidine derivative of imatinib is 30 times more potent than imatinib *in vitro* as an Abl inhibitor (IC50 = 25 nM) but is more selective, having activity similar to imatinib against c-Kit (IC50 = 90 nM) and PDGFR-β (IC50 = 72 nM) receptor kinases [29]. Like imatinib, nilotinib binds the inactive conformation of Abl. However, unlike imatinib it does not need to distort the kinase domain as much to achieve good binding.

In a phase I study of nilotinib, 92%, 17%, and 17% of imatinib-resistant patients with CML-CP achieved CHR,

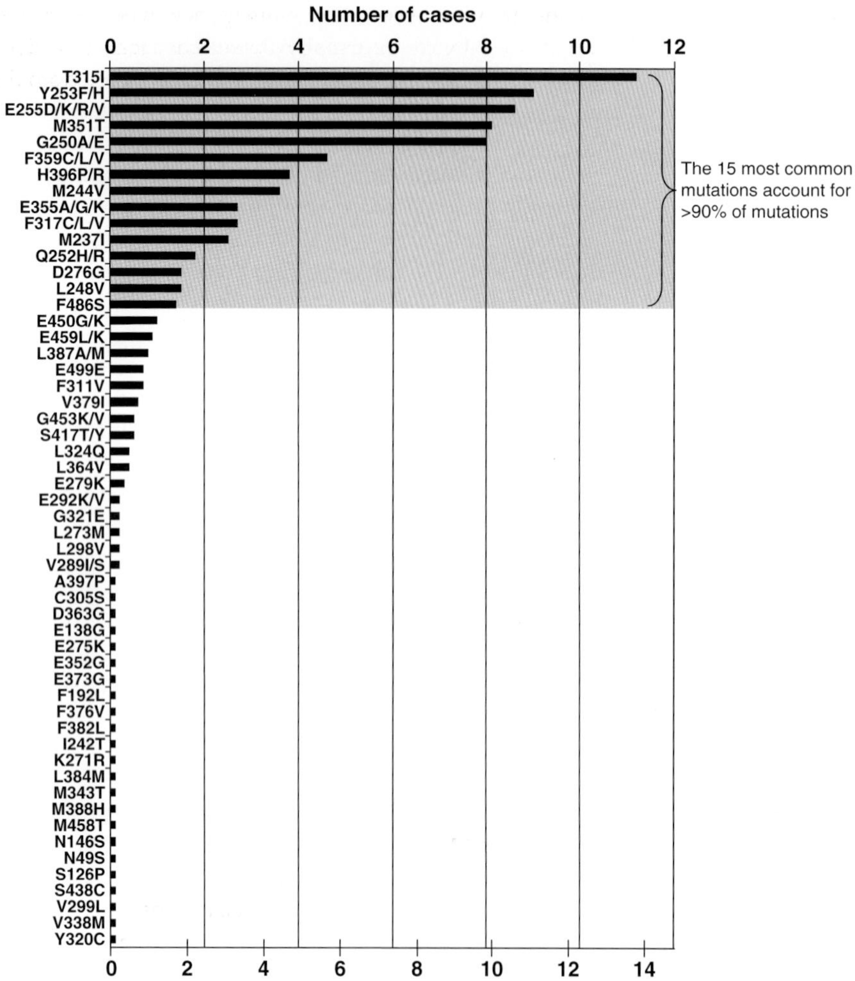

Figure 23.1 Incidence of mutations in immune-modulations treated patients: incidence of Bcr–Abl kinase domain mutations are arranged in the order of frequency. The 15 most common mutations account for >90% of mutations (shaded area).

McyR, and CCyR respectively [30]. These encouraging results were further confirmed in a phase II study of patients with CML-CP (n = 280) who were resistant (69%) or intolerant (31%) to imatinib [31]. At 6 months, CHR, MCyR, and CCyR were achieved in 74%, 48%, and 31% of patients, respectively. OS and PFS at 18 months were 91% and 64%. The MCyR rates were similar (47% and 48%, respectively) in imatinib-intolerant and resistant patients. Responses were obtained across all mutations except *T315I*; although patients with mutations appeared to have lower rates of response [31].

Dasatinib trials in imatinib-resistant/intolerant patients with chronic-phase chronic myeloid leukemia

Dasatinib (BMS-354825; Bristol-Myers Squibb, New York, USA) is a highly potent orally active TKI. It inhibits Bcr–Abl, the Src family, c-Kit, PDGFR, and ephrine receptor tyrosine kinases. It is over 300 times more potent than imatinib in *in vitro* cell proliferation assays and active against most of the imatinib-resistant mutants, except *T315I* [32].

In a phase I study of dasatinib, 92%, 45%, and 35% of imatinib-resistant/intolerant patients with CML-CP achieved CHR, MCyR and CcyR, respectively [33]. These promising results were further confirmed in a phase II study—90%, 55%, and 40% of imatinib-resistant patients (n = 288) achieved CHR, MCyR, and CcyR, respectively [33]. The responses were higher in imatinib-intolerant patients. CHR, MCyR, and CCyR were achieved in 94%, 80%, and 75% of imatinib-intolerant patients, respectively [33]. The MCyR was similar in patients with and without baseline mutations (59% vs. 58%) [34]. Estimated OS and PFS at 24 months was 94% and 80%, respectively [33]. In a phase III dose-optimization study, imatinib-resistant/intolerant patients with CML-CP (n = 670) were treated with four different schedules of dasatinib, including 100 mg daily, 50 mg twice daily, 140 mg daily, and 70 mg twice daily. Comparable CHR (86–90%), MCyR (54–59%), and CCyR (41–45%) were achieved in all four groups. Time to and duration of cytogenetic response were similar in all four groups. Compared with the 70 mg twice-daily regimen, dasatinib taken at 100 mg daily resulted in significantly lower rates of pleural effusions (16% vs. 7%), grade 3 to 4 thrombocytopenia (37% vs. 22%), and fewer patients required dose interruption (68% vs. 51%), reduction (55% vs. 30%), or discontinuation (23% vs. 16%) [35].

Bosutinib in imatinib-resistant/intolerant patients with chronic-phase chronic myeloid leukemia

Bosutinib (SKI-606) is an orally bioavailable dual Src/Abl inhibitor, 100–200-fold more potent (*in vitro*) than imatinib [36]. Unlike imatinib, bosutinib does not exhibit significant inhibition of c-Kit or PDGFR, which may result in a relatively favorable safety profile [36]. In a phase II study of imatinib-resistant or intolerant patients with CML-CP, 76% and 30% of patients achieved CHR and CcyR, respectively [37]. Responses were achieved in patients with and without P-loop mutations. The drug was well tolerated, with grade 3–4 nonhematologic and hematologic toxicities occurring in 5–10% of patients [37].

How to choose the tyrosine kinase inhibitor for imatinib-failure patients with chronic-phase chronic myeloid leukemia

Imatinib failure (primary resistance) is defined in the Leukemia Net recommendations as failure to achieve CHR by 3 months, any cytogenetic response by 6 months, MCyR by 12 months, or CCyR by 18 months [2]. These patients can be further subdivided into two groups. The first group of patients are those who tolerated the standard dose of imatinib (400 mg daily) but failed to achieve target responses. Patients in this group should be investigated further, including trough plasma imatinib level, compliance checks, and mutation analysis (less likely to be positive for mutation). Compliant patients with lower trough plasma imatinib levels may be treated with high-dose imatinib and observed closely, while patients with high trough plasma imatinib levels may benefit from switching to a second-line TKI. The second group of patients are those who could not tolerate full-dose imatinib in spite of appropriate supportive care and failed to achieve target response. Second-line TKI may be appropriate in some patients with recurrent non-hematologic toxicities at grade 3 or higher as there is minimal cross-intolerance (defined as the occurrence of ≥3 grade toxicity with dasatinib or nilotinib, which was previously reported in the same patient receiving imatinib) with dasatinib or nilotinib. However, the hematologic toxicities of second-line TKI are similar or higher than standard-dose imatinib, hence it may be more difficult to maintain therapeutic doses of TKI's in patients with significant hematologic toxicities.

Patients who lose a previously achieved response should initially have a repeat assay to confirm loss of response and a careful check of compliance. If loss of response is confirmed then the patient should be further investigated, including mutation analysis, bone marrow aspiration to assess disease progression, and cytogenetic analysis to detect additional chromosomal abnormality. Treatment options for patients who have lost previously achieved response (secondary resistance) but remained in CP include high-dose imatinib, second-line TKI, and allogeneic stem-cell transplantation (SCT). In a randomized study of imatinib-resistant patients, dasatinib resulted in significantly higher CHR (93% vs. 82%), CCyR (40% vs. 16%), and MMR (16% vs. 4%) compared with high-dose imatinib. Significantly more patients discontinued high-dose imatinib than dasatinib (82% vs. 28%, $P < 0.0001$), and most of the discontinuations (61%) in the high-dose imatinib group were a result of a lack of response or disease progression [28]. Moreover, high-dose imatinib is not a viable choice for patients who are intolerant to standard-dose imatinib or in patients who have mutations that are highly resistant to imatinib. As there are several effective second-line TKIs available, it may be reasonable to switch the patient on to another TKI in most cases of acquired resistance. The question of which second-line TKIs to select, dasatinib or nilotinib, is rather more difficult. In phase I and II trials both dasatinib and nilotinib demonstrated similar efficacy. We highlight some features that may help in decision-making.

Although studies on dasatinib and nilotinib have demonstrated similar responses in patients with and without baseline mutations, a closer look at the data reveals that responses vary with sensitivity of mutations as determined by *in vitro* analysis. Patients harboring native *BCR–ABL* or dasatinib-sensitive mutation (dasatinib IC50 <3 nM; *G250E*, *Y253F/H*, *M315T*, *E355G*, *F359V*, *V379I*, *L387M*, *H396P*, *H396R*, *M244V*) had comparable response rates. Whereas patients with mutations conferring intermediate sensitivity to dasatinib *in vitro* (IC50 3–60 nM; *Q252H*, *E255K/V*, *V299L*, and *F317L/V*) exhibited lower rates of MCyR (15–20% compared with 50–55% in patients with native *BCR–ABL*). None of the patients with the highly resistant mutation *T315I* responded to dasatinib [38]. Similarly, nilotinib responses also varied according to baseline mutations. In a phase II study of nilotinib, CHR (85% vs. 67%), MCyR (60% vs. 49%), and CCyR (45% vs. 29%) were higher in patients without baseline mutations compared with patients who had baseline mutations. Among patients with baseline mutations, responses differed according to *in vitro* sensitivity of mutant clones against nilotinib. Patients with sensitive mutations (IC50 <100 nM; *M244V*, *E275K*, *D276G*, *F317L*, *M351T*, *E355A*, *E355G*, and *L387M*) had response rates comparable with patients without baseline mutations. The response rates were lower in patients with less-sensitive mutations (IC50

201–800 nM, *Y253H*, *E255K*, *E255V*, and *F359C*), and none of the patients with highly resistant *T315I* (IC50 >10,000 nM) mutations responded [31]. In the same study, progression rates were higher among patients with baseline mutations compared with patients without baseline mutations (40% vs. 15%), and the majority of the patients (7/9) harboring *F359V* progressed during follow-up [39]. Hence, baseline mutations in imatinib-resistant/intolerant patients may guide further treatment selection.

For patients harboring mutations that are insensitive to nilotinib (eg, *Y253F*, *E255K*, and *F359C*), dasatinib may be a valid alternative. Similarly, for patients with mutants that have intermediate sensitivity to dasatinib (*F317L* and *V299L*), nilotinib may be a more suitable alternative. Allogeneic SCT for eligible patients is the preferred treatment for patients with the *T315I* mutation. Thus, *in vitro* mutation sensitivity data may be a useful guide. Nevertheless, there are limitations with these assays. *In vitro* sensitivity of mutant clones depends on the assay type and is based on a single-mutant clone; however, in some patients, there is more than one mutant clone or clones with multiple mutations. The ratio of mutant clones to native Bcr–Abl clones may vary within the same patient over a period of time. For such patients, *in vitro* mutation analysis may not be so helpful. Moreover, there are no IC50 data available for most patient mutations. Furthermore, around 40% of imatinib-resistant patients have no kinase-domain mutations to guide therapy selection.

Another issue that needs to be considered is the toxicity profile of second-generation TKI drugs. Nilotinib is more potent than imatinib, but non-hematologic toxicity is no more common than it is for imatinib. This may be because of the relative selectivity of nilotinib against Bcr–Abl (relative to other targets, such as the Src-family or c-Kit kinases). Toxicity profiles of nilotinib and imatinib are different, with minimal cross intolerance [31]. Most common adverse effects of nilotinib include skin rash (28%), nausea and pruritus (24% each), and headache and fatigue (19% each) [31]. The most common adverse effects of imatinib include superficial edema (55%), nausea (43%), musculoskeletal pain (36%), rash (34%), diarrhea (33%), and headache (31%) [40]. Hence, for patients with cardiac failure and/or imatinib-induced significant fluid-retention problems, nilotinib may be preferred over high-dose imatinib or dasatinib.

There are no randomized studies comparing dasatinib and nilotinib; however, data from different studies suggest that non-hematologic toxicities of dasatinib are different to nilotinib. Frequency of grade 3–4 neutropenia (33% vs. 29%) and thrombocytopenia (22% vs. 29%) were not significantly different between dasatinib- (100 mg daily) and nilotinib-treated patients. However, the non-hematologic toxicities (all grades) such as pleural effusion (7% vs. 1%), peripheral edema (14% vs.<1%), diarrhea (23% vs. 11%), and headache (30% vs. 19%) were more frequent in dasatinib-treated patients (100 mg daily) compared with nilotinib-treated patients [31,35].

The selection of appropriate second-line TKI for patients with imatinib failure can be based on the type of mutation(s), the patient's tolerance imatinib, and type of toxicities. Other features, such as patient-specific IC50 of dasatinib or nilotinib, may be helpful. However, these tests need to be proven in prospective studies. Treatment options for patients who failed imatinib treatment and progressed to AP or BC are discussed in the next section.

Therapeutic options against *T315I* mutations

The *T315I* mutation occurs in ~15% of imatinib-resistant patients with a mutation, and may be more frequently detected in patients with advanced CML and Ph^+ acute lymphoblastic leukemia (ALL) [24]. Survival of patients with the *T315I* mutation mostly depends on the stage of the disease. At 2 years, 87% of patients in CP with the *T315I* mutation were alive, and many patients had an indolent course [41]. Patients with the *T315I* mutation are resistant to imatinib, dasatinib, nilotinib, and bosutinib. Allogeneic SCT is a potentially curative treatment for these patients. PHA-739358 [42], KW-2449 [43], and homoharringtonine [44,45] are in early clinical testing for patients with *T315I* mutations. New classes of molecules including non-ATP-competitive inhibitors [46], inhibitors of Bcr–Abl *T315I* kinase downstream effectors are currently under preclinical evaluation.

How to monitor patients on second-generation tyrosine kinase inhibitors

Approximately 50% of imatinib-resistant patients treated with dasatinib or nilotinib will not achieve CCyR. Patients who were treated with second-line TKIs for imatinib failure and achieved MCyR at 12 months had a higher projected survival (97% vs. 84%, $P = 0.02$) for the next 12 months than patients who did not achieve MCyR. Similarly, more patients on second-line TKIs who did not achieve MCyR at 12 months progressed compared with patients who did achieve MCyR at 12 months (17% vs. 3%, $P = 0.003$) [47]. Hence, patients who did not achieve MCyR at 12 months could be considered for alternative therapy. The decision to switch will depend on the available options. Response at an earlier time point can predict the response to second-line TKIs at 12 months. Only 7% and 3% of patients who did not achieve minor cytogenetic response (MiCR) at 3 and 6 months achieved MCyR at 12 months. In contrast, 67% and 50% of patients who achieved MiCR at 3 and 6 months, respectively, achieved MCyR at 12 months [47].

Monitoring of patients on second-line TKIs is guided by the phase of disease and the reason for starting a second-generation TKI (imatinib intolerance or resistance). imatinib-intolerant or slow responding patients with CML-CP (patients who have demonstrated progressive drop in Ph^+ chromosomes and/or Bcr–Abl transcript but failed to achieve the target response) who were switched to a second-generation TKI can be monitored with a CBC every 2 weeks, RQ-PCR for *BCR–ABL* every 3 months, and bone marrow cytogenetic analysis at 6 months, 12 months, and then annually. Patients who lose previously achieved response (but maintained CP) and/or had rapidly rising Bcr–Abl levels or Ph chromosome metaphases should be monitored very closely by RQ-PCR for Bcr–Abl monthly, until a progressive fall is demonstrated, and then every 3 months. These patients may need bone marrow aspiration and cytogenetic analysis at 3, 6, and 12 months. Frequency of mutation analysis will depend on the baseline mutation status. Patients with baseline mutations probably need mutation analysis every 3 months or when there is a confirmed rise in Bcr–Abl transcripts or Ph^+ chromosomes. Patients without baseline mutations may not require regular mutation analysis unless the Bcr–Abl value at 3 months is >10% international scale. However, these suggestions are still tentative and may change with increasing experience in managing these patients.

Advanced-stage chronic myeloid leukemia

Advanced stage CML includes patients with AP and BC. Progression to advanced phase is associated with a marked worsening of prognosis with median survival of 1–2 years in AP and 3–6 months in BC.

Accelerated phase

The World Health Organization (WHO) [48], International Bone Marrow Transplant Registry (IBMTR), and M. D. Anderson Cancer Center (MDACC) [49] criteria for diagnosing AP differ and are summarized in Table 23.2. Clonal evolution (CE), defined as the appearance of additional chromosomal abnormality in the leukemic clone, is one of the criteria to define AP. CE occurs in 20–40% of patients in AP [49–51], and common chromosomal abnormalities include trisomy 8 (30–40%), isochromosome 17i (17q, 15–20%), and additional Ph chromosome (20–30%) [49]. Patients who were diagnosed as AP on the basis of CE have a much better outcome compared with patients who have other criteria of AP [52].

Treatment for patients with accelerated phase chronic myeloid leukemia

Patients in AP steadily progress to BC if untreated. The median survival of patients treated with only hydroxyurea was 1–2 years [49]. Kantarjian *et al.* reported a CHR in 25% of patients in AP treated with daunorubicin and high-dose cytarabine; however, the responses were transient and median survival was 8 months [53]. The response to interferon was also poor in patients in AP; only 20–30% patients achieved some hematologic response and cytogenetic response was rare [54,55]. A combination of cytarabine and interferon resulted in 50% and 5% of CHR and MCyR, respectively [55].

Table 23.2 Comparison of WHO, IBMTR, and MDACC diagnostic criteria for accelerated phase.

Criteria	WHO	IBMTR	MDACC
BM or PB blasts (%)	10–19%	≥10%	15–29%
Blasts + promyelocytes (%)	NA	>20%	>30%
PB or BM basophils (%)	≥20%	≥20%	≥20%
Platelets ($\times 10^9$/L)	Persistent platelets <100 × 10^9/L unrelated to therapy or ≥1000 × 10^9/L unresponsive to therapy	Persistent platelets <100 × 10^9/L unrelated to therapy or ≥1000 × 10^9/L unresponsive to therapy	Persistent platelets <100 × 10^9/L unrelated to therapy or
Cytogenetic	Clonal evolution	Clonal evolution	Clonal evolution
WBC count	Increasing WBC count unresponsive to therapy	WBC count difficult to control or doubling <5 days	NA
Splenomegaly	Increasing spleen size	Increasing spleen size	NA

According to the WHO: megakaryocytic proliferation that occurs in sizeable sheets and clusters, associated with marked reticulin or collagen fibrosis and/or severe granulocytic dysplasia, should be considered as suggestive of accelerated-phase chronic myeloid leukmeia only in association with other findings.

BM, bone marrow; IBMTR, International Bone Marrow Transplant Registry; MDACC, M. D. Anderson Cancer Center; PB, peripheral blood; WBC, white blood cell; WHO, World Health Organization.

In a phase II study of imatinib in patients in AP, higher CHR (37% vs. 27%), MCyR (28% vs. 16%), and CCyR (19% vs. 11%) were achieved with 600 mg daily compared with 400 mg daily [16]. imatinib 600 mg daily also resulted in higher OS at 12 months (78% vs. 65%) compared with 400 mg daily. Although imatinib responses were superior to historic controls (eg, interferon, hydroxyurea), 50% of imatinib-treated patients in AP progressed and 38% of patients died within 4 years of treatment [56]. Hence, it is crucial to monitor these patients closely and to identify poor responders early, particularly if transplant options are available. Patients in AP who achieved MCyR at 3 months had significantly better 3-year survival compared with patients who did not achieve MCyR at 3 months (85% vs. 52%, $P < 0.001$) [57].

In a phase I study of nilotinib, 46%, 27%, and 14% of imatinib-resistant patients with CML-AP achieved CHR, MCyR, and CcyR, respectively [30]. A phase II study of patients with CML-AP ($n = 136$) who were resistant (81%) or intolerant (19%) to imatinib also demonstrated the efficacy of nilotinib. CHR, MCyR, and CCyR were achieved in 26%, 29%, and 16% of patients, and the median duration of response was 15 months (Table 23.2). The estimated OS at 12 months was 79%. The rate of MCyR at 6 months was not significantly different in patients with and without baseline mutations (21% and 36%, respectively) [58]. Nilotinib was well tolerated, and median-dose intensity was 99% of the intended dose. Grade 3–4 neutropenia and thrombocytopenia occurred in 21% and 35% of patients, respectively.

Dasatinib studies have also demonstrated efficacy in imatinib-resistant or intolerant patients in AP. In a phase I study of dasatinib, 45%, 27%, and 18% imatinib-resistant/intolerant patients with CML-AP achieved CHR, MCyR, and CcyR [59]. This was further confirmed in a phase II study of 161 patients with CML-AP [60]. CHR, MCyR, and CCyR were achieved in 39%, 33%, and 24% of patients, respectively. At 12 months, PFS and OS were 66% and 82%, respectively. Responses were achieved in all patients irrespective of their baseline mutation status (except *T315I*). Grade 3–4 neutropenia and thrombocytopenia were reported in 76% and 82% of patients [60].

In an ongoing phase I trial of bosutinib, CHR and MCyR were achieved in 4 of 14 (29%) and 3 of 9 (33%) evaluable patients with CML-AP [61].

INNO-404 is a dual Abl/Lyn kinase inhibitor that is 55 times more potent than imatinib *in vitro* and is active against most of the imatinib-resistant mutants except *T315I*. Unlike other second-line TKIs, INNO-406 demonstrates specific Lyn kinase activity with no or limited activity against other Src-family member kinases. Phase I studies are ongoing and early results show some activity in heavily pretreated patients with CML-AP and BC. Other drugs that have demonstrated some activity in patients in AP include homoharrington [62], decitabine [63], and farnesyl transferase inhibitors [64].

Allogeneic SCT can be curative in approximately 30–40% of these patients and therefore should be considered in patients with CML-AP [65–67]. At present, front-line therapy with imatinib (600 mg daily) is probably appropriate for all patients in AP who have not received prior imatinib therapy. Patients with CML-CP who progressed to AP while on imatinib therapy should be treated with second-generation TKIs (dasatinib or nilotinib) as a bridge to allogeneic SCT if donor is available. Phase II studies of dasatinib and nilotinib demonstrated similar efficacy in imatinib-resistant patients with AP. Hence, sensitivity of kinase domain mutations and adverse effects may guide the selection of second-line TKIs. However, these suggestions are still tentative.

Blast crisis

BC is characterized by the presence of ≥30% blasts in the peripheral blood or bone marrow or by the presence of extramedullary disease [68]. However, WHO diagnostic criteria for BC are different and are summarized in Table 23.3. The overall prognosis for patients with BC is poor, with a median survival of 3–12 months. With effective front-line therapy for CP, fewer patients will progress to AP or BC. In the IRIS study, 1.5, 2.8%, 1.6%, 0.9%, and 0.6% of patients progressed to AP or BC during the first, second, third, fourth, and fifth year of follow-up, respectively [1]. This suggests that the risk of transformation is maximal during the first 2 years of imatinib therapy and then progressively decreases. Moreover, patients who have achieved MMR by 12 months have 100% PFS by 60 months [1]. These data indicate that the depth of response during the first year of treatment determines their long-term outcome, and hence, with the availability of newer and more potent second-line TKIs for imatinib-resistant patients, the risk of disease progression may be further reduced. As BC remains incurable, a concern during treatment of patients in CP is the risk of sudden BC (sudden onset BC within 3 months of documented CHR), which

Table 23.3 Comparison of diagnostic criteria for blast crisis.

CML-blast crisis (one or more of the following)	
WHO criteria	MDACC and IBMTR criteria
BM and/or PB blast ≥20% Extramedullary blast proliferation or large foci or clusters of blast in the BM biopsy	BM and/or PB blast ≥30% Extramedullary infiltrates of leukemic cells outside liver or spleen

BM, bone marrow; IBMTR, International Bone Marrow Transplant Registry; MDACC, M. D. Anderson Cancer Center; PB, peripheral blood; WHO, World Health Organization.

may not allow time for alternative therapies. Sudden BC has been reported in 0.5–2.5% of patients treated with interferon. Kantarjian *et al.* reported 0.7% of sudden BC in a cohort of 541 patients with CML-CP treated with imatinib [69].

Approximately 50% of patients have myeloid blast crisis (MBC), 25% have lymphoid blast crisis (LBC), and 25% have an undifferentiated blast crisis [70]. Patients who have LBC tend to be younger than patients with MBC. The median survival of patients with LBC is 12 months, which is somewhat longer than patients with MBC (3–6 months) [71,72]. Other features that are associated with adverse prognosis include CE, a bone marrow blast >50%, and a platelet count $<50 \times 10^9$/L [72].

Nearly two-thirds of patients in BC have CE, and common chromosomal abnormalities include trisomy 8 (33%), isochromosome 17i(17q) 20%, trisomy 19 (12%) additional Ph chromosome (30%), trisomy 21 (7%), and monosomy 7 (5%) [73]. The mechanism of transformation to BC is not entirely understood. Differentiation arrest, genomic instability, telomere shortening, and loss of tumor-suppressor functions are involved in transformation. The differentiation arrest is by suppression of translation of the transcription factor CEBP-α. Bcr–Abl suppress translation of CEBP-α by increasing the stability of the transcriptional regulator, heterogeneous nuclear ribonucleoprotein E2 (HNRNPE2) [74]. The increased genomic instability in CML cells is the result of their reduced capacity to survey the genome for DNA damage and to correctly repair the DNA lesions, which leads to accumulation of deleterious mutations in genes that are essential for maintaining normal cell physiology. Mismatch repair is responsible for detecting misincorporated nucleotides, resulting in excision repair before point mutations occur and/or induction of apoptosis to avoid propagation of cells carrying excessive DNA lesions. Bcr–Abl kinase abrogates mismatch repair activity to inhibit apoptosis and induce mutated phenotype [75]. Impairment of tumor-suppressor genes, such as *TP53*, retinoblastoma 1, *CDKN2A*, and others [76–82] have been reported. Protein phosphatase 2a (PP2A) acts as a tumor suppressor in CML by antagonizing Bcr–Abl. The inactivation of PP2A is associated with disease progression. Bcr–Abl inhibits PP2A by post-transcriptional upregulation of SET, a phosphoprotein that functions as a physiologic inhibitor of PP2A [83].

Treatment for patients with blast crisis chronic myeloid leukemia

Before TKI, patients in BC were treated with intensive chemotherapy to allogeneic SCT or were palliated. AML-induction regimens (usually a combination of cytarabine and anthracyclines) were used to treat patients with myeloid, undifferentiated, and mixed-lineage BC. These regimens were associated with response rates of 20–30%; however, most responses were transient, with a median survival of 4–10 months [72,84,85]. In a single-institute study of non-lymphoid patients in BC, the response rates (26% vs. 28%) and survival (7 vs. 5 months) were similar with decitabine and intensive chemotherapy [84]. In another phase II study, low-dose decitabine induced a hematologic response in 84%, 41%, and 34% of imatinib-resistant patients with CML-CP, AP, and BC, respectively, although median duration of response was 3.5 months only [86].

In a phase II study of imatinib in patients with CML-BC (n = 260), CHR, MCyR, and CCyR were achieved in 8%, 16%, and 7% of patients, respectively (Table 23.4). The median survival was 7 months and estimated OS at 18 months was 20%. Patients with MCyR had a longer median OS compared with patients without MCyR (12 vs.

Table 23.4 Response to TKI therapy in patients with accelerated phase and blast crisis.

	CHR (%)	MCyR (%)	CCyR (%)	OS at 12 months	PFS at 12 months	Ref.
Accelerated-phase patients						
Imatinib 600 mg daily (n = 119)	37	28	19	78	67	Talpaz *et al.* [16]
Nilotinib (n = 119)	26	29	16	79	NA	le Coutre *et al.* [58]
Dasatinib (n = 174)	45	39	32	82	66	Guilhot *et al.* [60]
Blast crisis						
Imatinib (n = 260)	8	16	7	7 months	NA	Sawyers *et al.* [15]
Nilotinib in MBC (n = 119)	13	NA	NA	NA	NA	Giles *et al.* [87]
Nilotinib in LBC (n = 29)	26	NA	NA	NA	NA	Giles *et al.* [87]
Dasatinib in MBC (n = 109)	27	33	26	12 months	6.7 months	Cortes *et al.* [88]
Dasatinib in LBC (n = 48)	29	52	46	5 months	3 months	Cortes *et al.* [88]

Note: The data is pulled from different studies. Dasatinib and nilotinib study were conducted on imatinib failure patients.

CHR, Complete haematological response; CCyR, complete cytogenetic response; MCyR, Major cytogenetic response; NA, not available; OS, overall survival; PFS, progression free survival.

6 months) [15]. At the recommended dose of 600 mg, an estimated 7% of patients remained progression-free, and 14% patients were alive at 36 months after initiation of imatinib [57]. Poor survival in imatinib-treated patients in BC was also confirmed in another study; median OS and PFS were 7 and 3 months, respectively [89]. A combination of imatinib with low-dose cytarabine and idarubicin resulted in a 47% CHR with a median survival of 5 months in patients with MBC [90]. In a phase II study of a combination of imatinib and decitabine, hematologic response rates were higher (53% vs. 14%) in patients with CML-MBC without kinase domain mutations compared with patients with kinase domain mutations. However, median duration of hematologic response was only 18 weeks, and myelosuppression was the major adverse effect [91]. A combination of imatinib with hyper-CVAD was used to treat patients with CML-LBC and Ph^+ ALL. A complete response was achieved in 5 of 7 patients with CML-LBC. The addition of imatinib did not result in significant additional myelosuppression or non-hematologic toxicities [92]. These data suggest that imatinib as a single agent and in combination is not adequate to treat patients with BC.

In a phase I study of nilotinib, 42% and 21% of imatinib-resistant patients with BC achieved hematologic response and MCyR, respectively [30]. In a phase II study of nilotinib, a CHR was achieved in 13% of patients with MBC ($n = 87$) and 26% of patients with LBC ($n = 27$), respectively. However, 88% of patients discontinued treatment, mostly (53%) because of disease progression [87].

In a phase I study of dasatinib, CCyR was achieved in 29% of patients with MBC [59]; these results were subsequently confirmed. In a phase II study, major hematologic response (MHR), MCyR, and CCyR were achieved in 34%, 33%, and 26% of patients with MBC (n=109), respectively, and 31%, 52%, and 46% of patients with LBC ($n = 48$), respectively [88]. In the MBC group, CCyR was similar in patients with P-loop mutations (21%), with other mutations (25%), and without baseline mutations (22%). However, in LBC, the CCyR was lower in patients with P-loop mutations (27%) compared with patients with other mutations (43%) and no baseline mutations (50%). In spite of good cytogenetic response, duration of response was short. Median PFS and OS were 6.7 and 11.8 months in MBC and 3 and 5.3 months in LBC, respectively. During follow-up of this study, 59% of patients with MBC and 77% of patients with LBC progressed but >50% patients had died [88].

In an ongoing phase I trial of bosutinib, 25% and 33% of evaluable patients with BC achieved CHR and MCyR [61]. However, there were fewer patients and median follow-up was 2.3 months only.

The pursuit of a novel approach to effectively treat BC is continuing. There is increasing appreciation that an excess of proangiogenic factors, including vascular endothelial growth factor (VEGF), platelet-derived growth factors, and basic fibroblast growth factors are involved in the pathogenesis of leukemias [93–95]. Clinical trials with anti-VEGF monoclonal antibodies (bevacizumab) and receptor TKIs directed at the VEGF receptor family are currently being conducted. Other drugs that are in the early clinical phase are mTOR inhibitors, farnesyl transferase inhibitors, histone deacetylase inhibitors, homoharrington, arsenic trioxide, and bortezomib.

Allogeneic stem-cell transplantation for advanced-phase patients

Allogeneic SCT is the only potentially curative treatment for advanced-phase patients with CML, although results are significantly inferior than in CP. Survival following SCT is determined by various factors. Gratwohl *et al.* [96] developed a risk assessment score for the outcome of transplantation that involves five prognostic factors, including recipient age, disease stage at transplantation, donor type, donor–recipient gender combination, and the interval from diagnosis to transplantation. Disease phase at the time of transplantation remains the main determinant of transplant outcome. In the pre- imatinib era, 5-year survival of patients transplanted in first CP, AP, and BC was 50–80%, 30–40%, and 10–20%, respectively [66,67]. Patients in BC transplanted in the second CP (CP2) had a similar survival to patients in AP [66,67,97]. Visani *et al.* [98] also reported that achieving CP2 by induction chemotherapy prior to allogeneic SCT improves OS and DFS following transplant. However, some argue that achieving CP2 by chemotherapy might be selecting the best biologic group for allograft. Transplant-related mortality (TRM) was significantly higher among patients transplanted in AP and BC (20% and 60% at 1 and 3 years) compared with patients transplanted in CP1 or CP2 (12% and 20% at 1 and 3 years) [99].

Studies presented in the previous section demonstrated that imatinib, dasatinib, and nilotinib treatment can induce CHR and MCyR, and even CcyR, in some advanced-phase patients; however, these responses were short-lasting and relapses were very likely, particularly in patients with BC. Hence, TKI as monotherapy are not adequate to treat advanced-phase patients, especially patients with BC. The next question is can we use these TKIs as a bridge to SCT? Does imatinib prior to SCT increase post-SCT complications? As TKIs induce CP2 in some advanced disease patients (~50% of patients) [100,101] and there is evidence that transplanting in CP2 may lead to improved survival [98] compared with transplanting in BC, does TKI prior to SCT improve the survival of these patients?

Recently, survival and post-transplant complications of advanced-disease patients treated with imatinib prior to transplant were compared with patients who did not receive imatinib prior to SCT. imatinib treatment prior to SCT did not increase post-transplant toxicity, TRM, or non-relapse mortality [97,100,102–104]. There was no increase in hepatotoxicity, and engraftment was not delayed [97]. The effect of imatinib on acute graft-versus host disease (GVHD) and chronic GVHD is debatable. Most of the studies reported no difference in acute GVHD [97,100,102,104–106] while another group reported that there may be an increased acute GVHD [107] in imatinib-treated patients compared with historic controls. Chronic GVHD in imatinib pretreated patients were reported to be less common in some studies [97,100], but more common in another study [102], compared with historical control. Thus, current evidence would suggest that imatinib treatment prior to SCT does not increase post-SCT complications and hence can be used while searching for a suitable donor.

Most of the reported studies demonstrated that imatinib prior to SCT induces CP2 in ~40–50% of patients in AP and BC [97,100,103], and there is increasing evidence that patients transplanted in CP2 have fewer transplant-related complications and non-relapse mortality [98,100,102]. However, all these studies failed to demonstrate a survival advantage following SCT in imatinib pretreated patients compared with historic controls [97,100,102]. Post-SCT, median PFS, and OS of imatinib pretreated advanced-phase patients were 6 and 9 months, respectively [100], and 3-year OS ranged from 34% to 48% [97,102]. Oehler *et al.* reported similar post-SCT survival in patients who progressed from CP to advanced phase prior to SCT, advanced-phase patients returned back to CP, and those who did not respond to imatinib [97]. The possible explanation for the lack of survival benefit in patients who received imatinib prior to SCT may be that, in recent studies, more patients were transplanted with an unrelated donor compared with matched-related donors, which increases the non-relapse mortality. Secondly, imatinib allowed more patients to be transplanted who otherwise would not have had SCT.

Thus, there is no evidence that TKI therapy prior to SCT improved survival in advanced-phase patients. Clearly, the best management is to prevent disease progression to advanced phase. Patients who progress to advanced-phase CML or present with *de novo* advanced-phase disease can be treated with TKI until a suitable donor is available, and should progress to SCT as early as possible. There are no randomized studies comparing the effectiveness of imatinib, dasatinib and nilotinib in advanced-phase CML. When comparing different phase II studies, responses to dasatinib were higher compared with imatinib and nilotinib; however, responses to all TKIs were short-lived.

Recommendations for patients with *de novo* advanced-phase disease and blast crisis

Patients presenting with *de novo* AP should be treated with imatinib (600 mg daily) and monitored closely with RQ-PCR and mutation analysis every 3 months [21]. Donor search should be started at diagnosis, and patients with suitable donors should be considered for allogeneic SCT. Patients who subsequently develop imatinib resistance can be treated with second-line TKIs (dasatinib or nilotinib) as a bridge to transplantation. second-line TKIs are more potent and have demonstrated activity in imatinib-resistant patients; however, at present, there is no clinical data to support their use as front-line therapy.

Patients presenting with *de novo* BC should be treated with imatinib (600 mg daily) and proceed to allogeneic SCT if a suitable donor is available. Patients with CML-MBC who do not have a suitable matched donor can be treated with AML-like chemotherapy along with imatinib, and monitored closely by RQ-PCR, mutation analysis, and bone marrow examination. Patients with BC who subsequently develop imatinib resistance should be treated with second-generation TKIs (dasatinib or nilotinib). The selection between dasatinib or nilotinib can be guided by the mutation status of the patient and toxicity profile.

Conclusion

The majority of patients with newly diagnosed CML-CP respond to imatinib therapy; however, around 30% of patients fail imatinib treatment during the first 5 years of therapy. Hence, patients on imatinib treatment should be monitored closely. The majority of patients (~60%) with secondary resistance to imatinib have kinase domain mutations, and hence all patients with imatinib resistance should have kinase domain mutation studies. The selection of second-line TKIs depends on underlying mutation sensitivity, disease phase of patients, and the patient's toxicity profile. Fifty percent of imatinib-resistant patients will not achieve CCyR with a second-generation TKI, hence it is imperative to monitor these patients closely by RQ-PCR, bone marrow cytogenetics, and mutation analysis. At present, for patients with the *T315I* mutation, SCT is the only proven effective treatment option, although there are new drugs currently under evaluation.

Treatment of patients with advanced-phase CML is rather disappointing. Although some patients would respond to imatinib or second-generation TKI, most of the responses are short lived, and allogeneic SCT is the only curative treatment available for these patients. Hence, TKI may be used as bridge to SCT rather than monotherapy. Understanding the biology of advanced-phase CML will open new avenues for effective management.

References

1 Druker BJ, Guilhot F, O'Brien SG, *et al.* Five-year follow-up of patients receiving imatinib for chronic myeloid leukemia. *N Engl J Med* 2006;355:2408–17.

2 Baccarani M, Saglio G, Goldman J, *et al.* Evolving concepts in the management of chronic myeloid leukemia: recommendations from an expert panel on behalf of the European LeukemiaNet. *Blood* 2006;108:1809–20.

3 Shah NP. Loss of response to imatinib: mechanisms and management. *Hematology Am Soc Hematol Educ Program* 2005: 183–7.

4 White D, Saunders V, Lyons AB, *et al. In vitro* sensitivity to imatinib-induced inhibition of ABL kinase activity is predictive of molecular response in patients with de novo CML. *Blood* 2005;106:2520–6.

5 White D, Saunders V, Grigg A, *et al.* Measurement of *in vivo* Bcr–Abl kinase inhibition to monitor imatinib-induced target blockade and predict response in chronic myeloid leukemia. *J Clin Oncol* 2007;25:4445–51.

6 Kantarjian H, Talpaz M, O'Brien S, *et al.* High-dose imatinib mesylate therapy in newly diagnosed Philadelphia chromosome-positive chronic phase chronic myeloid leukemia. *Blood* 2004; 103:2873–8.

7 Kantarjian HM, Talpaz M, O'Brien S, *et al.* Dose escalation of imatinib mesylate can overcome resistance to standard-dose therapy in patients with chronic myelogenous leukemia. *Blood* 2003;101:473–5.

8 Larson RA, Druker BJ, Guilhot F, *et al.* Imatinib pharmacokinetics and its correlation with response and safety in chronic-phase chronic myeloid leukemia: a subanalysis of the IRIS study. *Blood* 2008;11:4022–8.

9 Thomas J, Wang L, Clark RE, Pirmohamed M. Active transport of imatinib into and out of cells: implications for drug resistance. *Blood* 2004;104:3739–45.

10 White DL, Saunders VA, Dang P, *et al.* OCT-1-mediated influx is a key determinant of the intracellular uptake of imatinib but not nilotinib (AMN107): reduced OCT-1 activity is the cause of low *in vitro* sensitivity to imatinib. *Blood* 2006;108:697–704.

11 White DL, Saunders VA, Dang P, *et al.* Most CML patients who have a suboptimal response to imatinib have low OCT-1 activity: higher doses of imatinib may overcome the negative impact of low OCT-1 activity. *Blood* 2007;110:4064–72.

12 Wang L, Giannoudis A, Lane S, Williamson P, Pirmohamed M, Clark RE. Expression of the uptake drug transporter hOCT1 is an important clinical determinant of the response to imatinib in chronic myeloid leukemia. *Clin Pharmacol Ther* 2008; 83:258–64.

13 Hughes TP, Kaeda J, Branford S, *et al.* Frequency of major molecular responses to imatinib or interferon alfa plus cytarabine in newly diagnosed chronic myeloid leukemia. *N Engl J Med* 2003;349:1423–32.

14 Hochhaus A, Druker B, Sawyers C, *et al.* Favorable long-term follow-up results over 6 years for response, survival, and safety with imatinib mesylate therapy in chronic-phase chronic myeloid leukemia after failure of interferon-alpha treatment. *Blood* 2008;111:1039–43.

15 Sawyers CL, Hochhaus A, Feldman E, *et al.* Imatinib induces hematologic and cytogenetic responses in patients with chronic myelogenous leukemia in myeloid blast crisis: results of a phase II study. *Blood* 2002;99:3530–9.

16 Talpaz M, Silver RT, Druker BJ, *et al.* Imatinib induces durable hematologic and cytogenetic responses in patients with accelerated phase chronic myeloid leukemia: results of a phase 2 study. *Blood* 2002;99:1928–37.

17 Hiwase DK, Saunders V, Hewett D, *et al.* Dasatinib cellular uptake and efflux in chronic myeloid leukemia cells: therapeutic implications. *Clin Cancer Res* 2008;14:3881–8.

18 Gorre ME, Mohammed M, Ellwood K, *et al.* Clinical resistance to STI-571 cancer therapy caused by *BCR–ABL* gene mutation or amplification. *Science* 2001;293:876–80.

19 Hochhaus A, Kreil S, Corbin AS, *et al.* Molecular and chromosomal mechanisms of resistance to imatinib (STI571) therapy. *Leukemia* 2002;16:2190–6.

20 Branford S, Rudzki Z, Walsh S, *et al.* High frequency of point mutations clustered within the adenosine triphosphate-binding region of BCR/ABL in patients with chronic myeloid leukemia or Ph-positive acute lymphoblastic leukemia who develop imatinib (STI571) resistance. *Blood* 2002;99:3472–5.

21 Branford S, Rudzki Z, Walsh S, *et al.* Detection of *BCR–ABL* mutations in patients with CML treated with imatinib is virtually always accompanied by clinical resistance, and mutations in the ATP phosphate-binding loop (P-loop) are associated with a poor prognosis. *Blood* 2003;102:276–83.

22 Cowan-Jacob SW, Guez V, Fendrich G, *et al.* Imatinib (STI571) resistance in chronic myelogenous leukemia: molecular basis of the underlying mechanisms and potential strategies for treatment. *Mini Rev Med Chem* 2004;4:285–99.

23 Shah NP, Nicoll JM, Nagar B, *et al.* Multiple Bcr–Abl kinase domain mutations confer polyclonal resistance to the tyrosine kinase inhibitor imatinib (STI571) in chronic phase and blast crisis chronic myeloid leukemia. *Cancer Cell* 2002;2:117–25.

24 Apperley JF. Part I: mechanisms of resistance to imatinib in chronic myeloid leukemia. *Lancet Oncol* 2007;8:1018–29.

25 Donato NJ, Wu JY, Stapley J, *et al.* Bcr–Abl independence and LYN kinase overexpression in chronic myelogenous leukemia cells selected for resistance to STI571. *Blood* 2003;101:690–8.

26 Gambacorti-Passerini C, Barni R, le Coutre P, *et al.* Role of alpha1 acid glycoprotein in the *in vivo* resistance of human *BCR–ABL*(+) leukemic cells to the abl inhibitor STI571. *J Natl Cancer Inst* 2000;92:1641–50.

27 Mahon FX, Belloc F, Lagarde V, *et al. MDR1* gene overexpression confers resistance to imatinib mesylate in leukemia cell line models. *Blood* 2003;101:2368–73.

28 Kantarjian H, Pasquini R, Hamerschlak N, *et al.* Dasatinib or high-dose imatinib for chronic-phase chronic myeloid leukemia after failure of first-line imatinib: a randomized phase 2 trial. *Blood* 2007;109:5143–50.

29 Weisberg E, Manley PW, Breitenstein W, *et al.* Characterization of AMN107, a selective inhibitor of native and mutant Bcr–Abl. *Cancer Cell* 2005;7:129–41.

30 Kantarjian H, Giles F, Wunderle L, *et al.* Nilotinib in imatinib-resistant CML and Philadelphia chromosome-positive ALL. *N Engl J Med* 2006;354:2542–51.

31 Kantarjian HM, Giles F, Gattermann N, *et al.* Nilotinib (formerly AMN107), a highly selective Bcr–Abl tyrosine kinase inhibitor, is effective in patients with Philadelphia chromosome-positive chronic myelogenous leukemia in chronic phase following imatinib resistance and intolerance. *Blood* 2007;110: 3540–6.

32 O'Hare T, Walters DK, Stoffregen EP, *et al. In vitro* activity of Bcr–Abl inhibitors AMN107 and BMS-354825 against clinically relevant imatinib-resistant Abl kinase domain mutants. *Cancer Res* 2005;65:4500–5.

33 Mauro MJ, Baccarani M, Cervantes F, *et al.* Dasatinib 2-year efficacy in patients with chronic-phase chronic myelogenous leukemia (CML-CP) with resistance or intolerance to imatinib (START-C). *J Clin Oncol* 2008;26, Abstract 7009.

34 Hochhaus A, Kantarjian HM, Baccarani M, *et al.* Dasatinib induces notable hematologic and cytogenetic responses in chronic-phase chronic myeloid leukemia after failure of imatinib therapy. *Blood* 2007;109:2303–9.

35 Shah NP, Kantarjian HM, Kim DW, *et al.* Intermittent target inhibition with dasatinib 100 mg once daily preserves efficacy and improves tolerability in imatinib-resistant and -intolerant chronic-phase chronic myeloid leukemia. *J Clin Oncol* 2008;26: 3204–12.

36 Puttini M, Coluccia AM, Boschelli F, *et al.* In vitro and in vivo activity of SKI-606, a novel Src-Abl inhibitor, against imatinib-resistant Bcr–Abl+ neoplastic cells. *Cancer Res* 2006; 66:11314–22.

37 Bruemmendorf TH, Cervantes F, Kim D, *et al.* Bosutinib is safe and active in patients (pts) with chronic phase (CP) chronic myeloid leukemia (CML) with resistance or intolerance to imatinib and other tyrosine kinase inhibitors. *J Clin Oncol* 2008;26, Abstract 7001.

38 O'Hare T, Eide CA, Deininger MW. Bcr–Abl kinase domain mutations, drug resistance, and the road to a cure for chronic myeloid leukemia. *Blood* 2007;110:2242–9.

39 Hughes T, Saglio G, Martinelli G, *et al.* Responses and disease progression in CML-CP patients treated with nilotinib after imatinib failure appear to be affected by the *BCR–ABL* mutation status and types. *Blood* 2007;110, Abstract 320.

40 O'Brien SG, Guilhot F, Larson RA, *et al.* Imatinib compared with interferon and low-dose cytarabine for newly diagnosed chronic-phase chronic myeloid leukemia. *N Engl J Med* 2003; 348:994–1004.

41 Jabbour E, Kantarjian H, Jones D, *et al.* Characteristics and outcomes of patients with chronic myeloid leukemia and *T315I* mutation following failure of imatinib mesylate therapy. *Blood* 2008;112:53–5.

42 Paquette R, Shah NP, Sawyers CL, *et al.* PHA-739358, an Aurora kinase inhibitor, induces clinical responses in chronic myeloid leukemia harboring *T315I* mutations of *BCR–ABL*. *Blood* 2007;110, Abstract 1030.

43 Cortes J, Roboz GJ, Kantarjian H, *et al.* A phase I dose escalation study of KW-2449, an oral multikinase inhibitor against FLT3, ABL, FGFR1, and Aurora in patients with relapsed/refractory AML, treatment resistant/intolerant CML, ALL, MDS. *Blood* 2007;110, Abstract 909.

44 Quintas-Cardama A, Kantarjian H, Garcia-Manero G, *et al.* Phase I/II study of subcutaneous homoharringtonine in patients with chronic myeloid leukemia who have failed prior therapy. *Cancer* 2007;109:248–55.

45 Khoury H, Michallet M, Corm S, *et al.* Safety and efficacy study of subcutaneous homoharringtonine (SC HHT) in imatinib (IM)-resistant chronic myeloid leukemia (CML) with the *T315I* mutation initial report of a phase II trial. *Blood* 2007;110, Abstract 1050.

46 Van Etten RA, Chan WW, Zaleskas VM, *et al.* DCC-2036. a novel switch pocket inhibitor of ABL tyrosine kinase with therapeutic efficacy against *BCR–ABL T315I* in vitro and in a CML mouse model. *Blood* 2007;110, Abstract 463.

47 Tam CS, Kantarjian H, Garcia-Manero G, *et al.* Failure to achieve a major cytogenetic response by 12 months defines inadequate response in patients receiving nilotinib or dasatinib as second or subsequent line therapy for chronic myeloid leukemia. *Blood* 2008;112:516–18.

48 Jaffe ES, Harris NL, Stein H, Vardiman JW. *Pathology and Genetics of Tumours of Haematopoietic and Lymphoid Tissues*. IARC Press: Lyon, 2001.

49 Kantarjian HM, Dixon D, Keating MJ, *et al.* Characteristics of accelerated disease in chronic myelogenous leukemia. *Cancer* 1988;61:1441–6.

50 Sokal JE, Gomez GA, Baccarani M, *et al.* Prognostic significance of additional cytogenetic abnormalities at diagnosis of Philadelphia chromosome-positive chronic granulocytic leukemia. *Blood* 1988;72:294–8.

51 Mitelman F. The cytogenetic scenario of chronic myeloid leukemia. *Leuk Lymphoma* 1993;11(Suppl.1):11–15.

52 Majlis A, Smith TL, Talpaz M, O'Brien S, Rios MB, Kantarjian HM. Significance of cytogenetic clonal evolution in chronic myelogenous leukemia. *J Clin Oncol* 1996;14:196–203.

53 Kantarjian HM, Talpaz M, Kontoyiannis D, *et al.* Treatment of chronic myelogenous leukemia in accelerated and blastic phases with daunorubicin, high-dose cytarabine, and granulocyte-macrophage colony-stimulating factor. *J Clin Oncol* 1992;10:398–405.

54 Kantarjian HM, Smith TL, O'Brien S, Beran M, Pierce S, Talpaz M. Prolonged survival in chronic myelogenous leukemia after cytogenetic response to interferon-alpha therapy. The Leukemia Service. *Ann Intern Med* 1995;122: 254–61.

55 Kantarjian HM, Keating MJ, Estey EH, *et al.* Treatment of advanced stages of Philadelphia chromosome-positive chronic myelogenous leukemia with interferon-alpha and low-dose cytarabine. *J Clin Oncol* 1992;10:772–8.

56 Kantarjian H, Talpaz M, O'Brien S, *et al.* Survival benefit with imatinib mesylate therapy in patients with accelerated-phase chronic myelogenous leukemia–comparison with historic experience. *Cancer* 2005;103:2099–108.

57 Silver RT, Talpaz M, Sawyers CL, *et al.* Four years of follow-up of 1027 patients with late chronic phase (L-CP), accelerated phase (AP), or blast crisis (BC) chronic myeloid leukemia (CML) treated with imatinib in three large phase II trials. *Blood* 2004;104, Abstract 23.

58 le Coutre P, Ottmann OG, Giles F, *et al.* Nilotinib (formerly AMN107), a highly selective Bcr–Abl tyrosine kinase inhibitor, is active in patients with imatinib-resistant or -intolerant accelerated-phase chronic myelogenous leukemia. *Blood* 2008; 111:1834–9.

59 Talpaz M, Shah NP, Kantarjian H, *et al.* Dasatinib in imatinib-resistant Philadelphia chromosome-positive leukemias. *N Engl J Med.* 2006;354:2531–41.

60 Guilhot F, Apperley J, Kim DW, *et al.* Dasatinib induces significant hematologic and cytogenetic responses in patients with imatinib-resistant or -intolerant chronic myeloid leukemia in accelerated phase. *Blood* 2007;109:4143–50.

61 Gambacorti-Passerini C, Kantarjian HM, Bruemmendorf T, *et al.* Bosutinib (SKI-606) demonstrates clinical activity and is well tolerated among patients with AP and BP CML and Ph+ ALL. *Blood* 2007;110, Abstract 473.

62 Quintas-Cardama A, Kantarjian HM, Garcia-Menaro G, *et al.* A phase II study of intravenous (IV) homoharringtonine (HHT) and imatinib (IM) in patients (pts) with chronic myeloid leukemia (CML). *Blood* 2006;11:616a.

63 Kantarjian HM, O'Brien SM, Estey E, *et al.* Decitabine studies in chronic and acute myelogenous leukemia. *Leukemia* 1997;11(Suppl.1):S35–6.

64 Thomas D, Cortes J, O'Brien S, *et al.* R115777, a farnesyl transferase inhibitor (FTI), has signficant antileukemia activity in patients with chronic myeloid leukemia. *Blood* 2001;98: 727a.

65 Griesshammer M, Arnold R, Bangerter M, *et al.* Chronic myeloid leukemia in accelerated phase: treatment results with conventional chemotherapy and allogeneic bone marrow transplantation in 96 patients. *Eur J Haematol* 1998;6:7–13.

66 Clift RA, Storb R. Marrow transplantation for CML: the Seattle experience. *Bone Marrow Transplant* 1996;17(Suppl.3):S1–3.

67 Horowitz MM, Rowlings PA, Passweg JR. Allogeneic bone marrow transplantation for CML: a report from the International Bone Marrow Transplant Registry. *Bone Marrow Transplant* 1996;17(Suppl.3):S5–6.

68 Faderl S, Talpaz M, Estrov Z, Kantarjian HM. Chronic myelogenous leukemia: biology and therapy. *Ann Intern Med* 1999;131:207–19.

69 Jabbour E, Kantarjian H, O'Brien S, *et al.* Sudden blastic transformation in patients with chronic myeloid leukemia treated with imatinib mesylate. *Blood* 2006;107:480–2.

70 Griffin JD, Todd RF, 3rd, Ritz J, *et al.* Differentiation patterns in the blastic phase of chronic myeloid leukemia. *Blood* 1983;61:85–91.

71 Kantarjian HM, Shan J, Smith T, *et al.* Response to therapy is independently associated with survival prolongation in chronic myelogenous leukemia in the blastic phase. *Cancer* 2001;92:2501–7.

72 Wadhwa J, Szydlo RM, Apperley JF, *et al.* Factors affecting duration of survival after onset of blastic transformation of chronic myeloid leukemia. *Blood* 2002;99:2304–9.

73 Johansson B, Fioretos T, Mitelman F. Cytogenetic and molecular genetic evolution of chronic myeloid leukemia. *Acta Haematologica* 2002;107:76–94.

74 Perrotti D, Cesi V, Trotta R, *et al.* Bcr–Abl suppresses C/EBPalpha expression through inhibitory action of hnRNP E2. *Nat Genet* 2002;30:48–58.

75 Stoklosa T, Poplawski T, Koptyra M, *et al.* Bcr–Abl inhibits mismatch repair to protect from apoptosis and induce point mutations. *Cancer Res* 2008;68:2576–80.

76 Feinstein E, Cimino G, Gale RP, *et al.* *p53* in chronic myelogenous leukemia in acute phase. *Proc Natl Acad Sci U S A* 1991;88:6293–7.

77 Ahuja HG, Jat PS, Foti A, Bar-Eli M, Cline MJ. Abnormalities of the retinoblastoma gene in the pathogenesis of acute leukemia. *Blood* 1991;78:3259–68.

78 Beck Z, Kiss A, Toth FD, *et al.* Alterations of *P53* and *RB* genes and the evolution of the accelerated phase of chronic myeloid leukemia. *Leuk Lymphoma* 2000;38:587–97.

79 Towatari M, Adachi K, Kato H, Saito H. Absence of the human retinoblastoma gene product in the megakaryoblastic crisis of chronic myelogenous leukemia. *Blood* 1991;78:2178–81.

80 Ahuja H, Bar-Eli M, Advani SH, Benchimol S, Cline MJ. Alterations in the *p53* gene and the clonal evolution of the blast crisis of chronic myelocytic leukemia. *Proc Natl Acad Sci U S A.* 1989;86:6783–7.

81 Sill H, Goldman JM, Cross NC. Homozygous deletions of the *p16* tumor-suppressor gene are associated with lymphoid transformation of chronic myeloid leukemia. *Blood* 1995;85: 2013–16.

82 Serra A, Gottardi E, Della Ragione F, Saglio G, Iolascon A. Involvement of the cyclin-dependent kinase-4 inhibitor (*CDKN2*) gene in the pathogenesis of lymphoid blast crisis of chronic myelogenous leukemia. *Br J Haematol* 1995;91:625–9.

83 Neviani P, Santhanam R, Trotta R, *et al.* The tumor suppressor PP2A is functionally inactivated in blast crisis CML through the inhibitory activity of the BCR/ABL-regulated SET protein. *Cancer Cell* 2005;8:355–68.

84 Sacchi S, Kantarjian HM, O'Brien S, *et al.* Chronic myelogenous leukemia in nonlymphoid blastic phase: analysis of the results of first salvage therapy with three different treatment approaches for 162 patients. *Cancer* 1999;86:2632–41.

85 Kantarjian HM, Cortes J, O'Brien S, *et al.* Imatinib mesylate (STI571) therapy for Philadelphia chromosome-positive chronic myelogenous leukemia in blast phase. *Blood* 2002;99: 3547–53.

86 Issa JP, Gharibyan V, Cortes J, *et al.* Phase II study of low-dose decitabine in patients with chronic myelogenous leukemia resistant to imatinib mesylate. *J Clin Oncol* 2005;23:3948–56.

87 Giles FJ, Larson RA, Kantarjian HM, *et al.* Nilotinib in patients with philadelphia chromosome-positive (Ph+) chronic myelogenous leukemia in blast crisis (CML-BC) who are resistant or intolerant to imatinib. *Blood* 2007;110, Abstract 1025.

88 Cortes J, Rousselot P, Kim DW, *et al.* Dasatinib induces complete hematologic and cytogenetic responses in patients with imatinib-resistant or -intolerant chronic myeloid leukemia in blast crisis. *Blood* 2007;109:3207–13.

89 Aoki E, Kantarjian H, O'Brien S, *et al.* Correlation of different responses to imatinib on survival of patients (pts) with chronic myelogenous leukemia (CML) in accelerated (AP) and blast phase (BP). *Blood* 2005;106, Abstract 1103

90 Quintas-Cardama A, Kantarjian H, Garcia-Manero G, *et al.* A pilot study of imatinib, low-dose cytarabine and idarubicin for patients with chronic myeloid leukemia in myeloid blast phase. *Leuk Lymphoma* 2007;48:283–9.

91 Oki Y, Kantarjian HM, Gharibyan V, *et al.* Phase II study of low-dose decitabine in combination with imatinib mesylate in patients with accelerated or myeloid blastic phase of chronic myelogenous leukemia. *Cancer* 2007;109:899–906.

92 Thomas D, Cortes J, Giles F, *et al.* Combination of hyper-CVAD with imatinib mesylate for Philadelphia-positive adult acute lymphoblastic leukemia or chronic myelogenous leukemia in lymphoid blast phase. *Blood* 2001;98:803, Abstract 3340.

93 Thomas DA, Estey E, Giles FJ, *et al.* Single agent thalidomide in patients with relapsed or refractory acute myeloid leukemia. *Br J Haematol* 2003;123:436–41.

94 Verstovsek S, Lunin S, Kantarjian H, *et al.* Clinical relevance of VEGF receptors 1 and 2 in patients with chronic myelogenous leukemia. *Leuk Res* 2003;27:661–9.

95 Verstovsek S, Kantarjian H, Manshouri T, *et al.* Prognostic significance of cellular vascular endothelial growth factor expression in chronic phase chronic myeloid leukemia. *Blood* 2002;99:2265–7.

96 Gratwohl A, Hermans J, Goldman JM, *et al.* Risk assessment for patients with chronic myeloid leukemia before allogeneic blood or marrow transplantation. Chronic Leukemia Working Party of the European Group for Blood and Marrow Transplantation. *Lancet* 1998;352:1087–92.

97 Oehler VG, Gooley T, Snyder DS, *et al.* The effects of imatinib mesylate treatment before allogeneic transplantation for chronic myeloid leukemia. *Blood* 2007;109:1782–9.

98 Visani G, Rosti G, Bandini G, *et al.* Second chronic phase before transplantation is crucial for improving survival of blastic phase chronic myeloid leukemia. *Br J Haematol* 2000;109: 722–8.

99 Crawley C, Szydlo R, Lalancette M, *et al.* Outcomes of reduced-intensity transplantation for chronic myeloid leukemia: an analysis of prognostic factors from the Chronic Leukemia Working Party of the EBMT. *Blood* 2005;106:2969–76.

100 Deininger M, Schleuning M, Greinix H, *et al.* The effect of prior exposure to imatinib on transplant-related mortality. *Haematologica* 2006;91:452–9.

101 Lee SJ, Kukreja M, Wang T, *et al.* Impact of prior imatinib mesylate on the outcome of hematopoietic cell transplantation for chronic myeloid leukemia. *Blood* 2008;112:3500–7.

102 Lee SJ, Kukreja M, Wang T, *et al.* Impact of prior imatinib mesylate on the outcome of hematopoietic cell transplantation for chronic myeloid leukemia. *Blood* 2008;112:3500–7.

103 Bornhauser M, Kroger N, Schwerdtfeger R, *et al.* Allogeneic hematopoietic cell transplantation for chronic myelogenous leukemia in the era of imatinib: a retrospective multicentre study. *Eur J Haematol* 2006;76:9–17.

104 Shimoni A, Kroger N, Zander AR, *et al.* Imatinib mesylate (STI571) in preparation for allogeneic hematopoietic stem cell transplantation and donor lymphocyte infusions in patients with Philadelphia-positive acute leukemias. *Leukemia* 2003;17:290–7.

105 Zaucha JM, Prejzner W, Giebel S, *et al.* Imatinib therapy prior to myeloablative allogeneic stem cell transplantation. *Bone Marrow Transplant* 2005;36:417–24.

106 Wassmann B, Pfeifer H, Scheuring U, *et al.* Therapy with imatinib mesylate (Glivec) preceding allogeneic stem cell transplantation (SCT) in relapsed or refractory Philadelphia-positive acute lymphoblastic leukemia (Ph+ALL). *Leukemia* 2002;16: 2358–65.

107 Zander AR, Zabelina T, Renges H, *et al.* Pretreatment with Glivec increases transplant-related mortality after allogeneic transplant. *Blood* 2003;102:468a.

Part 7
Chronic Lymphocytic Leukemia

Chapter 24
Chronic Lymphocytic Leukemia: Pathophysiology, Diagnosis and Manifestations, and Prognostic Markers

Thorsten Zenz, Hartmut Döhner, and Stephan Stilgenbauer
Department of Internal Medicine III, University of Ulm, Ulm, Germany

Introduction

Chronic lymphocytic leukemia (CLL) is a chronic lymphoproliferative disorder of the B lymphocytes. Small lymphocytic lymphoma (SLL) is considered to be the same disease in a non-leukemic form [1]. The progressive accumulation of monoclonal B lymphocytes leads to leukocytosis, lymphadenopathy, hepatosplenomegaly, and marrow failure, and is sometimes associated with autoimmune disease. The pathophysiology, diagnosis, and manifestations, as well as different ways of assessing the prognosis, will be reviewed in this chapter.

Pathophysiology

The most noteworthy abnormality among laboratory findings in CLL is lymphocytosis in the peripheral blood (and bone marrow). It has been suggested that CLL cells are defective in apoptosis, which leads to the accumulation of malignant B cells. Most CLL cells are in a resting state, and it appears that CLL is more a disease of inhibited apoptosis than strong proliferation. Strong expression of BCL-2 is a hallmark of CLL and one of the factors responsible for defects in apoptosis. Additional survival functions are mediated by the activation of several signaling pathways. More recently it has been shown that CLL cells display a significant proliferative activity, suggesting that there is a proliferative pool (reviewed in [2]). While cells with a proliferative history can be found in the blood, proliferation of CLL cells is most prominent in specific areas in lymph nodes and bone marrow, the proliferation centers (PCs). In these PCs, the CLL cells are in close contact and may interact with $CD4^+$ T cells and follicular dendritic cells. The cellular interactions in the PC may be essential for the survival and proliferation of the CLL clone. Indeed, when CLL cells are cultured alone *in vitro* they die after only a few days, but stimulation of particular signaling pathways, for example via different cytokines, or co-culturing with stromal cells can increase survival strongly. Thus, cellular interactions in the microenvironment of PC appear to be essential for the survival and expansion of CLL cells. Based on studies assessing the proliferative "history" of CLL cells as derived from the assessment of telomere length, CLL cells have been shown to exhibit a shorter telomere length than normal B cells. In addition, particularly short telomeres have been associated with poor-risk categories of CLL, suggesting that variable proliferative capacity exists [3].

Leukemias: Principles and Practice of Therapy, 1st edition. Edited by S. Faderl and H. Kantarjian.

Genomic aberrations

It is important to note that balanced translocations—as opposed to other lymphoid malignancies such as mantle cell lymphoma or follicular lymphoma—are very rare in CLL. It has therefore been difficult to link the deregulation of a single gene to the development of CLL. Genomic aberrations can, however, be identified in about 80% of CLL cases by fluorescence *in situ* hybridization (FISH) with a disease-specific probe set, and these aberrations usually consist of losses or gains of larger chromosomal regions [4]. The most common recurrent chromosomal abnormalities are deletions 13q, 11q, 17p, 6q, and trisomy 12 [4]. The single most common aberration in CLL is the deletion of a critical region in 13q14, which is found in 50–60% of patients with CLL. Specific genomic aberrations have provided some insights into the pathogenesis of the disease by pointing to candidate genes (17p13: *TP53*, 11q22–q23: *ATM*, and most likely other candidate genes), while for other loci (eg, 13q14) the precise role of possible tumor suppressors has not been fully elucidated. Recent work has implicated different micro-RNAs (miRNAs) in CLL. miRNAs are a class of small non-coding RNAs that modulate the expression of target mRNAs. Two miRNAs were recently identified to be located in the critical region of the 13q14 deletion [5]. Further analysis of micro-RNA profiles from patients with CLL have shown some miRNAs to be overexpressed (miR-21, miR-155), while others showed decreased expression (miR-15a/16 in cases of CLL with biallelic deletion of 13q14). The cases with monoallelic deletion had normal miR15-a/16 levels. The growing understanding of miRNA expression profiles and functional consequences of single miRNA deregulation is likely to extend our understanding of CLL. Further and definite evidence for the pathogenic meaning of the 13q14 MDR and miR-15a/miR-16-1 has been shown recently by generating a mouse model deleting the DLEU2/miR-15a/16-1 cluster [6]. Mice presenting deletions of the MDR or with sole miR-15a/16-1 deletion developed clonal B cell lymphoproliferation.

Other models for the pathogenetic link between deletion 13q14 and CLL have been brought forward. A complex epigenetic regulatory tumor-suppressor mechanism in the commonly deleted region of chromosomal band 13q14.3 has been described that would lead to deregulation of not only a single gene but also deregulation that may control gene expression of the whole region [7].

Immune repertoire of chronic lymphocytic leukemia

Normal B cells can follow two different maturation pathways. The response of follicular B cells to antigens requires help from T cells, and this process takes place in the germinal center. T cell-dependent antigenic stimulation invariably induces somatic IGHV gene mutations in follicular B cells. B cells that have undergone this process, and thereby passed through the germinal center, are called post-germinal center B cells. In contrast, marginal-zone B cells respond to antigens without T-cell participation. T cell-independent antigenic stimulation may or may not induce gene mutations in marginal-zone B cells, and in this process IGHV gene mutations occur outside of typical germinal-center structures (reviewed in [8]).

One of the most important molecular genetic parameters to dissect pathogenic and prognostic subgroups of CLL is the mutation status of the IGHV genes (reviewed in [8]). Since somatically mutated IGHV genes can be observed in about half of all cases of CLL (largely depending on the stage and activity of the disease), a separation was made into two different groups: one with unmutated IGHV genes, initially assumed to originate from pregerminal center cells, and another group with mutated IGHV genes, initially thought to originate from postgerminal center cells. This observation by itself is a remarkable finding as it is different from other B-cell lymphomas. In addition, the presence or absence of somatic mutations is associated with particular IGHV gene usage. Specific alleles of the IGHV*1-69* gene and the IGHV*4-39* gene have an unmutated profile. One particular IGHV gene, the *VH3-21* gene, shows strikingly homologous IGHV and *IgLV* gene rearrangements and is associated with poor prognosis, whether expressed in a mutated or unmutated form.

More than 20% of patients with CLL carry stereotypic B-cell receptors. These results point to a common antigen epitope that is recognized by these highly homologous molecules. As noted above, the extent of similarity varies among different groups of patients, but these characteristics differ from the much broader diversity found in B cells from people without leukemia, also suggesting that the antigen(s) recognized by CLL cells from different patients may, in fact, be identical. These findings are particularly striking since, given the huge number of possible combinations of *V* gene segments that can encode antigen-binding domains, one would not expect to find two cases of CLL with such structurally similar B-cell receptors in over 1 million cases. Therefore, a limited set of particular antigens may promote the development or maintenance of leukemic cells in CLL. The search to identify this possible common antigen is ongoing, but currently the antigen(s) is/are unknown. Bacterial, viral, and environmental antigens or autoantigens have been suggested to cause clonal expansion [8].

B cells from patients with CLL who have mutated IGHV genes are less capable of triggering apoptosis, survival, or proliferation, presumably owing to defective B-cell receptor (BCR) signaling. When IGHV gene mutations develop, they can lead to the abrogation of the polyreactivity of the B-cell receptors and thereby change their ability to bind the original antigen or autoantigen. Alternatively, or additionally, these mutations could result in anergy as a result of excessive BCR stimulation because of the acquisition of more avid receptors. Differences in the signals received through the B-cell receptors and other receptors may determine the extent of clonal expansion, and thus may influence the clinical course [8].

Cell of origin/normal counterpart

The malignant B cells of CLL do not quite resemble a normal B-lymphocyte subpopulation. Based on the expression of CD5, which is a hallmark of a distinct B-cell subset in mice, and perhaps also humans, the origin of CLL being $CD5^+$ naïve B cells has initially been proposed. However, because CD5 can be upregulated on B cells by stimulation, the expression of CD5 may or may not point to the cell of origin. Evidence from recent gene expression profiling studies indicated a close relationship of both mutated and unmutated CLL to memory or marginal-zone B cells. The pivotal studies showed strikingly similar gene expression profiles in the different subgroups with mutated and unmutated IGHV status, which show very different clinical behaviors. The comparison of CLL profiles with those of purified normal B-cell subpopulations indicates that the common CLL profile is more related to memory B cells than to those derived from naïve B cells, $CD5^+$ B cells, or germinal center centroblasts and centrocytes (reviewed in [9]).

The similar expression profile also suggests that the consequences or even the mechanism of transformation may be similar, irrespective of IGHV mutation status. As noted above, it has also been proposed that unmutated and mutated CLL clones derive from antigen-activated B cells. The mutated CLL clones may either derive from classic germinal center reactions where T-cell-dependent immune responses take place and somatic hypermutation of *IgV* genes occurs, or they may derive from T-cell-independent immune responses, which may, in some instances, also involve hypermutation of *IgV* genes.

Diagnosis and manifestations

Nowadays, most patients are diagnosed while asymptomatic because of abnormal complete blood counts. Although the absolute blood lymphocyte threshold for diagnosing CLL has been placed at >5000/μL, a large majority of patients present with counts as high as 200,000/μL. As CLL is the most common leukemia in the western world, it will be at the top of the list for the differential diagnosis of significant lymphocytosis. The morphology and immunophenotype usually allow relative ease in diagnosing CLL, but in atypical cases histology or cytogenetic findings may be needed. If the blood lymphocyte phenotype is clearly that of typical B-CLL, CLL can be diagnosed if the blood B-lymphocyte count is >5000/μL; below this value in asymptomatic patients a diagnosis of monoclonal B lymphocytosis (MBL) should be made [10]. Anemia and thrombocytopenia may be observed at the time of initial diagnosis. Low hemoglobin (<11 or 10 g/dL) and/or platelet levels (<100,000/μL) are observed at the time of diagnosis in about 20–30% of patients, and are a sign of more advanced disease and predict for poorer prognosis [11,12]. Autoimmune hemolytic anemia (AIHA) is a common complication in CLL. The direct antiglobulin test (DAT, Coombs test) may be positive at some time during the course of the disease in about one-third of cases, and overt AIHA occurs in 5–15% of cases. In a recent analysis within the UK CLL4 trial, the pretreatment incidence of a positive DAT was 14% and 10% developed AIHA. Interestingly, the presence of AIHA or a positive DAT predicted for reduced overall survival (OS) [13]. Autoimmune thrombocytopenia occurs in 2–3% of patients with CLL. Significant degrees of hypogammaglobulinemia and neutropenia may result in an increased predisposition of patients with CLL to major bacterial infections. In addition, the use of purine analogs as treatment for CLL has resulted in an increased incidence of opportunistic infections. Infections or autoimmune complications such as hemolytic anemia, thrombocytopenia, or pure red cell aplasia may be the first manifestation of the disease.

Approximately 5–10% of patients present with typical "B" symptoms of lymphoma. The most consistently abnormal finding on physical examination of a patient with CLL is lymphadenopathy, present in 50–90% of patients among various series. Lymph node enlargement may be generalized or localized and very variable in size. When nodes are extremely enlarged, they may be easily discernible by simple inspection, and bulky lymphadenopathy is associated with the 11q deletion [14].

The spleen is the second most frequently enlarged lymphoid organ. It may be palpably enlarged in up to 50% of cases. The extent of the enlargement varies and may occupy the entire left side of the abdomen and pelvis, crossing the midline. As is the case with enlarged lymph nodes, an enlarged spleen in CLL is usually painless, but, when enlarged significantly, can often lead to discomfort or fullness. Enlargement of the liver may be noted at the time of initial diagnosis of CLL in 15–25% of cases. The liver in CLL generally is not greatly enlarged. In addition to palpably enlarged peripheral lymph nodes, liver, and spleen, virtually any other lymphoid tissue in the body may be enlarged at diagnosis, such as Waldeyer ring or the tonsils. In contrast to other lymphomas, gastrointestinal mucosal involvement is rarely seen in CLL. Similarly, meningeal leukemia is also unusual in CLL at the time of initial presentation. Skin lesions are the most commonly involved non-lymphoid organ lesions (in <5% of cases), and other cutaneous lesions in CLL can be vasculitis or paraneoplastic pemphigus. Membranoproliferative glomerulonephritis (MPGN) has occasionally been described in CLL as in other lymphoproliferative diseases.

Morphology

The malignant cell in B-CLL has the appearance of a normal mature small lymphocyte. There are uniform populations of small lymphocytes [1]. The nucleus almost fills the entire cell. The nuclear chromatin is clumped and a nucleolus is usually not discernible. In addition to the typical small cells, a small proportion of cells may consist of larger lymphocytes with a wider cytoplasm and a visible nucleolus. These "prolymphocytes" may account for a minority of the overall population of lymphocytes in B-CLL (usually <10%). Most of the other conditions associated with blood lymphocytosis, such as leukemic mantle cell leukemia, prolymphocytic leukemia, or hairy cell leukemia, have their own characteristic morphologic features distinct from CLL. The diagnosis can usually be made by the peripheral blood smear and should be confirmed by immunophenotyping. Commonly flattened or smudged cells are found (Gumprecht phenomenon, reviewed in [15]).

The characteristic findings on the bone marrow aspirate smear include increased cellularity, with lymphocytes often accounting for the majority of all nucleated cells. Usually, a bone marrow biopsy examination is not required for establishing a diagnosis of CLL but it is warranted to clarify the reason for cytopenias, has some prognostic value, and is needed for remission assessment [10].

Histology

In addition to an increased percentage of mature-appearing lymphocytes in the smears of the bone marrow aspirate, there are three types of infiltrative patterns of lymphocytes that are recognized in trephine biopsy specimens of the bone marrow: nodular, interstitial, and diffuse. As was noted above, B-cell CLL and SLL are considered to be the same disease with different manifestations [1]. The diagnosis of SLL is made via a lymph node biopsy in a patient without peripheral lymphocytosis, while CLL is usually diagnosed through examination of the peripheral blood and bone marrow in patients with lymphocytosis. The histopathologic lymph node findings in SLL and CLL are identical and consist of a diffusely effaced nodal architecture with few residual germinal centers [1].

Immunophenotyping

There are three major sets of phenotypic findings classical of B-CLL lymphocytes (reviewed in [15]):

1 Surface membrane immunoglobulin is expressed at extremely low levels in CLL (SmIg weak). The immunoglobulin is most often IgM or both IgM and IgD, and only a single immunoglobulin light chain is expressed, confirming the clonal nature of these cells.

2 Expression of the B-cell-associated antigens CD23, CD19, and CD20, with a characteristically low expression of CD20 compared with other B-cell lymphomas.

3 Coexpression of CD5, a T cell-associated antigen, together with the B-cell markers.

Based on these key findings, the diagnosis of CLL is usually relatively simple. In addition, CLL cells are usually negative for cyclin D1 and CD10. FMC7, CD22, and CD79b are usually negative or weakly expressed. Cases with an unmutated IGHV mutation status have been reported to be CD38 positive, although the correlation is imperfect [16,17]. A scoring system for differentiating CLL from other B-cell lymphoproliferative diseases has been devised based on the above immunophenotypic findings. Each of the following cellular characteristics is scored with one point [15]: staining for surface immunoglobulin is weakly positive; $CD5^+$; $CD23^+$; CD79b or CD22 is weakly positive; and $FMC7^-$. A score of 4 or 5 had an accuracy of >95% for the diagnosis of CLL, while most of the other non-CLL B-cell lymphoproliferative diseases had scores of 0–2 [15].

Differential diagnosis

There are several malignant lymphoproliferative disorders, which may be similar to CLL in its clinical presentation, particularly leukemic mantle cell lymphoma (MCL), follicular lymphoma (FL), and other non-Hodgkin lymphoma (NHL) [15]. However, in contrast to the phenotypic features of CLL, the amount of surface membrane immunoglobulin is abundant in most lymphomas and, with the exception of MCL, the lymphocytes are usually $CD5^-$.

Work-up and staging

Historically, the staging for patients with CLL has been based on thorough clinical examination and complete blood count. This work-up was supplemented by clinical chemistry and, in some cases, a Coombs test to investigate hemolysis. With the advent of more intensive treatment regimens, including the use of monoclonal antibodies, serology for viruses (eg, hepatitis) should also be investigated if treatment is planned. Ultrasound has been widely used, but is not needed to ascertain patients to the clinical stage groups according to the Binet and Rai staging systems. An overview of the updated guidelines for the diagnosis and pretreatment evaluation has recently summarized the current work-up in CLL (Table 24.1) [10].

The Rai system is based upon a hierarchical grouping of disease manifestations of blood and bone marrow (lymphocytosis/Rai 0), enlarged lymph nodes (lymphadenopathy Rai I), spleen and liver (Rai II), bone marrow failure (anemia, Rai III), and thrombocytopenia (Rai IV) [12]. The median survival times from the time of diagnosis in the series of patients studied by Rai *et al.* were 150 months for stage 0, 101 months for stage I, 71 months for stage II, and only 9 months in stages III and IV. There were only three distinct actuarial survival patterns and it has been impractical to stratify patients in five categories. As with the Binet system, the staging system was modified to consist of three groups: low risk (0), intermediate risk (I and II), and high risk (III and IV). The Binet staging system takes into consideration five sites of involvement: cervical, axillary, inguinal lymph nodes (each area is counted as one whether it is unilateral or bilateral), spleen, and liver. Patients are classified according to the number of involved sites plus the pres-

Table 24.1 Overview of the current guidelines for the diagnosis and assessment of patients with chronic lymphocytic leukemia according to the updated National Cancer Institute guidelines (modified) [10].

Diagnosis of CLL	General practice	Clinical trial
Complete blood count and differential count	+	+
Immunophenotyping of lymphocytes	+	+
Assessment prior to treatment		
History and physical, performance status	+	+
Complete blood count and differential	+	+
Marrow aspirate and biopsy	+	+
Serum chemistry	+	+
Serum immunoglobulin	+	+
Direct antiglobulin test	+	+
Chest radiograph	+	+
History/work-up of infection	+	+
Cytogenetics (FISH) for $13q^-$, $11q^-$, $17p^-$, 12^+, 6q–	(+)[a]	+
IGHV mutational status, ZAP-70, and CD38	(+/–)	+
CT scan of chest, abdomen, and pelvis	–	+
MRI, lymphangiogram, gallium scan, PET scans	–	–
Abdominal ultrasound	(+/–)	–

CLL, chronic lymphocytic leukemia; CT, computed tomography; FISH, fluorescence *in situ* hybridization; MRI, magnetic resonance imaging; PET, positron emission tomography.
[a]FISH for $17p^-$ should be performed at treatment indication.

ence of anemia (hemoglobin <10 g/dL) and/or thrombocytopenia (platelets <100,000/μL) [13]:

- Stage A—fewer than three involved lymphoid sites.
- Stage B—three or more involved lymphoid sites.
- Stage C—presence of anemia and/or thrombocytopenia.

This system is of great value in stratifying patients with survival curves corresponding to the Rai low-risk, intermediate-risk, and high-risk groups, respectively.

Radiological assessment

As with nodal NHL, CT scans have now entered the scene of staging for CLL, and the advantages of a precise lymph node assessment appear self evident. This is particularly important if a patient is entered into a clinical trial in which CT of the abdomen, pelvis, and chest are recommended as baseline studies. Such studies provide an objective measure of the size of the liver, spleen, and retroperitoneal nodes for comparison with subsequent re-examinations to determine the level of clinical response from protocol-based therapy. The recent update on the guidelines for the diagnosis and treatment of CLL suggests using CT scans for response assessment in clinical trials [10].

Positron emission tomography (PET) is generally of no value in CLL, but it might be helpful when the transformation of CLL into a more aggressive lymphoma variant (Richter transformation) is thought to have occurred.

Prognosis

A highly variable clinical course characterizes CLL. Treatment has traditionally been used for advanced stage or symptomatic disease. Over recent years, highly effective approaches, such as the combination of antibodies with chemotherapy and allogeneic stem cell transplantation, are used in the treatment of patients with CLL. The improved response rate comes at the price of increased toxicity and therefore the definition of prognostic subgroups becomes increasingly important. Molecular prognostic markers have been discovered and some of these are now used to stratify patients to different treatment options.

Clinical stage according to Binet and Rai

The standard clinical procedures to estimate prognosis in CLL are the staging systems developed by Rai and Binet [11,12]. These systems rely on physical examination and a simple blood count. The prognostic impact of these staging systems was confirmed in many independent studies. However, there is still heterogeneity in the course of the disease for patients within a single-stage group. Biologic risk factors such as the IGHV mutation status and genomic aberrations have the power to identify subgroups of patients with poor prognosis among clinical groups of patients. Both parameters have been shown in multivariate analyses to provide prognostic information independently of the clinical stage [17,18].

Markers of tumor burden

Apart from the clinical staging systems, other easily assessable parameters of disease activity and tumor burden, such as the lymphocyte count, the lymphocyte doubling time, the serum levels of LDH, and the bone marrow infiltration pattern, have been shown to be of prognostic relevance in CLL. Elevated levels of LDH and high lymphocyte counts are associated with disease activity. In multivariate analyses, including clinical (age, stage, etc) and genetic (*VH* status, genomic aberrations, etc) variables, these parameters were independent prognostic factors [4]. Although partially correlated with clinical stage, the lymphocyte doubling time was shown to have a clear prognostic significance by itself: lymphocyte doubling time of ≤12 months identifies a population of patients with poor prognosis, a doubling time >12 months is indicative of good prognosis. Not surprisingly, a short lymphocyte doubling time predicts rapid disease progression in patients in the early clinical stages. Another marker for tumor burden, the lymphocyte infiltration of the bone marrow, has been evaluated for its impact on prognosis. Several studies showed that cases with diffuse bone marrow infiltration had a poorer prognosis than cases presenting with a nodular pattern. In a more recent analysis, the bone marrow infiltration pattern was associated with progression-free survival (PFS), but not OS, and was not an independent prognostic factor [19]. A number of serologic parameters, including beta2-microglobulin (β2-M), thymidine kinase (TK), and soluble CD23 (sCD23), have been shown to provide information about the patients' outcomes. TK levels correlate with the proliferative activity of CLL cells and elevated levels predict disease progression in CLL. In a recent study, TK appeared to detect a subgroup of patients with early non-smoldering CLL at risk of rapid disease progression and provided independent prognostic information on PFS. CD23 is a functionally relevant surface molecule on B-CLL cells. High levels of the soluble form of CD23 (sCD23) at initial diagnosis were linked with disease progression in early-stage B-CLL. Furthermore, sCD23 was associated with a diffuse bone marrow infiltration pattern, a short lymphocyte doubling time, and elevated serum TK levels.

β2-M is an extracellular protein that is non-covalently associated with the class I major histocompatibility complex (MHC). Its serum levels show a correlation with the clinical staging systems according to Binet and Rai. Recently, a prognostic normogram based on a retrospective analysis from the MDACC has been developed, including age, β2-M, absolute lymphocyte count, sex, Rai stage, and number of involved lymph node groups [20].

IGHV mutational status and surrogate markers

As noted above, CLL cells may show mutated or unmutated IGHV genes. The definition of IGHV mutated or unmutated CLL relies on an arbitrarily defined threshold of 98% homology to the most similar germ-line gene. Importantly, it could be demonstrated that the IGHV mutation status is clinically highly relevant as it predicts risk of disease progression and outcome in untreated patients with CLL [16,17,21,22]. While CLL with unmutated IGHV follows an unfavorable course with rapid progression, CLL with mutated IGHV often shows slow progression and long survival. Figure 24.1 depicts the survival curves for patients distributed over all stages (n = 300) and separately for patients diagnosed with Binet stage A disease (n = 189) from our single-center cohort. Furthermore, independent of the mutation status, the usage of specific IGHV genes such as *V3-21* is associated with an inferior outcome [22].

As the determination of IGHV mutation status is technically demanding, a search for "surrogate markers," that is parameters that are strongly correlated with IGHV mutation status, is ongoing. Among these surrogate markers, ZAP-70, a molecule usually involved in T-cell receptor signaling that was identified in gene expression profiling studies, is most widely used. It was shown that the measurement of ZAP-70 levels by fluorescent activated cell sorter (FACS) could separate the distinct prognostic groups of patients with Binet stage A CLL with similar clinical behavior and great overlap to the groups segregated by IGHV mutation profile [23]. In all patients in whom at least 20% of the leukemic cells were positive for ZAP-70, IGHV was unmutated, whereas IGHV mutations were found in 21 of 24 patients in whom <20% of the leukemic cells were positive for ZAP-70.

As with any prognostic marker, the relation of new prognostic markers must be related to other markers known to impact on outcome in order to define its independence from or dependence on other factors. A number of studies have shown a strong association between high ZAP-70 expression and unmutated IGHV genes. However, discordance of ZAP-70 expression and IGHV mutation status occurred in up to 25% of cases [24]. The proportion of discordant cases is particularly high in the distinct subgroups with *V3-21* usage and 17p or 11q deletion (39%). The IGHV mutation status, *V3-21* usage, and presence of high-risk genomic aberrations (17p or 11q deletion), but not ZAP-70 expression, were identified as independent prognostic factors. Nonetheless, the association of ZAP-70 and IGHV mutation status was strong in cases without additional genetic high-risk features (no 17p or 11q deletion, no *V3-21* usage), and the majority of *V3-21* cases showed high ZAP-70 expression irrespective of the IGHV mutation status. If high-risk genomic aber-

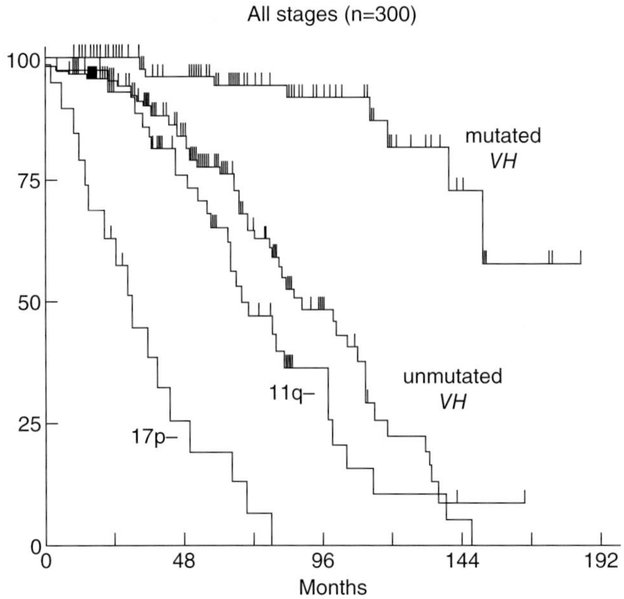

Figure 24.1 Prognostic relevance of genomic aberrations in chronic lymphocytic leukemia, and IGHV mutation status in chronic lymphocytic leukemia. Survival probabilities among patients in the following genetic categories: 17p deletion ($17p^-$ irrespective of IGHV mutation status), 11q deletion ($11q^-$ irrespective of IGHV mutation status), unmutated IGHV (homology ≥98% and no $17p^-$ or $11q^-$), and mutated IGHV (homology <98% and no $17p^-$ or $11q^-$). (a) Among all 300 patients estimated median survival times were: 17p deletion 30 m, 11q deletion 70 m, IGHV ≥ 98% 89m, and IGHV <98% not reached (54% survival at 152 m); (b) In Binet A patients only (n = 189) estimated median survival times were: 17p deletion 36 m, 11q deletion 68 m, IGHV ≥ 98% 86 m, and IGHV < 98% not reached (52% survival at 152 m). m, months.

rations (17p or 11q deletion) are present, it appears to be important to consider this presence in addition to the prognostic impact of the IGHV status and ZAP-70 status for the prediction of the clinical course. In the absence of high-risk genomic aberrations, the IGHV status and ZAP-70 status may have a similar prognostic impact, and might therefore be alternately applied. In addition to the prognostic consequences, the data provide evidence for a theoretic model of ZAP-70 expression in the pathogenesis of CLL, in which active BCR signaling stimulates the malignant clone. A survival advantage for CLL cells as a result of the BCR-related interaction with unknown antigens could explain the signs of antigen-selection pressure, such as restricted IGHV gene usage. In contrast, 17p or 11q deletions that affect critical cancer genes may lead to an inherent survival advantage independently of ZAP-70 or BCR-mediated effects in CLL cells [24]. A problem concerning ZAP-70 determination in clinical practice is the challenge in the standardization of a FACS assay for its measurement.

In the gene expression studies a number of other genes have been identified with differential expression in the IGHV mutated and unmutated subgroups, suggesting that expression levels of these genes may be used to simplify IGHV mutational assessment by use of "surrogate marker(s)" [25]. In a recent study, 10 genes were tested with real-time quantitative polymerase chain reaction (RQ-PCR) in unpurified samples from 130 patients with CLL [25]. In multivariate logistic regression analysis expression levels of LPL, ZAP-70, *ADAM29*, and *SEPT10* were the most predictive for IGHV mutational status. In univariate analysis, the expression of LPL was the best predictor, and in a multivariate analysis LPL expression remained a significant predictor.

While the study of the IGHV mutational status has greatly enhanced our understanding of the disease and increased our ability to separate prognostic subgroups in CLL, the role of the IGHV mutational status in guiding therapy is currently unresolved and treatment decisions should not be based on outside clinical trials.

Genomic aberrations and chronic lymphocytic leukemia

Specific chromosomal aberrations can be detected by FISH, not only in dividing cells but also in interphase nuclei, an approach referred to as interphase cytogenetics. FISH can identify genomic aberrations in about 80% of CLL cases with a disease-specific comprehensive probe set [4]. The most common recurrent chromosomal abnormalities are deletions 13q, 11q, 17p, 6q, and trisomy 12

(55%, 18%, 7%, 7%, and 16%, respectively) [4]. Five prognostic categories have been defined in a statistical model showing very poor survival in patients with 17p deletion (median survival 32), poor survival for patients with 11q deletion (79 months), and better survival for patients with 12q trisomy, normal karyotype, and 13q deletion as the sole abnormality (114, 111, and 133 months, respectively). It is important to note that there are some differences with regard to the occurrence of high-risk ($17p^-$, $11q^-$, unmutated IGHV) and low-risk ($13q^-$ single, mutated IGHV) markers in different clinical situations. High-risk cytogenetic aberrations are more likely to be found in more advanced disease and after therapy, suggesting that reassessment of chromosomal abnormalities may be useful during the course of disease and also providing further evidence for the biologic significance [26]. The prognostic impact of genomic aberrations is now reproduced in prospective clinical trials with very similar results [18]. In addition, specific genomic aberrations have been associated with disease characteristics such as marked lymphadenopathy (11q deletion) and resistance to treatment with conventional chemotherapy ($17p^-$), further documenting the importance of genomic aberrations on the course of CLL [14,27]. Although the group of patients with 17p deletion is quite small in early stages and at first-line treatment, the detection of this chromosome aberration is important because these patients are unlikely to respond to chemotherapy. The poor prognosis of this subgroup has been confirmed in clinical trials with a significantly inferior outcome with regard to OS after first-line therapy with alkylating agents and purine analogs [18,28]. There is a growing consensus that cytogenetics by FISH should be obtained (at least for $17p^-$) in every patient before therapy is given [10]. Cases with 17p deletion account for a large proportion of the fludarabine refractory cases. One logical consequence of the central role of 17p deletion in refractory disease is a growing interest in therapies that act independently of p53.

With the genomic aberrations and the IGHV mutation status, two separate genetic parameters of prognostic relevance are available and they appear to be correlated. Unfavorable aberrations ($11q^-$, $17p^-$) occur more frequently in unmutated IGHV, and favorable aberrations ($13q^-$ single) occur more frequently in the mutated IGHV subgroup [4,17,24]. This unbalanced distribution of genomic aberrations emphasizes the different biologic background of the CLL subgroups with mutated or unmutated IGHV but only partly explains their different clinical course. About two-thirds of cases of unmutated IGHV CLL show no unfavorable genomic aberrations, indicating a differential influence of these factors. The IGHV mutation status, 17p deletion, 11q deletion, age, leukocyte count, and LDH were identified as independent prognostic factors regarding OS. When the IGHV mutation status and 11q/17p aberrations are included in a prognostic model, the clinical stage of disease according to the Rai or Binet systems may not be identified as an independent prognostic factor [24]. Therefore, four subgroups of CLL with markedly differing survival probabilities can be defined by the IGHV mutation status, 11q deletion, and 17p deletion. Based on these studies it appears that IGHV mutation status and genomic aberrations are among the strongest currently available parameters and are of independent value to predict outcome in CLL (Figure 24.1).

In recent years, molecular and cellular markers have helped to elucidate major pathogenic aspects of CLL. More importantly, for the treatment of patients, molecular genetics has helped to predict the prognosis of CLL. The development of molecular genetic techniques has proven pivotal in helping to subdivide CLL into distinct clinical subgroups and identify patients with specific clinical manifestations, for example rapid disease progression (unmutated IGHV), massive lymphadenopathy ($11q^-$), or resistance to therapy ($17p^-$). Patients with these genetic abnormalities may be candidates for clinical trials investigating alternate treatments and allogeneic stem-cell transplantation. The near future is likely to bring greater insight into the prognosis and molecular basis of CLL as new techniques, including high-resolution SNP arrays, genome wide methylation, and miRNA profiling methods, can now be used in larger patient cohorts.

References

1 Jaffe ES, Harris NL, Stein H, Vardiman JW, (eds). *World Health Organization Classification of Tumours. Pathology and Genetics of Tumors of Haematopoietic and Lymphoid Tissues*. IARC Press: Lyon, 2001.
2 Chiorazzi N. Cell proliferation and death: forgotten features of chronic lymphocytic leukemia B cells. *Best Pract Res Clin Haematol* 2007;20:399–413.
3 Roos G, Kröber A, Grabowski P, *et al*. Short telomeres are associated with genetic complexity, high-risk genomic aberrations, and short survival in chronic lymphocytic leukemia. *Blood* 2008;111:2246–52.
4 Dohner H, Stilgenbauer S, Benner A, *et al*. Genomic aberrations and survival in chronic lymphocytic leukemia. *N Engl J Med* 2000;343:1910–16.
5 Mertens D, Wolf S, Tschuch C, *et al*. Allelic silencing at the tumor-suppressor locus 13q14.3 suggests an epigenetic tumor-suppressor mechanism. *Proc Natl Acad Sci U S A* 2006;103: 7741–6.
6 Klein U, Lia M, Crespo M, *et al*. The DLEU2/miR-15a/16-1 cluster controls B cell proliferation and its deletion leads to chronic lymphocytic leukemia. *Cancer Cell* 2010;17:28–40.
7 Lagos-Quintana M, Rauhut R, Lendeckel W, Tuschl T. Identification of novel genes coding for small expressed RNAs. *Science* 2001;294:853–8.
8 Chiorazzi N, Rai KR, Ferrarini M. Chronic lymphocytic leukemia. *N Engl J Med* 2005;352:804–15.

9 Klein U, Dalla-Favera R. New insights into the phenotype and cell derivation of B cells in chronic lymphocytic leukemia. *Curr Top Microbiol Immunol* 2005;294:31–49.

10 Hallek M, Cheson BD, Catovsky D, *et al.* Guidelines for the diagnosis and treatment of chronic lymphocytic leukemia: a report from the International Workshop on Chronic Lymphocytic Leukemia (IWCLL) updating the National Cancer Institute-Working Group (NCI-WG) 1996 guidelines. *Blood* 2008;111:5446–56.

11 Rai, KR, Sawitsky, A, Cronkite, EP, *et al.* Clinical staging of chronic lymphocytic leukemia. *Blood* 1975;46:219.

12 Binet J-L, Auquier A, Dighiero G, *et al.* A new prognostic classification of chronic lymphocytic leukemia derived from a multivariate survival analysis. *Cancer* 1981;48:198.

13 Dearden C, Wade R, Else M, *et al.* The prognostic significance of a positive direct antiglobulin test in chronic lymphocytic leukemia—a beneficial effect of the combination of fludarabine and cyclophosphamide on the incidence of hemolytic anemia. *Blood* 2008;111:1820–6.

14 Döhner H, Stilgenbauer S, James MR, *et al.* 11q deletions identify a new subset of B-cell chronic lymphocytic leukemia characterized by extensive nodal involvement and inferior prognosis. *Blood* 1997;89:2516–22

15 Matutes E, Wotherspoon A, Catovsky D. Differential diagnosis in chronic lymphocytic leukemia. *Best Pract Res Clin Haematol* 2007;20:367–84.

16 Damle RN, Wasil T, Fais F, *et al.* Ig V gene mutation status and CD38 expression as novel prognostic indicators in chronic lymphocytic leukemia. *Blood* 1999;94:1840–7.

17 Kröber A, Seiler T, Benner A, *et al.* V(H) mutation status, CD38 expression level, genomic aberrations, and survival in chronic lymphocytic leukemia. *Blood* 2002;100:1410–16.

18 Catovsky D, Richards S, Matutes E, *et al.* Assessment of fludarabine plus cyclophosphamide for patients with chronic lymphocytic leukemia (the LRF CLL4 Trial): a randomised controlled trial. *Lancet* 2007;370:230–9.

19 Bergmann MA, Eichhorst B, Busch R, *et al.* Prospective evaluation of prognostic parameters in early stage chronic lymphocytic leukemia (CLL): Results of the CLL1-protocol of the German CLL Study Group (GCLLSG). *Blood* (ASH Annual Meeting Abstracts) 2007;110:625.

20 Wierda WG, O'Brien S, Wang X, *et al.* Prognostic nomogram and index for overall survival in previously untreated patients with chronic lymphocytic leukemia. *Blood* 2007;109:4679–85.

21 Hamblin TJ, Davis Z, Gardiner A, *et al.* Unmutated Ig V(H) genes are associated with a more aggressive form of chronic lymphocytic leukemia. *Blood* 1999;94:1848–54.

22 Tobin G, Thunberg U, Johnson A, *et al.* Somatically mutated Ig V(H)3–21 genes characterize a new subset of chronic lymphocytic leukemia. *Blood* 2002;99:2262–4.

23 Crespo M, Bosch F, Villamor N, *et al.* ZAP-70 expression as a surrogate for immunoglobulin-variable-region mutations in chronic lymphocytic leukemia. *N Engl J Med* 2003;348:1764–75.

24 Krober A, Bloehdorn J, Hafner S, *et al.* Additional genetic high-risk features such as 11q deletion, 17p deletion, and V3-21 usage characterize discordance of ZAP-70 and VH mutation status in chronic lymphocytic leukemia. *J Clin Oncol* 2006;24:969–75.

25 van't Veer MB, Brooijmans AM, Langerak AW, *et al.* The predictive value of lipoprotein lipase for survival in chronic lymphocytic leukemia. *Haematologica* 2006;91:56–63.

26 Stilgenbauer S, Sander S, Bullinger L, *et al.* Clonal evolution in chronic lymphocytic leukemia: acquisition of high-risk genomic aberrations associated with unmutated VH, resistance to therapy, and short survival. *Haematologica* 2007;92:1242–5.

27 Döhner H, Fischer K, Bentz M, *et al.* p53 gene deletion predicts for poor survival and non-response to therapy with purine analogs in chronic B-cell leukaemias. *Blood* 1995;85:1580–9.

28 Grever MR, Lucas DM, Dewald GW, *et al.* Comprehensive assessment of genetic and molecular features predicting outcome in patients with chronic lymphocytic leukemia: results from the US Intergroup Phase III Trial E2997. *J Clin Oncol* 2007; 25:799–804.

Chapter 25
Therapy of Chronic Lymphocytic Leukemia: Front-line and Salvage

Valentin Goede, Barbara Eichhorst, and Michael Hallek
Department I of Internal Medicine, University Hospital Cologne, Cologne, Germany

Introduction

Chronic lymphocytic leukemia (CLL) accounts for one-third of all leukemias of the western hemisphere. Despite its significant contribution to the burden of hematologic malignancy in Europe and North America, treatment options for CLL were rather limited until the early 1990s. Since then, the arsenal of therapeutic options has been constantly broadened by a shift from palliative alkylator-based chemotherapy toward modern chemoimmunotherapy with purine analogs and monoclonal antibodies.

However, this rapid development of novel therapeutic regimens has also complicated decision-making in clinical practice, because treatment is now to be tailored to the patient's individual age, physical fitness, and risk of disease progression or recurrence. This chapter aims to provide an overview of the current front-line and salvage treatment of CLL. Indications for therapy and choice of treatment are summarized in Tables 25.1 and 25.2 and will be discussed on the basis of the latest clinical trial results.

Indications for front-line therapy

Patients with newly diagnosed CLL are characterized by a highly variable course of their disease. Some patients will have asymptomatic "smoldering" CLL for many years. Others will experience early progression and need of treatment. In general, initiation of therapy should rely on criteria proposed by international guidelines [1,2].

Treatment is always indicated in patients with advanced-stage disease and concurrent bone marrow failure (Rai stage III or IV, Binet stage C) because overall survival is limited to 1–2 years with supportive treatment. In contrast, immediate therapy in patients with less advanced disease stages (Rai stage 0–II, Binet stage A or B) has failed to prolong overall survival so far [3,4]. Therefore, in routine practice and outside of a clinical trial, treatment of less-advanced CLL should be offered only to patients who present with at least one of the following symptoms: severe B symptoms (ie, weight loss of 10% or more within the previous 6 months, fever of >38°C, or night sweats without evidence of infection), extreme fatigue not attributable to other health problems, complications from massive lymphadenopathy, hepatomegaly or splenomegaly, lymphocyte doubling time of <6 months, and autoimmune anemia or thrombocytopenia that do not properly respond to corticosteroid therapy.

Recently, the traditional strategy of starting treatment solely in advanced or symptomatic CLL was challenged by the advent of novel prognostic markers that have been reported to be predictive for progression-free and overall survival [5]. Chromosomal aberrations, such as the 11q or 17p deletion, unmutated *IgVH* gene status, overexpression of ZAP-70 or CD38, and elevated serum levels of thymidine kinase or β2-microglobulin all have been found to be associated with an unfavorable course of the disease. It has been hypothesized that patients with non-advanced asymptomatic CLL but poor-risk markers may benefit from early front-line treatment. Indeed, ongoing trials are currently addressing the question of whether early intervention might be beneficial in this particular subgroup of patients (see, for example, [6]). However, definitive results from these trials are not yet available. Therefore, in the absence of clinical criteria for need of treatment, the presence of poor risk markers does not allow initiation therapy outside of a clinical trial [1,5].

Choice of front-line therapy

Options for front-line treatment of CLL range from single-agent chemotherapy to combined chemoimmunotherapy. None of these treatments has resulted in a definite cure for the disease so far and improvement of overall survival has not yet been conclusively demonstrated. With modern treatment regimens, however, remission rates of up to

---

Leukemias: Principles and Practice of Therapy, 1st edition. Edited by S. Faderl and H. Kantarjian.

Table 25.1 Indications for chronic lymphocytic leukemia treatment.

	Routine practice	Clinical trial
Front-line therapy		
(A) Advanced CLL (Rai III or IV, Binet C)	Yes	Yes
(B) Non-advanced CLL (Rai 0-II, Binet A or B)		
Symptomatic	Yes	Yes
Asymptomatic		
Unfavorable marker profile	No	Yes
Favorable marker profile	No	No
Salvage therapy		
(C) Relapsed CLL		
Symptomatic/active	Yes	Yes
Asymptomatic/inactive		
MRD positive	No	Yes
MRD negative	No	No

CLL, chronic lymphocytic leukemia; MRD, minimal residual disease.

Table 25.2 Choice of chronic lymphocytic leukemia treatment.

	Clinical routine	Clinical trial
Front-line therapy		
Younger patient, physically fit patient[a]	FC	FCR, PCR, BR
Poor-risk patient		
17p deletion (lack of p53)	—[b]	A, allo-HSCT
11q deletion	—[b]	FCR, PCR, A
Elderly patient, physically unfit patient	CLB	dF, dFC, B, PCR
Salvage therapy		
Late relapse (remission duration >1 year)	Repeat first-line	—
Early relapse (remission duration <1 year)		
Younger patient	—[b]	FCR, BR, A, FA, FCA
Elderly patient	—[b]	dF, dFC, B, CHOP
Poor-risk patient, refractory disease	—[b]	A, FA, FCA, CFAR, allo-HSCT

A, alemtuzumab; allo-HSCT, allogeneic hematopoietic stem-cell transplantation; B, bendamustine; C, cyclophosphamide; CLB, chlorambucil; d, dose-reduced; F, fludarabine; H, doxorubicin; O, oncovin; P, prednisolone (for HOP) or pentostatin (for PCR); R, rituximab.
[a]Category includes patients with ZAP-70$^+$ or CD38$^+$, increased serum tyrosine kinase or beta-2 microglobulin, and unmutated *IgVH*.
[b]Enroll in clinical trial whenever possible.

95% are observable and the duration of remission can be extended to 4–5 years. Both response and toxicity rates vary remarkably between the diverse front-line treatments. Hence, the choice of front-line therapy should be carefully tailored to a patient's individual disease- and host-related risk profile. The following sections outline the role of currently available treatment options for the front-line setting.

Current role of alkylator-based chemotherapy

Until the late 1980s, the alkylating drug chlorambucil was widely applied either as a single agent or in combination with prednisolone. Monochemotherapy with chlorambucil yields overall response rates of 37–72%, but complete remissions are rare (0–7%) and relapse generally occurs earlier than with purine analogs (median progression-free survival: 9–18 months) [7–11].

Although alkylator-based therapy with chlorambucil is no longer the treatment of choice in younger and physically fit patients, currently available trial results suggest that chemotherapy with chlorambucil remains a preferable option in the elderly and in the medically unfit patient [11]: despite the fact that complete remissions are not observed with chlorambucil in patients >65 years old, progression-free and overall survival are both similar to purine analog monochemotherapy.

Bendamustine is a type of purine analog/alkylator hybrid drug that is also active in CLL. The latest results from a randomized phase III trial indicate that front-line therapy with bendamustine is safe and highly effective [10]. Bendamustine induced complete remissions in 30% and overall remissions in 68% of treatment-naïve cases. Moreover, progression-free survival was significantly longer than with chlorambucil (22 vs. 9 months). However, it remains to be elucidated whether bendamustine is also superior to chlorambucil in elderly and physically unfit patients with primary CLL.

Current role of anthracycline-based chemotherapy

Front-line therapy of CLL with CHOP (cytoxan, hydroxyrubicin, oncovin, prednisone) or CAP (cyclophosphamide, adriamycin, prednisone) results in overall response rates of approximately 58–72%. However, in primary CLL both regimens did not prove to be superior to monochemotherapy with the purine analog fludarabine in terms of response induction, remission duration, overall survival, and toxicity [12,13]. Currently, anthracycline-based chemotherapy is no longer considered to be a treatment of choice in previously untreated CLL. Still, combination of CHOP with the monoclonal antibody rituximab (R-CHOP) is a valuable treatment option in transformed CLL (Richter transformation).

Current role of purine analog-based chemotherapy

The discovery of the purine-analog fludarabine in the late 1980s marked the beginning of a new era of CLL front-line therapy. Three phase III trials demonstrated that fludarabine is capable of inducing complete response rates of 20–40% and overall remission rates of 63–71% in treatment-naïve CLL [7,12,13]. Compared with alkylator-based treatment with chlorambucil, the median progression-free survival was extended to 25 months, but no effect on overall survival was observed. In a recent trial that exclusively enrolled patients of 65 years or older, fludarabine failed to prolong progression-free survival in comparison with chlorambucil (progression-free survival in both treatment arms: 18–19 months). The toxicity of both treatments was comparable except for myelotoxicity, which was more pronounced for fludarabine. Upon relapse, patients in the chlorambucil arm more frequently received salvage therapy than fludarabine-treated patients (26% vs. 12%) and responded well [11]. These findings and a recent meta-analysis comparing fludarabine with alkylator-based therapy [14] suggest that the benefit of single-agent treatment with fludarabine might have been overrated in the past.

Front-line treatment with fludarabine alone is used less often as trials combining the purine analog with cyclophosphamide (FC-regimen) suggested an increased efficacy of the combination treatment compared with purine analog monotherapy (see, for example, [15]). Recent phase III trials [16–18] confirmed that front-line treatment with FC indeed results in increased complete (22–39% vs. 6–15%) and overall response rates (70–95% vs. 50%–83%). The progression-free survival is significantly prolonged with FC (41–48 vs. 18–20 months). However, no advantage in overall survival could be demonstrated so far and, although easily manageable, toxicity with FC was higher than with fludarabine alone.

Based on sound phase III trial evidence, the FC regimen is currently considered to be the standard front-line treatment of CLL. The progression-free survival by far exceeds the duration of remissions with alkylator-based or purine analog-based monochemotherapy. The lack of overall survival improvement is probably not due to a lack of activity of FC itself. Recent data support the hypothesis that patients receiving FC as the first-line treatment may be less eligible for and benefit less from second-line therapies [19].

It must be emphasized that the superiority of FC in response and remission duration has so far been demonstrated mainly in younger patients. Patients >70 years old may also respond well to FC, but rates of life-threatening adverse events are higher and treatment is more frequently discontinued [20]. Consequently, in routine practice the combination treatment should be restricted to medically fit patients. Medically unfit patients of advanced age may receive front-line treatment with dose-adjusted FC when treated in the context of a clinical trial.

Besides fludarabine, the purine analogs cladribine and pentostatin also have been shown to be active in CLL. Cladribine has been successfully combined with cyclophosphamide, yielding response rates that are comparable to those with FC [21].

Current role of antibody-based immunotherapy and chemoimmunotherapy

The monoclonal antibody rituximab binds to the CD20 membrane protein on CLL cells, thereby resulting in CLL cell death. Single-agent treatment with rituximab has limited activity in CLL unless very high doses are used. Two pivotal phase II studies reported remission rates of 90–95%, with 50–70% of complete responses in treatment-naïve patients when fludarabine alone or fludarabine plus cyclophosphamide were combined with rituximab

(FR regimen, FCR regimen) [22,23]. Currently, front-line FCR is compared with FC in a randomized fashion within the CLL8 trial of the German CLL Study Group (GCLLSG). The recruitment was completed in 2006. In January 2008, the data-safety management board of the trial protocol informed the sponsor that, on the basis of the available data, the endpoint was reached and that FCR proved to be superior to FC. A careful analysis of these results and the examination of subgroups still have to be awaited, but this information suggests that FCR will be a new standard therapy for physically fit patients with CLL in the very near future. Currently, front-line treatment with FCR still should be carried out within the context of a clinical trial. Moreover, the treatment of elderly patients with FCR is accompanied by substantial toxicity if not properly tailored to the patient's burden of comorbidity and functional organ reserve [20]. Therefore, medically unfit patients of advanced age should not be considered to receive FCR as front-line therapy.

Apart from FCR, pentostatin plus cyclophosphamide [24] and bendamustine have also been successfully combined with rituximab to treat primary CLL (PCR regimen, BR regimen). Remission rates were comparable with those with FR and FCR. Of note, the PCR regimen has shown good antileukemic activity and relatively mild toxicity in elderly patients [25]. Future clinical trials are now under way to further optimize treatment with FCR or with other chemoimmunotherapeutic regimens (eg, FR, PCR, BR) that may be equally active but less toxic than FCR.

Alemtuzumab is a monoclonal antibody that binds to the CD52 protein of CLL cells and induces CLL cell apoptosis. In contrast to rituximab, treatment with alemtuzumab alone exerts marked antileukemic activity. A recent phase III trial demonstrated that treatment of primary CLL with alemtuzumab improves response rates (83% overall remissions, 24% complete remissions), progression-free survival, and time to alternative treatment (23 months) in comparison with traditional alkylator-based monochemotherapy [9].

In particular, front-line therapy of CLL with alemtuzumab is currently discussed to play a major role in patients presenting with a p53 dysfunction, which commonly is detected by fluorescence *in situ* hybridization (17p deletion). These patients have been recognized to respond poorly to monochemotherapy and combined chemoimmunotherapy with FC and eventually FCR. Until now, the monoclonal antibody alemtuzumab is the only drug that has been shown to be capable of overcoming p53-mediated refractoriness to standard therapeutic efforts [26]. Currently, there is not enough evidence to exclusively recommend the use of alemtuzumab for routine practice as the standard front-line treatment in poor-risk patients with lack of p53 function. Whenever possible, however, these patients should be included in a clinical trial with a research focus on the treatment of p53-lacking primary CLL. There is also increasing evidence that activity in patients with p53 dysfunction is not a unique feature of alemtuzumab. For instance, flavopiridol has also been shown to yield responses in such poor-risk patients [27].

Single-agent use of alemtuzumab has been applied to consolidate disease remission upon front-line therapy with FC or fludarabine alone [28]. Indeed, progression-free survival was longer with alemtuzumab consolidation treatment than with observation alone (not reached vs. 21 months). However, the occurrence of life-threatening infections due to sustained T-cell suppression neutralized the benefit of prolonged remission [29]. Integration of alemtuzumab-based consolidation in the front-line therapy of CLL is far from being established. Currently, future trials are ongoing to further explore the role and the administration schedule of alemtuzumab-based consolidation treatment.

Indications for salvage therapy

In routine practice, salvage treatment of relapse CLL should not be initiated before active or symptomatic disease (deterioration of blood counts, discomfort as a result of B symptoms, lymphadenopathy or hepatosplenomegaly, recurrent infections, and autoimmune disorders) has been clearly documented [1,2]. Minimal residual disease (MRD), which can be detected by flow cytometry or polymerase chain reaction, has been recognized to indicate CLL recurrence before the disease becomes clinically apparent. Based on these findings, it has been proposed to treat MRD in order to improve disease control by pre-emptively preventing the full remanifestation of relapsed CLL. At present, MRD treatment still remains an experimental strategy that needs further evaluation in prospective randomized trials. Outside of investigative trials, however, salvage therapy is not indicated until the patients present with the abovementioned clinical criteria [1].

Choice of salvage therapy

Salvage therapy of relapsed CLL has not been standardized so far. For patients with late relapses (response duration of >1 year upon traditional monochemotherapy and >2 years upon modern chemoimmunotherapy), the readministration of the front-line regimen is the treatment of choice.

Patients with shorter remission durations usually require therapy with alternative regimens. Monochemotherapy with chlorambucil was realized to be little effective in patients who previously had been treated with purine analog-based chemotherapy or chemoimmunotherapy. The alkylating drug bendamustine is active in relapsed or refractory CLL when applied either alone or in combination with other cytostatic drugs [30,31]. The anthracycline epirubicin showed remarkable activity in relapsed CLL when combined with fludarabine (FE regimen) [32], but has no superiority in comparison with the combined chemotherapy with FC (see, for example, [33]). Cytostatic drugs (fludarabine, fludarabine plus cyclophosphamide, pentostatin and bendamustine) have been successfully used in combination with the antibodies rituximab and alemtuzumab to treat relapsed CLL (FA regimen, CFAR regimen, FCR regimen, PCR regimen, BR regimen) [25,34–37]. Finally, both autologous and allogeneic hematopoietic stem-cell transplantation (HSCT) have been applied in relapsed or refractory CLL.

While autologous HSCT does not seem to yield better results than modern chemoimmunotherapies, allogeneic HSCT proved to be capable of completely eradicating the disease followed by long-lasting remissions and long-term survival [38]. However, myeloablative conditioning is associated with a transplant-related mortality (TRM) of up to 30–40% within 5 years after allogeneic HSCT, thereby offsetting the potential of the treatment modality to cure the disease [39–41]. Non-hematologic toxicity and organ failure, as well as graft-versus-host disease (GVHD) and infectious complications, account for the high rates of TRM after myeloablative conditioning. Promising results came from trials that used reduced-intensity conditioning (RIC), yielding lower rates of TRM (15–20% within 2–5 years post transplant by decreasing organ toxicity without affecting graft-versus-leukemia (GVL) activity [42–45].

As far as possible, patients suffering from recurrent CLL should be treated within clinical trials. The choice of treatment depends on several factors—nature and numbers of previously administered therapies, genetic risk, age, and physical fitness all must be taken into account. Early relapse after standard treatment with FC may be treated with chemoimmunotherapy (eg, FCR, BR, FA, FCA) or alemtuzumab alone. Patients who have refractory CLL (no response to front-line treatment) or relapsed CLL with a lack of p53 function should be enrolled in trials and receive a salvage regimen that includes alemtuzumab. Subsequent allogeneic HSCT with RIC should be strongly considered in younger and physically fit patients with refractory or relapsed disease and poor-risk factors, or generally in patients with p53 dysfunction, since in these patients durable remissions have not been observed with any other treatment modality. Elderly patients who relapse upon chlorambucil may be treated with low-dose fludarabine, low-dose FC, bendamustine, or CHOP. Those patients may also benefit from antibody monotherapy (rituximab, alemtuzumab) or other experimental approaches (eg, lenalidomide).

Perspective

Within the last few years, front-line and salvage therapy of CLL has undergone rapid changes by a constant growth of treatment options. Within the near future, treatment of primary and relapsed CLL will continue to develop and be further changed. For instance, results from ongoing phase III trials are expected to provide sound evidence for chemoimmunotherapy to be superior to the current standard front-line treatment, thereby improving outcome and, most importantly, overall survival in CLL. The definition of a standard front-line treatment for poor-risk patients and for physically unfit patients of advanced age remains a challenge. For both patient groups, separate trials are needed that are dedicated to the specific risk profile of these patients. New insights into the biology of CLL and mechanisms of drug action will help to develop new substances that are clinically active, and can be applied either alone or in combination with already existing regimens. The latest results from clinical trials are promising, and several agents, such as lenalidomide or flavopiridol, monoclonal antibodies (eg, lumiliximab, ofatumomab), or gene therapy (using CD40 ligand gene transfer), are expected to further improve both front-line and salvage treatment of CLL.

References

1 Hallek M, Cheson BD, Catovsky D, *et al.* Guidelines for the diagnosis and treatment of chronic lymphocytic leukemia: a report from the International Workshop on Chronic Lymphocytic Leukemia (IWCLL) updating the National Cancer Institute-Working Group (NCI-WG) 1996 guidelines. *Blood* 2008;111:5446–56.

2 Cheson BD, Bennett JM, Grever M, *et al.* National Cancer Institute-sponsored Working Group guidelines for chronic lymphocytic leukemia: revised guidelines for diagnosis and treatment. *Blood* 1996;87:4990–7.

3 Dighiero G, Maloum K, Desablens B, *et al.* Chlorambucil in indolent chronic lymphocytic leukemia. French Cooperative Group on Chronic Lymphocytic Leukemia. *N Engl J Med* 1998; 338:1506–14.

4 Shustik C, Mick R, Silver R, *et al.* Treatment of early chronic lymphocytic leukemia: intermittent chlorambucil versus observation. *Hematol Oncol* 1988;6:7–12.

5 Moreno C, Montserrat E. New prognostic markers in chronic lymphocytic leukemia. *Blood Rev* 2008;22:211–19.

6 Bergmann M, Eichhorst B, Busch R, *et al.* Early and risk-adapted therapy with fludarabine in high-risk Binet stage A CLL Patients prolongs progression free survival but not overall survival: results of the CLL1 protocol of the German CLL Study Group (GCLLSG). *Blood* (ASH Annual Meeting) 2007;110:2038.

7 Rai KR, Peterson BL, Appelbaum FR, *et al.* Fludarabine compared with chlorambucil as primary therapy for chronic lymphocytic leukemia. *N Engl J Med* 2000;343:1750–7.

8 Catovsky D, Richards S, Hillmen P. Early results from LRF CLL4: A UK multicenter randomized trial. *Blood* (ASH Annual Meeting Abstracts) 2005;106:716.

9 Hillmen P, Skotnicki AB, Robak T, *et al.* Alemtuzumab compared with chlorambucil as first-line therapy for chronic lymphocytic leukemia. *J Clin Oncol* 2007;25:5616–23.

10 Knauf K, Lissichkov T, Aldaoud A, *et al.* Bendamustine versus chlorambucil in treatment-naive patients with B-Cell chronic lymphocytic leukemia (B-CLL): results of an international phase III study. *Blood* (ASH Annual Meeting) 2007;110:2043.

11 Eichhorst B, Busch R, Stauch M, *et al.* No significant clinical benefit of first line therapy with fludarabine (F) in comparison to chlorambucil (Clb) in elderly patients (pts) with advanced chronic lymphocytic leukemia (CLL): results of a phase III study of the German CLL Study Group (GCLLSG). *Blood* (ASH Annual Meeting) 2007;110:629.

12 Leporrier M, Chevret S, Cazin B, *et al.* Randomized comparison of fludarabine, CAP, and ChOP in 938 previously untreated stage B and C chronic lymphocytic leukemia patients. *Blood* 2001;98:2319–25.

13 Johnson S, Smith AG, Loffler H, *et al.* Multicentre prospective randomized trial of fludarabine versus cyclophosphamide, doxorubicin, and prednisone (CAP) for treatment of advanced-stage chronic lymphocytic leukemia. The French Cooperative Group on CLL. *Lancet* 1996;347:1432–8.

14 Steurer M, Pall G, Richards S, *et al.* Purine antagonists for chronic lymphocytic leukemia. *Cochrane Database Syst Rev* 2006; 3:CD004270.

15 O'Brien SM, Kantarjian HM, Cortes J, *et al.* Results of the fludarabine and cyclophosphamide combination regimen in chronic lymphocytic leukemia. *J Clin Oncol* 2001;19:1414–20.

16 Eichhorst BF, Busch R, Hopfinger G, *et al.* Fludarabine plus cyclophosphamide versus fludarabine alone in first-line therapy of younger patients with chronic lymphocytic leukemia. *Blood* 2006;107:885–91.

17 Catovsky D, Richards S, Matutes E, *et al.* Assessment of fludarabine plus cyclophosphamide for patients with chronic lymphocytic leukemia (the LRF CLL4 Trial): a randomized controlled trial. *Lancet* 2007;370:230–9.

18 Flinn IW, Neuberg DS, Grever MR, *et al.* Phase III trial of fludarabine plus cyclophosphamide compared with fludarabine for patients with previously untreated chronic lymphocytic leukemia: US Intergroup Trial E2997. *J Clin Oncol* 2007;25: 793–8.

19 Catovsky D, Else M, Richards S, *et al.* The lack of survival differences in randomized trials in CLL may be related to the effect of second line therapies. A report from the LRF CLL4 trial. *Blood* (ASH Annual Meeting Abstracts) 2006;108:304.

20 Ferrajoli A, O'Brien S, Wierda W, *et al.* Treatment of patients with CLL 70 years old and older: a single center experience of 142 patients. *Leuk Lymph* 2005;46:S87.

21 Robak T, Blonski JZ, Gora-Tybor J, *et al.* Randomized comparison of cladribine with cyclophosphamide and fludarabine with cyclophosphamide in previously untreated progressive and symptomatic chronic lymphocytic leukemia: the interim analysis of PALG CLL3 trial. *Blood* (ASH Annual Meeting Abstracts) 2005;106:2121.

22 Byrd JC, Peterson BL, Morrison VA, *et al.* Randomized phase 2 study of fludarabine with concurrent versus sequential treatment with rituximab in symptomatic, untreated patients with B-cell chronic lymphocytic leukemia: results from Cancer and Leukemia Group B 9712 (CALGB 9712). *Blood* 2003;101:6–14.

23 Keating MJ, O'Brien S, Albitar M, *et al.* Early results of a chemoimmunotherapy regimen of fludarabine, cyclophosphamide, and rituximab as initial therapy for chronic lymphocytic leukemia. *J Clin Oncol* 2005;23:4079–88.

24 Kay NE, Geyer SM, Call TG, *et al.* Combination chemoimmunotherapy with pentostatin, cyclophosphamide, and rituximab shows significant clinical activity with low accompanying toxicity in previously untreated B chronic lymphocytic leukemia. *Blood* 2007;109:405–11.

25 Lamanna N, Kalaycio M, Maslak P, *et al.* Pentostatin, cyclophosphamide, and rituximab is an active, well-tolerated regimen for patients with previously treated chronic lymphocytic leukemia. *J Clin Oncol* 2006;24:1575–81.

26 Stilgenbauer S, Dohner H. Campath-1H-induced complete remission of chronic lymphocytic leukemia despite p53 gene mutation and resistance to chemotherapy. *N Engl J Med* 2002; 347:452–3.

27 Byrd JC, Lin TS, Dalton JT, *et al.* Flavopiridol administered using a pharmacologically derived schedule is associated with marked clinical efficacy in refractory, genetically high-risk chronic lymphocytic leukemia. *Blood* 2007;109:399–404.

28 Schweighofer C, Ritgen M, Eichhorst B, *et al.* Consolidation with alemtuzumab improves progression-free survival in patients with chronic lymphocytic leukemia (CLL) in first remission—long-term follow-up of a randomized phase III trial of the German CLL Study Group (GCLLSG). *Blood* (ASH Annual Meeting Abstracts) 2006;108:33.

29 Lin TS, Donohue KA, Lucas MS, *et al.* Consolidation therapy with subcutaneous (SC) alemtuzumab results in severe infectious toxicity in previously untreated CLL patients who achieve a complete response (CR) after fludarabine and rituximab (FR) induction therapy: interim safety analysis of the CALGB study 10101. *Blood* (ASH Annual Meeting Abstracts) 2007;110: 755.

30 Bergmann MA, Goebeler ME, Herold M, *et al.* Efficacy of bendamustine in patients with relapsed or refractory chronic lymphocytic leukemia: results of a phase I/II study of the German CLL Study Group. *Haematologica* 2005;90:1357–64.

31 Koppler H, Heymanns J, Pandorf A, *et al.* Bendamustine plus mitoxantrone–a new effective treatment for advanced chronic lymphocytic leukemia: results of a phase I/II study. *Leuk Lymphoma* 2004;45:911–13.

32 Rummel MJ, Kafer G, Pfreundschuh M, *et al.* Fludarabine and epirubicin in the treatment of chronic lymphocytic leukemia: a German multicenter phase II study. *Ann Oncol* 1999;10:183–8.

33 O'Brien S, Moore JO, Boyd TE, *et al.* Randomized phase III trial of fludarabine plus cyclophosphamide with or without oblimersen sodium (Bcl-2 antisense) in patients with relapsed or refractory chronic lymphocytic leukemia. *J Clin Oncol* 2007; 25:1114–20.

34 Elter T, Borchmann P, Schulz H, *et al.* Fludarabine in combination with alemtuzumab is effective and feasible in patients with relapsed or refractory B-cell chronic lymphocytic leukemia: results of a phase II trial. *J Clin Oncol* 2005;23:7024–31.

35 Wierda WG, Obrien S, Ferrajoli A, *et al.* Salvage therapy with combined cyclophosphamide (C), fludarabine (F), alemtuzumab (A), and rituximab (R) (CFAR) for heavily pre-treated patients with CLL. *Blood* (ASH Annual Meeting Abstracts) 2005;106:719.

36 Wierda W, O'Brien S, Wen S, *et al.* Chemoimmunotherapy with fludarabine, cyclophosphamide, and rituximab for relapsed and refractory chronic lymphocytic leukemia. *J Clin Oncol* 2005; 23:4070–8.

37 Fischer K, Stilgenbauer S, Schweighofer C, *et al.* Bendamustine in combination with rituximab (BR) for patients with relapsed chronic lymphocytic leukemia (CLL): a multicentre phase II trial of the German CLL Study Group (GCLLSG). *Blood* (ASH Annual Meeting) 2007.

38 Dreger P, Corradini P, Kimby E, *et al.* Indications for allogeneic stem cell transplantation in chronic lymphocytic leukemia: the EBMT transplant consensus. *Leukemia* 2007;21:12–17.

39 Moreno C, Villamor N, Colomer D, *et al.* Allogeneic stem-cell transplantation may overcome the adverse prognosis of unmutated VH gene in patients with chronic lymphocytic leukemia. *J Clin Oncol* 2005;23:3433–8.

40 Pavletic SZ, Khouri IF, Haagenson M, *et al.* Unrelated donor marrow transplantation for B-cell chronic lymphocytic leukemia after using myeloablative conditioning: results from the Center for International Blood and Marrow Transplant research. *J Clin Oncol* 2005;23:5788–94.

41 Pavletic ZS, Arrowsmith ER, Bierman PJ, *et al.* Outcome of allogeneic stem cell transplantation for B cell chronic lymphocytic leukemia. *Bone Marrow Transplant* 2000;25:717–22.

42 Caballero D, Garcia-Marco JA, Martino R, *et al.* Allogeneic transplant with reduced intensity conditioning regimens may overcome the poor prognosis of B-cell chronic lymphocytic leukemia with unmutated immunoglobulin variable heavy-chain gene and chromosomal abnormalities (11q- and 17p-). *Clin Cancer Res* 2005;11:7757–63.

43 Dreger P, Ritgen M, Bottcher S, *et al.* The prognostic impact of minimal residual disease assessment after stem cell transplantation for chronic lymphocytic leukemia: is achievement of molecular remission worthwhile? *Leukemia* 2005;19: 1135–8.

44 Schetelig J, Thiede C, Bornhauser M, *et al.* Evidence of a graft-versus-leukemia effect in chronic lymphocytic leukemia after reduced-intensity conditioning and allogeneic stem-cell transplantation: the Cooperative German Transplant Study Group. *J Clin Oncol* 2003;21:2747–53.

45 Sorror ML, Maris MB, Sandmaier BM, *et al.* Hematopoietic cell transplantation after nonmyeloablative conditioning for advanced chronic lymphocytic leukemia. *J Clin Oncol* 2005;23: 3819–29.

Chapter 26
The Role of Stem-cell Transplantation in Chronic Lymphocytic Leukemia

Simon Hallam and John G. Gribben
Barts and the London School of Medicine and Dentistry, Queen Mary University of London, London, UK

Introduction

Despite recent advances, conventional chemoimmunotherapy regimens appear unable to cure chronic lymphocytic leukemia (CLL). However, in most patients with CLL, disease presents in later life and follows an indolent course for which aggressive therapies are not warranted. Optimal management of the significant minority of patients with rapidly progressive CLL is challenging, and these patients remain very likely to die as a result of their disease. It is possible to identify patients with poor-risk features at diagnosis, or early in their disease course, so that alternate strategies incorporating stem-cell transplantation (SCT) can be considered. Nonetheless, optimal patient selection and timing of SCT is not yet clear from available study data. Recruitment of appropriate patients into well-designed clinical trials is vital to evaluate the role of SCT in CLL, particularly in the light of promising results with novel chemoimmunotherapy combinations alone.

Autologous stem-cell transplantation is feasible and has a low treatment-related mortality (TRM), but disease relapse appears inevitable. In the absence of other treatment modalities currently capable of inducing long-term survival, the treatment of choice for younger patients with poor-risk CLL may well be allogeneic SCT. The optimal strategy for allogeneic SCT in CLL is not entirely clear. Myeloablative conditioning results in very high TRM and may only be suitable for a small proportion of high-risk patients. A clinically significant graft-versus-leukemia effect in CLL has been demonstrated through reduced-intensity conditioning (RIC) SCT and donor lymphocyte infusion (DLI). As SCT strategies evolve in an attempt to minimize TRM and prolong survival, optimal patient selection and timing of transplantation remain to be the biggest challenges for the clinician.

Leukemias: Principles and Practice of Therapy, 1st edition. Edited by S. Faderl and H. Kantarjian.

Patient selection for stem-cell transplantation

The natural history of CLL varies enormously between patients. It is imperative that patients with indolent disease are not exposed to the risks of aggressive therapies. Similarly, we should strive not to miss opportunities for early disease control in those who are likely to otherwise die from rapidly progressive CLL. As our understanding of the pathophysiology of CLL has improved, a number of prognostic biomarkers have been identified to supplement previously validated clinical predictors. However, as treatments evolve the ongoing relevance of each prognostic factor must be re-addressed. Studies attempting to address the safety and efficacy of SCT in CLL have consistently used "high-risk" patient groups. Given the relatively high morbidity and mortality of SCT procedures, the accurate identification of such high-risk patients using a number of clinical and biologic characteristics should be a high priority for the treating clinician.

The pattern of bone marrow involvement (diffuse vs. nodular or interstitial) has prognostic significance [1]. Atypical lymphocyte morphology, with increased number of prolymphocytes, is also an independent factor associated with an adverse prognosis [2]. A lymphocyte doubling time (LDT) of <12 months in untreated patients predicts a progressive course [3]. Biochemical indices of tumor-cell proliferation have also been correlated with clinical outcome, including beta-2-microglobulin [4], Ki67 [5], p27 [6], and thymidine kinase [7]. Conventional cytogenetic analysis only detects chromosome aberrations in 40–50% of cases; however, when using fluorescence *in situ* hybridization (FISH), abnormalities are detected in >80% of patients with CLL [8]. The most frequent changes observed are 13q deletion, 11q deletion, trisomy 12q, and 17p deletion. Patients with 17p and 11q deletions have more advanced disease, shorter time to requirement for therapy, and poorer prognosis than those without these deletions. The presence of 17p deletion predicts for treatment failure with alkylating agents and fludarabine and short survival times. In multivariate analysis, 11q and 17p deletions provided independent adverse prognostic information. These findings have implications for the design of risk-adapted treatment strategies, including the selection of patients for SCT [9].

Patients with CLL who have unmutated immunoglobulin variable (*IgV*) region genes have poor prognoses compared with those whose immunoglobulin genes are mutated [10,11]. It has been suggested that higher levels of expression of CD38 are associated with unmutated *IgV* genes [10]. On multivariate analysis, high levels of expression of CD38 on B-cell CLL cells were associated with more rapid progression of disease and poor response to therapy [12,13]. A multivariate analysis was performed examining the prognostic significance of genetic abnormalities at presentation, clinical stage, lymphocyte morphology, CD38 expression, and *IgV* gene status in 205 patients with CLL [14]. Deletion of chromosome 11q23, absence of a deletion of chromosome 13q14, atypical lymphocyte morphology, and >30% CD38 expression were significantly associated with the presence of unmutated *IgV* genes. Advanced stage, male sex, atypical morphology, >30% CD38 expression, trisomy 12, deletion of chromosome 11q23, loss or mutation of the *p53* gene, and unmutated *IgV* genes were all poor prognostic factors in the univariate analysis in this study. However, *IgV* gene mutational status, loss or mutation of the *p53* gene, and clinical stage retained prognostic significance in a multivariate analysis [14]. Expression of ZAP70 has been examined as a surrogate for *IgV* mutational status, and is also associated with poor prognosis in CLL [15–17].

Management strategies in chronic lymphocytic leukemia

Evidence of a survival benefit from treatment is available only for patients with advanced-stage CLL (Rai III and IV or Binet B and C). Initiating treatment for early-stage disease is justified only by the presence of disease-associated morbidity such as troublesome lymphadenopathy or constitutional symptoms, and is not indicated for a high circulating lymphocyte count alone.

Traditional treatment regimens involve alkylating agents such as chlorambucil alone, cyclophosphamide, adriamycin, and prednisone (CAP), or cytoxan, hydroxyrubicin, oncovin, and prednisone (CHOP). Improved response rates are seen with purine analogs, particularly fludarabine, when compared with alkylating agents [18–20]. First-line therapy with fludarabine alone has not produced an overall survival (OS) benefit, partly because those treated initially with alkylating agents often respond well to purine analogs as second-line therapy. The combination of fludarabine with cyclophosphamide has been shown in randomized trials to increase response rates and produce a longer duration of response than fludarabine alone [21,22]. Incorporating the monoclonal anti-CD20 antibody rituximab into an FCR combination appears to further improve response rates and duration of response [23,24].

The management of relapsed CLL is an evolving field, which currently defies a clear consensus. Combination chemoimmunotherapy produces the best response rates [25], yet the optimal regimen should be tailored for individual circumstances. The aims and selection of treatment are dependent upon several clinical factors. Age, performance status, previous treatments, the extent and duration of response to such treatments, and time from last treatment appear to be critical. In addition, the goal of therapy, whether aggressive or palliative, should be established. There is no evidence to date that any available chemoimmunotherapy combination is curative and patients invariably relapse again and subsequently develop resistance to chemotherapy, often with the loss of function of p53 [26]. Once refractory to purine analogs the median survival has been reported as <1 year [27]. The humanized anti-CD52 monoclonal antibody alemtuzumab is approved for treating fludarabine refractory CLL. In the pivotal study of alemtuzumab in 93 such patients, the overall response rate was 33%, although only 2% of patients achieved complete remission (CR) [28]. The median time to progression for responders was 9.5 months, and there was an improvement in survival in responding patients at 32 months compared with 16 months for all patients. Of note, alemtuzumab appears to have activity against cases that are unresponsive to chemotherapy because of the presence of *p53* mutations [29,30]. Despite often effecting hematologic responses, alemtuzumab has relatively poor activity against bulky lymphadenopathy. Alemtuzumab has shown benefit when used in combination with fludarabine [31,32]. Studies are also examining the role of alemtuzumab treatment after chemotherapy to clear residual disease [33], and this may be an effective way to obtain autologous peripheral blood stem cells free from contamination with CLL [34]. Given the limited survival benefits achieved with the above agents in the face of aggressive and/or relapsing CLL in a younger patient, there is currently likely to be a role for hematopoietic SCT.

Role of transplantation in chronic lymphocytic leukemia

Several studies have attempted to ascertain whether SCT might offer the potential of cure or reversal of chemotherapy resistance in CLL. Largely a disease of later life, with a median age of presentation between 65 and 70 years, most patients with CLL are insufficiently robust to consider such an approach with its attendant morbidity and mortality. However, 40% of patients with CLL are aged <60 years and 12% are aged <50 years at the time of diagnosis. Unlike older patients, who often eventually die of causes unrelated to CLL, >90% of younger patients die because of CLL itself [35]. As such, this group might benefit the most and suffer the least morbidity and mortality from more aggressive approaches incorporating SCT. The various strategies for employing SCT in CLL are explored below.

Autologous stem-cell transplantation

There has been no prospective study directly comparing the outcome after conventional therapy with that obtained after autologous SCT, although a retrospective matched-pair analysis suggested a survival advantage for autologous SCT [36]. As induction regimens have evolved, it would now be useful to look at the new chemoimmunotherapeutic regimens in direct comparison with autologous SCT.

A number of phase II studies have reported the outcome following autologous SCT for CLL [37–43] (Table 26.1). The approach is feasible in CLL with a TRM of between 2% and 10% [42,43]. Encouraging early results were reported in patients with chemosensitive disease [37], whereas patients transplanted in relapse or with chemoresistant disease had poor outcome [38]. In a study of 16 patients undergoing autologous SCT, at a median follow-up of 41 months eight had relapsed and six had died (three from progressive CLL) [41]. Other groups have observed better results. In 18 patients with CLL, including early-stage disease, autologous SCT was performed in 13 individuals, only one of whom had relapsed at the time of publication [40]. Eight heavily pretreated patients received autologous SCT with partially purged $CD34^+$ peripheral blood stem cells, and although four patients remained in CR, the median follow-up was only 9 months [39]. The experience in Finland has been updated recently for 72 patients autografted in five centers between 1995 and 2005 [44]. The median age was 57 (range 38–69 years) with a median time from diagnosis of 32 months (range 6–181 months). The median number of prior therapies was one. The most commonly used conditioning regimen was total body irradiation (TBI) and cyclophosphamide ($n = 38$, 53%). There were no early TRMs and 37% had relapsed or progressed after a median follow-up of 28 months. The projected median progression-free survival (PFS) and OS were 48 months and 95 months, respectively.

A pilot study from the Medical Research Council (MRC) enrolled previously untreated patients and followed them prospectively to assess the feasibility of performing autologous SCT [42]. Only 65 of 115 patients (56%) entered into the study were able to proceed to autologous SCT after initial therapy with fludarabine. Only one patient died from early transplant-related complications, and the CR rate after transplantation was 74% (48/65). The 5-year OS was 77.5% and the 5-year PFS was 51.5%. None of the variables examined at study entry were predictive of either OS or PFS. Out of 20 patients available for analysis, 16 achieved a molecular CR in the first 6 months following transplantation. Detectable molecular disease by polymerase chain reaction (PCR) was highly predictive of disease recurrence. Of concern, 5 of 65 (8%) patients developed post-transplant acute myeloid leukemia

Table 26.1 Autologous transplantation for chronic lymphocytic leukemia.

Number of patients	Transplant-related mortality	Ongoing complete remission	Median follow-up (months)	Reference
137	5 early 13 MDS/AML 15 other cancer	67	78	Gribben *et al.* [43]
77	0	50	28	Jantunen *et al.* [44]
65	1 early 5 MDS/AML	45	36	Milligan *et al.* [42]
16	2	5	37	Pavletic *et al.* [41]
13	0	12	19	Dreger *et al.* [40]
11	1	2	10	Khouri *et al.* [38]
8 20 enrolled 12 stem cells collected	0	5	36	Sutton *et al.* [82]
5	0	4	9	Itala *et al.* [39]

AML, acute myeloid leukemia; MDS, myelodysplastic syndrome.

(AML)/myelodysplastic syndrome (MDS). This equates to a 5-year actuarial risk of developing MDS/AML post-autologous SCT of 12.4% (95%; confidence interval 2.5–24%). None of the potential risk factors analyzed were predictive. The group postulates that potential causative factors may be fludarabine, low cell dose, and use of TBI in the conditioning regimen. This finding has been supported by the long-term outcome reported in a series from the Dana Farber Cancer Institute, which reported an actuarial incidence of MDS/AML in patients with CLL post autograft of 12% at 8 years [43]. Such late effects of SCT may be under reported, as many recent studies necessarily have relatively short follow-up.

Although the early TRM is low after autologous SCT, there is a high incidence of opportunistic infections in patients with CLL compared with other patient populations. Whether this is due to disease-related immune defects in patients with CLL or is secondary to the immune-suppressive effects of treatment is unknown. Patients have a better outcome when they are treated early in the course of the disease and when they have less tumor burden. By extrapolation of this principle, it might be considered beneficial to transplant selected high-risk patients in first complete or partial remission. One difficulty in selecting high-risk patients is that these patients may also have an adverse outcome even after SCT. The immunoglobulin gene mutation status maintains its poor prognostic significance after autologous transplantation [45], although it appears that this can be overcome using allogeneic SCT [46,47]. A randomized trial proposed by the European Bone Marrow Transplant Group should help to address this issue. The timing of the harvesting of the cells, and whether they should be harvested in first remission and kept until later in the treatment course, also needs to be further investigated. It is not always possible to collect enough $CD34^+$ cells, especially in heavily pretreated patients [48], and an interval of at least 3 months should be allowed between the last dose of fludarabine and stem-cell collection [49].

Relapse of disease remains the major problem after autologous SCT, and patients continue to relapse years later [50]. A number of methods, including multiparameter flow cytometry analysis [51] and PCR [52], are being used to investigate whether persistence of MRD will predict which patients will relapse following transplant in CLL. Molecular remissions can be achieved in more than two-thirds of patients, but these are not durable [42,52–54] and most patients who achieve CR after autologous SCT will eventually relapse. Detectable molecular disease post transplant is, however, highly predictive of clinical recurrence [42].

One of the major concerns in autologous transplantation is that reinfusion of tumor cells may theoretically contribute to the risk of relapse. Numerous groups have attempted to improve outcome by "purging" the graft. The techniques most frequently employed utilize either negative selection using B-cell monoclonal antibodies to deplete tumor cells from the graft or positive selection of stem cells using CD34 antibodies. Unfortunately, these methods remain inefficient at removing CLL cells [52]. Purging also results in loss of stem cells. If there has been difficulty in obtaining a sufficiently large harvest, as seen in 50% of cases in the MRC pilot study, purging cannot be performed. This problem could be addressed by attempting *in vivo* purging using alemtuzumab or rituximab as part of the conditioning regime. In this way, high-dose alemtuzumab was used in one arm of the CLL3 trial from the German CLL Study Group, with unexpected consequences [55]. Sixteen patients were treated in this arm and received a median dose of alemtuzumab of 103 mg. A high incidence of initially unexplained skin rashes led to further analysis. Twelve of 16 patients (87%) developed a skin rash between 43 and 601 days after autologous SCT, and in seven of these patients a diagnosis of graft-versus-host disease (GVHD) could be made compared with no cases in the TBI/cyclophosphamide-only conditioned patients. Autologous GVHD is an autoimmune syndrome initiated by autologous effector T cells that recognize self-major histocompatibility complex (MHC) class II antigens and is usually self-limiting. In this case, however, all cases required immunosuppression and the median duration was 517 days (range 60–867 days). The trial was discontinued as a result of the high non-relapse mortality. However, of note, the addition of alemtuzumab led to improved disease control at the molecular level. It is interesting that the use of alemtuzumab in combination with other immunosuppressants prior to allogeneic SCT results in effective prevention of GVHD. In this situation, it was postulated that the markedly immunosuppressive regimen depleted regulatory CD4 and CD8 T cells and natural killer (NK) cells, allowing the subsequent development of autoimmune disease. The patients receiving alemtuzumab/TBI/cyclophosphamide had a severe CD8 lymphopenia in the first year after SCT. The authors recommend that future trials investigating *in vivo* purging with alemtuzumab should use a less immunosuppressive conditioning regimen such as BEAM and avoid the use of TBI.

The concept of using alemtuzumab for *in vivo* purging should perhaps not yet be discarded. When used at a modification from the standard doses (10 mg subcutaneously three times per week for 6 weeks) in 34 patients who had expressed a clinical response to a fludarabine-based regimen, the CR rate improved from 35% to 79.5%, with 56% achieving eradication of MRD [56]. Peripheral blood stem cell (PBSC) collection was subsequently successfully performed in 92% of patients. Eighteen patients underwent autologous SCT, with 17 remaining in CR at a median follow-up of 14.5 months post SCT.

Myeloablative allogeneic stem-cell transplantation

Allogeneic SCT attempts to supplement the dose-intensification effect of autologous transplant by adding cellular immune therapy to generate a graft-versus-leukemia (GVL) effect. This introduces the potential for better disease control and possibly cure, but at the price of greater toxicity. The morbidity and mortality of allogeneic SCT mostly relate to organ failure caused by the combination of the conditioning regimen and both acute and chronic GVHD (aGVHD and cGVHD, respectively). The risk of life-threatening infection is increased by both GVHD and the immune-suppressive treatment employed to control GVHD.

The feasibility of allogeneic SCT in CLL was first demonstrated in 1988 in eight patients, five of whom were alive and in CR after a median follow-up of 27 months post SCT [57]. The high TRM rate was apparent from registry data, with rates of 46–50% reported [58]. Despite the high TRM, patients who survive can have long-term disease control [37,58–61] (Table 26.2). Among 25 patients with CLL who underwent allogeneic SCT at the Fred Hutchinson Cancer Center [61], 14 developed grades 2–4 aGVHD and 10 developed clinical extensive cGVHD. Non-relapse mortality at day 100 was unacceptably high at 57% for the seven patients conditioned with busulphan and cyclophosphamide, and 17% for the 18 patients conditioned with TBI-containing regimens. Actuarial survival at 5 years for the 25 patients was 32%. All patients who received busulphan and cyclophosphamide died within 3 years of transplant. For the 14 patients transplanted since 1992 and who received TBI, actuarial 5-year OS is 56%, suggesting that long-term DFS might be achieved in this disease.

However, there are no data from randomized trials demonstrating improved outcome with dose intensification. Indeed, the major advantage of the use of allogeneic SCT appears to be the potential for a GVL effect. A strong GVL effect was noted, with those developing a- or cGVHD having near-complete protection from relapse [62]. This effect can be exploited by infusion of donor lymphocytes following allografting (Figure 26.1) [43,63] or after

Table 26.2 Myeloablative allogeneic transplantation for chronic lymphocytic leukemia.

Number	Transplant-related mortality	Severe graft-versus-host disease	Ongoing complete remission	Median follow-up (months)	Reference
54	25	18	24	27	Michellet *et al.* [58]
25	1 early 5 late	5	13 8 after DLI	78	Gribben *et al.* [43]
25	7	56	9	60	Doney *et al.* [61]
23	8	47	14	24	Pavletic *et al.* [60]
15	5	26	8	35	Khouri *et al.* [67]

DLI, donor lymphocyte infusions.

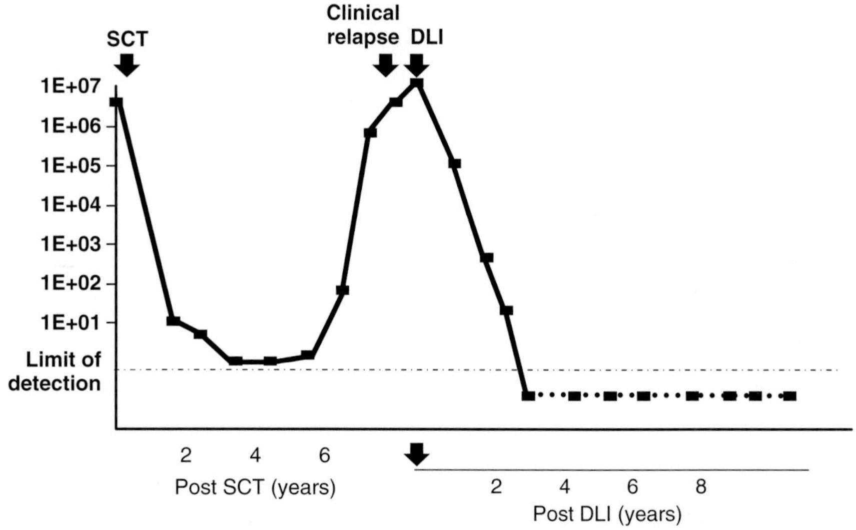

Figure 26.1 Response to donor lymphocyte infusion in chronic lymphocytic leukemia. Quantitive real-time PCR analysis of levels of disease following T-cell depleted allogeneic stem-cell transplantation (SCT). Donor lymphocyte infusion (DLI) administered as sole therapy after clinical evidence of relapse induced subsequent achievement of complete response and eradication for polymerase chain reaction detectable disease. Adapted from Gribben *et al.* [43].

cessation of immunosuppressive therapy [64]. Studies are under way addressing the number of lymphocytes required and the optimal timing of donor lymphocyte infusions after allogeneic SCT in this and other hematologic malignancies.

As human leukocyte antigen (HLA)-matched sibling allogeneic transplants are only possible in one-quarter of all potential recipients, the use of unrelated donor stem cells has been investigated. Among 38 heavily pretreated patients, 11 were alive and disease-free at a median of 6 years [65]. The 5-year OS rate was 33%, TRM was 38%, and the disease progression rate was 32%. Of note, 45% developed grade 2–4 aGVHD and 85% had cGVHD. The authors concluded that lasting remissions could be achieved but that the high TRM illustrated that unrelated HLA-mismatched donors should be avoided.

Comparison of autologous versus allogeneic stem-cell transplantation

Registry data have suggested that, although durable responses were being achieved after allogeneic SCT, survival was worse than after autologous SCT with a 3-year probability of survival reported as 45% for allogeneic SCT and 87% for autologous SCT [66]. Studies from the M. D. Anderson Cancer Center, however, have suggested improved outcome after allogeneic SCT compared with autologous transplant [38]. Of 14 patients with CLL refractory to or relapsed after chemotherapy with fludarabine, 13 (87%) achieved CR post transplant. At the time of reporting, nine patients (53%) remained alive and in CR with a median follow-up of 36 months [67], suggesting that allogeneic hematopoietic transplantation can induce durable remission even in patients with CLL refractory to fludarabine. There are no studies directly comparing the outcome of autologous SCT with allogeneic SCT. In a phase II study at the Dana Farber Cancer Institute (Figure 26.2), 162 patients with high-risk CLL were enrolled in a study between 1989 and 1999 in which 25 patients with an HLA-matched sibling donor underwent T-cell depleted allogeneic transplant and 137 with no sibling donor underwent B-cell purged autologous transplantation [43]. The 100-day mortality was 4% in both autologous and allogeneic SCT groups, although later TRM had a major impact on outcome. With a median follow-up of 6.5 years there was no difference in OS of 58% after autologous SCT and 55% after allogeneic SCT. PFS was significantly longer following autologous SCT than T-cell depleted allogeneic SCT, but no significant differences were observed in disease recurrence or deaths without recurrence according to type of transplant.

Reduced-intensity conditioned allogeneic stem-cell transplantation

The rationale of reduced-intensity conditioned (RIC) allogeneic SCT is to exploit the GVL effect while attenuating the significant morbidity and mortality associated with myeloablative conditioning. Study data indicate that RIC regimens do indeed appear to be associated with a

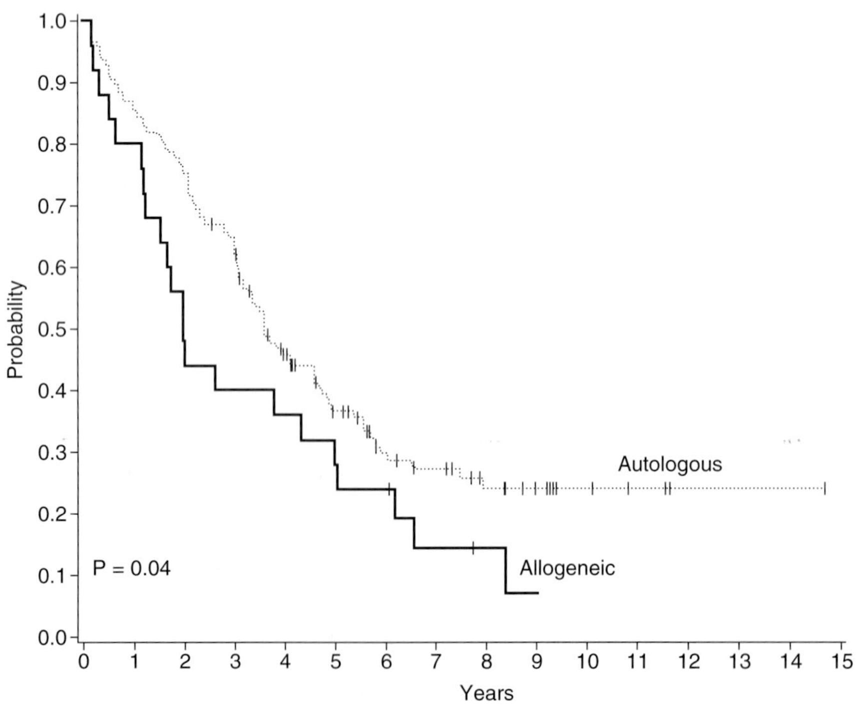

Figure 26.2 Progression-free survival after autologous and T-cell depleted allogeneic stem-cell transplantation. Adapted from Gribben *et al.* [43].

decreased mortality and could thus expand the age range that might benefit from the GVL effect [68–75]. Patients in these studies were often heavily pretreated and refractory to therapy. Despite this, the majority demonstrated donor engraftment with a high CR rate. Survival was improved in patients transplanted while they still had chemosensitive disease. These studies provide strong evidence for a clinically significant GVL effect in CLL. Current research is addressing the amount of pre- and post-transplant immunosuppression required to eventually establish a full donor chimerism following RIC SCT. It should be stressed that these procedures are currently investigational in nature. Although the acute morbidity and mortality appear significantly lower than high-dose conditioning regimens with allogeneic transplantation, the longer-term results are awaited. Further benefit could potentially be gained by separating the beneficial GVL effects of allogeneic SCT from the detrimental effects of GVHD. One such approach would be to target tumor-specific antigens, and *ex vivo* expansion of fluorescent activated cell sorter (FACS) isolated donor-derived T lymphocytes has allowed the infusion of peptide-specific cells with the potential to target CLL cells directly. Such experimental approaches hold great interest when considering future allogeneic SCT strategies.

To examine whether RIC decreases TRM after allogeneic SCT for CLL, the outcome of 73 patients treated with RIC was compared with that of 82 matched patients from the European Group for Blood and Marrow Transplantation Registry (EBMTR) database who had undergone standard myeloablative conditioning for CLL during the same time period [76]. Patients undergoing RIC had a significant reduction of TRM but a higher incidence of relapse. There was no significant difference in OS or EFS between the two groups.

Outcomes have been reported after RIC allogeneic SCT for 64 patients with advanced CLL using the Fred Hutchinson Cancer Research Center multi-institutional protocol using related ($n = 44$) or unrelated ($n = 20$) donors (Figure 26.3) [73]. As shown in Table 26.3, the median age was 56 years (range 44–69 years). The majority of patients were fludarabine refractory. TRM at 100 days was 11% and 22% by 2 years with significant GVHD. At a median follow-up of 24 months, 39 patients were alive and 25 were in CR. Two-year OS was 60% and disease-free survival was 52%. Although complications were higher in the patients with unrelated donors, there were higher CR and lower relapse rates than with related SCT, suggesting more effective GVL activity from the unrelated donors. These results have recently been updated, and at a median 5-year follow-up PFS was 39% and OS was 50% [75]. A similar high rate of GVHD was seen in a smaller group of Australian patients [77].

The incidence of GVHD can be reduced by the use of alemtuzumab in the conditioning regimen, with a consequent reduction in TRM. Unfortunately, it also delays post-SCT immune reconstitution, increases the risk of infective complications, and potentially impairs the GVL effect. This impaired antitumor response may necessitate the early use of DLI post SCT [78]. A study by the British Society of Bone Marrow Transplantation (BSBMT) used alemtuzumab with fludarabine and melphalan as the conditioning regimen [79]. Forty-one consecutive patients were treated, 24 had HLA-matched sibling donors, and 17 had unrelated volunteer donors (four mismatched). The conditioning regimen had significant antitumor effects, and 100% of patients with chemosensitive disease and 86% with chemorefractory disease attaining CR or partial remission (PR). The TRM rate was 26%, OS was 51%, and relapse risk was 29% at 2 years. GVHD rates were relatively low, with aGVHD occurring in 17 patients (41%) and cGVHD in 13 patients (33%). The unexpectedly high TRM rate was due to a high incidence of fungal and viral infections. What emerged from this study was the clear adverse prognostic factor of fludarabine refractoriness. This group of patients had a 2-year OS of only 31%.

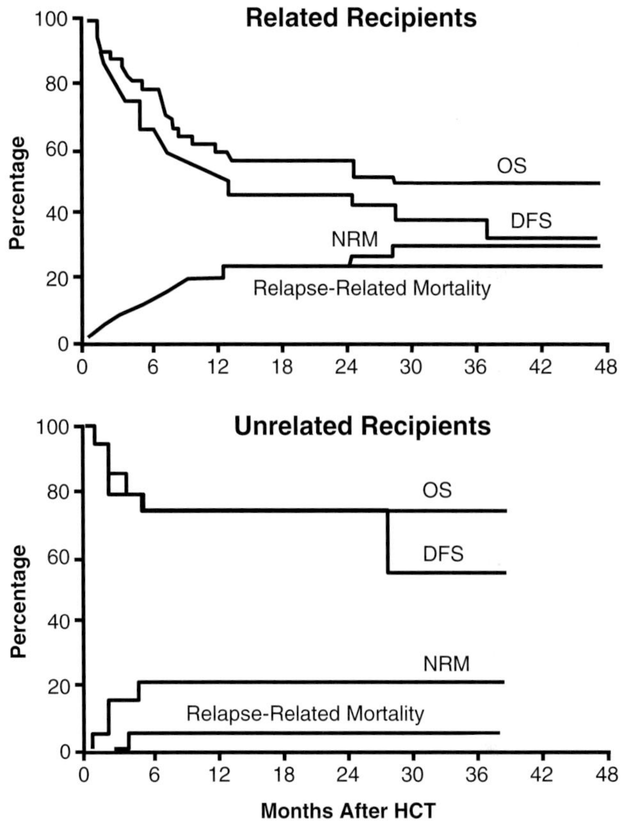

Figure 26.3 Outcome after reduced-intensity conditioning allogeneic stem-cell transplantation for chronic lymphocytic leukemia. DFS, disease-free survival; NRM, non-relapse mortality; OS, overall survival. Adapted from Sorror *et al.* [75].

Table 26.3 Reduced-intensity conditioned allogeneic stem-cell transplantation for chronic lymphocytic leukemia.

n	Age in years (range)	Prior regimens (range)	Chemotherapy refractory	Donor (includes mismatch) (%)	Transplant-related mortality (%)	Graft-versus-host disease(%)		Survival (%/year)	Reference
						Acute grade 2–4	Chronic extensive		
30	50 (12–63)	3 (0–8)	47%	50 related, 50 unrelated	13 overall	56	21	OS 72/2, PFS 67	Schetelig *et al.* [68]
77	54 (30–66)	3 (0–8)	33%, 10 prior auto-SCT	81 related	18/12 m	34	58	OS 72/2, PFS 56	Dreger *et al.* [72]
82	56 (42–72)	4	87%	63 related, 37 unrelated 31 unrelated	25 overall 22 overall	55	49 related 53 unrelated	OS 50/5, PFS 45	Sorror *et al.* [75]
39	57 (34–70)	3 (2–8)	Not stated 87% "active" disease	90 related, 10 unrelated	2 at 100 d	45	58	OS 48/4, PFS 44	Khouri *et al.* [83]
46	53 (35–67)	5 (1–10)	57%, 10 prior auto-SCT	33 related, 67 unrelated	17 overall	34	43	OS 54/2, PFS 34	Brown *et al.* [74]
41	54 (37–67)	3 (1–8)	27%,11 prior auto-SCT	58 related, 42 unrelated	5 at 100 d 26 overall	10 (grade 3–4)	33 after DLI	OS 51/2, PFS 45	Delgado *et al.* [79]

auto-SCT, autologous stem-cell transplantation; DLI, donor lymphocyte infusions; PFS, progression-free survival; OS, overall survival.

It has been demonstrated that patients with unmutated CLL who have undergone autologous SCT have a poor outcome [36,45]. This adverse event can be overcome with the use of allogeneic SCT [47]. Among 50 patients who underwent SCT, 34 had unmutated immunoglobulin variable heavy chain genes (*IgVH*) (14 underwent allogeneic SCT and 20 underwent autologous SCT) and 16 had mutated *IgVH* genes (nine underwent allogeneic SCT and seven underwent autologous SCT). There was no difference in CR rate between the type of transplantation and *IgVH* mutational status. After a median follow-up of 5 years, autologous SCT resulted in a significantly higher relapse rate than allogeneic SCT in both mutational groups. Thus, the GVL effect of allogeneic SCT may overcome the negative impact of unmutated *VH* gene status on outcome. Myeloablative conditioning may not be required for this effect. In 30 patients with poor-prognosis CLL as defined by the mutational status of *VH* genes and cytogenetic abnormalities ($11q^-$, $17p^-$) who had undergone RIC allogeneic, OS and event-free survival were 90% and 92%, respectively, and was not significantly different to that seen in the good-prognosis group [80].

European Group for Blood and Marrow Transplantation guidelines

The EBMT have established guidelines outlining indications for allogeneic SCT in CLL [81]. The guidelines conclude that there is evidence supporting the efficacy of allogeneic SCT in CLL and that this approach is indicated for selected high-risk patients. Precisely what factors are defined as high risk are not clear, but patients with *p53* deletions or mutations are considered to be candidates in first remission, and ongoing studies are assessing the impact of biomarkers including *IgVH* mutational status and cytogenetic abnormalities to identify patients at sufficiently high risk to merit consideration for transplant in first remission. The consensus of the EBMT working group was that allogeneic SCT was recommended early in the disease course for young patients with CLL who fail to achieve CR or who progress within 12 months after purine analogs, and those who relapse within 24 months after having achieved a response with purine analog-based combination therapy or autologous transplantation. It is clear that neither of these categories requires assessment of biologic risk factors, and ongoing prospective clinical studies will be required to determine the specific risk factors that identify patients at sufficiently high risk to merit the use of allogeneic SCT in first CR. However, there is consensus that patients requiring treatment who have *p53* abnormalities have a sufficiently poor prognosis to merit transplantation in first response. This should be considered early in the disease course to avoid the development of refractory disease. The indications for these approaches are shown in Table 26.4.

Table 26.4 Role of stem-cell transplantation in CLL.

Autologous SCT	No defined role Clinical trial only
Myeloablative allogeneic SCT	Chemorefractory disease in young patients
RIC allogeneic SCT	Incomplete response to first-line therapy Short duration of response after purine analog-containing regimens Richter transformation *p53* mutation at first treatment Other "high risk" in clinical trials

CLL, chronic lymphocytic leukemia; SCT, stem-cell transplantation.

Conclusions

The role, if any, of autologous SCT in CLL is not clear, and guidelines for its use in routine clinical practice do not exist. Autologous transplantation appears not to overcome the poor prognosis conferred by unmutated *VH* genes or poor-risk cytogenetic abnormalities. Allogeneic SCT should certainly be considered in these patients. Myeloablative regimens currently offer no survival advantage over autologous procedures. As such, the major clinical and research focus with respect to SCT in CLL is on the use of RIC allogeneic strategies.

Despite encouraging initial results, we are still in the position where the follow-up of most clinical trials is too short to assess whether RIC allogeneic SCT can cure CLL. Future approaches to the management of this disease must take into account the balance between the increased morbidity and mortality of SCT in CLL with the curative potential that these approaches may offer. Clearly, the indications for SCT in CLL will evolve as both transplant and non-transplant approaches to treating this disease develop. Continued enrollment of appropriate patients into well-designed clinical trials is vital for further progress.

References

1 Rozman C, Montserrat E, Rodriguez-Fernandez JM, *et al.* Bone marrow histologic pattern–the best single prognostic parameter in chronic lymphocytic leukemia: a multivariate survival analysis of 329 cases. *Blood* 1984;64:642–8.

2 Oscier DG, Matutes E, Copplestone A, *et al.* Atypical lymphocyte morphology: an adverse prognostic factor for disease progression in stage A CLL independent of trisomy 12. *Br J Haematol* 1997;98:934–9.

3 Montserrat E, Sanchez-Bisono J, Vinolas N, Rozman C. Lymphocyte doubling time in chronic lymphocytic leukemia: analysis of its prognostic significance. *Br J Haematol* 1986;62: 567–75.

4 Fayad L, Keating MJ, Reuben JM, *et al.* Interleukin-6 and interleukin-10 levels in chronic lymphocytic leukemia: correlation with phenotypic characteristics and outcome. *Blood* 2001; 97:256–63.

5 Cordone I, Matutes E, Catovsky D. Monoclonal antibody Ki-67 identifies B and T cells in cycle in chronic lymphocytic leukemia: correlation with disease activity. *Leukemia* 1992;6:902–6.

6 Vrhovac R, Delmer A, Tang R, Marie JP, Zittoun R, Ajchenbaum-Cymbalista F. Prognostic significance of the cell cycle inhibitor p27Kip1 in chronic B-cell lymphocytic leukemia. *Blood* 1998; 91:4694–700.

7 Hallek M, Langenmayer I, Nerl C, *et al.* Elevated serum thymidine kinase levels identify a subgroup at high risk of disease progression in early, nonsmoldering chronic lymphocytic leukemia. *Blood* 1999;93:1732–7.

8 Dohner H, Stilgenbauer S, Benner A, *et al.* Genomic aberrations and survival in chronic lymphocytic leukemia. *N Engl J Med* 2000;343:1910–16.

9 Stilgenbauer S, Bullinger L, Lichter P, Dohner H. Genetics of chronic lymphocytic leukemia: genomic aberrations and V(H) gene mutation status in pathogenesis and clinical course. *Leukemia* 2002;16:993–1007.

10 Damle RN, Wasil T, Fais F, *et al.* Ig V gene mutation status and CD38 expression as novel prognostic indicators in chronic lymphocytic leukemia. *Blood* 1999;94:1840–7.

11 Hamblin TJ, Davis Z, Gardiner A, Oscier DG, Stevenson FK. Unmutated Ig V(H) genes are associated with a more aggressive form of chronic lymphocytic leukemia. *Blood* 1999;94: 1848–54.

12 Del Poeta G, Maurillo L, Venditti A, *et al.* Clinical significance of CD38 expression in chronic lymphocytic leukemia. *Blood* 2001;98:2633–9.

13 Ibrahim S, Keating M, Do KA, *et al.* CD38 expression as an important prognostic factor in B-cell chronic lymphocytic leukemia. *Blood* 2001;98:181–6.

14 Oscier DG, Gardiner AC, Mould SJ, *et al.* Multivariate analysis of prognostic factors in CLL: clinical stage, IGVH gene mutational status, and loss or mutation of the p53 gene are independent prognostic factors. *Blood* 2002;100:1177–84.

15 Crespo M, Bosch F, Villamor N, Bellosillo B, *et al.* ZAP-70 expression as a surrogate for immunoglobulin-variable-region mutations in chronic lymphocytic leukemia. *N Engl J Med* 2003; 348:1764–75.

16 Rassenti LZ, Huynh L, Toy TL, *et al.* ZAP-70 compared with immunoglobulin heavy-chain gene mutation status as a predictor of disease progression in chronic lymphocytic leukemia. *N Engl J Med* 2004;351:893–901.

17 Orchard JA, Ibbotson RE, Davis Z, *et al.* ZAP-70 expression and prognosis in chronic lymphocytic leukemia. *Lancet* 2004;363: 105–11.

18 Johnson S, Smith AG, Loffler H, *et al.* Multicentre prospective randomised trial of fludarabine versus cyclophosphamide, doxorubicin, and prednisone (CAP) for treatment of advanced-stage chronic lymphocytic leukaemia. The French Cooperative Group on CLL. *Lancet* 1996;347:1432–8.

19 Rai KR, Peterson BL, Appelbaum FR, *et al.* Fludarabine compared with chlorambucil as primary therapy for chronic lymphocytic leukemia. *N Engl J Med* 2000;343:1750–7.

20 Leporrier M, Chevret S, Cazin B, *et al.* Randomized comparison of fludarabine, CAP, and ChOP in 938 previously untreated stage B and C chronic lymphocytic leukemia patients. *Blood* 2001;98:2319–25.
21 Eichhorst BF, Busch R, Hopfinger G, *et al.* Fludarabine plus cyclophosphamide versus fludarabine alone in first-line therapy of younger patients with chronic lymphocytic leukemia. *Blood* 2006;107:885–91.
22 Grever MR, Lucas DM, Dewald GW, *et al.* Comprehensive assessment of genetic and molecular features predicting outcome in patients with chronic lymphocytic leukemia: results from the US Intergroup Phase III Trial E2997. *J Clin Oncol* 2007;25:799–804.
23 Byrd JC, Rai K, Peterson BL, *et al.* Addition of rituximab to fludarabine may prolong progression-free survival and overall survival in patients with previously untreated chronic lymphocytic leukemia: an updated retrospective comparative analysis of CALGB 9712 and CALGB 9011. *Blood* 2005;105: 49–53.
24 Keating MJ, O'Brien S, Albitar M, *et al.* Early results of a chemoimmunotherapy regimen of fludarabine, cyclophosphamide, and rituximab as initial therapy for chronic lymphocytic leukemia. *J Clin Oncol* 2005;23:4079–88.
25 Wierda W, O'Brien S, Wen S, *et al.* Chemoimmunotherapy with fludarabine, cyclophosphamide, and rituximab for relapsed and refractory chronic lymphocytic leukemia. *J Clin Oncol* 2005; 23:4070–8.
26 Dohner H, Fischer K, Bentz M, *et al.* p53 gene deletion predicts for poor survival and non-response to therapy with purine analogs in chronic B-cell leukemias. *Blood* 1995;85:1580–9.
27 Keating MJ, O'Brien S, Kontoyiannis D, *et al.* Results of first salvage therapy for patients refractory to a fludarabine regimen in chronic lymphocytic leukemia. *Leuk Lymphoma* 2002;43: 1755–62.
28 Keating MJ, Flinn I, Jain V, *et al.* Therapeutic role of alemtuzumab (Campath-1H) in patients who have failed fludarabine: results of a large international study. *Blood* 2002;99:3554–61.
29 Stilgenbauer S, Dohner H. Campath-1H-induced complete remission of chronic lymphocytic leukemia despite p53 gene mutation and resistance to chemotherapy. *N Engl J Med* 2002; 347:452–3.
30 Lozanski G, Heerema NA, Flinn IW, *et al.* Alemtuzumab is an effective therapy for chronic lymphocytic leukemia with p53 mutations and deletions. *Blood* 2004;103:3278–81.
31 Kennedy B, Rawstron A, Carter C, *et al.* Campath-1H and fludarabine in combination are highly active in refractory chronic lymphocytic leukemia. *Blood* 2002;99:2245–7.
32 Elter T, Borchmann P, Schulz H, *et al.* Fludarabine in combination with alemtuzumab is effective and feasible in patients with relapsed or refractory B-cell chronic lymphocytic leukemia: results of a phase II trial. *J Clin Oncol* 2005;23:7024–31.
33 Wendtner CM, Ritgen M, Schweighofer CD, *et al.* Consolidation with alemtuzumab in patients with chronic lymphocytic leukemia (CLL) in first remission–experience on safety and efficacy within a randomized multicenter phase III trial of the German CLL Study Group (GCLLSG). *Leukemia* 2004;18:1093–101.
34 Montillo M, Tedeschi A, Rossi V, *et al.* Successful CD34+ cell mobilization by intermediate-dose Ara-C in chronic lymphocytic leukemia patients treated with sequential fludarabine and Campath-1H. *Leukemia* 2004;18:57–62.
35 Montserrat E, Gomis F, Vallespi T, *et al.* Presenting features and prognosis of chronic lymphocytic leukemia in younger adults. *Blood* 1991;78:1545–51.
36 Dreger P, Stilgenbauer S, Benner A, *et al.* The prognostic impact of autologous stem cell transplantation in patients with chronic lymphocytic leukemia: a risk-matched analysis based on the VH gene mutational status. *Blood* 2004;103:2850–8.
37 Rabinowe SN, Soiffer RJ, Gribben JG, *et al.* Autologous and allogeneic bone marrow transplantation for poor prognosis patients with B-cell chronic lymphocytic leukemia. *Blood* 1993; 82:1366–76.
38 Khouri IF, Keating MJ, Vriesendorp HM, *et al.* Autologous and allogeneic bone marrow transplantation for chronic lymphocytic leukemia: preliminary results. *J Clin Oncol* 1994;12: 748–58.
39 Itala M, Pelliniemi TT, Rajamaki A, Remes K. Autologous blood cell transplantation in B-CLL: response to chemotherapy prior to mobilization predicts the stem cell yield. *Bone Marrow Transplant* 1997;19:647–51.
40 Dreger P, von Neuhoff N, Kuse R, *et al.* Early stem cell transplantation for chronic lymphocytic leukemia: a chance for cure? *Br J Cancer* 1998;77:2291–7.
41 Pavletic ZS, Bierman PJ, Vose JM, *et al.* High incidence of relapse after autologous stem-cell transplantation for B-cell chronic lymphocytic leukemia or small lymphocytic lymphoma. *Ann Oncol* 1998;9:1023–6.
42 Milligan DW, Fernandes S, Dasgupta R, *et al.* Results of the MRC pilot study show autografting for younger patients with chronic lymphocytic leukemia is safe and achieves a high percentage of molecular responses. *Blood* 2005;105:397–404.
43 Gribben JG, Zahrieh D, Stephans K, *et al.* Autologous and allogeneic stem cell transplantation for poor risk chronic lymphocytic leukemia. *Blood* 2005;106:4389–96.
44 Jantunen E, Itala M, Siitonen T, *et al.* Autologous stem cell transplantation in patients with chronic lymphocytic leukemia: the Finnish experience. *Bone Marrow Transplant* 2006; 37:1093–8.
45 Ritgen M, Lange A, Stilgenbauer S, *et al.* Unmutated immunoglobulin variable heavy-chain gene status remains an adverse prognostic factor after autologous stem cell transplantation for chronic lymphocytic leukemia. *Blood* 2003;101: 2049–53.
46 Ritgen M, Stilgenbauer S, von Neuhoff N, *et al.* Graft-versus-leukemia activity may overcome therapeutic resistance of chronic lymphocytic leukemia with unmutated immunoglobulin variable heavy-chain gene status: implications of minimal residual disease measurement with quantitative PCR. *Blood* 2004;104:2600–2.
47 Moreno C, Villamor N, Colomer D, *et al.* Allogeneic stem-cell transplantation may overcome the adverse prognosis of unmutated VH gene in patients with chronic lymphocytic leukemia. *J Clin Oncol* 2005;23:3433–8.
48 Sala R, Mauro FR, Bellucci R, *et al.* Evaluation of marrow and blood haemopoietic progenitors in chronic lymphocytic leukemia before and after chemotherapy. *Eur J Haematol* 1998;61: 14–20.
49 Michallet M, Thiebaut A, Dreger P, *et al.* Peripheral blood stem cell (PBSC) mobilization and transplantation after fludarabine therapy in chronic lymphocytic leukemia (CLL): a report of the European Blood and Marrow Transplantation (EBMT) CLL

subcommittee on behalf of the EBMT Chronic Leukaemias Working Party (CLWP). *Br J Haematol* 2000;108:595–601.

50 Dreger P, Montserrat E. Autologous and allogeneic stem cell transplantation for chronic lymphocytic leukemia. *Leukemia* 2002;16:985–92.

51 Rawstron AC, Kennedy B, Evans PA, *et al.* Quantitation of minimal disease levels in chronic lymphocytic leukemia using a sensitive flow cytometric assay improves the prediction of outcome and can be used to optimize therapy. *Blood* 2001; 98:29–35.

52 Provan D, Bartlett-Pandite L, Zwicky C, *et al.* Eradication of polymerase chain reaction-detectable chronic lymphocytic leukemia cells is associated with improved outcome after bone marrow transplantation. *Blood* 1996;88:2228–35.

53 Schey S, Ahsan G, Jones R. Dose intensification and molecular responses in patients with chronic lymphocytic leukemia: a phase II single centre study. *Bone Marrow Transplant* 1999;24: 989–93.

54 Schultze JL, Donovan JW, Gribben JG. Minimal residual disease detection after myeloablative chemotherapy in chronic lymphatic leukemia. *J Mol Med* 1999;77:259–65.

55 Zenz T, Ritgen M, Dreger P, *et al.* Autologous graft-versus-host disease-like syndrome after an alemtuzumab-containing conditioning regimen and autologous stem cell transplantation for chronic lymphocytic leukemia. *Blood* 2006;108:2127–30.

56 Montillo M, Tedeschi A, Miqueleiz S, *et al.* Alemtuzumab as consolidation after a response to fludarabine is effective in purging residual disease in patients with chronic lymphocytic leukemia. *J Clin Oncol* 2006;24:2337–42.

57 Michallet M, Corront B, Hollard D, Gratwohl A, Domingo A, Burnett S. Allogeneic bone marrow transplantation in chronic lymphocytic leukemia: report from the European Cooperative Group for bone marrow transplantation (8 cases). *Nouv Rev Fr Hematol* 1988;30:467–70.

58 Michallet M, Archimbaud E, Bandini G, *et al.* HLA-identical sibling bone marrow transplantation in younger patients with chronic lymphocytic leukemia. European Group for Blood and Marrow Transplantation and the International Bone Marrow Transplant Registry. *Ann Internal Med* 1996;124:311–15.

59 Khouri I, Champlin R. Allogenic bone marrow transplantation in chronic lymphocytic leukemia. *Ann Intern Med* 1996;125: 780–7.

60 Pavletic ZS, Arrowsmith ER, Bierman PJ, *et al.* Outcome of allogeneic stem cell transplantation for B cell chronic lymphocytic leukemia. *Bone Marrow Transplant* 2000;25:717–22.

61 Doney KC, Chauncey T, Appelbaum FR. Allogeneic related donor hematopoietic stem cell transplantation for treatment of chronic lymphocytic leukemia. *Bone Marrow Transplant* 2002;29: 817–23.

62 Toze CL, Galal A, Barnett MJ, *et al.* Myeloablative allografting for chronic lymphocytic leukemia: evidence for a potent graft-versus-leukemia effect associated with graft-versus-host disease. *Bone Marrow Transplant* 2005;36:825–30.

63 Rondon G, Giralt S, Huh Y, *et al.* Graft-versus-leukemia effect after allogeneic bone marrow transplantation for chronic lymphocytic leukemia. *Bone Marrow Transplant* 1996;18:669–72.

64 de Magalhaes-Silverman M, Donnenberg A, Hammert L, *et al.* Induction of graft-versus-leukemia effect in a patient with chronic lymphocytic leukemia. *Bone Marrow Transplant* 1997;20: 175–7.

65 Pavletic SZ, Khouri IF, Haagenson M, *et al.* Unrelated donor marrow transplantation for B-cell chronic lymphocytic leukemia after using myeloablative conditioning: results from the Center for International Blood and Marrow Transplant research. *J Clin Oncol* 2005;23:5788–94.

66 Horowitz M, Montserrat, E, Sobocinski, K, Giralt, S, Khouri, IF, Schmitz, N. Haemopoietic stem cell transplantation for chronic lymphocytic leukemia. *Blood* 2000;96(Suppl.1): Abstract 2245.

67 Khouri IF, Przepiorka D, van Besien K, *et al.* Allogeneic blood or marrow transplantation for chronic lymphocytic leukemia: timing of transplantation and potential effect of fludarabine on acute graft-versus-host disease. *Br J Haematol* 1997;97:466–73.

68 Schetelig J, Thiede C, Bornhauser M, *et al.* Reduced non-relapse mortality after reduced intensity conditioning in advanced chronic lymphocytic leukemia. *Ann Hematol* 2002;81(Suppl .2): S47–8.

69 Schetelig J, Thiede C, Bornhauser M, *et al.* Evidence of a graft-versus-leukemia effect in chronic lymphocytic leukemia after reduced-intensity conditioning and allogeneic stem-cell transplantation: the Cooperative German Transplant Study Group. *J Clin Oncol* 2003;21:2747–53.

70 Khouri IF, Keating M, Korbling M, *et al.* Transplant-lite: induction of graft-versus-malignancy using fludarabine-based nonablative chemotherapy and allogeneic blood progenitor-cell transplantation as treatment for lymphoid malignancies. *J Clin Oncol* 1998;16:2817–24.

71 Khouri IF, Saliba RM, Giralt SA, *et al.* Nonablative allogeneic hematopoietic transplantation as adoptive immunotherapy for indolent lymphoma: low incidence of toxicity, acute graft-versus-host disease, and treatment-related mortality. *Blood* 2001;98:3595–9.

72 Dreger P, Brand R, Hansz J, *et al.* Treatment-related mortality and graft-versus-leukemia activity after allogeneic stem cell transplantation for chronic lymphocytic leukemia using intensity-reduced conditioning. *Leukemia* 2003;17:841–8.

73 Sorror ML, Maris MB, Sandmaier BM, *et al.* Hematopoietic cell transplantation after nonmyeloablative conditioning for advanced chronic lymphocytic leukemia. *J Clin Oncol* 2005;23: 3819–29.

74 Brown JR, Kim HT, Li S, *et al.* Predictors of improved progression-free survival after nonmyeloablative allogeneic stem cell transplantation for advanced chronic lymphocytic leukemia. *Biol Blood Marrow Transplant* 2006;12:1056–64.

75 Sorror ML, Storer BE, Sandmaier BM, *et al.* Five-year follow-up of patients with advanced chronic lymphocytic leukemia treated with allogeneic hematopoietic cell transplantation after nonmyeloablative conditioning. *J Clin Oncol* 2008;26: 4912–20.

76 Dreger P, Brand R, Milligan D, *et al.* Reduced-intensity conditioning lowers treatment-related mortality of allogeneic stem cell transplantation for chronic lymphocytic leukemia: a population-matched analysis. *Leukemia* 2005;19:1029–33.

77 Hertzberg M, Grigg A, Gottlieb D, *et al.* Reduced-intensity allogeneic haemopoietic stem cell transplantation induces durable responses in patients with chronic B-lymphoproliferative disorders. *Bone Marrow Transplant* 2006;37:923–8.

78 Morris E, Thomson K, Craddock C, *et al.* Outcomes after alemtuzumab-containing reduced-intensity allogeneic transplantation regimen for relapsed and refractory non-Hodgkin lymphoma. *Blood* 2004;104:3865–71.

79 Delgado J, Thomson K, Russell N, *et al.* Results of alemtuzumab-based reduced-intensity allogeneic transplantation for chronic lymphocytic leukemia: a British Society of Blood and Marrow Transplantation Study. *Blood* 2006;107:1724–30.
80 Caballero D, Garcia-Marco JA, Martino R, *et al.* Allogeneic transplant with reduced intensity conditioning regimens may overcome the poor prognosis of B-cell chronic lymphocytic leukemia with unmutated immunoglobulin variable heavy-chain gene and chromosomal abnormalities (11q- and 17p-). *Clin Cancer Res* 2005;11:7757–63.
81 Dreger P, Corradini P, Kimby E, *et al.* Indications for allogeneic stem cell transplantation in chronic lymphocytic leukemia: the EBMT transplant consensus. *Leukemia* 2007;21:12–17.
82 Sutton L, Maloum K, Gonzalez H, *et al.* Autologous hematopoietic stem cell transplantation as salvage treatment for advanced B cell chronic lymphocytic leukemia. *Leukemia* 1998;12:1699–707.
83 Khouri IF. Reduced-intensity regimens in allogeneic stem-cell transplantation for non-Hodgkin lymphoma and chronic lymphocytic leukemia. *Hematology Am Soc Hematol Educ Program* 2006:390–7.

Chapter 27
Special Situations: Management of Elderly Patients and Chronic Lymphocytic Leukemia in Transformation

Wei-Gang Tong and Alessandra Ferrajoli
University of Texas M. D. Anderson Cancer Center, Houston, Texas, USA

Management of chronic lymphocytic leukemia in transformation

Introduction

Richter syndrome (RS, also known as Richter transformation) is named after Dr. Maurice Richter, who first identified the syndrome in 1928 in a patient with chronic lymphocytic leukemia (CLL) in whom fatal generalized lymphadenopathy and hepatosplenomegaly developed rapidly [1]. RS is defined as the clinicopathologic transformation of CLL to an aggressive high-grade lymphoproliferative disease. The most commonly encountered histology in patients with RS is diffuse large B-cell lymphoma (DLBCL) [1], which accounts for about 65–70% of RS cases. Other, less common, histologies include Hodgkin disease (15%) [2], prolymphocytic leukemia (15–20%) [3], acute lymphoblastic leukemia (ALL) (<1%) [4], hairy cell leukemia [5], and aggressive T-cell lymphoma [6]. RS is a rare complication of CLL, occurring in about 2–9% of cases. A study found that the 20-year actuarial risk of RS in patients with CLL was about 20% [7,8]. Another study of a series of 185 consecutive previously untreated patients with CLL showed that the median time from diagnosis of CLL to development of RS was about 23 months [9,10]. The clinical outcome in patients with RS is dismal and is characterized by a short overall survival (OS) duration after diagnosis, ranging from 5 to 8 months even with aggressive chemotherapy [11–13].

Biology of Richter syndrome

The large cells in patients with RS may either arise through transformation of the original CLL clones or represent a new neoplasm. Researchers have yet to establish any risk factors for RS in patients with CLL. However, studies have shown that clonal evolution of CLL cells may be triggered by viral infections, which are common in patients with CLL because of their immunosuppression [14,15]. Several prognostic factors in patients with CLL have been associated with an increased risk of transformation. One study found that an advanced Rai stage, hemoglobin level <12 g/dL, elevated lactate dehydrogenase (LDH) level, and elevated beta-2 microglobulin (β2–MG) levels were associated with increased risk of transformation. In addition, a multivariate analysis identified lymph node size >3 cm (hazard ratio = 6.5; $P = 0.001$) and absence of del(13q14) (hazard ratio = 9.07; $P < 0.001$) as independent prognostic factors for RS [9]. Furthermore, acquisition of new cytogenetic abnormalities and genetic mutations is also associated with progression and transformation of CLL. Mutations of various tumor-suppressor and cell cycle-regulatory genes appear to be associated with RS, and *p53* gene mutations were found in about 60% of patients with RS [16]. Studies have implicated mutation of the DNA repair gene $p21^{WAF1}$ in RS, and mutations of $p21^{WAF1}$ and *p53* coexisted more frequently in patients with RS than in those with CLL. Other investigators have detected abnormalities of the other cell cycle-regulatory genes, such as mutations of $p16^{INK4A}$, loss of *p27* expression, and deletion of the retinoblastoma gene in patients with RS [17–19], but none of these genetic changes appears to be a predominant factor responsible for transformation. It is likely that these genetic changes may cause CLL cells to proliferate and consequently facilitate the acquisition of new genetic abnormalities, which leads to their transformation to RS cells.

Clinical features and diagnosis of Richter syndrome

Patients with RS typically present with a history of CLL/small lymphocytic lymphoma (SLL) and sudden clinical deterioration. They usually report worsening of systemic symptoms (such as fever, night sweats, and weight loss), rapid enlargement of lymph nodes or increased splenomegaly and/or hepatomegaly, and elevated LDH levels [20,21]. Patients with RS may also occasionally present

Leukemias: Principles and Practice of Therapy, 1st edition. Edited by S. Faderl and H. Kantarjian.

with extranodal disease involving the central nervous system (CNS), gastrointestinal tract, eyes, skin, or testes. In a report on a series of 3986 patients with CLL/SLL from 1975 to 2005, Tsimberidou *et al.* [22] found biopsy- or fine-needle aspiration-proven RS in 148 patients (3.7%). Clinical features associated with RS in this study included elevated serum LDH levels (82%), progressive lymphadenopathy (64%), worsening systemic symptoms (59%), presence of a monoclonal gammopathy (44%), and extranodal involvement (41%). Diagnosis of RS is best established by biopsy of enlarged lymph nodes or other involved extranodal sites [23], and the histologic diagnosis will further specify the histologic subtype. Imaging studies such as positron emission tomography (PET) and CT are increasingly used for diagnosis and staging of RS, and imaging results often correlate with the histologic findings of bone marrow or lymph node biopsy. Overall, PET/CT has exhibited a sensitivity of 91% and specificity of 80% for specific diagnosis of RS in patients with CLL [24].

Treatment of Richter syndrome

Although there have been numerous published studies on treatments for RS, a consensus on the best therapeutic approach for this disease is still lacking. The most commonly used approach includes chemotherapeutic regimens originally designed for *de novo* DLBCL or ALL. The response rates for these aggressive therapies ranges from 5% to 43%, with complete response (CR) rates ranging from 5% to 38% and median survival durations of only 5–8 months [11–13,22]. Chemoimmunotherapy (CIT) with monoclonal antibodies followed by allogeneic stem cell transplantation (allo-SCT) as postremission therapy has been an effective treatment strategy.

Tsimberidou *et al.* [13] reported on a phase II study with the combination of fludarabine, cytarabine, cyclophosphamide, cisplatin, and granulocyte macrophage colony-stimulating factor (GM-CSF) in patients with RS. This regimen induced CR in only 1 of 16 (6%) patients, and had significant toxic effects. The same group has also studied the efficacy and tolerability of radioimmunotherapy in patients with RS. Specifically, they evaluated yttrium-90-labeled ibritumomab tiuxetan (Zevalin), a radiolabeled monoclonal antibody that selectively targets radiation to $CD20^+$ B cells. In a trial of seven patients with RS no responses occurred, and all of the patients experienced disease progression. This approach was associated with severe hematologic toxic effects consisting of prolonged grade 3–4 thrombocytopenia and neutropenia [25].

In a phase I–II study of 20 patients with RS, combination therapy with oxaliplatin, fludarabine, cytarabine, and rituximab (OFAR) resulted in an overall response (OR) rate of 50% [26]. This regimen was well tolerated, as hematologic toxic effects occurred but were not prolonged. Interestingly, this regimen was also well tolerated and effective in elderly patients with RS, with an OR rate of 50% in 14 patients >70 years old.

Dabaja *et al.* [12] investigated the combination of fractionated cyclophosphamide, vincristine, liposomal daunorubicin, and dexamethasone (hyper-CVXD) in patients with RS. The median number of cycles the patients received was three (range 1–8). Six patients (20%) died during treatment, with a CR rate of 38% and OR rate of 41%. The median survival duration was 10 months overall, 19 months in patients who achieved a CR and only 3 months in patients who did not have a CR ($P = 0.0008$). Tsimberidou *et al.* [11] subsequently reported the results with the administration of hyper-CVXD plus rituximab with GM-CSF support alternating with methotrexate and cytarabine plus rituximab with GM-CSF support to 30 patients with RS. Use of this regimen resulted in CR in 18% and partial response (PR) in 22% of the patients, with an OR rate of 41%. The 12-month failure-free survival rate was 27%, and the OS rate was 39% after a median follow-up duration of 7.5 months and maximum follow-up duration of 15.2 months.

Rodriguez *et al.* [27] evaluated the use of high-dose chemotherapy followed by allo-SCT in eight patients with RS who had received a median of four previous treatments. The median interval from the initial diagnosis of CLL/SLL to transformation was 48 months. Six patients received transplants from matched sibling donors, and two patients who had previously undergone autologous SCT received transplants from matched-unrelated donors. The 30-day mortality rate was 38%; five patients died from transplant-related toxic effects. The three surviving patients were in remission at 14, 47, and 67 months, respectively. These data suggest that even in heavily treated patients with RS, long-term survival can be achieved in a proportion of patients who undergo stem-cell transplantion.

In the same large retrospective review of 3986 patients with CLL/SLL who presented to the University of Texas M. D. Anderson Cancer Center from 1975 to 2005 described above, 204 patients (5.1%) had possible RS based on their clinical features, and 148 patients (3.7%) had biopsy or fine-needle aspiration-proven RS [22]. Treatment included chemotherapy alone or CIT with rituximab. The chemotherapy regimens included hyper-CVXD with or without rituximab; cyclophosphamide, doxorubicin, vincristine, and prednisone (CHOP) with or without rituximab; etoposide, methylprednisolone, high-dose cytarabine, and cisplatin (ESHAP); mesna, ifosfamide, mitoxantrone, and etoposide (MINE); and fludarabine, cyclophosphamide, and rituximab (FCR). The OR rate in 130 assessable patients was 39%, and the investigators found no difference in OR rate between the patients who received treatment with and without rituximab ($P = 0.2$). In a multivariate analysis, factors predicting longer survival durations were Zubrod performance statuses of 0–1 ($P = 0.006$), LDH levels no more than 1.5 times the upper limit of normal ($P = 0.003$), platelet counts of at least 100,000/μL ($P = 0.01$), tumor size of no more than 5 cm ($P = 0.02$), and fewer than two prior therapies ($P = 0.02$). Twenty of these patients underwent SCT. Patients who underwent allo-SCT as postremission therapy had longer survival durations than patients who experienced remission but received no additional therapy and patients who underwent allo-SCT or autologous SCT as salvage therapy ($P = 0.019$).

In rare cases, patients with CLL/SLL may experience transformation to a Hodgkin disease variant. In a retrospective analysis of 1011 patients with CLL, the researchers found classic RS in 1.8% of cases and a Hodgkin disease variant in 0.4% [28]. Patients with a Hodgkin disease variant generally present with a more advanced stage of disease and have a worse prognosis compared with patients with true Hodgkin disease [29]. Data on the optimal treatment in such patients are limited, although they usually respond to the standard therapies for Hodgkin disease such as doxorubicin, bleomycin, vinblastine, and dacarbazine (ABVD), or mechlorethamine, vincristine, procarbazine, and prednisone (MOPP), with and without radiotherapy [29–31].

Patients with RS who present with CNS involvement usually also have disseminated disease; the treatments in these patients often include systemic or intrathecal chemotherapy or radiation therapy. The role of radiation therapy is usually palliative, although it has a role in controlling compression syndromes that arise from bulky disease. Prophylactic intrathecal therapy and radiotherapy may be useful in some patients who are at high risk for involvement of the CNS, such as those with involvement of more than one extranodal site and increased LDH levels [32,33].

Conclusions

For patients with CLL or SLL, RS is a rare complication that usually has a poor prognosis. More studies are needed to identify prognostic factors that can predict risk of transformation, and may allow intervention at a time when patients still have chemosensitive disease. Recent development of specific therapeutic strategies for RS have shown promise, as improvements are likely to emerge with increased understanding of the biology of the disease and from intensive treatment. Patients with RS who have high-risk features should be offered participation in investigational studies evaluating new agents or combination regimens. Myeloablative or non-myeloablative allo-SCT may offer benefits and prolong survival in some patients [34,35], and should be considered as postremission therapy in young patients with good performance statuses and available donors.

Management of chronic lymphocytic leukemia in elderly patients

Introduction

About 3–5/100,000 individuals annually are affected by CLL, making it one of the most common hematologic malignancies. With a median age at diagnosis of 72 years, the incidence of CLL is dramatically increased in patients >65 years old to 22–30/100,000 per year [36–38]. Despite its high incidence and the size of the patient population, elderly patients with CLL are under-represented in most clinical trials. The median ages of patients enrolled in large clinical trials evaluating various front-line treatments ranges from 58 years to 66 years [39–41]. Also, elderly patients with CLL often present with advanced-stage disease and relevant comorbidities or other malignancies that often limit their therapeutic options and treatment tolerability [42–46]. This further limits the eligibility of elderly patients with relapsed disease or those who have responded after receiving standard treatment regimens for clinical trials evaluating novel agents, as most of these types of clinical studies have traditionally required patients to have good performance statuses and normal organ function [47–49].

Epidemiology of chronic lymphocytic leukemia in the elderly

Several published studies have evaluated the incidence and age distribution of patients with newly diagnosed CLL in the general population as well as in patients referred to large tertiary treatment centers [50,51]. In particular, Wierda *et al.* [52] reported on a series of 2216 consecutive patients with CLL/SLL who presented to the M. D. Anderson Cancer Center between 1985 and 2005. In this series, 30% of the patients were 60–69 years old and 16% were >70 years old. The 5-year survival rate was significantly decreased with increasing age from 86% in patients <60 years to 74% in patients 60–69 years old and only 59% in patients >70 years old. Another large study from the Mayo Clinic reported by Thurmes *et al.* [42] reviewed 1195 patients with newly diagnosed CLL between 1995 and 2006. The median age of this group of patients was 68 years; two-thirds of the patients were >60 years old, and one-quarter were >75 years old. One or more comorbidities were present in 89% of the patients at the time of the CLL diagnosis, and 46% patients had at least one major comorbidity. Advanced Rai stage ($P < 0.0001$) and age (1.056/year increase; $P < 0.0001$) were the only factors associated with OS in multivariate analysis. Data from the National Cancer Institute's Surveillance Epidemiology and End Results (SEER) program referring to the 1995–2005 years showed that 70% of all patients with CLL in the US population were >65 years old, 43% were >75 years old, and 13% were >85 years old [53].

Prognostic factors in elderly patients with chronic lymphocytic leukemia

Studies have shown that CLL is clearly a heterogeneous disease, not only at the clinical level, but also at the molecular and cellular levels. Rai [54] and Binet [55] staging, the clinical staging systems that were introduced almost three decades ago, have been effective in classifying patients into different risk categories. These systems have provided a foundation on which clinicians build their management and therapeutic decisions. However, these systems have limitations in accurately predicting the course of the disease and do not take into account new discoveries regarding the molecular and cytogenetic features of the disease.

Over the past decade, researchers have developed several novel prognostic factors for patients with CLL, but their prognostic significance for elderly patients has not been studied. In the landmark study by Dohner *et al.* [56], reported a decade ago, genomic aberrations were independent predictors of disease progression and survival in patients with CLL. The chromosomal abnormalities associated with poor prognosis for CLL include 17p deletion ($P < 0.001$) and 11q deletion ($P = 0.004$). Other established prognostic factors for CLL, including the *IgVH* mutational status [57,58]; level of ZAP-70 [59,60] and CD38 [61,62] expression; and cytogenetic abnormalities such as 17p deletion, 13q deletion and trisomy 12 have not been shown to be associated with patient age [56,63]. In the case of 11q deletion, it appears to be associated with age in a statistically significant manner ($P = 0.02$) as the negative prognostic impact of 11q deletion diminishes in patients >55 years old. In a review of 1577 patients with CLL who presented to the M. D. Anderson Cancer Center from 1970 to 2000, 48% were >60 years old, and 17% were >70 years old (unpublished data). In this population, elderly patients (defined as age ≥70 years) presented with more significant anemia, higher β2–MG, worse performance statuses, and more advanced Rai stages than younger patients. Multivariate analysis showed that age, albumin level, total white blood cell count, and performance status were significantly associated with inferior OS in these patients.

Several large retrospective and prospective analyses have shown that comorbidities have significant prognostic value in elderly patients with CLL [42,46]. Thurmes *et al.* [42] evaluated the comorbidities in 1195 patients with newly diagnosed CLL with a median age of 68 years. At the time of CLL diagnosis, the patients had a median of two comorbidities and took a median of two prescription medications daily. Of these patients, 14% had a second malignancy diagnosed prior to or simultaneously with CLL. The presence of one or more major comorbidities at the time of diagnosis was associated with reduced OS durations ($P = 0.04$) in univariate analysis, although the survival curves did not separate until approximately 6 years after diagnosis. Shanafelt *et al.* [46] conducted an international survey of 1482 patients with CLL to assess their quality of life. About half of the patients were >60 years old, and 72% had at least one comorbid health condition; the number of comorbidities increased with more advanced age. Advanced age and the extent of comorbidities have been associated with poor overall quality of life in both univariate and multivariate analyses. Wierda *et al.* [51] identified age, β2–MG, absolute lymphocyte count, sex, Rai stage, and number of involved lymph node groups as independent prognostic factors for survival. They constructed a weighted prognostic model, or normogram, predictive of 5- and 10-year survival probability and estimated the median survival duration using these six characteristics. This prognostic model may help researchers and clinicians with clinical decision-making as well as clinical research and clinical trial design for CLL.

Treatment strategies for elderly patients with chronic lymphocytic leukemia

Although the development of front-line treatment regimens and novel agents for CLL has improved significantly over the past decade, few data on the efficacy and tolerability of these regimens in elderly patients or those with significant comorbidities have been published (Table 27.1). For elderly patients with good performance statuses, no major comorbidities, and relatively long life expectancies, the goal of treatment should be CR and prolonged survival. For elderly patients with poor performance statuses and significant comorbidities, the goal is to improve quality of life via supportive care or use of low-intensity chemotherapeutic regimens and prevent complications or mortality associated with the treatment.

Alkylating agent- and purine analog-based chemotherapeutic regimens

Chlorambucil is often used as the first-line treatment of CLL in elderly patients and those with comorbid conditions for many years, but no data are available on the various doses and schedules of this agent and their tolerance and efficacy in older patients.

The introduction of purine analogs such as fludarabine in the treatment of CLL has improved the CR and OR rates beyond those seen with alkylating agents, such as chlorambucil and cyclophosphamide [64,65]. Clinical studies of fludarabine have shown improved CR, OR, and progression-free survival (PFS) rates, but no improvement in OS in patients with CLL [65]. Recent data from several phase II clinical trials in which fludarabine was combined with cyclophosphamide and/or rituximab demonstrated high response rates and long PFS durations, but not OS [66,67]. For patients with advanced-stage CLL requiring treatment, treatment selection is largely based on age, performance status, and presence of comorbid conditions, and the treatment consists of either

Table 27.1 Summary of published studies on elderly patients with chronic lymphocytic leukemia.

Reference	Regimen	Indication	Number	Age (years)	Responses	Survival and response durations	Adverse events
Shvidel *et al.* [48]	F, FC, and FCM	Salvage	32	>65	OR rate, 59%; no CRs, 3 nPRs, 16 PRs	Median time to progression, 7 months; median survival duration, <30 months	8 patients with neutropenic fever, 14 patients with severe infection; only 10 patients (31%) completed treatment
Forconi *et al.* [70]	Oral FC	Front-line/ salvage	26	>65	OR rate, 92%; CR rate, 46%	Median EFS duration, 48 months	8 patients with myelosuppression
Eichhorst *et al.* [69]	F versus Ch	Front-line	206	>64	F: OR rate, 86% (7% CR rate); Ch: OR rate, 59% (no CRs)	F: PFS duration, 18.7 months; OS duration, 45.9 months; Ch: PFS duration, 17.8 months; OS duration, 63.3 months	Minimal toxicity reported
Keating *et al.* [49]	FCR	Front-line	30	>70	OR rate, 87%; CR rate, 47%	Median survival duration, 48 months	50% G3–4 myelosuppression, 10% G3–4 infection; 40% completed 6 cycles
Wierda *et al.* [41]	FCR	Salvage	39	>70	OR rate, 69% (18% CR, 10% nPR, and 41% PR rate); 8% early deaths	Median survival duration, 24 months	50% G3–4 myelosuppression, 25% G3–4 infection; 20% completed 6 cycles
Shanafelt *et al.* [81]	PCR	Front-line	18	>70	OR rate, 83%; CR rate, 39%; no difference in patients <70 years old	EFS duration, 30 months; no difference in patients <70 years old	61% G3–4 myelosuppression, 22% non-hematologic toxicity; 78% completed 6 cycles
Ferrajoli *et al.* [74]	R plus GM-CSF	Front-line/ salvage	48	>70	OR rate, 56% (68% front-line, 31% salvage)	Median response duration, 18+ months	No G3–4 infection, 28% G1 injection site reactions with GM-CSF
Keating *et al.* [75]	Alemtuzumab	Salvage	26	>70	OR rate, 31% (1 CR, 7 PRs)	Median time to progression, 9.5 months; median OS, 32 months for responders	81% infusion-related toxic effects, 55% infection; 7 reactivation of CMV
Pitini *et al.* [77]	Alemtuzumab	Front-line	48	74[a]	CR rate, 7%; PR rate, 33%	PFS duration, 12 months; OS duration, 30 months for responders	Four patients with reactivation of CMV, 4 patients with G3 anemia, 19 patients with G3–4 neutropenia
Hillmen *et al.* [76]	Alemtuzumab versus Ch	Front-line	53	>65	OR rate, 76% for alemtuzumab versus 56% for Ch	Median PFS duration, 12.5 months	15% G3–4 infusion-related toxic effects, 15.6% symptomatic CMV infection
Ferrajoli *et al.* [84]	Lenalidomide	Front-line	43	>65	OR rate, 54%; SD 40%	N/A	26% G3–4 myelosuppression, 44% tumor flare reactions; 2 patients discontinued owing to toxic effects

[a]Median age.

Ch, chlorambucil; CMV, cytomegalovirus; CR, complete remission; EFS, event-free survival; F, fludarabine; FC, fludarabine plus cyclophosphamide; FCM, fludarabine, cyclophosphamide, and mitoxantone; FCR, fludarabine, cyclophosphamide, and rituximab; G, grade; GM-CSF, granulocyte macrophage colony-stimulating factor; N/A, not available; nPR, nodular partial response; OR, overall response; PCR, pentostatin, cyclophosphamide, and rituximab; PR, partial remission; R, rituximab; SD, stable disease;.

chlorambucil-based monotherapy or fludarabine-based combination regimens. Fludarabine-based regimens are feasible in young patients who can tolerate chemotherapy, but elderly patients and those who have comorbid conditions do not tolerate these regimens well and thus often receive chlorambucil [68].

Whereas fludarabine and fludarabine-based combination regimens can be delivered safely to elderly patients who have good performance statuses with modestly increased myelosuppression and no increases in severe infectious complications or treatment-related mortality, elderly patients with poor performance statuses may have higher incidences of opportunistic infections.

Researchers in the German CLL Study Group reported that elderly patients with CLL did not have a significant clinical benefit of first-line therapy with fludarabine over that with chlorambucil [69]. In this study, 206 elderly patients (>64 years) with CLL were randomly allocated to receive six courses of fludarabine or chlorambucil for up to 12 months. The OR rate in the fludarabine group (86%) was higher than that in the chlorambucil group (59%), but the PFS durations were similar at 18.7 and 17.8 months, respectively. No survival advantage was seen with fludarabine group, the main reason for which appears to be poor response to salvage therapy after initial failure.

Shvidel *et al.* [48] reported on the results of fludarabine-based salvage chemotherapy in 32 previously treated patients >65 years old. The regimens used included fludarabine alone, fludarabine plus cyclophosphamide (FC), and fludarabine, cyclophosphamide, and mitoxantrone (FCM). The OR rate was 59% with no CR, three (9%) nodular PR (nPR), and 16 (50%) PRs. Only 10 patients (32%) completed the entire treatment program because of poor compliance due to toxicity. This small experience compared poorly with a younger group of patients treated with the same program. The authors highly recommended dose reduction of fludarabine and appropriate use of myeloid growth factors and prophylactic antibiotics in this group of patients.

Forconi *et al.* [70] studied the FC regimen given orally at reduced doses in 26 patients >65 years old (median age 71 years) in both the front-line and relapse setting who were thought to be unfit for conventional treatments. They received oral fludarabine at 25 mg/m^2 per day and oral cyclophosphamide at 120 mg/m^2 per day for four consecutive days every 4 weeks for a maximum of four cycles. Twenty-four patients (92%) had a response, with 12 (46%) having a CR. Non-hematologic toxicity was mild, and myelosuppression occurred in eight patients (31%). The median event-free survival (EFS) duration was 48 months with a median follow-up duration of 24 months. This experience appeared to be favorable in elderly patients who cannot benefit from more aggressive treatments, and was easy to administer on an outpatient basis.

Monoclonal antibodies and chemoimmunotherapy

Rituximab is a chimeric monoclonal anti-CD20 antibody that has shown remarkable activity in patients with non-Hodgkin lymphoma in both the front-line and relapse setting [71]. Studies have tested the use of single-agent rituximab in patients with previously untreated CLL, resulting in an OR rate of 58% and CR rate of 9% [72,73]. Ferrajoli *et al.* [74] designed a non-chemotherapeutic approach for CLL, administering rituximab plus GM-CSF as both front-line and salvage treatment in patients >70 years old. The rationale for this study was based on *in vitro* evidence that GM-CSF was able to upregulate CD20 expression in CLL cells. The treatment consisted of subcutaneous administration of GM-CSF at a dose of 250 µg on days 1 and 3 in a priming fashion and then three times a week over 8 weeks. Rituximab was administered at a standard dose (375 mg/m^2) intravenously on day 4 and then weekly over 4 weeks. Patients who had at least a 50% improvement in absolute lymphocyte count could undergo a second cycle according to this program. The OR rate was 68% (6% CR, 6% nPR, and 56% PR) in 32 untreated patients and 31% (6% CR, 6% nPR, and 19% PR) in 16 previously treated patients. The median response duration was 18 months or more. Despite the fact that the patients in this study did not receive routine antibiotic prophylaxis, no grade 3–4 infections were observed.

Alemtuzumab is a humanized monoclonal anti-CD52 antibody that has been investigated in both front-line and relapse treatment of patients with CLL. In one study of 93 heavily pretreated fludarabine-refractory patients with CLL with a median age of 66 years (range 31–86 years), treatment with alemtuzumab resulted in an OR rate of 33% and a CR rate of 2% in 26 patients >70 years old. The median time to progression was 9.5 months in responders, and the median OS duration was 16 months in all patients and 32 months in responders [75]. Toxic effects of alemtuzumab-based therapy included infusion-related toxicity (81%), transient cytopenia, and infections (55%), with reactivation of cytomegalovirus seen in seven patients. In another study comparing alemtuzumab with chlorambucil as initial therapy for CLL [76], an OR rate of 83% (24% CR) for alemtuzumab and 55% (2% CR) for chlorambucil was observed, and in patients >65 years old the OR rate was 76% for alemtuzumab and 56% for chlorambucil ($P = 0.04$) with similar PFS.

Subcutaneous alemtuzumab had been studied as first-line therapy in 48 elderly patients (median age 74 years) with deletion of 17p [74,77]. Alemtuzumab was given as a subcutaneous injection at 10 mg, three times a week for up to 18 weeks (a significantly lower dose than the more commonly used dose of 30 mg). Three patients (7%) achieved a CR and 16 (33%) a PR. The median PFS duration was 11.8 months in the responders, whereas the median OS duration was longer (30.0 months) in the responders than in the non-responders (12.5 months). The therapy was well tolerated except for some mild reactions at local injection sites. Four patients experienced transient reactivation of cytomegalovirus; they recovered without specific treatment. Also, four patients had grade 3 anemia, and 19 patients had grade 3–4 neutropenia. Therefore, the authors conclude that this regimen seems to be particularly effective and has a favorable toxicity profile in elderly patients with unfavorable cytogenetics.

Two independent studies investigated combination therapy with alemtuzumab and rituximab. In the first, Faderl *et al.* [78] administered rituximab to 32 patients at 375 mg/m^2 weekly for 4 weeks and alemtuzumab in a loading-dose schedule of 3, 10, and 30 mg on 3 consecutive days during week 1, followed by 30 mg on days 3 and 5 of weeks 2–4. Twenty patients (63%) had a response, with two (6%) patients having a CR. In the second study, Nabhan *et al.* [79] administered a similar regimen to 12 patients with CLL at a median age of 70 years (range 53–73 years) who had experienced failure of previous purine analog-based therapy. All 12 patients obtained normalization of peripheral blood lymphocytosis within a median of 23.5 days without any treatment-related mortality. Therefore, this combination also appeared to be safe, feasible, and active in elderly patients with refractory disease.

Various investigators have studied the chemoimmunotherapy combination FCR in untreated patients with CLL as well as patients with relapsed and refractory CLL [41,49,80]. Both univariate and multivariate analyses showed that the CR rate was significantly associated with a young age ($P < 0.05$) in patients who received this regimen. Of 224 patients receiving FCR as front-line therapy, only 30 (13%) were >70 years old [49]. Early discontinuation of therapy was commonly associated with advanced age (>65 years). The CR rates with this regimen were 80%, 68%, and 47% and the OR rates were 96%, 96%, and 87% in patients <55, 55–69, and >70 years old, respectively. Dose reductions were required in 35 patients, and the incidence was significantly higher in patients >60 years old and in patients with pretreatment Rai stage IV disease ($P = 0.01$). When FCR was given as salvage therapy in 39 patients >70 years old, the OR rate was 69% (18% CR, 10% nPR, and 41% PR), with three (8%) early deaths. Grade 3–4 myelosuppression occurred in 50% and grade 3–4 infections occurred in 25% of these patients. Only 40% of untreated and 20% of previously treated patients >70 years old were able to complete the intended six cycles of treatment, mainly because of prolonged mylosuppresion [41].

Shanafelt *et al.* [81] reported on the outcome of 18 patients aged ≥70 years among 64 patients with CLL treated with pentostatin, cyclophosphamide, and rituximab (PCR) regimen. Fourteen patients (78%) completed the intended six cycles of treatment. Although patients aged 70 and older were more likely to have their doses delayed during treatment, the incidences of grade 3–4 hematologic and non-hematologic toxicity and infectious complications did not differ from the entire group. No significant differences were observed in OR (83% vs. 93%; $P = 0.34$) or CR (39% vs. 41%; $P = 0.86$) in patients >70 years old and those <70 years old. This small experience suggested that PCR is an effective, well-tolerated regimen in elderly patients with CLL.

Novel therapeutic agents for chronic lymphocytic leukemia

Lenalidomide

Lenalidomide (Revlimid®) is a derivative of thalidomide shown to have immunomodulatory activity that has been used in the treatment of myelodysplastic syndrome and multiple myeloma. Based on the clinical efficacy of lenalidomide in patients with relapsed or refractory CLL [82,83], Ferrajoli *et al.* [84] designed a phase II study to evaluate its efficacy and tolerability as initial therapy for CLL in patients >65 years old. All of the patients received lenalidomide orally at a starting daily dose of 5 mg, which could be titrated up by 5-mg increments every 28 days to a maximum daily dose of 25 mg. Forty-three patients with a median age of 72 years (range 66–85 years) received treatment, 18 (42%) of whom with Rai stage III–IV disease have been reported so far in an early analysis. Thirty-five of the patients evaluable for response received treatment for at least 3 months: 19 patients (54%) had a PR, 14 patients (40%) had stable disease, and two patients (6%) had disease progression after 4 and 5 months, respectively. Treatment with lenalidomide rapidly reduced the number of circulating lymphocytes in these patients, with 47% having a blood CR and 38% having a blood PR. Grade 3–4 neutropenia and thrombocytopenia occurred in 10 patients (26%), and infections occurred in three patients (8%). Furthermore, grade 1–2 tumor-flare reactions occurred in 17 patients (44%) and were managed using oral steroids in symptomatic patients. This study is ongoing, 37 patients (84%) are still receiving treatment and two patients discontinued treatment after 6 and 8 months, respectively, because of toxic effects (rash and fatigue). No mortality was associated with this treatment. These early results indicated that lenalidomide given as continuous therapy at a starting daily dose of 5 mg followed by slow-dose escalation was safe and well tolerated as initial therapy for elderly patients with CLL.

Ofatumumab

Researchers are developing several new-generation anti-CD20 antibodies for treatment of CLL. One of these is ofatumumab, a fully humanized monoclonal anti-CD20 antibody that is currently in clinical trials. Administration of single-agent ofatumumab at the highest dose level resulted in an OR rate of 50% (42% PR and 8% nPR) in a phase I–II study [85]. Several phase III trials are investigating ofatumumab in combination with fludarabine and cyclophosphamide in both the front-line and salvage setting.

Oblimersen

Oblimersen is an antisense oligonucleotide that can downregulate *BCL-2* mRNA and Bcl-2 protein expression in CLL cells [86]. O'Brien *et al.* [87] reported on a randomized phase III study of the FC regimen with and without oblimersen given in 241 patients with relapsed CLL after a fludarabine-containing regimen; more than half were >65 years old. Overall, 20 patients (17%) in the FC–oblimersen group versus eight patients (7%) in the FC-only group had a CR or nPR ($P = 0.025$). Oblimersen did not increase the incidence of FC-associated myelosuppression, whereas tumor lysis syndrome and cytokine-release reactions occurred less frequently.

Flavopiridol

Flavopiridol is a cyclin-dependent kinase inhibitor that induces cell-cycle arrest and apoptosis in patients with B-cell malignancies. Phelps *et al.* [88] studied administration of this agent as a 30-min bolus followed by a 4-h infusion in 52 patients with relapsed CLL at a median age of 60 years (range 38–84 years). Twenty-one patients (40%) had a PR, with a median PFS duration of 12 months. Grade 3–4 neutropenia and tumor lysis syndrome were the most common severe toxic effects and usually occurred in patients with advanced disease [88,89].

Stem-cell transplantation

Use of allo-SCT after high-dose chemotherapy is an effective tool in the treatment of CLL. However, the widespread use of this approach has several limitations. First, because CLL occurs generally in elderly, often debilitated, patients, only a minority of patients can be considered for this approach. Second, the treatment-related mortality rate for allo-SCT is considerably high, ranging from 15% to 22% even with reduced-intensity or non-myeloablative conditioning regimens. Currently, the major focus has been the non-myeloablative allo-SCT, particularly in elderly patients. Using this approach with the FCR regimen, Khouri *et al.* [90] administered treatment to 39 patients with a median age of 57 years (range 34–70 years). The median time from CLL diagnosis to transplantation was 4.5 years, and all patients had recurrent advanced disease after treatment with fludarabine- and rituximab-based regimens. Of 38 evaluable patients in this study, 27 (71%) achieved a CR. The estimated OS and PFS rates at 4-years after transplant were 48% and 44%, respectively. Multivariate analysis showed that disease chemorefractory at the time of transplantation ($P = 0.01$) and mixed T-cell chimerism on day 90 after transplant ($P = 0.02$), but not ZAP-70 status, were correlated with risk of progression after transplantation.

Supportive care in elderly patients with chronic lymphocytic leukemia

Supportive care plays an important role in the management of elderly patients with CLL. Elderly patients often present with advanced-stage disease, poor performance statuses, comorbidities, disease-associated complications, impaired organ function, or poor nutritional statuses. These factors decrease their ability to tolerate aggressive CLL therapy. Patients with CLL, especially if elderly, often present with more severe immunodeficiency and an increased risk of infection because of hypogammaglobulinemia [91]. There has been a direct correlation between low levels of immunoglobulin G and the severity and frequency of bacterial infections, so prophylactic intravenous use of immunoglobulins may be beneficial in selected groups of patients [92]. Adequate hematopoietic growth factor support during treatment can help recovery of bone marrow function and minimize the infectious complications associated with treatment. In addition, elderly patients usually present with impaired renal function and decreased creatinine clearance. Therefore, adequate hydration, urinary alkalinization, and treatment with allopurinol should be used regularly in these patients to prevent the development of tumor lysis syndrome and deterioration of renal function during treatment, especially in patients with high white blood cell counts. Administration of rasburicase in patients who have high levels of uric acid or cannot tolerate allopurinol may also be indicated [93]. Patients who receive adequate supportive care also can better tolerate aggressive regimens and complete the intended treatment.

Conclusions

Despite the fact that elderly patients represent the largest population of patients with CLL, they have been underrepresented in most clinical trials evaluating novel agents or combination regimens. The best CLL treatment strategies have yet to be defined for this group of patients, and there is a growing need for specially designed programs. The goal of therapy for CLL in elderly patients depends on several factors, including patient age, performance status, disease stage, prognostic factors, and comorbidities. In elderly patients with poor performance statuses and significant comorbidities, physicians should favor regimens with favorable toxicity profiles. In elderly patients with good performance statuses and no significant comorbidities, combinations of CIT, rituximab and alemtuzumab, lenalidomide, or other novel agents may be administered with proper monitoring and dose modifications. The conduction of a larger number of clinical trials testing treatment regimens specifically designed for elderly patients should be encouraged and will provide valuable information in this patient population.

References

1 Richter M. Generalized reticular cell sarcoma of lymph nodes associated with lymphatic leukemia. *Am J Pathol* 1928;4: 285–92.

2 Brecher M, Banks PM. Hodgkin's disease variant of Richter's syndrome. Report of eight cases. *Am J Clin Pathol* 1990;93: 333–9.

3 Melo JV, Catovsky D, Gregory WM, Galton DA. The relationship between chronic lymphocytic leukemia and prolymphocytic leukemia. IV. Analysis of survival and prognostic features. *Br J Haematol* 1987;65:23–9.

4 Pistoia V, Roncella S, Di Celle PF, *et al.* Emergence of a B-cell lymphoblastic lymphoma in a patient with B-cell chronic lymphocytic leukemia: evidence for the single-cell origin of the two tumors. *Blood* 1991;78:797–804.

5 Duchayne E, Delsol G, Kuhlein E, *et al.* Hairy cell transformation of a B-cell chronic lymphocytic leukemia: a morphological, cytochemical, phenotypic and molecular study. *Leukemia* 1991; 5:150–5.

6 Lee A, Skelly ME, Kingma DW, Medeiros LJ. B-cell chronic lymphocytic leukemia followed by high grade T-cell lymphoma. An unusual variant of Richter's syndrome. *Am J Clin Pathol* 1995;103:348–52.

7 Tsimberidou AM, Keating MJ. Richter syndrome: biology, incidence, and therapeutic strategies. *Cancer* 2005;103:216–28.

8 Nakamura N, Abe M. Richter syndrome in B-cell chronic lymphocytic leukemia. *Pathol Int* 2003;53:195–203.

9 Rossi D, Cerri M, Capello D, *et al.* Biological and clinical risk factors of chronic lymphocytic leukemia transformation to Richter syndrome. *Br J Haematol* 2008;142:202–15.

10 Rossi D, Gaidano G. Richter syndrome: molecular insights and clinical perspectives. *Hematol Oncol* 2009;27:1–10.

11 Tsimberidou AM, Kantarjian HM, Cortes J, *et al.* Fractionated cyclophosphamide, vincristine, liposomal daunorubicin, and dexamethasone plus rituximab and granulocyte-macrophage-colony stimulating factor (GM-CSF) alternating with methotrexate and cytarabine plus rituximab and GM-CSF in patients with Richter syndrome or fludarabine-refractory chronic lymphocytic leukemia. *Cancer* 2003;97:1711–20.

12 Dabaja BS, O'Brien SM, Kantarjian HM, *et al.* Fractionated cyclophosphamide, vincristine, liposomal daunorubicin (daunoXome), and dexamethasone (hyperCVXD) regimen in Richter's syndrome. *Leuk Lymphoma* 2001;42:329–37.

13 Tsimberidou AM, O'Brien SM, Cortes JE, *et al.* Phase II study of fludarabine, cytarabine (Ara-C), cyclophosphamide, cisplatin and GM-CSF (FACPGM) in patients with Richter's syndrome or refractory lymphoproliferative disorders. *Leuk Lymphoma* 2002;43:767–72.

14 Thompson MP, Kurzrock R. Epstein-Barr virus and cancer. *Clin Cancer Res* 2004;10:803–21.

15 Ansell SM, Li CY, Lloyd RV, Phyliky RL. Epstein-Barr virus infection in Richter's transformation. *Am J Hematol* 1999;60: 99–104.

16 Gaidano G, Ballerini P, Gong JZ, *et al.* *p53* mutations in human lymphoid malignancies: association with Burkitt lymphoma and chronic lymphocytic leukemia. *Proc Natl Acad Sci U S A* 1991;88:5413–17.

17 Pinyol M, Cobo F, Bea S, *et al.* *p16(INK4*a) gene inactivation by deletions, mutations, and hypermethylation is associated with transformed and aggressive variants of non-Hodgkin's lymphomas. *Blood* 1998;91:2977–84.

18 Martinez JC, Piris MA, Sanchez-Beato M, *et al.* Retinoblastoma (Rb) gene product expression in lymphomas. Correlation with Ki67 growth fraction. *J Pathol* 1993;169:405–12.

19 Cobo F, Martinez A, Pinyol M, *et al.* Multiple cell cycle regulator alterations in Richter's transformation of chronic lymphocytic leukemia. *Leukemia* 2002;16:1028–34.

20 Robertson LE, Pugh W, O'Brien S, *et al.* Richter's syndrome: a report on 39 patients. *J Clin Oncol* 1993;11:1985–9.

21 Swords R, Bruzzi J, Giles F. Recent advances in the diagnosis and therapy of Richter's syndrome. *Med Oncol* 2007;24:17–32.

22 Tsimberidou AM, O'Brien S, Khouri I, *et al.* Clinical outcomes and prognostic factors in patients with Richter's syndrome treated with chemotherapy or chemoimmunotherapy with or without stem-cell transplantation. *J Clin Oncol* 2006;24: 2343–51.

23 Foucar K, Rydell RE. Richter's syndrome in chronic lymphocytic leukemia. *Cancer* 1980;46:118–34.

24 Bruzzi JF, Macapinlac H, Tsimberidou AM, *et al.* Detection of Richter's transformation of chronic lymphocytic leukemia by PET/CT. *J Nucl Med* 2006;47:1267–73.

25 Tsimberidou AM, Murray JL, O'Brien S, Wierda WG, Keating MJ. Yttrium-90 ibritumomab tiuxetan radioimmunotherapy in Richter syndrome. *Cancer* 2004;100:2195–200.

26 Tsimberidou AM, Wierda WG, Plunkett W, *et al.* Phase I-II study of oxaliplatin, fludarabine, cytarabine, and rituximab combination therapy in patients with Richter's syndrome or fludarabine-refractory chronic lymphocytic leukemia. *J Clin Oncol* 2008;26:196–203.

27 Rodriguez J, Keating MJ, O'Brien S, Champlin RE, Khouri IF. Allogeneic haematopoietic transplantation for Richter's syndrome. *Br J Haematol* 2000;110:897–9.

28 Mauro FR, Foa R, Giannarelli D, *et al.* Clinical characteristics and outcome of young chronic lymphocytic leukemia patients: a single institution study of 204 cases. *Blood* 1999;94:448–54.

29 Alliot C, Tabuteau S, Desablens B. Hodgkin's disease variant of Richter's syndrome: complete remission of the both malignancies after 14 years. *Hematology* 2003;8:229–31.

30 Juneja S, Carney D, Ellis D, Januszewicz EH, Wolf M, Prince HM. Hodgkin's disease type Richter's syndrome in chronic lymphocytic leukemia. *Leukemia* 1999;13:826–7.

31 Fayad L, Robertson LE, O'Brien S, *et al.* Hodgkin's disease variant of Richter's syndrome: experience at a single institution. *Leuk Lymphoma* 1996;23:333–7.

32 Saad ED, Thomas DA, O'Brien S, *et al.* Progressive multifocal leukoencephalopathy with concurrent Richter's syndrome. *Leuk Lymphoma* 2000;38:183–90.

33 van Besien K, Ha CS, Murphy S, *et al.* Risk factors, treatment, and outcome of central nervous system recurrence in adults with intermediate-grade and immunoblastic lymphoma. *Blood* 1998;91:1178–84.

34 Khouri IF, Keating M, Korbling M, *et al.* Transplant-lite: induction of graft-versus-malignancy using fludarabine-based nonablative chemotherapy and allogeneic blood progenitor-cell transplantation as treatment for lymphoid malignancies. *J Clin Oncol* 1998;16:2817–24.

35 Khouri IF, Saliba RM, Giralt SA, *et al.* Nonablative allogeneic hematopoietic transplantation as adoptive immunotherapy for indolent lymphoma: low incidence of toxicity, acute

graft-versus-host disease, and treatment-related mortality. *Blood* 2001;98:3595–9.
36 Jemal A, Siegel R, Ward E, *et al*. Cancer statistics, 2008. *CA Cancer J Clin* 2008;58:71–96.
37 Apelgren P, Hasselblom S, Werlenius O, Nilsson-Ehle H, Andersson PO. Evaluation of clinical staging in chronic lymphocytic leukemia- population-based study. *Leuk Lymphoma* 2006;47:2505–16.
38 Diehl LF, Karnell LH, Menck HR. The American College of Surgeons Commission on Cancer and the American Cancer Society. The National Cancer Database report on age, gender, treatment, and outcomes of patients with chronic lymphocytic leukemia. *Cancer* 1999;86:2684–92.
39 Eichhorst B, Goede V, Hallek M. Treatment of elderly patients with chronic lymphocytic leukemia. *Leuk Lymphoma* 2009;50: 171–8.
40 Faderl S, Ferrajoli A, Frankfurt O, Pettitt A. Treatment of B-cell chronic lymphocytic leukemia with nonchemotherapeutic agents: experience with single-agent and combination therapy. *Leukemia* 2009;23:457–66.
41 Wierda W, O'Brien S, Wen S, *et al*. Chemoimmunotherapy with fludarabine, cyclophosphamide, and rituximab for relapsed and refractory chronic lymphocytic leukemia. *J Clin Oncol* 2005; 23:4070–8.
42 Thurmes P, Call T, Slager S, *et al*. Comorbid conditions and survival in unselected, newly diagnosed patients with chronic lymphocytic leukemia. *Leuk Lymphoma* 2008;49:49–56.
43 Tsimberidou AM, Wen S, McLaughlin P, *et al*. Other malignancies in chronic lymphocytic leukemia/small lymphocytic lymphoma. *J Clin Oncol* 2009;27:904–10.
44 Balducci L, Extermann M. Management of cancer in the older person: a practical approach. *Oncologist* 2000;5:224–37.
45 Piccirillo JF, Tierney RM, Costas I, Grove L, Spitznagel EL, Jr. Prognostic importance of comorbidity in a hospital-based cancer registry. *JAMA* 2004;291:2441–7.
46 Shanafelt TD, Bowen D, Venkat C, *et al*. Quality of life in chronic lymphocytic leukemia: an international survey of 1482 patients. *Br J Haematol* 2007;139:255–64.
47 Wierda W, O'Brien S, Faderl S, *et al*. A retrospective comparison of three sequential groups of patients with recurrent/refractory chronic lymphocytic leukemia treated with fludarabine-based regimens. *Cancer* 2006;106:337–45.
48 Shvidel L, Shtalrid M, Bairey O, *et al*. Conventional dose fludarabine-based regimens are effective but have excessive toxicity in elderly patients with refractory chronic lymphocytic leukemia. *Leuk Lymphoma* 2003;44:1947–50.
49 Keating MJ, O'Brien S, Albitar M, *et al*. Early results of a chemoimmunotherapy regimen of fludarabine, cyclophosphamide, and rituximab as initial therapy for chronic lymphocytic leukemia. *J Clin Oncol* 2005;23:4079–88.
50 Wierda WG, O'Brien S, Wang X, *et al*. Characteristics associated with important clinical end points in patients with chronic lymphocytic leukemia at initial treatment. *J Clin Oncol* 2009;27:1637–43.
51 Wierda WG, O'Brien S, Wang X, *et al*. Prognostic nomogram and index for overall survival in previously untreated patients with chronic lymphocytic leukemia. *Blood* 2007;109:4679–85.
52 Tsimberidou AM, Wen S, O'Brien S, *et al*. Assessment of chronic lymphocytic leukemia and small lymphocytic lymphoma by absolute lymphocyte counts in 2,126 patients: 20 years of experience at the University of Texas M.D. Anderson Cancer Center. *J Clin Oncol* 2007;25:4648–56.
53 Ries LAG MD, Krapcho M, Stinchcomb DG, *et al*, (eds.). *SEER Clinical Statistics Review, 1975–2005*. National Cancer Institute: Bethesda, MD, 2008.
54 Rai KR, Sawitsky A, Cronkite EP, Chanana AD, Levy RN, Pasternack BS. Clinical staging of chronic lymphocytic leukemia. *Blood* 1975;46:219–34.
55 Binet JL, Auquier A, Dighiero G, *et al*. A new prognostic classification of chronic lymphocytic leukemia derived from a multivariate survival analysis. *Cancer* 1981;48:198–206.
56 Dohner H, Stilgenbauer S, Benner A, *et al*. Genomic aberrations and survival in chronic lymphocytic leukemia. *N Engl J Med* 2000;343:1910–16.
57 Hamblin TJ, Davis Z, Gardiner A, Oscier DG, Stevenson FK. Unmutated *Ig V(H)* genes are associated with a more aggressive form of chronic lymphocytic leukemia. *Blood* 1999;94: 1848–54.
58 Damle RN, Wasil T, Fais F, *et al*. *Ig V* gene mutation status and CD38 expression as novel prognostic indicators in chronic lymphocytic leukemia. *Blood* 1999;94:1840–7.
59 Crespo M, Bosch F, Villamor N, *et al*. ZAP-70 expression as a surrogate for immunoglobulin-variable-region mutations in chronic lymphocytic leukemia. *N Engl J Med* 2003;348: 1764–75.
60 Orchard JA, Ibbotson RE, Davis Z, *et al*. ZAP-70 expression and prognosis in chronic lymphocytic leukemia. *Lancet* 2004;363: 105–11.
61 Ibrahim S, Keating M, Do KA, *et al*. CD38 expression as an important prognostic factor in B-cell chronic lymphocytic leukemia. *Blood* 2001;98:181–6.
62 Del Poeta G, Maurillo L, Venditti A, *et al*. Clinical significance of CD38 expression in chronic lymphocytic leukemia. *Blood* 2001;98:2633–9.
63 Shanafelt TD, Jelinek D, Tschumper R, *et al*. Cytogenetic abnormalities can change during the course of the disease process in chronic lymphocytic leukemia. *J Clin Oncol* 2006;24:3218–9, Author reply 9–20.
64 Keating MJ, O'Brien S, Lerner S, *et al*. Long-term follow-up of patients with chronic lymphocytic leukemia (CLL) receiving fludarabine regimens as initial therapy. *Blood* 1998;92:1165–71.
65 Rai KR, Peterson BL, Appelbaum FR, *et al*. Fludarabine compared with chlorambucil as primary therapy for chronic lymphocytic leukemia. *N Engl J Med* 2000;343:1750–7.
66 O'Brien SM, Kantarjian HM, Cortes J, *et al*. Results of the fludarabine and cyclophosphamide combination regimen in chronic lymphocytic leukemia. *J Clin Oncol* 2001;19:1414–20.
67 Flinn IW, Byrd JC, Morrison C, *et al*. Fludarabine and cyclophosphamide with filgrastim support in patients with previously untreated indolent lymphoid malignancies. *Blood* 2000; 96:71–5.
68 Robak T. Therapy of chronic lymphocytic leukemia with purine nucleoside analogues: facts and controversies. *Drugs Aging* 2005;22:983–1012.
69 Eichhorst BF, Busch R, Stauch M, *et al*. No significant clinical benefit of first line therapy with fludaravine (F) in comparison with chlorambucil (Clb) in elderly patients (pts) with advanced chronic lymphocytic leukemia (CLL): Results of a Phase III study of the German CLL Study Group (GCLLSG). *Blood* 2007; 194a:629.

70 Forconi F, Fabbri A, Lenoci M, *et al*. Low-dose oral fludarabine plus cyclophosphamide in elderly patients with untreated and relapsed or refractory chronic lymphocytic leukemia. *Hematol Oncol* 2008;26:247–51.

71 McLaughlin P, Grillo-Lopez AJ, Link BK, *et al*. Rituximab chimeric antiCD20 monoclonal antibody therapy for relapsed indolent lymphoma: half of patients respond to a four-dose treatment program. *J Clin Oncol* 1998;16:2825–33.

72 Hainsworth JD, Litchy S, Barton JH, *et al*. Single-agent rituximab as first-line and maintenance treatment for patients with chronic lymphocytic leukemia or small lymphocytic lymphoma: a phase II trial of the Minnie Pearl Cancer Research Network. *J Clin Oncol* 2003;21:1746–51.

73 Huhn D, von Schilling C, Wilhelm M, *et al*. Rituximab therapy of patients with B-cell chronic lymphocytic leukemia. *Blood* 2001;98:1326–31.

74 Ferrajoli A, O'Brien S, Faderl S, *et al*. The combination of rituximab and GM-CSF in elderly patients with chronic lymphocytic leukemia (CLL). *J Clin Oncol* 2006;24:6602.

75 Keating MJ, Flinn I, Jain V, *et al*. Therapeutic role of alemtuzumab (Campath-1H) in patients who have failed fludarabine: results of a large international study. *Blood* 2002;99:3554–61.

76 Hillmen P, Skotnicki AB, Robak T, *et al*. Alemtuzumab compared with chlorambucil as first-line therapy for chronic lymphocytic leukemia. *J Clin Oncol* 2007;25:5616–23.

77 Pitini V, Arrigo C, Naro C, *et al*. Subcutaneous low-dose alemtuzumab as first line therapy for elderly CLL patients with deletion of 17p. *J Clin Oncol* 2008;26:7048.

78 Faderl S, Thomas DA, O'Brien S, *et al*. Experience with alemtuzumab plus rituximab in patients with relapsed and refractory lymphoid malignancies. *Blood* 2003;101:3413–15.

79 Nabhan C, Patton D, Gordon LI, *et al*. A pilot trial of rituximab and alemtuzumab combination therapy in patients with relapsed and/or refractory chronic lymphocytic leukemia (CLL). *Leuk Lymphoma* 2004;45:2269–73.

80 Tam CS, O'Brien S, Wierda W, *et al*. Long-term results of the fludarabine, cyclophosphamide, and rituximab regimen as initial therapy of chronic lymphocytic leukemia. *Blood* 2008; 112:975–80.

81 Shanafelt TD, Lin T, Geyer SM, *et al*. Pentostatin, cyclophosphamide, and rituximab regimen in older patients with chronic lymphocytic leukemia. *Cancer* 2007;109:2291–8.

82 Chanan-Khan A, Miller KC, Musial L, *et al*. Clinical efficacy of lenalidomide in patients with relapsed or refractory chronic lymphocytic leukemia: results of a phase II study. *J Clin Oncol* 2006;24:5343–9.

83 Ferrajoli A, Lee BN, Schlette EJ, *et al*. Lenalidomide induces complete and partial remissions in patients with relapsed and refractory chronic lymphocytic leukemia. *Blood* 2008;111: 5291–7.

84 Ferrajoli A, O'Brien S, Wierda WG, *et al*. Lenalidomide as initial treatment of elderly patients with chronic lymphocytic leukemia (CLL). *Blood* (ASH Annual Meeting Abstracts) 2008; 112:45.

85 Coiffier B, Lepretre S, Pedersen LM, *et al*. Safety and efficacy of ofatumumab, a fully human monoclonal antiCD20 antibody, in patients with relapsed or refractory B-cell chronic lymphocytic leukemia: a phase 1–2 study. *Blood* 2008;111: 1094–100.

86 O'Brien SM, Cunningham CC, Golenkov AK, Turkina AG, Novick SC, Rai KR. Phase I to II multicenter study of oblimersen sodium, a Bcl-2 antisense oligonucleotide, in patients with advanced chronic lymphocytic leukemia. *J Clin Oncol* 2005;23:7697–702.

87 O'Brien S, Moore JO, Boyd TE, *et al*. Randomized phase III trial of fludarabine plus cyclophosphamide with or without oblimersen sodium (Bcl-2 antisense) in patients with relapsed or refractory chronic lymphocytic leukemia. *J Clin Oncol* 2007; 25:1114–20.

88 Phelps MA, Lin TS, Johnson AJ, *et al*. Clinical response and pharmacokinetics from a phase I study of an active dosing schedule of flavopiridol in relapsed chronic lymphocytic leukemia. *Blood* 2008;113:2637–45.

89 Byrd JC, Lin TS, Dalton JT, *et al*. Flavopiridol administered using a pharmacologically derived schedule is associated with marked clinical efficacy in refractory, genetically high-risk chronic lymphocytic leukemia. *Blood* 2007;109:399–404.

90 Khouri I, Saliba RM, Keating M, *et al*. ZAP-70 status may not predict outcome after non-myeloablative allogeneic transplantation (NMY) in patients with chronic lymphocytic leukemia (CLL) who failed conventional chemotherapy. *Blood* 2005;106: 577a.

91 Shanafelt TD, Call TG. Current approach to diagnosis and management of chronic lymphocytic leukemia. *Mayo Clin Proc* 2004; 79:388–98.

92 Dearden C. Disease-specific complications of chronic lymphocytic leukemia. *Hematology Am Soc Hematol Educ Program* 2008;2008:450–6.

93 Bosly A, Sonet A, Pinkerton CR, *et al*. Rasburicase (recombinant urate oxidase) for the management of hyperuricemia in patients with cancer: report of an international compassionate use study. *Cancer* 2003;98:1048–54.

Part 8
Other Leukemic Disorders

Chapter 28
Hairy Cell Leukemia

Farhad Ravandi
University of Texas M. D. Anderson Cancer Center, Houston, Texas, USA

Introduction

Hairy cell leukemia (HCL) is an uncommon and indolent lymphoid neoplasm that is historically highly significant owing to the evolution of its therapy. The development of effective agents such as nucleoside analogs and monoclonal antibodies has transformed the disease into one of the most curable h[illegible] ... s. The combi- ... al antibodies ... ay improve ... to molecular ... this highly ... ing of other, ... 1–5].

... years (range ... lastic B cells ... nfiltrate the ... ally, lymph ... -sized lym- ... ucleoli and ... ble for the ... tions [6,8]. ... plenic mar- ... tween this

... penia and ... de signifi- ... mbocyto- ... en in 60%; these cytopenias can be severe and life-threatening and are probably multifactorial, with the more important factors being hypersplenism and marrow infiltration by the disease [11]. In most patients, circulating hairy cells are scant and sometimes absent. Bone marrow involvement can be interstitial or patchy with the infiltrate characterized by widely spaced nuclei owing to the abundant cytoplasm, which gives rise to the commonly described "fried egg" appearance [6]. Occasionally, an increase in the bone marrow reticulin fibrosis, as well as significant loss of the hematopoietic elements, leads to a "dry tap" [6,8]. Combined expression of DBA.44 and tartrate-resistant phosphatase (TRAP) by immunohistochemical analysis is highly specific and useful for arriving at a diagnosis [12,13]. More recently, immunostaining for annexin A1 (ANAX1) has been reported to be very specific for HCL [14]. Splenomegaly is present in the majority of patients and can be greatly enlarged in >20% of cases [10,11]. Clinically significant lymphadenopathy is uncommon and present only in the advanced stages of the disease. Hepatomegaly is uncommon, but the liver is almost always involved with a mononuclear infiltrate. Other clinical features include a predisposition to infections and an association with autoimmune disorders [11]. A higher incidence of second malignancies in HCL, even before the administration of therapy, has been reported, although the data are inconclusive [11].

A variant form of HCL has been described, which is a rare disorder accounting for approximately 10% of cases and occurring in the older population (median age 71 years) [6,7,15,16]. Patients often have an elevated white blood cell (WBC) count (>10 × 10^9/L) including atypical hairy cells with prolymphocytic features. Splenomegaly and cytopenias are present in the majority of patients, and the pattern of bone marrow and splenic involvement is similar to HCL but different from prolymphocytic leukemia and SMZL [7,17].

Recent studies have provided new clues as to the cell of origin in HCL. It has been traditionally thought that HCL is a clonal expansion of mature B cells with light chain-restricted surface immunoglobulin expression and the unusual expression of multiple immunoglobulin heavy-chain isotypes with predominance of Immunoglobulin G3 [18,19]. More recently, the existence of clonally related multiple isotypes in individual hairy cells was demonstrated, suggesting the generation of isotypes through RNA splicing [2]. It was postulated that hairy cells are arrested at a stage of isotype switching where RNA processing may precede deletional recombinations [2,3].

Leukemias: Principles and Practice of Therapy, 1st edition. Edited by S. Faderl and H. Kantarjian.

In the majority of patients with HCL, the leukemic cells express mutated immunoglobulin heavy-chain variable gene (V_H), suggesting their origin from a post-germinal center (GC) antigen-experienced memory B cell [3,20]. Other groups have demonstrated the existence of a population of patients with HCL with unmutated V_H genes, thereby contesting the notion of a post-GC cell of origin [21]. An origin within the GC is supported by the existence of patients with multiple and clonally related surface immunoglobulin isotypes consistent with an arrest at the stage of isotype switching within the GC [2]. Gene expression profiling experiments have not demonstrated the existence of different subsets of HCL, and high-density genome-wide DNA profiling demonstrated a remarkably stable genomic profile in patients with HCL [1,4]. Furthermore, when compared with the gene expression profiles of purified normal B-cell populations including those of pre-GC (naïve), GC, and post-GC (memory) B cells, the HCL profile resembled that of memory B cells [1].

Cells in HCL have a characteristic immunophenotype (Table 28.1) [22]. They express B-cell-associated antigens CD19, CD20, CD22, FMC7, and CD79a, but typically lack CD79b, CD5, CD10, and CD23 expression. No single marker is specific for distinguishing HCL from other B-cell neoplasms; however, the antigens CD11c, CD103, and the interleukin 2 (IL-2) receptor α-subunit (CD25) are typically expressed in HCL [6]. Bright expression of CD22 and CD20 are also seen [22,23]. CD52 has been reported to be universally expressed in the patients evaluated [24]. HCL-variant cases lack CD25 and may also lack CD103 but express other HCL-associated antigens.

Several cytogenetic abnormalities have been reported in HCL, but no one abnormality is consistently present [25,26]. Few cytogenetic studies have been reported owing to the rarity of the disease, difficulty in obtaining marrow samples, and low responsiveness of hairy cells to common mitogens. Chromosome 5 and 14 abnormalities, deletions and mutations of *p53*, as well as overexpression of cyclin-D1, have been reported [25–29].

Treatment of hairy cell leukemia

Significant advances in the therapy for HCL over the last 25 years have led to survival curves that are not significantly different from age-matched cohorts without the disease [30]. Historically, splenectomy was the treatment of choice for HCL and resulted in significant improvements in cytopenias, which were limited in duration [31]. More recently, interferon α (IFN-α) and nucleoside analogs such as 2-chlorodeoxyadenosine (2-CDA or cladribine) and 2-deoxycoformycin (DCF or pentostatin) have been successfully used to treat patients with HCL.

IFN-α produces a response rate of >80%; however, most were partial responses (PRs) and were of limited duration [32–34]. Cladribine has been very effective, with overall response rates ranging from 75% to 100% after a single course of the drug administered by continuous infusion daily for 7 days (Table 28.2) [47]. Schedules using a 2-h infusion on five consecutive days have been associated with an equal efficacy and tolerance [48,49]. More recently, 132 patients with untreated HCL were randomized to receive cladribine either on five consecutive days or a novel schedule of six weekly doses [46]. The complete remission rates, overall response rates, progression-free and overall survival, and incidence of grade 3 and 4 infections were the same in the two arms of the study [46]. Despite the very high response rate to cladribine, responses are not universal and a significant proportion of patients relapse. Saven *et al.* [36] reported the long-term outcome of 358 patients with HCL who were followed for a median of 52 months. Twenty-six percent of patients relapsed at a median of 29 months. Goodman *et al.* [37] described 209 patients treated with cladribine with a follow-up period of at least 7 years. Although the overall response rate was 100%, 76 (37%) patients relapsed after their first course of cladribine, with a median time to relapse of 42 months [37]. Importantly, there was no obvious plateau on the time-to-treatment failure curve. The authors concluded that it is unclear what proportion

Table 28.1 Immunophenotypic features of selected B-cell neoplasms.

Disease	Sig	CD5	CD10	CD11c	CD20	CD22	CD23	CD25	CD103
CLL	+/–	++	–	–/+	+/–	–/+	++	–/+	–
B-PLL	++	+	–	–/+	+/–	+	+/–	–	–
HCL	+/–	–	–	++	+	++	–	+	++
HCLv	+/–	–/+	–	++	+	+	–/+	–	–/+
MCL	+	++	–	–	+	+	–/+	–	–
SMZL	+	–/+	–/+	+	+	+	–/+	–	–
FL	+	–	+	–	++	+	–	–	–

CLL, chronic lymphocytic leukemia; B-PLL, B-prolymphocytic leukemia; FL: follicular lymphoma; HCL, hairy cell leukemia; HCLv, hairy cell leukemia variant; MCL, mantle cell lymphoma; SMZL, splenic marginal zone lymphoma.

Table 28.2 Selected trials of cladribine in hairy cell leukemia.

Reference	Evaluable patients (*n*)	Complete response (%)	Partial response (%)	Overall response (%)
Cheson *et al.* [35]	861	50	37	87
Saven *et al.* [36]	349	91	7	98
Goodman *et al.* [37]	207	95	5	100
Tallman *et al.* [38]	50	80	18	98
Chadha *et al.* [39]	85	79	21	100
Hoffman *et al.* [40]	49	76	24	100
Estey *et al.* [41]	46	78	11	89
Dearden *et al.* [42]	45	84	16	100
Juliusson *et al.* [43]	16	75	0	75
Zinzani *et al.* [44]	37	81	19	100
Jehn *et al.* [45]	44	98	2	100
Robak *et al.* [46][a]	132	76.72	19.19	95.91

[a]Numbers reported for the two arms of a randomized study.

Table 28.3 Selected trials of pentostatin in hairy cell leukemia.

Reference	Evaluable patients (*n*)	Complete response (%)	Partial response (%)	Overall response (%)
Kraut *et al.* [51]	23	87	4	91
Johnston *et al.* [52]	28	89	11	100
Dearden *et al.* [42]	165	82	15	97
Catovsky *et al.* [53]	148	74	22	96
Grever *et al.* [54]	154	76	3	79
Rafel *et al.* [55]	78	72	16	88
Ribeiro *et al.* [56]	49	44	52	96
Maloisel *et al.* [57]	230	79	17	96

of patients, if any, will be cured. Several recent publications have confirmed the high response rate of patients with HCL treated with cladribine [39–44]. Jehn *et al.* [45] described a 12-year follow-up of 44 patients (including 11 with prior therapy before receiving cladribine) who received cladribine at a dosage of 0.1 mg/kg/day by continuous infusion for 7 days. The complete response (CR) rate was 98%, and at a median follow-up of 8.5 years (range 0.1–12.2 years) 17 patients had relapsed. Eight of nine patients re-treated with cladribine responded a second time. The overall survival at 12 years was 79% [45]. Zinzani *et al.* [44] reported their long-term follow-up of 37 patients treated with one of two regimens of cladribine. Twenty-one patients received cladribine at 0.14 mg/kg/day by a 2-h infusion for 5 days, whereas 16 patients were treated with a once-weekly dose of cladribine at 0.14 mg/kg for 5 weeks [44]. A CR rate of 81% with an overall response rate of 100% was reported, with no difference between the two schedules. After a median follow-up of 122 months (range 54–156 months), the overall relapse rate was about 30% for both groups. The projected 13-year overall and relapse-free survival rates were 96% and 52%, respectively [44]. Chadha and colleagues [39] at Northwestern University treated 86 consecutive patients with cladribine administered at 0.1 mg/kg/day by continuous infusion over 24 h for 7 days. A CR rate of 79% as well as a PR rate of 21% was noted. The progression-free survival after 12 years was 54%. At a median follow-up of 9.7 years (range 0.3–13.8 years), 31 (36%) patients relapsed. Twenty-three relapsed patients were treated with a second course of cladribine, and 12 (52%) achieved a CR with seven (30%) achieving a PR. The overall survival after 12 years was 87% [39]. The authors suggested that the lower CR rate in this study was due to their more stringent criteria for response, with the requirement for resolution of splenomegaly and lymphadenopathy by CT scan as criteria for CR. We have recently reported an estimated 10-year and 20-year survival of 84% and 65% among 176 patients receiving cladribine as their first therapy [50].

Similar results have been achieved using pentostatin (Table 28.3) [58]. Overall CR rates of 44–89% have been reported with pentostatin administered at a dose of 2–4 mg/m^2 every 2 weeks [58]. Dearden *et al.* [42] found that 82% of 165 patients with HCL achieved a CR with pentostatin, and compared their outcome with of 45 patients treated with cladribine who achieved a similar response rate. Relapse rates were 24% with pentostatin and 29% with cladribine after median follow-up of 71 and 45 months, respectively. They suggested a longer remission duration with pentostatin [42]. However, with further follow-up there appears to be no difference between the two agents with regards to disease-free survival [59]. Flinn *et al.* [60] described the long-term follow-up of 241 patients treated with pentostatin either as initial therapy or after failure of IFN-α. The 5- and 10-year event-free survival rates were 85% and 67%, respectively. Maloisel *et al.* [57] reported the long-term follow-up of 230 evaluable patients with HCL treated with pentostatin. Pentostatin was the first-line agent in 84 patients. A CR rate of 79% with an overall response rate of 96% was reported. With a median follow-up of 63.5 months (range 0.39–138.4 months), 34 of 220 responding patients (15%) had relapsed. The estimated 5-year and 10-year disease-free survival was 88% and 69%, respectively, and the estimated 5-year overall survival was 89% [57].

The above data indicate that, despite excellent responses, there is a definite relapse rate associated with therapy of HCL with both cladribine and pentostatin, and the relapse-free survival does not appear to plateau. Wheaton *et al.* noted that detection of minimal residual disease (MRD) by immunohistochemistry (using anti-CD45RO, anti-CD20, and DBA.44) in paraffin-imbedded bone marrow sections of 39 patients with HCL in CR after receiving cladribine was predictive of relapse [61]. More sensitive methods of MRD detection, such as immunophenotyping by flow cytometry and analysis for consensus primer polymerase chain reaction (cpPCR) of antigen receptor genes, have been evaluated recently and can be used to monitor the disease course [62].

Multiple therapeutic options have become available for patients with relapsed HCL. A number of reports have demonstrated the efficacy of the monoclonal antibody rituximab in treating these patients (Table 28.4). Rituximab is a monoclonal antibody directed against the pan-B-cell antigen CD20, which is brightly expressed on the surface of hairy cells [23]. Nieva *et al.* [63] reported their experience in 24 patients with HCL in whom cladribine therapy was failing. Rituximab was administered at 375 mg/m^2 once weekly for 4 weeks. The CR rate was 13% and the PR rate was 13% for an OR rate of 25%. No unusual toxicity was reported [63]. Lauria *et al.* [64] treated 10 patients with relapsed/progressed HCL with a similar regimen of rituximab and reported one CR and four PRs (OR 50%). In a study by Hagberg *et al.* [65], 11 patients with HCL (including three previously untreated patients) were treated with rituximab at 375 mg/m^2 weekly for 4 weeks. The OR rate was 64% with six CRs and one PR (including one CR in an untreated patient). Thomas *et al.* used an extended dosing regimen and administered rituximab at 375 mg/m^2 weekly for eight doses to 15 patients with relapsed/refractory HCL [66]. They reported a response rate of 80% including eight CRs (52%), two CRs with MRD (13%), and two (13%) PRs [66]. Rituximab has been evaluated for the eradication of MRD assessed by flow cytometry and cpPCR; whether such elimination of MRD can translate to a longer relapse-free survival is unclear [67,68]. Furthermore, it may be potentially possible to improve the outcome by concomitant administration of rituximab and a nucleoside analog for the initial treatment of patients [69,70].

Another potential treatment option for patients with relapsed HCL is BL22, a recombinant immunotoxin containing an anti-CD22 variable domain fused to a truncated pseudomonas endotoxin [71]. In a dose-escalation study, 16 patients who were resistant to cladribine were treated with BL22 by intravenous infusion every other day for a total of three doses. Eleven patients achieved a CR and two a PR. The three non-responders had either pre-existing neutralizing antibodies or received low doses of the immunotoxin. Toxicity included a cytokine-release syndrome and development of a reversible hemolytic-uremic syndrome in two patients [71]. CD52 is also expressed on the surface of hairy cells, and a recent anecdotal report of a response to alemtuzumab has been published [24,72].

Conclusions

Significant progress in the treatment of HCL has resulted in a survival expectation similar to the age-matched individuals without the disease. Further attempts at improv-

Table 28.4 Reported trials of rituximab in hairy cell leukemia.

Reference	Patients (*n*)	No prior therapy (*n*)	Complete response (%) (Untreated)	Partial response (%)	Overall response (%)
Lauria *et al.* [64]	10	0	10	40	50
Hagberg *et al.* [65]	11	3	55 (33)	10	65
Nieva *et al.* [63]	24	0	13	13	26
Thomas *et al.* [66]	15	0	66	13	80

ing disease-free survival are likely to be centered on better identification of minimal residual leukemia by PCR, flow cytometry, and serum levels of soluble surface-markers such as CD25 and CD22 [73]. Use of relatively non-toxic monoclonal antibodies in this setting and for the treatment of relapse is under investigation.

References

1 Basso K, Liso A, Tiacci E, *et al*. Gene expression profiling of hairy cell leukemia reveals a phenotype related to memory B cells with altered expression of chemokine and adhesion receptors. *J Exp Med* 2004;199:59–68.

2 Forconi F, Sahota SS, Raspadori D, Mockridge CI, Lauria F, Stevenson FK. Tumor cells of hairy cell leukemia express multiple clonally related immunoglobulin isotypes via RNA splicing. *Blood* 2001;98:1174–81.

3 Forconi F, Sahota SS, Raspadori D, *et al*. Hairy cell leukemia: at the crossroad of somatic mutation and isotype switch. *Blood* 2004;104:3312–17.

4 Forconi F, Poretti G, Kwee I, *et al*. High density genome-wide DNA profiling reveals a remarkably stable profile in hairy cell leukemia. *Br J Haematol* 2008;141:622–30.

5 Galiegue-Zouitina S, Delestre L, Dupont C, Troussard X, Shelley CS. Underexpression of RhoH in hairy cell leukemia. *Cancer Res* 2008;68:4531–40.

6 Foucar K, Catovsky D. Hairy cell leukemia. In: Jaffe ES, Harris NL, Stein H, Vardiman JW, (eds). *World Health Organization Classification of Tumors: Tumors of Hematopoietic and Lymphoid Tissues*. IARC Press: Lyon, 2001. pp.138–41.

7 Matutes E, Wotherspoon A, Catovsky D. The variant form of hairy-cell leukemia. *Best Pract Res Clin Haematol* 2003;16: 41–56.

8 Bethel KJ, Sharpe RW. Pathology of hairy-cell leukemia. *Best Pract Res Clin Haematol* 2003;16:15–31.

9 Bouroncle BA. Leukemic reticuloendotheliosis (hairy cell leukemia). *Blood* 1979;53:412–36.

10 Golomb HM, Catovsky D, Golde DW. Hairy cell leukemia: a clinical review based on 71 cases. *Ann Intern Med* 1978;89: 677–83.

11 Kraut EH. Clinical manifestations and infectious complications of hairy-cell leukemia. *Best Pract Res Clin Haematol* 2003;16: 33–40.

12 Hoyer JD, Li CY, Yam LT, Hanson CA, Kurtin PJ. Immunohistochemical demonstration of acid phosphatase isoenzyme 5 (tartrate-resistant) in paraffin sections of hairy cell leukemia and other hematologic disorders. *Am J Clin Pathol* 1997;108:308–15.

13 Went PT, Zimpfer A, Pehrs AC, *et al*. High specificity of combined TRAP and DBA.44 expression for hairy cell leukemia. *Am J Surg Pathol* 2005;29:474–8.

14 Falini B, Tiacci E, Liso A, *et al*. Simple diagnostic assay for hairy cell leukemia by immunocytochemical detection of annexin A1 (ANXA1). *Lancet* 2004;363:1869–70.

15 Catovsky D, O'Brien M, Melo JV, Wardle J, Brozovic M. Hairy cell leukemia (HCL) variant: an intermediate disease between HCL and B prolymphocytic leukemia. *Semin Oncol* 1984;11: 362–9.

16 Sainati L, Matutes E, Mulligan S, *et al*. A variant form of hairy cell leukemia resistant to alpha-interferon: clinical and phenotypic characteristics of 17 patients. *Blood* 1990;76:157–62.

17 Cessna MH, Hartung L, Tripp S, Perkins SL, Bahler DW. Hairy cell leukemia variant: fact or fiction. *Am J Clin Pathol* 2005; 123:132–8.

18 Burns GF, Cawley JC, Worman CP, *et al*. Multiple heavy chain isotypes on the surface of the cells of hairy cell leukemia. *Blood* 1978;52:1132–47.

19 Kluin-Nelemans HC, Krouwels MM, Jansen JH, *et al*. Hairy cell leukemia preferentially expresses the IgG3-subclass. *Blood* 1990;75:972–5.

20 Vanhentenrijk V, Tierens A, Wlodarska I, Verhoef G, Wolf-Peeters CD. *V(H)* gene analysis of hairy cell leukemia reveals a homogeneous mutation status and suggests its marginal zone B-cell origin. *Leukemia* 2004;18:1729–32.

21 Thorselius M, Walsh SH, Thunberg U, Hagberg H, Sundstrom C, Rosenquist R. Heterogeneous somatic hypermutation status confounds the cell of origin in hairy cell leukemia. *Leuk Res* 2005;29:153–8.

22 Robbins BA, Ellison DJ, Spinosa JC, *et al*. Diagnostic application of two-color flow cytometry in 161 cases of hairy cell leukemia. *Blood* 1993;82:1277–87.

23 Ginaldi L, De Martinis M, Matutes E, Farahat N, Morilla R, Catovsky D. Levels of expression of CD19 and CD20 in chronic B cell leukaemias. *J Clin Pathol* 1998;51:364–9.

24 Quigley MM, Bethel KJ, Sharpe RW, Saven A. CD52 expression in hairy cell leukemia. *Am J Hematol* 2003;74:227–30.

25 Sambani C, Trafalis DT, Mitsoulis-Mentzikoff C, *et al*. Clonal chromosome rearrangements in hairy cell leukemia: personal experience and review of literature. *Cancer Genet Cytogenet* 2001;129:138–44.

26 Zuzel M, Cawley JC. The biology of hairy cells. *Best Pract Res Clin Haematol* 2003;16:1–13.

27 Wu X, Ivanova G, Merup M, *et al*. Molecular analysis of the human chromosome 5q13.3 region in patients with hairy cell leukemia and identification of tumor suppressor gene candidates. *Genomics* 1999;60:161–71.

28 Vallianatou K, Brito-Babapulle V, Matutes E, Atkinson S, Catovsky D. *p53* gene deletion and trisomy 12 in hairy cell leukemia and its variant. *Leuk Res* 1999;23:1041–5.

29 Konig EA, Kusser WC, Day C, *et al*. *p53* mutations in hairy cell leukemia. *Leukemia* 2000;14:706–11.

30 Golomb HM. Hairy cell leukemia: treatment successes in the past 25 years. *J Clin Oncol* 2008;26:2607–9.

31 Zakarija A, Peterson LC, Tallman MS. Splenectomy and treatments of historical interest. *Best Pract Res Clin Haematol* 2003; 16:57–68.

32 Quesada JR, Reuben J, Manning JT, Hersh EM, Gutterman JU. Alpha interferon for induction of remission in hairy-cell leukemia. *N Engl J Med* 1984;310:15–18.

33 Golomb HM, Ratain MJ, Fefer A, *et al*. Randomized study of the duration of treatment with interferon alfa-2B in patients with hairy cell leukemia. *J Natl Cancer Inst* 1988;80:369–73.

34 Berman E, Heller G, Kempin S, Gee T, Tran LL, Clarkson B. Incidence of response and long-term follow-up in patients with hairy cell leukemia treated with recombinant interferon alfa-2a. *Blood* 1990;75:839–45.

35 Cheson BD, Sorensen JM, Vena DA, *et al*. Treatment of hairy cell leukemia with 2-chlorodeoxyadenosine via the Group C

protocol mechanism of the National Cancer Institute: a report of 979 patients. *J Clin Oncol* 1998;16:3007–15.
36 Saven A, Burian C, Koziol JA, Piro LD. Long-term follow-up of patients with hairy cell leukemia after cladribine treatment. *Blood* 1998;92:1918–26.
37 Goodman GR, Burian C, Koziol JA, Saven A. Extended follow-up of patients with hairy cell leukemia after treatment with cladribine. *J Clin Oncol* 2003;21:891–6.
38 Tallman MS, Hakimian D, Rademaker AW, *et al.* Relapse of hairy cell leukemia after 2-chlorodeoxyadenosine: long-term follow-up of the Northwestern University experience. *Blood* 1996;88:1954–9.
39 Chadha P, Rademaker AW, Mendiratta P, *et al.* Treatment of hairy cell leukemia with 2-chlorodeoxyadenosine (2-CdA):long-term follow-up of the Northwestern University experience. *Blood* 2005;106:241–6.
40 Hoffman MA, Janson D, Rose E, Rai KR. Treatment of hairy-cell leukemia with cladribine: response, toxicity, and long-term follow-up. *J Clin Oncol* 1997;15:1138–42.
41 Estey EH, Kurzrock R, Kantarjian HM, *et al.* Treatment of hairy cell leukemia with 2-chlorodeoxyadenosine (2-CdA). *Blood* 1992;79:882–7.
42 Dearden CE, Matutes E, Hilditch BL, Swansbury GJ, Catovsky D. Long-term follow-up of patients with hairy cell leukemia after treatment with pentostatin or cladribine. *Br J Haematol* 1999;106:515–19.
43 Juliusson G, Liliemark J. Rapid recovery from cytopenia in hairy cell leukemia after treatment with 2-chloro-2′-deoxyadenosine (CdA): relation to opportunistic infections. *Blood* 1992;79:888–94.
44 Zinzani PL, Tani M, Marchi E, *et al.* Long-term follow-up of front-line treatment of hairy cell leukemia with 2-chlorodeoxyadenosine. *Haematologica* 2004;89:309–13.
45 Jehn U, Bartl R, Dietzfelbinger H, Haferlach T, Heinemann V. An update:12-year follow-up of patients with hairy cell leukemia following treatment with 2-chlorodeoxyadenosine. *Leukemia* 2004;18:1476–81.
46 Robak T, Jamroziak K, Gora-Tybor J, *et al.* Cladribine in a weekly versus daily schedule for untreated active hairy cell leukemia: final report from the Polish Adult Leukemia Group (PALG) of a prospective, randomized, multicenter trial. *Blood* 2007;109:3672–5.
47 Goodman GR, Beutler E, Saven A. Cladribine in the treatment of hairy-cell leukemia. *Best Pract Res Clin Haematol* 2003;16: 101–16.
48 Damasio EE, Resegotti L, Masoudi B, *et al.* Five day intermittent vs seven day continuous 2-chlorodeoxyadenosine infusion for the treatment of hairy cell leukemia. A study by Italian Group for the Hairy Cell leukemia. *Recenti Prog Med* 1998;89:68–73.
49 Robak T, Blasinska-Morawiec M, Blonski J, *et al.* 2-chlorodeoxyadenosine (cladribine) in the treatment of hairy cell leukemia and hairy cell leukemia variant: 7-year experience in Poland. *Eur J Haematol* 1999;62:49–56.
50 Ravandi-Kashani F, Kantarjian H, Faderl S, *et al.* Long term follow-up of patients with hairy cell leukemia (HCL). *Blood* 2004;104:Abstract 3474.
51 Kraut EH, Bouroncle BA, Grever MR. Pentostatin in the treatment of advanced hairy cell leukemia. *J Clin Oncol* 1989;7: 168–72.
52 Johnston JB, Eisenhauer E, Wainman N, Corbett WE, Zaentz SD, Daeninck PJ. Long-term outcome following treatment of hairy cell leukemia with pentostatin (Nipent): a National Cancer Institute of Canada study. *Semin Oncol* 2000;27:32–6.
53 Catovsky D, Matutes E, Talavera JG, *et al.* Long term results with 2′deoxycoformycin in hairy cell leukemia. *Leuk Lymphoma* 1994;14(Suppl.1):109–13.
54 Grever M, Kopecky K, Foucar MK, *et al.* Randomized comparison of pentostatin versus interferon alfa-2a in previously untreated patients with hairy cell leukemia: an intergroup study. *J Clin Oncol* 1995;13:974–82.
55 Rafel M, Cervantes F, Beltran JM, *et al.* Deoxycoformycin in the treatment of patients with hairy cell leukemia: results of a Spanish collaborative study of 80 patients. *Cancer* 2000;88: 352–7.
56 Ribeiro P, Bouaffia F, Peaud PY, *et al.* Long term outcome of patients with hairy cell leukemia treated with pentostatin. *Cancer* 1999;85:65–71.
57 Maloisel F, Benboubker L, Gardembas M, *et al.* Long-term outcome with pentostatin treatment in hairy cell leukemia patients. A French retrospective study of 238 patients. *Leukemia* 2003;17:45–51.
58 Grever MR, Doan CA, Kraut EH. Pentostatin in the treatment of hairy-cell leukemia. *Best Pract Res Clin Haematol* 2003;16: 91–9.
59 Else M, Osuji N, Giudice ID, *et al.* Pentostatin and cladribine in hairy cell leukemia- a retrospective comparison of a large series with long follow up. *Blood* 2004;104:Abstract 3472.
60 Flinn IW, Kopecky KJ, Foucar MK, *et al.* Long-term follow-up of remission duration, mortality, and second malignancies in hairy cell leukemia patients treated with pentostatin. *Blood* 2000;96:2981–6.
61 Wheaton S, Tallman MS, Hakimian D, Peterson L. Minimal residual disease may predict bone marrow relapse in patients with hairy cell leukemia treated with 2-chlorodeoxyadenosine. *Blood* 1996;87:1556–60.
62 Sausville JE, Salloum RG, Sorbara L, *et al.* Minimal residual disease detection in hairy cell leukemia. Comparison of flow cytometric immunophenotyping with clonal analysis using consensus primer polymerase chain reaction for the heavy chain gene. *Am J Clin Pathol* 2003;119:213–17.
63 Nieva J, Bethel K, Saven A. Phase 2 study of rituximab in the treatment of cladribine-failed patients with hairy cell leukemia. *Blood* 2003;102:810–13.
64 Lauria F, Lenoci M, Annino L, *et al.* Efficacy of antiCD20 monoclonal antibodies (Mabthera) in patients with progressed hairy cell leukemia. *Haematologica* 2001;86:1046–50.
65 Hagberg H, Lundholm L. Rituximab, a chimeric antiCD20 monoclonal antibody, in the treatment of hairy cell leukemia. *Br J Haematol* 2001;115:609–11.
66 Thomas DA, O'Brien S, Bueso-Ramos C, *et al.* Rituximab in relapsed or refractory hairy cell leukemia. *Blood* 2003;102: 3906–11.
67 Ravandi F, Jorgensen JL, O'Brein SM, *et al.* Eradication of minimal residual disease in hairy cell leukemia. *Blood* 2008; 107:4658–62.
68 Cervetti G, Galimberti S, Andreazzoli F, *et al.* Rituximab as treatment for minimal residual disease in hairy cell leukemia: extended follow-up. *Br J Haematol* 2008;43:296–8.

69 Else M, Osuji N, Forconi F, *et al*. The role of rituximab in combination with pentostatin or cladribine for the treatment of recurrent/refractory hairy cell leukemia. *Cancer* 2007;110: 2240–7.

70 Forconi F, Toraldo F, Sozzi E, Amato T, Raspadori D, Lauria F. Complete molecular remission induced by concomitant cladribine–rituximab treatment in a case of multi-resistant hairy cell leukemia. *Leuk Lymphoma* 2007;48: 2441–3.

71 Kreitman RJ, Wilson WH, Bergeron K, *et al*. Efficacy of the antiCD22 recombinant immunotoxin BL22 in chemotherapy-resistant hairy-cell leukemia. *N Engl J Med* 2001;345:241–7.

72 Fietz T, Rieger K, Schmittel A, Thiel E, Knauf W. Alemtuzumab (Campath 1H) in hairy cell leukemia relapsing after rituximab treatment. *Hematol J* 2004;5:451–2.

73 Matsushita K, Margulies I, Onda M, Nagata S, Stetler-Stevenson M, Kreitman RJ. Soluble CD22 as a tumor marker for hairy cell leukemia. *Blood* 2008.;112:2272–7.

Chapter 29
Therapeutic Approaches to the Mature T-cell Lymphoproliferative Leukemias

Nnenna Osuji and Claire Dearden
Royal Marsden NHS Foundation Trust and Institute of Cancer Research, Surrey, UK

Introduction

Mature T-cell disorders are a rare and heterogeneous group of disorders that globally show poor response to treatment and short survival. Geographic predilection is well documented for many of these diseases and reflects, in part, the etiologic association of viruses such as the human T-cell leukemia virus (HTLV-1) and Epstein–Barr virus (EBV). Diagnosis of T-cell leukemias, as endorsed by the World Health Organization (WHO), is based on a multiparameter approach that encompasses clinical presentation, peripheral blood count and morphology, immunohistochemistry, flow cytometry, cytogenetics, and molecular genetics. Unlike B-cell disorders, there is no single defining chromosomal abnormality that underscores the diagnosis and pathogenesis of these diseases. This, in conjunction with the rarity of these disorders, hinders any targeted therapeutic approach. Many treatment recommendations are therefore based on small case series, phase II trials, and expert opinions. An important aspect in advancing treatment of T-cell disorders is adopting an international approach to diagnosis, documentation, trial design, and entry in order to recruit sufficient patient and clinicopathologic data to inform robust choices. This paper summarizes and updates treatment options for mature natural killer (NK)/T-cell leukemias, including T-cell prolymphocytic leukemia (T-PLL), T-cell large granular lymphocyte (T-LGL) leukemia, NK-cell leukemias, and adult T-cell leukemia/lymphoma (ATLL), and addresses recent descriptions of clinicopathologies and pathogeneses of these disorders so as to better understand the approaches to their management.

T-cell prolymphocytic leukemia

Initial definitions of a disorder akin to B-cell prolymphocytic leukemia but associated with E-rosetting of lymphocytes heralded the discovery of this aggressive leukemia [1,2] that accounts for 2% of small lymphocytic leukemias in the over 30 age group. High white cell counts ($>100 \times 10^9$/L in over half of all cases), splenomegaly, lymphadenopathy, serous effusions, and dermal lymphoid infiltrates are commonly seen in T-PLL [3,4]. Complex cytogenetic abnormalities are common, and frequently involve chromosome 14q32.1, including inv(14)(q11;q32) and t(14;14)(q11;q32) [5], which lead to deregulation and activation of the *TCL1* gene and overexpression of the Tcl-1 protein. Tcl-1 and its homolog MTCP1 (t(X;14)(q28;q11) (Figure 29.1) induce T-cell leukemia in transgenic murine models [6,7]. Tcl-1 plays a role in T- and B-cell growth and survival, including resistance to receptor-mediated apoptosis [8–10].

The median age at onset of T-PLL in adults is 65 years, and a slight male predominance is seen. In the majority of cases, prolymphocytes are medium-sized cells containing mature nuclear chromatin and prominent nucleoli in a nuclear outline, which may be regular or irregular. Basophilic cytoplasm with cytoplasmic blebs is a conspicuous feature. Small cell and cerebriform variants are described [11]. Regardless of the morphologic variant, all cases display an aggressive disease with similar immunophenotypes and cyogenetics. Prolymphocytes show a post-thymic profile with TdT$^-$, CD1a$^-$, CD2$^+$, CD3$^+$ (may be mCD3$^-$, cCD3$^+$), CD5$^+$, and CD7$^+$ expression. CD4$^+$ CD8$^-$ is most commonly seen (65% of cases); however, CD4$^+$ CD8$^+$ and CD4$^-$ CD8$^+$ are also common at 21% and 13%, respectively [11,12]. A cohort of patients may present with relatively indolent disease [12–15] although progression is invariable after a median of 33 months [15]. In these instances a watch and wait approach can be adopted. Previous treatment approaches, including splenectomy and/or alkylating agents used singly or in combination [12,16,17], have demonstrated limited efficacy and have largely been abandoned. Median survival is historically reported to be 7 months [12] in patients receiving conventional chemotherapy; however, survival has increased following the introduction of relatively newer agents including the purine analogs and the anti-CD52 antibody (alemtuzumab; campath-1H).

Leukemias: Principles and Practice of Therapy, 1st edition. Edited by S. Faderl and H. Kantarjian.

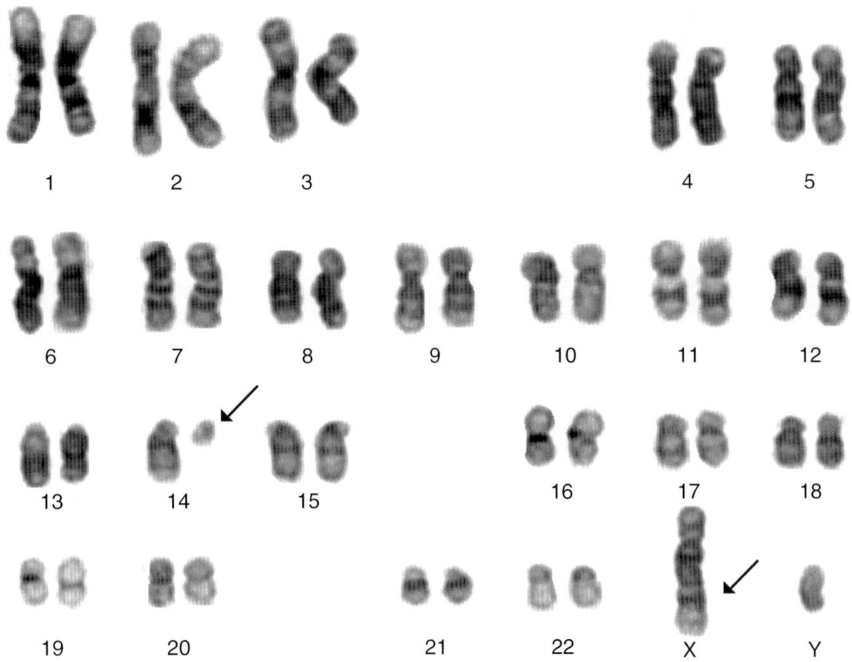

Figure 29.1 Conventional cytogenetics from a patient with T-cell prolymphocytic leukemia showing the t (14,X) translocation that results in the dysregulation of the proto-oncogene *MTCP1*.

Purine and pyrimidine analogs

The purine analogs fludarabine, cladribine, and pentostatin (DCF) share a similar chemical structure and mechanism of action, with effects on both quiescent and proliferating cells [18]. Anecdotal reports and case series have documented the efficacy of DCF in T-PLL [19–21]. This was first described by el'Agnaf *et al.* [19] who reported on two patients receiving DCF at 5 mg/m^2, one of whom remained in remission for over 1 year. A subsequent larger study (n = 55) of DCF in patients with T-PLL reported response rates of 45%, with 9% complete remissions (CRs) and a median response duration of 6 months [20]. Unlike standard approaches to the use of DCF in hairy cell leukemia, initial doses were given weekly for 4 weeks and then every 2 weeks to maximial response. Interestingly, no significant difference in response rate was observed between previously treated and untreated patients, rendering this agent a versatile option in treatment of T-PLL. A prospective phase II trial conducted by the EORTC (Leukemia Cooperative Group of the European Organisation for Research and Treatment of Cancer) used a similar dose schedule in six patients with previously treated T-PLL and reported response rates of 33% but no CR [21]. Equally positive results have been reported with cladribine, although study numbers are smaller [22,23]. The best results were obtained in untreated patients. More recent successes with gemcitabine [24] and purine analog combinations [25] have been reported. These agents have proven to be effective and relatively safe in patients with T-PLL when used as initial or salvage therapy.

Monoclonal antibody therapy

Expression of CD52 (the exact role of which remains undefined) is high on both normal and malignant T-cells. Ginaldi *et al.* [26] show that, by using semiquantitative flow cytometry, expression of this molecule is highest on T-PLL cells versus normal T-cells, and that these differences in antigen expression may indicate a trend toward higher response rates to treatment with the monoclonal anti-CD52 antibody, alemtuzumab. Alemtuzumab induces both complement-dependent cytotoxicity and antibody-dependent cytotoxicity [27,28], although other mechanisms of apoptosis, for example caspase-independent processes, are also implicated [29,30]. An initial anecdote of CR in a patient with T-PLL treated with alemtuzumab [29] was substantiated by a number of case series and prospective studies spanning a total of >150 patients with predominantly relapsed or refractory disease [31–35]. Anti-CD52 treatment proved effective as salvage therapy. Treatment was largely administered intravenously at a dose of 30 mg daily for 3 days per week following initial dose escalation. Re-treatment with alemtuzumab was able to induce second responses in patients relapsing after initial alemtuzumab therapy. As with the use of alemtuzumab in B-cell disorders, the best responses were observed in patients with blood, bone marrow, and splenic disease as opposed to patients with hepatic, central nervous system (CNS), or serous effusions [36]. Alemtuzumab was administered to 39 pretreated patients with T-PLL in a phase II multicenter study [32]. The results pointed to a higher overall response (76%) and CR (60%) than had previously been documented with any other treatment in this disorder. The depth of response was positively associated with prolongation of survival. Factors associated with non-response included third space effusions, liver involvement, and CNS involvement. Similar results were obtained in an American retrospective study of 76 pretreated patients, with an overall response rate (ORR) of 50% and a CR of 37.5% [33]. Although the response rates were superior, these remained finite, and stem-cell transplantation (SCT) in first remission was advocated in order to sustain response.

Treatment with alemtuzumab is not, however, without risk. Alemtuzumab causes prolonged T-cell depletion with significant immunosuppression and infective complications, as reported in approximately 13% of patients [33]. Prophylaxis for pneumocystis and herpetic infections is required both during treatment and for a protracted period after, and screening for cytomegalovirus (CMV) reactivation is advocated. The use of alemtuzumab in heavily pretreated, often elderly, patients is associated with an increased risk of infectious and other treatment-related complications. Used as first-line therapy, response rates are superior, with 100% CR rates achieved and a median response duration of 10 months (range 2–25 months) [37]. Tolerability is enhanced by such upfront use. This antibody has revolutionized the treatment of T-PLL, improving median survival from around 7 months to >2 years (Figure 29.2), and is now accepted as the standard.

German researchers from the chronic lymphocytic leukemia study group (GCLLSG) have reported on alemtuzumab as consolidation therapy after combination FCM (fludarabine, cyclophosphomide, and mitoxantrone) treatment [33] (T-PLL-1 protocol) following a 1–3-month washout period in treatment-naïve patients with T-PLL [25]. This approach increased ORR from 66% among 18 patients, including 12 treatment-naïve patients, to 87%, with a median overall survival of 19.2 months. A combination of alemtuzumab with purine analogs is also reported [38] with significantly better survival when compared with conventional chemotherapy. Such combinations do, however, increase the potential for opportunistic infections.

Stem-cell transplantation

Despite the success of newer agents in T-PLL, responses are not sustained and consolidation with autologous or allogeneic SCT has been adopted for patients with aggressive disease [39–43] in order to prolong survival. While autologous SCT can increase disease-free survival, one-third of such patients relapse [44,45]. Allogeneic SCT offers the potential for cure. Myeloablative approaches are challenging and often limited by advanced age, comorbidities, and poor performance status in addition to inherent transplant-related mortality. Reduced-intensity conditioning approaches were first described in a single case report [40], and while this patient relapsed and died 5 months post transplant, other researchers have documented long-term progression-free survival [43,46] using this approach.

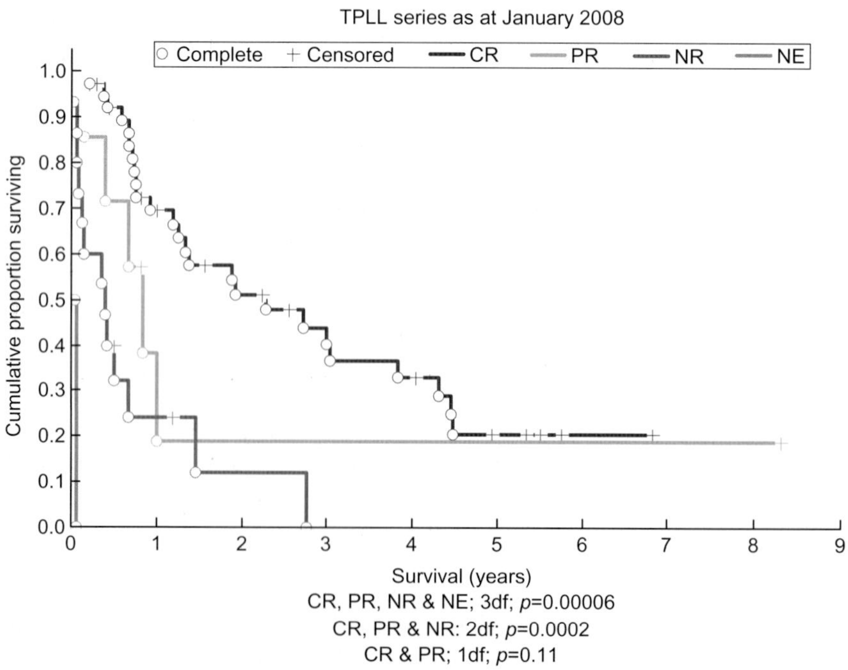

Figure 29.2 Kaplan-Meier survival curves from 54 patients with T-cell prolymphocytic leukemia (T-PLL) treated with alemtuzumab as first-line therapy or for relapsed/refractory disease showing results by response to treatment. CR, complete response; NE, non-evaluable; NR, no response; PR, partial response.

Monoclonal anti-CD52 antibody has emerged as the gold standard for treatment of patients with T-PLL. Such treatment should be consolidated by SCT where feasible. The use of alemtuzumab upfront is associated with superior response rates. This approach may improve the tolerability of the agent. Other agents, such as the purine analogs, remain a versatile option and may be used sequentially or concomitantly with alemtuzumab. Anti-infective prophylaxis and CMV monitoring is essential.

T-cell large granular lymphocyte leukemia

This disorder is becoming increasingly recognized. The median age at diagnosis is 60 years with equal gender predilection. The term "LGL leukemia" was first coined by Loughran [47] and later adopted into the WHO classification of tumors of the hematopoietic and lymphoid tissues [48]. This is a clonal lymphoproliferative condition derived from T cells that show a mature post-thymic phenotype. Most cases involve $CD8^+$ cytotoxic T cells; however, rarer incidences of $CD4^+$, $CD4^+$ $CD8^+$, and even $CD4^-$ $CD8^-$ disease are reported [49,50]. Aberrant expression of NK antigens is seen [50]. More recently, skewed expression of killer immunoglobulin-like receptors (KIRs) has also been described [49,51,52]. Although the etiology of this condition has not been fully elucidated, chronic activation of T cells by an autoreactive or viral antigen is believed to be involved in its pathogenesis [53–56]. This is evidenced in part by the non-random clonal selection demonstrated by the sequencing of the variable β (Vb)-chain complementarity determining region 3 (CDR3) [56] and by association with other immune-mediated bone marrow-failure syndromes. A polyclonal autoimmune response may represent the initiating element and explain the increased association of autoimmune disorders, including rheumatoid arthritis, systemic lupus erythematosus, Hashimoto's thyroiditis [47,57–59], and immune-mediated cytopenias. Preclinical studies also describe dysregulation of several intracellular signaling pathways, including the Fas/Fas ligand [60], phosphatidylicnositol-3 kinase (PI3K) [61], and mitogen-activated protein kinase/extracellular signal-regulated kinase/Ras (MAPK/ERK/Ras) [62], which may account for the inherent resistance to apoptosis in LGL cells *in vitro* [63]. The distortion of the Ras pathway [62] has led to the adoption of newer therapeutic strategies using farnesyl transferase inhibitors.

Unlike related mature T-cell disorders, T-LGL leukemia has a good median survival in excess of 10 years [64]. Although most cases of T-cell LGL leukemia are indolent, about 60% of patients will become symptomatic at some point in their disease [63,65]. Neutropenia, seen in 80% of patients and severely ($<0.5 \times 10^9$/L) in approximately 45% [47,49,64], remains the main indication for treatment. Possible mechanisms for neutropenia include deregulated Fas/Fas ligand-induced apoptosis of myeloid cells, immune complex or antibody-mediated neutrophil destruction, hypersplenism, or direct inhibition of myeloid maturation [49,64,66]. The aim of treatment in this disease also differs from its counterparts in that the objective has been primarily to alleviate cytopenias rather than necessarily eliminate the malignant clone.

Treatment data for T-cell LGL leukemia are derived from retrospective and prospective case series and single-institution studies. Asymptomatic patients are managed by careful observation [47,64]. Indications for treatment include recurrent infections, severe neutropenia, symptomatic anemia or thrombocytopenia, massive splenomegaly, and systemic features. Symptomatic improvement may occur despite failure to normalize neutrophil counts, and cytopenias may improve without eradication of the malignant clone [64,67,68].

Immunosuppressants

Immunosuppression using weekly methotrexate, oral cyclosporine, or low-dose cyclophosphamide have all proved effective in alleviating cytopenias, while more cytotoxic approaches such as CHOP (cytoxan, hydroxyrubicin, oncovin, and prednisone) have a limited effect [69]. Up to half of all patients treated with the single agent methotrexate achieve a CR that is sustained with continued treatment [68,70,71]. This treatment is well tolerated. Cyclophosphamide at 50–100 mg per day is an effective therapeutic alternative, with successes reported in many cases including patients with pure red cell aplasia [68,72]. Cyclosporine at 5–10 mg/kg per day also shows good efficacy [67,68,73,74], with a growing evidence base in the literature. HLA-DR4 status has been suggested to predict for response to cyclosporine in T-cell LGL leukemia [73]. CD26 expression has also been theorized to be prognostic in this disorder [75]. There are no randomized controlled trials directly comparing these agents, which are believed to act via immunomodulatory rather than cytotoxic mechanisms. The choice of agent may thus be dictated by patient- and/or center-specific features. Cyclosporine, methotrexate, and cyclophosphamide are all relatively disadvantaged by the need for long-term maintenance. Appropriate monitoring of blood counts, renal function, liver function, lung function, and/or cyclosporine levels is needed. Therapeutic cyclosporine levels are variable and dose may be titrated to response in the absence of toxicity [67,68]. Initial responses to these agents may be sluggish, and therapeutic trials should thus span at least 4 months before being abandoned [64,68]. Cross-resistance among these agents, which have all demonstrated good overall safety, efficacy, and tolerability in the majority of patients, is absent. While long-term treatment appears safe, reports of second malignancies [68] taken in conjunction with the intrinsic potential for high-grade transformation in T-cell LGL leukemia [76] raise a note of caution.

Purine analogs

The purine analogs including fludarabine, cladribine, and pentostatin have also demonstrated efficacy in T-cell LGL leukemia [20,77] and have the advantage of being administered as single, discrete courses without the need for long-term maintenance therapy. As such, they offer potentially attractive alternatives for younger symptomatic patients with T-cell LGL leukemia. Appropriate anti-infective prophylaxis is needed. Ma *et al.* [78] and Tse *et al.* [79] report on the successful use of combination chemotherapy with fludarabine, dexamethasone, and mitoxantrone in T-cell LGL leukemia.

Monoclonal antibodies

High CD52 expression on T-cell LGLs [80] support the anecdotally reported success of alemtuzumab in refractory disease [69,81,82], although long-term maintenance-type regimens have been applied in some instances with associated cost and immunosuppression implications. Other monoclonal antibodies, including anti-CD2 (Siplizumab; MedImmune, Gaitherburg, MD) and the humanized MiK-β 1 monoclonal antibody (anti-CD122—the β subunit of both interleukin 2 and interleukin 15 receptors) are being evaluated in phase I studies for T-cell LGL leukemia and other T-cell disorders. Both interleukin 2 and interleukin 15 are thought to impact on the proliferation, survival, and activity of LGLs [83,84]. Though well tolerated, MiK-β 1 monoclonal antibody treatment for T-cell LGL leukemia did not result in amelioration of cytopenias in any of the 12 patients treated with this agent, despite a downregulation of surface receptors seen in seven patients [85]. SCT has been described in a few anecdotal reports [86]. Conditioning and graft-versus-host disease (GVHD) prophylaxis regimens in these reports have been heavily immunosuppressive in nature and may thus have contributed to the responses observed. Initial growth factor and/or steroid therapy remain an option, and synergy has been described with both erythropoietin and colony stimulating factors when used in combination with immunosuppressive agents [68,73,87]. Long-term steroid therapy should be avoided owing to adverse effects. It is largely accepted that splenectomy, in the absence of splenic bulk and/or immune thrombocytopenia, has little to add to the management of T-cell LGL leukemia and often induces transient responses in the neutrophil count at the expense of increasing lymphocytosis [88,89].

$CD56^+$ variants

CD56 expression is thought to define a subgroup of T-cell LGL leukemia with younger age at onset, more aggressive disease evolution, and shorter survival [90–94]. Conventional management with combination systemic chemotherapy is said to be ineffective for this variant. Data available from limited studies suggest better results for $CD56^+$ variants using acute lymphoblastic leukemia (ALL)-type induction therapy consolidated with SCT in first remission [94].

Trials

There are few current phase II trials assessing treatment approaches for T-cell LGL leukemia. The National Cancer Institute (NCI)-sponsored Eastern Cooperative Oncology Group E5998 trial is evaluating the use of methotrexate at $10\,mg/m^2$/week with or without a tapering dose of prednisolone at 1 mg/kg in T-cell LGL leukemia with severe neutropenia or symptomatic anemia. Crossover to cyclophosphamide at 100 mg daily is offered to patients who fail to respond after 4 months. Another NCI-sponsored phase II trial looks at the efficacy of the farnesyl transferase inhibitor tipifarnib in symptomatic patients with T-cell LGL leukemia.

There remains no optimum standard of therapy for T-cell LGL leukemia. Active monitoring is appropriate in almost half of all patients who may be asymptomatic. Treatment is often indicated for cytopenias, usually neutropenia. The most common and successful reported approaches involve the use of low-dose methotrexate or cyclosporine, although agents such as the purine analogs and newer approaches, including the monoclonal antibodies, should not be discounted. As far as possible a collaborative research approach should be adopted to the management of this disorder. Aggressive $CD56^+$ T-cell LGL leukemia may warrant more intensive ALL-type treatment in order to induce remission, and SCT should be used in first remission.

Natural killer-cell leukemias

Natural killer-cell leukemias are surface $CD3^-$ disorders usually associated with a poor prognosis, and are common among younger patients of Asian descent [49,95]. These disorders show a germ-line T-cell receptor configuration, and detection of clonality has been difficult until recently when skewed expression of the KIRs on the surface of leukemic NK cells provided a surrogate marker of clonality [51,96,97]. The WHO classification of hematolymphoid malignancies recognizes three categories of NK-cell neoplasms, including blastic NK-cell lymphoma, aggressive NK-cell leukemia [98], and extranodal NK/T-cell lymphoma nasal-type. In addition, the WHO describes, although does not officially recognize, a more indolent, chronic form of NK-cell leukemia, which is thought to be reactive in most instances [98]. Aggressive NK-cell leukemia was originally described by Fernandez *et al.* [99] and

Koizumi *et al.* [100], then further established by Imamura *et al.* [101], Song *et al.* [102], and Suzuki *et al.* [103], and is diagnosed by the presence of LGLs showing $sCD3^-$, $CD3e^{+/-}$, leukemia $CD56^+/CD16^-/+$, $CD57^-$ phenotype with germ-line configuration of the T-cell receptor, and *IgH* genes. An association with EBV with clonal episomal viral integration is described, suggesting possible etiologic significance [104–106]. A rapidly progressive clinical course with B symptoms, hepatosplenomegaly, and lymphadenopathy [107] is seen, with hepatic dysfunction, disseminated intravascular coagulopathy, and hemophagocytic syndrome common particularly in the latter phases of the disease. Median overall survival is 2 months [103]. The influence of a number of cytokines, including CXCR1, CCR5 [108], IFN-α, TNF-α [109], Fas ligand [110], and interleukin 8 [111], are associated with the clinical manifestations observed. As with $CD56^+$ aggressive T-cell LGL leukemia, standard combination cytotoxic chemotherapy proves ineffective [112]. This may be partially explained by the presence of the multidrug resistance gene-encoded P-glycoprotein (P-gp) on the cell membrane. This P-gp extrudes various cytotoxic agents such as the vinca-alkaloids and anthracyclines [113,114]. Intensive ALL-like therapies that utilize P-gp unrelated agents such as methotrexate and ifosfamide are a better initial approach consolidated with SCT in first remission for patients achieving good responses to induction therapy [115]. Certainly for the nasal NK-cell lymphoma-related disorder, low asparaginase synthetase activity and high *in vitro* sensitivity to L-asparaginase [116] has been associated with successful anecdotal treatment of this disorder with single agent L-asparaginase [117]. Etoposide-containing regimens are also effective based on *in vitro* sensitivity data [118] and clinical data in pediatric EBV-related hemophagocytic syndromes [119]. Single-case reports also show efficacy for purine analogues [120].

Conversely, the more indolent proliferation of NK-LGLs, variably termed chronic NK-cell lymphocytosis, presents with incidental circulating NK-cell lymphocytosis without B symptoms, organomegaly, or lymphadenopathy. Cytopenias are less common and less severe than in T-cell LGL leukemia [121] and the disease is characterized by persistence of an expanded NK-cell LGL component in the blood for >6 months [121,122]. This disorder is considered to be reactively driven [123] although abnormal NK-receptor phenotypic expression has been documented [97]. Spontaneous regression may be seen, and rarely transformation to the aggressive NK-cell leukemia may occur. Treatment approaches are similar, with the vast majority of patients requiring simple surveillance. Where indicated for cytopenias, immunosuppressive approaches to treatment may be used.

There are limited data available on the management of patients with rarer NK-cell leukemias. Aggressive NK-cell leukemia warrants ALL-type induction therapy with the use of SCT as consolidation for responders, while chronic NK-cell lymphocytosis is usually asymptomatic and managed similarly to T-cell LGL leukemia.

Adult T-cell leukemia/lymphoma

A clear epidemiologic distribution is seen with ATLL, with most patients located in south–western Japan, the Caribbean, South America, Papua New Guinea, and intertropical Africa [124]. This distribution parallels that of HTLV-I, the etiologic agent in ATLL. HTLV-I may be transmitted from mother to infant, through sexual intercourse, and via blood products. Lifetime risks of developing ATLL are small (2–5%) with a long latency period [125]. ATLL is seen more commonly when HTLV-I is acquired in early life [126]. This presents a useful, preventive approach to the management of this disorder. ATLL cells show characteristic morphologic appearances (flower-like nuclei), express CD4 and CD25 on their surface membranes, and show monoclonal integration of the HTLV-I proviral DNA. Four distinct clinical presentations are reported, including acute, lymphoma, chronic, and smoldering subtypes [127]. Acute and lymphoma types show an aggressive disease course with limited therapeutic successes, while chronic and smouldering variants are more indolent. In the latter cases, initial treatment may be deferred until progression is seen. Major challenges in treating patients with ATLL relate not only to the intrinsic tumor resistance to conventional chemotherapies, but also to the inherently immunocompromised state of patients with associated potentially life-threatening opportunistic infections, including *Pneumocytis jiroveci, Candida, Cytomegalovirus,* and *Strongyloides stercoralis* [128]. Chemotherapy resistance is multifactorial with the expression of P-glycoproteins [129], lung resistance-related protein [130], antiapoptotic proteins [131,132], and activation of proliferation and survival signals [133,134]. Methods of safely bypassing these resistance mechanisms are crucial to achieving treatment success in this poor-prognosis disease. Management adopts a tripartite approach with disease control, virus suppression, and consolidation of response. CNS prophylaxis should be considered, particularly for acute and lymphoma subtypes.

Conventional chemotherapy

Combination cytotoxic therapy is utilized for patients with acute and lymphoma-type ATLL. Cumulative results from a number of prospective clinical trials run by the Japanese Clinical Oncology Group (JCOG) have utilized various vinca alkaloid-based combinations with or without etoposide or cisplatin with good effect and prolongation of survival to >1 year. The optimum suggested approach based on the LSG1 trial used VCAP (vincristine, cyclophosphamide, doxorubicin, and prednisolone)/AMP (doxorubicin, ranimustine, and prednisolone)/VECP (vindesine, etoposide, carboplatin, and prednisolone) in largely younger patients with a good performance status [135]. Other reported chemotherapy combinations including RCM (vindesine, adriamycin, pirarubicin, cyclophosphamide, etoposide, ranimustine, methotrexate, peplomycin, prednisolone) [136], OPEC (vincristine, etoposide, prednisolone, and cyclophosphamide)/MPEC (methotrexate, etoposide, prednisolone, and cyclophosphamide) [137] and ATL-G-SCF (vincristine, vindesine, adriamycin, mitoxantrone, cylcophosphamide, etoposide, ranimustine, and prednisolone with G-CSF support) [138] have also yielded some success in a more elderly, less fit patient cohort, although none of these combinations have equalled the survival benefits reported by JCOG. These regimens share a basis of more frequent cycles of chemotherapy (given weekly), an approach that the authors believe may offer greater advantages in achieving and maintaining disease control in ATLL. G-CSF support is usually needed to facilitate chemotherapy. Analogous to these regimens are the more commonly used PMitCEBO(M) and, more recently, CHOP-14. The latter combination has demonstrated a 66% overall response (25% CR) among 61 patients with a median survival of 13 months [135]. Three-year overall survival post-CHOP-14 treatment for ATLL is 12.7% with a median survival of 10.9 months [139], while those of the more potent VCAP/VECP combination were 23.6% and 12.7 months, respectively. Intrathecal prophylaxis with methotrexate and prednisolone is essential since CNS disease is present in 10–25% of patients with ATLL [140,141].

Etoposide is emerging as a useful drug used singly or in combination [137,142]. Matsushita *et al.* [137] suggest an oral regimen utilizing etoposide at 25 mg daily with prednisolone at 10 mg, and report superior results to some multidrug regimens. Other drugs used with variable success in ATLL include the purine analogs pentostatin [20,143,144] and cladribine [145], which show modest activity, and ironotecan, which, when used alone, induced responses in 5 of 13 patients with refractory ATLL including one CR [146]. The oral topoisomerase II inhibitor (MST-16) shows some promise in the treatment of naïve and pretreated patients with ATLL, with responses seen in 9 of 23 patients, including one CR [147].

Antiretroviral therapy

The single agent interferon (IFN) shows modest *in vitro* activity [148,149] and there are anecdotal reports of clinical response [150–153]; however, no significant benefit was seen with IFN-α in a prospective clinical trial of patients with acute and lymphoma-type ATLL. This agent may be beneficial in cutaneous ATLL lesions [151].

Use of antiretroviral therapy with zidovudine (AZT) and IFN-α, as reported in a number of phase I/II studies, induces a high response rate with enhanced survival [154–158]. Toxicity is manageable and largely hematologic in nature. Median time to response for use of this combination upfront in ATLL is 60 days (range 10–250 days) [157], and recent consensus suggests that the use of combination cytotoxic therapy to reduce tumor burden prior to initiation AZT and IFN-α therapy may improve therapeutic outcomes in patients with progressive and/or aggressive disease. This combination is thought to work not just by reducing HTLV-I proviral loads but may also have an antiangiogenic effect by reducing plasma vascular endothelial growth factor (VEGF) levels in patients with ATLL [159]. AZT is also thought to inhibit the elevated telomerase activity seen in ATLL-infected cells [160–162], thereby enhancing activity of anticancer agents [163–166]. There is some suggestion that progressive telomerase shortening induced by AZT is followed by increased production of $p14^{ARF}$, a pro-apoptotic agent, as well as activation and stabilization of p53 [167].

Stem-cell transplantation

Autologous SCT offers little benefit in ATLL because of early relapse [168]; however, retrospective analyses suggest that allogeneic SCT may prolong survival [169,170]. Median leukemia-free survival among 10 patients with ATLL post-allogeneic SCT was 17.5 months. Graft-versus-leukemia effects are thought to be crucial here, with relapses seen in cases where GVHD was absent [169], re-attainment of responses in relapsed patients when immunosuppressive therapy is withdrawn or donor lymphocytes are infused [171], and increases in Tax-specific cytotoxic T-lymphocytes in patients with ATLL post SCT are seen [172]. Matched-related donors may be limited because of HTLV-I infection [173], which may potentially result in donor-derived T-cell leukemia post transplantation [174]. Matched-unrelated donor transplantation, despite higher transplant-related mortality, remains feasible [175]; however, many patients with ATLL are older and reduced-intensity conditioning regimens are being prospectively evaluated with greater efficacy and tolerability reported [176].

Monoclonal antibodies

Molecules expressed on ATLL cells such as CD4, CD25, and CD52 are attractive targets for therapy. CD25 especially has been investigated. This interleukin 2 receptor alpha molecule is not expressed on normal resting cells. Initial reports of murine anti-CD25 inducing responses in patients with acute and chronic ATLL without significant toxicity caused optimism. Treatment failures were postulated to occur in aggressive disease where IL-2-independent ATLL cells were thought to be proliferating

[177]. An yttrium-90 conjugated anti-CD25 antibody was therefore utilized and did indeed result in improved event-free survival as opposed to the naked antibody compound. Toxicity was marked with grade 3 hepatotoxicity and myelosuppression [178]. Other anti-CD25 antibodies/conjugates, including the humanized daclizumab [179], the pseudomonas–exotoxin conjugate [180], and IL-2 fused with the diphtheria toxin denileukin [181], showed some efficacy, although availability of these agents is variable. Anti-CD52 antibody alemtuzumab [182,183], anti-CD2 MoAb siplizumab [184], and anti-CD4 antibody zanolimumab [185] have been reported among small numbers of patients in preliminary studies. The risk of opportunistic infections such as cytomegalovirus reactivation and development of EBV-associated lymphoproliferative disorders should be considered when depleting normal T cells that express these target molecules in a patient who is already intrinsically immunocompromised. The CC chemokine receptor 4 (CCR4) is frequently expressed on ATLL cells. A clinical study investigating the use of chimeric anti-CCR4 antibody (KM2760) is currently under way in Japan [186,187]. *In vitro* activity of an anti-transferrin receptor, MoAb [188], is also a promising prospect for future clinical studies.

NF-κB-directed treatment

NF-κB activation has been reported in ATLL cells [189,190]. Unfortunately, the success of bortezomib, a potent NF-κB inhibitor, in inducing cell death in HTLV-I-associated cell lines and in murine models when used in combination with anti-CD25 [191,192] has not always translated into clinical success [193]. However, the histone deacetylase inhibitor depsipeptide successfully inhibits NF-κB in ATLL and induces apoptosis [194].

Arsenic trioxide is most commonly used in treating acute promyelocytic leukemia, and has been used in ATLL with or without IFN-α, inducing responses in approximately 50% of patients with relapsed/refractory disease [195,196], although patient numbers were small in these series. Such responses are more likely when arsenic trioxide is combined with IFN-α [195], and are thought to be restricted to patients with moderately aggressive relapsed or refractory ATLL as opposed to those with rampantly progressive disease [196]. The side-effects are manageable and are mainly hematologic or neurologic in nature. Less common, although severe, events include infection and effects on the QT interval. Arsenic trioxide switches off the NF-κB pathway and, when combined with IFN-α, specifically reverses two distinct gene networks essential for the survival of HTLV-I-infected leukemic cells [197–199]. This inhibition may be enhanced *in vitro* by compounds such as docosahexaenoic acid and emodin [200].

These agents warrant further elucidation either alone or in combination.

Other aspects of management

Appropriate caution must be addressed to managing associated and underlying complications seen in ATLL. One such complication is hypercalcemia (present in 70% of patients), which may be severe, and all those presenting with ATLL should be tested for this disorder. Hypercalcemia should be treated with aggressive hydration, intravenous bisphosphonate, and glucocorticoids. Infective complications are an important cause of morbidity and mortality in ATLL. The *Pneumocystis jiroveci* infection is commonly seen in patients with ATLL [201] and may be exacer-bated by treatment itself. Standard prophylaxis with cotrimoxazole/sulfamethoxazole is advocated.

On a global level, prevention remains a cornerstone in managing this condition. A vital aspect in the management of this disorder is the identification of family members with the HTLV-I virus. While the lifetime risk of developing ATLL remains small, other HTLV-I associated conditions may be diagnosed earlier and transmission of the virus by vertical means or breastfeeding may be reduced.

Initial treatment with combination chemotherapy, preferably administered on a 1–2-weekly cycle, is advantageous in achieving disease control. Antiretroviral therapy is an integral part of controlling the disease and maintaining response. Curative options should be sought where appropriate, using SCT in first response. Family members should be screened to reduce further viral transmission, to diagnose other associated pathologies, and to identify possible matched-related donors. Alemtuzumab offers a useful therapeutic alternative particularly for refractory disease and/or in the presence of p53 abnormalities. This agent also benefits from a maintenance-type administrative schedule, which may help to hold the disease in remission while SCT is arranged.

Conclusion

Despite the clinicopathologic heterogeneity seen between and within the leukemias of mature T cell origin, a uniting theme is the lack of response to chemotherapy and the need for therapeutic agents to be delivered with increasing regularity and/or maintenance-type schedules to sustain responses. Multistage pathogenic processes often limit the utility of conventional agents/approaches, and therapeutic progress has been attained by specifically targeting surface molecules, etiologic agents, and/or methods of bypassing mechanisms of resistance. Interestingly, active surveillance is a well-recognized initial strategy for many of these leukemias. Treatment decisions for aggressive T/NK-cell leukemias should be comprehensive from the outset and should anticipate methods for consolidation so that remission induction can be suitably refined to maximize efficacy but minimize treatment-related toxicities, which may subsequently thwart opportunities for SCT. Therapeutic advances have been hampered by the rarity of these disorders and the singular approaches to clinical studies. Universal frameworks for investigating and treating these uncommon malignancies will help to optimize treatment decisions.

References

1 Catovsky D, Galetto J, Okos A, Galton DA, Wiltshaw E, Stathopoulos G. Prolymphocytic leukemia of B and T cell type. *Lancet* 1973;2:232–4.

2 Galton DA, Goldman JM, Wiltshaw E, Catovsky D, Henry K, Goldenberg GJ. Prolymphocytic leukemia. *Br J Haematol* 1974;27:7–23.

3 Cao TM, Coutre SE. T-cell prolymphocytic leukemia: update and focus on alemtuzumab (Campath-1H). *Hematology* 2003; 8:1–6.

4 Ravandi F, Kantarjian H, Jones D, Dearden C, Keating M, O'Brien S. Mature T-cell leukemias. *Cancer* 2005;104:1808–18.

5 Brito-Babapulle V, Pomfret M, Matutes E, Catovsky D. Cytogenetic studies on prolymphocytic leukemia. II. T cell prolymphocytic leukemia. *Blood* 1987;70:926–31.

6 Virgilio L, Lazzeri C, Bichi R, *et al*. Deregulated expression of *TCL1* causes T cell leukemia in mice. *Proc Natl Acad Sci U S A* 1998;95:3885–9.

7 Gritti C, Dastot H, Soulier J, *et al*. Transgenic mice for MTCP1 develop T-cell prolymphocytic leukemia. *Blood* 1998;92: 368–73.

8 Laine J, Kunstle G, Obata T, Sha M, Noguchi M. The protooncogene *TCL1* is an Akt kinase coactivator. *Mol Cell* 2000;6: 395–407.

9 Kang SM, Narducci MG, Lazzeri C, *et al*. Impaired T- and B-cell development in *Tcl1*-deficient mice. *Blood* 2005;105: 1288–94.

10 Shen RR, Ferguson DO, Renard M, *et al*. Dysregulated *TCL1* requires the germinal center and genome instability for mature B-cell transformation. *Blood* 2006;108:1991–8.

11 Catovksy D, Ralfkiaer E, Muller-Hermelink HK. T-cell prolymphocytic leukemia. In: Jaffe ES, Harris NL, Stein H, Vardiman JW, (eds). *Classification of Tumors Pathology and Genetics of Tumors of Hematopoietic and Lymphoid Tissues*. IARC Press: Lyon, 2001. pp.195–6.

12 Matutes E, Brito-Babapulle V, Swansbury J, *et al*. Clinical and laboratory features of 78 cases of T-prolymphocytic leukemia. *Blood* 1991;78:3269–74.

13 Domingo-Domenech E, Gonzalez-Barca E, Salar A, Claros AD, Granena A. Indolent course as presentation in t-prolymphocytic leukemia. *Br J Haematol* 1999;105:840.

14 Hoyer JD, Ross CW, Li CY, *et al*. True T-cell chronic lymphocytic leukemia: a morphologic and immunophenotypic study of 25 cases. *Blood* 1995;86:1163–9.

15 Garand R, Goasguen J, Brizard A, *et al*. Indolent course as a relatively frequent presentation in T-prolymphocytic leukemia. Groupe Francais d'Hematologie Cellulaire. *Br J Haematol* 1998;103:488–94.

16 Newland AC, Turnbull AL, Bainbridge D, Jenkins GC. Complete remission in T-cell prolymphocytic leukemia. *Br J Haematol* 1980;45:513–14.

17 Taylor HG, Butler WM, Rhoads J, Karcher DS, Detrick-Hooks B. Prolymphocytic leukemia: treatment with combination chemotherapy to include doxorubicin. *Cancer* 1982;49: 1524–9.

18 Robak T, Korycka A, Kasznicki M, Wrzesien-Kus A, Smolewski P. Purine nucleoside analogs for the treatment of hematological malignancies: pharmacology and clinical applications. *Curr Cancer Drug Targets* 2005;5:421–44.

19 el'Agnaf MR, Ennis KE, Morris TC, Robertson JH, Markey G, Alexander HD. Successful remission induction with deoxycoformycin in elderly patients with T-helper prolymphocytic leukemia. *Br J Haematol* 1986;63:93–104.

20 Mercieca J, Matutes E, Dearden C, MacLennan K, Catovsky D. The role of pentostatin in the treatment of T-cell malignancies: analysis of response rate in 145 patients according to disease subtype. *J Clin Oncol* 1994;12:2588–93.

21 Dohner H, Ho AD, Thaler J, *et al*. Pentostatin in prolymphocytic leukemia: phase II trial of the European Organization for Research and Treatment of Cancer Leukemia Cooperative Study Group. *J Natl Cancer Inst* 1993;85:658–62.

22 Palomera L, Domingo JM, Agullo JA, Soledad Romero M. Complete remission in T-cell prolymphocytic leukemia with 2-chlorodeoxyadenosine. *J Clin Oncol* 1995;13:1284–5.

23 Delannoy A. 2-chloro-2'-deoxyadenosine:clinical applications in hematology. *Blood Rev* 1996;10:148–66.

24 Sallah S, Wan JY, Nguyen NP. Treatment of refractory T-cell malignancies using gemcitabine. *Br J Haematol* 2001;113: 185–7.

25 Hopfinger G, Raymonde B, Eichhorst B, *et al*. T-PLL 1 protocol of the German CLL Study Group (GCLLSG)—A prospective phase II trial of fludarabine phosphate, mitoxantrone and cyclophosphamide (FMC) followed by alemtuzumab consolidation in T-PLL. *Blood* 2007;110:2039.

26 Ginaldi L, De Martinis M, Matutes E, *et al*. Levels of expression of CD52 in normal and leukemic B and T cells: correlation with *in vivo* therapeutic responses to Campath-1H. *Leuk Res* 1998;22:185–91.

27 Ravandi F, O'Brien S. Alemtuzumab. *Expert Rev Anticancer Ther* 2005;5:39–51.

28 Robak T. Alemtuzumab in the treatment of chronic lymphocytic leukemia. *BioDrugs* 2005;19:9–22.

29 Smolewski P, Szmigielska-Kaplon A, Cebula B, *et al*. Proapoptotic activity of alemtuzumab alone and in combination with rituximab or purine nucleoside analogs in chronic lymphocytic leukemia cells. *Leuk Lymphoma* 2005;46:87–100.

30 Mone AP, Cheney C, Banks AL, *et al*. Alemtuzumab induces caspase-independent cell death in human chronic lymphocytic leukemia cells through a lipid raft-dependent mechanism. *Leukemia* 2006;20:272–9.

31 Pawson R, Dyer MJ, Barge R, *et al*. Treatment of T-cell prolymphocytic leukemia with human CD52 antibody. *J Clin Oncol* 1997;15:2667–72.

32 Dearden CE, Matutes E, Cazin B, *et al*. High remission rate in T-cell prolymphocytic leukemia with CAMPATH-1H. *Blood* 2001;98:1721–6.

33 Keating MJ, Cazin B, Coutre S, *et al*. Campath-1H treatment of T-cell prolymphocytic leukemia in patients for whom at

least one prior chemotherapy regimen has failed. *J Clin Oncol* 2002;20:205–13.
34 Ferrajoli A, O'Brien SM, Cortes JE, *et al.* Phase II study of alemtuzumab in chronic lymphoproliferative disorders. *Cancer* 2003;98:773–8.
35 McCune SL, Gockerman JP, Moore JO, *et al.* Alemtuzumab in relapsed or refractory chronic lymphocytic leukemia and prolymphocytic leukemia. *Leuk Lymphoma* 2002;43:1007–11.
36 Robak T, Robak P. Current treatment options in prolymphocytic leukemia. *Med Sci Monit* 2007;13:RA69–80.
37 Dearden CE, Matutes E, Cazin B, Catovsky D. Very high response rates in previously untreated T-cell prolymphocytic leukemia patients receiving alemtuzumab therapy. *Blood* 2003;102:644.
38 Ravandi F, Gandhi V. Novel purine nucleoside analogs for T-cell-lineage acute lymphoblastic leukemia and lymphoma. *Expert Opin Investig Drugs* 2006;15:1601–13.
39 Murase K, Matsunaga T, Sato T, *et al.* Allogeneic bone marrow transplantation in a patient with T-prolymphocytic leukemia with small-intestinal involvement. *Int J Clin Oncol* 2003;8: 391–4.
40 Garderet L, Bittencourt H, Kaliski A, *et al.* Treatment of T-prolymphocytic leukemia with nonmyeloablative allogeneic stem cell transplantation. *Eur J Haematol* 2001;66:137–9.
41 Collins RH, Pineiro LA, Agura ED, Fay JW. Treatment of T prolymphocytic leukemia with allogeneic bone marrow transplantation. *Bone Marrow Transplant* 1998;21:627–8.
42 Shvidel L, Shtalrid M, Klepfish A, Haran M, Berrebi A. Successful autologous stem cell transplantation in aggressive prolymphocytic leukemia. *Am J Hematol* 2000;63:230–1.
43 Tanimoto TE, Hirano A, Nagafuji K, *et al.* Mismatched unrelated cord blood transplantation in a patient with T-cell prolymphocytic leukemia. *Leukemia* 2005;19:679–81.
44 Krishnan B, Matutes E, Dearden C. Prolymphocytic leukemias. *Semin Oncol* 2006;33:257–63.
45 Krishnan B, Swansbury J, Cazin B, *et al.* Clinical outcome of stem cell transplantation (SCT) in patients with T cell prolymphocytic leukemia (T-PLL) previously treated with alemtuzumab: a multicentre experience. *Blood* (ASH Annual Meeting Abstracts) 2005;106:1127.
46 Curtin NJ, Schwarer AP. Nonmyeloablative peripheral blood stem cell transplant for T-cell prolymphocytic leukemia complicated by fulminant haemolysis and acute renal failure at engraftment secondary to minor ABO incompatibility. *Clin Lab Haematol* 2005;27:206–8.
47 Loughran TP, Jr. Clonal diseases of large granular lymphocytes. *Blood* 1993;82:1–14.
48 Chan WC, Catovsky D, Foucar K, Monserrat E. T-cell large granular lymphocyte leukemia. In: Jaffe ES, Harris NL, Stein H, Vardiman JW, (eds). *Pathology and Genetics of Tumors of Hematopoietic and Lymphoid Tissues.* IARC Press: Lyon, 2001. pp.197–8.
49 Lamy T, Loughran TP, Jr. Clinical features of large granular lymphocyte leukemia. *Semin Hematol* 2003;40:185–95.
50 Semenzato G, Zambello R, Starkebaum G, Oshimi K, Loughran TP, Jr. The lymphoproliferative disease of granular lymphocytes: updated criteria for diagnosis. *Blood* 1997;89: 256–60.
51 Morice WG, Kurtin PJ, Leibson PJ, Tefferi A, Hanson CA. Demonstration of aberrant T-cell and natural killer-cell antigen expression in all cases of granular lymphocytic leukemia. *Br J Haematol* 2003;120:1026–36.
52 Fischer L, Hummel M, Burmeister T, Schwartz S, Thiel E. Skewed expression of natural-killer (NK)-associated antigens on lymphoproliferations of large granular lymphocytes (LGL). *Hematol Oncol* 2006;24:78–85.
53 Zambello R, Trentin L, Facco M, *et al.* Analysis of the T cell receptor in the lymphoproliferative disease of granular lymphocytes: superantigen activation of clonal CD3+ granular lymphocytes. *Cancer Res* 1995;55:6140–5.
54 O'Keefe CL, Plasilova M, Wlodarski M, *et al.* Molecular analysis of TCR clonotypes in LGL: a clonal model for polyclonal responses. *J Immunol* 2004;172:1960–9.
55 Kanchan K, Loughran TP, Jr. Antigen-driven clonal T cell expansion in disorders of hematopoiesis. *Leuk Res* 2003;27: 291–2.
56 Wlodarski MW, O'Keefe C, Howe EC, *et al.* Pathologic clonal cytotoxic T-cell responses: nonrandom *Nature* of the T-cell-receptor restriction in large granular lymphocyte leukemia. *Blood* 2005;106:2769–80.
57 Loughran TP, Jr., Deeg HJ, Storb R. Morphologic and phenotypic analysis of canine natural killer cells: evidence for T-cell lineage. *Cell Immunol* 1985;95:207–17.
58 Sampalo Lainz A, Lopez-Gomez M, Jimenez-Alonso J. [Proliferation of large granular lymphocytes in patients with systemic lupus erythematosus]. *Rev Clin Esp* 1995;195: 373–9.
59 Starkebaum G. Chronic neutropenia associated with autoimmune disease. *Semin Hematol* 2002;39:121–7.
60 Lamy T, Liu JH, Landowski TH, Dalton WS, Loughran TP, Jr. Dysregulation of CD95/CD95 ligand-apoptotic pathway in CD3(+) large granular lymphocyte leukemia. *Blood* 1998;92: 4771–7.
61 Schade AE, Powers JJ, Wlodarski MW, Maciejewski JP. Phosphatidylinositol-3-phosphate kinase pathway activation protects leukemic large granular lymphocytes from undergoing homeostatic apoptosis. *Blood* 2006;107:4834–40.
62 Epling-Burnette PK, Bai F, Wei S, *et al.* ERK couples chronic survival of NK cells to constitutively activated Ras in lymphoproliferative disease of granular lymphocytes (LDGL). *Oncogene* 2004;23:9220–9.
63 Lamy T, Loughran TP, Jr. Current concepts: large granular lymphocyte leukemia. *Blood Rev* 1999;13:230–40.
64 Sokol L, Loughran TP, Jr. Large granular lymphocyte leukemia. *Oncologist* 2006;11:263–73.
65 Pandolfi F, Loughran TP, Jr., Starkebaum G, *et al.* Clinical course and prognosis of the lymphoproliferative disease of granular lymphocytes. A multicenter study. *Cancer* 1990;65: 341–8.
66 Liu JH, Wei S, Lamy T, *et al.* Chronic neutropenia mediated by fas ligand. *Blood* 2000;95:3219–22.
67 Sood R, Stewart CC, Aplan PD, *et al.* Neutropenia associated with T-cell large granular lymphocyte leukemia: long-term response to cyclosporine therapy despite persistence of abnormal cells. *Blood* 1998;91:3372–8.
68 Osuji N, Matutes E, Tjonnfjord G, *et al.* T-cell large granular lymphocyte leukemia: A report on the treatment of 29 patients and a review of the literature. *Cancer* 2006;107:570–8.
69 Osuji N, Matutes E, Wotherspoon A, Catovsky D. Lessons from a case of T-cell large granular lymphocytic leukemia

suggesting that immunomodulatory therapy is more effective than intensive treatment. *Leuk Res* 2005;29:225–8.
70 Loughran TP, Jr., Kidd PG, Starkebaum G. Treatment of large granular lymphocyte leukemia with oral low-dose methotrexate. *Blood* 1994;84:2164–70.
71 Hamidou MA, Sadr FB, Lamy T, Raffi F, Grolleau JY, Barrier JH. Low-dose methotrexate for the treatment of patients with large granular lymphocyte leukemia associated with rheumatoid arthritis. *Am J Med* 2000;108:730–2.
72 Dhodapkar MV, Lust JA, Phyliky RL. T-cell large granular lymphocytic leukemia and pure red cell aplasia in a patient with type I autoimmune polyendocrinopathy: response to immunosuppressive therapy. *Mayo Clin Proc* 1994;69:1085–8.
73 Battiwalla M, Melenhorst J, Saunthararajah Y, *et al.* HLA-DR4 predicts haematological response to cyclosporine in T-large granular lymphocyte lymphoproliferative disorders. *Br J Haematol* 2003;123:449–53.
74 Gabor EP, Mishalani S, Lee S. Rapid response to cyclosporine therapy and sustained remission in large granular lymphocyte leukemia. *Blood* 1996;87:1199–200.
75 Dang NH, Aytac U, Sato K, *et al.* T-large granular lymphocyte lymphoproliferative disorder: expression of CD26 as a marker of clinically aggressive disease and characterization of marrow inhibition. *Br J Haematol* 2003;121:857–65.
76 Matutes E, Wotherspoon AC, Parker NE, Osuji N, Isaacson PG, Catovsky D. Transformation of T-cell large granular lymphocyte leukemia into a high-grade large T-cell lymphoma. *Br J Haematol* 2001;115:801–6.
77 Witzig TE, Weitz JJ, Lundberg JH, Tefferi A. Treatment of refractory T-cell chronic lymphocytic leukemia with purine nucleoside analogs. *Leuk Lymphoma* 1994;14:137–9.
78 Ma SY, Au WY, Chim CS, *et al.* Fludarabine, mitoxantrone and dexamethasone in the treatment of indolent B- and T-cell lymphoid malignancies in Chinese patients. *Br J Haematol* 2004; 124:754–61.
79 Tse E, Chan JC, Pang A, *et al.* Fludarabine, mitoxantrone and dexamethasone as first-line treatment for T-cell large granular lymphocyte leukemia. *Leukemia* 2007;21:2225–6.
80 Osuji N, Del Giudice I, Matutes E, *et al.* CD52 expression in T-cell large granular lymphocyte leukemia-Implications for treatment with alemtuzumab. *Leuk Lymphoma* 2005;46:723–7.
81 Rosenblum MD, LaBelle JL, Chang CC, Margolis DA, Schauer DW, Vesole DH. Efficacy of alemtuzumab treatment for refractory T-cell large granular lymphocytic leukemia. *Blood* 2004;103:1969–71.
82 Ru X, Liebman HA. Successful treatment of refractory pure red cell aplasia associated with lymphoproliferative disorders with the antiCD52 monoclonal antibody alemtuzumab (Campath-1H). *Br J Haematol* 2003;123:278–81.
83 Lamy T, Loughran TP. Large granular lymphocyte leukemia. *Cancer Control* 1998;5:25–33.
84 Aprile JA, Russo M, Pepe MS, Loughran TP, Jr. Activation signals leading to proliferation of normal and leukemic CD3+ large granular lymphocytes. *Blood* 1991;78:1282–5.
85 Morris JC, Janik JE, White JD, *et al.* Preclinical and phase I clinical trial of blockade of IL-15 using Mikbeta1 monoclonal antibody in T cell large granular lymphocyte leukemia. *Proc Natl Acad Sci U S A* 2006;103:401–6.
86 Toze CL, Shepherd JD, Connors JM, *et al.* Allogeneic bone marrow transplantation for low-grade lymphoma and chronic lymphocytic leukemia. *Bone Marrow Transplant* 2000;25: 605–12.
87 Lamy T, LePrise PY, Amiot L, *et al.* Response to granulocyte-macrophage colony-stimulating factor (GM-CSF) but not to G-CSF in a case of agranulocytosis associated with large granular lymphocyte (LGL) leukemia. *Blood* 1995;85:3352–3.
88 Loughran TP, Jr., Starkebaum G, Clark E, Wallace P, Kadin ME. Evaluation of splenectomy in large granular lymphocyte leukemia. *Br J Haematol* 1987;67:135–40.
89 Gentile TC, Loughran TP, Jr. Resolution of autoimmune hemolytic anemia following splenectomy in CD3+ large granular lymphocyte leukemia. *Leuk Lymphoma* 1996;23:405–8.
90 Gentile TC, Uner AH, Hutchison RE, *et al.* CD3+, CD56+ aggressive variant of large granular lymphocyte leukemia. *Blood* 1994;84:2315–21.
91 Macon WR, Williams ME, Greer JP, *et al.* Natural killer-like T-cell lymphomas: aggressive lymphomas of T-large granular lymphocytes. *Blood* 1996;87:1474–83.
92 Passetto Falcao R, Pinto Simoes B, Garcia AB, Fonseca BA, Terra Filho J. Aggressive variant of morphologically typical T large granular lymphocyte leukemia/lymphoma lacking NK cell markers. *Acta Haematol* 2000;104:110–14.
93 Tordjman R, Macintyre E, Emile JF, *et al.* Aggressive acute CD3+, CD56- T cell large granular lymphocyte leukemia with two stages of maturation arrest. *Leukemia* 1996;10:1514–19.
94 Alekshun TJ, Tao J, Sokol L. Aggressive T-cell large granular lymphocyte leukemia: a case report and review of the literature. *Am J Hematol* 2007;82:481–5.
95 Cheung MM, Chan JK, Wong KF. Natural killer cell neoplasms: a distinctive group of highly aggressive lymphomas/ leukemias. *Semin Hematol* 2003;40:221–32.
96 Zambello R, Falco M, Della Chiesa M, *et al.* Expression and function of KIR and natural cytotoxicity receptors in NK-type lymphoproliferative diseases of granular lymphocytes. *Blood* 2003;102:1797–805.
97 Zambello R, Semenzato G. Natural killer receptors in patients with lymphoproliferative diseases of granular lymphocytes. *Semin Hematol* 2003;40:201–12.
98 Chan W C, Wong KF, Jaffe ES, Ralfiaer E. Aggressive NK-cell leukemia. In: Jaffe ES, Harris NL, Stein H, Vardiman JW, (eds). *Pathology and Genetics of Tumours of Haematopoietic and Lymphoid Tissues*. IARC Press: Lyon, 2001. pp.198–200.
99 Fernandez LA, Pope B, Lee C, Zayed E. Aggressive natural killer cell leukemia in an adult with establishment of an NK cell line. *Blood* 1986;67:925–30.
100 Koizumi S, Seki H, Tachinami T, *et al.* Malignant clonal expansion of large granular lymphocytes with a Leu-11+, Leu-7- surface phenotype: *in vitro* responsiveness of malignant cells to recombinant human interleukin 2. *Blood* 1986;68:1065–73.
101 Imamura N, Kusunoki Y, Kawa-Ha K, *et al.* Aggressive natural killer cell leukemia/lymphoma: report of four cases and review of the literature. Possible existence of a new clinical entity originating from the third lineage of lymphoid cells. *Br J Haematol* 1990;75:49–59.
102 Song SY, Kim WS, Ko YH, Kim K, Lee MH, Park K. Aggressive natural killer cell leukemia: clinical features and treatment outcome. *Haematologica* 2002;87:1343–5.
103 Suzuki R, Suzumiya J, Nakamura S, *et al.* Aggressive natural killer-cell leukemia revisited: large granular lymphocyte leukemia of cytotoxic NK cells. *Leukemia* 2004;18:763–70.

104 Chan JK, Sin VC, Wong KF, *et al*. Nonnasal lymphoma expressing the natural killer cell marker CD56: a clinicopathologic study of 49 cases of an uncommon aggressive neoplasm. *Blood* 1997;89:4501–13.

105 Kawa-Ha K, Ishihara S, Ninomiya T, *et al*. CD3-negative lymphoproliferative disease of granular lymphocytes containing Epstein–Barr viral DNA. *J Clin Invest* 1989;84:51–5.

106 Siu LL, Chan JK, Kwong YL. Natural killer cell malignancies: clinicopathologic and molecular features. *Histol Histopathol* 2002;17:539–54.

107 Oshimi K, Yamada O, Kaneko T, *et al*. Laboratory findings and clinical courses of 33 patients with granular lymphocyte-proliferative disorders. *Leukemia* 1993;7:782–8.

108 Makishima H, Ito T, Asano N, *et al*. Significance of chemokine receptor expression in aggressive NK cell leukemia. *Leukemia* 2005;19:1169–74.

109 Lay JD, Tsao CJ, Chen JY, Kadin ME, Su IJ. Upregulation of tumor necrosis factor-alpha gene by Epstein–Barr virus and activation of macrophages in Epstein–Barr virus-infected T cells in the pathogenesis of hemophagocytic syndrome. *J Clin Invest* 1997;100:1969–79.

110 Kato K, Ohshima K, Ishihara S, Anzai K, Suzumiya J, Kikuchi M. Elevated serum soluble Fas ligand in natural killer cell proliferative disorders. *Br J Haematol* 1998;103:1164–6.

111 Makishima H, Ito T, Momose K, *et al*. Chemokine system and tissue infiltration in aggressive NK-cell leukemia. *Leuk Res* 2007;31:1237–45.

112 Ruskova A, Thula R, Chan G. Aggressive natural killer-cell leukemia: report of five cases and review of the literature. *Leuk Lymphoma* 2004;45:2427–38.

113 Yamaguchi M, Kita K, Miwa H, *et al*. Frequent expression of P-glycoprotein/MDR1 by nasal T-cell lymphoma cells. *Cancer* 1995;76:2351–6.

114 Egashira M, Kawamata N, Sugimoto K, Kaneko T, Oshimi K. P-glycoprotein expression on normal and abnormally expanded natural killer cells and inhibition of P-glycoprotein function by cyclosporin A and its analog, PSC833. *Blood* 1999; 93:599–606.

115 Okamura T, Kishimoto T, Inoue M, *et al*. Unrelated bone marrow transplantation for Epstein–Barr virus-associated T/NK-cell lymphoproliferative disease. *Bone Marrow Transplant* 2003;31:105–11.

116 Ando M, Sugimoto K, Kitoh T, *et al*. Selective apoptosis of natural killer-cell tumors by l-asparaginase. *Br J Haematol* 2005;130:860–8.

117 Yong W, Zheng W, Zhang Y, *et al*. L-asparaginase-based regimen in the treatment of refractory midline nasal/nasal-type T/NK-cell lymphoma. *Int J Hematol* 2003;78:163–7.

118 Uno M, Tsuchiyama J, Moriwaki A, *et al*. *In vitro* induction of apoptosis for nasal angiocentric natural killer cell lymphoma-derived cell line, NK-YS, by etoposide and cyclosporine A. *Br J Haematol* 2001;113:1009–14.

119 Imashuku S. Advances in the management of hemophagocytic lymphohistiocytosis. *Int J Hematol* 2000;72:1–11.

120 Osuji N, Matutes E, Morilla A, Del Giudice I, Wotherspoon A, Catovsky D. Prolonged treatment response in aggressive natural killer cell leukemia. *Leuk Lymphoma* 2005;46:757–63.

121 Tefferi A, Li CY, Witzig TE, Dhodapkar MV, Okuno SH, Phyliky RL. Chronic natural killer cell lymphocytosis: a descriptive clinical study. *Blood* 1994;84:2721–5.

122 Oshimi K, Kawa K, Nakamura S, *et al*. NK-cell neoplasms in Japan. *Hematology* 2005;10:237–45.

123 Nash R, McSweeney P, Zambello R, Semenzato G, Loughran TP, Jr. Clonal studies of CD3- lymphoproliferative disease of granular lymphocytes. *Blood* 1993;81:2363–8.

124 Takatsuki K. Discovery of adult T-cell leukemia. *Retrovirology* 2005;2:16.

125 Takatsuki K, Yasunaga J, Matsuoka M. *AT and HTLV-I related diseases. Adult T-cell leukemia*. Oxford University Press: New York, 1994.

126 Cleghorn FR, Manns A, Falk R, *et al*. Effect of human T-lymphotropic virus type I infection on non-Hodgkin's lymphoma incidence. *J Natl Cancer Inst* 1995;87:1009–14.

127 Shimoyama M. Diagnostic criteria and classification of clinical subtypes of adult T-cell leukemia-lymphoma. A report from the Lymphoma Study Group (1984–87). *Br J Haematol* 1991;79: 428–37.

128 Tashiro T, Yamasaki T, Nagai H, Kikuchi H, Nasu M. Immunological studies on opportunistic infection and the development of adult T-cell leukemia. *Intern Med* 1992;31: 1132–6.

129 Kuwazuru Y, Hanada S, Furukawa T, *et al*. Expression of P-glycoprotein in adult T-cell leukemia cells. *Blood* 1990;76: 2065–71.

130 Ohno N, Tani A, Uozumi K, *et al*. Expression of functional lung resistance–related protein predicts poor outcome in adult T-cell leukemia. *Blood* 2001;98:1160–5.

131 Nicot C, Mulloy JC, Ferrari MG, *et al*. HTLV-1 p12(I) protein enhances STAT5 activation and decreases the interleukin-2 requirement for proliferation of primary human peripheral blood mononuclear cells. *Blood* 2001;98:823–9.

132 Mori N, Fujii M, Cheng G, *et al*. Human T-cell leukemia virus type I tax protein induces the expression of antiapoptotic gene *Bcl-xL* in human T-cells through nuclear factor-kappaB and c-AMP responsive element binding protein pathways. *Virus Genes* 2001;22:279–87.

133 Takemoto S, Mulloy JC, Cereseto A, *et al*. Proliferation of adult T cell leukemia/lymphoma cells is associated with the constitutive activation of JAK/STAT proteins. *Proc Natl Acad Sci U S A* 1997;94:13897–902.

134 Tomita M, Kikuchi A, Akiyama T, Tanaka Y, Mori N. Human T-cell leukemia virus type 1 tax dysregulates beta-catenin signaling. *J Virol* 2006;80:10497–505.

135 Yamada Y, Tomonaga M, Fukuda H, *et al*. A new G-CSF-supported combination chemotherapy, LSG15, for adult T-cell leukemia-lymphoma: Japan Clinical Oncology Group Study 9303. *Br J Haematol* 2001;113:375–82.

136 Uozumi K, Nakahara K, Takatsuka Y, *et al*. Granulocyte colony-stimulating factor in the combination chemotherapy for adult T-cell leukemia (ATL). *Leuk Lymphoma* 1998;29: 407–14.

137 Matsushita K, Matsumoto T, Ohtsubo H, *et al*. Long-term maintenance combination chemotherapy with OPEC/MPEC (vincristine or methotrexate, prednisolone, etoposide and cyclophosphamide) or with daily oral etoposide and prednisolone can improve survival and quality of life in adult T-cell leukemia/lymphoma. *Leuk Lymphoma* 1999;36:67–75.

138 Taguchi H, Kinoshita KI, Takatsuki K, *et al*. An intensive chemotherapy of adult T-cell leukemia/lymphoma: CHOP followed by etoposide, vindesine, ranimustine, and mitoxantrone

with granulocyte colony-stimulating factor support. *J Acquir Immune Defic Syndr Hum Retrovirol* 1996;12:182–6.
139 Tsukasaki K, Fukushima T, Utsunomiya A, *et al.* Phase III study of VCAP-AMP-VECP vs. biweekly CHOP in aggressive adult T-cell leukemia-lymphoma (ATLL): Japan Clinical Oncology Group Study, JCOG9801. *Blood* 2005;106:812.
140 Teshima T, Akashi K, Shibuya T, *et al.* Central nervous system involvement in adult T-cell leukemia/lymphoma. *Cancer* 1990;65:327–32.
141 Dungerwalla M, Osuji N, Waldman AD, *et al.* Isolated central nervous system involvement in adult T-cell lymphoma/leukemia. *Br J Haematol* 2005;130:511–15.
142 Kojima H, Hori M, Shibuya A, Nagasawa T, Miwa M, Abe T. Successful treatment of a patient with adult T-cell leukemia by daily oral administration of low-dose etoposide. Decrease in the amount of HTLV-I proviral DNA revealed by the polymerase chain reaction method. *Cancer* 1993;72: 3614–17.
143 Tsukasaki K, Tobinai K, Shimoyama M, *et al.* Deoxycoformycin–containing combination chemotherapy for adult T-cell leukemia-lymphoma: Japan Clinical Oncology Group Study (JCOG9109). *Int J Hematol* 2003;77:164–70.
144 Tobinai K, Shimoyama M, Inoue S, *et al.* Phase I study of YK-176 (2′-deoxycoformycin) in patients with adult T-cell leukemia-lymphoma. The DCF Study Group. *Jpn J Clin Oncol* 1992;22:164–71.
145 Tobinai K, Uike N, Saburi Y, *et al.* Phase II study of cladribine (2-chlorodeoxyadenosine) in relapsed or refractory adult T-cell leukemia-lymphoma. *Int J Hematol* 2003;77:512–17.
146 Tsuda H, Takatsuki K, Ohno R, *et al.* Treatment of adult T-cell leukemia-lymphoma with irinotecan hydrochloride (CPT-11). CPT-11 Study Group on Hematological Malignancy. *Br J Cancer* 1994;70:771–4.
147 Ohno R, Masaoka T, Shirakawa S, *et al.* Treatment of adult T-cell leukemia/lymphoma with MST-16, a new oral antitumor drug and a derivative of bis(2,6-dioxopiperazine). The MST-16 Study Group. *Cancer* 1993;71:2217–21.
148 Bazarbachi A, El-Sabban ME, Nasr R, *et al.* Arsenic trioxide and interferon-alpha synergize to induce cell cycle arrest and apoptosis in human T-cell lymphotropic virus type I-transformed cells. *Blood* 1999;93:278–83.
149 Mahieux R, Pise-Masison C, Gessain A, *et al.* Arsenic trioxide induces apoptosis in human T-cell leukemia virus type 1- and type 2-infected cells by a caspase-3-dependent mechanism involving Bcl–2 cleavage. *Blood* 2001;98:3762–9.
150 Tamura K, Makino S, Araki Y, *et al.* A case of CD4+/CD8- adult T-cell leukemia with good response to interferon-beta terminating as a CD4+/CD8+ adult T-cell lymphoma. *Leuk Res* 1987; 11:665–8.
151 Takemori N, Hirai K, Onodera R, Saito N, Watanabe S, Namiki M. Splenectomy followed by local injections of interferon-alpha is effective for treating cutaneous-type adult T-cell leukemia/lymphoma. *Br J Dermatol* 1993;129:746–7.
152 Fujiwara H, Arima N, Akasaki Y, *et al.* Interferon-alpha therapy following autologous peripheral blood stem cell transplantation for adult T cell leukemia/lymphoma. *Acta Haematol* 2002;107:213–19.
153 Tamura K, Makino S, Araki Y, Imamura T, Seita M. Recombinant interferon beta and gamma in the treatment of adult T-cell leukemia. *Cancer* 1987;59:1059–62.
154 Matutes E, Taylor GP, Cavenagh J, *et al.* Interferon alpha and zidovudine therapy in adult T-cell leukemia lymphoma: response and outcome in 15 patients. *Br J Haematol* 2001;113: 779–84.
155 Hermine O, Wattel E, Gessain A, Bazarbachi A. Adult T cell leukemia: a review of established and new treatments. *BioDrugs* 1998;10:447–62.
156 Hermine O, Bouscary D, Gessain A, *et al.* Brief report: treatment of adult T-cell leukemia-lymphoma with zidovudine and interferon alfa. *N Engl J Med* 1995;332:1749–51.
157 Hermine O, Allard I, Levy V, Arnulf B, Gessain A, Bazarbachi A. A prospective phase II clinical trial with the use of zidovudine and interferon-alpha in the acute and lymphoma forms of adult T-cell leukemia/lymphoma. *Hematol J* 2002;3:276–82.
158 Gill PS, Harrington W, Jr., Kaplan MH, *et al.* Treatment of adult T-cell leukemia-lymphoma with a combination of interferon alfa and zidovudine. *N Engl J Med* 1995;332:1744–8.
159 Kchour G, Makhoul NJ, Mahmoudi M, *et al.* Zidovudine and interferon-alpha treatment induces a high response rate and reduces HTLV-1 proviral load and VEGF plasma levels in patients with adult T-cell leukemia from North East Iran. *Leuk Lymphoma* 2007;48:330–6.
160 Uchida N, Otsuka T, Arima F, *et al.* Correlation of telomerase activity with development and progression of adult T-cell leukemia. *Leuk Res* 1999;23:311–16.
161 Sinha-Datta U, Horikawa I, Michishita E, *et al.* Transcriptional activation of hTERT through the NF-kappaB pathway in HTLV-I-transformed cells. *Blood* 2004;104:2523–31.
162 Kubuki Y, Suzuki M, Sasaki H, *et al.* Telomerase activity and telomere length as prognostic factors of adult T-cell leukemia. *Leuk Lymphoma* 2005;46:393–9.
163 Strahl C, Blackburn EH. Effects of reverse transcriptase inhibitors on telomere length and telomerase activity in two immortalized human cell lines. *Mol Cell Biol* 1996;16:53–65.
164 Mo Y, Gan Y, Song S, *et al.* Simultaneous targeting of telomeres and telomerase as a cancer therapeutic approach. *Cancer Res* 2003;63:579–85.
165 Brown T, Sigurdson E, Rogatko A, Broccoli D. Telomerase inhibition using azidothymidine in the HT-29 colon cancer cell line. *Ann Surg Oncol* 2003;10:910–15.
166 Savaraj N, Wu C, Wangpaichitr M, *et al.* Overexpression of mutated MRP4 in cisplatin resistant small cell lung cancer cell line: collateral sensitivity to azidothymidine. *Int J Oncol* 2003; 23:173–9.
167 Datta A, Nicot C. Telomere attrition induces a DNA double-strand break damage signal that reactivates p53 transcription in HTLV-I leukemic cells. *Oncogene* 2008;27:1135–41.
168 Tsukasaki K, Maeda T, Arimura K, *et al.* Poor outcome of autologous stem cell transplantation for adult T cell leukemia/lymphoma: a case report and review of the literature. *Bone Marrow Transplant* 1999;23:87–9.
169 Utsunomiya A, Miyazaki Y, Takatsuka Y, *et al.* Improved outcome of adult T cell leukemia/lymphoma with allogeneic hematopoietic stem cell transplantation. *Bone Marrow Transplant* 2001;27:15–20.
170 Fukushima T, Miyazaki Y, Honda S, *et al.* Allogeneic hematopoietic stem cell transplantation provides sustained long-term survival for patients with adult T-cell leukemia/lymphoma. *Leukemia* 2005;19:829–34.

171 Ishikawa T. Current status of therapeutic approaches to adult T-cell leukemia. *Int J Hematol* 2003;78:304–11.

172 Harashima N, Kurihara K, Utsunomiya A, *et al*. Graft-versus-Tax response in adult T-cell leukemia patients after hematopoietic stem cell transplantation. *Cancer Res* 2004;64: 391–9.

173 Momita S, Ikeda S, Amagasaki T, *et al*. Survey of antihuman T-cell leukemia virus type I antibody in family members of patients with adult T-cell leukemia. *Jpn J Cancer Res* 1990;81: 884–9.

174 Tamaki H, Matsuoka M. Donor-derived T-cell leukemia after bone marrow transplantation. *N Engl J Med* 2006;354:1758–9.

175 Kato K, Kanda Y, Eto T, *et al*. Allogeneic bone marrow transplantation from unrelated human T-cell leukemia virus-I-negative donors for adult T-cell leukemia/lymphoma: retrospective analysis of data from the Japan Marrow Donor Program. *Biol Blood Marrow Transplant* 2007;13:90–9.

176 Okamura J, Utsunomiya A, Tanosaki R, *et al*. Allogeneic stem-cell transplantation with reduced conditioning intensity as a novel immunotherapy and antiviral therapy for adult T-cell leukemia/lymphoma. *Blood* 2005;105:4143–5.

177 Tendler CL, Greenberg SJ, Burton JD, *et al*. Cytokine induction in HTLV-I associated myelopathy and adult T-cell leukemia: alternate molecular mechanisms underlying retroviral pathogenesis. *J Cell Biochem* 1991;46:302–11.

178 Waldmann TA, White JD, Carrasquillo JA, *et al*. Radioimmunotherapy of interleukin-2R alpha-expressing adult T-cell leukemia with Yttrium-90-labeled antiTac. *Blood* 1995;86:4063–75.

179 Osborne GE, Pagliuca A, Ho A, du Vivier AW. Novel treatment of Sezary-like syndrome due to adult T-cell leukemia/lymphoma with daclizumab (humanized antiinterleukin-2 receptor alpha antibody). *Br J Dermatol* 2006;155:617–20.

180 Kreitman RJ, Wilson WH, White JD, *et al*. Phase I trial of recombinant immunotoxin antiTac(Fv)-PE38 (LMB-2) in patients with hematologic malignancies. *J Clin Oncol* 2000;18: 1622–36.

181 Di Venuti G, Nawgiri R, Foss F. Denileukin diftitox and hyper-CVAD in the treatment of human T-cell lymphotropic virus 1-associated acute T-cell leukemia/lymphoma. *Clin Lymphoma* 2003;4:176–8.

182 Mone A, Puhalla S, Whitman S, *et al*. Durable hematologic complete response and suppression of HTLV-1 viral load following alemtuzumab in zidovudine/IFN-{alpha}-refractory adult T-cell leukemia. *Blood* 2005;106:3380–2.

183 Ravandi F, Faderl S. Complete response in a patient with adult T-cell leukemia (ATL) treated with combination of alemtuzumab and pentostatin. *Leuk Res* 2006;30:103–5.

184 Janik JE, Morris JC, Stetler-Stevenson M, *et al*. Phase I trial of siplizumab in CD2-positive lymphoproliferative disease. *J Clin Oncol* (Meeting Abstracts) 2005;23:2533.

185 d'Amore F, Relander T, Hagberg H, *et al*. HuMax-CD4 (Zanolimumab), a fully human monoclonal antibody: early results of an ongoing clinical trial in CD4+ peripheral T-cell lymphoma of non-cutaneous type. *Blood* (ASH Annual Meeting Abstracts) 2005;106:3354.

186 Yoshie O, Fujisawa R, Nakayama T, *et al*. Frequent expression of CCR4 in adult T-cell leukemia and human T-cell leukemia virus type 1-transformed T cells. *Blood* 2002;99:1505–11.

187 Ishida T, Inagaki H, Utsunomiya A, *et al*. CXC chemokine receptor 3 and CC chemokine receptor 4 expression in T-cell and NK-cell lymphomas with special reference to clinicopathological significance for peripheral T-cell lymphoma, unspecified. *Clin Cancer Res* 2004;10:5494–500.

188 Callens C, Moura IC, Lepelletier Y, *et al*. Recent advances in adult T-cell leukemia therapy: focus on a new antitransferrin receptor monoclonal antibody. *Leukemia* 2008;22:42–8.

189 Ballard DW, Bohnlein E, Lowenthal JW, Wano Y, Franza BR, Greene WC. HTLV-I tax induces cellular proteins that activate the kappa B element in the IL-2 receptor alpha gene. *Science* 1988;241:1652–5.

190 Mori N, Fujii M, Ikeda S, *et al*. Constitutive activation of NF-kappaB in primary adult T-cell leukemia cells. *Blood* 1999; 93:2360–8.

191 Satou Y, Nosaka K, Koya Y, Yasunaga JI, Toyokuni S, Matsuoka M. Proteasome inhibitor, bortezomib, potently inhibits the growth of adult T-cell leukemia cells both in vivo and in vitro. *Leukemia* 2004;18:1357–63.

192 Nasr R, El-Sabban ME, Karam JA, *et al*. Efficacy and mechanism of action of the proteasome inhibitor PS-341 in T-cell lymphomas and *HTLV-I* associated adult T-cell leukemia/lymphoma. *Oncogene* 2005;24:419–30.

193 Strauss SJ, Maharaj L, Hoare S, *et al*. Bortezomib therapy in patients with relapsed or refractory lymphoma: potential correlation of in vitro sensitivity and tumor necrosis factor alpha response with clinical activity. *J Clin Oncol* 2006;24:2105–12.

194 Mori N, Matsuda T, Tadano M, *et al*. Apoptosis induced by the histone deacetylase inhibitor FR901228 in human T-cell leukemia virus type 1-infected T-cell lines and primary adult T-cell leukemia cells. *J Virol* 2004;78:4582–90.

195 Hermine O, Dombret H, Poupon J, *et al*. Phase II trial of arsenic trioxide and alpha interferon in patients with relapsed/refractory adult T-cell leukemia/lymphoma. *Hematol J* 2004;5: 130–4.

196 Ishitsuka K, Suzumiya J, Aoki M, Ogata K, Hara S, Tamura K. Therapeutic potential of arsenic trioxide with or without interferon-alpha for relapsed/refractory adult T-cell leukemia/lymphoma. *Haematologica* 2007;92:719–20.

197 Ishitsuka K, Ikeda R, Utsunomiya A, *et al*. Arsenic trioxide induces apoptosis in HTLV-I infected T-cell lines and fresh adult T-cell leukemia cells through CD95 or tumor necrosis factor alpha receptor independent caspase activation. *Leuk Lymphoma* 2002;43:1107–14.

198 El-Sabban ME, Nasr R, Dbaibo G, *et al*. Arsenic-interferon-alpha-triggered apoptosis in HTLV-I transformed cells is associated with tax down-regulation and reversal of NF-kappa B activation. *Blood* 2000;96:2849–55.

199 Nasr R, Rosenwald A, El-Sabban ME, *et al*. Arsenic/interferon specifically reverses 2 distinct gene networks critical for the survival of HTLV-1-infected leukemic cells. *Blood* 2003;101: 4576–82.

200 Brown MJ, Nijhara R, Hallam JA, *et al*. Chemokine stimulation of human peripheral blood T lymphocytes induces rapid dephosphorylation of ERM proteins, which facilitates loss of microvilli and polarization. *Blood* 2003;102:3890–9.

201 Yoshioka R, Yamaguchi K, Yoshinaga T, Takatsuki K. Pulmonary complications in patients with adult T-cell leukemia. *Cancer* 1985;55:2491–4.

Chapter 30
Philadelphia Chromosome-negative Myeloproliferative Neoplasms

Ruben A. Mesa[1] *and Srdan Verstovsek*[2]
[1]Mayo Clinic Arizona, Scottsdale, Arizona, USA
[2]University of Texas M. D. Anderson Cancer Center, Houston, Texas, USA

Myeloproliferative neoplasms

Philadelphia chromosome-negative (Ph^-) myeloproliferative neoplasms (MPNs) are a pathophysiologically interrelated group of clonal hematopoietic stem cell disorders that include polycythemia vera (PV), essential thrombocythemia (ET), primary myelofibrosis (PMF), hypereosinophilic syndrome/chronic eosinophilic leukemia (HES/CEL), and systemic mast cell disease (SMCD) [1–4]. MPNs have a cumulative incidence of approximately eight cases per 100,000 persons per year and have a median age at onset of approximately 60 years (however, patients <50 years of age are still commonly seen) [5]. Clinically, early in the disease course patients with MPN are at risk of thrombohemorrhagic complications and with progression can develop profound cytopenias, hepatosplenomegaly, eventually culminating in leukemic transformation. An MPN can lead to premature death, with the most aggressive entity, myelofibrosis (MF), having a median survival of 5–7 years [6]. Patients may have primary myelofibrosis (PMF) and additionally may develop MF in the advanced phases of PV and ET; the latter complications are known as post-PV MF and post-ET MF, respectively. Even in the absence of MF, patients with PV and ET may have compromised survivals compared with age-matched controls [7]. The sources of mortality in ET and PV are the short-term risk of thrombohemorrhagic complications and the long-term risk of leukemic transformation, as well as development of post-ET/PV MF with their attendant cytopenias [7].

Patients with MPN suffer from a full range of disease-associated symptoms, some of which are shared with patients with other chronic leukemias and other malignancies and some of which are unique to the disorders themselves. Symptoms that are particularly associated, and sometimes uniquely so, with MPNs include a risk of both thrombosis and/or bleeding, especially in patients with ET and PV. These symptoms have a range of manifestations. In the setting of acute venous thrombosis, one can be left with deep venous thrombosis or post-phlebitic symptoms of the legs including pain, chronic peripheral edema, and other such difficulties of a similar nature. Chronic pulmonary emboli, which can arise in these patients, can lead to short-term morbidity from arrhythmia, but also to long-term problems including pulmonary hypertension, chronic dyspnea, and a general compromise in cardiac or lung function. Vascular events can also be more subtle. Individuals with extremes of either erythrocytosis or thrombocytosis, even in the absence of frank thrombosis, can have compromised microvascular circulation and have periods that are described by patients as confusion, lack of ability to concentrate, migraine headaches, and visual disturbances. Hemorrhagic symptoms can range from acute gastrointestinal bleeding to more chronic bleeding events from esophageal varices or gastrointestinal sources that can lead to, or exacerbate, chronic anemia and all of the challenges with dyspnea and fatigue that anemia can bring.

The presence of itching or pruritus is very common across the spectrum of MPNs and particularly among those individuals with PV. These individuals classically have aquagenic pruritus, meaning that the itching in the skin is most prominent after exposure to water and drying. The itching can occur in the absence of exposure to water. It is felt that this is potentially associated with histamine release and other cytokine mediators in the skin. Other skin sensations can include painful microvascular circulation, a difficulty known to occur with erythromelalgia. Patients with MPNs can suffer from significant constitutional symptoms including a loss of lean muscle mass or a cachexia, which we feel is potentially associated with underlying disease manifestations that have a selective predisposition for the consumption of lean muscle mass. Additionally, they can have fevers and night sweats that are likely cytokine-driven in association with the underlying myeloid process. MPNs are characterized by

Leukemias: Principles and Practice of Therapy, 1st edition. Edited by S. Faderl and H. Kantarjian.

increases in circulating white blood cells, and, in the case of PMF, a variety of immature myeloid cells. This can lead to the development of sequestration of these cells or extramedullary hematopoiesis (EMH), which particularly can lead to significant splenomegaly and/or hepatomegaly. The splenomegaly can be sufficient to cause significant early satiety, pain, abdominal bloating, difficulty with finding a comfortable position, difficulties with bending over, portal hypertension, worsening of peripheral edema, and a whole constellation of symptoms including painful splenic infarcts. EMH can develop in a variety of organs, and it has been found everywhere from in the pericardium causing pericardial effusions to in the spinal canal causing cord compression to in the lungs causing pulmonary hypertension, all of which can lead to a very significant symptomatic burden in these groups of patients (Table 30.1).

The discovery of several key MPN-associated mutations has broadened the therapeutic horizons for these disorders significantly [8], starting with the discovery of the *JAK2-V617F* mutation [9–12] in the 14th exon of JAK2, to the now 10 mutations described in the 12th exon of JAK2. Additionally, five mutations thus far have been identified in the thrombopoietin receptor MPL. All of these mutations are diagnostically very helpful. They are primarily present in patients with MPNs and not in normal reactive controls, but, more importantly, they all seem to play at least a partial role in the development of myeloproliferation and lead to constitutive activation of cellular proliferation in these patients. All of these mutations seem to feed into a final common pathway of cellular activation through the PI3 kinase pathway, the STAT pathway, and the MAP kinase pathway [8].

Essential thrombocythemia and polycythemia vera

Currently available therapies are rarely able to alter the natural history of disease in ET and PV, although they may offer symptom palliation or decrease the risk of vascular events. Given these limitations, how should patients with ET and PV be optimally managed? When a diagnosis of an ET and PV is established or suspected, patients need to be stabilized and immediate coagulopathies from severe erythrocytosis, thrombocytosis, or thrombotic/bleeding events must be urgently addressed. Management decisions will then depend on the estimation of the treating clinician of overall disease prognosis and the separate estimation of individual patient risk of vascular events. In patients with ET and PV, the patients at high risk for vascular events are those who have had a prior vascular event or are >60 years of age; low-risk patients lack either of these features (and also have a platelet count $<1000 \times 10^9/L$). Patients with ET and PV classified as intermediate risk are those who are under 60 years old, those who have not had a prior event, but do have cardiovascular risk factors. Potential newly identified vascular risk factors include leukocytosis of $>15 \times 10^9/L$ at diagnosis in PV [13] or a high *JAK2-V617F* mutation allele burden in ET and MPNs [13,14]. How these new factors should be included in modeling ET and PV vascular risk is not yet known and requires further study.

The immediate therapeutic concerns for patients with ET and PV at presentation are both an adequate prophylaxis against vascular events and, when possible, palliation of symptoms. The management of patients with PV includes control of erythrocytosis (by phlebotomy) and, when no contraindication exists, the use of low-dose aspirin [15]. The degree to which a patient needs to be phlebotomized has been questioned, with traditional dogma suggesting a goal hematocrit of <42% for women and 45% for men. However, recent retrospective analysis of vascular events of patients on the ECLAP trial (European Collaborative Low Dose Aspirin Trial) has suggested that modestly higher targets (perhaps hematocrits of up to 55%) may not increase the risk of vascular events [16]. Whether the goal hematocrit should be changed for PV needs to be addressed by appropriately designed trials.

Table 30.1 Self-reported constitutional symptoms in 1179 patients with myeloproliferative neoplasms.

Symptom	PV (%) (*n* = 405)	ET (%) (*n* = 304)	MF (%) (*n* = 456)	Total (%) (*n* = 1179)
Fatigue	85	72	84	81
Bone pain	65	40	50	53
Fever	49	41	56	50
Pruritus	43	41	47	44
Night sweats	13	9	18	14
Symptomatic splenomegaly	10	7	20	13
Weight loss (>10%)	4	9	7	6

ET, essential thrombocythemia; MF, myelofibrosis; PV, polycythemia vera.

What about myelosuppressive therapy for managing ET and PV? Hydroxyurea was shown in a randomized fashion to aid in the prevention of thrombotic events in patients with high-risk ET [17]. The UK MRC (United Kingdom Medical Research Council) PT-1 (primary thrombocythemia 1) trial compared, in a randomized fashion, hydroxyurea and anagrelide (both along with low-dose aspirin) for patients with ET and found hydroxyurea plus aspirin to be superior in regards to preventing arterial events, hemorrhage, and transformation to post-ET MF [18]. Therefore, the standard front-line therapy for high-risk patients with ET and PV who require platelet-lowering therapy is hydroxyurea. Although concerns linger about whether hydroxyurea accelerates an MPN toward leukemic transformation, this has never been proven [19]. Pegylated interferon 2 alpha (PEG-IFN-2-α) has shown clinical activity and may be more tolerable than traditional IFN, for especially PV [20]. How interferon compares with hydroxyurea for control of vascular events has not yet been studied in a randomized fashion. Current attempts at palliating symptoms in patients with ET and PV can include therapies for pruritus (antihistamines and selective serotonin reuptake inhibitors), erythromelalgia (aspirin), and fatigue (exercise).

The most straightforward target of JAK2 inhibition is PV (with 99% of patients having a mutation somewhere in JAK2), and preliminary results of trials with XL019 [21], CEP-701 (Cephalon, Frazer, PA) [22], and ITF2347 [23] show preliminary activity in decreasing erythrocytosis. However, these trials are too early in their accrual and analyses to form a conclusion on their efficacy. Interestingly, in PV, the agent that has shown an ability to lead to significant reductions in *JAK2-V617F* allele burdens in 30–40% of patients (including complete molecular remissions) is pegylated IFN-2α (Pegasys). Recently reported outcomes from trials from Europe [24] and the USA [25] have both confirmed these observations. Intriguingly, even patients on hydroxyurea (who have had an excellent clinical response) may have significant reductions in mutant allele burden [26].

Myelofibrosis

Deciding on a treatment plan for patients with MF requires both an assessment of disease impact at diagnosis and an accurate assessment of prognosis. To aid in decision-making, the International Working Group for Myelofibrosis Research and Treatment (IWG-MRT) recently published an International Prognostic Scoring System for MF (IPSS-MF) that can help distinguish the prognosis in patients with MF. The IPSS-MF defines four risk groups with prognoses ranging from a median of 27 months to 135 months [27]. Currently, no therapy has been shown to be curative, alter natural history, or prolong survival in patients with an MPN, with the exception of allogeneic stem-cell transplantation, for which few patients are eligible owing to age and comorbidity. However, allogeneic stem-cell transplantation provides a 58% 3-year survival with a 32% non-relapse mortality rate [28]. Outcomes are perhaps slightly better with reduced-intensity conditioning regimens [29], but further studies are needed. Therefore, a key question after MF has been diagnosed is whether the patient is a suitable candidate for allogeneic transplantation. Given that no other therapy has led to cure or has been proven to confer a survival advantage in MF, all other non-transplantation forms of therapy must be considered palliative in nature and intent.

Observation is most appropriate for those patients with low-risk PMF. Observation requires continued vigilance of the patient's disease status for disease progression to a point where (i) a standard medical therapy or clinical trial would be appropriate or (ii) a stem-cell transplant would be considered. Current medical therapies for MF should be considered in two distinct tiers. Tier 1 consists predominantly of oral agents with (usually) modest toxicities. Cytopenias have improved in subsets of patients with erythropoietin supplementation [30], androgens [31], and/or corticosteroids. Similarly, the uses of non-specific myelosuppressive regimens such as oral hydroxyurea [32] and cladribine [33] have been reported to provide palliative reduction in painful splenomegaly. Early reports of phase I trials of JAK2 inhibitors indicate that these may also provide medical therapy of splenomegaly. Tier 2 includes more aggressive approaches, suitable for patients with severe splenomegaly or involvement of other organs by EMH (ie, lungs, ascites, etc.). In those patients, a more intensive intravenous myelosuppressive approach may be warranted. The choice of both initial and subsequent therapies should be based on the ability to tolerate myelosuppression (Table 30.2).

Hydroxyurea

Hydroxyurea is an oral myelosuppressive agent that is active in decreasing splenomegaly in MF [34]. It is the most common initial medical therapy used in patients with MF (with an estimated response rate of <50% for splenomegaly, although very little prospective clinical trial data exist). However, there are several limitations to the use of this agent for this indication in MF. First, hydroxyurea rarely induces a complete resolution of splenomegaly or even an IWG-MRT clinical improvement for splenomegaly (ie, >50% improvement sustained for at least 2 months) [42]. Nevertheless, more modest reductions in splenomegaly may benefit some patients with MF. Second, splenomegaly is not as responsive to hydroxyurea (compared with thrombocytosis) and might require a higher dose (ie, 2–3 g/day). Third, particularly at higher doses, hydroxyurea therapy may potentially exacerbate cytopenias.

Table 30.2 Medical therapy for myelofibrosis (available medications).

Agent	Administration route	Dose/schedule	Response rate	Additional efficacy	Toxicities	Reference
Tier 1						
Hydroxyurea	Oral	500–3000 mg (daily)	40–50%	None	Myelosuppression Skin ulcers	[34]
Busulfan	Oral	2–4 mg (daily)	Variable	None	Myelosuppression Leukemia	[60]
Melphalan	Oral	2.5 mg (3 × weekly)	67%	None	Myelosuppression Leukemia	[36]
Interferon 2 alpha	Subcutaneous	0.5–1.0 × 10^6 units (3 × weekly)	Limited data: 75% with small spleens Fewer with larger	None	Myelosuppression Depression	[61]
Thalidomide +/– prednisone taper	Oral	50 mg (daily)	19%	Anemia Thrombocytopenia	Neuropathy Sedation Myeloproliferation	[39]
Lenalidomide +/– prednisone taper	Oral	5–10 mg (daily)	33%	Anemia Thrombocytopenia	Myelosuppression Rash Diarrhea	[62]
Tier 2						
Cladribine (2-CdA)	Intravenous	5 mg/m^2/day (5 days monthly)	56%	None	Myelosuppression	[24]
Daunorubicin	Intravenous	60 mg/m^2 (days 1–3)	N/A	None	Myelosuppression Cardiotoxicity	–
5-Azacytidine	Subcutaneous	75 mg/m^2 (days 1–7) (monthly)	21%	Anemia	Myelosuppression Gastrointestinal	[45, 46]
Decitabine	Subcutaneous	20 mg/m^2 (days 1–5) (monthly)	N/A		Myelosuppression	–

Oral alkylators

Alkylators such as melphalan and busulfan can alleviate splenomegaly in some patients with MF but with potential myelosuppression and increased the risk of blastic transformation. In one study, melphalan (eg, 2.5 mg of oral melphalan three times per week) reduced the size of the spleen in 66% of patients; however, 26% of the study cohort [36] developed acute leukemia. Busulfan may also be utilized [43] and was used in the related myeloproliferative disorder of chronic myeloid leukemia in the pre-imatinib era.

Immunomodulatory inhibitory drugs

The group of immunomodulatory, cytokine inhibitory, and antiangiogenic agents collectively known as IMIDs have been able to palliate primarily cytopenias (anemia and thrombocytopenia) in MF, but may also reduce splenomegaly. Based on this potential combination of effects, patients with concurrent cytopenias and splenomegaly should be considered for an IMID.

Low-dose (ie, 50 mg/day) thalidomide with a prednisone taper (THAL-PRED regimen) [44] achieves significant responses in MF for anemia (67%), thrombocytopenia (75%), and splenomegaly (33%). Subsequently, lenalidomide (LEN) (a second-generation IMID) was evaluated in 68 patients with symptomatic MF, with overall response rates of 22% for anemia, 33% for splenomegaly, and 50% for thrombocytopenia [39]. Mirroring the activity of LEN in del(5q) myelodysplastic syndromes (MDS), patients with MF with an abnormality of chromosome 5 seem to respond best to this agent [45].

Interferon alpha

Therapy with IFN-α has been utilized in patients with MF based on its cytoreductive properties, and this agent has been active in patients with PV [24]. However, clinical trials of IFN-α in MF with standard preparations [46] and PEG-IFN-α-2b [47] have demonstrated poor patient tolerance and negligible response rates. In one study, subcutaneous PEG-IFN-α-2b (PEG-Intron) was administered weekly to 36 patients with Ph⁻ MPNs [47], and none of the patients with MF responded.

Cladribine

Palliative benefit from the purine nucleoside analog, 2-chlorodeoxyadenosine (2-CdA), has been reported in patients with MF [33]. 2-CdA has been administered as four to six monthly cycles of treatment with either 0.1 mg/kg/day administered intravenously by continuous infusion for 7 days or 5 mg/m^2 administered intravenously over 2 h for 5 consecutive days. In the Mayo Clinic experience, we observed responses in 55%, 50%, 55%, and 40% of patients for organomegaly, thrombocytosis, leukocytosis, and anemia, respectively. Responses were frequently durable and lasted for a median of 6 months after discontinuation of treatment.

Hypomethylating agents

The two hypomethylating agents approved for MDS, azacitidine (AZA) and decitabine, have both been tested in MF to improve cytopenias, splenomegaly, or delay blastic transformation. Recent trials of AZA (75 mg/m^2/day administered for either 5 or 7 days) [48, 49] showed a 21% response rate for splenomegaly in MF, exclusively in the 7-day regimen. Decitabine is in the early stages of testing in MF, and trials are ongoing. Both the frequent visits required for the administration of these hypomethylating agents and the myelosuppression that is their most common adverse effect limits the use of these therapies in MF.

Therapeutic splenectomy in myelofibrosis

The experience with splenectomy in MF dates back to the beginning of the 20th century [35]. Progressive surgical series demonstrated a significant, but slowly decreasing, perioperative mortality rate owing to improvements in surgical technique, antimicrobials, and patient selection. Although splenectomy can be helpful for improving the symptoms in patients with MF, it seems to have no clear outcome on patient survival nor any impact in the disease course or its intramedullary manifestations. We recently analyzed three decades of experience of palliative splenectomy in MF from the Mayo Clinic to see if better control of post-splenectomy thrombocytosis, modern operative techniques, and supportive care have diminished morbidity and mortality [37]. Although meaningful improvements in symptoms can be observed in 30–50% of patients, complication rates (27.7%; 6.7% fatal) are sobering and require close perioperative management and careful choice of candidates.

Radiation for myelofibrosis

For patients with MF, EMH, regardless of location, is exquisitely sensitive to external-beam radiotherapy. Sites frequently irradiated in patients with MF include the lungs [50] (where EMH can contribute to pulmonary hypertension), paraspinal masses [51], or the spleen. Splenomegaly can be palliated by external-beam radiotherapy, but benefit is typically transient and myelosuppression can be severe. Several reports have described the palliative benefit to external-beam radiation in improving symptomatic splenomegaly in MF [52,53]. Experience from the Mayo Clinic [52] includes a group of 23 patients with MF who received a median radiation course of 277 cGy in a median of eight fractions. An objective decrease in spleen size was noted in 94% of patients; however, 44% of patients experienced post-treatment cytopenias (26% were severe; 13% fatal). Splenic radiation also seemed to increase morbidity and mortality of subsequent splenectomy when undertaken. This latter effect seems related to the development of splenic adhesions to the abdominal wall and surrounding viscera, leading to greater complexity with subsequent attempts at surgical extirpation. Additionally, delayed hemorrhage in irradiated areas in which the spleen had to be bluntly dissected away from other structures was common.

JAK2 inhibitors

The discovery of several key MPN-associated mutations has broadened the therapeutic horizons for MF significantly [8]. Discovery of the *JAK2-V617F* mutation in the 14th exon of JAK2 was followed by the now 10 mutations described in the 12th exon of JAK2. Additionally, five constitutively activating mutations thus far have identified in the thrombopoietin receptor, MPL, which signals through JAK2. All of these mutations seem to feed into a final common pathway of cellular activation through the PI3 kinase pathway, the STAT pathway, and the MAP kinase pathway [8].

The most mature clinical experience for a JAK2 inhibitor is for INCB018424 (Incyte Co., Wilmington, DE), which is selective against JAK1 and JAK2. This agent leads to a significant reduction in splenomegaly and dramatic improvement in constitutional symptoms with toxicities of thrombocytopenia and anemia [54]. Additional drugs being tested include the selective JAK2 inhibitor, TG101348 (TarGen, San Francisco) [55], the selective JAK2 inhibitor XL019 (Exelexis, San Francisco, CA) [56], CEP-701 (a tyrosine kinase inhibitor of JAK2 and FLT3) (Cephalon, Frazer, PA) [22], and ITF2357 (histone deacetylase inhibitor) (Italfarmaco, Italy) [23]. With each agent, preliminary results also report improvements in splenomegaly and symptoms in patients with MF, although variable toxicities are seen (gastrointestinal, neuropathy). They all share the potential for causing anemia and/or thrombocytopenia. No JAK2 inhibitor has yet reported a significant ability to improve cytopenias, fibrosis, or histologic changes associated with MF.

Hypereosinophilic syndrome and chronic eosinophilic leukemia

Hypereosinophilic syndrome is a rare hematologic disorder characterized by the overproduction of eosinophils in the bone marrow, eosinophilia, tissue infiltration, and end-organ damage by eosinophil infiltration and secretion of mediators. The diagnosis of HES is based on marked eosinophilia (absolute eosinophil count $>1.5 \times 10^9/L$), chronic course (>6 months), exclusion of other evident etiologies for eosinophilia (eg, parasitic infestations, allergic diseases, Hodgkin disease, and metastatic cancer), and signs and symptoms of eosinophil-mediated tissue injury (eg, cardiomyopathy, gastroenteritis, pneumonitis, cutaneous lesions, sinusitis, neurologic and ophtalmologic manifestations, and vasculitis) [57]. Over the last few years, considerable insights with regards to the pathogenesis of HES have been gained that have highlighted the marked heterogeneity of patients with this disorder. A diagnosis of "true" HES according to the World Health Organization (WHO) is predicated upon the demonstration of absence of any molecular or cytogenetic features of clonality or any bone marrow findings suggesting an abnormal population of mast cells, monocytosis, or evidence of trilineage myeloproliferation or dysplasia. It is now clear that there are at least three distinct groups of patients among those previously diagnosed as having "idiopathic" HES. First, a subset of patients have been reclassified as having "clonal" eosinophilia or CEL upon the discovery of the Fip1-like 1–platelet-derived growth-factor receptor alpha (FIP1L1–PDGFRα) fusion transcript. Second, there is a subset of patients with HES, in whom no evidence of clonality can be demonstrated with currently available techniques, which must still be considered "idiopathic." However, it is well documented that cases of "idiopathic" HES presenting in the absence of any distinct cytogenetic abnormalities can ulteriorly evolve into acute leukemia or aggressive forms of myeloproliferative disorders. This group is often called myeloproliferative variant of HES. Third, a final subset of patients carry an abnormal T-cell population (helper Th2 lymphocytes), detectable either by flow cytometry or polymerase chain reaction (PCR), that produces interleukin 5 (IL-5), a cytokine required for the growth and differentiation of eosinophils. This group is frequently referred to as a lymphoproliferative variant of "idiopathic" HES. This likely incomplete division has had direct implications regarding treatment options for these patients. Hence, the distinction between clonal and idiopathic eosinophilia is not conspicuous in many instances, which does not necessarily imply monoclonal proliferation of eosinophils in the HES, but rather highlights the absence of such evidence. CEL is defined as an HES phenotype associated with either a molecular/cytogenetic clonal marker or excess myeloblasts in the blood (>2%) or bone marrow (>5%) [58]. Molecularly defined CEL is characterized by mutations involving *PDGFRA* (located on chromosome 4q12), *PDGFRB* (located on chromosome 5q31-q32), and *FGFR1* (located on chromosome 8p11).

Males are primarily affected by HES, and clinical manifestations include pruritus, urticaria, angioedema, erythematous papules, valvular disease, mural thrombi, cardiomyopathy, sensorimotor polyneuropathies, mononeuritis multiplex, isolated central nervous system vasculitis, optic neuritis, acute transverse myelitis, pulmonary infiltrates, pleural effusion, hepatosplenomegaly, gastroenteritis, sclerosing cholangitis, cytopenias, bone marrow fibrosis, and thrombotic angiopathy [59]. HES is a potentially fatal disease, with a reported 10-year survival of <50% [60].

The initial evaluation of "HES" should include bone marrow examination with both cytogenetic and molecular (ie, fluorescence *in situ* hybridization [FISH] or real-time PCR for *FIP1L1-PDGFRA*) studies. A diagnosis of either HES or idiopathic eosinophilia is made only after all causes of clonal eosinophilia are excluded. Also, in all cases, T-cell immunophenotyping and T-cell-receptor antigen gene rearrangement analysis should be performed and if either clonal or immunophenotypically aberrant T cells are discovered, a diagnosis of lymphoproliferative variant of HES is preferred. Initial evaluation should also include echocardiogram, chest radiograph, pulmonary function tests, and measurement of serum troponin levels. Increased levels of serum cardiac troponin have been shown to correlate with the presence of cardiomyopathy in HES [61].

In general, treatment for HES is not indicated in the asymptomatic patient with normal troponin and no evidence of organ damage. The first-line drug of choice for symptomatic HES is prednisone (starting dose of 1 mg/kg/day). Most patients respond to this regimen but relapse is inevitable during steroid taper [62]. The second-line drug of choice is IFN-α (starting dose 3 million units three times per week) [38]. Patients intolerant to IFN-α can be treated with hydroxyurea instead (starting dose 500 mg twice daily) [62]. In true HES (ie, *FIP1L1/PDGFRA*$^-$), treatment with imatinib is unlikely to produce durable remissions [40]. Alemtuzumab, a monoclonal antibody that targets the CD52 antigen expressed by eosinophils, has been reported as active therapy in refractory cases [41].

There are currently three distinct types of molecularly defined CEL: *PDGFRA*, *PDGFRB*, and *FGFR1* rearranged. *PDGFRA* is usually rearranged by an interstitial deletion involving chromosome 4q12 (*FIP1L1-PDGFRA*) but can also be activated by chromosomal translocations; examples include *KIF5B-PDGFRA*, t(4:10)(q12;p11),

BCR–PDGFRA, t(4;22)(q12;q11), and *CDK5RAP2-PDGFRA*, ins(9;4)(q33;q12q25) [57]. The prevalence of *FIP1L1-PDGFRA* among patients with eosinophilia is low, and reported mutational frequencies in large studies ranges from 10% to 15% [63]. *FIP1L1-PDGFRA* can be detected by either FISH or PCR-based assays. Imatinib at 100 mg per day is the treatment of choice for *FIP1L1-PDGFRA*$^{+}$ CEL or other clonal eosinophilia and induces a complete hematologic and molecular remission in almost all affected patients [64]. Therefore, it is of utmost therapeutic relevance to perform peripheral blood screening for *FIP1L1-PDGFRA*, using either FISH or RT-PCR, in all patients with primary eosinophilia. Minimal residual disease after imatinib therapy can be assessed by quantitative molecular analysis. As has been the case with *PDGFRA*-rearranged cases, imatinib therapy produces complete hematologic remission in *PDGFRB*-rearranged clonal eosinophilia [65]. *PDGFRB*-rearranged cases are readily identifiable by cytogenetic testing where rearrangements of chromosome 5 are involved (5q31–q32). *FGFR1* translocations are usually associated with a clinical phenotype with features of both an aggressive eosinophilia-associated MPN and T-cell lymphoblastic lymphoma [66]. The composite syndrome is known as either the 8p11 myeloproliferative syndrome (EMS) or stem-cell leukemia lymphoma syndrome (SCLL). At present, drug therapy is ineffective and allogeneic stem-cell transplantation should be considered as soon as the particular diagnosis is established.

Systemic mast cell disease

Mastocytosis is a heterogeneous group of disorders characterized by clonal expansion of mast cells (MC) and their excessive accumulation in various organs such as skin, bone marrow, gastrointestinal tract, lymph nodes, liver, and spleen. Clinical course can range from no/minimal symptoms to diffuse systemic involvement with multiorgan failure. Mastocytosis has been classified into seven subtypes by the 2001 WHO guidelines: cutaneous mastocytosis, indolent systemic mastocytosis (ISM), SM with an associated clonal hematologic non-MC-lineage disease (SM-AHNMD); aggressive SM (ASM); MC leukemia; MC sarcoma; and extracutaneous mastocytoma [67]. SM is defined by the presence of one major and one minor, or three minor, diagnostic criteria (Box 30.1). Patients with SM are further characterized with regard to the presence of so called "B" and "C" findings (assessing disease burden and disease aggressiveness, respectively) (Box 30.2). Patients with SM with no findings are identified as ISM, those with B findings as smoldering SM (SSM, a subtype of ISM with possibly more aggressive clinical course) [68], and those with C findings as ASM. New WHO guidelines, due out this year, redefine mastocytosis

Box 30.1 World Health Organization diagnostic criteria for systemic mastocytosis.

Major criteria

1 Multifocal, dense infiltrates of mast cells (≥15 mast cells in aggregates) in bone marrow biopsy sections and/or in other extracutaneous organ(s)

Minor criteria

1 >25% mast cells in bone marrow or other extracutaneous organ(s) that show an atypical morphology (typically spindle shaped)
2 c-*KIT* mutation at codon 816 is present in extracutaneous tissues
3 Mast cells in bone marrow coexpress CD117 and either CD2, CD25, or both (by flow cytometry)
4 Serum tryptase persistently is ≥20 ng/mL (not accounted for in patients with an associated clonal hematologic non-mast cell disorder)

A diagnosis of systemic mastocytosis requires the fulfillment of either one major criterion and one minor criterion or three minor criteria.

Box 30.2 B findings and C findings in systemic mastocytosis.

B findings: indication of high mast-cell burden and expansion of the genetic defect into various myeloid lineages

1 Infiltration grade of mast cells in bone marrow >30% on histology and serum total tryptase levels >200 ng/mL
2 Hypercellular bone marrow with loss of fat cells, discrete signs of dysmyelopoiesis without substantial cytopenias, or World Health Organization criteria for myelodysplastic syndrome or myeloproliferative disorder
3 Organomegaly: palpable hepatomegaly, splenomegaly, or lymphadenopathy (>2 cm on CT or ultrasound) without impaired organ function

C findings: indication of impaired organ function because of mast-cell infiltration (confirmed by biopsy in most patients)

1 Cytopenia(s): absolute neutrophil count <1000/µL, or hemoglobin <10 g/dL, or platelets <100,000/µL
2 Hepatomegaly with ascites and impaired liver function
3 Palpable splenomegaly with hypersplenism
4 Malabsorption with hypoalbuminemia and weight loss
5 Skeletal lesions: large osteolyses or/and severe osteoporosis causing pathologic fractures
6 Life-threatening organomegaly in other organ systems that definitively is caused by an infiltration of the tissue by neoplastic mast cells

as "mast-cell disease", with SM as a subtype with bone marrow involvement [69].

Symptoms of mastocytosis can be divided into those caused by MC mediator release and those caused by MC organ infiltration.

1 Symptoms of mediator release: vasoactive mediators (histamine, leukotrienes, heparin, prostaglandins) released from MC can lead to itching, flushing, lightheadedness, syncope, palpitations, diarrhea, heartburn, fatigue, and headache. MC degranulation can be exacerbated by infections, alcohol, exercise, and medications.

2 Symptoms of organ infiltration: skin involvement can occur as cutaneous mastocytosis or as cutaneous manifestation of SM. Urticaria pigmentosa is the most common skin manifestation, characterized by reddish-brown macules and papules. Nodular and plaque-like lesions can occur. Associated pruritus is exacerbated by local friction, spicy food, and temperature changes. Scratching of affected skin characteristically leads to development of urticaria and erythema (Darier sign). Gastrointestinal involvement can present as chronic diarrhea, steatorrhea, malabsorbtion, and ascites. Anemia is the most common hematologic abnormality because of bone marrow infiltration, and peripheral eosinophilia is seen in around 20% of patients [70]. Bone pain and fractures can occur as a result of MC mediator-induced abnormal bone turnover or from direct destruction of the bones by invading MCs [71].

Diagnosis of SM is based on a set of diagnostic criteria (Table 30.1) but primarily relies on the identification of neoplastic MC in various organs. Bone marrow examination is imperative for SM diagnosis as most adults with mastocytosis have underlying bone marrow involvement. Bone marrow examination also helps to diagnose any underlying AHNMD. Neoplastic MC are characteristically spindle shaped and present in multifocal aggregates. Unlike normal MC, neoplastic MC expresses surface markers CD2 and/or CD25. Serum tryptase levels and urinary histamine levels (both released by MC) are typically elevated. KIT gene *D816V* mutation screening should be considered for all patients with MS as it is present in approximately 90% of cases.

There is a lack of effective treatment for SM and standard treatments have been aimed at symptom control. These include the use of oral antihistamines and MC stabilizers like cromolyn sodium [72]. Patients should avoid specific factors that can trigger MC degranulation, like emotional stress, cold exposure, alcohol use, strenuous exercise, and use of non-steroidal anti-inflammatory drugs. Both sedating (hydroxyzine, diphenhydramine) and non-sedating second generation H1 antihistamines (cetrizine, loratidine, desloratidine, fexofenadine) can be used to alleviate pruritus and itching. As both H1 and H2 receptors are present in skin (85% of cutaneous histamine receptors are H1 and 15% are H2), the addition of an H2 blocker (ranitidine, famotidine) should be considered for patients not responding to H1 antihistamines alone.

Cromolyn sodium has been shown to be beneficial in patients with gastrointestinal symptoms (diarrhea, vomiting, abdominal pain). Short courses of prednisone can be considered for patients with severe symptoms not controlled with other supportive medications, or for those with malabsorbtion and ascites. Topical cromoglycates, topical corticosteroids, and PUVA (psoralen-ultraviolet A) therapy has been used for some patients with cutaneous manifestations. Patients with history of anaphylaxis or cardiovascular collapse should carry an EpiPen for epinephrine self-administration. For patients with osteoporosis, bisphosphonate therapy (pamidronate at 90 mg intravenously per month) should be considered. Cytoreductive therapies (IFN-α-2b and cladribine) are usually reserved for patients with ASM, or occasionally patients with ISM with uncontrolled symptoms or with severe osteoporosis. Casassus *et al.* [73] reported a multicenter trial in 20 patients with SM (16 ASM, four ISM) with use of IFN-α-2b (starting dose of 1 million units subcutaneously daily, dose escalated to 5 million units/m^2/day depending on tolerance). Thirteen patients (65%) who completed 6 months of treatment responded (seven partial, six minor, no complete responses). However, many patients experienced undesirable side-effects. The combination of IFN-α-2b plus prednisone has also been used [74]. Few reports have documented the efficacy of cladribine in SM. In a multicenter study, all 10 patients treated with cladribine (0.13 mg/kg/day for 5 days repeated every 4–6 weeks) showed improvement in MC-mediated signs and symptoms [75]. In the largest series so far of 33 patients, use of cladribine led to a major response in 24 patients (and a minor response in another two patients) [76]. In this study, the mean time to best response was 4 months and mean duration of response was 16 months. Myelosuppression is the main treatment-related side-effect in patients treated with cladribine.

Novel treatments targeting the mutated KIT tyrosine kinase are being investigated in clinical studies. KIT is a tyrosine kinase receptor, encoded by the *c-KIT* gene located on chromosome 4q12 in humans [77]. The binding of a stem-cell factor (SCF, KIT ligand) to KIT leads to receptor dimerization and phosphorylation of the downstream signaling molecules. KIT plays an important role in normal hematopoiesis. KIT expression declines in hematopoietic cell lines with maturation except in MC. Furitsu *et al.* [78] were the first to show that KIT was constitutively activated and expressed in the absence of SCF in an MC line derived from a patient with MC leukemia. A point mutation, *D816V* (substitution of valine for aspartate at codon 816, *Asp816Val*), in the tyrosine kinase domain of the KIT receptor has been described in >90% of adult patients with SM using a sensitive PCR-based assay. Other KIT mutations involving tyrosine kinase, juxtamembrane, and transmembrane domains have been described in sporadic cases. Sporadic KIT mutations (*F522C, K509I, V560G,* and *del419*) have been shown to be imatinib-sensitive in isolated cases [79]. Imatinib at a dose of 400 mg daily is approved by the Food and Drug Administration in the USA for adult patients with ASM without the KIT *D816V* mutation or with an unknown KIT mutational status. Several medications targeting the KIT *D816V* mutant are currently being investigated as therapy for SM.

An important subgroup of patients with SM with imatinib responsiveness is the group with *FIP1L1–PDGFRα* mutation. Peripheral blood eosinophilia is seen in approximately 20% of patients with SM (SM-eos), and bone marrow eosinophilia has been reported in 19–33% of patients [70]. For patients with the *FIP1L1–PDGFRα* mutation, imatinib at 100 mg daily is the treatment of choice as it eliminates the disease in almost all cases [80]. Imatinib is currently approved in the USA for patients with ASM associated with eosinophilia (starting dose 100 mg daily with dose escalation to 400 mg daily if there is an insufficient response and an absence of side-effects).

References

1 Adamson JW, Fialkow PJ. The pathogenesis of myeloproliferative syndromes. *Br J Hematol* 1978;38:299–303.

2 Dameshek W. Some speculations on the myeloproliferative syndrome. *Blood* 1951;6:372–5.

3 Gilbert. The spectrum of myeloproliferative disorders. *Med Clin North Am* 1973;57:355–93.

4 Tefferi A, Thiele J, Orazi A, *et al.* Proposals and rationale for revision of the World Health Organization diagnostic criteria for polycythemia vera, essential thrombocythemia, and primary myelofibrosis: recommendations from an ad hoc international expert panel. *Blood* 2007;110:1092–7.

5 Mesa RA, Silverstein MN, Jacobsen SJ, Wollan PC, Tefferi A. Population-based incidence and survival figures in essential thrombocythemia and agnogenic myeloid metaplasia: an Olmsted County Study, 1976–1995. *Am J Hematol* 1999;61:10–15.

6 Dupriez B, Morel P, Demory JL, *et al.* Prognostic factors in agnogenic myeloid metaplasia: a report on 195 cases with a new scoring system [see comments]. *Blood* 1996;88:1013–18.

7 Passamonti F, Rumi E, Pungolino E, *et al.* Life expectancy and prognostic factors for survival in patients with polycythemia vera and essential thrombocythemia. *Am J Med* 2004;117:755–61.

8 Pardanani A. JAK2 inhibitor therapy in myeloproliferative disorders: rationale, preclinical studies and ongoing clinical trials. *Leukemia* 2008;22:23–30.

9 Baxter EJ, Scott LM, Campbell PJ, *et al.* Acquired mutation of the tyrosine kinase JAK2 in human myeloproliferative disorders. *Lancet* 2005;365:1054–61.

10 Levine RL, Wadleigh M, Cools J. Activating mutation in the tyrosine kinase JAK2 in polycythemia vera, essential thrombocythemia, and myelofibrosis with myeloid metaplasia. *Cancer Cell* 2005;7:387–97.

11 Kralovics R, Passamonti F, Buser AS, *et al.* A gain-of-function mutation of *JAK2* in myeloproliferative disorders. *N Engl J Med* 2005;352:1779–90.

12 James C, Ugo V, Le Couedic JP, *et al.* A unique clonal *JAK2* mutation leading to constitutive signaling causes polycythaemia vera. *Nature* 2005;434:1144–8.

13 Landolfi R, Di Gennaro L, Barbui T, *et al.* Leukocytosis as a major thrombotic risk factor in patients with polycythemia vera. *Blood* 2007;109:2446–52.

14 Vannucchi AM, Antonioli E, Guglielmelli P, *et al.* Prospective identification of high-risk polycythemia vera patients based on *JAK2(V617F)* allele burden. *Leukemia* 2007;21:1952–9.

15 Landolfi R, Marchioli R, Kutti J, *et al.* Efficacy and safety of low-dose aspirin in polycythemia vera. *N Engl J Med* 2004; 350:114–24.

16 Di Nisio M, Barbui T, Di Gennaro L, *et al.* The haematocrit and platelet target in polycythemia vera. *Br J Haematol* 2007;136: 249–59.

17 Cortelazzo S, Finazzi G, Ruggeri M, *et al.* Hydroxyurea for patients with essential thrombocythemia and a high risk of thrombosis. *N Engl J Med* 1995;332:1132–6.

18 Harrison CN, Campbell PJ, Buck G, *et al.* Hydroxyurea compared with anagrelide in high-risk essential thrombocythemia. *N Engl J Med* 2005;353:33–45.

19 Finazzi G, Caruso V, Marchioli R, *et al.* Acute leukemia in polycythemia vera: an analysis of 1638 patients enrolled in a prospective observational study. *Blood* 2005;105:2664–70.

20 Kiladjian JJ, Cassinat B, Turlure P, *et al.* High molecular response rate of polycythemia vera patients treated with pegylated interferon alpha-2a. *Blood* 2006;108:2037–40.

21 Paquette R, Sokol L, Shah NP, *et al.* A phase I study of XL019, a selective JAK2 inhibitor, in patients with polycythemia vera. *Blood* (ASH Annual Meeting Abstracts) 2008;112:971.

22 Moliterno AR, Roboz GJ, Carroll M, Luger S, Hexner E, Bensen-Kennedy DM. An open-label study of CEP-701 in patients with JAK2 V617F-positive polycythemia vera and essential thrombocytosis. *Blood* (ASH Annual Meeting Abstracts) 2008; 112:44.

23 Rambaldi A, Dellacasa CM, Salmoiraghi S, *et al.* A phase 2A study of the histone-deacetylase inhibitor ITF2357 in patients with Jak2V617F positive Chronic myeloproliferative neoplasms. *Blood* 2008;112:44–5.

24 Kiladjian JJ, Cassinat B, Chevret S, *et al.* Pegylated interferon-alfa-2a induces complete hematologic and molecular responses with low toxicity in polycythemia vera. *Blood* 2008;112: 3065–72.

25 Quintas-Cardama A, Kantarjian HM, Garcia-Manero G, *et al.* Pegylated interferon-ALFA-2A (PEG-IFN-{alpha}–2A; PEGASYS) therapy renders high clinical and molecular response rates in patients with essential thrombocythemia (ET) and polycythemia Vera (PV). *Blood* (ASH Annual Meeting Abstracts) 2008;112:246.

26 Besses C, Alvarez-Larran A, Martinez-Aviles L, Longaron R, Serrano S, Bellosillo B. Major hematological response is the main factor for achieving a major molecular response in JAK2V617F-positive essential thrombocythemia and polycythemia vera patients treated with hydroxyurea. *Blood* (ASH Annual Meeting Abstracts) 2008;112:246–7.

27 Cervantes F, Dupriez B, Pereira A, *et al.* New prognostic scoring system for primary myelofibrosis based on a study of the International Working Group for Myelofibrosis Research and Treatment. *Blood* 2009;113:2895–901.

28 Deeg HJ, Gooley TA, Flowers ME, *et al.* Allogeneic hematopoietic stem cell transplantation for myelofibrosis. *Blood* 2003; 102:3912–18.

29 Rondelli D, Barosi G, Bacigalupo A, *et al.* Allogeneic hematopoietic stem cell transplantation with reduced intensity conditioning in intermediate or high risk patients with myelofibrosis with myeloid metaplasia. *Blood* 2005;105:4115–19.

30 Cervantes F, Alvarez-Larran A, Hernandez-Boluda JC, Sureda A, Torrebadell M, Montserrat E. Erythropoietin treatment of the anaemia of myelofibrosis with myeloid metaplasia: results in 20 patients and review of the literature. *Br J Haematol* 2004; 127:399–403.

31 Cervantes F, Hernandez-Boluda JC, Alvarez A, Nadal E, Montserrat E. Danazol treatment of idiopathic myelofibrosis with severe anemia. *Haematologica* 2000;85:595–9.

32 Lofvenberg E, Wahlin A, Roos G, Ost A. Reversal of myelofibrosis by hydroxyurea. *Eur J Haematol* 1990;44:33–8.

33 Faoro LN, Tefferi A, Mesa RA. Long-term analysis of the palliative benefit of 2-chlorodeoxyadenosine for myelofibrosis with myeloid metaplasia. *Eur J Haematol* 2005;74:117–20.

34 Lofvenberg E, Wahlin A. Management of polycythaemia vera, essential thrombocythaemia and myelofibrosis with hydroxyurea. *Eur J Haematol* 1988;41:375–81.

35 Hickling RA. Splenectomy in myeloid metaplasia. *QJM* 1937; 30:253.

36 Petti MC, Latagliata R, Spadea T, *et al.* Melphalan treatment in patients with myelofibrosis with myeloid metaplasia. *Br J Haematol* 2002;116:576–81.

37 Mesa RA, Nagorney DS, Schwager S, Allred J, Tefferi A. Palliative goals, patient selection, and perioperative platelet management: outcomes and lessons from 3 decades of splenectomy for myelofibrosis with myeloid metaplasia at the Mayo Clinic. *Cancer* 2006;107:361–70.

38 Butterfield JH, Gleich GJ. Interferon-alpha treatment of six patients with the idiopathic hypereosinophilic syndrome. *Ann Intern Med* 1994;121:648–53.

39 Tefferi A, Cortes J, Verstovsek S, *et al.* Lenalidomide therapy in myelofibrosis with myeloid metaplasia. *Blood* 2006;108: 1158–64.

40 Pardanani A, Brockman SR, Paternoster SF, *et al.* FIP1L1–PDGFRA fusion: prevalence and clinicopathologic correlates in 89 consecutive patients with moderate to severe eosinophilia. *Blood* 2004;104:3038–45.

41 Verstovsek S, Tefferi A, Kantarjian H, *et al.* Alemtuzumab therapy for hypereosinophilic syndrome and chronic eosinophilic leukemia. *Clin Cancer Res* 2009;15:368–73.

42 Tefferi A, Barosi G, Mesa RA, *et al.* International Working Group (IWG) consensus criteria for treatment response in myelofibrosis with myeloid metaplasia, for the IWG for Myelofibrosis Research and Treatment (IWG-MRT). *Blood* 2006; 108:1497–503.

43 Silver RT, Jenkins DE, Jr., Engle RL, Jr. Use of testosterone and busulfan in the treatment of myelofibrosis with myeloid metaplasia. *Blood* 1964;23:341–53.

44 Mesa RA, Steensma DP, Pardanani A, *et al.* A phase 2 trial of combination low-dose thalidomide and prednisone for the treatment of myelofibrosis with myeloid metaplasia. *Blood* 2003;101:2534–41.

45 Tefferi A, Lasho TL, Mesa RA, Pardanani A, Ketterling RP, Hanson CA. Lenalidomide therapy in del(5)(q31)-associated myelofibrosis: cytogenetic and JAK2V617F molecular remissions. *Leukemia* 2007;21:1827–8.

46 Tefferi A, Elliot MA, Yoon SY, *et al.* Clinical and bone marrow effects of interferon alfa therapy in myelofibrosis with myeloid metaplasia. *Blood* 2001;97:1896.

47 Verstovsek S, Lawhorn, K, Giles, F, *et al.* PEG-Intron for myeloproliferative diseases: an update of ongoing phase II study. *Blood* 2004;104: Abstract 633.

48 Quintás-Cardama A, Tong W, Kantarjian H, *et al.* A phase II study of 5-azacitidine for patients with primary and post essential thrombocythemia/polcythemia vera myelofibrosis. *Leukemia* 2008;22:965–70.

49 Mesa RA, Verstovsek S, Rivera C, *et al.* 5-Azacitidine has limited therapeutic activity in myelofibrosis. *Leukemia* 2008; 23:180–2.

50 Steensma DP, Hook CC, Stafford SL, Tefferi A. Low-dose, single-fraction, whole-lung radiotherapy for pulmonary hypertension associated with myelofibrosis with myeloid metaplasia. *Br J Haematol* 2002;118:813–16.

51 Koch CA, Li CY, Mesa RA, Tefferi A. Nonhepatosplenic extramedullary hematopoiesis: associated diseases, pathology, clinical course, and treatment. *Mayo Clin Proc* 2003;78: 1223–33.

52 Elliott MA, Chen MG, Silverstein MN, Tefferi A. Splenic irradiation for symptomatic splenomegaly associated with myelofibrosis with myeloid metaplasia. *Br J Hematol* 1998;103: 505–11.

53 Bouabdallah R, Coso D, Gonzague-Casabianca L, Alzieu C, Resbeut M, Gastaut JA. Safety and efficacy of splenic irradiation in the treatment of patients with idiopathic myelofibrosis: a report on 15 patients. *Leuk Res* 2000;24:491–5.

54 Verstovsek S, Kantarjian HM, Pardanani AD, *et al.* The JAK inhibitor, INCB018424, demonstrates durable and marked clinical responses in primary myelofibrosis (PMF) and post-polycythemia/essential thrombocythemia myelofibrosis (Post PV/ETMF). *Blood* 2008;112:622.

55 Pardanani AD, Gotlib J, Jamieson C, *et al.* A phase I study of TG101348, an orally bioavailable JAK2-selective inhibitor, in patients with myelofibrosis. *Blood* 2008;112:97.

56 Shah NP, Olszynski P, Sokol L, *et al.* A phase I study of XL019, a selective JAK2 inhibitor, in patients with primary myelofibrosis, post-polycythemia vera, or post-essential thrombocythemia myelofibrosis. *Blood* (ASH Annual Meeting Abstracts) 2008; 112:44.

57 Tefferi A, Patnaik MM, Pardanani A. Eosinophilia: secondary, clonal and idiopathic. *Br J Haematol* 2006;133:468–92.

58 Bain BJ. Relationship between idiopathic hypereosinophilic syndrome, eosinophilic leukemia, and systemic mastocytosis. *Am J Hematol* 2004;77:82–5.

59 Fauci AS, Harley JB, Roberts WC, Ferrans VJ, Gralnick HR, Bjornson BH. NIH conference. The idiopathic hypereosinophilic syndrome. Clinical, pathophysiologic, and therapeutic considerations. *Ann Intern Med* 1982;97:78–92.

60 Lefebvre C, Bletry O, Degoulet P, *et al.* [Prognostic factors of hypereosinophilic syndrome. Study of 40 cases]. *Ann Med Interne (Paris)* 1989;140:253–7.

61 Pitini V, Arrigo C, Azzarello D, *et al.* Serum concentration of cardiac Troponin T in patients with hypereosinophilic syndrome treated with imatinib is predictive of adverse outcomes. *Blood* 2003;102:3456–7; Author reply 3457.

62 Parrillo JE, Fauci AS, Wolff SM. Therapy of the hypereosinophilic syndrome. *Ann Intern Med* 1978;89:167–72.

63 Pardanani A, Ketterling RP, Li CY, *et al.* FIP1L1-PDGFRA in eosinophilic disorders: prevalence in routine clinical practice, long-term experience with imatinib therapy, and a critical review of the literature. *Leuk Res* 2006;30:965–70.

64 Jovanovic JV, Score J, Waghorn K, *et al.* Low-dose imatinib mesylate leads to rapid induction of major molecular responses and achievement of complete molecular remission in FIP1L1-PDGFRA positive chronic eosinophilic leukemia. *Blood* 2007; 109:4635–40.

65 Apperley JF, Gardembas M, Melo JV, *et al.* Response to imatinib mesylate in patients with chronic myeloproliferative diseases with rearrangements of the platelet-derived growth factor receptor beta. *N Engl J Med* 2002;347:481–7.

66 Macdonald D, Reiter A, Cross NC. The 8p11 myeloproliferative syndrome: a distinct clinical entity caused by constitutive activation of FGFR1. *Acta Haematol* 2002;107:101–7.

67 Valent P, Horny HP, Escribano L, *et al.* Diagnostic criteria and classification of mastocytosis: a consensus proposal. *Leuk Res* 2001;25:603–25.

68 Valent P, Akin C, Sperr WR, Horny HP, Metcalfe DD. Smouldering mastocytosis: a novel subtype of systemic mastocytosis with slow progression. *Int Arch Allergy Immunol* 2002; 127:137–9.

69 Tefferi A, Vardiman JW. Classification and diagnosis of myeloproliferative neoplasms: The 2008 World Health Organization criteria and point-of-care diagnostic algorithms. *Leukemia* 2008; 22:14–22.

70 Lawrence JB, Friedman BS, Travis WD, Chinchilli VM, Metcalfe DD, Gralnick HR. Hematologic manifestations of systemic mast cell disease: a prospective study of laboratory and morphologic features and their relation to prognosis. *Am J Med* 1991;91:612–24.

71 Chiappetta N, Gruber B. The role of mast cells in osteoporosis. *Semin Arthritis Rheum* 2006;36:32–6.

72 Worobec AS. Treatment of systemic mast cell disorders. *Hematol Oncol Clin North Am* 2000;14:659–87, vii.

73 Casassus P, Caillat-Vigneron N, Martin A, *et al.* Treatment of adult systemic mastocytosis with interferon-alpha: results of a multicentre phase II trial on 20 patients. *Br J Haematol* 2002; 119:1090–7.

74 Hauswirth AW, Simonitsch-Klupp I, Uffmann M, *et al.* Response to therapy with interferon alpha-2b and prednisolone in aggressive systemic mastocytosis: report of five cases and review of the literature. *Leuk Res* 2004;28:249–57.

75 Kluin-Nelemans HC, Oldhoff JM, Van Doormaal JJ, *et al.* Cladribine therapy for systemic mastocytosis. *Blood* 2003;102: 4270–6.

76 Lortholary O, Vargaftig J, Feger F, *et al.* Efficacy and safety of cladribine in adult systemic mastocytosis: a French multicenter study of 33 patients. *Blood* 2004;104:190a.

77 Yarden Y, Kuang WJ, Yang-Feng T, *et al.* Human proto-oncogene *c-kit*: a new cell surface receptor tyrosine kinase for an unidentified ligand. *Embo J* 1987;6:3341–51.

78 Furitsu T, Tsujimura T, Tono T, *et al.* Identification of mutations in the coding sequence of the proto-oncogene *c-kit* in a human mast cell leukemia cell line causing ligand-independent activation of *c-kit* product. *J Clin Invest* 1993;92:1736–44.

79 Quintas-Cardama A, Aribi A, Cortes J, Giles FJ, Kantarjian H, Verstovsek S. Novel approaches in the treatment of systemic mastocytosis. *Cancer* 2006;107:1429–39.

80 Pardanani A, Ketterling RP, Brockman SR, *et al.* CHIC2 deletion, a surrogate for FIP1L1–PDGFRA fusion, occurs in systemic mastocytosis associated with eosinophilia and predicts response to imatinib mesylate therapy. *Blood* 2003;102:3093–6.

Part 9
General Treatment Principles and Clinical Developments

Chapter 31
Management of Emergencies in Leukemias

Olga Frankfurt
Northwestern University Feinberg School of Medicine, Robert H. Lurie Comprehensive Cancer Center, Chicago, Illinois, USA

Introduction

The clinical manifestations of leukemias may vary from mild non-specific symptoms, such as progressive malaise, fever and fatigue, to severe life-threatening complications requiring immediate medical intervention.

Hyperleukocytosis and leukostasis

Hyperleukocytosis, generally defined as circulating white blood cell (WBC) count exceeding 50,000–100,000/μL, is seen more commonly in specific leukemic subtypes. In acute lymphoblastic leukemia (ALL), the hyperleukocytosis (10–30%) is associated with T-cell phenotype, 11q23, and t(9; 22) chromosomal rearrangements. In acute myeloid leukemia (AML), 5–29% of adults, and an even higher percentage of children, will present with hyperleukocytosis (5–12%, WBC count >100,000/μL; 15–29%, WBC count >50,000/μL). It occurs more commonly with myelomonocytic (M4) and monocytic (M5) French–American–British (FAB) subtypes, the microgranular variant of acute promyelocytic leukemia (APL) (M3), 11q23, inv16 (p13;q22) and chromosome 6 abnormalities, internal tandem duplication of the FLT3 (FLT3-ITD) gene, and expression of lung resistance protein (LRP) [1–3]. In ALL, hyperleukocytosis is associated with poor long-term outcome and survival but does not appear to have a major impact on early mortality, unless the WBC count is >250,000/μL [4,5]. In AML, hyperleukocytosis is associated with an increased likelihood of early mortality and induction death; however, its influence on the long-term outcome remains controversial [6–13].

Leukostasis is a clinicopathologic syndrome occurring as a result of diffuse occlusion of tissue microvasculature by the leukemic blasts. It is an uncommon but potentially lethal feature of acute leukemias, causing respiratory failure, intracranial bleeding, and acute renal failure. Several factors, such as hyperleukocytosis, peculiar rheologic properties of the leukemic blasts, as well as activation of adhesion cell-surface molecules for endothelium and cell–cell interactions, contribute to the development of the leukostasis. Although hyperleukocytosis may occur more commonly in patients with ALL, those with AML are more likely to suffer serious complications and death attributed to leukostasis, indicating that factors other than leukocytosis contribute to the leukostasis (Plate 31.1) [14]. Symptomatic leukostasis is rare among patients with chronic myeloid (CML) and chronic lymphocytic (CLL) leukemias (Figure 31.1) [1, 6,14–16].

In vitro studies demonstrate that an increased expression of adhesion molecules by the endothelial cells and of the corresponding receptors in the myeloblasts contribute to leukostasis. Myeloblasts, via production of TNFα (tumor necrosis factor α) and IL-1β (interleukin 1 β) cytokines, upregulate the expression of ICAM-1 (intracellular adhesion molecule 1), VCAM-1 (vascular cell adhesion molecule 1), P-selectin, and E-selectin by the endothelial cells. These cytokines enable the endothelial cells to recruit additional myeloblasts, forming a self-perpetuating cycle in which more cells are trapped in microcirculation [15]. It was also shown that CD11b, a receptor of ICAM-1 and ICAM-2, was highly expressed on M4 and M5 myeloblasts. Recent data indicate that expression of CD56/NCAM (detected by the immunophenotyping) is associated with the development of leukostasis in M4 and M5 subtypes of AML [16]. Of interest, high CD56 expression also correlated with poor response to leukapheresis [17].

Additionally, the stiffness of myeloid blasts, as measured by atomic force microscopy, is 18 times that of lymphoid blasts and six times of that of normal neutrophils [18]. This difference in deformability of the cells may, at least partially, explain the increased frequency of leukostasis in AML compared with ALL.

In most cases, whole blood viscosity is not likely to contribute to the development of leukostasis. It has been

Leukemias: Principles and Practice of Therapy, 1st edition. Edited by S. Faderl and H. Kantarjian.

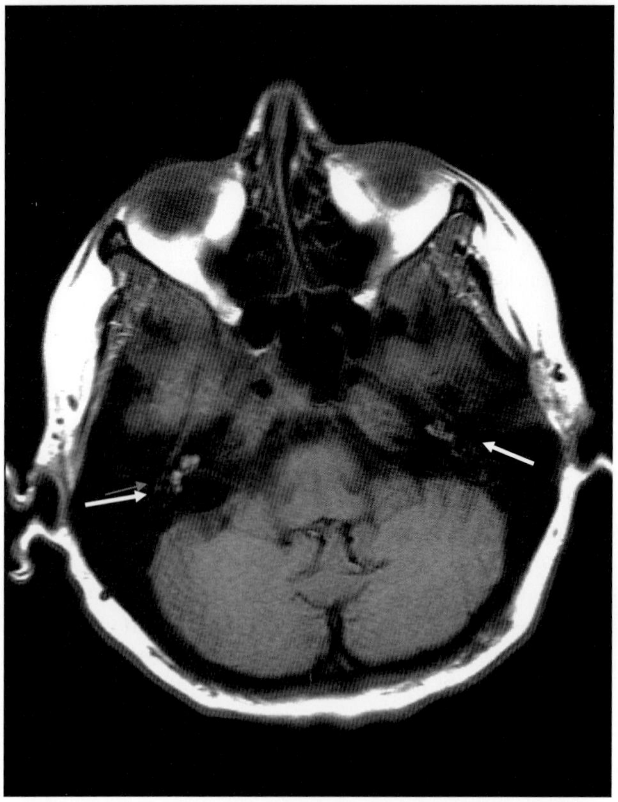

Figure 31.1 Bilateral cochlea bleed in a patient with chronic-phase chronic myeloid leukemia (CML) and a white blood cell (WBC) count of 850,000/μL, who presented with gradual loss of hearing and balance. Precontrast axial T1-weighted brain magnetic resonance imaging reveals a hyperintense signal bilaterally in the cochleae and vestibules (arrows).

estimated that the whole blood viscosity is affected only when the leukocrit reaches 20–25%, corresponding to 400,000–600,000/μL in AML and 500,000–1000,000/μL in ALL, levels that are rarely reached. However, blood transfusion must be administered with great care and only when absolutely required (hemoglobin <7 g/dL) to avoid increasing hematocrit (fractional erythrocyte volume), and consequently the whole blood viscosity, and to avoid potentiating the symptoms related to leukostasis.

The presence of symptoms suggestive of leukostasis, such as headache, blurred vision, dyspnea and hypoxia, constitute a medical emergency, and efforts should be made to lower WBC count rapidly. This is typically accomplished by the initiation of leukapheresis in conjunction with hydroxyurea, hydration, and electrolyte management while rapid preparations for the administration of definitive cytotoxic therapy are made. Historically, leukapheresis has been used in patients with WBC count >100,000/mL in AML and >100,000–200,000/mL in ALL and neurologic and pulmonary symptoms suggestive of leukostasis [19].

It remains controversial as to whether reduction in peripheral blood count by leukapheresis results in improved mortality, and there are no data to indicate that the outcome is improved in asymptomatic patients [2,20]. Despite the absence of definitive answers and because of the relative safety of the procedure, physicians are reluctant to withhold leukapheresis when leukostasis-related complications are encountered. This approach may not apply to patients with APL (or a variant) as leukapheresis may exacerbate the coagulopathy and increase the risk of bleeding.

Complications of leukapheresis include bleeding at the site of catheter placement, line-related infections, citrate-induced hypocalcemia, and rarely anaphylactoid reaction and bronchospasm. Patients may require platelet transfusion before the catheter placement to minimize the risk of bleeding. Citrate, present in the anticoagulant, binds to free calcium in the patient's plasma, leading to low free-calcium levels and, consequently, paresthesias and muscle cramps. Administration of calcium before the leukapheresis helps to alleviate these symptoms. Corticosteroids and bronchodilators should be at the patient's bedside to counteract the pulmonary complications.

Hydroxyurea may be administered simultaneously with, or in place of, leukapheresis. For 50–100mg/kg per day in three or four divided doses, it is expected to reduce the leukocyte counts by 50–60% within 48 h. Preliminary results of a randomized clinical trial demonstrated no survival advantage of leukapheresis over hydroxyurea in patients with AML and hyperleukocytosis [21]. Supportive measures aimed at volume resuscitation and electrolyte management (see section on Tumor lysis syndrome) should be instituted immediately.

Hyperleukocytosis may cause factitious laboratory results. Glucose and oxygen levels may be abnormally low owing to their utilization by the large number of leukocytes [22,23]. Rapid processing of the sample after collection may help avoid factitious hypoglycemia. Pulse oximetry rather than arterial blood gas will help to evaluate hypoxemia. Release of potassium from the malignant cells may cause hyperkalemia. Collecting the sample to ensure minimal trauma, optimal storage conditions and rapid analysis, and removing the plasma after high-speed centrifugation, will help to establish the actual potassium level. A discrepancy of 0.3 mEq/L between serum and plasma potassium will secure the diagnosis of factitious hyperkalemia.

Metabolic complications

Severe metabolic disturbances may accompany the initial diagnosis and therapy of acute and, less commonly, chronic leukemias [24]. Metabolic abnormalities account for significant morbidity and mortality in patients with leukemia if it is not recognized early and if they are not treated appropriately.

Tumor lysis syndrome

Tumor lysis syndrome (TLS) is a metabolic disorder characterized by hyperuricemia, hyperkalemia, hyperphosphatemia and secondary hypocalcemia, and occurs as a result of the release of intracellular contents during rapid tumor cell destruction. Such electrolyte abnormalities may lead to the development of oliguric renal failure due to the tubular precipitation of urate and calcium phosphate crystals, fatal cardiac arrhythmias, hypocalcemic tetany, and seizures.

Several TLS classification systems (Hande–Garrow, Cairo–Bishop) separate patients into groups based on the presence of laboratory and clinical evidence of TLS (Box 31.1 and Box 31.2). Recently, a European consensus on the management of TLS has updated and modified the TLS classification [25]. Laboratory TLS is defined by the occurrence of two or more of the following values from 3 days before to 7 days after the start of anticancer therapy:

1 uric acid—increase by more than 25% from baseline, or value of >476 mmol/L (8 mg/dL);
2 potassium—increase by more than 25% from baseline, or >6 mmol/L (6 mEq/L);
3 phosphorus—increase by more than 25% from baseline, or >1.45 mmol/L (4.5 mg/dL) in adults and >2.1 mmol/L (6.5 mg/dL) in children;
4 calcium—decrease by more than 25% from baseline, or ≤1.75 mmol/L (7 mg/dL).

Clinical TLS is defined by the presence of the above-mentioned laboratory TLS and at least one of the following clinical features: renal insufficiency, cardiac arrhythmia, and seizure. Utilization of the glomerular filtration rate (GFR) instead of elevated creatinine level has been proposed as a measure of renal insufficiency, as the latter could be influenced by the patient age, volume status, and muscle mass. Several formulas (Modification of Diet in Renal Disease Study group and Cockroft and Gault equation) can be utilized to assess the GFR (Figure 31.2). Grading of the clinical TLS ranges form I to IV and corresponds with the highest grade of the observed clinical complications (Table 31.1) [25].

All of the patients with hematologic malignancies are at risk of developing TLS, which may occur spontaneously or after initiation of systemic chemotherapy [26]. Tumor burden (reflected by the high WBC count of over 50,000/μL), extensive bone marrow involvement, and elevated serum lactate dehydrogenase (LDH), are the main predictors for the development of acute TLS (ATLS) [27]. Certain patient characteristics, such as baseline hyperuricemia, renal insufficiency, obstructive uropathy and advanced age, predispose to the development of TLS [27]. Among cytotoxic therapy, those with cycle-specific

Box 31.1 Cairo-Bishop Definition of Laboratory tumor lysis syndrome.

Uric acid	>8.0 mg/dL or 25% increase from baseline
Potassium	>6.0 mg/dL or 25% increase from baseline
Phosphorus	>6.5 mg/dL (children)
	>4.5 mg/dL (adults) or 25% increase from baseline
Calcium	≤7.0 mg/dL (adults) or 25% decrease from baseline

Reprinted with permission from Blackwell Publishing Ltd. Cairo MS, Bishop M. Tumor lysis syndrome: new therapeutic strategies and classification. *Br J Haematol.* 2004;127:3–11.

Box 31.2 Cairo-Bishop Definition of Clinical tumor lysis syndrome.

Creatinine: >1.5 ULN
Cardiac arrhythmia/sudden death
Seizure

Reprinted with permission from Blackwell Publishing Ltd. Cairo MS, Bishop M. Tumor lysis syndrome: new therapeutic strategies and classification. *Br J Haematol.* 2004;127:3–11.

MDRD formula

eGFR (mL/min/1.73m^2) = 175 x serum creatinine (mmol/L) x 0.0113)$^{-1.154}$ x Age (years)$^{-0.203}$ x (0.742 if female)

Race multiplier 1 for all except black for whom it is 1.212.

Cockroft and Gault equation

Estimated creatinine clearance = (140-age (years)) x weight (kg) x 1.2 x (0.85 if female) serum creatinine (mmol/L)

Figure 31.2 Modification of Diet in Renal Disease Study Group Formula and Cockroft and Gault Equation.

Table 31.1 Grading of clinical tumor lysis syndrome [25].

	I	II	III	IV
Renal failure	sCr 1.5 UNL or CrCl 30–45 mL/min	sCr 1.5–3 UNL or CrCl 10–30 mL/min	sCr 1.5–3 UNL or CrCl 10–20 mL/min	sCr >6 UNL or CrCl < 10 mL/min
Cardiac arrhythmia	Intervention not indicated	Non-urgent intervention indicated	Symptomatic and incompletely controlled or controlled with device (eg, defibrillator)	Life-threatening (eg, arrhythmia associated with CHF, hypotension, syncope, shock)
Seizure	None	One brief generalized seizure; seizures are well controlled with anticonvulsive drugs or are infrequent focal motor seizures not interfering with ADL	Seizure in which consciousness is altered; poorly controlled seizure disorder with breakthrough generalized seizures despite medical intervention	Seizure of any kind which is prolonged, repetitive, or difficult to control (eg, status epilepticus, intractable epilepsy)

Reprinted with permission from Tosi P, Barosi G, Lazzaro C, *et al.* Consensus conference on the management of tumor lysis. *Haematologica* 2008;93:1877–85.

CrCl, creatinine clearance; sCr, serum creatinine; UNL, upper normal limit.

mechanism of action, such as cytarabine and etoposide, are more frequently associated with TLS [28]. Therapy with corticosteroids, monoclonal antibodies (rituximab, alemtuzumab, gemtuzumab ozogamicin), intrathecal methotrexate (rare), thalidomide, lenalidomide and flavopiridol (in CLL), hydroxyurea, fludarabine, and imatinib, among others, can cause TLS [29–34]. In a univariate retrospective analysis of 194 patients with AML undergoing induction chemotherapy hyperuricemia, elevated creatinine levels, elevated LDH levels, male gender, and history of CMMoL were significant predictors of TLS [35]. In a multivariate analysis, serum creatinine levels, serum urate levels, and male gender remained significant predictors, and all three variables were utilized to create a scoring system ranging from 0 to 10. The higher the score, the higher the specificity and probability of TLS (0.99 specificity and 78% probability) [35].

Prevention of TLS is the best strategy. Administering vigorous intravenous hydration (approximately $3\,L/m^2$ per day), maintaining adequate urine output (>100 mL/m^2 per hour) which may require addition of a diuretic, monitoring fluid balance, weight and electrolytes, administering allopurinol, rasburicase or both, avoiding nephrotoxic agents (contrast media, non-steroidal antiinflammatory drugs [NSAIDs], nephrotoxic antibiotics) and drugs that inhibit uric acid excretion (probenecid, aspirin, and thiazide) remain the standard therapies for management of TLS. Urine alkalization is currently not uniformly recommended to prevent renal damage (see section on Hyperuricemia, below).

Hyperuricemia

Hyperuricemia, defined as a serum uric acid >8.0mg/day or 25% increase from baseline 3 days before to 7 days after the initiation of chemotherapy, more commonly develops 48–72 h after initiation of therapy [36]. The major route of urate clearance is through the proximal renal tubules, and is mediated by specialized transporters, such as urate–anion exchanger urate transporter 1 (URAT-1), efflux transporter OATv1, efflux pump MRP4, Tamm–Harsfall protein–uromodulin, and UAT/galectin-9, making the kidneys the main organ affected by high urate levels [27,37]. Certain polymorphisms of specific urate transporters may influence the development of hyperuricemia and TLS, and they may help explain the development of TLS despite adequate prophylactic measures.

Although urine alkalinization (urine pH > 7) historically has been recommended for the prophylaxis and treatment of ATLS, it remains controversial [38]. As maximum uric acid solubility occurs at the pH of 7.5, alkalinization of urine promotes the urinary excretion of the urate. However, solubility of urate precursors—xanthine and hypoxanthine—is dramatically reduced at such a pH, leading to the development of urinary xanthine crystals and xanthine obstructive uropathy [38,39].

A xanthine analog, allopurinol, which competitively inhibits xanthine oxidase and the conversion of xanthine and hypoxanthine to uric acid, has been demonstrated to effectively decrease the formation of uric acid and reduce the incidence of uric acid obstructive uropathy [40,41]. It is typically administered at a dose of 300–600 mg/day (max. 800 mg/day). Allopurinol, however, has several significant limitations. Firstly, allopurinol only prevents further uric acid formation and has no effect of already existing uric acid. Secondly, administration of allopurinol increases the serum levels of the purine precursors, xanthine, and hypoxanthine, which may lead to xanthine nephropathy and obstructive uropathy [40,42]. Thirdly, allopurinol reduces the degradation of other purines, including 6-mercaptopurine (6-MP) and azathioprine, requiring 50–70% of their dose reduction [42]. Additionally, in patients with renal insufficiency, the dose of allopurinol needs to be adjusted to avoid the drug accumulation of the drug and its metabolites.

An alternative to preventing uric acid formation by inhibiting xanthine oxidase with allopurinol is to promote the catabolism of uric acid to much more soluble allantoin by urate oxidase [43]. Urate oxidase is an endogenous enzyme commonly found in many mammalian species, but not in humans, due to a nonsense mutation in the coding region of the urate oxidase encoding gene [44]. A non-recombinant urate oxidase, extracted from *Aspergillus flavus*, has been demonstrated to reduce uric acid levels in patients at risk of TLS [45–47]. Subsequently, the gene coding for the urate oxidase was isolated from the *A. flavus* species and expressed in the yeast *Saccharomyces cerevisiae* strain to yield large quantities of the pure recombinant form of urate oxidase [48]. Recombinant urate oxidase (rasburicase) was demonstrated to be a safe and effective alternative to allopurinol in several multicenter clinical trials [41,48–50]. In a randomized clinical trial, rasburicase was shown to significantly reduce uric acid levels compared with allopurinol [41]. Although the recommended dose of rasburicase is 0.15–0.2 mg/kg per day for 5 days, at Northwestern University an excellent control of hyperuricemia was achieved with a lower dose of 3 mg/day. Administration of 3 mg of rasburicase to 18 patients with hyperuricemia secondary to leukemia/lymphoma resulted in the normalization of the uric acid in 11 patients with just a single dose of rasburicase, in six patients with two doses, and in one patient with three doses [51]. Although no randomized clinical trials comparing the efficacy of rasburicase and allopurinol in adults have been published, randomized studies in the pediatric population have demonstrated superiority of rasburicase in terms of reduction in level of uric acid, absence of TLS, and requirement for dialysis [41,49]. Rasburicase is contraindicated in patients with methemoglobinemia, G6PD deficiency, or other disorders that can potentially cause hemolytic anemia. Rasburicase may also cause bronchospasm, and the risk of hypersensitivity reaction has been 1% in published studies [41,52,53]. Patients with ALL, who either present with or are at high risk of developing TLS (high tumor burden with WBC count $>50 \times 10^9$/L, high LDH, or mediastinal mass; elevated uric acid level; renal infiltration with leukemic cells, or renal insufficiency), are good candidates for rasburicase therapy [42].

Hypocalcemia and hyperphosphatemia

Hypocalcemia, defined as a corrected serum calcium level ≤7.0 mg/dL or a 25% decrease from baseline 3 days before or 7 days after the initiation of chemotherapy, is one of the most dangerous sequelae of TLS, reported in <5% patients with acute leukemia at diagnosis. Hyperphosphatemia is defined as serum phosphate level ≥4.5 mg/dL or a 25% increase from baseline 3 days before or 7 days after the initiation of chemotherapy. Symptoms related to hyperphosphatemia manifest indirectly through its effect on calcium and may result in potentially lethal cardiac (ventricular arrhythmias, heart block) and neurologic (hallucination, seizures, coma) sequelae [54,55]. Both electrolyte abnormalities more commonly occur 24–48 h after the initiation of chemotherapy. Several mechanisms contribute to hyperphosphatemia in TLS, including increased endogenous release as a result of massive tumor breakdown, impaired glomerular filtration secondary to urate nephropathy/nephrocalcinosis-induced renal insufficiency and decreased ability of malignant cells to utilize available endogenous phosphate. Hyperphosphatemia may lead to elevated calcium and phosphate solubility product, which in turn will lead to calcium phosphate precipitates causing both organ damage and further hypocalcemia. In an asymptomatic patient with laboratory evidence of hypocalcemia and hyperphosphatemia, calcium replacement is not recommended because it may precipitate metastatic calcifications [54]. However, in a patient with symptomatic hypocalcemia, calcium gluconate may be carefully administered to correct the clinical symptoms. Appropriate management of hypocalcemia includes electrocardiogram monitoring and avoiding medications known to prolong QT interval. Hydration with intravenous fluids containing no phosphorus and no calcium products, and administration of phosphate binder aluminum hydroxide (50–100 mg/kg per day) will aid in decreasing the phosphorus level. Cases of recalcitrant hyperphosphatemia and hypocalcemia will require hemodialysis [39].

Hyperkalemia

Hyperkalemia, defined by a serum potassium level of >6 mEq/L or a 25% increase from baseline 3 days before or 7 days after the initiation of chemotherapy, caused by massive cellular degradation, may precipitate significant neuromuscular (muscle weakness, cramps, paresthesias) and potentially life-threatening cardiac abnormalities (asystole, ventricular tachycardia, and ventricular fibrillation) [54]. It most commonly occurs 6–72 h after the initiation of chemotherapy. In the cardiac tissue, depending on the extent of hyperkalemia, a variety of electrocardiographic changes may occur, including peaked T wave (>5 mm) with a K^+ level of 6–7 mEq/L; the QRS complex widening and a smaller amplitude of P wave with serum K^+ of 7–8 mEq/L; fusion of QRS complexes with the T wave forming sine waves, with serum K^+ of 8–9 mEq/L; and, ultimately, atrioventricular dissociation, ventricular tachycardia, or ventricular fibrillation and death when serum K^+ levels are >9 mEq/L [56]. Typically, patients become symptomatic once serum K^+ exceeds 6 mEq/L. Coexisting renal insufficiency, metabolic acidosis, and

K^+-sparing diuretics may exacerbate hyperkalemia, and must be considered and corrected. Patients should be treated with oral sodium–potassium exchange resin, such as Kayexalate, 15–30g every 6h and/or combined glucose–insulin therapy [57]. Calcium gluconate is helpful for stabilization of the cardiac membrane; however, it may be administered with extreme caution in a setting of hypercalcemia or hyperphosphatemia to avoid calcium phosphate precipitation (see section Hypocalcemia and Hyperphosphatemia, above).

Pseudohyperkalemia may occur in patients with leukocytosis (WBC count >100,000/μL). It occurs as a result of mechanical lysis of WBCs during phlebotomy or ionic shift following coagulation of blood in the vial. Evaluation of plasma K^+ level and sending the sample in the arterial blood gas (ABG) tube (for *stat* processing) may result in more accurate K^+ level evaluation.

Monitoring and therapy of TLS

No studies have been published investigating the optimal monitoring strategy for patients at risk of, and those who developed, TLS. Serum electrolytes should be monitored several times a day, depending on the severity of the clinical condition and degree of metabolic abnormality. It has been routine practice at Northwestern University in patients at high risk of TLS to monitor levels of LDH, uric acid, sodium, potassium, creatinine, blood urea nitrogen, phosphorus, and calcium every 12h for the first 3 days and every 24h subsequently. In patients who develop evidence of TLS, the above parameters are measured every 6h until stabilization and then daily. Electrocardiograms are obtained and cardiac rhythm is monitored while the electrolytes are corrected, and then it is monitored daily until resolution of TLS. Vital parameters, such as heart rate, blood pressure, urine output, and respiratory rate, are obtained every 6–8h.

Therapy of patients with TLS involves the same modalities as prophylaxis. Intravenous hydration and rasburicase should be administered to all patients (without obvious contraindications, such as hemolytic anemia) with laboratory or clinical TLS. Rasburicase should be considered in patients with a high risk of TLS and with rapid worsening of biochemical parameters that may lead to TLS. Although it was traditionally recommended to initiate hydration 48h before the beginning of chemotherapy, the use of rasburicase with subsequent rapid degradation of uric acid allows for the shorter interval if necessary. Urine output should be maintained at least at 100mL/h. In patients without evidence of obstructive uropathy, once euvolemic status is achieved, loop diuretics (or mannitol) may be added.

Hyperphosphatemia can be treated with aluminum hydroxide at 50–100mg/kg per day administered in four divided doses either orally or via a nasogastric tube. Asymptomatic hypocalcemia does not require intervention. If symptoms are noted, a dose of calcium gluconate 50–100mg/kg can be administered and cautiously repeated if necessary. Hyperkalemia is managed with oral sodium–potassium exchange resin, such as Kayexalate, 15–30g every 6h and a combination of insulin (0.1 unit/kg) and glucose (25% dextrose 2mL/kg). Calcium gluconate may be useful for the management of hypokalemia-induced cardiac arrhythmia.

Early hemodialysis may be required in patients who are developing oliguric renal failure, recalcitrant electrolyte disturbances, volume overload unresponsive to diuresis, and overt uremic symptoms such as pericarditis and encephalopathy. Daily dialysis is recommended considering the continuous release into the blood stream of electrolytes and metabolites from lysed leukemic cells. Patients who are hemodynamically unstable may benefit from continuous renal replacement therapy.

Lactic acidosis

Primary leukemia-induced lactic acidosis is a rare, yet potentially fatal, event characterized by low arterial pH resulting from the accumulation of blood lactate. It has been suggested that lactic acidosis occurring in the setting of hematologic malignancy is associated with an extremely poor prognosis [58]. Lactate, the end product of anaerobic glycolysis, is metabolized to glucose by the liver and kidneys. Because leukemic cells have a high rate of glycolysis, even in the presence of oxygen, and because they produce a large quantity of lactate, lactic acidosis may result from an imbalance between lactate production and hepatic lactate utilization [58]. Several factors may contribute to the high rate of glycolysis. Overexpression or aberrant expression of glycolytic enzymes such as hexokinase, the first rate-limiting enzyme in the glycolytic pathway, allows tumor cells to proliferate rapidly and survive for prolonged periods [59,60]. Although insulin normally regulates the expression of this enzyme, insulin-like growth factors (IGFs) that are overexpressed by malignant leukemic cells can mimic insulin activity [61–63].

Lactic acidosis is frequently associated with TLS, and its extent is correlated with the severity of TLS. There is laboratory evidence to suggest that loss of mitochondrial function induced by cytotoxic therapy leads to compensatory glycolysis and, subsequently, to lactate accumulation and acidosis [64]. In a review of 25 cases of lactic acidosis attributed to underlying malignancy, more than two-thirds were associated with leukemia and lymphoma [65]. Twenty-five cases of lactic acidosis associated with acute leukemia have been reported [58]. Typically, patients with lactic acidosis present with weakness, tachycardia, nausea, mental status changes, hyperventilation, and hypotension, which may progress to frank shock as acidosis worsens. Laboratory studies demonstrate decreased blood pH (<7.37), a widened anion gap (>18mEq/L), and low serum bicarbonate.

The most important therapy for lactic acidosis is the treatment of the underlying leukemia. The role of sodium bicarbonate in the treatment of lactic acidosis remains controversial. The deleterious effect of severe acidemia on cardiovascular function can potentially be ameliorated by sodium bicarbonate administration; however, no study has shown a convincing survival advantage for alkali therapy in this condition [66]. In addition, there are several reports suggesting that administration of sodium bicarbonate may increase lactate and carbon dioxide production, impair oxygen delivery, and worsen lactic acidosis [67]. Hemodialysis and hemofiltration with bicarbonate-based replacement fluid have been reported as successful therapy for severe lactic acidosis and have not been associated with malignancy [68,69]. Hemofiltration with bicarbonate-based replacement fluid used in a patient with lactic acidosis and underlying acute leukemia resulted in rapid correction of acidosis; however, only after the initiation of chemotherapy did the plasma lactate level decrease [58].

Hypercalcemia

Severe hypercalcemia is a rare serious manifestation of acute leukemia, reported in <5% of patients at diagnosis [55]. Patients may experience severe malaise, anorexia, diffuse abdominal pain, constipation, emesis, polyuria and polydipsia, and changes in mental status (hallucination, psychosis, somnolence, and coma). Shortening of the QT interval, tachycardia, and arrhythmia may be present. Both humoral and local mechanisms have been implicated in the pathogenesis of hypercalcemia in leukemias [70]. Paraneoplastic production of parathyroid hormone-related protein is thought to be responsible for hypercalcemia via humoral effect, whereas osteolytic skeletal metastasis and cytokines, such as TNF-α, IL-6 and IL-2, may be responsible for local osteolytic hypercalcemia [71,72]. Occasionally, a combination of high calcium and phosphorus level leads to the calcinosis cutis syndrome—an aberrant deposition of calcium salts in the skin [73].

The combination of hydration, loop diuretics, intravenous bisphosphonates, corticosteroids, and calcitonin is usually sufficient to achieve adequate control of hypercalcemia [74]. Pamidronate (90 mg), ibandronate (4 mg), or zoledronate (4 mg) administered as a single infusion is expected to restore normocalcemia within 5 days in 80% of the patients. Because of the potential nephrotoxicity, bisphosphonates are administered slowly, in large volume, and may require dose reduction. Patients who do not respond to bisphosphonate infusions should be considered for additional therapy with gallium nitrate, which is a potent inhibitor of bone resorbtion [75]. Randomized double-blinded studies have demonstrated superiority of gallium nitrate compared with calcitonin, etidronate, and pamidronate for acute treatment of resistant hypercalcemia. Administered as a continuous intravenous infusion at a dose of 200 mg/m^2 per day over 24 h for up to 5 days, gallium nitrate induces normocalcemia in 70–90% of patients [76]. Whether the recently introduced oral formulation can be a substitute for the parenteral form remains to be determined. If the above-mentioned interventions are not successful, calcitonin may be administered. However, dramatic responses typically are not seen and resistance to that treatment develops rapidly. Hemodialysis is the ultimate therapy for life-threatening recalcitrant hypercalcemia.

Cutaneous lesions are usually resistant to the initial therapy, causing significant morbidity. Patients experience severe resting and mechanical pain usually requiring a combination of morphine, tricyclic antidepressants, and antiinflammatory medications for adequate pain control. Cases of calcinosis cutis have been described to resolve over a period of time, once control of the calcium and phosphate levels have been established, which would imply successful therapy for the underlying leukemia [77,78].

Mediastinal mass/superior vena cava syndrome

Patients with ALL (particularly T-cell ALL [T-ALL]), may present with symptoms of cough, dyspnea, stridor, or dysphagia from tracheal and esophageal compression by a mediastinal mass (15% of patients). More than 27% of children who present with mediastinal mass have acute airway compromise [79]. Compression of the great vessels by a bulky mediastinal mass also may lead to the life-threatening superior vena cava (SVC) syndrome. In addition to the above-mentioned symptoms, the patient may develop cyanosis, facial edema, increased intracranial pressure, and syncope. Presence of mediastinal mass causing SVC syndrome in patients with AML has been reported [80,81].

The prognosis of patients with SVC syndrome is strongly correlated with the prognosis of underlying disease. Diagnosis of primary condition should be established promptly, and therapy with steroids (dexamethasone 4–8 mg four times daily), chemotherapy, and/or radiation should be initiated without a delay. Other medical measures such as head elevation and oxygen administration, which can reduce cardiac output and venous pressure, might be helpful. When the therapeutic goal is only palliation of SVC syndrome, or if emergent treatment of the venous obstruction is required, direct opening of the occlusion with endovascular stenting and angioplasty with possible thrombolysis should provide prompt relief of symptoms [82]. Rarely, the mediastinal mass does not consist of the leukemic cells. An association between AML (megakaryocytic and AML with isochromosome 12) and mediastinal germ-cell tumor (also with isochromosome 12) has been reported [83,84].

Management of bleeding complications in leukemias

Patients with leukemia have an increased risk of bleeding for a variety of reasons, including alterations in platelet number and function, clotting factor deficiencies, presence of circulating anticoagulants, and defects in vascular integrity (Table 31.2). Optimal management of hemorrhagic complications requires full understanding and characterization of the hemostatic defect. Clinical history and physical examination will reveal site, extent, and tempo of the bleeding. Petechia, ecchymosis, and mucosal hemorrhage are typically seen in a setting of thrombocytopenia, platelet function defect, and acquired von Willebrand disease [85]. Skin and muscle hematomas are common in a setting of deficiencies or inhibitors of clotting factors. Persistent oozing from the venipuncture sites is characteristic for disseminated intravascular coagulation (DIC). Bleeding gums and epistaxis are seen with excessive fibrinolysis. Periprocedural bleeding occurs with impairment in any phase of coagulation. Pertinent laboratory studies include platelet count and morphologic evaluation of the peripheral smear (and a bone marrow biopsy), a platelet function test (for platelet count exceeding 100,000/μL), the activated partial thromboplastin time (aPTT), the prothrombin time (PT), fibrinogen, D-dimer (or fibrinogen degradation products if available), and a clot lysis test. Presence of a defect in the intrinsic or extrinsic coagulation cascades as determined by the PT and aPTT may require mixing studies to indicate whether clotting factor deficiency or inhibitor is present.

Table 31.2 Management of acute hemorrhage in patients with leukemia.

Blood component	Problem	Therapy
Platelets	Thrombocytopenia	Platelet transfusions
	Platelet dysfunction	DDAVP, platelet transfusions
Clotting factors	Vitamin K deficiency	Vitamin K, oral, factor IV, or subcutaneous
	Autoantibodies: FVII, FIX	rFVII or FEIBA
	von Willebrand factor	DDAVP, IVIg
Fibrinogen	Hypo/ dysfibrinogenemia	Cryoprecipitate
	DIC	Cryoprecipitate, platelets
	Hyperfibrinolysis	ε-Aminocaproic acid, tranexamic acid

DDAVP, desmopressin; DIC, disseminated intravascular coagulation; rFVII—recombinant activated factor VII; FEIBA, factor VII inhibitor bypassing activity, IVIg, intravenous immunoglobulins. Adapted with permission from Seminars in Thrombosis and Hemostasis. Green D. Management of bleeding complications of hematologic malignancies. *Semin Thromb Hemost* 2007;33:427–34.

Thrombocytopenia is the major cause of bleeding in patients with leukemia. In a study of 256 patients with AML (excluding those with APL), the degree of thrombocytopenia correlated well with the severity of bleeding [86]. Presence of high fever and infections were associated not only with the increased risk of bleeding, but also with the blunted response to platelet transfusions. A higher hemoglobin level in that study was associated with the decreased risk of bleeding [86].

In patients with acute leukemia, the threshold level for platelet transfusions typically is 10,000/μL in the absence of active bleeding [87–91]. However, transfusions are indicated at higher platelet levels in a setting of bleeding, high fever, hyperleukocytosis, rapidly decreasing platelets, and associated coagulation abnormalities. The hemostatic benefits, post-transfusion increments, and adverse events are similar between random-donor and single-donor platelets. Although random-donor platelets are less costly, single-donor platelets may be preferred to avoid sensitization to multiple donor antigens. If possible, platelet products should be leukoreduced to avoid alloimmunization in patients who will require repeated transfusion for prolonged periods. In the absence of a vascular defect or in the presence of coagulopathy, failure to achieve hemostasis should prompt the evaluation of incremental platelets increase after transfusion. If there is no platelet increase 1 hour after transfusion, alloimmunization and hypersplenism are suspected etiologies [92]. If there is a satisfactory increase at 1 hour but the platelet count is back to baseline at 24h after the transfusion, fever, infection, or consumption due to continuous bleeding, DIC (sepsis and endotoxins), or release of procoagulants (APL) may be responsible. A patient is considered refractory if at least two ABO-compatible platelets doses, stored less than 72h fail to produce adequate (20–40,000/μL) platelet increase [93]. Increasing the dose of platelets or transfusing filtered apheresis platelets may be effective in some patients [94,95]. If these measures are not effective, platelet antibody testing for human leukocyte antigen (HLA) should be performed. Platelet transfusions from the donors who are HLA-A and HLA-B compatible may then be selected. If this is not feasible, histocompatible platelet donors may be identified using platelet cross-matching techniques. If, despite those efforts, patients continue to bleed and platelet count remains low, administration of recombinant factor FVIIa may control hemorrhage.

Fresh frozen plasma (FFP) is rarely indicated in treatment of bleeding complications in leukemias; hypofibrinogenemia is better managed with cryoprecipitate, owing to the higher fibrinogen concentration, whereas factor deficiency is treated with specific factor concentrates. Low levels of factors II, VII, IX, and X suggested vitamin K deficiency, which is remedied by the oral (2.5 mg) or intravenous (5–10 mg) vitamin K.

In a setting of excessive fibrinolysis, occurring as a result of impaired thrombin generation and deficient or defective antiplasmin or plasminogen activator inhibitor type 1 owing to thrombocytopenia, impaired hepatic protein synthesis, or excessive protein catabolism, ε-aminocaproic acid, and tranexamic acid may decrease bleeding, particularly from mucous membranes. ε-aminocaproic acid is administered either orally at a dose up to 5 g every 6 h or intravenously in 5 g bolus over 20 min followed by the 1 g/h rate. The dose should not exceed 30 g/day, as it may result in impaired platelet function and bleeding. Tranexamic acid is administered every 8 h at the oral dose of 25 mg/kg or intravenous dose of 10 mg/kg. In addition to bradycardia and hypotension occurring with rapid infusion of ε-aminocaproic acid, headache, nausea, dizziness, and rarely seizures have been reported. However, the most serious side-effect is thrombosis, particularly when administered to patients with DIC or concurrently with other clotting factor concentrates, estrogens, or all-trans-retinoic acid [96,97].

Disseminated intravascular coagulation

Disseminated intravascular coagulation is a known complication of acute leukemias and has been reported in about 10–16% of patients with ALL at presentation and 36–78% during remission induction therapy, and in about one-third of patients with AML [98–100]. Patients with ALL who develop DIC tend to have higher WBC counts (77,900/μL vs. 9400/μL) and a higher frequency of palpable spleen than patients who do not develop DIC. Patients with ALL who developed DIC after the initiation of chemotherapy had a lower platelet level and higher level of the E-fragment of serum fibrinogen–fibrin degradation products (FDPs) at presentation, suggesting that they already had DIC before the initiation of therapy. These findings indicate that perhaps patients with high WBC counts, higher FDP levels, low platelet counts, and splenomegaly at presentation require closer monitoring for DIC after the initiation of chemotherapy. Despite high prevalence of DIC, hemorrhagic symptoms usually are mild; however, serious hemorrhage occurs in 20% of patients with laboratory evidence of DIC [101]. In a recent retrospective analysis of 161 non-M3 patients with AML, hyperleukocytosis, high levels of C-reactive protein (CRP), and LDH, as well as negative expression of CD13, CD19, CD34, and HLA-DR, were associated with the occurrence of DIC. On multivariate logistic-regression analysis, hyperleukocytosis, high CRP level, negative expression of CD13 and HLA-DR, and normal karyotype or 11q23 abnormality were independent factors associated with DIC. An etiologic link between CD34 expression and DIC was suggested [100].

The best way to treat DIC is to treat the underlying leukemia. However, exacerbation of DIC may occur during induction therapy and with ATLS. The coagulation profile must be obtained at the time of diagnosis and repeated frequently, especially when laboratory evidence of DIC is detected, to guide the replacement therapy. Theoretical concerns for exacerbating DIC with blood products have not been substantiated clinically, and hemostatic competence to avoid severe bleeding must be maintained. It is reasonable to keep aPTT at about 1.5 times the normal level with FFP, platelets at about 50,000/μL with platelet transfusions, and fibrinogen level over 100 mg/dL with cryoprecipitate. Heparin therapy is rarely indicated in the patient with ALL and DIC, unless thrombosis is evident. If required, heparin levels should be followed to avoid over- or undertreating the patient.

L-asparaginase and coagulopathy

L-asparaginase, an enzyme from bacteria that destroys the amino acid asparagine, required primarily by leukemic cells, is an important component of combination chemotherapy for patients with ALL. L-asparaginase can produce depletion of many of the hemostatic, anticoagulant, and fibrinolytic factors, such as fibrinogen, factors VII, VIII, IX, X, and XI, antithrombin III, protein C and S, and plasminogen, with an associated risk of both thrombosis and hemorrhage [102–104]. These effects are likely a result of the decreased protein synthesis by the liver, rather than clotting factor consumption or the production of abnormal molecules [103,105]. This reduction of the synthesis of the clotting factors appears to be proportional to the elimination of asparagine from the plasma, and normalizes as soon as L-asparaginase is discontinued [106].

Despite the marked reductions in fibrinogen (factors VII, VIII, IX, X, and XI), excessive bleeding is rare, at least partially because of the concurrent impaired synthesis (to 30% of normal levels) of anticoagulant proteins (antithrombin, protein C, protein S, and plasminogen), predisposing to thrombosis [103,107]. Central nervous system (CNS) thrombosis occurs in approximately 4% of adult patients with ALL, usually 2–3 weeks after the initiation of therapy with L-asparaginase. Although most patients recover without significant neurologic consequences, death and permanent neurologic defects have been reported [108–110]. Although the risk of thrombosis is greatest during remission induction phase of chemotherapy with L-asparaginase, it may occur at any stage of therapy [111].

There are no prospective data to suggest a fibrinogen level at which replacement is required. It is reasonable to temporarily discontinue the L-asparaginase when fibrinogen level decreases to 50–70 mg/dL. However, in general, we do not recommend fibrinogen replacement therapy in an asymptomatic patient, regardless of fibrinogen level. Prophylactic use of FFP was ineffective in preventing the decrease in antithrombin III level induced by L-asparaginase [112]. When clinically significant bleeding occurs or if the patient is required to undergo surgical procedure, therapy with cryoprecipitate is usually successful in correcting the hemostatic defect [107]. In a setting of L-asparaginase therapy, the presence of an inherited hypercoagulable state, such as factor V Leiden or the prothrombin gene mutation, was shown to increase the risk of thrombosis in some studies [113] but not in others [114]. The presence of the antiphospholipid antibody increases the risk of thrombosis in patients treated with L-asparaginase [114].

Management of acute promyelocytic leukemia-associated coagulopathy

A life-threatening coagulopathy is a distinguishing feature of acute promyelocytic leukemia (APL). Approximately 70–80% of patients with newly diagnosed or relapsed APL have either laboratory or clinical evidence of coagulopathy, and, historically, 10–30% die from fatal hemorrhage, most commonly involving the CNS [115–120]. The pathogenesis of the coagulopathy includes DIC, fibrinolysis, and proteolysis [121,122]. Severe bleeding complications at presentation and during induction do not necessarily correlate with homeostatic parameters, but appear to be proportional to the initial WBC count [123]. The typical laboratory features, consistent with both DIC and hyperfibrinolysis, include thrombocytopenia, prolongation of PTT, PT, thrombin time (TT), increased levels of FDP, and hypofibrinogenemia [124,125]. However, normal levels of antithrombin III, protein C, and platelets survival, as well as severe bleeding in a setting of normal PT and PTT in APL patients, suggest a more complex process than DIC alone [125,126]. Several procoagulant mediators have been implicated in the APL-associated coagulopathy. The levels of gene expression and transcription of tissue factor, a major procoagulant responsible for initiation of coagulation cascade, leading to thrombin generation and fibrin formation, are elevated in the APL blasts [127,128]. Cancer procoagulant, a cysteine proteinase enzyme that initiates coagulation via direct activation of factor X in the absence of factor VII, is also preferentially expressed in APL blasts [129,130]. The levels of the cytokines, such as interleukin-1 (IL-1), tumor necrosis factor (TNF) and vascular permeability factor (VPF), able to initiate coagulation via induction of tissue factor in endothelial cell and monocytes, are elevated in patients with APL.

Excessive fibrinolysis is also an important factor in APL coagulopathy [131,132]. Plasminogen and α_2-plasmin inhibitor levels are reduced in patients with APL [133]. Furthermore, leukemic promyelocytes release plasminogen activators that cleave plasminogen and initiate fibrinolysis. Circulating tissue-type plasminogen activator (t-PA) and decreased level of circulating plasminogen activator inhibitor type 1 (PAI-1) have been reported in some patients with APL [133]. APL cells also contain elastases that inactivate α_2-plasmin inhibitor [134].

Annexin-VIII is one of the proteins that binds phospholipids and has both anticoagulant and phospholipase-A inhibitory properties [135]. The Annexin-VIII gene is expressed to a greater degree in cells from patients with APL than from patients with other subtypes of AML [136]. Annexin-VIII is highly expressed in the APL cell line,NB-4 and is significantly reduced after exposure to all-trans-retinoic acid (ATRA). Annexin-II is a co-receptor for plasminogen and t-PA, and it is expressed at higher levels on the surface of promyelocytes than for other AML subtypes, leading to an increased fibrinolytic potential [137–139]. Plasmin- and elastase-induced degradation of von Willebrand factor may contribute to the hemostatic defect in APL [140].

Successful remission induction with ATRA and arsenic trioxide (ATO) is accompanied by rapid resolution of clinical bleeding. Frequently, biochemical evidence of coagulopathy disappears as well, although elevated plasma levels of sensitive markers of clotting activation may persist [141–143]. Although ATRA therapy results in the resolution of coagulopathy, it may paradoxically induce thrombosis in a small proportion of patients with APL [144,145]. ATRA-associated thrombosis typically occurs 1–3 weeks after the initiation of therapy, at the time when the coagulopathy has been corrected, and it can involve multiple organs, including the heart, brain, lungs, and spleen [146–148]. Antifibrinolyic agents such as tranexamic acid have been shown to increase the risk of this potentially fatal complication [96,149]. Interestingly, the ATO-induced thrombosis in patients with APL has not been reported.

In addition to initiation of APL-specific ATRA- or ATO-based regimens, aggressive blood product support is imperative to combat the coagulopathy (Box 31.3). Platelet transfusions may be required several times per day with the goal of achieving platelet counts of 30–50,000/μL. It has been the routine practice at Northwestern University to maintain the fibrinogen level above 100 mg/dL using cryoprecipitate administration. Anticoagulation (heparin and low molecular weight heparin) and antifibrinolytic agents (ε-aminocaproic acid and tranexamic acid) are not used prophylactically. Although in the past heparin was used with the intent to inhibit thrombin formation, retrospective analysis conducted in the pre-ATRA era failed to show any advantage of its administration [118]. Several

Box 31.3 Guidelines for the Management of acute promyelocytic leukemia-associated coagulopathy.

Initiate ATRA therapy as soon as diagnosis is suspected based on clinical and morphologic presentation

Close monitoring of hematologic parameters (CBC, DIC panels, fibrinogen)

Aggressive correction of thrombocytopenia to maintain platelets >30–50,000/µL

Aggressive correction of hypofibrinogenemia to maintain fibrinogen >100 mg/dL

No routine use of anticoagulation

No routine use of antifibrinolytic agents

In a setting of leukocytosis, chemotherapy should be administered in combination with ATRA

CBC, complete blood count; DIC, disseminated intravascular coagulation.

small studies suggested a role for antifibrinolytic therapy in APL-associated coagulopathy; larger retrospective and prospective trials failed to show any advantage [143,150]. No prospective randomized trial of anticoagulation in APL has ever been conducted.

Neurologic complications

The precise mechanism of neuroleukemia remains to be elucidated; however, leukemic cells can gain access to the CNS in various ways. They can reach the subarachnoid space from the bone marrow of the skull via bridging veins, enter cerebrospinal fluid (CSF) via the choroid plexus, invade cerebellar parenchyma via the brain capillaries, or directly infiltrate the leptomeninges via bony lesions of the skull [151]. They can also grow alongside nerve roots and invade the subarachnoid space through the neural foramina [151].

At diagnosis, 5–10% of adult patients with ALL and <1% of patients with AML have evidence of leukemic involvement of the CNS [109,152–157]. Only a fraction will have clinical symptoms indicative of CNS disease. In ALL, patients with T-cell phenotype, leukocytosis (WBC count >100,000/µL), and the presence of mediastinal mass are at a higher risk of CNS leukemia. In AML, M4 and M5 FAB subtypes have the higher risk of CNS involvement [158]. Additionally, a syndrome of CNS involvement and diabetes insipidus has been reported in patients with monosomy 7 and inversion 16 chromosomal abnormalities [159–161]. CNS involvement may manifest as generalized headache and papilledema from elevated intracranial pressure, visual impairment due to the unilateral and bilateral optic nerve infiltration (as well as direct ocular involvement via infiltration of the orbit, retina, iris, cornea, and conjunctiva), trigeminal neuralgia secondary to seventh cranial nerve infiltration, leukemic meningitis, transverse myelopathy, and epidural spinal cord compression [162–164]. In a study of 36 patients with neuroleukemia (46 episodes of CNS involvement), 21.7% of the episodes involved the cranial nerves, most commonly the bulbar motor, facial, and optic nerves [165]. CT or MRI, the latter being a more sensitive test, will document cerebral edema, cranial nerve involvement, and meningeal spread. In the absence of increased intracranial pressure, lumbar puncture may be performed, and analysis of CSF by cytology, smear review, and flow cytometry should be conducted. The significance of the above-mentioned symptoms must be recognized immediately, and chemotherapy with systemic and intrathecal methotrexate or cytarabine, glucocorticoids (eg, dexamethasone 8 mg every 8 h), and radiation therapy should be administered promptly in hopes to prevent permanent damage. Although patients with cranial nerve involvement will likely require radiation therapy, the optimal protocol for radiation administration is yet to be determined. A total radiation dose of 3000 cGy, with 1000–1500 cGy of it applied to the nerve sheath and the cranial base has been recommended [166]. In the case of intracranial hemorrhage, glucocorticoids do not relieve intracranial pressure, and decompressive surgery might be indicated.

Rarely, a myelosarcoma (chloroma) or crashed vertebrae from direct leukemic infiltration compress the spinal cord, causing back pain. It may be localized, radicular or both, aggravated by straining, coughing and recumbency, and followed by sensory and motor dysfunction (weakness, loss of sphincter control, and paralysis). The diagnosis is established by neurologic exam and MRI. Plain radiographs are usually not helpful. A CT scan might be performed in patients for whom MRI is contraindicated. Treatment must be initiated promptly to avoid permanent damage. When decompression is delayed by >48 h after onset of paraplegia, the chance of neurologic recovery is dismal. Dexamethasone will relieve the edema in the affected regions and will have a direct antitumor effect in ALL. The mechanisms of action of dexamethasone is not completely understood; it has been shown to downregulate vascular endothelial growth factor expression in smooth muscle cells and to prevent cytoskeletal changes associated with increased vascular permeability [167–169]. Despite the established role of dexamethasone in management of spinal cord compression, the optimal doses and schedule are still debated [170,171]. Prompt initiation of chemotherapy aimed at cytoreduction alone or in combination with radiation therapy may achieve rapid results. Rarely, laminectomy or anterior decompression may be required.

Other organ involvement

Leukemic cells may infiltrate virtually any organ system, particularly in mature B-cell ALL (32%), T-cell ALL, and AML with monocytic differentiation, and they usually do not cause significant morbidity. However, patients presenting with diffuse abdominal pain require immediate surgical evaluation as morbidity and mortality rates from bowel perforation or spontaneous splenic rupture attributable to leukemic infiltrates are high [172–175]. In a series of 136 cases of spontaneous splenic rupture in patients with hematologic malignancies, 34% had acute leukemia and 18% had CML [173]. In another series of 53 cases of splenic rupture in patients with hematologic malignancies, 40% had acute leukemias and 18% had chronic leukemias [176]. Priapism due to leukostasis in corpora cavernosa and dorsal vein, and sacral involvement in acute leukemias, has been described [177,178]. In the pediatric population, leukemia is the most common cause of priapism. Decreased penile venous outflow and venous stasis of blood result in intracavernous blood acidosis and low oxygen tension, leading to the irreversible cellular damage and corporal fibrosis within 24–48h if emergent therapy is not instituted. Rapid cytoreduction with leukemia-specific chemotherapy, leukapheresis, or both is usually effective. Corporeal aspiration and irrigation with saline or dilute phenylephrine, creation of a shunt between the glans penis and corpora cavernosa, and radiation therapy have been used with varying degrees of success.

References

1 Porcu P, Cripe LD, Ng EW, *et al.* Hyperleukocytic leukemias and leukostasis: a review of pathophysiology, clinical presentation and management. *Leuk Lymphoma* 2000;39:1–18.

2 Maurer HS, Steinherz PG, Gaynon PS, *et al.* The effect of initial management of hyperleukocytosis on early complications and outcome of children with acute lymphoblastic leukemia. *J Clin Oncol* 1988;6:1425–32.

3 Frohling S, Schlenk RF, Breitruck J, *et al.* Prognostic significance of activating FLT3 mutations in younger adults (16 to 60 years) with acute myeloid Leukemia and normal cytogenetics: a study of the AML Study Group Ulm. *Blood* 2002;100: 4372–80.

4 Wetzler M, Dodge RK, Mrozek K, *et al.* Prospective karyotype analysis in adult acute lymphoblastic leukemia: the cancer and Leukemia Group B experience. *Blood* 1999;93:3983–93.

5 Hoelzer D, Thiel E, Loffler H, *et al.* Prognostic factors in a multicenter study for treatment of acute lymphoblastic leukemia in adults. *Blood* 1988;71:123–31.

6 Ventura GJ, Hester JP, Smith TL, Keating MJ. Acute myeloblastic Leukemia with hyperleukocytosis: risk factors for early mortality in induction. *Am J Hematol* 1988;27:34–7.

7 Appelbaum FR, Kopecky KJ. Long-term survival after chemotherapy for acute myeloid leukemia: the experience of the Southwest Oncology Group. *Cancer* 1997;80(Suppl.): 2199–204.

8 Bloomfield CD, Lawrence D, Byrd JC, *et al.* Frequency of prolonged remission duration after high-dose cytarabine intensification in acute myeloid Leukemia varies by cytogenetic subtype. *Cancer Res* 1998;58:4173–9.

9 Anderson JE, Kopecky KJ, Willman CL, *et al.* Outcome after induction chemotherapy for older patients with acute myeloid Leukemia is not improved with mitoxantrone and etoposide compared to cytarabine and daunorubic. In: a Southwest Oncology Group study. *Blood* 2002;100:3869–76.

10 Chen CC, Yang CF, Yang MH, *et al.* Pretreatment prognostic factors and treatment outcome in elderly patients with *de novo* acute myeloid Leukemia. *Ann Oncol* 2005;16:1366–73.

11 Gupta V, Chun K, Yi QL, *et al.* Disease biology rather than age is the most important determinant of survival of patients > or =60 years with acute myeloid Leukemia treated with uniform intensive therapy. *Cancer* 2005;103:2082–90.

12 Marbello L, Ricci F, Nosari AM, *et al.* Outcome of hyperleukocytic adult acute myeloid leukemia: a single-center retrospective study and review of literature. *Leuk Res* 2008;32: 1221–7.

13 Flasshove M, Meusers P, Schutte J, *et al.* Long-term survival after induction therapy with idarubicin and cytosine arabinoside for *de novo* acute myeloid leukemia. *Ann Hematol* 2000;79:533–42.

14 Byrd JC, Mrozek K, Dodge RK, *et al.* Pretreatment cytogenetic abnormalities are predictive of induction success, cumulative incidence of relapse, and overall survival in adult patients with de novo acute myeloid *leukemia*: results from Cancer and Leukemia Group B (CALGB 8461). *Blood* 2002;100: 4325–36.

15 Stucki A, Rivier AS, Gikic M, Monai N, Schapira M, Spertini O. Endothelial cell activation by myeloblasts: molecular mechanisms of leukostasis and leukemic cell dissemination. *Blood* 2001;97:2121–9.

16 Novotny JR, Nuckel H, Duhrsen U. Correlation between expression of CD56/NCAM and severe leukostasis in hyperleukocytic acute myelomonocytic leukemia. *Eur J Haematol* 2006;76:299–308.

17 Novotny JR, Muller-Beissenhirtz H, Herget-Rosenthal S, Kribben A, Duhrsen U. Grading of symptoms in hyperleukocytic leukemia: a clinical model for the role of different blast types and promyelocytes in the development of leukostasis syndrome. *Eur J Haematol* 2005;74:501–10.

18 Rosenbluth MJ, Lam WA, Fletcher DA. Force microscopy of nonadherent cells: a comparison of Leukemia cell deformability. *Biophys J* 2006;90:2994–3003.

19 Strauss RA, Gloster ES, McCallister JA, Jimenez JF, Neuberg RW, Berry DH. Acute cytoreduction techniques in the early treatment of hyperleukocytosis associated with childhood hematologic malignancies. *Med Pediatr Oncol* 1985;13:346–51.

20 Bunin NJ, Kunkel K, Callihan TR. Cytoreductive procedures in the early management in cases of leukemia and hyperleukocytosis in children. *Med Pediatr Oncol* 1987;15:232–5.

21 Kuo K, Callum J, Brandwein, J. Management of hyperleukocytosis in acute myelogenous leukemia using hydroxyurea rather than leukapheresis. *Blood* 2006;108.

22 Goodenow TJ, Malarkey WB. Leukocytosis and artifactual hypoglycemia. *JAMA* 1977;237:1961–2.

23 Canivet B, Squara P, Elbaze P, *et al* [*In vitro* glucose consumption in severe hyperleukocytosis. A cause of factitious hypoglycemia]. *Sem Hop* 1983;59:533–6.
24 O'Regan S, Carson S, Chesney RW, Drummond KN. Electrolyte and acid-base disturbances in the management of leukemia. *Blood* 1977;49:345–53.
25 Tosi P, Barosi G, Lazzaro C, *et al*. Consensus conference on the management of tumor lysis syndrome. *Haematologica* 2008.
26 Jasek AM, Day HJ. Acute spontaneous tumor lysis syndrome. *Am J Hematol* 1994;47:129–31.
27 Cairo MS, Bishop M. Tumour lysis syndrome: new therapeutic strategies and classification. *Br J Haematol* 2004;127:3–11.
28 McCroskey RD, Mosher DF, Spencer CD, Prendergast E, Longo WL. Acute tumor lysis syndrome and treatment response in patients treated for refractory chronic lymphocytic leukemia with short-course, high-dose cytosine arabinoside, cisplatin, and etoposide. *Cancer* 1990;66:246–50.
29 Sparano J, Ramirez M, Wiernik PH. Increasing recognition of corticosteroid-induced tumor lysis syndrome in non-Hodgkin's lymphoma. *Cancer* 1990;65:1072–3.
30 Simmons ED, Somberg KA. Acute tumor lysis syndrome after intrathecal methotrexate administration. *Cancer* 1991;67:2062–5.
31 Fer MF, Bottino GC, Sherwin SA, *et al*. Atypical tumor lysis syndrome in a patient with T cell lymphoma treated with recombinant leukocyte interferon. *Am J Med* 1984;77:953–6.
32 Yang H, Rosove MH, Figlin RA. Tumor lysis syndrome occurring after the administration of rituximab in lymphoproliferative disorders: high-grade non-Hodgkin's lymphoma and chronic lymphocytic leukemia. *Am J Hematol* 1999;62:247–50.
33 Hussain K, Mazza JJ, Clouse LH. Tumor lysis syndrome (TLS) following fludarabine therapy for chronic lymphocytic leukemia (CLL): case report and review of the literature. *Am J Hematol* 2003;72:212–15.
34 Seki JT, Al-Omar HM, Amato D, Sutton DM. Acute tumor lysis syndrome secondary to hydroxyurea in acute myeloid leukemia. *Ann Pharmacother* 2003;37:675–8.
35 Mato AR, Riccio BE, Qin L, *et al*. A predictive model for the detection of tumor lysis syndrome during AML induction therapy. *Leuk Lymphoma* 2006;47:877–83.
36 Davidson MB, Thakkar S, Hix JK, Bhandarkar ND, Wong A, Schreiber MJ. Pathophysiology, clinical consequences, and treatment of tumor lysis syndrome. *Am J Med* 2004;116: 546–54.
37 Ichida K, Hosoyamada M, Hisatome I, *et al*. Clinical and molecular analysis of patients with renal hypouricemia in Japan-influence of URAT1 gene on urinary urate excretion. *J Am Soc Nephrol* 2004;15:164–73.
38 Ten Harkel AD, Kist-Van Holthe JE, Van Weel M, Van der Vorst MM. Alkalinization and the tumor lysis syndrome. *Med Pediatr Oncol* 1998;31:27–8.
39 Jones DP, Mahmoud H, Chesney RW. Tumor lysis syndrome: pathogenesis and management. *Pediatr Nephrol* 1995;9: 206–12.
40 Spector T. Inhibition of urate production by allopurinol. *Biochem Pharmacol* 1977;26:355–8.
41 Goldman SC, Holcenberg JS, Finklestein JZ, *et al*. A randomized comparison between rasburicase and allopurinol in children with lymphoma or leukemia at high risk for tumor lysis. *Blood* 2001;97:2998–3003.
42 Beghini A, Ripamonti CB, Cairoli R, *et al*. KIT activating mutations: incidence in adult and pediatric acute myeloid leukemia, and identification of an internal tandem duplication. *Haematologica* 2004;89:920–5.
43 Brogard JM, Coumaros D, Franckhauser J, Stahl A, Stahl J. Enzymatic uricolysis: a study of the effect of a fungal urate-oxydase. *Rev Eur Etud Clin Biol* 1972;17:890–5.
44 Yeldandi AV, Yeldandi V, Kumar S, *et al*. Molecular evolution of the urate oxidase-encoding gene in hominoid primates: nonsense mutations. *Gene* 1991;109:281–4.
45 Masera G, Jankovic M, Zurlo MG, *et al*. Urate-oxidase prophylaxis of uric acid-induced renal damage in childhood leukemia. *J Pediatr* 1982;100:152–5.
46 Pui CH, Relling MV, Lascombes F, *et al*. Urate oxidase in prevention and treatment of hyperuricemia associated with lymphoid malignancies. *Leukemia* 1997;11:1813–16.
47 Noguera NI, Breccia M, Divona M, *et al*. Alterations of the FLT3 gene in acute promyelocytic leukemia: association with diagnostic characteristics and analysis of clinical outcome in patients treated with the Italian AIDA protocol. *Leukemia* 2002;16:2185–9.
48 Legoux R, Delpech B, Dumont X, *et al*. Cloning and expression in *Escherichia coli* of the gene encoding *Aspergillus flavus* urate oxidase. *J Biol Chem* 1992;267:8565–70.
49 Coiffier B, Mounier N, Bologna S, *et al*. Efficacy and safety of rasburicase (recombinant urate oxidase) for the prevention and treatment of hyperuricemia during induction chemotherapy of aggressive non-Hodgkin's lymphoma: results of the GRAAL1 (Groupe d'Etude des Lymphomes de l'Adulte Trial on Rasburicase Activity in Adult Lymphoma) study. *J Clin Oncol* 2003;21:4402–6.
50 Falanga A, Marchetti M, Barbui T. All-trans-retinoic acid and bleeding/thrombosis. *Pathophysiol Haemost Thromb* 2003;33 (Suppl. 1):19–21.
51 Trifilio S TM, Singhal S, Gordon L, Evens A, Mehta J. Low-Dose Recombinant Urate Oxidase (Rasburicase) is Effective in Hyperuricemia. 46th ASH Annual Meeting, 2004.
52 Pui CH, Mahmoud HH, Wiley JM, *et al*. Recombinant urate oxidase for the prophylaxis or treatment of hyperuricemia in patients With leukemia or lymphoma. *J Clin Oncol* 2001;19: 697–704.
53 Pui CH, Jeha S, Irwin D, Camitta B. Recombinant urate oxidase (rasburicase) in the prevention and treatment of malignancy-associated hyperuricemia in pediatric and adult patients: results of a compassionate-use trial. *Leukemia* 2001;15: 1505–9.
54 Jeha S. Tumor lysis syndrome. *Semin Hematol* 2001;38(Suppl 10):4–8.
55 Fukasawa H, Kato A, Fujigaki Y, Yonemura K, Furuya R, Hishida A. Hypercalcemia in a patient with B-cell acute lymphoblastic leukemia: a role of proinflammatory cytokine. *Am J Med Sci* 2001;322:109–12.
56 Mandal AK. Hypokalemia and hyperkalemia. *Med Clin North Am* 1997;81:611–39.
57 Kelly KM, Lange B. Oncologic emergencies. *Pediatr Clin North Am* 1997;44:809–30.
58 Sillos EM, Shenep JL, Burghen GA, Pui CH, Behm FG, Sandlund JT. Lactic acidosis: a metabolic complication of hematologic malignancies: case report and review of the literature. *Cancer* 2001;92:2237–46.

59 Mazurek S, Boschek CB, Eigenbrodt E. The role of phosphometabolites in cell proliferation, energy metabolism, and tumor therapy. *J Bioenerg Biomembr* 1997;29:315–30.

60 Mathupala SP, Rempel A, Pedersen PL. Aberrant glycolytic metabolism of cancer cells: a remarkable coordination of genetic, transcriptional, post-translational, and mutational events that lead to a critical role for type II hexokinase. *J Bioenerg Biomembr* 1997;29:339–43.

61 Elmlinger MW, Wimmer K, Biemer E, Blum WF, Ranke MB, Dannecker GE. Insulin-like growth factor binding protein 2 is differentially expressed in leukemic B- and T-cell lines. *Growth Regul* 1996;6:152–7.

62 Cohick WS, Clemmons DR. The insulin-like growth factors. *Annu Rev Physiol* 1993;55:131–53.

63 Werner H, LeRoith D. The role of the insulin-like growth factor system in human cancer. *Adv Cancer Res* 1996;68:183–223.

64 Tiefenthaler M, Amberger A, Bacher N, *et al.* Increased lactate production follows loss of mitochondrial membrane potential during apoptosis of human leukemia cells. *Br J Haematol* 2001;114:574–80.

65 Sculier JP, Nicaise C, Klastersky J. Lactic acidosis: a metabolic complication of extensive metastatic cancer. *Eur J Cancer Clin Oncol* 1983;19:597–601.

66 Stacpoole PW. Lactic acidosis: the case against bicarbonate therapy. *Ann Intern Med* 1986;105:276–9.

67 Avvisati G, Mandelli F, Petti MC, *et al.* Idarubicin (4-demethoxydaunorubicin) as single agent for remission induction of previously untreated acute promyelocytic leukemia: a pilot study of the Italian cooperative group GIMEMA. *Eur J Haematol* 1990;44:257–60.

68 Hingorani AD, Macdougall IC, Browne M, Walker RW, Tomson CR. Successful treatment of acute D-lactate encephalopathy by haemodialysis. *Nephrol Dial Transplant* 1993;8: 1283–5.

69 Barton IK, Streather CP, Hilton PJ, Bradley RD. Successful treatment of severe lactic acidosis by haemofiltration using a bicarbonate-based replacement fluid. *Nephrol Dial Transplant* 1991;6:368–70.

70 Schneider T, Seydlitz F, Zimmermann U, Sontag B, Boesken WH. [Life threatening hypercalcemia in a young man with ALL]. *Dtsch Med Wochenschr* 2001;126:7–11.

71 Lankisch P, Kramm CM, Hermsen D, Wessalowski R. Hypercalcemia with nephrocalcinosis and impaired renal function due to increased parathyroid hormone secretion at onset of childhood acute lymphoblastic leukemia. *Leuk Lymphoma* 2004;45:1695–7.

72 Esbrit P. Hypercalcemia of malignancy—new insights into an old syndrome. *Clin Lab* 2001;47:67–71.

73 Au WY, Fung A, Chim CS, *et al.* FLT3 aberrations in acute promyelocytic leukemia: clinicopathological associations and prognostic impact. *Br J Haematol* 2004;125:463–9.

74 Schmid I, Stachel D, Schon C, Bauer M, Haas RJ. Pamidronate and calcitonin as therapy of acute cancer-related hypercalcemia in children. *Klin Padiatr* 2001;213:30–4.

75 Bockman R. The effects of gallium nitrate on bone resorption. *Semin Oncol* 2003;30(Suppl 5):5–12.

76 Kakizuka A, Miller WH, Jr., Umesono K, *et al.* Chromosomal translocation t(15;17) in human acute promyelocytic leukemia fuses RAR alpha with a novel putative transcription factor, PML. *Cell* 1991;66:663–74.

77 Chaves Alvarez AJ, Herrera Saval A, Marquez Enriquez J, Camacho Martinez F. Metastatic calcinosis cutis in multiple myeloma. *Br J Dermatol* 2000;142:820–2.

78 Cochran RJ, Wilkin JK. An unusual case of calcinosis cutis. *J Am Acad Dermatol* 1983;8:103–6.

79 Bartlett JB, Dredge K, Dalgleish AG. The evolution of thalidomide and its IMiD derivatives as anticancer agents. *Nat Rev Cancer* 2004;4:314–22.

80 Gardella S, Cervantes F, Blade J, Sanchez Bisono J, Granena A, Rozman C. Acute myeloblastic leukemia presenting with superior vena cava syndrome due to mediastinal mass. *Acta Haematol* 1984;71:174–7.

81 Liu HW, Wong KL, Chan TY, Lau CC, Liang R. Superior vena cava syndrome: a rare presenting feature of acute myeloid leukemia. *Acta Haematol* 1988;79:213–16.

82 Schindler N, Vogelzang RL. Superior vena cava syndrome. Experience with endovascular stents and surgical therapy. *Surg Clin North Am* 1999;79:683–94, xi.

83 Nichols CR, Roth BJ, Heerema N, Griep J, Tricot G. Hematologic neoplasia associated with primary mediastinal germ-cell tumors. *N Engl J Med* 1990;322:1425–9.

84 Nichols CR, Hoffman R, Einhorn LH, Williams SD, Wheeler LA, Garnick MB. Hematologic malignancies associated with primary mediastinal germ-cell tumors. *Ann Intern Med* 1985; 102:603–9.

85 Federici AB. Acquired von Willebrand syndrome: an underdiagnosed and misdiagnosed bleeding complication in patients with lymphoproliferative and myeloproliferative disorders. *Semin Hematol* 2006;43(Suppl 1):S48–58.

86 Webert K, Cook RJ, Sigouin CS, Rebulla P, Heddle NM. The risk of bleeding in thrombocytopenic patients with acute myeloid leukemia. *Haematologica* 2006;91:1530–7.

87 Gmur J, Burger J, Schanz U, Fehr J, Schaffner A. Safety of stringent prophylactic platelet transfusion policy for patients with acute leukemia. *Lancet* 1991;338:1223–6.

88 Heckman KD, Weiner GJ, Davis CS, Strauss RG, Jones MP, Burns CP. Randomized study of prophylactic platelet transfusion threshold during induction therapy for adult acute leukemia: 10,000/microL versus 20,000/microL. *J Clin Oncol* 1997; 15:1143–9.

89 Rebulla P, Finazzi G, Marangoni F, *et al.* The threshold for prophylactic platelet transfusions in adults with acute myeloid leukemia. Gruppo Italiano Malattie Ematologiche Maligne dell'Adulto. *N Engl J Med* 1997;337:1870–5.

90 Wandt H, Frank M, Ehninger G, *et al.* Safety and cost effectiveness of a 10×10^9/L trigger for prophylactic platelet transfusions compared with the traditional $20 \times 10(9)$/L trigger: a prospective comparative trial in 105 patients with acute myeloid leukemia. *Blood* 1998;91:3601–6.

91 Wandt H, Ehninger G, Gallmeier WM. New strategies for prophylactic platelet transfusion in patients with hematologic diseases. *Oncologist* 2001;6:446–50.

92 Brubaker DB, Marcus C, Holmes E. Intravascular and total body platelet equilibrium in healthy volunteers and in thrombocytopenic patients transfused with single donor platelets. *Am J Hematol* 1998;58:165–76.

93 Schiffer CA, Anderson KC, Bennett CL, *et al.* Platelet transfusion for patients with cancer: clinical practice guidelines of the American Society of Clinical Oncology. *J Clin Oncol* 2001;19: 1519–38.

94 Slichter SJ, Davis K, Enright H, *et al.* Factors affecting post-transfusion platelet increments, platelet refractoriness, and platelet transfusion intervals in thrombocytopenic patients. *Blood* 2005;105:4106–14.

95 Heddle NM, Cook RJ, Tinmouth A, *et al.* A randomized controlled trial comparing standard- and low-dose strategies for transfusion of platelets (SToP) to patients with thrombocytopenia. *Blood* 2009;113:1564–73.

96 Brown JE, Olujohungbe A, Chang J, *et al.* All-trans retinoic acid (ATRA) and tranexamic acid: a potentially fatal combination in acute promyelocytic leukemia. *Br J Haematol* 2000;110: 1010–12.

97 Green D. Management of bleeding complications of hematologic malignancies. *Semin Thromb Hemost* 2007;33:427–34.

98 Abshire TC, Gold SH, Odom LF, Carson SD, Hathaway WE. The coagulopathy of childhood leukemia. Thrombin activation or primary fibrinolysis? *Cancer* 1990;66:716–21.

99 Sarris A, Cortes J, Kantarjian H, *et al.* Disseminated intravascular coagulation in adult acute lymphoblastic leukemia: frequent complications with fibrinogen levels less than 100 mg/dl. *Leuk Lymphoma* 1996;21:85–92.

100 Higuchi T, Mori H, Niikura H, Omine M, Okada S, Terada H. Disseminated intravascular coagulation in acute lymphoblastic *Leukemia* at presentation and in early phase of remission induction therapy. *Ann Hematol* 1998;76:263–9.

101 Sarris AH, Kempin S, Berman E, *et al.* High incidence of disseminated intravascular coagulation during remission induction of adult patients with acute lymphoblastic leukemia. *Blood* 1992;79:1305–10.

102 Bezeaud A, Drouet L, Leverger G, Griffin JH, Guillin MC. Effect of L-asparaginase therapy for acute lymphoblastic leukemia on plasma vitamin K-dependent coagulation factors and inhibitors. *J Pediatr* 1986;108(Pt 1):698–701.

103 Ramsay NK, Coccia PF, Krivit W, Nesbit ME, Edson JR. The effect of L-asparaginase of plasma coagulation factors in acute lymphoblastic leukemia. *Cancer* 1977;40:1398–401.

104 Priest JR, Ramsay NK, Bennett AJ, Krivit W, Edson JR. The effect of L-asparaginase on antithrombin, plasminogen, and plasma coagulation during therapy for acute lymphoblastic leukemia. *J Pediatr* 1982;100:990–5.

105 Bettigole RE, Himelstein ES, Oettgen HF, Clifford GO. Hypofibrinogenemia due to L-asparaginase: studies of fibrinogen survival using autologous 131-I-fibrinogen. *Blood* 1970; 35:195–200.

106 Nowak-Gottl U, Ahlke E, Klosel K, Jurgens H, Boos J. Changes in coagulation and fibrinolysis in childhood acute lymphoblastic leukemia re-induction therapy using three different asparaginase preparations. *Eur J Pediatr* 1997;156:848–50.

107 Cairo MS, Lazarus K, Gilmore RL, Baehner RL. Intracranial hemorrhage and focal seizures secondary to use of L-asparaginase during induction therapy of acute lymphocytic leukemia. *J Pediatr* 1980;97:829–33.

108 Gugliotta L, Mazzucconi MG, Leone G, *et al.* Incidence of thrombotic complications in adult patients with acute lymphoblastic leukemia receiving L-asparaginase during induction therapy: a retrospective study. The GIMEMA Group. *Eur J Haematol* 1992;49:63–6.

109 Benzon HT, Iqbal M, Tallman MS, Boehlke L, Russell EJ. Superior sagittal sinus thrombosis in a patient with postdural puncture headache. *Reg Anesth Pain Med* 2003;28:64–7.

110 Duru F, Ertem U, Dagdemir A, *et al.* Coexistence of life threatening chemotherapy related leukoencephalopathy, sagittal sinus thrombosis and multiple organ failure in a child with acute lymphoblastic leukemia: an unusual case with clinical recovery. *Leuk Lymphoma* 1997;26:377–85.

111 Castagnola C, Nozza A, Corso A, Bernasconi C. The value of combination therapy in adult acute myeloid leukemia with central nervous system involvement. *Haematologica* 1997;82: 577–80.

112 Halton JM, Mitchell LG, Vegh P, Eves M, Andrew ME. Fresh frozen plasma has no beneficial effect on the hemostatic system in children receiving L-asparaginase. *Am J Hematol* 1994;47:157–61.

113 Mauz-Korholz C, Junker R, Gobel U, Nowak-Gottl U. Prothrombotic risk factors in children with acute lymphoblastic leukemia treated with delayed *E. coli* asparaginase (COALL-92 and 97 protocols). *Thromb Haemost* 2000;83: 840–3.

114 Mitchell LG, Andrew M, Hanna K, *et al.* A prospective cohort study determining the prevalence of thrombotic events in children with acute lymphoblastic leukemia and a central venous line who are treated with L-asparaginase: results of the Prophylactic Antithrombin Replacement in Kids with Acute Lymphoblastic Leukemia Treated with Asparaginase (PARKAA) Study. *Cancer* 2003;97:508–16.

115 Gralnick HR, Bagley J, Abrell E. Heparin treatment for the hemorrhagic diathesis of acute promyelocytic leukemia. *Am J Med* 1972;52:167–74.

116 Cordonnier C, Vernant JP, Brun B, *et al.* Acute promyelocytic leukemia in 57 previously untreated patients. *Cancer* 1985;55: 18–25.

117 Kantarjian HM, Keating MJ, Walters RS, *et al.* The association of specific "favorable" cytogenetic abnormalities with secondary leukemia. *Cancer* 1986;58:924–7.

118 Rodeghiero F, Avvisati G, Castaman G, Barbui T, Mandelli F. Early deaths and antihemorrhagic treatments in acute promyelocytic leukemia. A GIMEMA retrospective study in 268 consecutive patients. *Blood* 1990;75:2112–17.

119 Head D, Kopecky KJ, Weick J, *et al.* Effect of aggressive daunomycin therapy on survival in acute promyelocytic leukemia. *Blood* 1995;86:1717–28.

120 Sanz MA, Jarque I, Martin G, *et al.* Acute promyelocytic leukemia. Therapy results and prognostic factors. *Cancer* 1988;61: 7–13.

121 Tallman MS, Kwaan HC. Reassessing the hemostatic disorder associated with acute promyelocytic leukemia. *Blood* 1992;79:543–53.

122 Barbui T, Finazzi G, Falanga A. The impact of all-trans-retinoic acid on the coagulopathy of acute promyelocytic leukemia. *Blood* 1998;91:3093–102.

123 Dally N, Hoffman R, Haddad N, Sarig G, Rowe JM, Brenner B. Predictive factors of bleeding and thrombosis during induction therapy in acute promyelocytic leukemia-a single center experience in 34 patients. *Thromb Res* 2005;116:109–14.

124 Gralnick HR, Sultan C. Acute promyelocytic leukemia: hemorrhagic manifestation and morphologic criteria. *Br J Haematol* 1975;29:373–6.

125 Bennett B, Booth NA, Croll A, Dawson AA. The bleeding disorder in acute promyelocytic leukemia: fibrinolysis due to u-PA rather than defibrination. *Br J Haematol* 1989;71:511–17.

126 Bennett JM, Catovsky D, Daniel MT, *et al*. Proposals for the classification of the acute leukaemias. French–American–British (FAB) co-operative group. *Br J Haematol* 1976;33: 451–8.
127 Bauer KA, Conway EM, Bach R, Konigsberg WH, Griffin JD, Demetri G. Tissue factor gene expression in acute myeloblastic leukemia. *Thromb Res* 1989;56:425–30.
128 Kubota T, Andoh K, Sadakata H, Tanaka H, Kobayashi N. Tissue factor released from leukemic cells. *Thromb Haemost* 1991;65:59–63.
129 Falanga A, Gordon SG. Isolation and characterization of cancer procoagulant: a cysteine proteinase from malignant tissue. *Biochemistry* 1985;24:5558–67.
130 Donati MB, Falanga A, Consonni R, *et al*. Cancer procoagulant in acute non lymphoid leukemia: relationship of enzyme detection to disease activity. *Thromb Haemost* 1990;64:11–16.
131 Call TG, Phyliky RL, Noel P, *et al*. Incidence of chronic lymphocytic leukemia in Olmsted County, Minnesota, 1935 through 1989, with emphasis on changes in initial stage at diagnosis. *Mayo Clin Proc* 1994;69:323–8.
132 Sterrenberg L, Haak HL, Brommer EJ, Nieuwenhuizen W. Evidence of fibrinogen breakdown by leukocyte enzymes in a patient with acute promyelocytic leukemia. *Haemostasis* 1985;15:126–33.
133 Wilson EL, Jacobs P, Dowdle EB. The secretion of plasminogen activators by human myeloid leukemic cells *in vitro*. *Blood* 1983;61:568–74.
134 Sakata Y, Murakami T, Noro A, Mori K, Matsuda M. The specific activity of plasminogen activator inhibitor-1 in disseminated intravascular coagulation with acute promyelocytic leukemia. *Blood* 1991;77:1949–57.
135 Hirata F, Schiffmann E, Venkatasubramanian K, Salomon D, Axelrod J. A phospholipase A2 inhibitory protein in rabbit neutrophils induced by glucocorticoids. *Proc Natl Acad Sci U S A* 1980;77:2533–6.
136 Chang KS, Wang G, Freireich EJ, *et al*. Specific expression of the annexin VIII gene in acute promyelocytic leukemia. *Blood* 1992;79:1802–10.
137 Hajjar KA, Jacovina AT, Chacko J. An endothelial cell receptor for plasminogen/tissue plasminogen activator. I. Identity with annexin II. *J Biol Chem* 1994;269:21191–7.
138 Menell JS, Cesarman GM, Jacovina AT, McLaughlin MA, Lev EA, Hajjar KA. Annexin II and bleeding in acute promyelocytic leukemia. *N Engl J Med* 1999;340:994–1004.
139 Zhang X, Zhou H, Wang J, et al. Arsenic trioxide, retinoic acid and Ara-c regulated the expression of annexin II on the surface of APL cells, a novel co-receptor for plasminogen/tissue plasminogen activator. *Thromb Res* 2002;106:63–70.
140 Federici AB, D'Amico EA. The role of von Willebrand factor in the hemostatic defect of acute promyelocytic leukemia. *Leuk Lymphoma* 1998;31:491–9.
141 Dombret H, Scrobohaci ML, Ghorra P, *et al*. Coagulation disorders associated with acute promyelocytic leukemia: corrective effect of all-trans retinoic acid treatment. *Leukemia* 1993;7:2–9.
142 Terada Y, Shindo T, Endoh A, Watanabe M, Fukaya T, Yajima A. Fetal arrhythmia during treatment of pregnancy-associated acute promyelocytic leukemia with all-trans retinoic acid and favorable outcome. *Leukemia* 1997;11:454–5.
143 Tallman MS, Brenner B, Serna Jde L, *et al*. Meeting report. Acute promyelocytic leukemia-associated coagulopathy, 21 January 2004, London, United Kingdom. *Leuk Res* 2005;29: 347–51.
144 Schneider W, Runde V, Aul C [From fatal hemorrhagic diathesis to life-threatening thrombosis risk. New complications of a "gentle" treatment of acute promyelocytic leukemias with all-trans-retinoic acid]. *Dtsch Med Wochenschr* 1991;116: 1971–5.
145 Tallman MS, Andersen JW, Schiffer CA, *et al*. All-trans-retinoic acid in acute promyelocytic leukemia. *N Engl J Med* 1997;337: 1021–8.
146 Runde V, Aul C, Heyll A, Schneider W. All-trans retinoic acid: not only a differentiating agent, but also an inducer of thromboembolic events in patients with M3 leukemia. *Blood* 1992; 79:534–5.
147 de Lacerda JF, do Carmo JA, Guerra ML, Geraldes J, de Lacerda JM. Multiple thrombosis in acute promyelocytic *Leukemia* after tretinoin. *Lancet* 1993;342:114–15.
148 Goldschmidt N, Gural A, Ben Yehuda D. Extensive splenic infarction, deep vein thrombosis and pulmonary emboli complicating induction therapy with all-trans-retinoic acid (ATRA) for acute promyelocytic leukemia. *Leuk Lymphoma* 2003;44:1433–7.
149 Hashimoto S, Koike T, Tatewaki W, *et al*. Fatal thromboembolism in acute promyelocytic leukemia during all-trans retinoic acid therapy combined with antifibrinolytic therapy for prophylaxis of hemorrhage. *leukemia* 1994;8:1113–15.
150 Schwartz BS, Williams EC, Conlan MG, Mosher DF. Epsilon-aminocaproic acid in the treatment of patients with acute promyelocytic leukemia and acquired alpha-2-plasmin inhibitor deficiency. *Ann Intern Med* 1986;105:873–7.
151 Pui CH, Howard SC. Current management and challenges of malignant disease in the CNS in pediatric leukemia. *Lancet Oncol* 2008;9:257–68.
152 Lazarus HM, Richards SM, Chopra R, *et al*. Central nervous system involvement in adult acute lymphoblastic leukemia at diagnosis: results from the international ALL trial MRC UKALL XII/ECOG E2993. *Blood* 2006;108: 465–72.
153 Reman O, Pigneux A, Huguet F, *et al*. Central nervous system involvement in adult acute lymphoblastic *Leukemia* at diagnosis and/or at first relapse: results from the GET-LALA group. *Leuk Res* 2008;32:1741–50.
154 Larson RA, Dodge RK, Burns CP, *et al*. A five-drug remission induction regimen with intensive consolidation for adults with acute lymphoblastic leukemia: cancer and leukemia group B study 8811. *Blood* 1995;85:2025–37.
155 Kantarjian HM, O'Brien S, Smith TL, *et al*. Results of treatment with hyper-CVAD, a dose-intensive regimen, in adult acute lymphocytic leukemia. *J Clin Oncol* 2000;18:547–61.
156 Cortes J, O'Brien SM, Pierce S, Keating MJ, Freireich EJ, Kantarjian HM. The value of high-dose systemic chemotherapy and intrathecal therapy for central nervous system prophylaxis in different risk groups of adult acute lymphoblastic leukemia. *Blood* 1995;86:2091–7.
157 Petersdorf SH, Kopecky KJ, Head DR, *et al*. Comparison of the L10M consolidation regimen to an alternative regimen including escalating methotrexate/L-asparaginase for adult acute

lymphoblastic leukemia: a Southwest Oncology Group Study. *Leukemia* 2001;15:208–16.

158 Byrd JC, Edenfield WJ, Shields DJ, Dawson NA. Extramedullary myeloid cell tumors in acute nonlymphocytic leukemia: a clinical review. *J Clin Oncol* 1995;13:1800–16.

159 Castagnola C, Morra E, Bernasconi P, Astori C, Santagostino A, Bernasconi C. Acute myeloid leukemia and diabetes insipidus: results in 5 patients. *Acta Haematol* 1995;93:1–4.

160 Holmes R, Keating MJ, Cork A, *et al*. A unique pattern of central nervous system leukemia in acute myelomonocytic leukemia associated with inv(16)(p13q22). *Blood* 1985;65: 1071–8.

161 Glass JP, Van Tassel P, Keating MJ, Cork A, Trujillo J, Holmes R. Central nervous system complications of a newly recognized subtype of leukemia: AMML with a pericentric inversion of chromosome 16. *Neurology* 1987;37: 639–44.

162 Schattner A, Kozack N, Sandler A, Shtalrid M. Facial diplegia as the presenting manifestation of acute lymphoblastic leukemia. *Mt Sinai J Med* 2001;68:406–9.

163 Mayo GL, Carter JE, McKinnon SJ. Bilateral optic disk edema and blindness as initial presentation of acute lymphocytic leukemia. *Am J Ophthalmol* 2002;134:141–2.

164 Pui CH. Central nervous system disease in acute lymphoblastic leukemia: prophylaxis and treatment. *Hematology Am Soc Hematol Educ Program* 2006:142–6.

165 Beslac-Bumbasirevic L, Boskovic D, Tomin D, Colovic M, Kovacevic M, Bumbasirevic V. [neuroleukemia in adults]. *Srp Arh Celok Lek* 1996;124:82–6.

166 Leibel SA PT. *Textbook of radiation oncology*. Philadelphia: WB Saunder;1998.

167 Criscuolo GR, Balledux JP. Clinical neurosciences in the decade of the brain: hypotheses in neuro-oncology. VEG/PF acts upon the actin cytoskeleton and is inhibited by dexamethasone: relevance to tumor angiogenesis and vasogenic edema. *Yale J Biol Med* 1996;69:337–55.

168 Nauck M, Karakiulakis G, Perruchoud AP, Papakonstantinou E, Roth M. Corticosteroids inhibit the expression of the vascular endothelial growth factor gene in human vascular smooth muscle cells. *Eur J Pharmacol* 1998;341:309–15.

169 Nauck M, Roth M, Tamm M, *et al*. Induction of vascular endothelial growth factor by platelet-activating factor and platelet-derived growth factor is downregulated by corticosteroids. *Am J Respir Cell Mol Biol* 1997;16:398–406.

170 Loblaw DA, Laperriere NJ. Emergency treatment of malignant extradural spinal cord compression: an evidence-based guideline. *J Clin Oncol* 1998;16:1613–24.

171 Greenberg HS, Kim JH, Posner JB. Epidural spinal cord compression from metastatic tumor: results with a new treatment protocol. *Ann Neurol* 1980;8:361–6.

172 Storti S, Marra R, Pagano L, *et al*. Emergency abdominal surgery in patients with acute leukemia and lymphoma. *Ital J Surg Sci* 1988;18:361–3.

173 Giagounidis AA, Burk M, Meckenstock G, Koch AJ, Schneider W. Pathologic rupture of the spleen in hematologic malignancies: two additional cases. *Ann Hematol* 1996;73:297–302.

174 Goddard SL, Chesney AE, Reis MD, *et al*. Pathological splenic rupture: a rare complication of chronic myelomonocytic leukemia. *Am J Hematol* 2007;82:405–8.

175 Rhee SJ, Sheena Y, Imber C. Spontaneous rupture of the spleen: a rare but important differential of an acute abdomen. *Am J Emerg Med* 2008;26:733 e5–6.

176 Bauer TW, Haskins GE, Armitage JO. Splenic rupture in patients with hematologic malignancies. *Cancer* 1981;48: 2729–33.

177 Ferrara F, D'Ambrosio V, Di Noto R, Mele G, Giovine S, Romano L. Spontaneous splenic rupture in a patient with acute lymphoblastic leukemia of Burkitt type. *Leuk Lymphoma* 1998;29:613–16.

178 Choo-Kang LR, Jones DM, Fehr JJ, Eskenazi AE, Toretsky JA. Cerebral edema and priapism in an adolescent with acute lymphoblastic leukemia. *Pediatr Emerg Care* 1999;15:110–12.

Chapter 32
Management of Infectious Complications in Patients with Leukemia

Marcio Nucci[1,2], *Nair Bijay*[1], *and Elias Anaissie*[1]
[1] Myeloma Institute for Research and Therapy, University of Arkansas for Medical Sciences, Little Rock, Arkansas, USA
[2] University Hospital, Federal University of Rio de Janeiro, Rio de Janeiro, Brazil

Introduction

The prognosis of patients with leukemia has markedly improved as a result of the introduction of novel antileukemic therapies, including allogeneic hematopoietic stem-cell transplantation (HSCT). These treatments induce severe alterations in host defense mechanisms, and, as a consequence, patients are at great risk of developing opportunistic infections, which frequently cause treatment failure or delay and/or death. Critical to the optimal management of patients with leukemia is the understanding of the time of development, presentation, etiology, diagnosis, and treatment of these infections.

Risk and epidemiology of infections in patients with leukemia

The risk of infection in leukemic patients is the result of the interaction between host, pathogen and environmental exposure. Infections occur when an imbalance develops between the weakened protective defense mechanisms of the host and the virulence factors of the offending pathogen.

Host-related factors

Immunodeficiency is the key risk factor for infection in patients with leukemia. It is caused by the underlying disease itself and its therapy, and may involve breakdown in skin and mucous membrane barriers, qualitative and quantitative defects in various arms of the immune system—including innate immunity (neutropenia, neutrophil dysfunction)—impaired production of immunoglobulins, and defective cell-mediated immunity (CMI). Although patients usually have deficits in various arms of the immune system, the nature of the pathogens causing infection is frequently determined by the immunodeficiency that is predominant at a given time (Tables 32.1 and 32.2). This interrelationship between the immunosuppressive effect of antineoplastic therapies and the causative pathogens can be appreciated in the setting of chronic lymphocytic leukemia (CLL). Untreated patients are susceptible to infection caused by encapsulated bacteria because of disease-related immunodeficiencies, including hypogammaglobulinemia [1]. However, the defective CMI that results from therapy with purine analogs and alemtuzumab causes infections with other pathogens, such as cytomegalovirus (CMV), varicella-zoster virus (VZV), and *Aspergillus* spp. [1–6]. Similarly, infections after therapy for acute myeloid leukemia (AML)/myelodsyplastic syndrome (MDS) are associated with the prolonged and profound neutropenia induced by myelosuppressive regimens [7]. Thus, a key principle in the assessment of the risk for infection is the understanding that patients with leukemia represent a heterogeneous group with respect to risk of infection—with the most important host factors being the net state of immunosuppression, tissue damage and organ dysfunction, and the immunogenetic and pharmacogenetic profiles (Table 32.3).

The net state of immunosuppression represents the cumulative effect of all immunosuppressive conditions caused by the underlying disease, previous and current therapies, comorbidities, infections with immunomodulating viruses such as cytomegalovirus (CMV), iron overload and, in allogeneic HSCT recipients, the presence of severe graft-versus-host disease (GVHD) and its therapy. Achievement of remission is usually critical in reducing the net state of immunosuppression, as is the control of GVHD [8–10]. The disruption of alimentary tract mucosal barriers caused by mucotoxic regimens and gut GVHD increases the risk of infection by facilitating the translocation of colonizing microorganisms into the bloodstream [11,12]. Likewise, dysfunction of renal, hepatic, and respiratory systems increase the risk for infection [13–15].

A role for immunogenetics and pharmacogenomics of antineoplastic drugs is being increasingly recognized.

Leukemias: Principles and Practice of Therapy, 1st edition. Edited by S. Faderl and H. Kantarjian.

Table 32.1 Immunodeficiencies associated with leukemia and its treatment.

	Disruption of skin and mucous membranes	Hypogammaglobulinemia	T-cell mediated immunodeficiency	Neutropenia and neutrophil dysfunction
Immunodeficiency associated with untreated underlying disease				
Acute leukemia and myelodysplasia				
Acute lymphoid leukemia	+	+	+++	++
Acute myeloid leukemia	+	+	+	+++
Myelodysplasia	–	–	–	+/+++
Chronic myeloid leukemia				
Chronic phase[a]	–	–	–	–
Accelerated phase	+	–	+	–
Blast crisis	+	+	++	+++
Other leukemias				
Adult T-cell leukemia/lymphoma	+	+	+++	+
Chronic lymphocytic leukemia	–	++	++	+
Large granular lymphocyte leukemia	–	–	+	++
Hairy cell leukemia	–	++	++	++
Immunodeficiency associated with treatment				
Corticosteroids	+	–	+++	+
Cytotoxic chemotherapy	–/++++[b]	+/++	+/+++[b]	–/+++[b]
Monoclonal antibodies	–	+/++	+/+++	+/++
Use of catheters	+++	–	–	–
Allogeneic transplantation	+/+++[c]	++	+++	+/+++[c]

–, none; +, mild; ++, moderate; +++, severe; ++++, very severe.

[a]No significant immunodeficiency in untreated patients.

[b]Immunodeficiency varies according to the type and dose intensity of the chemotherapeutic regimen.

[c]Severity of mucositis and neutropenia depend on the intensity of the conditioning regimen; duration of neutropenia also depends on the stem cell dose infused and *in vitro* manipulation of the stem cell product.

These genetic variations relate to the amount of drug exposure and hence risk for immunosuppression and tissue damage. An example is thiopurine methyltransferase (TPMT), an enzyme responsible for the degradation of two antileukemic agents, azathioprine and mercaptopurine. Patients with complete TPMT deficiency are at a much higher risk of potentially fatal hematologic toxicity than heterozygotes [16,17]. Genetic variations with other antileukemic agents are currently undergoing investigation.

Similarly, the role of host response to opportunistic pathogens is being explored. Polymorphisms in genes linked to Toll-like receptor 1 and 4, interleukin 10, tumor necrosis factor α (TNF-α), and mannose-binding lectin have been associated with an increased risk for various infections, including invasive aspergillosis and candidiasis [18–23], in patients with hematologic malignancies [24–26].

Most infections among patients with acute leukemia occur in the context of rapidly developing, profound (<100 neutrophils/μL) and prolonged (>14 days) neutropenia [27]. The trend of the neutrophil count is also an important determinant of infection outcome; a rapidly rising count is associated with a more favorable prognosis than one that continuously decreases or fails to normalize.

Qualitative abnormalities in neutrophil and other phagocytic cell functions resulting from the underlying disease and/or its therapies include inhibition of phagocytosis and granulocyte bactericidal activity [28–33]. Neutrophil chemotaxis is impaired in HSCT recipients treated for severe GVHD, as exemplified by decreased tissue neutrophils in patients with invasive pulmonary aspergillosis (IPA; similar to neutropenic states), despite adequate circulating neutrophil counts [34].

Lymphopenia and monocytopenia are considered independent risk factors for infection. In a series of 73 patients with hairy cell leukemia (HCL), 11 developed severe infections, and a lymphocyte count <1000/mm^3 (but not neutropenia) was the only risk factor identified [35]. In another study, monocytopenia, lymphopenia, and neutropenia independently predicted invasive mold infections (IMIs) among allogeneic HSCT recipients [36]. Lymphopenia has also been associated with an increased risk for CMV pneumonia [37] and respiratory syncytial

Table 32.2 Pathogens likely to cause infection in patients with hematologic malignancies according to immunodeficiency.

	Disruption of skin and mucous membranes	Hypogammaglobulinemia	T-cell mediated immunodeficiency	Neutropenia and neutrophil dysfunction
Bacteria				
Gram-positive cocci				
Coagulase-negative staphylococci	+++	–	–	++
Staphylococcus aureus	+++	–	–	++
Viridans streptococci	+++	–	–	++
Enterococci	++	–	–	++
Streptococcus pneumoniae	–	+++	–	–
Gram-positive bacilli				
Bacillus spp.	++	–	+	++
Corynebacterium jeikeium	++	–	+	++
Listeria monocytogenes	–	–	+++	–
Gram-negative bacilli				
Enterobacteriaceae[a]	++	–	–	+++
Pseudomonas aeruginosa	++	–	–	+++
Other non-fermentative bacteria[b]	++	–	–	+++
Salmonella spp.	+	+	++	+
Legionella spp.	–	++	++	–
Anaerobes				
Clostridium difficile	++	–	–	++
Clostridium septicum	++	–	–	++
Fungi				
Yeasts				
Candida spp.,[c] mucosal disease	+	–	+++	–
Candida spp.,[c] invasive disease	++	–	–	+++
Cryptococcus neoformans	–	–	+++	–
Trichosporon spp.	++	–	+	++
Molds				
Aspergillus spp.[d]	–	–	++	+++
Fusarium spp.	–/+	–	++	+++
Zygomycetes	–	–	++	+++
Scedosporium spp.	–	–	++	+++
Agents of phaeohyphomycosis	–	–	+	+
Other				
Pneumocystis jirovecii	–	–	+++	–
Histoplasma capsulatum	–	–	+++	–
Viruses				
Herpes simplex	++	–	+++	++
Varicella-zoster	–	–	+++	–
Cytomegalovirus	–	–	+++	–
Epstein–Barr virus	–	+	+++	–
Respiratory viruses[e]	+	+	++	–
Hepatitis A, B and C	–	+	+	–
Parvovirus B 19	–	++	++	–
Parasites				
Strongyloides stercoralis	–	–	++	–
Toxoplasma gondii	–	–	++	–
Cryptosporidium parvum	–	+	++	–
Mycobacteria				
Mycobacterium tuberculosis	–	–	+++	–
Rapid growing mycobacteria	++	–	+	–
Mycobacterium avium complex	–	–	+++	–

–, none; +, occasional; ++, frequent; +++, very frequent.

[a]Most frequent: *Escherichia coli, Klebsiella pneumoniae, Enterobacter* spp.

[b]Most frequent: *Acinetobacter* spp., *Stenotrophomonas maltophilia.*

[c]Most frequent: *C. albicans, C. glabrata, C. tropicalis, C. parapsilosis.*

[d]Most frequent: *A. fumigatus* (~90%), *A. flavus, A. terreus, A. niger.*

[e]Most frequent: respiratory syncytial virus, metapneumovirus, influenza A and B, parainfluenza 1–3, adenovirus, rhinovirus, coronavirus.

Table 32.3 Risk factors for infection in patients with leukemia.

1. Net state of immunosuppression
Older age
Refractory malignancy
Neutropenia
Related to the underlying disease (mostly acute leukemia)
Related to the treatment (intensity of myelosuppressive regimens)
T-cell mediated immunodeficiency
Related to the underlying disease (lymphoid malignancies)
Related to the treatment (extensive previous therapy, especially with high doses of corticosteroids, nucleoside analogs [eg, fludarabine, cladribine], monoclonal antibodies [eg, alemtuzumab], and reactivation of immunomodulatory viruses [cytomegalovirus])
Splenectomy
2. Patient's genetic profile
Pharmacogenomics (genetic variations in metabolism of antineoplastic drugs, potentially increasing toxicity)
Polymorphism of genes related to innate immunity (eg, Toll-like receptor 1 and 4, Interleukin 10 and 15, mannose-binding lectin)
3. Organ dysfunction
Oral and gastrointestinal mucositis (intensive chemotherapeutic regimens)
Skin breakdown (catheters, invasive procedures)
Renal insufficiency
Pulmonary dysfunction
Liver dysfunction
4. Exposure to pathogens
Colonization by potential pathogens (eg, Gram-positive and Gram-negative bacteria, yeasts)
Environmental exposure (eg, bacteria, molds, mycobacteria)
Reactivation of latent infection (eg, mycobacteria, viruses, *Toxoplasma gondii*)

virus (RSV) disease in patients with hematologic malignancies [38–40]. Patients with defective CMI are at greater risk for infections caused by intracellular pathogens, such as *Mycobacterium tuberculosis*, *Nocardia*, *Salmonella* spp., *Listeria*, *Cryptococcus neoformans*, *Histoplasma capsulatum*, *Pneumocystis jirovecii*, herpes simplex virus (HSV), VZV, and CMV (Table 32.2) [4,28–33,37,38,41–45]. Defective CMI may result from the underlying disease (eg, adult T-cell leukemia/lymphoma [ATLL]), but is most typically induced by various therapies, including purine analogs, alemtuzumab, corticosteroids, and other agents used to treat GVHD.

A significant impairment in B-cell function with hypogammaglobulinemia is associated with risk for infection with encapsulated bacteria [41]. Splenectomy also results in hypogammaglobulinemia, with an increased risk for such infections [46]. Additional risk factors for infection include older age, disruption of skin integrity (indwelling catheters, bone marrow biopsies), malnutrition, hyperglycemia, and iron overload (Table 32.3) [35,36,47,48].

Epidemiologic exposure to pathogens

Colonization by potential pathogens

The oral microbial flora includes viridans streptococci and anaerobic bacteria. Accordingly, patients with severe oral mucositis are at increased risk for infections with these pathogens [49,50]. Similarly, patients with severe intestinal mucositis are more likely to develop infection with common gut colonizers, such as *Escherichia coli*, *Klebsiella* spp., *Pseudomonas aeruginosa*, and *Candida* spp. [12]. By suppressing the endogenous microbial flora of the gut and skin, broad-spectrum antimicrobial agents facilitate the overgrowth of resistant bacteria and fungi [51,52], and hence the risk of infections by these organisms.

Exposure to environmental pathogens

Exposure to environmental pathogens is an important mode of acquisition of infection in patients with leukemia. Exposure can be airborne (*Aspergillus* spp. and other molds, respiratory viruses and others) [53–55], waterborne (*Legionella* spp., *Fusarium* spp., *Aspergillus* spp. and others) [56–59], or via the hands of healthcare workers (bacteria, *Candida* spp.) [60].

Pathogens of importance to patients with leukemia

Bacteria

The majority of bacterial infections in neutropenic patients with leukemia are caused by Gram-positive organisms (staphylococci [coagulase-negative and *S. aureus*], viridans *Streptococcus* and the enterococci), Gram-negative bacteria (including the Enterobacteriaceae *Escherichia coli*, *Klebsiella* spp. and *Enterobacter* spp.), and the non-fermentative bacteria (*Pseudomonas aeruginosa, Acinetobacter* spp. and *Stenotrophomonas maltophilia*) [61].

Considerable shifts in the spectrum of bacterial infections have occurred over time as a result of antimicrobial prophylaxis, therapy with more severely mucotoxic drugs [62], and the widespread use of intravascular catheters. Until the late 1980s, Gram-positive and Gram-negative organisms were equally distributed as causes of bloodstream infections. The introduction of quinolone prophylaxis was associated with a significant reduction in Gram-negative infections, but at the cost of an increase in infections caused by Gram-positive bacteria. A re-emergence of bacteremia by resistant Gram-negative organisms has been recently observed [63], including quinolone-resistant Enterobacteriaceae [64], extended-spectrum β-lactamase (ESBL)-producing bacteria (Enterobacteriaceae, *P. aeruginosa, Acinetobacter* spp., and others) [65], and multi-drug-resistant *P. aeruginosa* [66]. Infections by resistant Gram-positive organisms have also been noted with vancomycin-resistant enterococci, and nosocomial and community-acquired methicillin-resistant *S. aureus* (MRSA) [67,68]. A more serious problem in neutropenic patients with leukemia is the marked increase in *Clostridium difficile* colitis [69,70].

Great variability exists, between and within countries, in the etiology of bacterial infections and their susceptibility profiles [71], and an intimate knowledge of the local epidemiology remains critical when applying antimicrobial therapy.

Bacterial infections may also occur in patients with normal neutrophil counts, such as with hypogammaglobulinemia in untreated CLL and with chronic GVHD. Sinusitis and pneumonia are frequent particularly with *S. pneumoniae* and *H. influenzae*. Of concern is the increasing resistance of *S. pneumoniae* to penicillin and other β-lactam antibiotics, macrolides, tetracyclines, trimethoprim–sulfamethoxazole (TMP–SMX) and the quinolones [72].

Fungi

The epidemiology of invasive fungal infections (IFIs) has changed dramatically over the past 30 years. Autopsy studies of patients with leukemia indicate a steady increase in the incidence of IFIs, from 10% in the mid-1950s to 30% by the mid-1960s [73], and to 40% by the end of the 1970s [74]. In the 1980s, patients at risk for IFIs were those undergoing remission induction for AML and HSCT recipients early during pre-engraftment, and *Candida* spp. were the most frequent pathogens [75]. With the introduction of fluconazole prophylaxis, the incidence of candidiasis decreased dramatically, with a shift in species distribution: fewer infections due to *C. albicans* and *C. tropicalis*, but more infections caused by *C. glabrata* and *C. krusei* [76]. The incidence of invasive pulmonary aspergillosis (IPA) also increased, with >90% of cases accounted for by *A. fumigatus* [77], although infections by non-*fumigatus Aspergillus*—which tend to exhibit higher MICs for amphotericin B—have been increasingly reported. In a recent series of 40 cancer patients of IPA, 70% were caused by non-*fumigatus Aspergillus*, mostly *A. flavus* and *A. terreus* [78]. Molds, such as *Fusarium* spp., *Scedosporium* spp. and the Zygomycetes, have also emerged as significant pathogens in this population [79].

The population at risk for IFIs has expanded, with many infections occurring in non-neutropenic patients, especially among allogeneic HSCT recipients with severe GVHD, and heavily pretreated CLL patients receiving salvage therapies with purine analogs and/or alemtuzumab.

Without prophylaxis, *Pneumocystis jirovecii* pneumonia (PJP) is particularly frequent in children receiving chemotherapy for acute lymphocytic leukemia (ALL) [80] and among patients with severely defective CMI.

Viruses

Most viral diseases in patients with leukemia represent reactivation of latent infection, particularly with HSV, VZV and CMV [81], the respiratory viruses (Influenza A and B, parainfluenza 1–3, RSV, metapneumovirus, adenovirus), and Hepatitis A (HAV), B (HBV) and C (HCV) viruses. Epstein–Barr virus (EBV), Parvovirus B-19, and herpes simplex virus 6 (human herpesvirus 6; HHV-6) may cause disease among patients with leukemia who are severely immunosuppressed and who have undergone allogeneic HSCT [81].

In the absence of acyclovir prophylaxis, most patients with leukemia will develop symptomatic HSV mucocutaneous infection during therapy [82]. Tracheobronchitis, pneumonia, esophagitis, and hepatitis may rarely occur, and dissemination is only seen in patients with severely defective CMI [81].

Among HSCT recipients, reactivation of HHV-6 is common and has been associated with graft failure. Skin rash (at times resembling GVHD), pneumonitis, encephalitis, and hepatitis may rarely occur [83,84].

Before the introduction of ganciclovir, CMV infection was the most serious infection in patients with leukemia who were CMV seropositive and were undergoing HSCT [85]. Reactivation typically occurs after engraftment and manifests as fever, cytopenias, liver dysfunction or as CMV disease (eg, lungs, gut, eye). Preemptive treatment guided by the results of sensitive and reliable techniques for monitoring viral replication (antigen detection and/or polymerase chain reaction [PCR]) has markedly reduced the burden of CMV disease [86], although disease still occurs because of undetectable viral shedding (eg, gut infection) [86]. CMV reactivation may also occur in patients with ALL and in patients with CLL receiving alemtuzumab [2].

Without acyclovir prophylaxis, reactivation of VZV is common and can be complicated with severe post-herpetic neuralgia. Visceral dissemination (pneumonitis, meningoencephalitis, and hepatitis) may rarely occur in severely immunocompromised patients [87].

The respiratory viruses may cause disease in patients with leukemia, including HSCT recipients [81], and their timing and frequency vary according to their prevalence in the community.

Infection by HBV and HCV in leukemic patients may be chronic and persistent. Among HSCT recipients, previous infection by these viruses increases the risk for the sinusoidal obstruction syndrome, and, in the case of HCV, cirrhosis may also develop. However, the most frequent manifestation of viral reactivation is hepatitis, which can result in significant treatment delays and may be fatal [81].

Patients with leukemia undergoing haplo-identical or unrelated allogeneic HSCT are at increased risk for EBV-associated post-transplant lymphoproliferative disease, which may remain asymptomatic or manifest as extra nodal disease in the gut, liver, and central nervous system (CNS) [88,89]. Among HSCT recipients, BK virus infections may present as asymptomatic viral excretion or as severe hemorrhagic cystitis, and rarely nephritis or encephalitis [90].

Progressive multifocal leukoencephalopathy caused by JC polyoma virus may occur among severely immunosuppressed patients (eg, HSCT), but it has also been reported among patients with CLL receiving rituximab [91].

Parasites

Parasitic infections develop in the setting of severely defective CMI. Although infrequent in the setting of leukemia, toxoplasmosis may be very severe, causing encephalitis and pneumonitis [92,93]. *Strongyloides stercoralis* rarely causes a fatal disseminated syndrome with intestinal larval invasion and bacterial superinfection [94].

Mycobacteria

The incidence of tuberculosis in patients with leukemia is low, even in highly endemic regions. In a study of 917 patients with hematologic malignancies from Brazil, the prevalence of tuberculosis was 2.6% only; risk factors were an underlying disease associated with significant impairment in CMI (eg, receipt of fludarabine and corticosteroids) and malnutrition [95]. In a study from Spain, the incidence of tuberculosis was significantly higher than in the general population among allogeneic but not autologous HSCT recipients [96].

Infection caused by atypical mycobacteria may occur in the context of severe defects in CMI (*M. avium*), or as catheter-related infection in neutropenic patients (rapidly growing mycobacteria *M. fortuitum* and *M. chelonei*) [97].

Common clinical infectious syndromes

The common sites of infections in neutropenic patients with leukemia are upper and lower respiratory tract (25% each) followed by skin and soft tissue (20%), perianal region (5%), and urinary and gastrointestinal tracts (5% each).

Upper respiratory tract infections

Gingivostomatitis, acute necrotizing ulcerative gingivitis, and periodontal infections are common after chemotherapy, and may serve as the portal of entry for various pathogens that cause local, regional, and/or hematogenous infections. Thrush (oropharyngeal candidiasis) typically presents as a pseudomembrane (or rarely as hyperplastic or erythematous lesions) and angular cheilitis and is typically caused by *C. albicans*. The infection may extend to the esophagus. Fluconazole prophylaxis has markedly decreased the rate of oral thrush; however, breakthrough infections caused by *C. glabrata* and *C. krusei* may develop [76]. Occasionally other fungi, such as *Aspergillus* spp. and the Zygomycetes may cause oral, usually necrotic lesions [98–100].

Herpes simplex virus is the most common cause of stomatitis in patients with leukemia [101] and may be difficult to distinguish from chemotherapy-induced mucositis. Large, painful ulcerations may be seen in addition to the more typical vesicular lesions. HSV infections predispose tissues to bacterial and fungal superinfections [102]. Pharyngitis can be caused by the respiratory viruses and group A β-hemolytic streptococci, and it resembles treatment-induced mucositis [103]. The infection may progress to pneumonia. Failure to respond to standard treatment should raise concerns about the presence of peritonsillar, parapharyngeal or retropharyngeal abscesses.

Acute laryngitis presents with hoarseness and occasionally airway obstruction [104]. Agents include the respiratory viruses, followed by *Streptococcus* spp. and *Moraxella catarrhalis* [105,106], and rarely by *Candida* spp. and *Aspergillus* spp. [107–109]. Patients with laryngotracheitis may present with rhinorrhea, hoarseness, sore throat, cough, fever, and sometimes dyspnea with inspiratory stridor due to airway obstruction. The most common agents are HSV and *S. aureus*, and rarely *Aspergillus* spp. [110,111].

Epiglottitis is a life-threatening condition which may cause acute airway obstruction. It presents as fever, sore throat, dysphagia, and odynophagia. Respiratory distress and stridor may rapidly develop. Causative agents are *H. influenzae* type B, *S. aureus*, streptococci, *C. albicans*, *M. catarrhalis*, and the respiratory viruses [112].

Otitis externa is usually caused by *P. aeruginosa*, *S. aureus*, and rarely *Aspergillus* spp., whereas otitis media may be severe and recurrent in patients with leukemia [113,114]. Mastoiditis should be considered in patients with prolonged and refractory symptoms of otitis media, or when suppurative intracranial infections develop without apparent focus. Acute mastoiditis may be caused by group A β-hemolytic streptococci, *S. pneumoniae, S. aureus,* and *P. aeruginosa,* and less commonly *H. influenzae, M. catarrhalis,* and anaerobes. Various bacteria and fungi have been associated with chronic mastoiditis [115].

Sinusitis is common in patients with leukemia, usually following a viral upper respiratory tract infection (URI), and less commonly following dental infection. Frontal headache, dry cough, nasal discharge, and postnasal dripping are common presenting features. The angioinvasive nature of fungal sinusitis manifests as necrotic ulcers and epistaxis.

The most common agents of acute sinusitis are *S. pneumoniae, H. influenzae, M. catarrhalis,* anaerobes, and *P. aeruginosa,* whereas anaerobes, *S. aureus,* and viridans streptococci are associated with chronic bacterial sinusitis [103]. Sinusitis is a frequent manifestation of IMIs including aspergillosis, fusariosis, and zygomycosis [116–119].

Lower respiratory tract infections

Pneumonia is a serious infection in patients with leukemia. The clinical and radiologic findings do not offer a clue to the etiology, and chest radiography frequently fails to yield an early diagnosis, even in symptomatic patients. High-resolution computerized tomography (CT) is helpful in establishing the diagnosis and extent of infection, and may at times offer clues to its etiology.

In neutropenic patients, the most frequent causes of bacterial pneumonia are *K. pneumoniae, P. aeruginosa, S. aureus,* and viridans streptococci, and the concomitant occurrence of pneumonia and bacteremia is associated with poor prognosis [120,121]. A life-threatening pneumonia with respiratory failure and shock is known to occur with viridans streptococcal bacteremia following high-dose cytarabine [49]. Whether the syndrome is caused by the bacteria or the cytokine storm associated with severe mucositis remains unclear.

Community-acquired pathogens (*S. pneumoniae, H. influenzae, M. pneumoniae, Legionella* spp.) account for most bacterial pneumonias in non-neutropenic patients with leukemia. The risk of pneumonia is increased with pre-existing pulmonary disease and/or hypogammaglobulinemia [122].

Fungal pneumonia is predominantly caused by *Aspergillus* spp. and may develop among patients with profound and prolonged neutropenia (eg, remission induction for AML/MDS) and non-neutropenic patients who have severely defective CMI (eg, allogeneic HSCT patients with severe GVHD). The risk for IPA among AML patients was calculated at 1% per day early during neutropenia, but increased to 4.3% per day after 24 to 36 days [123]. In a large series of IFIs in patients with hematologic malignancies, 69% of cases of IPA developed in patients with AML, and two-thirds occurred during neutropenia that followed remission induction for newly diagnosed or relapsed patients [124].

In neutropenic patients, the classic clinical picture of IPA (and other IMIs) consists of persistent or recurrent fever, dry cough, and pleuritic chest pain [125–127]. A characteristic CT finding is the halo sign: a nodule surrounded by a ground-glass opacity [128]. The halo sign is then rapidly replaced by non-specific infiltrates [129], followed by the air-crescent sign which typically is noted after hematopoeitic recovery and IPA response [130].

Among non-neutropenic patients, IPA manifestations are subtle and non-specific. In a series of 22 cases of IMIs (18 IPA), shortness of breath was the most frequent finding (64%), whereas fever, cough and chest pain were only observed in 32%, 23%, and 14% of cases, respectively [131]. The halo sign is rarely seen in these patients, who typically have air space consolidations or nodules. Bacterial pneumonia may coexist with IPA [132].

The respiratory viruses may cause pneumonia in patients with leukemia, and they occur predominantly during the winter season. In HSCT recipients, URI precedes RSV pneumonia in >80% of cases [133].

Pneumonia due to *P. jirovecii* may develop in patients who are not compliant with TMP–SMX prophylaxis and in recipients of less-effective regimens [134]. The typical clinical picture is that of a rapidly evolving (over 1 week) bilateral pneumonia with fever, cough, and dyspnea. Chest CT reveals bilateral interstitial infiltrates or ground-glass attenuation [43]. Patients at risk include those with severely depressed CMI, such as in ALL, multiply relapsed AML/MDS, CLL therapy with high doses of corticosteroids, purine analogs and/or alemtuzumab, and patients with HCL or ATL (Table 32.2) [43].

Among HSCT recipients, CMV pneumonia presents with shortness of breath and hypoxemia. Bilateral ground-glass attenuation, patchy alveolar infiltrates, or small nodules may be seen on chest CT scan [135].

A broad list of additional pathogens may cause pneumonia in patients with leukemia, including *Toxoplasma gondii, Strongyloides stercoralis, Mycobacterium tuberculosis, Nocardia* spp., and others.

Skin and soft tissue infections

Skin infection in patients with leukemia may be primary or secondary. Gram-positive cocci (group A streptococci and *S. aureus*) account for most primary skin infections. These infections may rarely be caused by Gram-positive bacilli, the Enterobacteriaceae, or *P. aeruginosa.* Secondary (metastatic) skin infections are more common during neutropenia and may be caused by a large number of pathogens, including *P. aeruginosa*, HSV and VZV, and several fungi (*Candida* spp., *Aspergillus* spp., *Fusarium* spp. and others). The clinical characteristics of cutaneous lesions (appearance, location/distribution, and timing) may help in establishing the etiology. A dermatomal distribution of papular/vesicular lesions in patients with severe CMI dysfunction is diagnostic of VZV.

Several lesions may be seen during neutropenia. For example, perirectal cellulitis suggests infections by Gram-negative bacteria and anaerobes [136], whereas extremity cellulitis (toe/finger) usually implies fusariosis [137]. Ecthyma gangrenosum-like lesions can be caused by *P. aeruginosa* (early during neutropenia) or by molds (especially *Fusarium* spp., during later phases) [138,139]. Papular or nodular skin lesions are seen in approximately 8% of patients with candidemia, particularly with *C. tropicalis* [140]. A remarkable feature of invasive–disseminated fusariosis is the high frequency of skin lesions (>75% of patients) [116], usually multiple erythematous papular or nodular and painful, and frequently with central necrosis (ecthyma gangrenosum-like). Target lesions (a thin rim of erythema surrounding the papular or nodular components) may occur in 10% of patients. Lesions at different stages of evolution (papules, nodules, and necrotic lesions) may be present in one-third of patients [139].

Hematogenous infections

Approximately 20–25% of febrile neutropenic patients with leukemia develop bacteremia [61], the etiology of which varies according to local epidemiology, prophylactic practices, and the underlying disease and its therapy. When complicated by organ involvement (especially pneumonia), bacteremia carries a poor prognosis. With the exception of a few organisms, such as coagulase-negative staphylococci, almost any pathogen may cause overwhelming sepsis. Blood cultures should always be obtained in patients with fever and neutropenia, and the recovery of any known pathogen should be considered significant until proven otherwise.

Candida spp. and *Fusarium* spp. are the most frequent fungi recovered from the bloodstream of neutropenic patients. Fluconazole prophylaxis has reduced the frequency of candidemia with a shift in species distribution (see section on Fungi) [76]. Hematogenous candidiasis during neutropenia is usually acute, evolving over days with skin lesions and systemic inflammatory response syndrome, but may evolve in chronic disseminated candidiasis (previously known as hepatosplenic candidiasis), which extends over several weeks and is characterized by refractory fever, abdominal complaints and elevated serum alkaline phosphatase levels. Deep-seated abscesses of the liver, spleen, kidneys, and lungs can be seen on ultrasound, CT scan, or magnetic resonance imaging (MRI) [141].

Infections of the gastrointestinal tract

The gastrointestinal tract is frequently a source of infection in neutropenic patients with leukemia.

Esophagitis may be treatment-related or infectious, caused by fungi such as *Candida* spp., viruses, particularly HSV and CMV, and Gram-negative bacteria. In the absence of fluconazole and acyclovir prophylaxis, patients with esophagitis should be empirically treated with intravenous fluconazole and acyclovir.

Abdominal pain is frequent in neutropenic patients with leukemia and may be due to chemotherapy-induced gastrointestinal mucositis (also known as neutropenic enterocolitis [NEC] and typhlitis) and *C. difficile*-associated diarrhea (CDAD)/colitis, both of which manifest with fever, abdominal pain with or without rebound tenderness, abdominal distension, and diarrhea. Thickening of the bowel wall by abdominal ultrasound, CT, or MRI confirms the diagnosis [142–144]. The pathogenesis of NEC involves chemotherapy-induced mucositis with microbial invasion by Enterobacteriaceae, *P. aeruginosa*, enterococci, C. *septicum*, and *Candida* spp. [145]. The incidence of CDAD is increasing among patients with leukemia. In a study of 134 patients with AML receiving 301 chemotherapy courses, CDAD was documented in 18% of patients [70], and leukemia was an independent risk factor for CDAD in a retrospective study of 36,086 hospitalized patients in the USA [69].

Perirectal cellulitis typically develops in the setting of prolonged and profound neutropenia, and is associated with aerobic and anaerobic Gram-negative bacilli and enterococci [146]. Perirectal mucositis, hemorrhoids and anal fissures, and rectal manipulation are known predisposing factors. Disseminated strongyloidiasis presents with diarrhea, abdominal pain, fever, cough, and rapidly evolving septic shock, but is very rare even in endemic regions [147]. Pancreatitis may be drug induced (eg, L-asparaginase) [148], or rarely caused by atypical VZV infection [149]. Right upper quadrant pain may result from an acute distension of the liver capsule in patients with sinusoidal obstruction syndrome who have undergone HSCT.

Hepatic infections may be caused by various pathogens (hepatitis viruses, HSV, CMV, EBV, Coxsackie-B, adenovirus, and fungi). Hepatic involvement with *Candida* spp. is seen in chronic disseminated candidiasis. Infection with other fungi and with *Bartonella henselae* may have a similar presentation [150].

Infections of the central nervous system

Infections of the CNS in patients with leukemia include meningitis, encephalitis, and meningoencephalitis; these may develop in various settings, such as with severe defects in CMI, severe and prolonged neutropenia, or the presence of prosthetic devices such as Ommaya reservoirs.

Meningitis or meningoencephalitis in patients with defective CMI are usually caused by *C. neoformans* [151–153], *L. monocytogenes*, *T. gondii* [154] and HSV, and rarely VZV, HHV-6 and JC virus [2,91,93,146,151,154]. The clinical presentation varies according to type (meningitis, encephalitis or meningoencephalitis), location, and disease tempo (acute, subacute or chronic). The diagnosis relies on a careful history and physical examination, a comprehensive analysis of the cerebrospinal fluid (CSF) by direct exam, culture, antigen detection and PCR, imaging (CT scan and MRI), and sometimes brain biopsy.

Cryptococcosis manifests as subacute or chronic meningoencephalitis, with headache, memory loss, personality changes, and fever. The diagnosis is established by direct exam (India ink) and culture of the CSF, and by antigen detection in the CSF and/or serum [155]. Listeriosis presents as acute or subacute meningitis, at times with focal neurologic signs [5]. The diagnosis is confirmed by culture of CSF and/or blood [156].

Involvement of the CNS by *Aspergillus* spp. and other molds may occur as a result of hematogenous dissemination or direct extension from sinusitis [157,158]. New-onset seizures and focal neurologic signs may be the presenting features.

Other sites

The genitourinary tract is rarely the source of infection in patients with leukemia, with Gram-negative bacilli and enterococci accounting for most infections. Diagnosis relies on recovering the organism. Urinary leukocytes may be absent in neutropenic patients. Candiduria is frequent in hospitalized patients, but usually represents colonization only [159]. Among HSCT recipients, BK virus hemorrhagic cystitis is relatively frequent [90,160–162].

Infectious endocarditis is rare in patients with leukemia (<1%) but is associated with a high mortality rate [163].

Infections in special hosts

Infection in patients with acute myelogenous leukemia

Neutropenia, chemotherapy-induced gastrointestinal mucositis, and failure to achieve hematologic remission are the dominant risk factors for infection in patients with AML/MDS (Tables 32.3 and 32.4). Therefore, infections occur almost exclusively after induction or consolidation therapy.

Infections that are more likely to occur in patients with AML/MDS are bacteremia due to viridans *Streptococcus* spp. (high-dose cytarabine) [164], NEC/typhlitis (severely mucotoxic regimens) [145], and invasive mold infections (prolonged and severe neutropenia) [165]. Fever may also be a manifestation of AML/MDS; this diagnosis, however, can be entertained only after excluding an infectious etiology [166].

Infection in patients with acute lymphocytic leukemia

The period at risk for infection in patients with ALL is much longer than with AML/MDS. In the early postinduction phase, neutropenia, mucositis, and failure to achieve remission are the main risk factors for infection (Tables 32.3 and 32.4). With achievement of remission and

Table 32.4 Risk for infections in neutropenic patients with leukemia.

Factor	Low risk	High risk
Age	Younger (<40 years)	Older (>70 years)
Performance status	Good	Poor
Comorbidities[a]	Absent	Present
Disease status	Complete remission	Active or relapsed
Relapse vs. first induction	First induction	Relapse
Probability of achieving complete remission[b]	High	Low
History of latent infections (eg, CMV, aspergillosis)	No	Yes
Colonization with resistant bacteria	No	Yes
Chemotherapy dose density/dose intensity[c]	Low	High
Pharmacogenomics—metabolism of antineoplastic drugs	Poor metabolizer	Fast metabolizer
Pharmacogenetics—polymorphisms in innate immunity[d]	Favorable	Unfavorable

[a]Important comorbidities: renal failure, hepatic failure, chronic lung disease, malnutrition, iron overload.

[b]Factors impacting the probability of achieving complete remission include: acute lymphocytic leukemia—age, initial white blood cell count, cytogenetics, immunophenotype, rapidity of cytoreduction. Acute myeloid leukemia—advanced age, de novo vs. secondary leukemia, before previous myelodysplasia, cytogenetics, gene mutation profile.

[c]Dose intensity and dose density (with rapidly cycling courses) relate to the likelihood of inducing severe mucositis and prolonged neutropenia.

[d]Polymorphisms in genes linked to Toll-like receptor 1 and 4, Interleukin 10 and 15, transforming growth factor TGF-β, tumor necrosis factor α, mannose-binding lectin, and lung surfactant proteins SPA-2 increase the risk of aspergillosis and candidiasis.

initiation of maintenance therapy, T-cell immunodeficiency becomes the main risk factor for infection and persists throughout the duration of treatment and for long periods after the end of treatment; hence PJP prophylaxis and monitoring for infections associated with defective CMI are critical.

Patients with ATL have severe T-cell immunodeficiency early in the course of disease and are at greater risk for CMI-associated infections, including disseminated strongyloidiasis, toxoplasmosis, CMV, PJP, listeriosis, leprosy, and tuberculosis (Tables 32.1 and 32.2) [167–171].

Infection in patients with chronic myeloid leukemia

The introduction of tyrosine-kinase inhibitors (TKIs) in the treatment of chronic myeloid leukemia (CML) brought a new era for this disease. Accordingly, infectious complications in patients with CML are now uncommon, although reports of tuberculosis, VZV, hepatitis B, and parvovirus B-19 infections in patients receiving TKIs suggest that these agents impair host defenses [172–176]. *In vitro* and *in vivo* studies indicate that TKIs reduce the capacity to induce a cytotoxic T-cell response, cause lymphopenia and hypogammaglobulinemia, and impair CD8 T-cell responses [177–179].

Infection in patients with chronic lymphocytic leukemia

More than 50% of patients with CLL suffer recurrent infections, and infection accounts for up to 60–80% of deaths resulting from CLL [41]. This increased risk is the result of the interplay between the immune defects inherent to CLL, and the therapies given to control the disease. The risk increases with advanced disease and multiple treatment courses, and the disease appears to be, in some reports, directly related to the severity of hypogammaglobulinemia (Table 32.5) [1,180]. Hypogammaglobulinemia occurs in virtually all patients with CLL, and various treatment regimens further impair host defenses, particularly purine analogs and alemtuzumab. Such patients are at greater risk for infections caused by pathogens associated with defective CMI, including HSV, VZV, CMV, *Listeria, Nocardia, Cryptococcus, M. tuberculosis, Candida* spp., *Aspergillus* and others [1–3,5,6,41,95,151,154,180].

The timing of infections in patients receiving purine analogs varies according to the extent of previous therapy. Most infections occur early, usually during the first 6 weeks of treatment, and many are caused by neutropenia-related opportunistic pathogens, including bacteria, HSV and *Candida* spp. Late infections (particularly after repeated therapies with purine analogs) include opportunistic pathogens associated with depressed CMI (Table 32.2) [41]. The risk and severity of infection in recipients of purine analogs vary according to whether these agents are used as frontline therapy (rate of infection ~35%), or in previously treated patients (~50%), whether they are used alone (~30%) or in combination with other agents (~40%), and, most importantly, whether optimal antimicrobial prophylaxis is provided (~10–15% rate of infection) [1,41].

In patients receiving alemtuzumab as primary treatment, the risk of infection is low with appropriate prophylaxis. However, the risk increases significantly in heavily pretreated patients. Pathogens include bacteria (*L. monocytogenes*, others), viruses (particularly HSV/VZV and CMV), fungi (*Aspergillus* spp., *C. neoformans*, and *P. jirovecii*), and, less commonly, protozoa (*T. gondii, C. parvum, Acanthamoeba*) and mycobacteria (Table 32.2) [1].

Table 32.5 Risk assessment of infection in patients with chronic lymphocytic leukemia.

Factor	Low risk	High risk
Age	Younger (<40 years)	Older (>70 years)
Performance status	Good	Poor
Comorbidities[a]	Absent	Present
Disease stage	Rai I–II	Advanced stage (III–IV)
Disease status	Controlled	Refractory[b]
Disease prognostic features (poor-prognosis chronic lymphocytic leukemia[c])	No	Yes
Previous chemotherapy	No	Extensive
Recent receipt of purine analogs, alemtuzumab, and/or high dose corticosteroids	No	Yes
Hypogammaglobulinemia	Absent	Present
Neutropenia (<500/mm^3)	Absent	Present
CD4 cytopenia: absolute CD4 count <50/mm^3	Absent	Present
History of latent infections (eg, aspergillosis, tuberculosis, cytomegalovirus)	No	Yes
Colonization with resistant bacteria	No	Yes
Appropriate antimicrobial prophylaxis	No	Yes

[a]Important comorbidities: renal failure, low serum albumin.

[b]Refractoriness to purine analogs carries a high risk for infection.

[c]Poor prognosis defined by mutational status of immunoglobulin VH gene and chromosomal abnormalities.

Management of infection

Neutropenic patients

Risk assessment

The risk assessment group comprises mostly patients with acute leukemia and MDS undergoing remission induction, intensive consolidation, or salvage treatment. Risk assessment includes a detailed medical history with an emphasis on potentially latent infections (VZV, aspergillosis, tuberculosis), assessment of marrow reserve (especially in elderly patients), and comorbidities (renal and liver function, iron overload), and the characteristics of the underlying disease and planned therapy (Tables 32.3 and 32.4).

Prophylactic measures

Prophylactic measures in neutropenic patients with leukemia include antibacterial, antifungal, and antiviral prophylaxis (Table 32.6), the use of growth factors to accelerate neutrophil recovery, and general measures to prevent exposure to potential pathogens.

Table 32.6 Dosage schedule of antimicrobial agents used in the prophylaxis and treatment of infection in patients with leukemia.

Disease	Prophylaxis	Treatment
Bacterial infections		
Neutropenic	Quinolone (QL)[a,b]	Antipseudomonal β-lactam antibiotic[a,c]
Non-neutropenic	TMP–SMX—800 mg/160 mg p.o. daily or daily QL[d]	Broad spectrum antibiotic (QL[b], β-lactam, other).[d] If QL not used in prophylaxis, add a QL or macrolide[e] for pneumonia[c,d]
Clostridium Difficile diarrhea	Consider metronidazole prophylaxis (500 mg p.o. t.i.d.) if history of CDAD[f]	Metronidazole 500 mg p.o. t.i.d. or vancomycin 125 mg p.o. q.i.d.[a]—treat for 2–4 weeks
Tuberculosis	Isoniazid 300 mg p.o. daily[f]	Various regimens
Fungal infections		
Invasive candidiasis	Fluconazole 200–400 mg p.o. daily[a]	Echinocandin (caspofungin 70 mg i.v. loading dose and 50 mg per day; micafungin 100 mg i.v. per day; anidulafungin 200 mg i.v. loading dose and 100 mg i.v. per day)[a]
Invasive aspergillosis	Posaconazole 200 mg t.i.d.[a]	Voriconazole (6 mg/kg i.v. b.i.d. loading dose and 4 mg/kg i.v. per day or 300 mg p.o. b.i.d.)[a]
Oral and/or esophageal candidiasis	Clotrimazole troches (10 mg, five times daily) or fluconazole 100–200 mg p.o. daily[a]	Fluconazole 200–400 mg p.o. daily for 7–10 days[a]
Pneumocystis jirovecii pneumonia	TMP–SMX 800 mg/160 mg p.o. daily or twice weekly,[a] pentamidine 300 mg aerosol monthly,[a] dapsone 100 mg p.o. daily,[d] atovaquone 1500 mg p.o. daily[d]	TMP–SMX 15–20 mg/kg of trimethoprim i.v. daily[d] or pentamidine 4 mg/kg i.v. daily[d]–treat for 3 weeks and give secondary prophylaxis
Viral infections		
Herpes simplex	Acyclovir 200—400 mg p.o. b.i.d. or t.i.d.,[a] valacyclovir 500 mg p.o. t.i.d.[a] or famciclovir 500 mg p.o. t.i.d.[a]	7–14 days of acyclovir 250 mg/m^2 i.v. t.i.d.,[a] valacyclovir 1 g p.o. t.i.d.,[a] or famciclovir 500 mg p.o. b.i.d.[a]
Herpes zoster	Acyclovir 400 mg p.o. b.i.d. or t.i.d.,[a] valacyclovir 500 mg p.o. t.i.d.,[a] or famciclovir 500 mg p.o. t.i.d.[a]	7–14 days of acyclovir 500 mg/m^2 i.v. t.i.d.,[a] valacyclovir 1 g p.o. t.i.d.,[a] or famciclovir 500 mg p.o. b.i.d.[a]
Cytomegalovirus	Ganciclovir 5 mg/kg i.v. b.i.d.,[a] valganciclovir 900 mg/d p.o.,[a] or foscarnet 60 mg/kg i.v. b.i.d.[a]	14–21 days of ganciclovir 5 mg/kg i.v. b.i.d., valganciclovir p.o. 900 mg b.i.d., or foscarnet 90 mg/kg i.v. b.i.d.
Influenza virus	Oseltamivir—75 mg p.o. daily for the duration of the Influenza season; zanamivir is more appropriate in the presence of viral resistance.	Oseltamivir 75 mg p.o. b.i.d. for 5–7 days; use zanamivir when viral resistance is documented.

[a]Recommendation based on randomized clinical trials.
[b]Includes ciprofloxacin—500 mg p.o. b.i.d., levofloxacin—500 mg p.o. daily, moxifloxacin—400 mg p.o. daily, others.
[c]Antipseudomonal β-lactam antibiotics: ceftazidime, cefepime, piperacillin–tazobactam, imipenem or meropenem.
[d]Recommendation based on cohort studies or case series.
[e]Erythromycin 500 mg p.o. b.i.d., azythromycin 500 mg/day p.o. or i.v., or clarithromycin 500 mg b.i.d. p.o. or i.v.
[f]Recommendation based on expert advice.
Unless otherwise stated, the duration of treatment depends on clinical response and persistence or resolution of immunosuppression; Antibiotic choices should be dictated by local epidemiologic factors.
b.i.d., twice daily; CDAD, *Clostridium difficile*-associated diarrhea; p.o., *per os*; q.i.d., four times daily; t.i.d., three times daily; TMP–SMX, trimethoprim–sulfamethoxazole.

Antibacterial prophylaxis

Prophylaxis with quinolones has been associated with a reduction in the frequency of fever and infections, including Gram-negative bacteremia, and in infection-related mortality [181]. A major concern, however, is the potential to induce resistance. A meta-analysis suggested that patients receiving quinolone prophylaxis had a nonsignificant increase in colonization by quinolone-resistant bacteria [182]. However, the decision to use quinolone prophylaxis should be based on local epidemiology. When used, the quinolones are usually started with chemotherapy and continued until marrow recovery or onset of febrile neutropenia.

Antifungal prophylaxis

Prophylaxis for invasive candidiasis is effective in AML/MDS patients undergoing induction or postinduction chemotherapy, and in allogeneic HSCT recipients [183]. The drug of choice is fluconazole [184]. Fluconazole prophylaxis should also be given to patients with ALL undergoing therapy with regimens known to cause severe mucositis and prolonged neutropenia.

Antimold prophylaxis with posaconazole was as effective as fluconazole in preventing candidiasis in patients with AML/MDS receiving induction therapy [185]. A reduction in IPA and in fungal-related mortality was also noted. However, most cases of IPA in the fluconazole arm were diagnosed on the basis of positive serum *Aspergillus* galactomannan. Hence, the lower rate of IPA in posaconazole-treated patients could be due to the known decreased sensitivity of subacute with mold-active azoles. Posaconazole prophylaxis in this setting should be balanced against our significantly improved ability for the early detection of IFIs using serial chest CT scans and serum biomarkers such as subacute and 1,3-beta-D-glucan (BDG) [186], and the undesirable consequences of prophylaxis (toxicities, drug–drug interactions, costs, and emergence of resistance).

Antiviral prophylaxis

Prevention of HSV reactivation is indicated in all patients with leukemia receiving chemotherapy. Acyclovir is the most frequently used drug, but valacyclovir and famciclovir are equally effective [187]. Preventing influenza virus infections is important and is best accomplished by vaccinating healthcare workers, caregivers, and household members, and by providing patients with neuraminidase inhibitor prophylaxis such as oseltamivir during the influenza season [188].

Growth factors

Three meta-analyses examined the role of prophylactic colony-stimulating factors (CSFs) in patients with acute leukemia; in children with ALL, the use of CSFs significantly reduced the number of febrile episodes, infectious episodes, and length of hospitalization but without an impact on duration of neutropenia, delays in chemotherapy, or survival [189]. In children and adults with ALL and in adults with AML/MDS, prophylactic CSFs decreased the duration of neutropenia but without consistent effect on infectious complications or duration of hospitalization [190], whereas no effect on survival rates was observed among patients with AML [191].

Management of febrile neutropenic patients

Work-up for infection

Work-up for infection includes medical history and physical examination, with emphasis on common sites of infection in neutropenic patients (ie, the respiratory and gastrointestinal tract and skin). Risk factors for severe complications (and hence need for hospitalization) in febrile neutropenic patients are shown in Table 32.7. Blood tests include complete blood counts, immature reticulocyte fraction [192], C-reactive protein [193], serum albumin, liver and renal function tests, and cultures of blood and other clinically relevant sites. Chest and sinus CT scans should be obtained when respiratory symptoms are present. Empiric antibiotics should be immediately started and may include ceftazidime, cefepime, piperacillin–tazobactam, imipenem, or meropenem. Knowledge of the local epidemiology, including most common pathogens and susceptibility patterns, should guide the selection of antimicrobial therapy.

Table 32.7 Risk factors for complications in patients with acute leukemia and febrile neutropenia.

Hemodynamic instability
Hypotension (systolic blood pressure <90 mmHg of >10% below baseline)
Increase in pulse rate (>110/min or >10% from baseline)
Orthostatic hypotension (>10%)
Severe infections present
Pneumonia
Bacteremia
Typhlitis/enterocolitis/perirectal abscess
Severe infection likely
Highly elevated or rapidly increasing levels of serum C-reactive protein
Uncontrolled leukemia
Older age (>65 years)
Severe (<100/mm^3) and prolonged (>10 days) neutropenia expected
Severe alimentary tract mucositis (oral, esophageal, lower gastrointestinal)
Organ/metabolic dysfunction
Significant organ dysfunction (respiratory, renal, hepatic, cardiac [and/or arrhythmias])
Altered mental status and/or witnessed syncopal episode/seizure
Profound weakness

Modifications of the antibiotic regimen

Fever usually resolves in 4–5 days among patients with undocumented infection, and 5 days or longer when clinically or microbiologically documented infection is present. Therefore, empiric therapy should only be changed if there is evidence of clinical deterioration or of a newly documented infection that is not optimally treated with the empiric regimen. Modifications may include the addition of antianaerobic agents in patients with NEC/typhlitis, a glycopeptide in patients with documented Gram-positive bacterial infection, and oral vancomycin or metronidazole for those with CDAD. Empiric antifungal therapy for persistent fever has been replaced by a preemptive strategy based on serial monitoring with subacute and/or BDG. These circulating antigens are released by *Aspergillus* (and, in the case of BDG, other fungi as well) during infection, and abnormal levels may be detected before the clinical manifestations. Both tests perform well in neutropenic patients, with a negative predictive value of >95%, suggesting that they are particularly useful at ruling out the diagnosis of IFI [194,195].

Non-neutropenic patients

Risk assessment

Risk assessment of non-neutropenic patients should take into account the most important risk factors for infection in these patients. A common scenario for infection among patients with non-neutropenic leukemia is that seen with CLL which will be used as an example (Table 32.5).

Prophylactic measures

Prophylaxis against encapsulated bacteria should be given to all patients with CLL with either a respiratory quinolone (levofloxacin or moxifloxacin) or TMP–SMX (Table 32.6). These patients should also receive acyclovir prophylaxis for HSV and VZV.

Reactivation of CMV infection occurs in 15–30% of CLL patients receiving alemtuzumab-containing regimens and peaks at the time of the T-cell count nadir (between weeks 3 and 6). Preemptive therapy based on weekly testing for CMV viremia (preferably by PCR) prevents progression to potentially fatal CMV disease [196]. Measures to prevent influenza virus infections are similar to those recommended for patients with neutropenia [188].

In patients with CLL treated with chlorambucil, prophylactic intravenous immunoglobulin (400 mg/kg every 3 weeks) decreases the risk of mild and moderate bacterial infections [197]. Lower doses appear equally effective [198]. Considering the high cost of intravenous immunoglobulin and the availability of less-expensive and more effective antibiotics, intravenous immunoglobulin should only be given to patients with immunoglobulin G levels ≤500 mg/dL and with recurrent infections despite appropriate antibiotic prophylaxis [1]. The appropriate duration of antimicrobial prophylaxis in patients with CLL receiving purine analog and/or alemtuzumab is unclear. However, because patients who achieve a major response have a lower risk for infection, prophylaxis could be discontinued 2–3 months after the completion of therapy in such patients, particularly if they do not display other high-risk features for infection (Table 32.5).

Vaccination of patients with CLL may decrease infections due to *H. influenzae* type B, *S. pneumoniae*, and influenza virus. However, response to vaccination is highly variable in patients with CLL and is always lower than in control subjects [199].

Management of febrile patients

Fever in patients with CLL should be considered of infectious origin until proven otherwise. Sinopulmonary infections caused by encapsulated bacteria predominate in patients who are untreated and in those receiving chlorambucil [1]. Because *S. pneumoniae* infection may be rapidly fatal, prompt empiric antibiotic therapy for febrile patients is recommended. In the absence of neutropenia, cefuroxime, penicillins with β-lactamase inhibitors, or macrolides may be given. Neutropenic patients should receive a respiratory quinolone or a broad-spectrum β-lactam antibiotic such as cefepime, a carbapenem, or piperacillin-tazobactam (Table 32.6).

The investigation of fever in patients treated with fludarabine or alemtuzumab should include a search for CMI-associated infections (HSV, VZV, CMV, listeriosis, cryptococcosis, tuberculosis, and others) (Table 32.2). Likewise, empiric antimicrobial therapy should cover the most likely pathogens. For example, mucocutaneous lesions suggest HSV or VZV infection, whereas neurologic findings should prompt investigation for listeriosis, cryptococcosis, and toxoplasmosis. Evaluation of CMV infection is always recommended in alemtuzumab-treated patients [1].

Acknowledgments

The authors woudl like to acknowledge financial support from the Conselho Nacional de Desenvolvimento Científico e Tecnológico (CNPq), Brazil, grant 200425/2009–9 (Marcio Nucci).

References

1 Anaissie E. *Infectious complications in patients with chronic lymphocytic Leukemia*. In: O'Brien S, Gribben JG (eds). Chronic lymphocytic leukemia Informa Healthcare, New York, 2008: 261–292.

2 Elter T, Vehreschild JJ, Gribben J, Cornely OA, Engert A, Hallek M. Management of infections in patients with chronic

lymphocytic leukemia treated with alemtuzumab. *Ann Hematol* 2009;88:121–132.
3 Gill S, Carney D, Ritchie D, *et al.* The frequency, manifestations, and duration of prolonged cytopenias after first-line fludarabine combination chemotherapy. *Ann Oncol* 2010;21: 331–4.
4 Park SH, Choi SM, Lee DG, *et al.* Infectious complications associated with alemtuzumab use for allogeneic hematopoietic stem cell transplantation: comparison with antithymocyte globulin. *Transpl Infect Dis* 2009;11, 413–23.
5 Anaissie E, Kontoyiannis DP, Kantarjian H, Elting L, Robertson LE, Keating M. Listeriosis in patients with chronic lymphocytic leukemia who were treated with fludarabine and prednisone. *Ann Intern Med* 1992;117:466–9.
6 Anaissie EJ, Kontoyiannis DP, O'Brien S, *et al.* Infections in patients with chronic lymphocytic leukemia treated with fludarabine. *Ann Intern Med* 1998;129:559–66.
7 Sung L, Gamis A, Alonzo TA, *et al.* Infections and association with different intensity of chemotherapy in children with acute myeloid leukemia. *Cancer* 2009;115:1100–8.
8 Alousi AM, Weisdorf DJ, Logan BR, *et al.* Etanercept, mycophenolate, denileukin, or pentostatin plus corticosteroids for acute graft-versus-host disease: a randomized phase 2 trial from the Blood and Marrow Transplant Clinical Trials Network. *Blood* 2009;114, 511–17.
9 Martinez C, Solano C, Ferra C, Sampol A, Valcarcel D, Perez-Simon JA. Alemtuzumab as treatment of steroid-refractory acute graft-versus-host disease: results of a phase II study. *Biol Blood Marrow Transplant* 2009;15:639–42.
10 Thin L, Macquillan G, Adams L, *et al.* Acute graft-versus-host disease after liver transplant: novel use of etanercept and the role of tumor necrosis factor alpha inhibitors. *Liver Transpl* 2009;15:421–6.
11 Grazziutti ML, Dong L, Miceli MH, *et al.* Oral mucositis in myeloma patients undergoing melphalan-based autologous stem cell transplantation: incidence, risk factors, and a severity predictive model. *Bone Marrow Transplant* 2006;38: 501–6.
12 Nucci M, Anaissie E. Revisiting the source of candidemia: skin or gut? *Clin Infect Dis* 2001;33:1959–67.
13 Cesana C, Nosari AM, Klersy C, *et al.* Risk factors for the development of bacterial infections in multiple myeloma treated with two different vincristine–adriamycin–dexamethasone schedules. *Haematologica* 2003;88:1022–8.
14 Kuderer NM, Dale DC, Crawford J, Cosler LE, Lyman GH. Mortality, morbidity, and cost associated with febrile neutropenia in adult cancer patients. *Cancer* 2006;106:2258–66.
15 Marcolini JA, Malik S, Suki D, Whimbey E, Bodey GP. Respiratory disease due to parainfluenza virus in adult leukemia patients. *Eur J Clin Microbiol Infect Dis* 2003;22:79–84.
16 Yates CR, Krynetski EY, Loennechen T, *et al.* Molecular diagnosis of thiopurine S-methyltransferase deficiency: genetic basis for azathioprine and mercaptopurine intolerance. *Ann Intern Med* 1997;126:608–14.
17 Relling MV, Hancock ML, Rivera GK, *et al.* Mercaptopurine therapy intolerance and heterozygosity at the thiopurine S-methyltransferase gene locus. *J Natl Cancer Inst* 1999;91: 2001–8.
18 Kesh S, Mensah NY, Peterlongo P, *et al.* TLR1 and TLR6 polymorphisms are associated with susceptibility to invasive aspergillosis after allogeneic stem cell transplantation. *Ann N Y Acad Sci* 2005;1062:95–103.
19 Sainz J, Hassan L, Perez E, *et al.* Interleukin-10 promoter polymorphism as risk factor to develop invasive pulmonary aspergillosis. *Immunol Lett* 2007;109:76–82.
20 Sainz J, Perez E, Hassan L, *et al.* Variable number of tandem repeats of TNF receptor type 2 promoter as genetic biomarker of susceptibility to develop invasive pulmonary aspergillosis. *Hum Immunol* 2007;68:41–50.
21 Granell M, Urbano-Ispizua A, Suarez B, *et al.* Mannan-binding lectin pathway deficiencies and invasive fungal infections following allogeneic stem cell transplantation. *Exp Hematol* 2006; 34:1435–41.
22 van der Graaf CA, Netea MG, Morre SA, *et al.* Toll-like receptor 4 Asp299Gly/Thr399Ile polymorphisms are a risk factor for *Candida* bloodstream infection. *Eur Cytokine Netw* 2006;17:29–34.
23 Carvalho A, Pasqualotto AC, Pitzurra L, Romani L, Denning DW, Rodrigues F. Polymorphisms in toll-like receptor genes and susceptibility to pulmonary aspergillosis. *J Infect Dis* 2008; 197:618–21.
24 Lambourne J, Agranoff D, Herbrecht R, *et al.* Association of mannose-binding lectin deficiency with acute invasive aspergillosis in immunocompromised patients. *Clin Infect Dis* 2009;49:1486–91.
25 Vekemans M, Robinson J, Georgala A, *et al.* Low mannose-binding lectin concentration is associated with severe infection in patients with hematological cancer who are undergoing chemotherapy. *Clin Infect Dis* 2007;44:1593–1601.
26 Schlapbach LJ, Aebi C, Otth M, *et al.* Serum levels of mannose-binding lectin and the risk of fever in neutropenia pediatric cancer patients. *Pediatr Blood Cancer* 2007;49:11–16.
27 Bodey GP, Buckley M, Sathe YS, Freireich EJ. Quantitative relationships between circulating leukocytes and infection in patients with acute leukemia. *Ann Intern Med* 1966;64: 328–40.
28 Fumarulo R, Riccardi S, Pantaleo R, Coluccia M, Giordano D, Aresta M. *In vitro* cisplatin effects on phagocyte functions. *Int J Cancer* 1985;35:777–80.
29 Pickering LK, Cleary TG, Kletzel M, Wang YM, Parra MM. Modulation of polymorphonuclear leukocyte function by doxorubicin (Adriamycin) and alpha tocopherol (vitamin E). *J Clin Lab Immunol* 1983;11:95–100.
30 Pickering LK, Ericsson CD, Kohl S. Effect of chemotherapeutic agents on metabolic and bactericidal activity of polymorphonuclear leukocytes. *Cancer* 1978;42:1741–6.
31 Pickering LK, Anderson DC, Choi S, Feigin RD. Leukocyte function in children with malignancies. *Cancer* 1975;35: 1365–71.
32 Martin S, Baldock SC, Ghoneim AT, Child JA. Defective neutrophil function and microbicidal mechanisms in the myelodysplastic disorders. *J Clin Pathol* 1983;36:1120–8.
33 Child JA, Cawley JC, Martin S, Ghoneim AT. Microbicidal function of the neutrophils in hairy-cell leukemia. *Acta Haematol* 1979;62:191–8.
34 Stergiopoulou T, Meletiadis J, Roilides E, *et al.* Host-dependent patterns of tissue injury in invasive pulmonary aspergillosis. *Am J Clin Pathol* 2007;127:349–55.
35 Damaj G, Kuhnowski F, Marolleau JP, Bauters F, Leleu X, Yakoub-Agha I. Risk factors for severe infection in patients

with hairy cell leukemia: a long-term study of 73 patients. *Eur J Haematol* 2009;83:246–50.
36 Garcia-Vidal C, Upton A, Kirby KA, Marr KA. Epidemiology of invasive mold infections in allogeneic stem cell transplant recipients: biological risk factors for infection according to time after transplantation. *Clin Infect Dis* 2008;47: 1041–50.
37 Torres HA, Aguilera E, Safdar A, *et al*. Fatal cytomegalovirus pneumonia in patients with haematological malignancies: an autopsy-based case–control study. *Clin Microbiol Infect* 12008; 4:1160–6.
38 El Saleeby CM, Somes GW, Devincenzo JP, Gaur AH. Risk factors for severe respiratory syncytial virus disease in children with cancer: the importance of lymphopenia and young age. *Pediatrics* 2008;121:235–43.
39 Chemaly RF, Ghosh S, Bodey GP, *et al*. Respiratory viral infections in adults with hematologic malignancies and human stem cell transplantation recipients: a retrospective study at a major cancer center. *Medicine* (Baltimore) 2006;85:278–87.
40 Nichols WG, Guthrie KA, Corey L, Boeckh M. Influenza infections after hematopoietic stem cell transplantation: risk factors, mortality, and the effect of antiviral therapy. *Clin Infect Dis* 2004;39:1300–6.
41 Morrison VA. Infectious complications in patients with chronic lymphocytic leukemia: pathogenesis, spectrum of infection, and approaches to prophylaxis. *Clin Lymphoma Myeloma* 2009;9:365–70.
42 Al-Anazi KA, Al-Jasser AM, Evans DA. Infections caused by mycobacterium tuberculosis in patients with hematological disorders and in recipients of hematopoietic stem cell transplant, a twelve year retrospective study. *Ann Clin Microbiol Antimicrob* 2007;6:16.
43 Bollee G, Sarfati C, Thiery G, *et al*. Clinical picture of *Pneumocystis jiroveci* pneumonia in cancer patients. *Chest* 2007;132:1305–10.
44 Cibickova L, Horacek J, Prasil P, *et al*. Cerebral toxoplasmosis in an allogeneic peripheral stem cell transplant recipient: case report and review of literature. *Transpl Infect Dis* 2007;9: 332–5.
45 Novitzky N, Rouskova A. Infectious complications following T-cell depleted hematopoietic stem-cell transplantation. *Cytotherapy* 2001;3:165–73.
46 Jirillo E, Mastronardi ML, Altamura M, *et al*. The immunocompromised host: immune alterations in splenectomized patients and clinical implications. *Curr Pharm Des* 2003;9, 1918–23.
47 Sala A, Pencharz P, Barr RD. Children, cancer, and nutrition—A dynamic triangle in review. *Cancer* 2004;100:677–87.
48 Shoham S, Han G, Granek T, Walsh T, Magee MF. Association between blood glucose levels and development of candidemia in hospitalized patients. *Endocr Pract* 2009;15:111–15.
49 Paganini H, Staffolani V, Zubizarreta P, Casimir L, Lopardo H, Luppino V. Viridans streptococci bacteremia in children with fever and neutropenia: a case–control study of predisposing factors. *Eur J Cancer* 2003;39:1284–9.
50 Ulstrup AK, Hartzen SH. Leptotrichia buccalis: a rare cause of bacteremia in non-neutropenic patients. *Scand J Infect Dis* 2006;38:712–16.
51 Samonis G, Maraki S, Anatoliotakis N, *et al*. Effects of erythromycin, clarithromycin, roxithromycin and azithromycin on murine gut colonization by *Candida albicans*. *Med Mycol* 2002;40:139–42.
52 van der WD, de Vries-Hospers HG, Welling GW. The influence of antibiotics on gut colonization. *J Antimicrob Chemother* 1986;18(Suppl. C):155–8.
53 Vonberg RP, Gastmeier P. Nosocomial aspergillosis in outbreak settings. *J Hosp Infect* 2006;63:246–254.
54 Wilder-Smith A, Low JG. Risk of respiratory infections in health care workers: lessons on infection control emerge from the SARS outbreak. *Southeast Asian J Trop Med Public Health* 2005;36:481–8.
55 Gerberding JL. Nosocomial transmission of opportunistic infections. *Infect Control Hosp Epidemiol* 1998;19:574–7.
56 Anaissie EJ, Stratton SL, Dignani MC, *et al*. Pathogenic molds (including *Aspergillus* species) in hospital water distribution systems: a 3-year prospective study and clinical implications for patients with hematologic malignancies. *Blood* 2003;101: 2542–6.
57 Anaissie EJ, Stratton SL, Dignani MC, *et al*. Pathogenic *Aspergillus* species recovered from a hospital water system: a 3-year prospective study. *Clin Infect Dis* 2002;34:780–9.
58 Anaissie EJ, Kuchar RT, Rex JH, *et al*. Fusariosis associated with pathogenic fusarium species colonization of a hospital water system: a new paradigm for the epidemiology of opportunistic mold infections. *Clin Infect Dis* 2001;33: 1871–8.
59 Brulet A, Nicolle MC, Giard M, *et al*. Fatal nosocomial *Legionella pneumophila* infection due to exposure to contaminated water from a washbasin in a hematology unit. *Infect Control Hosp Epidemiol* 2008;29:1091–3.
60 Harbarth S. Nosocomial transmission of antibiotic-resistant microorganisms. *Curr Opin Infect Dis* 2001;14:437–42.
61 Feld R. Bloodstream infections in cancer patients with febrile neutropenia. *Int J Antimicrob Agents* 2008;32(Suppl. 1):S30–3.
62 Zinner SH. Changing epidemiology of infections in patients with neutropenia and cancer: emphasis on gram-positive and resistant bacteria. *Clin Infect Dis* 1999;29:490–4.
63 Garnica M, Maiolino A, Nucci M. Factors associated with bacteremia due to multidrug-resistant Gram-negative bacilli in hematopoietic stem cell transplant recipients. *Braz J Med Biol Res* 2009;42:289–93.
64 Cattaneo C, Quaresmini G, Casari S, *et al*. Recent changes in bacterial epidemiology and the emergence of fluoroquinolone-resistant *Escherichia coli* among patients with haematological malignancies: results of a prospective study on 823 patients at a single institution. *J Antimicrob Chemother* 2008;61:721–8.
65 Trecarichi EM, Tumbarello M, Spanu T, *et al*. Incidence and clinical impact of extended-spectrum-beta-lactamase (ESBL) production and fluoroquinolone resistance in bloodstream infections caused by *Escherichia coli* in patients with hematological malignancies. *J Infect* 2009;58:299–307.
66 Nouer SA, Nucci M, de-Oliveira MP, Pellegrino FL, Moreira BM. Risk factors for acquisition of multidrug-resistant *Pseudomonas aeruginosa* producing SPM metallo-beta-lactamase. *Antimicrob Agents Chemother* 2005;49:3663–7.
67 Rolston KV. Challenges in the treatment of infections caused by gram-positive and gram-negative bacteria in patients with cancer and neutropenia. *Clin Infect Dis* 2005;40(Suppl. 4): S246–52.

68 Dubberke ER, Hollands JM, Georgantopoulos P, *et al.* Vancomycin-resistant enterococcal bloodstream infections on a hematopoietic stem cell transplant unit: are the sick getting sicker? *Bone Marrow Transplant* 2006;38:813–19.

69 Dubberke ER, Reske KA, Yan Y, Olsen MA, McDonald LC, Fraser VJ. *Clostridium difficile*-associated disease in a setting of endemicity: identification of novel risk factors. *Clin Infect Dis* 2007;45:1543–9.

70 Schalk E, Bohr UR, Konig B, Scheinpflug K, Mohren M. Clostridium difficile-associated diarrhoea, a frequent complication in patients with acute myeloid leukemia. *Ann Hematol* 2009;89:9–14.

71 Maschmeyer G, Haas A. The epidemiology and treatment of infections in cancer patients. *Int J Antimicrob Agents* 2008;31: 193–7.

72 Reinert RR. The antimicrobial resistance profile of *Streptococcus pneumoniae*. *Clin Microbiol Infect* 2009;15(Suppl. 3):7–11.

73 Bodey GP. Fungal infections complicating acute leukemia. *J Chronic Dis* 1966;19:667–87.

74 Pizzo PA, Robichaud KJ, Wesley R, Commers JR. Fever in the pediatric and young adult patient with cancer. A prospective study of 1001 episodes. *Medicine (Baltimore)* 1982; 61:153–165.

75 Bodey G, Bueltmann B, Duguid W, *et al.* Fungal infections in cancer patients: an international autopsy survey. *Eur J Clin Microbiol Infect Dis* 1992;11:99–109.

76 Abi-Said D, Anaissie E, Uzun O, Raad I, Pinzcowski H, Vartivarian S. The epidemiology of hematogenous candidiasis caused by different *Candida* species. *Clin Infect Dis* 1997;24: 1122–8.

77 Wald A, Leisenring W, van Burik JA, Bowden RA. Epidemiology of *Aspergillus* infections in a large cohort of patients undergoing bone marrow transplantation. *J Infect Dis* 1997;175: 1459–66.

78 Torres HA, Rivero GA, Lewis RE, Hachem R, Raad II, Kontoyiannis DP. Aspergillosis caused by non-fumigatus *Aspergillus* species: risk factors and *in vitro* susceptibility compared with *Aspergillus fumigatus*. *Diagn Microbiol Infect Dis* 2003;46:25–28.

79 Nucci M. Emerging moulds: *Fusarium*, *Scedosporium* and *Zygomycetes* in transplant recipients. *Curr Opin Infect Dis* 2003;16:607–12.

80 Hughes WT, Price RA, Kim HK, Coburn TP, Grigsby D, Feldman S. *Pneumocystis carinii* pneumonitis in children with malignancies. *J Pediatr* 1973;82:404–15.

81 Wade JC. Viral infections in patients with hematological malignancies. *Hematology Am Soc Hematol Educ Program* 2006: 368–374. Review.

82 Khan SA, Wingard JR. Infection and mucosal injury in cancer treatment. *J Natl Cancer Inst Monogr* 2001:31–36. Review.

83 Ljungman P, Singh N. Human herpesvirus-6 infection in solid organ and stem cell transplant recipients. *J Clin Virol* 2006;37 (Suppl. 1):S87–91.

84 Zerr DM. Human herpesvirus 6 and central nervous system disease in hematopoietic cell transplantation. *J Clin Virol* 2006; 37(Suppl. 1):S52–6.

85 Winston DJ, Ho WG, Champlin RE. Cytomegalovirus infections after allogeneic bone marrow transplantation. *Rev Infect Dis* 1990;12(Suppl. 7):S776–92.

86 Boeckh M, Ljungman P. How we treat cytomegalovirus in hematopoietic cell transplant recipients. *Blood* 2009;113: 5711–19.

87 Partridge DG, McKendrick MW. The treatment of varicella-zoster virus infection and its complications. *Expert Opin Pharmacother* 2009;10:797–812.

88 Landgren O, Gilbert ES, Rizzo JD, *et al.* Risk factors for lymphoproliferative disorders after allogeneic hematopoietic cell transplantation. *Blood* 2009;113:4992–5001.

89 Hou HA, Yao M, Tang JL, *et al.* Poor outcome in post transplant lymphoproliferative disorder with pulmonary involvement after allogeneic hematopoietic SCT:13 years' experience in a single institute. *Bone Marrow Transplant* 2009;l 43:315–21.

90 Gorczynska E, Turkiewicz D, Rybka K, *et al.* Incidence, clinical outcome, and management of virus-induced hemorrhagic cystitis in children and adolescents after allogeneic hematopoietic cell transplantation. *Biol Blood Marrow Transplant* 2005;11: 797–804.

91 Carson KR, Focosi D, Major EO, *et al.* Monoclonal antibody-associated progressive multifocal leucoencephalopathy in patients treated with rituximab, natalizumab, and efalizumab: a Review from the Research on Adverse Drug Events and Reports (RADAR) Project. *Lancet Oncol* 2009;10, 816–24.

92 Martino R, Cordonnier C. Toxoplasmosis following allogeneic hematopoietic stem cell transplantation. *Bone Marrow Transplant* 2003;31:617–18.

93 Martin SI, Marty FM, Fiumara K, Treon SP, Gribben JG, Baden LR. Infectious complications associated with alemtuzumab use for lymphoproliferative disorders. *Clin Infect Dis* 2006;43: 16–24.

94 Segarra-Newnham M. Manifestations, diagnosis, and treatment of *Strongyloides stercoralis* infection. *Ann Pharmacother* 2007;41:1992–2001.

95 Silva FA, Matos JO, de QMF, Nucci M. Risk factors for and attributable mortality from tuberculosis in patients with hematologic malignances. *Haematologica* 2005;90:1110–15.

96 de la Camara R, Martino R, Granados E, *et al.* Tuberculosis after hematopoietic stem cell transplantation: incidence, clinical characteristics and outcome. Spanish Group on Infectious Complications in Hematopoietic Transplantation. *Bone Marrow Transplant* 2000;26:291–8.

97 Cordonnier C, Martino R, Trabasso P, *et al.* Mycobacterial infection: a difficult and late diagnosis in stem cell transplant recipients. *Clin Infect Dis* 2004;38:1229–36.

98 Myoken Y, Sugata T, Kyo T, *et al.* Invasive *Aspergillus* stomatitis in patients with acute leukemia: report of 12 cases. *Clin Infect Dis* 2001;33:1975–80.

99 Mohammed S, Sahoo TP, Jayshree RS, Bapsy PP, Hema S. Sinooral zygomycosis due to *Absidia corymbifera* in a patient with acute leukemia. *Med Mycol* 2004;42:475–8.

100 Jones AC, Bentsen TY, Freedman PD. Mucormycosis of the oral cavity. *Oral Surg Oral Med Oral Pathol* 1993;75:455–60.

101 Miller CS, Redding SW. Diagnosis and management of orofacial herpes simplex virus infections. *Dent Clin North Am* 1992;36:879–95.

102 Degre M. Interaction between viral and bacterial infections in the respiratory tract. *Scand J Infect Dis Suppl* 1986;49:140–5.

103 Morrison VA, Pomeroy C. Upper respiratory tract infections in the immunocompromised host. *Semin Respir Infect* 1995;10: 37–50.

104 Au WY, Tsang TY, Lie AK, *et al.* (2002) Speechless after bone marrow transplantation: a rare complication of parainfluenza virus related group in an adult. *Leuk Lymphoma* 43: 421–2.

105 Ernst-Kruis MR, Rutgers MI, Revesz T, Wolfs TF, Fleer A, Geelen SP. [Invasive infection with Moraxella catarrhalis in two children with lymphatic leukemia and granulocytopenia]. *Ned Tijdschr Geneeskd* 2003;147:1126–8.

106 Vernham GA, Crowther JA. Acute myeloid leukemia presenting with acute *Branhamella catarrhalis* epiglottitis. *J Infect* 1993;26:93–5.

107 Cole S, Zawin M, Lundberg B, Hoffman J, Bailey L, Ernstoff MS. *Candida epiglottitis* in an adult with acute nonlymphocytic leukemia. *Am J Med* 1987;82:662–4.

108 Barnes C, Berkowitz R, Curtis N, Waters K. *Aspergillus* laryngotracheobronchial infection in a 6-year-old girl following bone marrow transplantation. *Int J Pediatr Otorhinolaryngol* 2001;59:59–62.

109 Vrabec DP. Fungal infections of the larynx. *Otolaryngol Clin North Am* 1993;26:1091–14.

110 Krenke R, Kolkowska-Lesniak A, Palynyczko G, Prochorec-Sobieszek M, Konopka L. Ulcerative and pseudomembranous *Aspergillus* tracheobronchitis in a patient with acute myeloid leukemia. *Int J Hematol* 2009;89:257–8.

111 Warman M, Lahav J, Feldberg E, Halperin D. Invasive tracheal aspergillosis treated successfully with voriconazole: clinical report and review of the literature. *Ann Otol Rhinol Laryngol* 2007;116:713–16.

112 Lee AC, Lam SY. Life threatening acute epiglottitis in acute leukemia. *Leuk Lymphoma* 2002;43:665–7.

113 Arcand P, Cerat J, Spenard JR. Acute otomastoiditis in the leukemic child. *J Otolaryngol* 1989;18:380–3.

114 Wolff LJ. Necrotizing otitis externa during induction therapy for acute lymphoblastic leukemia. *Pediatrics* 1989;84: 882–5.

115 Stanley RJ, McCaffrey TV, Weiland LH. Fungal mastoiditis in the immunocompromised host. *Arch Otolaryngol Head Neck Surg* 1988;114:198–9.

116 Nucci M, Anaissie EJ, Queiroz-Telles F, *et al.* Outcome predictors of 84 patients with hematologic malignancies and *Fusarium* infection. *Cancer* 2003;98:315–19.

117 Pagano L, Offidani M, Fianchi L, *et al.* Mucormycosis in hematologic patients. *Haematologica* 2004;89:207–14.

118 Todd T, Besser M, Gudgin E, *et al.* (2008) Invasive fungal sinusitis in patients treated with fludarabine. *J Infect* 2008;56: 156–8.

119 Vlaardingerbroek H, van der FM, Borgstein JA, Lequin MH, van dS, I. Fatal *Aspergillus* rhinosinusitis during induction chemotherapy in a child with acute lymphoblastic leukemia. *J Pediatr Hematol Oncol* 2009;31:367–9.

120 Ramzi J, Mohamed Z, Yosr B, *et al.* Predictive factors of septic shock and mortality in neutropenic patients. *Hematology* 2007; 12:543–8.

121 Gonzalez-Barca E, Fernandez-Sevilla A, Carratala J, *et al.* Prognostic factors influencing mortality in cancer patients with neutropenia and bacteremia. *Eur J Clin Microbiol Infect Dis* 1999;18:539–44.

122 Vento S, Cainelli F, Temesgen Z. Lung infections after cancer chemotherapy. *Lancet Oncol* 2008;9:982–92.

123 Gerson SL, Talbot GH, Hurwitz S, Strom BL, Lusk EJ, Cassileth PA. Prolonged granulocytopenia: the major risk factor for invasive pulmonary aspergillosis in patients with acute leukemia. *Ann Intern Med* 1984;100:345–51.

124 Pagano L, Caira M, Candoni A, *et al.* The epidemiology of fungal infections in patients with hematologic malignancies: the SEIFEM-2004 study. *Haematologica* 2006;91:1068–75.

125 Gerson SL, Talbot GH, Lusk E, Hurwitz S, Strom BL, Cassileth PA. Invasive pulmonary aspergillosis in adult acute leukemia: clinical clues to its diagnosis. *J Clin Oncol* 1985;3: 1109–16.

126 Nucci M, Anaissie E. Emerging fungi. *Infect Dis Clin North Am* 2006;20:563–79.

127 Chamilos G, Marom EM, Lewis RE, Lionakis MS, Kontoyiannis DP. Predictors of pulmonary zygomycosis versus invasive pulmonary aspergillosis in patients with cancer. *Clin Infect Dis* 2005;41:60–6.

128 Hruban RH, Meziane MA, Zerhouni EA, Wheeler PS, Dumler JS, Hutchins GM. Radiologic–pathologic correlation of the CT halo sign in invasive pulmonary aspergillosis. *J Comput Assist Tomogr* 1987;11:534–6.

129 Caillot D, Couaillier JF, Bernard A, *et al.* Increasing volume and changing characteristics of invasive pulmonary aspergillosis on sequential thoracic computed tomography scans in patients with neutropenia. *J Clin Oncol* 2001;19:253–9.

130 Gefter WB, Albelda SM, Talbot GH, Gerson SL, Cassileth PA, Miller WT. Invasive pulmonary aspergillosis and acute leukemia. Limitations in the diagnostic utility of the air crescent sign. *Radiology* 1985;157:605–10.

131 Shaukat A, Bakri F, Young P, *et al.* Invasive filamentous fungal infections in allogeneic hematopoietic stem cell transplant recipients after recovery from neutropenia: clinical, radiologic, and pathologic characteristics. *Mycopathologia* 2005;159: 181–8.

132 Alangaden GJ, Wahiduzzaman M, Chandrasekar PH. Aspergillosis: the most common community-acquired pneumonia with gram-negative bacilli as copathogens in stem cell transplant recipients with graft-versus-host disease. *Clin Infect Dis* 2002;35:659–64.

133 Boeckh M. The challenge of respiratory virus infections in hematopoietic cell transplant recipients. *Br J Haematol* 2008;143: 455–67.

134 Rodriguez M, Fishman JA. Prevention of infection due to *Pneumocystis* spp. in human immunodeficiency virus-negative immunocompromised patients. *Clin Microbiol Rev* 2004;17: 770–82, table.

135 Horger MS, Pfannenberg C, Einsele H, *et al.* Cytomegalovirus pneumonia after stem cell transplantation: correlation of CT findings with clinical outcome in 30 patients. *AJR Am J Roentgenol* 2006;187:W636–43.

136 Angel C, Patrick CC, Lobe T, Rao B, Pui CH. Management of anorectal/perineal infections caused by *Pseudomonas aeruginosa* in children with malignant diseases. *J Pediatr Surg* 1991;26:487–92.

137 Boutati EI, Anaissie EJ. Fusarium, a significant emerging pathogen in patients with hematologic malignancy: ten years' experience at a cancer center and implications for management. *Blood* 1997;90:999–1008.

138 Fergie JE, Patrick CC, Lott L. *Pseudomonas aeruginosa* cellulitis and ecthyma gangrenosum in immunocompromised children. *Pediatr Infect Dis J* 1991;10:496–500.

139 Nucci M, Anaissie E. Cutaneous infection by *Fusarium* species in healthy and immunocompromised hosts: implications for diagnosis and management. *Clin Infect Dis* 2002;35: 909–20.

140 Bae GY, Lee HW, Chang SE, *et al.* Clinicopathologic review of 19 patients with systemic candidiasis with skin lesions. *Int J Dermatol* 2005;44:550–5.

141 Masood A, Sallah S. Chronic disseminated candidiasis in patients with acute leukemia: emphasis on diagnostic definition and treatment. *Leuk Res* 2005;29:493–501.

142 Alioglu B, Avci Z, Ozcay F, Arda S, Ozbek N. Neutropenic enterocolitis in children with acute leukemia or aplastic anemia. *Int J Hematol* 2007;86:364–8.

143 Cloutier RL. Neutropenic enterocolitis. *Emerg Med Clin North Am* 2009;27:415–22.

144 Mullassery D, Bader A, Battersby AJ, *et al.* Diagnosis, incidence, and outcomes of suspected typhlitis in oncology patients—experience in a tertiary pediatric surgical center in the United Kingdom. *J Pediatr Surg* 2009;44:381–5.

145 Davila ML. Neutropenic enterocolitis: current issues in diagnosis and management. *Curr Infect Dis Rep* 2007;9: 116–20.

146 Barnes SG, Sattler FR, Ballard JO. Perirectal infections in acute leukemia. Improved survival after incision and debridement. *Ann Intern Med* 1984;100:515–18.

147 Lam CS, Tong MK, Chan KM, Siu YP. Disseminated strongyloidiasis: a retrospective study of clinical course and outcome. *Eur J Clin Microbiol Infect Dis* 2006;25:14–18.

148 Treepongkaruna S, Thongpak N, Pakakasama S, Pienvichit P, Sirachainan N, Hongeng S. Acute pancreatitis in children with acute lymphoblastic leukemia after chemotherapy. *J Pediatr Hematol Oncol* 2009;31:812–15.

149 van der Werff ten Bosch JE, Kollen WJ, Ball LM, *et al.* Atypical varicella zoster infection associated with hemophagocytic lymphohistiocytosis. *Pediatr Blood Cancer* 2009;53: 226–8.

150 Meyer MH, Letscher-Bru V, Waller J, Lutz P, Marcellin L, Herbrecht R. (2002) Chronic disseminated *Trichosporon asahii* infection in a leukemic child. *Clin Infect Dis* 2002;35: e22–5.

151 Bassetti M, Repetto E, Mikulska M, *et al.* Cryptococcus neoformans fatal sepsis in a chronic lymphocytic leukemia patient treated with alemtuzumab: case report and review of the literature. *J Chemother* 2009;21:211–14.

152 Dincol G, Kahraman R. *Cryptococcus neoformans* meningitis in a patient with hairy cell leukemia. *Am J Hematol* 2006;81:387.

153 Malhotra P, Chauhan S, Bhatt P, *et al.* Cryptococcal meningitis in acute lymphoblastic leukemia. *J Assoc Physicians India* 2004;52:831–2.

154 Bacchu S, Fegan C, Neal J. Cerebral toxoplasmosis in a patient with chronic lymphocytic leukemia treated with fludarabine. *Br J Haematol* 2007;139:349.

155 Saha DC, Xess I, Jain N. Evaluation of conventional & serological methods for rapid diagnosis of cryptococcosis. *Indian J Med Res* 2008;127:483–8.

156 Doganay M. Listeriosis: clinical presentation. *FEMS Immunol Med Microbiol* 2003;35:173–5.

157 Pagano L, Girmenia C, Mele L, *et al.* Infections caused by filamentous fungi in patients with hematologic malignancies. A report of 391 cases by GIMEMA Infection Program. *Haematologica* 2001;86:862–70.

158 Scully EP, Baden LR, Katz JT. Fungal brain infections. *Curr Opin Neurol* 2008;21:347–52.

159 Kauffman CA. Candiduria. *Clin Infect Dis* 2005;41(Suppl. 6):S371–6.

160 Cheuk DK, Lee TL, Chiang AK, Ha SY, Lau YL, Chan GC. Risk factors and treatment of hemorrhagic cystitis in children who underwent hematopoietic stem cell transplantation. *Transpl Int* 2007;20:73–81.

161 Giraud G, Bogdanovic G, Priftakis P, *et al.* The incidence of hemorrhagic cystitis and BK-viruria in allogeneic hematopoietic stem cell recipients according to intensity of the conditioning regimen. *Haematologica* 2006;91:401–4.

162 Hatakeyama N, Suzuki N, Yamamoto M, *et al.* Detection of BK virus and adenovirus in the urine from children after allogeneic stem cell transplantation. *Pediatr Infect Dis J* 2006;25: 84–5.

163 Kuruvilla J, Forrest DL, Lavoie JC, *et al.* Characteristics and outcome of patients developing endocarditis following hematopoietic stem cell transplantation. *Bone Marrow Transplant* 2004;34:969–73.

164 Okamoto Y, Ribeiro RC, Srivastava DK, Shenep JL, Pui CH, Razzouk BI. Viridans streptococcal sepsis: clinical features and complications in childhood acute myeloid leukemia. *J Pediatr Hematol Oncol* 2003;25:696–703.

165 Pagano L, Caira M, Candoni A, *et al.* Invasive aspergillosis in patients with acute myeloid leukemia: SEIFEM-2008 registry study. *Haematologica* 2010;95:644–50.

166 Bow EJ. Neutropenic fever syndromes in patients undergoing cytotoxic therapy for acute leukemia and myelodysplastic syndromes. *Semin Hematol* 2009;46:259–68.

167 Marcos LA, Terashima A, Dupont HL, Gotuzzo E. Strongyloides hyperinfection syndrome: an emerging global infectious disease. *Trans R Soc Trop Med Hyg* 2008;102: 314–18.

168 Maciel E, Siqueira I, Queiroz AC, Melo A. *Toxoplasma gondii* myelitis in a patient with adult T-cell leukemia-lymphoma. *Arq Neuropsiquiatr* 2000;58: 1107–9.

169 Oshima Y, Nishida K, Kawazoye S, *et al.* Successful treatment of cytomegalovirus colitis with ganciclovir in a patient with adult T cell leukemia lymphoma: case report. *J Chemother* 1999;11: 215–19.

170 Arakaki N, Higa F, Tateyama M, *et al.* Concurrent infection with *Legionella pneumophila* and *Pneumocystis carinii* in a patient with adult T cell leukemia. *Intern Med* 1999;38: 160–3.

171 Marsh BJ. Infectious complications of human T cell leukemia/ lymphoma virus type I infection. *Clin Infect Dis* 1996;23: 138–45.

172 Ikeda K, Shiga Y, Takahashi A, *et al.* Fatal hepatitis B virus reactivation in a chronic myeloid leukemia patient during imatinib mesylate treatment. *Leuk Lymphoma* 2006;47: 155–7.

173 Mattiuzzi GN, Cortes JE, Talpaz M, *et al.* (2003) Development of Varicella-Zoster virus infection in patients with chronic myelogenous leukemia treated with imatinib mesylate. *Clin Cancer Res* 2003;9: 976–80.

174 Durosinmi MA, Ogbe PO, Salawu L, Oyekunle AA. Herpes zoster complicating imatinib mesylate for gastrointestinal stromal tumour. *Singapore Med J* 2007;48: e16–18.
175 Daniels JM, Vonk-Noordegraaf A, Janssen JJ, Postmus PE, van AR. Tuberculosis complicating imatinib treatment for chronic myeloid leukemia. *Eur Respir J* 2009;33: 670–2.
176 Garcia-Munoz R, Galar A, Moreno C, *et al.* Parvovirus B19 acute infection and a reactivation of cytomegalovirus and herpesvirus 6 in a chronic myeloid leukemia patient during treatment with dasatinib (BMS-354825). *Leuk Lymphoma* 2007;48: 2461–4.
177 Appel S, Boehmler AM, Grunebach F, *et al.* Imatinib mesylate affects the development and function of dendritic cells generated from $CD34^+$ peripheral blood progenitor cells. *Blood* 2004;103: 538–44.
178 Steegmann JL, Moreno G, Alaez C, *et al.* Chronic myeloid leukemia patients resistant to or intolerant of interferon alpha and subsequently treated with imatinib show reduced immunoglobulin levels and hypogammaglobulinemia. *Haematologica* 2003;88: 762–8.
179 Sinai P, Berg RE, Haynie JM, Egorin MJ, Ilaria RL, Jr., Forman J. Imatinib mesylate inhibits antigen-specific memory CD8 T cell responses *in vivo*. *J Immunol* 2007;178: 2028–37.
180 Robertson TI. Complications and causes of death in B cell chronic lymphocytic leukemia: a long term study of 105 patients. *Aust N Z J Med* 1990;20: 44–50.
181 Gafter-Gvili A, Fraser A, Paul M, Leibovici L. Meta-analysis: antibiotic prophylaxis reduces mortality in neutropenic patients. *Ann Intern Med* 2005;142: 979–95.
182 Gafter-Gvili A, Paul M, Fraser A, Leibovici L. Effect of quinolone prophylaxis in afebrile neutropenic patients on microbial resistance: systematic review and meta-analysis. *J Antimicrob Chemother* 2007;59: 5–22.
183 Marr KA, Bow E, Chiller T, *et al.* Fungal infection prevention after hematopoietic cell transplantation. *Bone Marrow Transplant* 2009;44: 483–7.
184 Bow EJ, Laverdiere M, Lussier N, Rotstein C, Cheang MS, Ioannou S. Antifungal prophylaxis for severely neutropenic chemotherapy recipients: a meta analysis of randomized-controlled clinical trials. *Cancer* 2002;94: 3230–46.
185 Cornely OA, Maertens J, Winston DJ, *et al.* Posaconazole vs. fluconazole or itraconazole prophylaxis in patients with neutropenia. *N Engl J Med* 2007;356: 348–59.
186 Maertens J, Huysmans G, Theunissen K. Early diagnosis and preemptive therapy of pulmonary mold infections in high-risk patients. *Curr Infect Dis Rep* 2008;10: 459–65.
187 Yahav D, Gafter-Gvili A, Muchtar E, *et al.* Antiviral prophylaxis in haematological patients: systematic review and meta-analysis. *Eur J Cancer* 2009;45:1131–48.
188 Anaissie E. Prophylaxis of infections in hematopoietic cell transplant recipients. UpToDate, 2008. Available at: www.uptodate.com/patients/content/topic.do?topicKey=~CC2Lt3dnd_wwn2
189 Sasse EC, Sasse AD, Brandalise S, Clark OA, Richards S. Colony stimulating factors for prevention of myelosupressive therapy induced febrile neutropenia in children with acute lymphoblastic leukemia. *Cochrane Database Syst Rev* 2005; CD004139.
190 Holdsworth MT, Mathew P. (2001) Efficacy of colony-stimulating factors in acute leukemia. *Ann Pharmacother* 35: 92–108.
191 Wang J, An L, Chen S, *et al.* Prophylactic use of granulocyte colony-stimulating factor after chemotherapy does not affect survival rate in acute myeloid leukemia: a meta-analysis. *Acta Haematol* 121, 2009;223–6.
192 Grazziutti ML, Dong L, Miceli MH, *et al.* Recovery from neutropenia can be predicted by the immature reticulocyte fraction several days before neutrophil recovery in autologous stem cell transplant recipients. *Bone Marrow Transplant* 2006;37: 403–9.
193 Fassas AB, Miceli MH, Grazzlutti M, Dong L, Barlogie B, Anaissie E. Serial measurement of serum C-reactive protein levels can identify patients at risk for severe complications following autologous stem cell transplantation. *Leuk Lymphoma* 2005;46: 1159–61.
194 Pfeiffer CD, Fine JP, Safdar N. Diagnosis of invasive aspergillosis using a galactomannan assay: a meta-analysis. *Clin Infect Dis* 2006;42: 1417–27.
195 Senn L, Robinson JO, Schmidt S, *et al.* 1,3-Beta-D-glucan antigenemia for early diagnosis of invasive fungal infections in neutropenic patients with acute leukemia. *Clin Infect Dis* 2008;46: 878–85.
196 Keating M, Coutre S, Rai K, *et al.* Management guidelines for use of alemtuzumab in B-cell chronic lymphocytic leukemia. *Clin Lymphoma* 2004;4: 220–7.
197 Intravenous immunoglobulin for the prevention of infection in chronic lymphocytic leukemia. A randomized, controlled clinical trial. Cooperative Group for the Study of Immunoglobulin in Chronic Lymphocytic Leukemia. *N Engl J Med* 1988;319: 902–7.
198 Molica S, Musto P, Chiurazzi F, *et al.* Prophylaxis against infections with low-dose intravenous immunoglobulins (IVIG) in chronic lymphocytic leukemia. Results of a crossover study. *Haematologica* 1996;81: 121–6.
199 Sinisalo M, Aittoniemi J, Kayhty H, Vilpo J. Vaccination against infections in chronic lymphocytic leukemia. *Leuk Lymphoma* 2003;44: 649–52.

Chapter 33
Transfusion Support and Hematopoietic Growth Factors

Paolo Rebulla
Center of Transfusion Medicine, Cellular Therapy, Foundation Ca'Granda Ospedale Maggiore Policlinico, Milano, Italy

Principles of blood transfusion

Blood donor recruitment and retention

The lack of clinically effective synthetic substitutes of blood and blood components demands straightforward attention by all health professionals to blood donor recruitment and retention. Although the latter activities currently represent a well-defined, specialized health-related profession being developed primarily at blood centers [1], it is important for clinicians to share with blood donor recruiters common cultural elements facilitating the renovation and maintenance of the required donor pool. This is particularly true considering increasing blood needs by hematology and oncology recipients, in turn related to the progressive increase of population age [2] and morbidity, to the implementation of additional, more stringent donor deferral criteria [3] and to the development of novel, more aggressive medical and surgical procedures.

The relation between the physician, the patient and his or her family, and their neighborhood represents a unique element in raising the awareness of blood donation as a key element of social responsibility. Particularly relevant in this regard are recent studies showing significant changes in blood donor social and demographic characteristics, motivations, and attitudes [4–6]. These studies indicate that traditional and valuable elements related to donor motivation and return, such as altruistic behavior, empathy and social responsibility, must be considered together with other categories, such as "having a good donation experience" and "having a convenient place to donate" [4]. Also, in the current era of the "safest blood," it is of utmost importance, particularly for long-term transfusion recipients, to rely on and expand the pool of repeat donors, who offer a higher infection safety margin compared with first-time donors [7].

Leukemias: Principles and Practice of Therapy, 1st edition. Edited by S. Faderl and H. Kantarjian.

Basic blood banking and blood component preparation procedures

For many years, in most developed countries, standard blood banking has been based on the collection of 450 mL whole blood donations from volunteer, non-remunerated, healthy blood donors denying behavioral or historical high-risk factors associated with transmission of infectious agents; their donation is screened with a battery of laboratory tests aimed at the identification of pathogen carriers. Whole blood collection is performed using commercial multiple plastic bag sets containing a citrate-based anticoagulant. Shortly after collection, whole blood units are fractionated with simple centrifugation procedures into three main blood components: red blood cells (RBCs), random donor platelets (RDPs), and fresh frozen plasma (FFP). RBCs, RDPs, and FFP must be stored at 2–6°C, 20–24°C, and below −18°C, respectively. Shelf life may vary slightly according to storage system and national regulations. Most procedures allow RBCs, RDPs, and FFP storage for 5–6 weeks, 5 or 7 days [8], and 3–24 months, respectively [9,10]. With regard to the cellular components, efficient and effective standard methods for RBC cryopreservation are available, whereas current procedures are not satisfactory and improvements are necessary for platelet cryopreservation.

A relevant proportion of plasma recovered from whole blood donations is used for the manufacture of immunoglobulins, coagulation factors and albumin. White blood cells (WBCs) present in RBCs and RDPs, which can cause untoward reactions in the recipients, can be removed by filtration [11], a procedure which has become standard in several countries. Depending on the patient's body size, RDPs are pooled before transfusion to obtain a clinically effective dose, usually one RDP concentrate per 10 kg of body weight [12].

In the USA, RDPs are obtained mainly with the sequence of a soft spin of whole blood to concentrate the platelets in the supernatant "platelet-rich" plasma (PRP), followed by a hard spin to reduce the PRP volume [13]. In Europe, RDPs are prepared primarily with the "buffy coat" procedure, which consists of whole blood hard centrifugation, buffy coat collection in a satellite bag, buffy coat pooling and dilution with an optimized crystalloid platelet additive solution (PAS), and finally soft spin to discard contaminating RBCs and WBCs in the bottom fraction and to recover the platelet concentrate as a pool in the supernatant [13]. Canada is progressively converting from a PRP to a buffy coat platelet production method [14].

Starting in the 1970s, the automated selective collection of individual blood components—a technology termed "apheresis"—has been developed and expanded in parallel to whole blood collection. Apheresis, currently applied primarily to the collection of one or two adult platelet doses from a single donor (single donor platelets, SDPs), is also used for the collection of peripheral blood stem cells (PBSCs), FFP, and, although less frequently, for the collection of lymphocytes and polymorphonuclear granulocytes (PMNs). PMNs have been successfully used in the past to treat septic patients unresponsive to antibiotic treatment [15,16]. Currently, PMNs represent an infrequently used blood component, owing to the availability of more effective antibiotics and to the high frequency of severe transfusion reactions in recipients.

Recently, novel apheresis procedures have been developed for the collection from healthy donors of different blood component combinations, including two units of RBCs, one unit of SDPs and one unit of FFP, one unit of RBCs and one unit of SDP, etc. [17]. Current highly sophisticated apheresis devices operate with very efficient protocols which permit the collection of SDPs with very low WBC contamination, thus avoiding the labor and expense of WBC reduction by filtration [18]. Therapeutic apheresis procedures have been successfully applied to the treatment of hyperviscosity syndromes developed by leukemic patients with hyperleukocytosis [19,20].

Details on the methods of preparation and content of blood components can be found in the North American "Technical Manual" of the AABB [9] and in the European "Guide to the Preparation, Use and Quality Assurance of Blood Components" [10]. Additional information can be found in reports of multicenter investigations aimed at comparing volumes and cellular contents of blood components prepared in different countries with different procedures [21].

Blood request and administration

Blood request and administration are critical start and end points of transfusion therapy which require careful attention to identify patient's clinical needs and to prevent transfusion of incorrect components to non-intended recipients. Critical control points of blood request and administration are positive patient identification with at least two identifiers (such as name and date of birth, name and code, etc.), accurate paper or electronic form completion, and multiple checks of samples and component bags labels [22]. Several standard procedures mandate that patient and product identification are made by two individuals to reduce the chance of transfusing a blood component different from that requested (eg, non-irradiated or non-leukoreduced RBCs or platelets) or of the requested component being given to a "wrong" recipient [23]. The occurrence of an incorrect blood component transfusion should trigger prompt investigations aimed at detecting a possible related error of a parallel unit being administered to another non-intended recipient because of exchange of units secondary to clerical or operational errors.

Several systems have been proposed and tested to improve patient, sample, and component identification [24], none being so effective, reliable, convenient, and inexpensive to become standard practice at national or international levels. In spite of the current limitations, the research and implementation of positive identification tools should be encouraged to improve patient safety and reduce legal consequences of errors along the blood transfusion chain.

Blood administration must be preceded and followed by registration of patients' vital signs and followed by the evaluation of transfusion outcome, both in clinical terms (resolution of bleeding, correction of symptoms of anemia) and through laboratory tests (hemoglobin concentration and platelet counts, correction of coagulation abnormalities, etc.).

Complications of blood transfusion

Blood transfusion can cause acute and delayed hemolysis, febrile, allergic and anaphylactic reactions, acute lung injury, circulatory overload, graft-versus-host disease, and donor to recipient transmission of viruses, bacteria and parasites. Moreover, chronic RBC recipients, such as those suffering from hemoglobinopathies and myelodysplastic syndromes, can develop hemosiderosis, which can be prevented by iron chelation. A proportion of transfusion recipients develop alloantibodies to red blood cells, white blood cells, and platelets, which may have a causative role in hemolysis, febrile reactions, and refractoriness to platelet transfusion, respectively [12,25,26].

Although most patients and some health professionals are more concerned of the risks of transmission of infectious agents through blood transfusion than of other side-effects, administrative and operational errors occurring during blood request, distribution, and administration currently generate greater risks to transfusion recipients than human immunodeficiency virus (HIV), hepatitis C virus (HCV), and hepatitis B virus (HBV) infections.

With regard to the infectious risks, several recent publications report similar tables on residual risks per million donations in different countries. During 1997–2001, in a sample of countries with high human development indices, including Canada [27], the USA [28], France [29],

Spain [30], and Italy [31], the HIV, HCV, and HBV residual risks of one infected unit entering the blood supply ranged from 0.10 to 1.95, from 0.35 to 16.64, and from 2.13 to 69.16 per million donations, respectively. With regard to HCV, it has been estimated that the adoption of nucleic acid testing, which reduces the window period in which infectious donors cannot be detected from 72 to 12 days, reduced the risk of transmission in Italy from 16.74 to 3.01 per million donations [32]. Recent risk evaluations in other countries have been reported in the literature [33–37].

The potential impact of different blood donor screening policies on residual risk should be determined in light of local data on the prevalence and incidence of infectious markers in the population. In fact, the main differences in the risks of viral infections transmitted by transfusions depend on the different prevalences and incidences of infection carriers in different geographical areas, on prevalent use of voluntary versus commercial and repeat versus first-time blood donors, on local resources and policies for blood donor screening, and on the ability of current commercial blood donor screening assays to identify viral variants that may be differently represented in selected areas of the globe. The straightforward improvement in the reduction of the infectious risks occurring during the last two decades, particularly in countries with adequate economical resources—in part triggered by the acquired immune deficiency syndrome (AIDS) epidemic—should be considered, remembering that 30 years ago about 30% of transfusion recipients could still develop post-transfusion icteric hepatitis [38]. Therefore, non-infectious complications have currently become relatively more frequent, as indicated by a recent analysis of the 1996–2003 reports from the Serious Hazards of Transfusion scheme, which indicate that "the risk of an error occurring during transfusion of a blood component is estimated at 1:16,500, an ABO incompatible transfusion at 1:100,000 and the risk of death as a result of an 'incorrect blood components transfused' (IBCT) is around 1:1,500,000" [39].

Other than viral pathogens, blood components—in particular platelets, which are stored at 20–24°C and are a critical therapeutic tool for the leukemic recipient—can also transmit bacterial infections [40]. Data from countries where routine hemovigilance systems are in place, such as the USA [41], France [42], UK [39], and Canada [43], indicate that about 1 in 3,000 platelet concentrates contain bacteria [44,45] and that bacterial sepsis was the second cause of fatal transfusion-associated untoward effects in the USA during 1990 and 1998 [46]. In most cases, bacteria enter the blood collection bag at the time of venipuncture together with a small skin biopsy containing a poorly disinfected pilonidal bulb. Although bacterial contamination of blood components can be a potential cause of severe consequences, and careful attention must be paid by operators to ensure proper component manipulation, storage and management, 80–90% of platelets originally contaminated with bacteria do not cause clinically evident harm because the bacterial load is small and the strain pathogenicity is low. This translates into an actual frequency of severe or fatal sepsis in about 1:25,000 platelet transfusion episodes (ie, about 1 in 8 transfusions containing at least one contaminated product) [44]. This complication may be particularly relevant for patients with leukemia who suffer from prolonged intervals of profoundly reduced immune competence.

Novel technologies have recently become commercially available, mostly for platelet and plasma components, which inactivate viruses, bacteria, and nucleated cells with a high degree of efficacy [47–51]. These technologies have the potential to inactivate unrecognized pathogens which may enter the blood supply, as was recently the case for West Nile virus and the Chykungunya virus [38]. Unfortunately, these technologies cause some degree of damage to the platelets and add significant cost to transfusion treatment [52–54]. In addition, several manufacturers have developed commercial methods for bacterial detection in platelet concentrates that have been routinely implemented in some countries. These technologies also require improvements as their sensitivity is still suboptimal in some cases and their use does not fit easily with the short lifespan of platelet concentrates [12,55,56].

Careful attention must be paid to the prompt detection of a complication called transfusion-associated acute lung injury (TRALI), which has been frequently overlooked in the past and the pathophysiology of which has been partially clarified in recent years. Although relatively infrequent, TRALI is associated with significant morbidity and mortality [57] and has also been described in leukemic patients [58]. A recent publication reports the consensus of a panel of experts on TRALI diagnostic criteria (Box 33.1) [59].

Practice of blood transfusion in leukemia

The leukemic blood recipient

On average, a patient suffering from acute myelogenous leukemia (AML) requires 41, 6, 15, and 33 units of RBCs, FFP, SDPs, and RDPs, respectively [60]. Based on these data, it can be estimated that the average blood transfusion support of patients suffering from acute leukemia requires the generous gift of about 100 blood donors per patient. These figures and the estimated numbers of 20,540 and 18,120 new cases of lymphocytic and myeloid leukemias, respectively, in the USA for 2008 [61] indicate that a significant amount of the national blood supply—15,288,000 whole blood/RBC units, in 2004—[62] is utilized to treat acute leukemia patients. Recent reports from

Box 33.1 TRALI recommended diagnostic criteria

1 TRALI criteria
- i ALI
  - a Acute onset
  - b Hypoxemia
    Research setting: PaO_2/FiO_2 <300 or SpO_2 <90% on room air
    Non-research setting: PaO_2/FiO_2 <300 or SpO_2 <90% on room air or other clinical evidence of hypoxemia
  - c Bilateral infiltrates on frontal chest radiograph
  - d No evidence of left atrial hypertension (ie, circulatory overload)
- ii No pre-existing ALI before transfusion
- iii During or within 6 h of transfusion
- iv No temporal relationship to an alternative risk factor for ALI

2 Possible TRALI
- i ALI
- ii No pre-existing ALI before transfusion
- iii During or within 6 h of transfusion
- iv A clear temporal relationship to an alternative risk factor for ALI

ALI, acute lung injury; TRALI, transfusion-associated acute lung injury.
With permission from Kleinman S, *et al.* (2004) *Transfusion* 44,1774–89.

Finland and Korea indicate that patients with leukemia use about 8–10% of the blood supply [63,64].

Use of blood components in leukemia

It is common practice in leukemia treatment to administer RBCs based on a "threshold" hemoglobin value of 7–9 g/dL, depending on the patient's ability to tolerate anemia. Two recent studies have evaluated a restrictive [65] and an augmented [66] RBC transfusion policy in leukemia. The former study was aimed at reducing RBC use and decreasing transfusion-associated costs and potential side-effects, whereas the latter explored the possible impact of an opposite strategy, (ie, if increased hematocrit values were associated with reduced bleeding). Although the former study demonstrated that the restrictive policy was well tolerated, no bleeding reduction was documented in the latter. It seems, therefore, appropriate to refer to a traditional hemoglobin threshold of 7–9 g/dL for RBC transfusion in leukemia, until novel information is collected.

As far as platelet support is concerned, current prevalent consensus supports a threshold of 10×10^9 platelets/L in stable patients and of 20×10^9 platelets/L in those with bleeding risk factors such as recent bleeding, high body temperature, infection, and rapid fall of the platelet count [67–71].

Similarly to other categories of chronic blood transfusion recipients, patients suffering from leukemia are more prone to becoming alloimmunized to red cell, white cell, and platelet antigens than occasional recipients of transfusion support, such as most surgical patients. Usually, alloimmunization to red cell antigens can be easily managed by the immunohematology laboratory of the blood transfusion service. More complex cases, such as mixtures of alloantibodies to different specificities or infrequent cases of alloimmunization to public antigens, may require consultation with an immunohematology reference laboratory. As red cell antibodies may cause not only acute, but also delayed, hemolytic transfusion reactions, the symptoms and laboratory signs of which may be less readily evident, it is very important to carefully investigate all cases of chronically transfused leukemic patients with unexpectedly low hemoglobin values.

Anti-human leukocyte antigen (anti-HLA) alloimmunization, which is associated with febrile reactions and refractoriness to random donor platelet support, is more frequent in female patients as a possible consequence of primary sensitization during pregnancy [68]. Patients with repeated febrile reactions must receive leukoreduced blood components, which is standard practice in countries where this policy has been adopted as a national rule. Leukoreduction is not only able to prevent most febrile reactions in sensitized patients, but is also considered by most experts equivalent to donor cytomegalovirus (CMV) seronegativity in preventing CMV transmission. Therefore, in consideration of the cumulative effect of leukoreduction, many hematology units have adopted a policy of universal leukoreduction for their patients also in countries lacking a national universal leukoreduction rule.

Mainly during the profound immune suppression associated with bone marrow transplantation, leukemic patients are at risk of developing transfusion-associated graft-versus-host disease, a complication due to the immune reaction of donor lymphocytes against recipient's skin, liver, gastrointestinal tract, and bone marrow. This complication can be distinguished from allogeneic transplantation graft-versus-host disease because the former, differently from the latter, is almost always associated with pancytopenia and is prevented by the administration of gamma-irradiated blood components. As the occurrence of transfusion-associated graft-versus-host disease is more frequent when the donor is HLA homozygous or haploidentical with the recipient, blood components must be gamma irradiated in any case in which the donor is a family member; there is a high likelihood that family members share an HLA haplotype.

Both the universal leukoreduction and universal gamma irradiation policies, although associated with increased cost, avoid the inadvertent administration of an untreated product to patients in need of leukoreduced or gamma-irradiated components.

Although RBC support is usually easily managed in leukemia, platelet transfusion is characterized by the occurrence of refractoriness to random donor support in 27% of leukemic recipients [68]. Refractoriness can be caused by immune and non-immune factors, most frequently represented by anti-HLA antibodies and fever, respectively, secondary to sepsis [68]. Patients with leukemia given non-leukoreduced or leukoreduced blood components develop alloimmune refractoriness in about 15% and 4–5%, respectively, of the cases [72]. Patients refractory to random donors need HLA-compatible platelets, which can be selected through HLA-typed donor registries or by cross-match [73]. The choice between the two systems, which show similar clinical efficacy if managed by expert clinicians and transfusion specialists, depends on local availability of HLA-typed donors and reliable laboratory assays for platelet cross-matching.

The clinical efficacy of platelet support is measured by the prevention or correction of bleeding. Patient monitoring is also based on the evaluation of the post-transfusion increment of the platelet count. This can be routinely determined 18–24 h after transfusion (ie, from the routine complete blood count carried out daily in most oncohematology recipients during their hospital admissions). For patients showing confirmed unexpected decrements of the post-transfusion platelet count increments, it is desirable to obtain earlier evaluations, which can be collected 10–60 minutes after transfusion. Accurate and elegant investigations in large adult leukemic patient series indicate average 10- to 60-minute increments of the platelet count of about 25×10^9 platelets/L in recipients of about 5–6 billion platelets per kilogram body weight. These increments usually fall to 50% at 18–24 h [68]. Large deviations from these average values are commonly seen in patients with leukemia as a result of comorbidity, splenomegaly, concurrent administration of drugs capable of reducing platelet lifespan and function in the circulation, and other detrimental factors [74].

Clinical uses of hematopoietic growth factors in leukemia

Erythropoietin (EPO), granulocyte and granulocyte-macrophage colony stimulating factors (G-CSFs and GM-CSFs) and thrombopoietin (TPO) have been used with the specific target of increasing the production of red cells, neutrophils, and platelets, respectively. Moreover, G-CSF is now used to mobilize hematopoietic progenitors into the circulation of healthy donors and patients in view of apheresis collection and allogeneic or autologous transplantation, respectively [75]. The clinical availability of G-CSF has favored a shift from the use of bone marrow to the use of mobilized peripheral blood as a more convenient source of hematopoietic progenitors. The clinical use of TPO has been discontinued early during safety and efficacy clinical trials because of its antigenicity. G-CSF and GM-CSF are also used to increase neutrophil counts during neutropenia associated with myeloablative therapy, although the demonstrated benefit of shortening the neutropenic phase has not been accompanied by increased patient survivals [76].

The use of EPO, after its initial application aimed at the correction of anemia secondary to renal disease, has been expanded to include the treatment of anemia associated with cancer. Concern has been raised by recent data demonstrating that several cancer cell lines show EPO receptors, [77] including malignant lymphoid and normal B and T cells, although the latter cell types did not show surface protein expression and no EPO-induced *in vitro* stimulation of tumor B cells was observed [78].

In spite of this apparent evidence of safety, prudent use of EPO has been recommended also in patients with cancer who are anemic because of increased risks of thromboembolic events [79,80].

Conclusions

Safe and effective blood transfusion for both medical and surgical patients requires the availability of high-quality blood components given by a sufficient number of motivated, properly selected, repeat blood donors screened with state of the art laboratory tests. Patients suffering from acute and chronic leukemia represent a category of transfusion recipients requiring special attention not only for their reduced immune competence, but also for the profound cytopenia which may occur during several phases of treatment. Although red blood cell replacement is usually uneventful, severe neutropenia and thrombocytopenia significantly increase the risks of infection and bleeding. Moreover, although prophylactic platelet support during thrombocytopenia does protect patients from severe hemorrhage in most cases, this component of supportive therapy is still imperfect as it is probably unnecessary in some cases and it becomes ineffective in some patients, who are then exposed to the occurrence of clinically relevant bleeding episodes. Similar to other pathologic conditions, but particularly so in leukemia, close cooperation between clinicians and transfusion medicine specialists is the cornerstone of effective transfusion support.

Acknowledgments

The author acknowledges the secretarial assistance of Dr. Giusy Baldocchi.

References

1 Davey RJ. The blood centre as a community health resource. *Vox Sang* 2006;91: 206–13.
2 Zou S, Musavi F, Notari EP, 4th, *et al.* Changing age distribution of the blood donor population in the United States. *Transfusion* 2008;48: 251–7.
3 Riley W, Schwei M, McCullough J. The United States' potential blood donor pool: estimating the prevalence of donor-exclusion factors on the pool of potential donors. *Transfusion* 2007;47: 1180–8.
4 Schlumpf KS, Glynn SA, Schreiber GB, *et al.* Factors influencing donor return. *Transfusion* 2008;48: 264–72.
5 Steele WR, Schreiber GB, Guiltinan A, *et al.* Role of altruistic behavior, empathetic concern, and social responsibility motivation in blood donation behavior. *Transfusion* 2008;48: 43–54.
6 Schreiber GB, Schlumpf KS, Glynn SA, *et al.* Convenience, the bane of our existence, and other barriers to donating. *Transfusion* 2006;46: 545–53.
7 Pillonel J, Barin F, Laperche S, *et al.* Human immunodeficiency virus type 1 incidence among blood donors in France, 1992 through 2006: use of an immunoassay to identify recent infections. *Transfusion* 2008;48: 1567–75.
8 Cardigan R, Williamson LM. The quality of platelets after storage for 7 days. *Transfus Med* 2003;13: 173–87.
9 Brecker ME. *AABB Technical Manual*, 15th edn. American Association of Blood Banks (AABB): Bethesda, MD, 2005.
10 The European Directorate for the Quality of Medicines. *Guide to the Preparation, Use and Quality Assurance of Blood Components*, 13th edn. Council of Europe Publishing: Strasbourg, 2007.
11 Dzik WH. Leukoreduction of blood components. *Curr Opin Hematol* 2002;9: 521–6.
12 Stroncek DF, Rebulla P. Platelet transfusions. *Lancet* 2007;370: 427–38.
13 Vassallo RR, Murphy S. A critical comparison of platelet preparation methods. *Curr Opin Hematol* 2006;13: 323–30.
14 Ramirez-Arcos S, Goldman M. Evaluation of pooled cultures for bacterial detection in whole blood-derived platelets. *Transfusion* 2005;45: 1275–9.
15 Stanworth SJ, Massey E, Hyde C, *et al.* Granulocyte transfusions for treating infections in patients with neutropenia or neutrophil dysfunction. *Cochrane Database Syst Rev* CD005339, 2005.
16 Briones MA, Josephson CD, Hillyer CD. Granulocyte transfusion: revisited. *Curr Hematol Rep* 2003;2: 522–7.
17 Popovsky MA. Multicomponent apheresis blood collection in the United States: current status and future directions. *Transfus Apher Sci* 2005;32: 299–304.
18 Seghatchian J. Platelet storage lesion: an update on the impact of various leukoreduction processes on the biological response modifiers. *Transfus Apher Sci* 2006;34: 125–30.
19 Blum W, Porcu P. Therapeutic apheresis in hyperleukocytosis and hyperviscosity syndrome. *Semin Thromb Hemost* 2007;33: 350–4.
20 Bug G, Anargyrou K, Tonn T, *et al.* Impact of leukapheresis on early death rate in adult acute myeloid leukemia presenting with hyperleukocytosis. *Transfusion* 2007;47: 1843–50.
21 Heaton WA, Rebulla P, Pappalettera M, *et al.* A comparative analysis of different methods for routine blood component preparation. *Transfus Med Rev* 1997;11: 116–29.
22 Murphy MF, Stearn BE, Dzik WH. Current performance of patient sample collection in the UK. *Transfus Med* 2004;14: 113–21.
23 Moore SB, Foss ML. Ordering blood for the wrong patient—getting inside the minds of ordering physicians. *Mayo Clin Proc* 2003;78: 1337–9.
24 Pagliaro P, Rebulla P. Transfusion recipient identification. *Vox Sang* 2006;91: 97–101.
25 Klein HG, Spahn DR, Carson JL. Red blood cell transfusion in clinical practice. *Lancet* 2007;370: 415–26.
26 Eder AF, Chambers LA. Noninfectious risks of blood transfusion. *Arch Pathol Lab Med* 2007;131: 708–18.
27 Chiavetta JA, Escobar M, Newman A, *et al.* Incidence and estimated rates of residual risk for HIV, hepatitis C, hepatitis B and human T-cell lymphotropic viruses in blood donors in Canada, 1990–2000. *CMAJ* 2003;169: 767–73.
28 Dodd RY, Notari EP, 4th, Stramer SL. Current prevalence and incidence of infectious disease markers and estimated window-period risk in the American Red Cross blood donor population. *Transfusion* 2002;42: 975–9.
29 Pillonel J, Laperche S, Saura C, *et al.* Trends in residual risk of transfusion-transmitted viral infections in France between 1992 and 2000. *Transfusion* 2002;42: 980–8.
30 Alvarez M, Oyonarte S, Rodrìguez PM, *et al.* Estimated risk of transfusion-transmitted viral infections in Spain. *Transfusion* 2002;42: 994–8.
31 Velati C, Romano L, Baruffi L, *et al.* Residual risk of transfusion-transmitted HCV and HIV infections by antibody-screened blood in Italy. *Transfusion* 2002;42: 989–93.

32 Gonzalez M, Règine V, Piccinini V, *et al.* Residual risk of transfusion-transmitted human immunodeficiency virus, hepatitis C virus, and hepatitis B virus infections in Italy. *Transfusion* 2005; 45: 1670–5.
33 Campos RH, Mbayed VA, Pineiro Y, Leone FG. Molecular epidemiology of hepatitis B virus in Latin America. *J Clin Virol* 2005;34(Suppl. 2): S8–13. Review.
34 Ouattara H, Siransy-Bogui L, Fretz C, *et al.* Residual risk of HIV, HVB and HCV transmission by blood transfusion between 2002 and 2004 at the Abidjan National Blood Transfusion Center. *Transfus Clin Biol* 2006;13: 242–5.
35 Zaller N, Nelson KE, Ness P, *et al.* Demographic characteristics and risks for transfusion-transmissible infection among blood donors in Xinjiang autonomous region, People's Republic of China. *Transfusion* 2006;46: 265–71.
36 Alfaresi MS, Elnazer AM, Alzaabi AS, *et al.* Transfusion transmitted virus in screened United Arab Emirates blood donors. *Saudi Med J* 2006;27: 58–62.
37 Maresch C, Schluter PJ, Wilson AD, *et al.* Residual infectious disease risk in screened blood transfusion from a high-prevalence population: Santa Catarina, Brazil. *Transfusion* 2008;48: 273–81.
38 Alter HJ. Pathogen reduction: a precautionary principle paradigm. *Transfus Med Rev* 2008;22: 97–102.
39 Stainsby D, Jones H, Asher D, *et al.* Serious hazards of transfusion: a decade of hemovigilance in the UK. *Transfus Med Rev* 2006;20: 273–82.
40 Eder AF, Kennedy JM, Dy BA, *et al.* Bacterial screening of apheresis platelets and the residual risk of septic transfusion reactions: the American Red Cross experience (2004–2006). *Transfusion* 2007;47: 1134–42.
41 Menitove JE. (1998) Hemovigilance in the United States of America. *Vox Sang* 1998;74: 447–55.
42 Andreu G, Morel P, Forestier F, *et al.* Hemovigilance network in France: organization and analysis of immediate transfusion incident reports from 1994 to 1998. *Transfusion* 2002;42: 1356–64.
43 Robillard P, Nawej KI, Jochem K. The Quebec hemovigilance system: description and results from the first two years. *Transfus Apher Sci* 2004;31: 111–22.
44 Blajchman MA, Beckers EA, Dickmeiss E, *et al.* Bacterial detection of platelets: current problems and possible resolutions. *Transfus Med Rev* 2005;19: 259–72.
45 Blajchman MA, Vamvakas EC. The continuing risk of transfusion-transmitted infections. *N Engl J Med* 2006;355: 1303–5.
46 Centers for Disease Control and Prevention (CDC). Fatal bacterial infections associated with platelet transfusions. United States 2004. *MMWR Weekly* 2005;54: 168–70.
47 Murphy S, Snyder E, Cable R, *et al.* Platelet dose consistency and its effect on the number of platelet transfusions for support of thrombocytopenia: an analysis of the SPRINT trial of platelets photochemically treated with amotosalen HCl and ultraviolet A light. *Transfusion* 2006;46: 24–33.
48 Snyder E, McCullough J, Slichter SJ, *et al.* Clinical safety of platelets photochemically treated with amotosalen HCl and ultraviolet A light for pathogen inactivation: the SPRINT trial. *Transfusion* 2005;45: 1864–75.
49 Slichter SJ, Raife TJ, Davis K, *et al.* Platelets photochemically treated with amotosalen HCl and ultraviolet A light correct prolonged bleeding times in patients with thrombocytopenia. *Transfusion* 2006;46: 731–40.
50 Corash L, Lin L. Novel processes for inactivation of leukocytes to prevent transfusion-associated graft-versus-host disease. *Bone Marrow Transplant* 2004;33: 1–7.
51 AuBuchon JP, Herschel L, Roger J, *et al.* Efficacy of apheresis platelets treated with riboflavin and ultraviolet light for pathogen reduction. *Transfusion* 2005;45: 1335–41.
52 Bell CE, Botteman MF, Gao X, *et al.* Cost-effectiveness of transfusion of platelet components prepared with pathogen inactivation treatment in the United States. *Clin Ther* 2003;25: 2464–86.
53 Moeremans K, Warie H, Annemans L. Assessment of the economic value of the INTERCEPT blood system in Belgium. *Transfus Med* 2006;16: 17–30.
54 Postma MJ, van Hulst M, De Wolf JT, *et al.* Cost-effectiveness of pathogen inactivation for platelet transfusions in the Netherlands. *Transfus Med* 2005;15: 379–87.
55 AuBuchon JP. The reliability of bacterial detection in platelets. *ISBT Science Series* 2006;1: 59–63.
56 Brecher ME, Hay SN, Rose AD, *et al.* Evaluation of BacT/ALERT plastic culture bottles for use in testing pooled whole blood-derived leukoreduced platelet-rich plasma platelets with a single contaminated unit. *Transfusion* 2005;45: 1512–17.
57 Goldman M, Webert KE, Arnold DM, *et al.* Proceedings of a consensus conference: towards an understanding of TRALI. *Transfus Med Rev* 2005;19: 2–31.
58 Fung YL, Williams BA. TRALI in 2 cases of leukemia. *J Pediatr Hematol Oncol* 2006;28: 391–4.
59 Kleinman S, Caulfield T, Chan P, *et al.* Toward an understanding of transfusion-related acute lung injury: statement of a consensus panel. *Transfusion* 2004;44: 1774–89.
60 Lopez-Plaza I, Weissfeld J, Triulzi DJ. The cost-effectiveness of reducing donor exposures with single-donor versus pooled random-donor platelets. *Transfusion* 1999;39: 925–32.
61 http://seer.cancer.gov/cgi-bin/csr/1975_2005/search.pl#results
62 Whitaker BI, Sullivan M. The 2005 National Blood Collection and Utilization Survey Report. US Department of Health and Human Services. Available from: http://www.aabb.org/apps/docs/05nbcusrpt.pdf (last accessed 22 May 2008)
63 Lim YA, Lee WG, Cho SR, *et al.* A study of blood usage by diagnoses in a Korean university hospital. *Vox Sang* 2004;86: 54–61.
64 Syrjälä MT, Kytöniemi I, Mikkolainen K, *et al.* Transfusion practice in Helsinki University Central Hospital: an analysis of diagnosis-related groups (DRG). *Transfus Med* 2001;11: 423–31.
65 Jansen AJ, Caljouw MA, Hop WC, *et al.* Feasibility of a restrictive red-cell transfusion policy for patients treated with intensive chemotherapy for acute myeloid leukemia. *Transfus Med* 2004;14: 33–8.
66 Webert KE, Cook RJ, Couban S, *et al.* A multicenter pilot-randomized controlled trial of the feasibility of an augmented red blood cell transfusion strategy for patients treated with induction chemotherapy for acute leukemia or stem cell transplantation. *Transfusion* 2008;48: 81–91.
67 Foss B, Bruserud O. Platelet functions and clinical effects in acute myelogenous leukemia. *Thromb Haemost* 2008;99: 27–37.

68 Slichter SJ, Davis K, Enright H, *et al.* Factors affecting post-transfusion platelet increments, platelet refractoriness, and platelet transfusion intervals in thrombocytopenic patients. *Blood* 2005;105: 4106–14.
69 Rebulla P, Finazzi G, Marangoni F, *et al.* The threshold for prophylactic platelet transfusions in adults with acute myeloid leukemia. Gruppo Italiano Malattie Ematologiche Maligne dell'Adulto. *N Engl J Med* 1997;337: 1870–5.
70 Schiffer CA, Anderson KC, Bennett CL, *et al.* Platelet transfusion for patients with cancer: clinical practice guidelines of the American Society of Clinical Oncology. *J Clin Oncol* 2001;19: 1519–38.
71 Friedmann AM, Sengul H, Lehmann H, *et al.* Do basic laboratory tests or clinical observations predict bleeding in thrombocytopenic oncology patients? A reevaluation of prophylactic platelet transfusions. *Transfus Med Rev* 2002;16: 34–45.
72 Slichter SJ. Leukocyte reduction and ultraviolet B irradiation of platelets to prevent alloimmunization and refractoriness to platelet transfusions. The Trial to Reduce Alloimmunization to Platelets Study Group. *N Engl J Med* 1997;337: 1861–9.
73 Rebulla P, Morelati F, Revelli N, *et al.* Outcomes of an automated procedure for the selection of effective platelets for patients refractory to random donors based on cross-matching locally available platelet products. *Br J Haematol* 2004;125:83–9.
74 Slichter SJ. Evidence-based platelet transfusion guidelines. *Hematology Am Soc Hematol Educ Program* 2007:172–8. Review.
75 Gutierrez-Delgado F, Bensinger W. Safety of granulocyte colony-stimulating factor in normal donors. *Curr Opin Hematol* 2001;8:155–60.
76 Ottmann OG, Bug G, Krauter J. Current status of growth factors in the treatment of acute myeloid and lymphoblastic leukemia. *Semin Hematol* 2007;44:183–92.
77 Phillips TM, Kim K, Vlashi E, *et al.* Effects of recombinant erythropoietin on breast cancer-initiating cells. *Neoplasia* 2007;9:1122–9.
78 Kokhaei P, Abdalla AO, Hansson L, *et al.* Expression of erythropoietin receptor and *in vitro* functional effects of epoietins in B-cell malignancies. *Clin Cancer Res* 2007;13:3536–44.
79 Bennett CL, Silver SM, Djulbegovic B, *et al.* Venous thromboembolism and mortality associated with recombinant erythropoietin and darbepoetin administration for the treatment of cancer-associated anemia. *JAMA* 2008;299:914–24.
80 Rizzo JD, Somerfield MR, Hagerty KL, *et al.* Use of epoetin and darbepoetin in patients with cancer: 2007 American Society of Clinical Oncology/American Society of Hematology clinical practice guideline update. *J Clin Oncol* 2008;26:132–49.

Chapter 34
New Designs for Clinical Trials: Acute Myeloid Leukemia as an Example

Elihu Estey
Fred Hutchinson Cancer Research Center, University of Washington School of Medicine, Seattle, Washington, USA

Introduction

For many years new drugs have been tested in three sequential phases. Phase I trials formally monitor toxicity (but not efficacy) and use a "3 + 3" rule to identify a drug's "maximum tolerated dose" (MTD). In phase II, efficacy (but not toxicity) is assessed in comparison with a historical standard; a Simon two-stage design is most commonly used for this purpose [1]. Phase III trials randomize patients among two or more different treatments, one of which is often "standard." Typically, these trials seek to detect differences in a single measure of efficacy, eg, complete remission or survival, specifying false-positive rates <5% (P-value <0.05) and false-negative rates <10–20%. The false-positive rate corresponds to "type I1" error and the false negative rate to "type II" error. The power of a trial is [1 minus false-negative rate] and thus is generally set at 80–90%.

A general problem with the phase I → II → III paradigm is that it ignores the complexity inherent in medical practice and the corresponding reality that physicians and patients are interested in more than one endpoint [2]. Many different types of such multiplicities arise in acute myeloid leukemia (AML) trials, including multivariate outcomes that may occur at different points during treatment, multiple courses of treatment and patient heterogeneity, in particular interactions between treatments and patient subgroups. As a simple example, a trial of a lower intensity therapy in AML may wish to improve survival while simultaneously not causing a decrease in the complete remission rate. Hence, both survival and complete remission need to be monitored, although in such a case, only survival often is. This level of complexity is likely to become increasingly common in AML therapeutics. In addition to failing to account for multiplicities, the commonly used 3 + 3 and the Simon two-stage designs have poor statistical properties ("operating characteristics"), thus failing to reliably accomplish their goals. Given these issues, it is not surprising that the statistical literature proposes many new designs as replacements for the conventional ones. This chapter details some of the problems with standard designs and describes alternatives. Because many of these alternatives are based on Bayesian (as opposed to p-value-based-) statistics, we begin with a description of the Bayesian paradigm.

Bayesian approach

The Bayesian approach [3] begins with parameters such as the probability of toxicity at a given dose, the probability of complete remission, or median survival time. When comparing two treatments, the parameter of interest might be the ratio (relative risk) between two such survival times. An important feature of the Bayesian paradigm is that parameters (denoted here as θ) are random quantities, with probability distributions describing one's uncertainty about them. Thus the Bayesian paradigm begins with a prior distribution, $p(\theta)$, that characterizes one's uncertainty about θ before observing any data. The second Bayesian quantity is the likelihood, L(data | θ), which describes the probability of observing any specified data given any value of θ. Examples of likelihoods include the binomial distribution for binary events and the "normal" ("bell-shaped") distribution for continuous variables. Bayesians combine the observed data with the prior to arrive at a "posterior" distribution of θ, which describes one's uncertainty about θ after observing the data. Specifically, Bayes's theorem arrives at the posterior by multiplying the prior by the likelihood of observing the data given the parameter:

$$p(\theta|\text{data}) \propto \text{L}(\text{data}|\theta) \times p(\theta)$$

Thus, the Bayesian paradigm bases inferences on the probabilities of the parameters' or hypotheses' given data, whereas conventional P-value-based methods do the reverse.

The proportionality symbol "∝" rather than "=" is used in the above expression because a multiplicative constant,

Leukemias: Principles and Practice of Therapy, 1st edition. Edited by S. Faderl and H. Kantarjian.

const(data), must be computed to ensure that the posterior takes on values between 0 and 1. That is,

$$p(\theta|\text{data}) = \text{const}(\text{data}) \times L(\text{data}|\theta) \times p(\theta)$$

Until recently, computation of const(data) was often technically difficult, making most of the Bayesian paradigm nothing more than a theoretical construct. However, the emergence of powerful computational technology has made the Bayesian paradigm a practical reality.

When making decisions or inferences based on accruing data, Bayes's theorem may be applied repeatedly, with the posterior at each stage becoming the prior for the next stage. The probability distributions in this sequence become increasingly informative about θ as the data accumulate. This process, which is known as "Bayesian learning," is especially useful in sequential data monitoring during a clinical trial. The current posterior probability distribution may be used to make a variety of interim decisions, including modifying doses, dropping an inferior treatment arm, unbalancing a randomization in favor of a treatment or treatments that have relatively superior performance, or terminating the trial early due to either superiority of a treatment or futility. Figure 34.1 illustrates the process of Bayesian learning in a setting where the parameter of interest is the probability of achieving complete remission in relapsed AML. The prior on θ is shown by the dotted line, and it reflects almost no knowledge of θ beyond the average value of 0.20. The dashed line is the posterior after observing five complete remissions in the first 10 patients. The solid line is the posterior after observing seven complete remissions in the next 30 patients, and it is based on the combined data consisting of 12 complete remissions in 40 patients. This illustrates how the posteriors become successively more informative as the data accumulate, and how they shift to reflect the overall average behavior of the data.

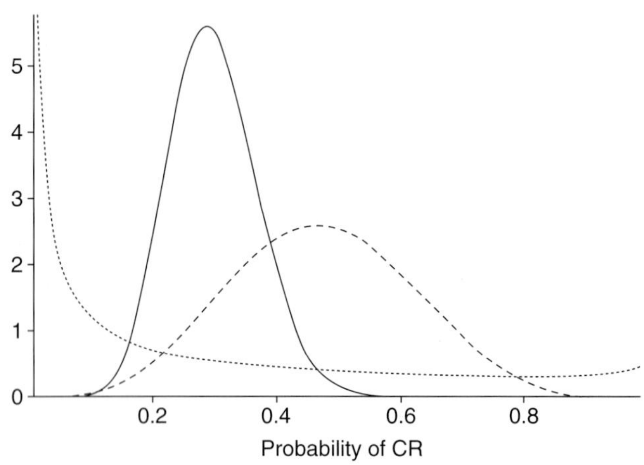

Figure 34.1 Bayesian probability distributions. The values on the vertical axis represent the weight assigned to each complete remission probability. Prior to treatment (dotted line), although the average complete remission rate is thought to be 20%, some credence is assigned to each probability of complete remission, After observing 5/10 complete remissions (dashed line), the average complete remission rate is close to 50%, and no credence is given to complete remission rates <10% or >90%, reflecting the impact of the observed data on the prior. After observing seven complete remissions in the next 30 patients, the average complete remission rate is approximately 30%, and no credence is given to a complete remission rate >60% (solid line).

The Bayesian approach is properly contrasted with the conventional approach, which, in particular, uses *P*-values as a basis for inferring strength of evidence [4,5]. Unlike Bayesians, who view θ as a random quantity, the standard ("frequentist") approach assumes that θ is fixed, but unknown. For a given frequentist test of hypothesis, the *P*-value is defined as the probability, under the null hypothesis, of observing a result as extreme, or more extreme, than that observed. Although some believe that the *P*-value is the probability that the null hypothesis is true given the observed data, this quantity is a Bayesian posterior probability, not a *P*-value. Calculation of a *P*-value involves both observed and unobserved data, because the definition of the *P*-value includes any data that might have been observed under a predetermined experimental design. An obvious logical flaw is that a given data set could give rise to two or more different *P*-values, depending on which design was intended. For observational data, where there is no experimental design, the *P*-value of a given test may be a wide variety of different quantities, depending on what sort of assumptions one makes about how the data arose and on the manner in which putative hypotheses are formulated.

As an example, assume that pairs of patients are treated, with one member of each pair randomly chosen to receive treatment A and the other receiving treatment B. If survival is longer for the patient treated with A, then a preference for A is recorded, and *vice versa*. The null hypothesis is that the probability of a preference for A over B is 1/2, that is, that the two treatments do not differ. Suppose that six pairs of patients have been treated and five preferences for A and one for B have been observed. If the investigator in fact planned to treat exactly six pairs of patients, then the *P*-value equals $6 \times (1/2)^5(1/2)^1 + (1/2)^6 = 0.11$, based on the binomial distribution. The first summand corresponds to the probability of observing the actual data, namely five preferences for A and one for B in six pairs, whereas the second summand represents the probability of the more extreme, but unobserved, case of six successes in six pairs. As with all *P*-values, these probabilities are computed under the null hypothesis. If, instead, the investigator originally planned to stop the trial once a single preference for B was observed, the *P*-value equals $(1/2)^5(1/2)^1 + (1/2)^6 = 0.03$, since with this design there is only one way that five preferences for A and one for B could have occurred. This simple illustration shows that, because *P*-values are based on both the observed data and unobserved, possible data, one's conclusions, such as whether one treatment is superior to another, depend in a fundamental way on completely arbitrary claims of how a given experiment *might* have been conducted.

Once a frequentist experimental design *is* specified, the investigator is permitted to look at the accruing data only if and when an interim test is specified by the design. If this constraint is violated, then the *P*-value must be adjusted upward to account for the fact that a false-positive decision might have been made. Indeed, many "group sequential" designs have been described to deal with the issue of interim analyses. Each design's statistical rules are constructed so that, accounting for the interim analyses, the overall false-positive probability (type I error) will be maintained below a desired level, typically, $P = 0.05$. In practice, this is done by performing the interim tests at *P*-values much smaller than 0.05. However, the same overall *P*-value can lead to different decisions depending on the particular design employed. Regardless of the type of boundary, however, the frequentist method *punishes the investigator for looking at data*. Consider a trial designed to have an overall type I error of 0.05. If the investigator looks at the data at any unplanned times and performs a test at each look, then it is possible that all of the planned 0.05 type I error has been spent before the trial is completed. Thus, when new data become available thereafter, the frequentist approach makes no allowance for using it along with the previous data! The same problem arises in a frequentist design for a trial in which the final planned test yields a *P*-value of 0.051, but additional data are subsequently obtained that strengthen the evidence in favor of a difference. The frequentist approach does not permit these subsequent data to be used, since they were not obtained as part of the planned experiment.

In contrast, Bayesian inference utilizes all of the available data, with inferences based on posterior probabilities computed from observed data. In particular, Bayesian inference does not involve unobserved data and is not affected by the experimental design. That is, the data enter inferences only through the likelihood function. Consequently, not only can posterior probabilities be used as an explicit measure of support for a hypothesis, but Bayesian inference makes more logical sense than frequentist inference. In the above example wherein pairs of patients are treated with A and B, taking a Bayesian approach, let θ denote the probability that a patient given A survives longer than a patient given B. If one assumes a non-informative prior for θ similar to that given in Figure 34.1 but with prior mean 1/2 rather than 0.20, then posterior probability ($\theta > 1/2$ | five preferences for A and one for B in six pairs) = 0.95. That is, given the observed data, the posterior probability that A is superior to B equals 0.95. Compare this with the frequentist statement "The probability is 0.03 of a result as extreme or more extreme than that observed, assuming there is no difference between therapies and based on the study's design that stops when one preference for B is observed," along with the ambiguity that the value 0.03 might be replaced by 0.11 if one changes the assumptions about what was intended at the start of the experiment. Given the indirect and complex nature of frequentist statements, many scientists believe that the *P*-value is the Bayesian posterior probability of the null hypothesis, which is not the case. This *de facto* situation provides a rather strong rationale for explicit use of Bayesian inference. Bayesian methods are especially useful for design and conduct of clinical trials because posterior probabilities can be updated at any time, there is no penalty if the investigator looks at the data, and the posterior can readily be used to compute predictive probabilities (unlike *P*-values). The Bayesian approach thus facilitates frequent data analyses and decisions. Its flexibility can be appreciated by contrasting the frequentist's need to do an entire additional trial if a large phase III trial has a final *P*-value = 0.06, whereas the Bayesian approach could simply continue the initial trial, if desired.

Phase 1: the 3 + 3 rule

The 3 + 3 design's simplicity is undoubtedly at least partially responsible for its popularity. Three patients are entered at a given dose. If none of these have dose-limiting toxicity (DLT) the next three are entered at the next higher dose level. If one of the first three experience DLT, three additional patients receive the same dose. If none of these three has DLT (DLT thus occurred in 1/6) the next three patients receive the next higher dose. In contrast, if two or more have DLT (DLT thus being observed in 2 of the 4–6 patients treated at the dose), the maximum tolerated dose is considered exceeded, the next cohort of three patients receive a lower dose, and the process is repeated. Similarly if two of the first three treated at a dose experience DLT, the next three are treated at a one dose level decrease. The fact that 1/6 is an acceptable level of toxicity but that 2/6 is not implies that an acceptable toxicity rate is 20–30%.

The most obvious problem with the 3 + 3 design is that the small sample sizes are statistically unreliable. For example, an exact 95% confidence interval about 0/3 is (0–0.71) and the corresponding interval about 1/6 is (0–0.64). Furthermore, decisions about how to proceed depend solely on observations made at the current dose level. Observations made at other dose levels are irrelevant. In contrast, Bayesian methods for dose finding, such as the continuous reassessment method (CRM), the modified CRM, or Bayesian logistic regression, use all available information [6]. For example the CRM begins with prior probabilities of toxicity at the different dose levels to be investigated in phase I. The first cohort of patients is treated at the level associated with a prior probability closest to 20–30%. As data accumulate, the posterior probabilities of toxicity at each dose may change, with each subsequent cohort treated at the dose associated with a posterior probability closest to 20–30%. A given dose may be revisited if it appears that all dose levels below it are consistently associated with probabilities of toxicity <20–30%. Given that it uses more information, it is not surprising that it has been repeatedly demonstrated in the statistical literature that, in contrast to Bayesian methods, the 3 + 3 has very poor operating characteristics and, accordingly, is unlikely to identify a dose that is "truly" associated with a probability of DLT of 20–30%, with truly referring to what would have been obtained had an infinite number of patients been treated at various doses; Table 34.1 provides an example. Various doses between 100 and 600 mg are associated with true probabilities of toxicity between 0.01 and 0.76, with the 200 mg doses associated with a true probability of 26%. Assume a trial in which a maximum of 36 patients will be enrolled in cohorts of three each. Table 34.1(a) indicates that Bayesian logistic regression (BLR) will correctly identify 300 mg as the dose for phase II in 72% of (4000) computer simulations of this scenario, whereas the 3 + 3 will identify 300 mg in only 41% of simulations. Furthermore, although more patients will be treated with the BLR than with the 3 + 3 (36 vs. 17), 58% of the patients will be treated at 300 mg versus only 29% of patients with the 3 + 3. As illustrated in this scenario, the 3 + 3 is prone to underestimate the MTD. It is also likely to conclude that there is no acceptable dose (Table 34.1b). Thus, contrasted with the 3 + 3, the BLR (or the CRM or modified CRM) is likely to require more patients to complete phase I but is also likely to be more reliable.

Failure to account for covariates in phase 1

If two of the first three patients at a given dose experience DLT, that dose is not re-visited regardless of whether the two patients were, for example, age 35 or age 65. As it is clinically intuitive, however, that on average a 65-year-old is more likely to incur DLT than a 35-year-old, this essentially universal practice ignores clinical reality. In a formal demonstration Rogatko *et al.* [7] performed multivariate analyses to assess independent risk factors for DLT in phase I trials of various drugs. With paclitaxel, weight loss but not dose was such a predictor, whereas, in the case of tipifarnib, alkaline phosphatase and albumin, but again not dose, were predictive, and, with irinotecan and tomudex, dose, a history of smoking, and alkaline phosphatase were independently associated with DLT. Thus, the current approach is not unlikely to declare a dose "too toxic" when toxicity reflects the type of patient treated rather than the dose administered. Similarly, a dose may be declared as safe only because the patients given that dose were unlikely to experience DLT. It follows that, rather than a single MTD, there may be different MTDs for different patients. Methods have been proposed that account for covariates in phase I trials that examine both toxicity and efficacy [8], as discussed below.

Combination phase I and phase II trials

Many oncologists believe that the purpose of a phase I trial is to determine a dose that can be administered safely in phase II trials. Again, this view ignores clinical reality. Specifically, patients enter phase I trials not to avoid toxicity, but to have a response. Furthermore, knowledge about toxicity is incomplete after completion of phase I consequent to the small sample sizes in the typical 3 + 3 study. These considerations suggest that it would be worthwhile to adaptively monitor both response and toxicity in hybrid phase I/II trials. Using a Bayesian approach, Thall *et al.* [9] proposed such a design. Let θ(R,D) denote the probability of response at dose d and θ (T,D) the probability of toxicity at dose d. In the initial, simplest formulation, patients could have response or toxicity but not both. Assume there are four dose levels, with the initial patients receiving dose level 1 and with a maximum sample size of 45. After each cohort of three patients is entered, a determination is made as to which of the four dose levels is acceptable, based on efficacy and toxicity.

Table 34.1 Operating characteristics[a] of Bayesian logistic regression (BLR) and 3 + 3 methods for dose finding in phase I

Dose	*100*	*200*	*300*	*400*	*500*	*600*	*None*
True PTox	*0.01*	*0.09*	*0.26*	*0.47*	*0.64*	*0.76*	–
BLR, percent MTD	0	21	72	6	0	0	
Number of patients	0	11	21	4	0	0	–
3 + 3, percent MTD	8	43	41	7	0	0	
Number of patients	4	5	5	3	0	0	–

Maximum sample size was 36, three patients per cohort.
MTD, maximum tolerated dose; PTox, probability of toxicity.
[a]4000 simulations.

For example, assume we are testing a new drug in patients receiving second salvage therapy for AML that relapsed after an initial remission of <6 months. As the historical response rate in this situation is 5%, we will say that a dose is unacceptable if it is very likely that it is associated with a response rate <12%, with the criterion probability 0.95 quantifying the term "very likely." Given that the 3 + 3 rule implicitly considers a toxicity rate of 2/6, but not 1/6, too great, we will also consider a dose unacceptable if it is very likely associated with a toxicity rate >30%; here the criterion probability 0.90 will quantify "very likely." If, at the time of entry of the next cohort, no dose is acceptable, the trial concludes; if more than one dose is acceptable the dose given the next cohort is that associated with the highest response rate.

As is always the case, the parameters above, such as the maximum sample size, cohort size, and criterion probabilities, are selected after examination of the design's operating characteristics in various clinical scenarios. Table 34.2(a) illustrates three such scenarios. In the first, the true response rate is 0.12 with each of the four doses, but toxicity increases with dose from 0.30 at the first dose to 0.75 at the fourth dose; thus only the first dose is acceptable. In the second scenario, both response and toxicity rates increase with dose, with the third and fourth doses acceptable. In the third scenario, although true rates of toxicity are <0.30 at each dose, true response rates are <0.12 at each dose; thus no dose is acceptable. Table 34.2(b) contrasts the phase I/II design with the 3 + 3 in each scenario. The table illustrates the probabilities that each method will correctly identify an acceptable dose (dose 1 in scenario 1, doses 3 and 4 in scenario 2 and no dose in scenario 3), based on 1000 computer simulations of each scenario. Although in scenario 1 this probability is only slightly higher with the phase I/II than with the 3 + 3, the number of patients treated at an acceptable dose is much higher with the phase I/II. The probabilities of correctly identifying an acceptable dose are much higher with the phase I/II than the 3 + 3 in scenarios 2 and 3. In the latter scenario, because it monitors only toxicity, the 3 + 3 identifies each dose as acceptable, whereas, because it monitors both efficacy and toxicity, the phase I/II finds no dose acceptable. It is certainly true that the phase I/II requires more patients than the 3 + 3. However, the trade-off is more accuracy in identification of acceptable doses. Furthermore, a more relevant comparison is of sample sizes in the phase I/II with the sample size in the 3 + 3 plus the sample size in the Simon two-stage phase design that follows the 3 + 3. Here, maximum sample sizes are less with the phase I/II.

Subsequent iterations of the phase I/II allow for both response and toxicity to occur in the same patient and account for covariates [8].

Simon two-stage design

The Simon two-stage design [1] is probably the most commonly used design for single-arm phase II trials. The "optimal" and the "minimax" versions differ slightly in number of patients entered in the first stage and after both stages. Many freely downloadable programs for the design are available (eg, http://www.edavar.com/). The investigator specifies a rate of no interest (known as p_0), typically corresponding to the historical rate, a rate of interest (p_1) typically 0.15–0.20 higher than the historical

Table 34.2 (a) and (b).Various dose outcome scenarios and operating characteristics in these scenarios of Bayesian phase I–II and 3 + 3 designs

(a)

D1		D2		D3		D4	
θ(R)	θ(T)	θ(R)	θ(T)	θ(R)	θ(T)	θ(R)	θ(T)
0.12	**0.3**	0.12	0.45	0.12	0.6	0.12	0.75
0.02	0.1	0.05	0.15	**0.15**	**0.25**	**0.2**	**0.3**
0.01	0.05	0.02	0.1	0.05	0.15	0.02	0.25

(b)

Case	Correct dose	Probability of selection		No. patients	
		Phase I–II	3 + 3	Phase I–II	3 + 3
1	1	0.54	0.49	40	8
2	3,4	0.89	0.35	44	13

θ(R), probability of response; θ(T), probability of toxicity.

rate, and false-positive and false-negative rates (typically 0.10). These parameters determine the number of patients treated in the first stage and the minimum number of responses needed to proceed to a second stage of specified number. After the latter is completed, a drug is accepted if the number of responses in both stages is greater than a specified minimum; they are rejected otherwise.

Although the design is quite practical, it is not without several problems, as first pointed out by Thall and Simon [10]. These authors noted that the design assumes p_0 to be a fixed value rather than a statistic. However, in most cases, an insufficient number of patients have received the historical treatment for this to be the case. As a consequence, the false-positive and false-negative rates are often considerably greater than the nominal values, such as 0.10. Obviously, the fewer the historical patients and thus the greater variance about the mean historical rate the greater the departure from these nominal values. Other substantive problems with the design are its failure to account for prognostic heterogeneity and for "trial effects."

Accounting for prognostic heterogeneity in phase II

It is commonly accepted that outcome following a given treatment for AML is influenced by several covariates. Principal among these is the karyotype of a patient's AML blasts [11].The past few years have seen the use of molecular techniques to expand knowledge of prognosis in patients with a normal karyotype. Examples of these techniques are detection of mutations in genes for FLT3 (FMS-like tyrosine kinase receptor 3), NPM (nucleophosmin), or CEBA and of overexpression of genes such as *BAALC* and *ERG*. It is estimated that use of such molecular methodology enables 75–80% of patients with a normal karyotype to be placed into a distinct prognostic group [12].

It is remarkable that, despite this increase in knowledge of prognostic factors, the Simon two-stage design is still in vogue, although it does not account for prognostic heterogeneity. Thus, it is quite plausible that inferences about a drug's activity have more to do with the patients given the drug than with the drug itself. For example, a trial of a new drug in older patients with untreated AML may stop not because the drug is inactive, but because the low response rate reflected entry of a preponderance of patients with particularly unfavorable cytogenetics. Similar to this false-negative case, a drug may be declared (falsely) positive because of entry of a higher than expected proportion of patients with a normal karyotype and no FLT3 mutation. Given that a limited number of patients are treated before a stopping rule is invoked, the chance of such an imbalance is not trivial. It might be argued that more patients should be treated before interim decisions are made. An extension of this view would favor separate Simon designs in patients with better and worse cytogenetics. However, this lengthens the trial and does not permit information learned from one prognostic group to potentially be applied to another.

As an alternative to the extremes of ignoring prognostic heterogeneity and of conducting separate phase II trials for various prognostic groups, Wathen *et al.* [13] proposed a method that accounts for treatment–subgroup interactions, specifically adaptively using data from the trial to estimate the degree to which the results in different subgroups can be combined. The method involves "hierarchical Bayes," so-called because there are two levels of prior probability distributions. The first is the usual probability of response to a drug in each of, for example, two prognostic groups. The second specifies the degree to which it is believed *a priori* that the data from the groups can be combined. As usual, these priors are updated as the trial proceeds. For example, if in an interim analysis complete remission rates in a better and worse cytogenetic group are 3/12 and 2/15, respectively, it would intuitively be more reasonable to combine the data than if the rates were 3/12 and 0/20.

An example of the design is provided by a hypothetical trial of a new drug in relapsed AML. Actual historical data indicated a response rate of 21% in 169 patients. This rate was 11% (118 patients) if initial complete remission duration was <1 year, but was 43% (51 patients) if initial complete remission duration was >1 year. The goal of the trial is to increase response rate to 31% (an absolute increase of 0.20) in the worse prognostic group and to 58% (an absolute increase of 15%) in the better prognostic group. As the historical data suggest that 69% of patients will be in the worse group, the overall targeted improvement is $[0.20 \times 0.69] + [0.15 \times 0.31] = 0.18$. Thus, a Simon two-stage design would set 21% as p_0 and $0.21 + 0.18 = 0.39$ as p_1. Setting the nominal false-positive and false-negative rates at 0.10, the Simon design would treat 22 patients in a first stage and the trial would stop if fewer than five responses occurred. If more than four responses occurred, an additional 21 patients would be enrolled and the drug declared a success if responses were seen in >12/43 patients. Thus, to make the proposed design (hereafter STI because it examines subgroup–treatment interactions) similar to the Simon two-stage, we specify that STI will also take its first look after 22 patients have been evaluated and will also set its false-negative rate at 0.10.

As usual, we compare the STI and Simon two-stage designs by examining their operating characteristics under a variety of clinical scenarios. In the first scenario (Table 34.3a) the new drug achieves its goal in the better but not the worse group. Thus, the correct decision is to reject the drug in the worse but not the better group. Because the Simon two-stage does not consider interactions between prognostic subgroups and treatment, it has the same probability (0.75) of rejecting the drug in both

Table 34.3 (a) and (b). Comparison of subgroup–treatment interactions (STI) and Simon two-stage (S2S) designs

(a)

Subgroup	True complete remission rate	Probability of rejection		Mean number of patients	
		STI	S2S	STI	S2S
Better	**0.58**	0.10	0.75	21	10
Worse	0.11	0.90	0.75	19	25

(b)

Subgroup	True complete remission rate	Probability of rejection		Mean number of patients	
		STI	S2S	STI	S2S
Better	0.43	0.5	0.26	13	11
Worse	0.31	0.1	0.26	27	30

groups. In contrast, the STI are less likely to reject the drug in the better group and more likely to reject it in the worse group. Furthermore, 52% of the patients treated with STI will be in the better group, versus only 29% with the Simon two-stage design. Table 34.3(b) illustrates a case in which the desired improvement occurs in the worse but not the better group. Again STI are more likely to accept and reject the drug in the appropriate subgroups. Although conducting separate Simon two-stage designed trials in better and worse subgroups corrects this problem, Simon two-stage's inability to allow results in one subgroup to affect the conduct of the trial in the other subgroup continues to result in a smaller proportion of treated patients belonging to the better or worse group as appropriate, given the disparate effects of drug in these groups. The failure of the Simon two-stage design to address prognostic heterogeneity is likely to become more acute as therapies are developed that are specific for distinct subgroups of patients, as, for example, seems to be the case with ATRA in *NPM*$^+$ *FLT3–ITD*$^-$ AML [14].

Accounting for trial effects in phase II and the need for comparison in phase II

As noted above, but as ignored by designs such as the 3 + 3 and Simon two-stage, the effect of a drug on outcome is the sum of the effect of the drug and the prognosis of the patients given the drug. The latter, in turn, is a sum of known prognostic covariates, such as age and cytogenetics, and less quantifiable prognostic covariates. These less quantifiable prognostic covariates are referred to as "trial effects" or "latent variables." For example, it is well known that many patients eligible for a trial are not entered. It is often suspected that the patients not entered "look worse" than the patients who are entered. Indeed, such selection bias is often thought to contribute to the difficulty reproducing initial "promising" results once a new drug becomes widely available. The principle underlying randomization is to eliminate the effect of such latent variables.

The importance of trial effects in phase II stems from the concept that phase II trials are inherently comparative [2]. That is, patients are interested in the effectiveness of a new drug but are more profoundly interested in the comparative effectiveness of the new drug compared with an old (standard) drug or to other new drugs. Indeed the idea of comparison in phase II trials is inherent in the Simon two-stage design's setting of a rate of no interest (p_0), as based on historical data. Under these circumstances, it seems desirable to emphasize comparison as early as possible in the drug development process and, in particular, in phase II rather than delaying efforts to compare until phase III.

Given the importance of comparison in phase II and the effect of latent variables on the ability to plausibly compare different treatments, the idea of randomization in phase II has received attention. In particular, randomized selection designs have been proposed [15]. The underlying concept is that many new drugs and their combinations are available for comparison with a standard, but that preclinical rationale provides relatively little guidance in selecting which new drug to compare with this standard. Thus a compelling preclinical rationale did not exist for many drugs that have nonetheless improved outcome in leukemia; examples are arsenic trioxide in acute promyelocytic leukemia (APL), fludarabine in chronic lymphocytic leukemia (CLL), and cladribine in hairy cell leukemia. In contrast, many drugs that were clinical failures were accompanied by what, at the time, seemed like unassailable rationales. Accepting that preclinical rationale is an imperfect guide to selecting new therapies, a Bayesian selection design proposes to randomize 45–80 patients among three to four therapies. Each therapy begins with the same previous probability distribution. As patients are treated, the priors are updated with these posteriors used to shut down accrual to an arm if, for example, the probability that its true response rate is >20% worse than a competing arm is high. At the end of the trial, the arm with the highest response rate is selected for further therapy, at times provided its response rate is also higher than some historical standard.

Such selection designs are often criticized as "underpowered phase III trials." And indeed, examination of selection designs' operating characteristics indicate that, in a scenario where three drugs have the same true response rate and the fourth provides an absolute 20% improvement, the probability of correctly selecting the fourth drug (that is, the probability that it will not stop early and the probability that it will have the highest response rate at the end of the trial) is only about 60%. This, of course, contrasts with the 80% power typical of randomized trials, involving, for example, a new drug versus a standard. However, it needs to be emphasized that the 80% is nominal. Specifically, it ignores the process by which the new drug was selected. Assuming that four potential new therapies are available for comparison with a standard, that each is equally likely to be useful clinically, and that preclinical rationale cannot substitute for clinical data in the selection process, it follows that the probability of correctly selecting the best drug is 25%. This 25% is ignored in the computation of 80% power; if it were not, the power of the trial would be 25% × 80% = 20%. Thus, the selection design's 60% probability of correct selection should be viewed not in relation to 80% power, but in relation to the 25% probability of correct selection that would obtain in the absence of the selection design. This issue is likely to become more pressing given the development of increasing numbers of new therapies, many of which can be administered with various schedules that might affect their efficacy and many of which can be combined in a myriad of ways with other new drugs. Under these circumstances, it is encouraging that Medical Research Council-sponsored trials in AML in the UK are employing selection designs rather than more conventional phase III designs.

Phase III trials and adaptive randomization

Typical phase III trials in AML enroll approximately 400 patients [16–18]. This number is required if relatively small differences between treatments are to be detected with a power of 80% and a false-positive rate of 5%. The large number mandates a trial of several years investigating a small number of therapies relative to the number available, as discussed in the preceding section. One way to reduce the number of patients and the time required for study completion is to aim for more medically significant gains. Thus, it might be argued that improvements in event-free survival (EFS) from 10% to 20% at 2 years, with a median EFS from 6 months to 12 months and with a complete remission rate of 50–65% (each specified in separate recent phase III trials in AML) [15–17], are not sufficient medically, as opposed to statistically, significant to justify the number of patients invested in the trial. The desire for more protection (95%) against a false-positive result than against a false-negative rate (80%) is also problematic. Although this formulation is generally applied to many different diseases, it seems to ignore medical reality. Thus, it is far more reasonable to justify a higher degree of protection against a false-positive result with a new drug in a disease in which standard treatment is routinely successful than in a disease like AML in which standard treatment is routinely unsuccessful, and thus in which the consequences of replacing standard therapy are much less.

Although randomized trials are the preferred method to minimize trial effects such as selection bias, it must be recognized that minimization applies only to the treatments being compared in the trial, thus potentially limiting the general applicability of phase III trials. Another issue is whether all randomized trials meet the acknowledged standard calling for identical benefit–risk ratios in each arm of the trial. Consider, for example, a randomized comparison of standard 3 + 7 therapy versus a new agent in older patients with untreated AML, including those with complex karyotypes. Although it is certainly possible that the new therapy may be worse than 3 + 7, the results with 3 + 7 are sufficiently poor that it is fair to ask whether the new therapy can be much worse and, more explicitly, whether the benefit–risk ratios are really identical. This situation occurs not infrequently. Adaptive randomization is an attempt to balance the need for randomization with the desire to limit exposure to an inferior treatment. Bayesian adaptive randomization accomplishes this by using interim data to compute the posterior probability that one treatment arm is better than another, unbalancing randomization in favor of the better treatment, and continuously repeating this process [19–20]. This contrasts with the standard *P*-value-based randomized trial in which interim analyses often only occur after 100 patients have received treatment. This practice almost certainly departs from the patients' assumption that physicians closely monitor data after each patient is treated. But of course, interim analyses can not be done more frequently if the final *P*-value of 0.05 is to be preserved at the end of the trial. As noted above, the Bayesian approach encourages interim analyses, making adaptive randomization feasible.

A trial adaptively randomizing patients over age 50 years with untreated AML among idarubicin and Ara-C (the standard), troxacitabine and Ara-C, and troxacitabine–idarubicin serves as an example [21]. The first 15 patients were to be randomized in a ratio of 1 : 1 : 1 among the three arms. As each patient after the 16th entered the trial we computed the posterior probability that the complete remission rate for idarubicin and Ara-C was >10% better than with troxacitabine and Ara-C or troxacitabine–idarubicin. If this probability was <15%, accrual to idarubicin and Ara-C was suspended. If, in contrast, the posterior probability was >85% of the complete remission rate with troxacitabine and Ara-C, or if troxacitabine–idarubicin was >10% worse with idarubicin and Ara-C, accrual to either troxacitabine and Ara-C or troxacitabine–idarubicin was suspended. Depending on results in arms that remained open, a closed arm could re-open. A maximum of 75 patients were to be randomized. The troxacitabine–idarubicin arm closed and remained closed after the first five patients failed to respond, whereas the troxacitabine and Ara-C arm closed and remained closed after the complete remission rate was 3/11, at which time the complete remission rate in the idarubicin and Ara-C arm was 10/18.

A principal perceived problem with adaptive randomization is the possibility of a false-negative result in the above case with troxacitabine and Ara-C or troxacitabine–idarubicin. One way to reduce the problem is to begin adaptive randomization only once 15–20 patients have been randomized equally among the various treatment arms. At any rate, it is, as always, critical to examine the operating characteristics of the design under different clinical scenarios. If clinicians feel these are unsatisfactory, the parameters above, such as the criterion probabilities of 15% and 85% or the number of patients to be fairly randomized, are changed until desirable operating characteristics are obtained. Table 34.4 illustrates 1000 computer simulations for two scenarios in the idarubicin and Ara-C versus troxacitabine and Ara-C versus troxacitabine–idarubicin trial. In the first, the true complete remission rates with troxacitabine and Ara-C, idarubicin and Ara-C, and troxacitabine–idarubicin are 50%, 40%, and 30%, respectively; hence, the correct conclusion is that troxacitabine and Ara-C is superior. As parameterized above, the probability was 80% that the design would reach the correct conclusion, corresponding to a power of 80%. In contrast, if the true complete remission rates were 30%, 40%, and 30% with troxacitabine and Ara-C, idarubicin and Ara-C, and troxacitabine–idarubicin, respectively, the probability that the design would correctly select idarubicin and Ara-C as superior was only 10%. Hence, in this case the design provided much more protection against a false negative (declaring troxacitabine and Ara-C or troxacitabine–idarubicin worse than idarubicin and Ara-C when they were not) than a false positive (declaring troxacitabine and Ara-C or troxacitabine–idarubicin superior to idarubicin and Ara-C when they were not). The false-positive rate could have been decreased by eliminating the requirement that, with a high probability, troxacitabine and Ara-C or troxacitabine–idarubicin may be at least 10% worse than idarubicin and Ara-C before either of these arms would close. However, this would have also increased the false-negative rate, contrary to the desire of the clinical investigators to maintain a low false-negative rate.

The consequences of adaptive randomization are relatively easy to depict. If the 34 patients who had been entered on the trial when both troxacitabine and Ara-C and troxacitabine–idarubicin arms were closed had been randomized without bias, 11 patients each would have received troxacitabine and Ara-C, troxacitabine–idarubicin, and idarubicin and Ara-C. With adaptive randomization, only 16, rather than 22, patients received the inferior troxacitabine and Ara-C or troxacitabine–idarubicin arms. Given these consequences, it seems likely that patients would prefer adaptive randomization to the current methods. However, implementation of adaptive randomization requires not only sophisticated computing, but also a relatively short time to observe the outcome of interest and, in particular, that patients do not often present for randomization before there has been sufficient opportunity to observe the outcome in previous patients.

Table 34.4 Operating characteristics for idarubicin and Ara-C (IA) vs. troxacitabine and Ara-C (TA) vs. troxacitabine–idarubicin (TI) trial

True complete remission rates (%)			Correct conclusion	Probability of correct conclusion (%)
TA	IA	TI		
50	40	30	TA superior	80
30	40	30	IA superior	10

References

1 Simon R. Optimal two-stage designs for phase 2 clinical trials. *Controlled Clin Trials* 1989;10:1–10.

2 Estey E, Thall PF. New designs for phase 2 trials. *Blood* 2003;102:442–8.

3 Berry DA, Stangl DK (eds). Bayesian Biostatistics. Marcel Dekker: New York, NY, 1996.

4 Goodman SA. Toward evidence-based medical statistics, 1: the *p*-value fallacy. *Ann Int Med* 1999;130:996–1004.

5 Goodman SA. Toward evidence-based medical statistics, 2: the Bayes factor. *Ann Int Med* 1999;130:1005–13.

6 O'Quigley J, Pepe M, Fisher L. Continual reassessment method: a practical design for phase 1 clinical trials in cancer. *Biometrics* 1990;46:33–48.

7 Rogatko A, Babb JS, Wang H, *et al.* Patient characteristics compete with dose as predictors of acute treatment toxicity in early phase clinical trials. *Clin Cancer Res* 2004;10: 4645–51.

8 Thall PF, Nguyen HQ, Estey E. Patient-specific dose finding based on bivariate outcomes and covariates. *Biometrics* 2008; 64:1126–36.

9 Thall PF, Estey E, Sung H. A new statistical method for dose-finding based on efficacy and toxicity in early phase clinical trials. *Invest New Drugs* 1999;17:155–67.

10 Thall PF, Simon R. Incorporating historical control data in planning phase 2 clinical trials. *Stat Med* 1990;9:215–28.

11 Estey E, Dohner H. Acute myeloid leukemia. *Lancet* 2006;368: 1894–907.

12 Mrozek K, Marcucci G, Paschka P, *et al.* Clinical relevance of mutations and gene-expression changes in adult acute myeloid leukemia with normal cytogenetics: are we ready for a prognostically prioritized molecular classification? *Blood* 2007;109: 431–8.

13 Wathen J, Thall PF, Cook J, Estey E. Accounting for patient heterogeneity in phase 2 clinical trials. *Stat Med* 2008;27: 2802–15.

14 Schlenk R, Dohner H, Kneba M, *et al.* Gene mutations and response to treatment with all-trans retinoic acid in elderly patients with acute myeloid leukemia. Results from the AMLSG Trial AML HD98B. *Haematologica* 2009;94:54–60.

15 Thall PF, Estey E. A Bayesian strategy for screening cancer treatments prior to phase 2 clinical evaluation. *Stat Med* 1993; 12:1197–211.

16 van der Holt B, Lowenberg B, Burnett A, *et al.* The value of the MDR1 reversal agent PSC-833 in addition to daunorubicin and cytarabine in the treatment of elderly patients with previously untreated acute myeloid leukemia, in relation to MDR1 status at diagnosis. *Blood* 2005;106:2646–54.

17 Rowe J, Neuberg D,, Friedenberg W, *et al.* A phase 3 study of three induction regimens and of priming with GM-CSF in older adults with acute myeloid leukemia: a trial by the Eastern Cooperative Oncology Group. *Blood* 2004;103:479–85.

18 Baer M, George S, Dodge R, *et al.* Phase 3 study of the multidrug resistance modulator PSC-833 in previously untreated patients 60 years of age and older with acute myeloid leukemia: Cancer and Leukemia Group B Study 9720. *Blood* 2002;100: 1224–32.

19 Berry D, Eick S. Adaptive assignment vs. balanced randomization in clinical trials: a decision analysis. *Stat Med* 1995;14: 231–46.

20 Thall PF, Wathen J. Practical Bayesian adaptive randomization in clinical trials. *Eur J Cancer* 2007;43:859–866.

21 Giles F, Kantarjian H, Cortes J, *et al.* Adaptive randomized study of idarubicin and cytarabine versus troxacitabine and cytarabine versus troxacitabine and idarubicin in untreated patients 50 years or older with adverse karyotype acute myeloid leukemia. *J Clin Oncol* 2003;21:1722–7.

Index

Notes
Pages numbers followed by "f" indicate figures: those followed by "t" indicate tables.

To save space in the index, the following abbreviations have been used:

ALL	acute lymphoblastic leukemia
AML	acute myeloid leukemia
APL	acute promyelocytic leukemia
ATLL	adult T-cell leukemia/lymphoma
B-ALL	B-cell acute lymphoblastic leukemia
CLL	chronic lymphocytic leukemia
CML	chronic myeloid leukemia
HSC	hematopoietic stem cell
HSCT	hematopoietic stem cell transplantation
LSCs	leukemic stem cells
MDS	myelodysplastic syndromes
T-ALL	T-cell acute lymphoblastic leukemia
TBI	total body irradiation
T-PLL	T-cell prolymphocytic leukemia

D

G